PHARMACOLOGY FOR NURSES

A PATHOPHYSIOLOGICAL APPROACH

PHARMACOLOGY FOR NURSES

A PATHOPHYSIOLOGICAL APPROACH

MICHAEL PATRICK ADAMS
Professor of Anatomy and Physiology
St. Petersburg College
Formerly Dean of Health Professions
Pasco-Hernando State College

CAROL QUAM URBAN
Director, School of Nursing
Associate Dean, College of Health and Human Services
Associate Professor
George Mason University

MOHAMED EL-HUSSEIN
Associate Professor, School of Nursing & Midwifery
Department of Health, Community & Education
Mount Royal University

JOSEPH OSUJI
Associate Professor, School of Nursing & Midwifery
Department of Health, Community & Education
Mount Royal University

SHIRLEY KING
Fellow, Canadian College of Neuropsychopharmacology
Professor Emeritus, Mount Royal School of Nursing
Mount Royal University

SECOND CANADIAN EDITION

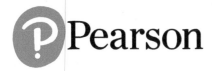

EDITORIAL DIRECTOR: Claudine O'Donnell
ACQUISITIONS EDITOR: Kimberley Veevers
MARKETING MANAGER: Michelle Bish
PROGRAM MANAGER: John Polanszky
PROJECT MANAGER: Jessica Mifsud
MANAGER OF CONTENT DEVELOPMENT: Suzanne Schaan
DEVELOPMENTAL EDITOR: Charlotte Morrison-Reed
MEDIA EDITOR: Charlotte Morrison-Reed
MEDIA DEVELOPER: Tiffany Palmer

PRODUCTION SERVICES: Cenveo® Publisher Services
PERMISSIONS PROJECT MANAGER: Shruti Jamadagni
PHOTO PERMISSIONS RESEARCH: Integra Publishing Services
TEXT PERMISSIONS RESEARCH: Integra Publishing Services
ART DIRECTOR: Alex Li
INTERIOR AND COVER DESIGNER: Anthony Leung
COVER IMAGE: Watchara/Shutterstock
VICE-PRESIDENT, CROSS MEDIA AND PUBLISHING
SERVICES: Gary Bennett

Pearson Canada Inc., 26 Prince Andrew Place, Don Mills, Ontario M3C 2T8.

ISBN-13: 978-0-13-357521-7

Library and Archives Canada Cataloguing in Publication

Adams, Michael, 1951-, author
    Pharmacology for nurses : a pathophysiological approach / Michael Patrick Adams, Leland Norman Holland, Paula Bostwick, Sheila E. King, Mohammed El-Hussein, Joseph Osuji. — Second Canadian edition.

ISBN 978-0-13-357521-7 (hardback)

1. Pharmacology—Textbooks. 2. Nursing—Textbooks. I. Title.

RM301.A33 2017   615.1   C2016-905770-4

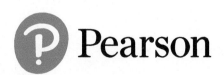

About the Authors

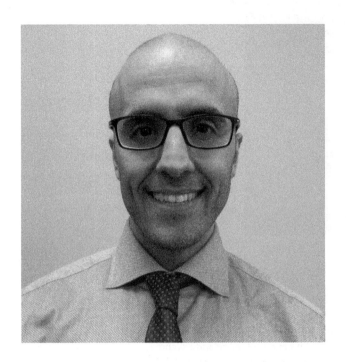

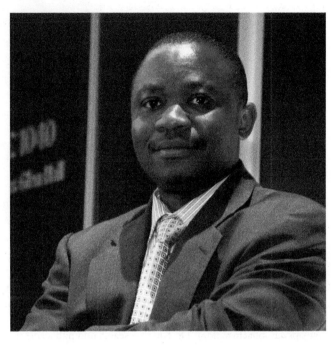

Mohamed Toufic El-Hussein, RN, BSN, MSN, PhD, is an
Associate Professor of Nursing in the Department of Health,
Community & Education at Mount Royal University in Calgary.
Dr. El-Hussein is a recipient of the distinguished teaching faculty
award in the Bachelor of Nursing program at Mount Royal
University, School of Nursing & Midwifery. He has initiated and
implemented several innovative teaching approaches that have
contributed immensely to the critical thinking, analytical, and
clinical skills of nursing students. Dr. El-Hussein's passion for
teaching emerged while working as a Registered Nurse in critical
care settings, where he was selected to facilitate and deliver
lectures in the Department of In-Service Education at different
hospitals. He completed his Master's in Critical Care and Trauma
at the University of KwaZulu-Natal, South Africa, and earned
a PhD in Nursing from the University of Calgary. His research
program focuses on clinical reasoning in nursing practice and the
use of innovative teaching strategies to enhance critical thinking
among nursing students. Dr. El-Hussein has authored several
publications and conference presentations that discuss clinical
reasoning processes and highlight innovative teaching strategies
designed to bridge the theory-practice gap in nursing and to help
students deconstruct and assimilate complex concepts.

Joseph Chinyere Osuji, RN, BScN, MN, PhD, is an Associate
Professor at the School of Nursing & Midwifery, Mount Royal
University, Calgary. His current teaching assignments are
Medical-Surgical Nursing, Pharmacology, Pathophysiology,
Community Health, and Chronic Disease Management. Dr. Osuji
has published widely and has authored and contributed chapters
on Medical/Surgical Nursing, Research Methods, and Chronic
Disease Management. He is interested in research questions that
deal with the social determinants of health, homelessness, social
justice and poverty, soft computing modelling and informatics,
teaching and learning processes in students, and clinical
reasoning among Registered Nurses. He has been published
in several peer-reviewed journals and has presented on related
topics in conferences, both locally and internationally. Dr. Osuji
is the proud husband of Mrs. Genevieve Osuji and the father of
three girls and two boys.

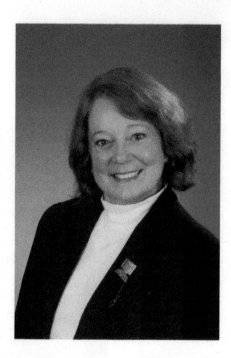

Shirley Linda King, RN, BN, MN, PhD, is a recipient of distinguished teaching and teaching excellence awards and teaches pharmacology in the Bachelor of Nursing program at Mount Royal School of Nursing. She has clinical experience in critical care and medical-surgical nursing. She is a member of several professional organizations, including the Canadian College of Neuropsychopharmacology. Dr. King's research and publications focus on the neuroendocrine and psychological effects of traumatic stress and factors that influence the subsequent development of post-traumatic stress disorder (PTSD) and depression. She has received major fellowship, research, and academic awards for her work. She is an early adopter, leader, researcher, and enthusiastic mentor in the innovative use of technology for teaching and learning and a recipient of PanCanadian Technology Awards.

Preface

When students are asked which subject in their nursing program is the most challenging, pharmacology always appears near the top of the list. The study of pharmacology demands that students apply knowledge from a wide variety of the natural and applied sciences. The successful prediction of drug action requires a thorough knowledge of anatomy, physiology, chemistry, and pathology, as well as knowledge of the social sciences of psychology and sociology. Current knowledge of drug actions, mechanisms, interactions, and legislation is mandatory for nurses to provide safe and effective care to their clients in all healthcare settings. Lack of proper application of pharmacology can result in immediate and direct harm to the client; therefore, the stakes in learning the subject are high.

Pharmacology can be made more understandable if the proper connections are made to knowledge learned in other disciplines. The vast majority of drugs in clinical practice are prescribed for specific diseases, yet many pharmacology texts fail to recognize the complex interrelationships between pharmacology and pathophysiology. When drugs are learned in isolation from their associated diseases or conditions, students have difficulty connecting pharmacotherapy to therapeutic goals and client wellness. The pathophysiology approach of this text gives the student a clearer picture of the importance of pharmacology to disease, and ultimately to client care. The approach and rationale of this text focus on a holistic perspective to client care, which clearly shows the benefits and limitations of pharmacotherapy in curing or preventing illness. Although challenging, the study of pharmacology is truly a fascinating, lifelong journey.

The new edition provides a unique Canadian perspective on pharmacotherapeutics, geared towards the education of Canadian undergraduate nursing students and their curriculum. During the editorial process, the text content was thoroughly reviewed and scrutinized by Canadian nurse educators and seasoned Canadian clinical pharmacists. The editors adapted the content accordingly to fit the Canadian nursing context. The technical review process helped ensure accurate information on Canadian drug names, and their respective doses and routes of administration, including common Canadian Trade names for drugs, and highlighting drugs that are exclusively available in Canada. Pregnancy categorization of drugs were updated based on Canadian standards. Finally tables and illustrations to help students better assimilate pharmacotherapeutic concepts were also added to the respective chapters.

Organization: A Body System and Disease Approach

Pharmacology for Nurses: A Pathophysiological Approach, 2nd Canadian Edition, is organized according to body systems (units) and diseases (chapters). This edition of the text has been expanded with new information. We have added many new chapters and included NCLEX Success Tips within each chapter to assist the student with making connections to the new NCLEX exam requirement for Canadian registered nurses. The first chapter in each unit (except in Units 1, 2, and 3) provides a brief discussion of the physiology of the corresponding body system. Each chapter provides complete information on the drug classifications used to treat the diseases discussed in that chapter. Specially designed headings cue students to each classification discussion.

The pathophysiology approach clearly places the drugs in context in terms of how they are used therapeutically. The student is able to easily locate all relevant anatomy, physiology, pathology, and pharmacology in the same chapter in which the drugs are discussed. This approach provides the student with a clear view of the connections between pharmacology, pathophysiology, and the nursing care learned in other clinical courses.

NCLEX Success Tips

The second Canadian edition of *Pharmacology for Nurses: A Pathophysiological Approach* includes more chapters to address the rapidly growing needs of students practising in the Canadian healthcare system. Before we started writing the text, we collected feedback from university professors, asking specifically about their experience using other pharmacology texts and their perceptions of an ideal text. These professors shared some of the challenges their students face while taking a pharmacology course. An emerging but immediate need that echoed at a national level was the need to prepare Canadian nursing students to pass the NCLEX exam. Although students can take NCLEX courses after graduation or just before taking the exam, we believe that early introduction of NCLEX format and concepts will give the students ample time to understand and assimilate these concepts. Our textbook, is the first nursing pharmacology text to incorporate NCLEX Success Tips.

We experienced challenges while trying to address all stakeholder concerns, as well as student needs, and at the same time keeping the text to a reasonable length. As a result, we reviewed several NCLEX texts and designed tips based on the NCLEX exam blueprints. We have presented the new content in a concise and succinct format and have used tables, figures, and illustrations to explain concepts.

Prototype Approach to Learning Drugs

The number of drugs available in clinical practice is staggering. To facilitate learning, we use prototype drugs and provide detailed introductions to the one or two most representative drugs in each classification. Students are less intimidated when they can focus their learning on one representative drug in each class. **Prototype Drug** boxes clearly describe these important medications. Within these boxes, the **actions and uses** of the drug are succinctly presented, including **administration alerts**, which highlight vital information related to the administration of that drug and treatment of overdose and antidotes when known. **Pharmacokinetics** information regarding the absorption, distribution, metabolism, excretion, and half-life of drugs is included when known. **Adverse effects and interactions** are also included when necessary.

Focused Coverage of the Nursing Process

This text features a focused approach to the nursing process, which allows students to quickly find the content that is essential for safe and effective drug therapy. **Nursing Considerations** sections appear within the discussion of each drug class. These sections discuss the major needs of the client, including general assessments, interventions, and client teaching for the classification. Client education discussions provide students with the essential information that they need to convey to their clients. **Integrated rationales** for nursing actions help students to learn the reasoning that is key to the development of critical thinking skills.

Nursing Process Focus charts provide a succinct, easy-to-read view of the most commonly prescribed drug classes for the disease. Need-to-know nursing actions are presented in a format that reflects the "flow" of the nursing process: nursing assessment, pattern identification and potential nursing diagnoses, planning, interventions, client education and discharge planning, and evaluation. Rationales for interventions are included in parentheses. The Nursing Process Focus charts identify clearly the nursing actions that are most important. Some prototype drugs have important nursing actions that are specific to that drug; in these instances, we provide a Nursing Process Focus chart in the text devoted solely to the prototype drug.

Holistic Pharmacology

Our new edition, examines pharmacology from a holistic perspective. The **Special Considerations** and **Lifespan Considerations** features present pharmacology and nursing issues related to **cultural, ethnic, age, gender,** and **psychosocial** aspects. These features remind students that a drug's efficacy is affected as much by its pharmacokinetics as by the uniqueness of the client. In addition, **pediatric** and **geriatric** considerations are integrated throughout the text.

Natural Therapies features present a popular herbal or dietary supplement that may be considered along with conventional drugs. Although the authors do not recommend the use of these alternative treatments in lieu of conventional medicines, many clients use complementary and alternative therapies and the nurse must become familiar with how they affect client health. **Herb-drug interactions** are also included within the Prototype Drug boxes when relevant. Non-pharmacological methods for controlling many diseases are also integrated into the chapters and include **lifestyle and dietary modifications.**

Learning Pharmacology Through Visuals

For nearly all students, learning is a highly visual process. This text incorporates generous use of artwork to illustrate and summarize key concepts. At the beginning of each unit, photographs are used to humanize the disease experience of clients. Vivid and colourful illustrations begin each chapter and help students to recall important concepts of anatomy and physiology for that body system. Pharmacotherapy illustrations provide students with a visual overview of a drug therapy process, showing specifically how the drug acts to counteract the effects of disease on the body.

The chapters on **Medication Incidents and Risk Reduction and Toxicology, Bioterrorism, and Emergency Preparedness** include important content on the promotion of client safety, management of medication incidents, and role of the nurse in situations that involve toxicity and biochemical emergencies.

Key Concepts outline what students should have learned in each chapter.

Scenarios with **Critical Thinking Questions** connect the student to a client at the end of most chapters. The student learns details about the client's health history and participates in critical thinking questions about the scenario. This allows for application of the knowledge obtained in the chapter.

NCLEX Practice Questions prepare students for course exams on chapter content and expose them to NCLEX-style questions. Answers and rationales are provided in Appendix A.

A Note about Terminology

The term *healthcare provider* is used to denote the physician, nurse practitioner, or any other health professional who is legally authorized to prescribe drugs.

Student Resources

The following resources have been developed in support of the text to help students in their learning of pharmacology.

MyNursingLab

Pearson eText. Pearson eText gives students access to the text whenever and wherever they have access to the Internet. eText pages look exactly like the printed text, offering powerful new functionality for students and instructors. Users can create notes, highlight text in different colours, create bookmarks, zoom, click hyperlinked words and phrases to view definitions, and view the text in single-page and two-page views. Pearson eText allows for quick navigation to key parts of the eText using a table of contents and provides full-text search. The eText may also offer links to associated media files, enabling users to access videos, animations, or other activities as they read the text.

Study Plan. Every chapter includes a two-part study plan with Practice Questions to help students identify the areas and topics that require more study and a Quiz to ensure that they have mastered the chapter content. Additional resources available to students through MyNursingLab include an NCLEX Study Quiz and access to Learning Catalytics.

Learning Catalytics. A "bring your own device" assessment and classroom activity system that expands the possibilities for student engagement. Using Learning Catalytics, you can deliver a wide range of auto-gradable or open-ended questions that test content knowledge and build critical thinking skills. Eighteen different answer types provide great flexibility, including graphical, numerical, textual input, and more.

Student Workbook (ISBN: 9780134636313)

The workbook contains a large number and variety of practice questions and learning activities, including fill in the blanks, matching, multiple choice, case studies, and dosage calculations.

Instructor Resources

To aid in teaching your pharmacology course, the following resources have been designed to support the text.

These instructor supplements are available for download from a password-protected section of Pearson Canada's online catalogue (catalogue.pearsoned.ca). Navigate to your text's catalogue page to view a list of the available supplements. Speak to your local Pearson sales representative for details and access.

The **Instructor's Resource Manual** includes:

- Learning Outcomes
- Suggested Classroom and Clinical Activities
- Summary of key points of each chapter

A comprehensive **PowerPoint Presentation** integrates lecture slides, images, and other resources.

A **Test Bank** with questions mapped to the chapter learning objectives is available.

Learning Solutions Managers

Pearson's Learning Solutions Managers work with faculty and campus course designers to ensure that Pearson technology products, assessment tools, and online course materials are tailored to meet your specific needs. This highly qualified team is dedicated to helping schools take full advantage of a wide range of educational resources, by assisting in the integration of a variety of instructional materials and media formats. Your local Pearson Education sales representative can provide you with more details on this service program.

Acknowledgments

Authoring the second Canadian edition of this text has been a major undertaking made possible by the contributions of many individuals. First, we would like to acknowledge the efforts of the authors of the first Canadian edition and those of *Pharmacology: Connections to Nursing Practice* (3rd U.S. Edition). Their work provided an excellent foundation for this text.

Thanks to the dedicated and talented team at Pearson Education Canada: acquisitions editor Kimberley Veevers; marketing manager Michelle Bish; developmental editor Charlotte Morrison-Reed; production editor Hardik Popli; designer Anthony Leung; and production manager Jessica Mifsud. Thanks also go to copy editor Susan Broadhurst and proofreader Upendra Prasad.

We would like to thank Kaitlyn Harnden, RPH, PharmD, CDE for her keen eye as she conducted the technical review of our book.

We also want to thank the reviewers for their invaluable feedback on drafts of this text:

Mary-Lou Bois, Conestoga College

Joanne Bouma, Mount Royal University, Calgary

Sandra Carless, University of Alberta

Spring Farrell, Dalhousie University

Karen Katsademas, Fanshawe College

Christa MacLean, Saskatchewan Polytechnic

Krista Patton, St. Lawrence College

Faith Richardson, Trinity Western University

Crystal Schauerte, Algonquin College

Joseph Osuji and Mohamed El-Husein

Learning Pharmacology in Context

The vast majority of drugs are prescribed for specific diseases, yet many pharmacology texts fail to recognize the complex inter-relationships between pharmacology and disease. Learning drugs in the context of their associated diseases will make it easier for you to connect pharmacotherapy to therapeutic goals and client wellness. The pathophysiology approach of this text gives you a clearer picture of the importance of pharmacology to disease and, ultimately, to nursing care.

▶ **NCLEX Success Tips** Addressing the need to prepare Canadian nursing students for the NCLEX exam, NCLEX Success Tips introduce the format and concepts of the NCLEX exam early enough to give students ample time to understand and assimilate them.

UNIT 5	Pharmacology of Alterations in the Central Nervous System

▶ **Prototype Drugs.** presents a quick way for you to see the classifications and prototypes that are covered in the chapter, organized by disorder drug class.

▶ **Prototype Approach and Prototype Drug Boxes.**
The number of drugs available in clinical practice is staggering. To help you learn them, we use a prototype approach in which we introduce the one or two most representative drugs in each classification in detail. It can be less intimidating to focus your learning on one representative drug in each class. **Prototype Drug** boxes clearly summarize these important medications, presenting:

- Actions and Uses
- Administration Alerts
- Pharmacokinetics (including onset of action, duration, half-life, and peak effect, when known)
- Adverse Effects and Interactions (with drugs, herbs, and food)

NCLEX Success Tips

The IV route does not involve absorption as a step after IV administration because it bypasses absorption barriers and results in an immediate systemic response. The fastest route of absorption is the inhalation route.

The body must absorb drugs that are administered PO, IM, sub Q, intradermally, or by nebulizer (metered dose inhaler) before the system can respond.

◀ **Disease and Body System Approach.** The organization by body systems (units) and diseases (chapters) clearly places the drugs in context in terms of how they are used therapeutically. You can easily locate all relevant anatomy, physiology, pathophysiology, and pharmacology in the same chapter in which we present complete information for the drug classifications used to treat the diseases in each chapter. This organization builds the connection between pharmacology, pathophysiology, and the nursing care you learn in your clinical nursing courses.

PROTOTYPE DRUG	Bethanechol (Duvoid)

Actions and Uses: Bethanechol is a direct-acting cholinergic that interacts with muscarinic receptors to cause actions typical of parasympathetic stimulation. Its effects are most noted in the digestive and urinary tracts, where it will stimulate smooth muscle contraction. These actions are useful in increasing smooth muscle tone and muscular contractions in the GI tract following general anesthesia. In addition, it is used to treat non-obstructive urinary retention in clients with atony of the bladder.

PROTOTYPE DRUG	Atropine

Actions and Uses: By occupying muscarinic receptors, atropine blocks the parasympathetic actions of acetylcholine and induces symptoms of the fight-or-flight response. Most prominent are increased heart rate, bronchodilation, decreased motility in the GI tract, mydriasis, and decreased secretions from glands. At therapeutic doses, atropine has no effect on nicotinic receptors in ganglia or skeletal muscle.

Providing a Nursing Focus

Once you understand how a drug works on the body—that is, its actions, therapeutic effects, potential side effects and interactions, and more—you begin to understand the "why" of the interventions you will take as a nurse. Each chapter guides you to the content that is essential in order for you to provide safe and effective drug therapy.

Nursing Considerations

The role of the nurse in dopaminergic therapy involves careful monitoring of the client's condition and providing education as it relates to the prescribed drug regimen. Prior to the initiation of drug therapy, the client's health history should be taken. Those with narrow-angle glaucoma, undiagnosed skin lesions, or history of hypersensitivity should not take dopaminergic agents. Dopaminergics should be used cautiously in clients with severe cardiac, renal, liver, or endocrine diseases; mood disorders; or a history of seizures or ulcers and in those who are pregnant or lactating. Initial lab testing should include a complete blood count and liver and renal function studies. These tests should be obtained throughout the treatment regimen. Baseline information should include vital signs (especially blood pressure), mental status, and symptoms of Parkinson's disease. Lastly, all other medications taken by the client should be fully evaluated for compatibility with dopaminergic agonists.

During initial treatment, blood pressure, pulse, and respirations should be closely monitored because these drugs may cause hypotension and tachycardia. Additional lab testing for diabetes and acromegaly should be done if the client is expected to take the drug long term. The nurse should especially monitor clients for excessive daytime sleepiness, eye twitching, involuntary movements, hand tremors, fatigue, anxiety, mood changes, confusion, agitation, nausea, vomiting, anorexia, dry mouth, and constipation. Muscle twitching and mood changes may indicate toxicity and should be reported at once. The nurse may need to assist clients with drug administration and activities of daily living, including ambulation, at least initially. It is normal for the client's urine and perspiration to darken in colour.

◀ **Nursing Considerations** appear within each drug class section and discuss the major needs of the client, including:

* General Assessments
* Interventions
* Lifespan Considerations
* Client Education for all drugs in that classification, when applicable

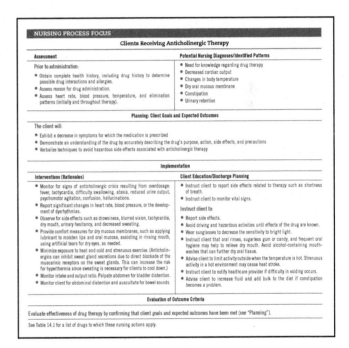

▲ **Nursing Process Focus** charts present need-to-know nursing actions in the nursing process—assessment, nursing diagnoses, planning, implementation with interventions and rationales, evaluation—and include client teaching and discharge planning.

▼ **Special Considerations** boxes present a variety of special issues related to ethnicity, gender, and psychosocial concerns that nurses must consider during drug therapy.

CONNECTIONS Special Considerations

◀ Enzyme Deficiency in Certain Ethnic Populations

Pharmacogenetics has identified a number of people who are deficient in the enzyme glucose-6-phosphate dehydrogenase (G6PD). This enzyme is essential in carbohydrate metabolism. Males of Mediterranean and African descent are more likely to express this deficiency. According to Carter (2012), G6PD deficiency is the most common enzyme deficiency worldwide. It is estimated to affect 400 million people worldwide. The disorder is caused by mutations in the DNA that encode for G6PD, resulting in one or more amino acid changes in the protein molecule. Following administration of certain drugs, such as primaquine, sulfonamides, and nitrofurantoin (Macrobid), an acute hemolysis of red blood cells occurs due to the breaking of chemical bonds in the hemoglobin molecule. Up to 50% of the circulating red blood cells may be destroyed. Genetic typing does not always predict toxicity; therefore, the nurse must observe clients carefully following the administration of these medications. Fortunately, there are good alternative choices for these medications.

Carter, S. M. (2012). *Glucose-6-phosphate dehydrogenase deficiency.* Retrieved from http://emedicine.medscape.com/article/200390-overview

▶ **Cultural Considerations** boxes explore issues specifically related to clients' cultural backgrounds, which may affect their responses to illness and their attitudes to drug therapy.

CONNECTIONS Cultural Considerations

◀ **Cultural Influences on Pain Expression and Perception**

How a person responds to pain and the type of pain management chosen may be culturally determined. Establishment of a therapeutic relationship is of the utmost importance in helping a client to attain pain relief. Respect the client's attitudes and beliefs about pain as well as their preferred treatment. An assessment of the client's needs, beliefs, and customs by listening, showing respect, and allowing the client to help develop and choose treatment options to attain pain relief is the most culturally sensitive approach.

When assessing pain, the nurse must remember that some clients may openly express their feelings and need for pain relief while others believe that the expression of pain symptoms, such as crying, is a sign of weakness. Pain management also varies according to cultural and religious beliefs. Traditional pain medications may or may not be the preferred method for pain control. For example, some Aboriginal peoples and some Asian Canadians may prefer to use alternative therapies such as herbs, thermal therapies, acupuncture, massage, and meditation. Prayer plays an important role within some Canadian cultural groups, including some African Canadians.

CONNECTIONS Lifespan Considerations

◀ **The Influence of Age on Pain Expression and Perception**

Pain control in both children and older adults can be challenging. Knowledge of developmental theories, the aging process, behavioural cues, subtle signs of discomfort, and verbal and nonverbal responses to pain are a must when it comes to effective pain management. Older clients may have a decreased perception of pain or simply ignore pain as a "natural" consequence of aging. Because these clients are frequently undermedicated, a thorough assessment is a necessity. As with adults, it is important that the nurse believe children's self-reports when assessing for pain. Developmentally appropriate pain rating tools are available and should be used on a continuous basis. Comfort measures should also be used.

When administering opioids for pain relief, always closely monitor older adults and children. Smaller doses are usually indicated, and side effects may be heightened. Closely monitor decreased respirations, LOC, and dizziness. Body weight should be taken prior to the start of opioid administration and doses calculated accordingly. Bed or crib rails should be kept raised, and the bed should be in the low position at all times to prevent injury from falls. Some opioids, such as meperidine, should be used cautiously in children. Many older adults take multiple drugs (polypharmacy); therefore, it is important to obtain a complete list of all medications taken and check for interactions.

◀ **Lifespan Considerations** boxes specifically address client care issues across the lifespan.

CONNECTIONS Natural Therapies

◀ **Valerian**

Valerian root (*Valeriana officinalis*) is a perennial native to Europe and North America that is an herbal choice for nervous tension and anxiety. This natural product promotes rest without affecting rapid eye movement (REM) sleep and has a reputation for calming an individual without causing side effects or discomfort. Its name comes from the Latin *valere*, which means "to be well." One thing that is *not well*, however, is its pungent odour, although many users claim that the smell is well worth the benefits. Valerian also is purported to reduce pain and headaches without the worry of dependency. There is no drug hangover, as is sometimes experienced with tranquilizers and sedatives. It is available as a tincture (alcohol mixture), tea, or extract. Sometimes it is placed in juice and consumed immediately before taking a nap or going to bed.

▶ **Natural Therapies** boxes present popular herbal or dietary supplements that clients may use along with conventional drugs. As a nurse, you need to assess clients to see if they are using any natural remedies that may have interactions with medications they are taking.

Teaching Through Visuals

For nearly all students, learning is a highly visual process. Therefore, we use numerous visuals to help you review the anatomy and physiology of body systems as well as understand the principles of drug action on the body.

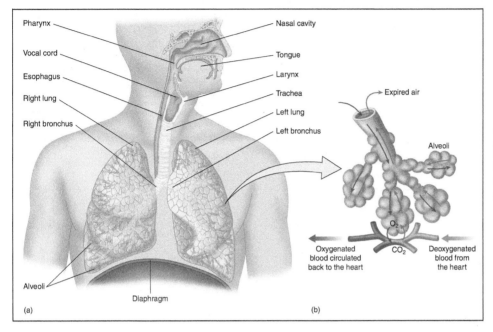

◄ **Vivid and Colorful Illustrations** help you to review specific anatomy, physiology, and pathophysiology for a body system and better understand the impact of disease on that system.

Putting It All Together

The tools at the end of each chapter and on **MyNursingLab** help you to test your understanding of the drugs and nursing care presented in that chapter. Using these tools will help you to succeed in your pharmacology course, in the clinical setting, on the NCLEX exam, and ultimately in your professional nursing practice.

► **Key Concepts Summary** provides expanded summaries of concepts that correlate to sections within the chapter. You can use this succinct summary to ensure that you understand the concepts before moving on to the next chapter. The numbering of these concepts helps you to easily locate that section within the chapter if you need further review.

CHAPTER

3   Understanding the Chapter

Key Concepts Summary

The numbered key concepts provide a succinct summary of the important points from the corresponding numbered section within the chapter. If any of these points are not clear, refer to the numbered section within the chapter for review.

3.1 Pharmacokinetics focuses on the movement of drugs throughout the body after they are administered. The four processes of pharmacokinetics are absorption, metabolism, distribution, and excretion.

3.2 The physiological properties of plasma membranes determine movement of drugs throughout the body.

3.3 Absorption is the process of moving a drug from the site of administration to the bloodstream. Absorption of a drug molecule depends on its size, lipid solubility, degree of ionization, and interactions with food or other medications.

3.4 Distribution represents how drugs are transported throughout the body. Distribution depends on the formation of drug-protein complexes and special

barriers such as the fetal-placental and blood-brain barriers.

3.5 Metabolism is a process that changes a drug's form and makes it more likely to be excreted. Changes in hepatic metabolism can significantly affect drug action.

3.6 Excretion processes remove drugs from the body. Drugs are primarily excreted by the kidneys but may be excreted by the lung or glands, or into bile.

3.7 The therapeutic response of most drugs depends on their concentration in the plasma. The difference between the minimum effective concentration and the toxic concentration is called the therapeutic range.

3.8 Plasma half-life represents the duration of action for most drugs.

3.9 Repeated dosing allows a plateau drug plasma level to be reached. Loading doses allow a therapeutic drug level to be reached rapidly.

▶ **NCLEX Practice Questions** allow you to test your knowledge. Answers are available in Appendix A at the end of your text. Select questions are also available for use in class with our Learning Catalytics tool.

NCLEX Practice Questions

1 A nurse is teaching a client about a newly prescribed medication. Which statement by the client would indicate the need for further medication education?

  a. "The liquid form of the drug will be absorbed faster than the tablets."

  b. "If I take more, I'll have a better response."

  c. "Taking this drug with food will decrease how much of it gets in my system."

  d. "I can consult my healthcare provider if I experience unexpected adverse effects."

2 A nurse is caring for several clients. Which client will the nurse anticipate to be most likely to experience an alteration in drug metabolism?

  a. A 3-day-old premature infant

  b. A 22-year-old pregnant female

  c. A 32-year-old man with kidney stones

  d. A 50-year-old executive with hypertension

3 A client is receiving multiple medications, including one drug specifically used to stimulate gastric peristalsis. What influence could this drug have on additional oral medications?

  a. Increased absorption

  b. Reduced excretion

  c. Decreased absorption

  d. Enhanced distribution

4 A client is being discharged from the hospital with a nebulizer for self-administration of inhalation medication. Which statement by the client would indicate to the nurse that client education has been successful?

  a. "Inhaled medications should only be taken in the morning."

  b. "Doses for inhaled medication are larger than for oral medication."

  c. "Medicines taken by inhalation produce a very rapid response."

  d. "Inhaled drugs are often rendered inactive by hepatic metabolic reactions."

5 A nurse is caring for a client with hepatitis and resulting hepatic impairment. The nurse would expect the duration of action of most of the client's medications to

  a. Decrease

  b. Improve

  c. Be unaffected

  d. Increase

See Answers to NCLEX Practice Questions in Appendix A.

▶ **Critical Thinking Questions** help you to apply the essential components of nursing care through case-based scenarios. Appendix B provides answers to these questions.

Critical Thinking Questions

1. What is the difference between therapeutic classification and pharmacological classification?

2. What classification is a barbiturate? Macrolide? Birth control pills? Laxatives? Folic acid antagonist? Antianginal agent?

3. What is a prototype drug, and what advantages does a prototype approach to studying pharmacology offer?

4. Why do nurses need to know all of this pharmacology?

See Answers to Critical Thinking Questions in Appendix B.

MyNursingLab

MyNursingLab engages students in higher-level thinking to move beyond knowledge acquisition to true learning through application of its unique "Review, Remember, Apply" Study Plan, Learning Catalytics, NCLEX Practice Tests, and additional Media Resources such as videos and animations.

Contents

UNIT

1

Fundamental Concepts and Principles of Pharmacology

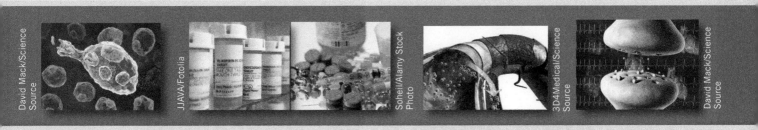

David Mack/Science Source · JJAVA/Fotolia · Soheil/Alamy Stock Photo · 3D4Medical/Science Source · David Mack/Science Source

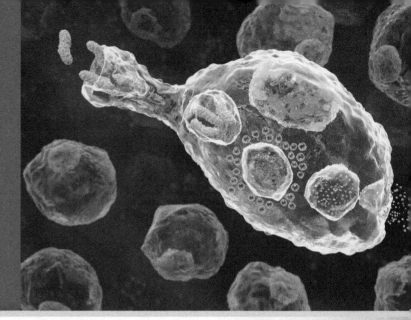
David Mack/Science Source

CHAPTER 1

Introduction to Pharmacology and Drug Regulations in Canada

LEARNING OUTCOMES

After reading this chapter, the student should be able to:

1. Define pharmacology.
2. Discuss the interdisciplinary nature of pharmacology.
3. Compare and contrast therapeutics and pharmacology.
4. Compare and contrast conventional drugs, biologics, and natural health products.
5. Identify the advantages and disadvantages of prescription and over-the-counter (OTC) drugs.
6. Identify key Canadian drug regulations that help to ensure the safety and efficacy of medications.
7. Discuss the role of Health Canada and the Health Products and Food Branch (HPFB) of Health Canada and its Therapeutic Products Directorate in the drug approval process.
8. Describe the stages of approval for therapeutic and biologic drugs in Canada.

CHAPTER OUTLINE

▸ Pharmacology: The Study of Medicines

▸ Pharmacology and Therapeutics

▸ Classification of Therapeutic Agents as Drugs, Biologics, or Natural Health Products

▸ Prescription and Over-the-Counter Drugs

▸ Drug Regulations and Standards

▸ Federal Drug Legislation

▸ Approval Process for Prescription Drugs

▸ Pricing and Access to Prescription Drugs Across Canada

More drugs are being prescribed to consumers than ever before. About 500 million prescriptions are dispensed each year in Canada. Each Canadian filled an average of 14 prescriptions in 2008, and in the year 2012–2013 Canadians spent about $23 billion on prescription medicine. The purpose of this chapter is to introduce the subject of pharmacology and to emphasize the role of government in ensuring that drugs, herbals, and other natural alternatives are safe and effective for public use.

Pharmacology: The Study of Medicines

1.1 Pharmacology is the study of medicines. It includes how drugs are administered and how the body responds.

The word **pharmacology** is derived from two Greek words: *pharmakon*, which means "medicine, drug," and *logos*, which means "study." Thus, pharmacology is most simply defined as the study of medicines.

Pharmacology is an expansive subject ranging from understanding how drugs are administered, to where they travel in the body, to the actual responses produced. To learn the discipline well, nursing students need a firm understanding of concepts from various foundation areas such as anatomy and physiology, chemistry, microbiology, and pathophysiology.

More than 10 000 brand name, generic, and combination agents are currently available. Each has its own characteristic set of therapeutic applications, interactions, side effects, and mechanisms of action. Many drugs are prescribed for more than one disease, and most produce multiple effects on the body. Further complicating the study of pharmacology is the fact that drugs may elicit different responses depending on individual client factors such as age, sex, body mass, health status, and genetics. Indeed, learning the applications of existing medications and staying current with new drugs introduced every year is an enormous challenge for the nurse. The task, however, is a critical one for both the client and the healthcare practitioner. If applied properly, drugs can dramatically improve quality of life. If applied improperly, the consequences can be devastating.

Pharmacology and Therapeutics

1.2 The fields of pharmacology and therapeutics are closely connected. Pharmacotherapy is the application of drugs to prevent disease and ease suffering.

A thorough study of pharmacology is important to healthcare providers who prescribe or administer drugs. Although federal and provincial laws sometimes limit the kinds of drugs marketed and the methods used to dispense them, *all* nurses are directly involved with client care and are active in educating, managing, and monitoring the proper use of drugs. This applies not only for nurses in clinics, hospitals, and home healthcare settings, but also for nurses who teach and for new students entering the nursing profession. In all of these cases, a thorough knowledge of pharmacology is necessary for them to perform their duties. As nursing students progress toward their chosen specialty, pharmacology is at the core of client care and is integrated into every step of the nursing process. As new drugs and research findings emerge, nurses are challenged to evaluate the information and incorporate relevant knowledge into evidence-based practice.

Another important area of study for the nurse, sometimes difficult to distinguish from pharmacology, is the study of therapeutics. Therapeutics is slightly different from the field of pharmacology, although the disciplines are closely connected. **Therapeutics** is the branch of medicine concerned with the prevention of disease and treatment of suffering. **Pharmacotherapy**, or **pharmacotherapeutics**, is the administration of drugs for the purpose of disease prevention or treatment and relief of suffering. Drugs are just one of many therapies available to the nurse for preventing or alleviating human suffering.

Classification of Therapeutic Agents as Drugs, Biologics, or Natural Health Products

1.3 Therapeutic agents may be classified as traditional drugs, biologics, or natural health products.

Substances applied for therapeutic purposes fall into one of the following three general categories:

- Drugs or medications
- Biologics
- Natural health products

A **drug** is a chemical agent capable of producing biological responses within the body. These responses may be desirable (therapeutic) or undesirable (adverse). A drug that is considered medically therapeutic is commonly referred to as a **medication**. Because drugs are defined so broadly, it is necessary to separate them from other substances that can alter the body's biological activities, such as foods, household products, and cosmetics. Agents such as antiperspirants, sunscreens, toothpastes, and shampoos might alter the body's biological activities, but they are not considered drugs or medications. Sometimes it is not clear whether a substance is a medication. For example, alcohol (beer, red wine) may be considered medically therapeutic when used in small amounts for cardiovascular effects, yet not be therapeutic when used in excess.

While most modern drugs are synthesized in a laboratory, **biologics** are agents naturally produced in animal cells, by microorganisms, or by the body itself. Examples of biologics include hormones, monoclonal antibodies, natural blood products and components, interferon, and vaccines. Biologics are used to treat a wide variety of illnesses and conditions.

Other therapeutic approaches include **natural health products (NHPs)** and complementary and alternative therapies. NHPs may include natural plant extracts, herbals, vitamins, minerals, and dietary supplements. NHPs are discussed in detail in Chapter 11. **Complementary and alternative therapies** include therapies such as acupuncture, hypnosis, biofeedback, and massage. Because of their growing popularity, herbal and alternative therapies are featured throughout this text. It is important to ensure that information related to home herbal remedies is shared with medical professionals, to ensure that the client does not receive two different forms of the same drug or drugs that may counteract the home remedy.

The nurse should support the client by facilitating an open discussion on the client's intent to use herbal remedy with the physician. This will make the client feel involved in the decisions related to his or her care. Remind the client that the herbs may interfere with current medications that he or she is taking.

NCLEX Success Tip

The nurse should ensure that pregnant women avoid any medication unless their physician instructs them to use it. This includes herbal remedies because their effects on the fetus have not been identified.

Prescription and Over-the-Counter Drugs

1.4 Drugs are available by prescription or over the counter. Prescription drugs require an order from a healthcare provider.

Legal drugs are obtained either by a prescription or over the counter (OTC). There are major differences between the two dispensing methods. To obtain prescription drugs, a qualified healthcare provider must give an order authorizing the client to receive the drug. The advantages to requiring an authorization are numerous. The healthcare provider has an opportunity to examine the client and determine a specific diagnosis. The practitioner can maximize therapy by ordering the proper drug for the client's condition and controlling the amount and frequency of drug to be dispensed. In addition, the healthcare provider has an opportunity to teach the client the proper use of the drug and what side effects to expect. In a few instances, a high margin of safety observed over many years can prompt a change in the status of a drug from prescription to OTC.

NCLEX Success Tips

Call the prescriber immediately if an order is difficult to read or for any questions about the order. Do not administer a medication that has an unclear order.

Under law, nurses are responsible for their own actions. For example, if a drug order is written incorrectly, the nurse who administers the incorrect order is responsible for the error.

In contrast to prescription drugs, OTC drugs do not require a prescription. In most cases, individuals may treat themselves safely if they carefully follow instructions included with the medication. If they do not follow these guidelines, OTC drugs can have serious adverse effects.

NCLEX Success Tip

Older adults commonly have multiple physicians and caregivers. The client needs to inform every doctor about all the medications being prescribed by all of them.

Individuals prefer to take OTC drugs for many reasons. They may be obtained more easily than prescription drugs. No appointment with a physician is required, thus saving time and money. Without the assistance of a healthcare provider, however, choosing the proper drug for a specific problem can be challenging for an individual. OTC drugs may react with foods, herbal products, prescription medications, or other OTC drugs. Individuals may not be aware that some drugs can impair their ability to function safely. Self-treatment is sometimes ineffective, and the potential for harm may increase if the disease is allowed to progress.

Drug Regulations and Standards

1.5 Drug regulations were created to protect the public from drug misuse and to assume continuous evaluation of safety and effectiveness.

Until the 19th century, there were few standards or guidelines to protect the public from drug misuse. The archives of drug regulatory agencies are filled with examples of early medicines, including rattlesnake oil for rheumatism; epilepsy treatment for spasms, hysteria, and alcoholism; and fat reducers for a slender, healthy figure. Many of these early concoctions proved ineffective, though harmless. At their worst, some contained hazardous levels of dangerous or addictive substances. It became quite clear that drug regulations were needed to protect the public.

Federal Drug Legislation

1.6 The regulatory agency responsible for ensuring that drugs are safe and effective is the Therapeutic Products Directorate of the Health Products and Food Branch of Health Canada.

The Health Products and Food Branch (HPFB) of **Health Canada** is responsible for ensuring that health products and

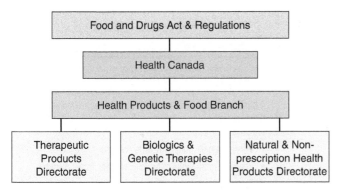

Figure 1.1 The governance structure for therapeutic products in Canada.

foods approved for sale to Canadians are safe and of high quality. The HPFB regulates the use of therapeutic products through directorates, as shown in Figure 1.1. The Therapeutic Products Directorate (TPD) authorizes marketing of a pharmaceutical drug or medical device once a manufacturer presents sufficient scientific evidence of the product's safety, efficacy, and quality as required by the Food and Drugs Act and Regulations. The Biologics and Genetic Therapies Directorate (BGTD) regulates biologic drugs (drugs derived from living sources) and radiopharmaceuticals. Products regulated by the BGTD include blood products, vaccines, tissues, organs, and gene therapy products. The Natural and Non-prescription Health Products Directorate (NNHPD) is the regulating authority for natural health products for sale in Canada. Natural health products and their regulation are presented in Chapter 11.

Approval Process for Prescription Drugs

1.7 Four levels of testing are required for therapeutic drugs and biologics. These progress from cellular and animal testing to use of the experimental drug in clients with the disease.

Preclinical investigation involves extensive laboratory research. Over a 3- to 5-year period, scientists perform many tests on human and microbial cells cultured in the laboratory. Studies are performed in different species of animals to examine the drug's effectiveness at different doses and to look for adverse effects. Extensive testing on cultured cells and in animals is essential because it allows scientists to predict whether the drug will cause harm to humans. Because laboratory tests do not always reflect the way a human will respond, preclinical investigation results are always inconclusive. Animal testing may overestimate or underestimate the actual risk to humans.

If the drug has a desirable effect and is safe for animals, a Clinical Trial Application (CTA) is made to Health Canada, requesting permission to start clinical trials. The CTA includes detailed information about the drug's ingredients and proposed mechanism of action, the results of animal testing, and the proposed methodology for the clinical trials.

The manufacturer of a newly developed drug applies for **patent protection** that gives the manufacturer the right to sell the drug without competition for 20 years. When a patent has expired, competing pharmaceutical companies are permitted to manufacture and sell generic (chemically identical) versions of the drug.

Clinical trials, the second stage of drug testing, take place in three phases. Clinical trials are the longest part of the drug approval process. In phase I, clinical investigators perform tests on 20 to 100 healthy volunteers to determine dosage and to assess how the drug is absorbed, metabolized, and excreted by the body. In phase II, 100 to 300 clients with the particular disease the drug is intended to treat are given the medication to determine proper dosage and side effects. In phase III, 1000 to 3000 clients with the disease are given the medication. To eliminate bias, a double-blind study is generally used in which clients and investigators do not know whether the treatment the client is receiving is the drug or a placebo. Only about 10% of investigational drugs tested will make it to phase III clinical trials. Clinical investigators from different medical specialties address concerns such as whether the drug is effective, worsens other medical conditions, interacts unsafely with existing medications, or affects one type of client more than others.

Clinical trials are an essential component of drug evaluations because of the variability of responses among clients. A clinical trial may be stopped if the drug is shown to be unsafe. In this case, the drug may be abandoned or may undergo further development. If the drug shows promise but precautions are noted, the process is delayed until the pharmaceutical company addresses the concerns. If a drug appears to have dramatic benefits and be without serious side effects, it may be fast-tracked through the Health Canada approval process. A Priority Review Process is in place and may permit a drug to be used even sooner in special cases, with careful monitoring.

A **New Drug Submission (NDS)** must be submitted before a drug is allowed to proceed to the next stage of the approval process. Health Canada receives about 80 NDSs for new drugs each year and approves about 10%. Health Canada reviews the submitted information and evaluates the drug's safety, efficacy, and quality. If Health Canada authorizes the drug to be marketed in Canada, a **Notice of Compliance (NOC)** and a **Drug Identification Number (DIN)** are issued to indicate official approval. The DIN must be displayed on the label of all prescription drugs, as shown in Figure 1.2. If there is insufficient evidence to support the safety, efficacy, or quality claims, authorization to market the drug will not be granted and a Notice of Deficiency or Notice of Non-Compliance is issued. Drug companies can then submit further information to support their claims and can appeal the decision not to authorize the drug.

Once drugs are marketed, the Marketed Health Products Directorate (MHPD) provides post-approval surveillance and regulation. Since clinical trials involve a limited number of individuals during a limited time period, they may detect only frequent or common adverse drug reactions (ADRs). It has been estimated that serious side effects may not be detected during clinical trials for as many as half of approved drugs. Under the Food and Drugs Act, manufacturers are required to continue to monitor the drug's safety and

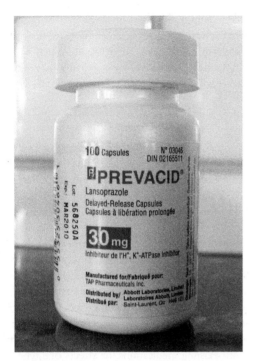

Figure 1.2   Example of a drug product labelled according to Canadian requirements: the generic drug name, Drug Identification Number, lot number, expiry date, and ingredients must be displayed.

Source: Shirley King

TABLE 1.1	Steps of Approval for Drugs Marketed in Canada
Step 1	Preclinical experiments in cultured cells, living tissue, and small animals are performed.
Step 2	A Clinical Trial Application (CTA) is submitted to Health Canada, followed by extensive clinical trials. Clinical trials are done in three phases: • Phase I: small group of healthy humans • Phase II: small group of humans with the target disorder • Phase III: large group of humans with the target disorder
Step 3	The pharmaceutical company completes a New Drug Submission (NDS) to Health Canada. This report details important safety and efficacy information, including testing data, how the drug product will be produced and packaged, expected therapeutic benefits, and adverse reactions.
Step 4	A committee of drug experts, including medical and drug scientists, reviews the NDS to identify potential drug benefits and risks.
Step 5	Health Canada reviews information about the drug product and passes on important details to healthcare practitioners and consumers.
Step 6	Health Canada issues a Notice of Compliance (NOC) and Drug Identification Number (DIN). Both are required for the manufacturer to market the drug product.
Step 7	Health Canada monitors the efficacy of the drug and any safety concerns after it has been marketed. This is done by regular inspection, notices, newsletters, and feedback from consumers and healthcare professionals.

effects and report undesirable effects to the MHPD. MHPD activities include reviewing product safety data, investigating complaints, monitoring product advertising, and communicating product-related risks to healthcare professionals and consumers. Nurses can subscribe to MedEffect Canada, an online service provided by Health Canada to quickly alert healthcare professionals about health product safety concerns. The Canadian Adverse Drug Reaction Information System (CADRIS) is a database of suspected adverse reactions to pharmaceuticals, biologics, and natural health products reported to Health Canada's Canadian Adverse Drug Reaction Monitoring Program (CADRMP). ADR reports are submitted voluntarily by health professionals or consumers. Only a small percentage of ADRs that occur are thought to be reported. Nurses play an important role in reporting ADRs and contributing to this database.

There are many sources of information about drugs marketed in Canada. Health Canada maintains an online **Drug Product Database** that is searchable by company, product name, active ingredient, DIN, or active ingredient group number. It is the most authoritative source of drugs marketed in Canada and contains listings for all human and veterinary drug products that have been assigned a DIN. The ***Compendium of Pharmaceuticals and Specialties* (CPS)** is a compilation of drug product monographs that are submitted by pharmaceutical manufacturers. Copies of the CPS are commonly available on nursing units, in pharmacies, and in physicians' offices. An online version (eCPS) is also readily available and accessible to healthcare practitioners. The contents are selected by the manufacturer and approved by Health Canada and frequently include information about product testing. Drug guides for nurses are published specifically to meet the need of nurses and their clients for accurate and concise information regarding drug action, desired and undesired effects,

application of the nursing process, client teaching, and other aspects of drug therapy.

The drug approval process in Canada is outlined in Table 1.1. Many similarities exist in how drugs are regulated in Canada and the United States. These include the fact that both governments have realized a need to monitor natural products, dietary supplements and herbs, and newly developed drug therapies. Many natural products do not need to go through as rigorous testing and often make it to market faster. Healthcare practitioners need to be aware that some clients may feel that just as they are taking "a natural product that it is safe or safer than a prescription product"—this is not always the case as often there is less data to come to this conclusion regarding these products.

Pricing and Access to Prescription Drugs Across Canada

1.8 Once criticized for being too slow, Health Canada has streamlined the process to get new drugs to market more quickly.

Access to new drugs may be further delayed and may vary among the provinces. Once Health Canada has approved drugs for marketing in Canada, each province and territory must decide which drugs to list on the provincial formulary and to reimburse under the provincial drug plan. A **formulary** is a list of drugs available for prescribing or dispensing. Although each province and territory must make its own final decision, the Common Drug Review (CDR) was established in 2002 to coordinate the jurisdictional review of new drugs and provide a listing recommendation. The CDR may require up to 6 months to make a recommendation. Generic and existing drugs are reviewed independently of the CDR by individual provinces, territories, and private insurers. Pharmacists in hospitals and other health agencies make decisions about which drugs from the provincial formulary to include in their own formularies.

The cost of drugs influences access. Public and private insurers have budgets and thus consider the cost of drugs in making decisions about whether to list patented medicines as well as other medicines in their formularies. The Patented Medicine Prices Review Board (PMPRB) is a quasi-judicial body that operates under the Patent Act and is independent of Health Canada. The PMPRB regulates the prices charged by manufacturers for patented medicines to ensure that they are not excessive in comparison to other countries. The PMPRB does not regulate nonpatented drugs. Generic drugs that are bioequivalent to the brand drug may be marketed once patents expire and the NOC is received. Generic drugs cost, on average, about 45% less than their brand name equivalents. Insurance coverage for approved drugs is a federal responsibility for a few special populations, such as veterans, Aboriginal peoples,

and members of the Royal Canadian Mounted Police and the Canadian Armed Forces. For all other Canadians, the provincial governments and private insurers determine which drugs will be covered under their drug benefit plans and what level of coverage will be provided.

Advertising is another factor that influences drug product awareness and access. Health Canada is the regulatory authority for drug advertising. Advertising Standards Canada (ASC) and the Pharmaceutical Advertising Advisory Board (PAAB) are responsible for ensuring that advertisements comply with rules set by Health Canada under the Food and Drugs Act and Regulations. Advertising in journals for healthcare providers may contain detailed drug information; however, unlike in the United States, Canada limits direct-to-consumer advertising of prescription medications. Direct-to-consumer advertising is not allowed for prescription drugs and drugs that treat or cure serious diseases.

Through a **Special Access Program (SAP)**, Health Canada provides access to drugs not currently approved in Canada for treatment of clients with serious or life-threatening conditions for whom conventional therapies are ineffective, unavailable, or unsuitable. Health Canada reviews the Special Access Request Form. If approved, Health Canada sends a Letter of Authorization to the drug manufacturer and the client's physician. Pharmaceutical companies have the right to decide whether, and under what conditions, to provide the drug to the client.

CHAPTER

1   **Understanding the Chapter**

Key Concepts Summary

The numbered key concepts provide a succinct summary of the important points from the corresponding numbered section within the chapter. If any of these points are not clear, refer to the numbered section within the chapter for review.

1.1 Pharmacology is the study of medicines. It includes how drugs are administered and how the body responds.

1.2 The fields of pharmacology and therapeutics are closely connected. Pharmacotherapy is the application of drugs to prevent disease and ease suffering.

1.3 Therapeutic agents may be classified as traditional drugs, biologics, or natural health products.

1.4 Drugs are available by prescription or over the counter. Prescription drugs require an order from a healthcare provider.

1.5 Drug regulations were created to protect the public from drug misuse and to assume continuous evaluation of safety and effectiveness.

1.6 The regulatory agency responsible for ensuring that drugs are safe and effective is the Therapeutic Products Directorate of the Health Products and Food Branch of Health Canada.

1.7 Four levels of testing are required for therapeutic drugs and biologics. These progress from cellular and animal testing to use of the experimental drug in clients with the disease.

1.8 Once criticized for being too slow, Health Canada has streamlined the process to get new drugs to market more quickly.

Chapter 1 Scenario

Gertrude Stone lives alone in the same house she has owned for 46 years. Although she is seldom sick, when she needs to see a healthcare provider she must ride the public bus system. The trip requires two bus transfers and can be tiring.

Because Gertrude lives only one block from a grocery store, she often self-medicates using OTC drugs. She strongly believes in the use of herbs, vitamins, and home remedies.

As a parish nurse, you assist with the health fair at a church where Gertrude is an active member.

Critical Thinking Questions

1. How would you respond to Gertrude about the safety of OTC drugs?
2. What are the advantages and disadvantages of OTC medications?
3. How can Gertrude be certain that OTC medications are safe for her?

See Answers to Critical Thinking Questions in Appendix B.

NCLEX Practice Questions

1 The nurse knows that governmental drug legislation requires the drug manufacturer to prove that a drug is both safe and

   a. Free of adverse effects and potential reactions

   b. Effective for a specified purpose

   c. Reasonable in cost and easily accessible

   d. Beneficial to various population groups

2 The drug research participant with a particular disease is taking part in an investigative study to examine the effects of a new drug. Previously, this drug was tested using healthy volunteers. The next phase of the clinical trial investigation in which the client will be participating is

   a. Phase 1

   b. Phase 2

   c. Phase 3

   d. Phase 4

3 When considering various drug therapies, the nurse knows that most drug testing and approval occurs with which population?

   a. Multiple population types and is usually safe for all clients

   b. Caucasian males and may not be safe for other populations

   c. Older adults and may be harmful to children and adolescents as well

   d. Animals, which verifies the drug's effectiveness in humans

4 The client requests that a refill prescription of a Schedule II controlled substance be telephoned to the drugstore. When responding to the client, the nurse would consider which factor? Refills of Schedule II drugs

   a. Are less costly than the original prescription

   b. Must be listened to by at least two people

   c. Are verified through the local RCMP drug enforcement office

   d. Are not permitted under federal law

5 The nurse knows that drugs subject to stricter regulations are those

   a. With a high potential for abuse or dependency

   b. That are most costly and difficult to produce

   c. With adverse effects and high occurrence of drug or food interactions

   d. That have taken years to be proven effective in the laboratory

See Answers to NCLEX Practice Questions in Appendix A.

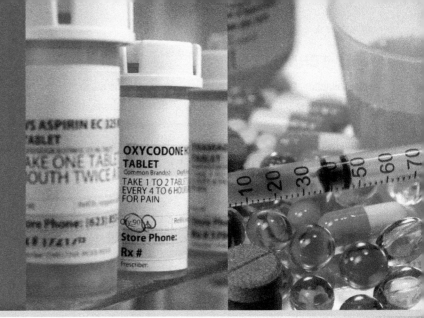

CHAPTER

2

Drug Classes and Schedules in Canada

LEARNING OUTCOMES

After reading this chapter, the student should be able to:

1. Explain what characterizes an ideal drug and how drugs are classified.

2. Explain the basis for placing drugs into therapeutic and pharmacological classes.

3. Discuss the prototype approach to drug classification.

4. Describe what is meant by a drug's mechanism of action.

5. Distinguish between a drug's chemical name, generic name, and trade name.

6. Explain why the use of generic names is preferred to trade names when referring to drugs.

7. Discuss why drugs are sometimes placed on a restrictive list and the controversy surrounding this issue.

8. Explain the meaning of a controlled substance.

9. Explain the Controlled Drugs and Substances Act (CDSA) of 1997 and the role of the Drug Strategy and Controlled Substances Programme (DSCSP) in controlling drug abuse and misuse.

10. Explain how drugs are scheduled according to Canada's Food and Drugs Act, the CDSA, and the Narcotic Control Regulations (NCR).

11. Identify the drug schedules, and give examples of drugs at each level.

12. Connect pharmacotherapy to nursing practice.

CHAPTER OUTLINE

▸ Characteristics of an Ideal Drug

▸ Therapeutic and Pharmacological Classification of Drugs

▸ Chemical, Generic, and Trade Names of Drugs

▸ Differences Between Brand Name Drugs and Their Generic Equivalents

▸ Drug Schedules

▸ Controlled Drugs and Substances

▸ Connecting Pharmacology to Nursing Practice

KEY TERMS

bioavailability, 12

chemical name, 11

combination drugs, 11

controlled substances, 13

dependence, 13

generic name, 11

indications, 10

mechanism of action, 10

pharmacological classification, 10

prototype drug, 11

therapeutic classification, 10

trade (proprietary or brand) name, 11

withdrawal, 13

The student beginning the study of pharmacology is quickly confronted with hundreds of drugs that have specific dosages, side effects, and mechanisms of action. Without a means of grouping or organizing this information, most students would be overwhelmed by the vast amounts of new information. It is recommended that students start with the notion of the ideal or "perfect" drug and understand what makes such drugs ideal and how they are classified. Drugs can be classified by a number of different methods that provide logical systems for identifying drugs and determining the limitations of their use. This chapter presents methods of grouping drugs by therapeutic or pharmacological classification and by drug schedules.

Characteristics of an Ideal Drug

2.1 The ideal drug is safe and effective.

An ideal drug is one that:

- Effectively treats, prevents, or cures the client's condition.
- Produces a rapid, predictable response at relatively low doses.
- Produces no adverse effects.
- Can be taken conveniently, usually by mouth.
- Can be taken infrequently, usually once a day, and for a short length of time.
- Is inexpensive and easily accessible.
- Is quickly eliminated by the body after it produces its beneficial effect.
- Does not interact with other medications or food.

After reading this description, it should appear clear to the student that there is really no such thing as a perfect drug. Some drugs meet most of the criteria, whereas others meet very few. At the very least, it is expected that all prescription drugs have some degree of effectiveness at treating or preventing a health condition. The conditions for which a drug is approved are its **indications**. Every prescription drug has at least one indication, and most have multiple indications. Some drugs are used for conditions for which they have not been approved; these are called unlabelled or off-label indications.

As a general rule, the more a medicine strays from the perfect drug profile, the less commonly it is used. This is because, whenever possible, healthcare providers strive to prescribe the most effective, safest, and most convenient medication for the client.

Therapeutic and Pharmacological Classification of Drugs

2.2 Drugs may be organized by their therapeutic or pharmacological classification.

One method of organizing drugs is based on their therapeutic usefulness in treating particular diseases. This is referred to as **therapeutic classification**. Drugs may also be organized by **pharmacological classification**. A drug's pharmacological classification refers to the way in which the drug works at the molecular, tissue, and body system level. Both types of classification are widely used in categorizing the thousands of available drugs. The key difference is that the therapeutic classification describes what is being treated by the drug, whereas the pharmacological classification describes how the drug acts.

Table 2.1 shows the method of therapeutic classification, using cardiac care as an example. Many different types of drugs affect cardiovascular function. Some drugs influence blood clotting, whereas others lower blood cholesterol or prevent the onset of stroke. Drugs may be used to treat elevated blood pressure, heart failure, abnormal rhythm, chest pain, heart attack, or circulatory shock. Therefore, drugs that treat cardiac disorders may be placed in several types of therapeutic classes, for example, anticoagulants, antihyperlipidemics, and antihypertensives.

A therapeutic classification need not be complicated. For example, it is appropriate to simply classify a medication as a "drug used for stroke" or a "drug used for shock." The key to therapeutic classification is to clearly state what a particular drug does clinically. Other examples of therapeutic classifications include antidepressants, antipsychotics, drugs for erectile dysfunction, and antineoplastics.

The pharmacological classification addresses a drug's **mechanism of action**, or *how* a drug produces its effect in the body. Table 2.2 shows a variety of pharmacological classifications, using hypertension as an example. A diuretic treats hypertension by lowering plasma volume. Calcium channel blockers treat this disorder by decreasing cardiac contractility. Other drugs block intermediates of the renin-angiotensin pathway. Notice that each example describes *how* hypertension might be controlled. A drug's pharmacological classification

TABLE 2.1 Organizing Drug Information by Therapeutic Classification

THERAPEUTIC FOCUS: CARDIAC CARE/DRUGS AFFECTING CARDIOVASCULAR FUNCTION

Therapeutic Usefulness	Therapeutic Classification
Inhibiting blood clotting	Anticoagulants
Lowering blood cholesterol	Antihyperlipidemics
Lowering blood pressure	Antihypertensives
Restoring normal cardiac rhythm	Antidysrhythmics
Treating angina	Antianginals

TABLE 2.2 Organizing Drug Information by Pharmacological Classification

FOCUS ON HOW A THERAPY IS APPLIED: PHARMACOTHERAPY FOR HYPERTENSION

Mechanism of Action	Pharmacological Classification
Lowering plasma volume	Diuretic
Blocking heart calcium channels	Calcium channel blocker
Blocking hormonal activity	Angiotensin-converting enzyme inhibitor
Blocking stress-related activity	Adrenergic antagonist
Dilating peripheral blood vessels	Vasodilator

properties. Although chemical names convey a clear and concise meaning about the nature of a drug, they are often complicated and difficult to remember or pronounce. For example, few nurses know the chemical name for diazepam: 7-chloro-1,3-dihydro-1-methyl-5-phenyl-2H-1,4-benzodiazepin-2-one. In only a few cases, usually when the name is brief and easy to remember will nurses use chemical names. Examples of useful chemical names include lithium carbonate, calcium gluconate, and sodium chloride.

More practically, drugs are sometimes classified by a *portion* of their chemical structure, known as the chemical group name. Examples are antibiotics such as fluoroquinolones and cephalosporins. Other common examples include phenothiazines, thiazides, and benzodiazepines. Although they may seem complicated when first encountered, knowledge of chemical group names will become invaluable as the nursing student begins to learn and understand major drug classes and actions.

The **generic name** (non-proprietary) describes the chemical substance or pharmacological property of a drug. A generic name is the proper name of the drug ingredient or the common name if the ingredient has no proper name. An International Nonproprietary Name (INN) identifies a generic name as unique. An INN is the only internationally accepted generic name. Drugs that do not have a defined chemical composition or structure or that cannot adequately be described due to mixtures of substances cannot be assigned an INN. In Canada, INNs are used exclusively when they exist. Because there is only one generic name for each drug, healthcare providers often use this name, and students generally must memorize it. Importantly, the use of generic names increases safety since they are unique, while trade names may look and sound alike.

A drug's **trade (proprietary or brand) name** is assigned by the company marketing the drug. The name is usually selected to be short and easy to remember. The trade name is sometimes called the product or brand name. The term *proprietary* suggests ownership. In Canada, a drug developer is given exclusive rights to name and market a drug for 20 years after a new drug application is submitted to Health Canada. Because it takes several years for a drug to be approved, the amount of time spent in approval is usually subtracted from the 20 years. For example, if it takes 7 years for a drug to be approved, competing companies will not be allowed to market a generic equivalent drug for another 13 years. The rationale is that the developing company should be allowed sufficient time to recoup the millions of dollars spent in research and development to design the new drug. After 20 years, competing companies may sell a generic equivalent drug, sometimes using a different trade name, which Health Canada must approve.

Trade names may be a challenge for students to learn because of the dozens of products with different names that contain similar ingredients. In addition, **combination drugs** contain more than one active generic ingredient. This poses a problem in trying to match one generic name with one trade name. As an example, refer to Table 2.3 and consider the drug diphenhydramine (generic name), also called Benadryl (one of many trade names). Diphenhydramine is an antihistamine. When looking for diphenhydramine, the nurse

is more specific than a therapeutic classification and requires an understanding of biochemistry and physiology. In addition, pharmacological classifications may be described with varying degrees of complexity, sometimes taking into account drugs' chemical names.

When classifying drugs, it is common practice to select a single drug from a class and compare all other medications to this representative drug. A **prototype drug** is the well-understood drug model with which other drugs in a pharmacological class are compared. By learning the prototype drug, students may predict the actions and adverse effects of other drugs in the same class. For example, by knowing the effects of penicillin V, students can extend this knowledge to the other drugs in the penicillin class of antibiotics. The original drug prototype is not always the most widely used drug in its class. Newer drugs in the same class may be more effective, have a more favourable safety profile, or have a longer duration of action. These factors may discourage healthcare providers from using the original prototype drug. In addition, healthcare providers and pharmacology texts sometimes differ as to which drug should be the prototype. In any case, becoming familiar with the drug prototypes and keeping up with newer and more popular drugs are essential parts of mastering drugs and drug classes.

Chemical, Generic, and Trade Names of Drugs

2.3 Drugs have chemical, generic, and trade names. A drug has only one chemical or generic name but may have multiple trade names.

A major challenge in studying pharmacology is learning thousands of drug names. Adding to this difficulty is the fact that most drugs have multiple names. The three basic types of drug name are chemical, generic, and trade.

Chemical names are assigned using standard nomenclature established by the International Union of Pure and Applied Chemistry (IUPAC). A drug has only one chemical name, which is sometimes helpful in predicting its physical and chemical

TABLE 2.3 Examples of Trade Name Products That Contain Popular Generic Substances

Generic Substance	Trade Names
Acetylsalicylic acid (ASA)	Asaphen, Asaphen E.C., Entrophen, Novasen
Diphenhydramine	Allerdryl, Allernix, Benadryl, Nytol, Nytol Extra Strength, Simply Sleep, Sominex
Ibuprofen	Advil, Motrin, Pamprin, Super Strength Motrin

may find it listed under many trade names, provided alone or in combination with other active ingredients. Ibuprofen and acetylsalicylic acid are also examples of drugs with many different trade names. The rule of thumb is that the active ingredients in a drug are described by their generic name. When referring to a drug, the generic name is usually written in lowercase, whereas the trade name is capitalized. As stated in the Food and Drug Regulations (FDR), a drug is identified on its inner and outer label by the trade name (if there is one) followed by the generic name.

Differences Between Brand Name Drugs and Their Generic Equivalents

2.4 Generic drugs are less expensive than brand name drugs, but they may differ in their bioavailability, which is the ability of the drug to reach its target tissue and produce its effect.

During its 20 years of exclusive rights to a new drug, the pharmaceutical company determines the price of the medication. Because there is no competition, the price is generally quite high. The developing company sometimes uses legal tactics to extend its exclusive rights since this can bring in hundreds of millions of dollars per year in profits for a popular medicine. Once the exclusive rights end, competing companies market the generic drug for less money, and consumer savings may be considerable. In some jurisdictions, pharmacists may routinely substitute a generic drug when the prescription calls for a brand name. In other jurisdictions, the pharmacist must dispense drugs exactly as written by the healthcare provider or obtain approval before providing a generic substitute.

The companies marketing brand name drugs often lobby aggressively against laws that might restrict the routine use of their brand name products. The lobbyists claim that significant differences exist between a trade name drug and its generic equivalent and that switching to the generic drug may be harmful for the client. Consumer advocates, on the other hand, argue that generic

substitutions should always be permitted because of the cost savings to clients.

Are there really differences between a brand name drug and its generic equivalent? The answer is unclear. Despite the fact that the dosages may be identical, drug formulations are not always the same. The two drugs may have different inert or added ingredients. For example, if in tablet form, the active ingredients may be more tightly compressed in one of the preparations.

The key to comparing brand name drugs and their generic equivalents lies in measuring the bioavailability of the two preparations. **Bioavailability** is the amount of drug that is absorbed into systemic circulation and therefore physiologically available to reach its target cells and produce its effect. Bioavailability may indeed be affected by inert or added ingredients and tablet compression. Anything that affects absorption of a drug, or its distribution to the target cells, can certainly affect drug action. Measuring peak drug concentration in plasma and how long a drug takes to exert its effect gives a crude measure of bioavailability. For example, if a client is in circulatory shock and it takes the generic equivalent drug 5 minutes longer to produce its effect, that difference is significant; however, if a generic medication for arthritis pain relief takes 45 minutes to act, compared with the brand name drug, which takes 40 minutes, it probably does not matter which drug is prescribed. As a general rule, bioavailability is of most concern when using critical care drugs and those with a narrow safety margin (therapeutic index, or TI).

The physician should base changes to drug dosages on creatinine clearance test results, which reflect the kidney's glomerular filtration rate; this factor is important because most drugs are excreted at least partially by the kidneys. The gastrointestinal (GI) absorption rate, TI, and liver function studies do not help to determine dosage change in a client with decreased renal function. Clients with decreased renal function should continue taking the brand name drug and *not* switch to a generic equivalent, unless approved by the healthcare provider. For most other drugs, the generic equivalent may be safely substituted for the trade name drug.

Drug Schedules

2.5 Drugs with a potential for abuse are categorized into schedules.

Throughout Canada, both prescription and non-prescription drugs must meet specific criteria for public distribution and use. Health Canada has established that all drugs used for medicinal purposes be grouped into the schedules summarized in Table 2.4. Drugs that require a prescription are listed in Schedule F of the FDR. In Canada, all Schedule F drugs must display "Pr" on the outside label of the product. Non-prescription drugs are provided according to guidelines and acts established by the respective Canadian provinces and territories. Pharmacies must monitor drugs used specifically to treat self-limiting discomforts such as cold, flu, and mild GI symptoms. Other non-prescription drugs may be sold without monitoring.

TABLE 2.4 Schedule System for Drugs Sold in Canada

Schedule	Description
Schedule I	Available only by prescription and provided by a pharmacist; includes the following: • All prescription drugs • Drugs with less potential for abuse: Schedule F • Controlled drugs: Schedule G • Narcotic drugs
Schedule II	Available only from a pharmacist; must be retained in an area with no public access
Schedule III	Available via open access in a pharmacy or pharmacy area (over the counter)
Unscheduled	Can be sold in any store without professional supervision

Canadian provinces and territories (except Quebec) use a national drug scheduling system to ensure consistent conditions of availability and sale among the provinces. Scheduling recommendations are made to provincial regulatory authorities by the National Drug Scheduling Advisory Committee (NDSAC). A set of factors is used to determine the schedule under which a drug can be sold. These factors include potential for dependency and abuse, adverse reactions, and interaction with other drugs. As illustrated in Table 2.4, Canada uses four categories (three schedules) for the sale of drugs.

Prescribers must follow standards of practice and legislation as set by national and provincial/territorial regulatory authorities. These authorities set out prescribing restrictions and the level of professional intervention and advice necessary for the safe and effective use of drugs by consumers. Nurse prescribers must obtain special permits from their provincial nursing associations. Nurses can visit the website of their provincial nursing association to assess current licensing requirements.

Controlled Drugs and Substances

2.6 Controlled substances are drugs whose use is restricted by the Controlled Drugs and Substances Act and the Narcotic Control Regulations. Canadian regulations restrict drugs with the potential for abuse and label them as *C* (controlled) or *N* (narcotic).

Some drugs and substances are frequently abused or have a high potential for addiction. Technically, addiction refers to the overwhelming feeling that drives someone to use a drug repeatedly. **Dependence** is a related term, often defined as a physiological or psychological need for a substance. Physical dependence refers to an altered physical condition caused by the nervous system adapting to repeated drug use. In this case, when the drug is no longer available, the individual experiences and shows physical signs of discomfort known as **withdrawal**. The nurse instructs the client to continue taking the controlled substance as prescribed to ensure a safe, slow tapering withdrawal from the substance. The client needs to follow the tapering schedule to ensure a safe withdrawal from controlled substance dependence.

In contrast, when an individual is psychologically dependent on a controlled substance, there are few signs of physical discomfort when the drug is withdrawn; however, the individual feels an intense and compelling desire to continue using the drug. These concepts are discussed in detail in Chapter 12.

Canada's Drug Strategy and Controlled Substances Programme (DSCSP) manages the 1997 Controlled Drugs and Substances Act (CDSA) and the Narcotic Control Regulations (NCR). Regulating drugs under the CDSA and the NCR protects the health and safety of Canadians by reducing the availability of substances on the illicit market that can alter mental processes and may produce harm to the health of an individual or to society when diverted or misused. These regulations control the import, production, export, distribution, and possession of narcotics and controlled substances. As a signatory to United Nations drug control conventions, Canada has an obligation to meet international requirements. Health Canada's Office of Controlled Substances (OCS) works to ensure that drugs and controlled substances are not diverted for illegal use.

The NCR governs the activities of manufacturers, pharmacies, hospitals, and healthcare professionals related to narcotic drugs. Licensed hospitals and other agencies must provide the required physical security measures for controlled substances in their possession and maintain records of all movements of controlled substances into and out of their inventory. Monitoring compliance with the NCR is the responsibility of Health Canada. Offences under the CDSA and NCR are subject to criminal prosecution.

In Canada, **controlled substances** are those drugs outlined in the CDSA Schedules. A healthcare provider may dispense these medications only to clients suffering from specific diseases or illnesses. Controlled drugs must be labelled clearly with the letter *C* on the outside of the container. Narcotic drugs must be labelled clearly with the letter *N* on the outside of the container. The CDSA Schedules include restricted drugs such as amphetamines, barbiturates, anabolic steroids, morphine, and cannabis. Hallucinogens that are not intended for human use, such as lysergic acid diethylamide and 3,4-methylenedioxy-N-methylamphetamine, better known as Ecstasy, are also listed in the CDSA Schedules. Examples of drugs grouped by CDSA Schedule are presented in Table 2.5.

Connecting Pharmacology to Nursing Practice

2.7 Pharmacology is intimately connected to nursing practice and is a key intervention.

Pharmacology is intimately connected to nursing practice and is a key intervention in relieving and preventing human suffering and illnesses. The importance of pharmacology to nursing practice

TABLE 2.5   Controlled Drugs and Substances Act Drug Schedules

Drug Schedule	Examples
I	opium, codeine, hydrocodone, morphine, oxycodone, methamphetamine, dextromethorphan, naloxone, ketamine, fentanyl
II	cannabis, cannabis resin
III	amphetamines (except methamphetamine)
IV	barbiturates, phenobarbital, thiopental, meprobamate, benzodiazepines, clozapine, anabolic steroids, testosterone, zolpidem
V	phenylpropanolamine
VI	ephedrine, ergotamine, lysergic acid diethylamide, pseudoephedrine
VII	cannabis, cannabis resin
VIII	cannabis, cannabis resin

cannot be overstated. Knowledge of pharmacology is at the core of client care and is integrated into the nursing process. The connection between pharmacology and clinical nursing practice is emphasized throughout this text. Indeed, pharmacology would not be an important science without its connections to client care and nursing practice.

Whether administering medications or supervising drug use, the nurse is expected to understand the pharmacotherapeutic principles for all medications received by each client. Given the large number of different drugs and the potential consequences of medication errors, this is indeed an enormous task. A major goal of this text is to prepare the nurse for the responsibilities of drug administration. Chapters 2 through 4 provide the legal and scientific bases for pharmacotherapeutics. The nurse's responsibilities include knowledge and understanding of the following:

- What drug is ordered
  - Name (generic and trade) and drug classification
  - Intended or proposed use
  - Effects on the body
  - Contraindications
  - Special considerations, such as how age, sex, weight, body fat distribution, genetic factors, and pathophysiological states affect pharmacotherapeutic response
  - Expected and potential adverse events
- Why the drug has been prescribed for this particular client
- How the drug is supplied by the pharmacy
- How the drug is to be administered, including dose ranges
- What nursing process considerations related to the drug apply to this client

Major goals in studying pharmacology are to eliminate medication errors and to limit the number and severity of adverse drug events. Many adverse effects are preventable. Professional nurses can routinely avoid many serious adverse drug effects in their clients by applying their experience and knowledge of pharmacotherapeutics to clinical practice. However, some adverse effects are not preventable. It is vital that the nurse be prepared to recognize and respond to potential adverse effects of medications. The nursing management of adverse effects and medication errors are discussed in Chapters 5 and 6, respectively.

NCLEX Success Tips

Check for client allergies to ordered medications and all of their ingredients.

Assess client condition in relation to the reason the medication is being ordered.

Check for interactions between all ordered medications; be aware of side effects (mild), adverse effects (more severe), and toxic effects (most harmful) associated with high doses.

Address client concerns about medications; don't administer any medication that the client questions until the order and dose are rechecked.

Source: Based on Hogan, M. (2012). *Comprehensive Review for NCLEX-RN. Reviews & Rationales* (2nd ed.). Upper Saddle River, NJ: Pearson Education.

Before any drug is administered, the nurse must obtain and process pertinent information regarding the client's medical history, physical assessment, disease processes, and learning needs and capabilities. Growth and developmental factors must always be considered. It is important to remember that a large number of variables influence a client's response to drugs throughout the lifespan. Having a firm understanding of these variables can increase treatment success. Chapters 8 through 11 of this text address these aspects of pharmacotherapy. For a nurse, knowledge of pharmacology is an ongoing, lifelong process that builds as a nurse is in practice and chooses specific clinical areas. It may seem daunting at first, but learning prototypes, recognizing key similarities in generic names, and always looking up unknown or new drugs will help to build this knowledge base.

Drugs are a form of medical intervention given to improve the client's condition or to prevent harm. Pharmacotherapy often begins when the client experiences signs and symptoms of diseases. A major role of the nurse is to design interventions that meet the desired health goals of the client. Pharmacotherapy is a critical intervention for many conditions. The rationale for pharmacotherapy is illustrated in Figure 2.1.

Despite its essential nature, the study of pharmacology should be viewed in the proper perspective. Drugs are just one of many tools available to the nurse for preventing or treating human suffering. Although pharmacology is a key intervention in many cases, nurses must use all healing sciences in treating their clients. The effectiveness of a drug in treating disease can never substitute for skilled, compassionate nursing care. Too much reliance on drug therapy can diminish the importance of the nurse-client relationship.

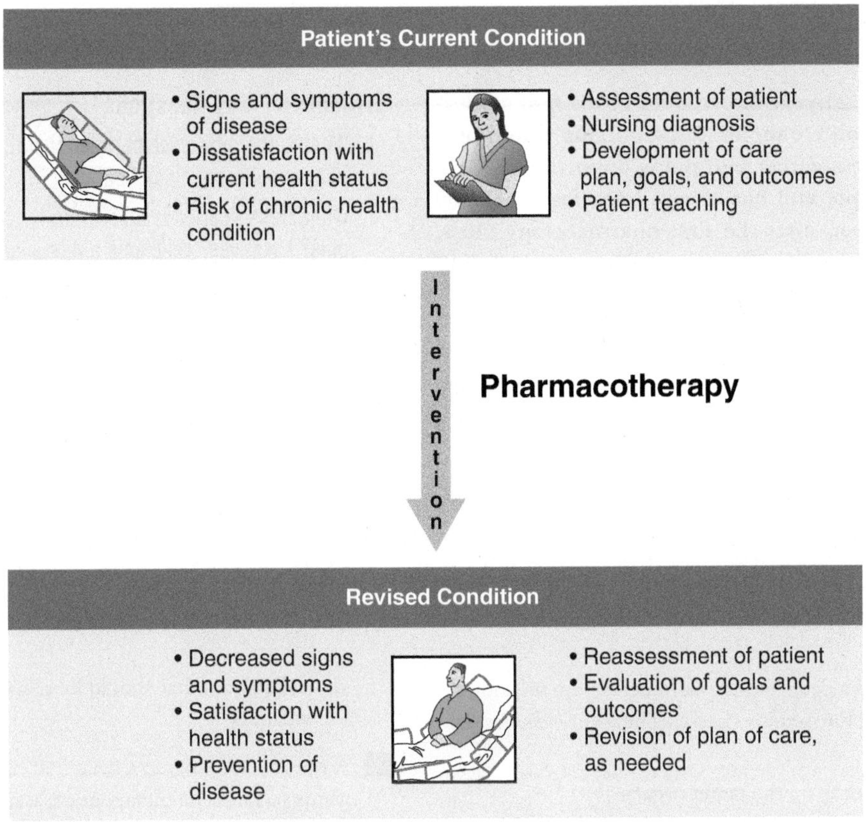

Patient's Current Condition

- Signs and symptoms of disease
- Dissatisfaction with current health status
- Risk of chronic health condition

- Assessment of patient
- Nursing diagnosis
- Development of care plan, goals, and outcomes
- Patient teaching

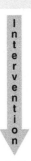
Intervention

Pharmacotherapy

Revised Condition

- Decreased signs and symptoms
- Satisfaction with health status
- Prevention of disease

- Reassessment of patient
- Evaluation of goals and outcomes
- Revision of plan of care, as needed

Figure 2.1 Rationale for pharmacotherapy: A partnership between the client and the healthcare provider.

CHAPTER

2

Understanding the Chapter

Key Concepts Summary

The numbered key concepts provide a succinct summary of the important points from the corresponding numbered section within the chapter. If any of these points are not clear, refer to the numbered section within the chapter for review.

2.1 The ideal drug is safe and effective.

2.2 Drugs may be organized by their therapeutic or pharmacological classification.

2.3 Drugs have chemical, generic, and trade names. A drug has only one chemical or generic name but may have multiple trade names.

2.4 Generic drugs are less expensive than brand name drugs, but they may differ in their bioavailability, which is the ability of the drug to reach its target tissue and produce its effect.

2.5 Drugs with a potential for abuse are categorized into schedules.

2.6 Controlled substances are drugs whose use is restricted by the Controlled Drugs and Substances Act and the Narcotic Control Regulations. Canadian regulations restrict drugs with the potential for abuse and label them as C (controlled) or N (narcotic).

2.7 Pharmacology is intimately connected to nursing practice and is a key intervention.

Chapter 2 Scenario

Josh Remming is a 23-year-old student in his first semester of nursing school. He thought that nursing would provide him with a great career and many opportunities. He enjoys helping people and has always been fascinated by health care. However, after the first pharmacology class, Josh is worried because there seems to be an overwhelming amount of content to learn in just one semester.

At the end of the class, Josh talks with other students who are also concerned and a bit anxious. Much of the conversation centres on lecture content provided by the professor. Following are some of the questions posed by Josh's classmates. How would you respond?

Critical Thinking Questions

1. What is the difference between therapeutic classification and pharmacological classification?
2. What classification is a barbiturate? Macrolide? Birth control pills? Laxatives? Folic acid antagonist? Antianginal agent?
3. What is a prototype drug, and what advantages does a prototype approach to studying pharmacology offer?
4. Why do nurses need to know all of this pharmacology?

See Answers to Critical Thinking Questions in Appendix B.

NCLEX Practice Questions

1 The nurse is using a drug handbook to determine the indications for the drug furosemide (Lasix). The term *indications* is defined as the
   a. Way a drug works on the target organs
   b. Amount of the drug to be administered
   c. Conditions for which a drug is approved
   d. Reason that the drug should not be given

2 While completing a client's health history, the nurse asks, "What medications do you take regularly?" Which drug names would the nurse expect the client to use in providing the answer?
   a. Chemical
   b. Generic
   c. Trade
   d. Standard

3 When providing nursing care for the client, the nurse understands that drugs are
   a. One of many tools available to prevent or treat human suffering
   b. The most important part of the therapeutic treatment plan
   c. Primarily the concern of the healthcare provider and not included in nursing care

   d. Substances that should be relied on for health and wellness

4 A nurse is looking up a drug that has been prescribed and wants to know its therapeutic classification. Which of the following indicates a therapeutic classification?
   a. Beta-adrenergic antagonist
   b. Antihypertensive
   c. Diuretic
   d. Calcium channel blocker

5 A nurse is asked by a family member, "They're giving Mom Motrin, but she takes Advil. Hasn't the wrong drug been ordered?" The nurse will respond, knowing that
   a. There has been an error in the order, so the nurse will contact the healthcare provider
   b. There may be a reason the healthcare provider is ordering a different drug
   c. Not all healthcare agencies buy the same generic drugs, and that may account for the difference
   d. Motrin and Advil are trade names for the same generic drug, ibuprofen

See Answers to NCLEX Practice Questions in Appendix A.

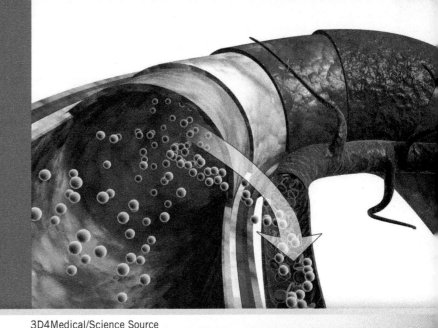

3D4Medical/Science Source

Pharmacokinetics

LEARNING OUTCOMES

After reading this chapter, the student should be able to:

1. Explain the applications of pharmacokinetics to clinical practice.
2. Identify the four components of pharmacokinetics.
3. Explain how substances travel across plasma membranes.
4. Discuss factors affecting drug absorption.
5. Explain the metabolism of drugs and its applications to pharmacotherapy.
6. Discuss how drugs are distributed throughout the body.
7. Describe how plasma proteins affect drug distribution.
8. Identify major processes by which drugs are excreted.
9. Explain how enterohepatic recirculation might affect drug activity.
10. Explain the applications of a drug's plasma half-life ($t_{1/2}$) to pharmacotherapy.
11. Explain how a drug reaches and maintains its therapeutic range in the plasma.
12. Differentiate between loading and maintenance doses.

CHAPTER OUTLINE

Medications are given to achieve a desirable effect. To do this, drugs must be able to reach their target cells in sufficient quantities, produce physiological or chemical changes, and then be removed from the body. This whole process is described as pharmacokinetics. Drugs are exposed to many barriers and destructive processes after they enter the body. Care that the nurse provides may influence biochemical and psychological responses in a client that affect how drugs move through the body and achieve their effects. The purpose of this chapter is to examine principles of pharmacokinetics and ways in which the nurse can influence pharmacokinetics through purposeful use of dietary modifications and other supportive therapies.

While seeking their target cells and attempting to pass through the various membranes, drugs are subjected to numerous physiological processes. For medications given by the enteral route, stomach acid and digestive enzymes often act to break down the drug molecules. Enzymes in the liver and other organs may chemically change the drug molecule to make it less or more active. If the drug is seen as foreign by the body, phagocytes may attempt to remove it, or an immune response may be triggered.

Pharmacokinetics: How the Body Handles Medications

3.1 Pharmacokinetics focuses on the movement of drugs throughout the body after they are administered. The four processes of pharmacokinetics are absorption, metabolism, distribution, and excretion.

The term **pharmacokinetics** is derived from the root words *pharmaco*, which means "medicines," and *kinetics*, which means "movement or motion." Pharmacokinetics is thus the study of drug movement throughout the body. In practical terms, it describes how the body handles medications. Pharmacokinetics is a core subject in pharmacology, and a firm grasp of this topic allows nurses to better understand and predict the actions and side effects of medications.

Drugs face numerous obstacles in reaching their target cells. For most medications, the greatest barrier is crossing the many membranes that separate the drug from its target cells. A drug taken by mouth, for example, must cross the plasma membrane of the mucosal cells of the gastrointestinal (GI) tract and that of the capillary endothelial cells to enter the bloodstream. To leave the bloodstream, the drug must again cross capillary cells, travel through interstitial fluid, and enter target cells by passing through their plasma membrane. Depending on the mechanism of action, the drug may also need to enter cellular organelles such as the nucleus, which are surrounded by additional membranes. Some of the membranes and barriers that many drugs must successfully penetrate before they can elicit a response are illustrated in Figure 3.1.

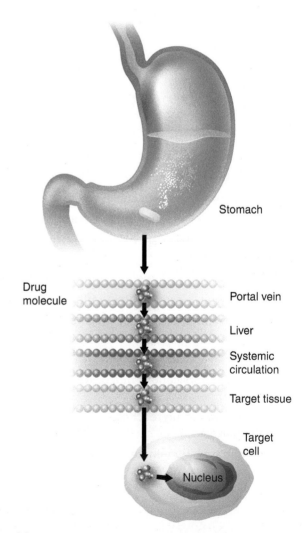

Figure 3.1 Barriers that a drug administered by the oral route must cross before interacting with a target cell.

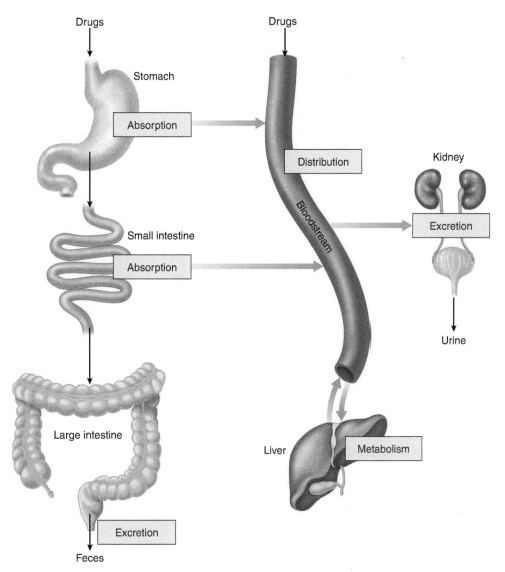

Figure 3.2 The four processes of pharmacokinetics: absorption, distribution, metabolism, and excretion.

The kidneys, large intestine, and other organs attempt to excrete the medication from the body.

These examples illustrate pharmacokinetic processes, or how the body handles medications. The many processes of pharmacokinetics are grouped into four categories—absorption, distribution, metabolism, and excretion—as illustrated in Figure 3.2.

The Passage of Drugs Through Plasma Membranes

3.2 The physiological properties of plasma membranes determine movement of drugs throughout the body.

Pharmacokinetic variables depend on the ability of a drug to cross plasma membranes. With few exceptions, drugs must penetrate these membranes to produce their effects. Like other chemicals, drugs primarily use two processes to cross body membranes: (1) **diffusion**, a type of **passive transport**, is the movement of

a substance from an area of higher concentration to an area of lower concentration, and (2) **active transport** is the movement of a substance against a concentration gradient or electrochemical gradient, which requires energy. Diffusion is best explained by the use of an example. When first administered, a drug given by the intravenous (IV) route is in high concentration in the blood but has not yet entered the tissues. The drug will move quickly by passive diffusion from its region of high concentration (blood) to a region of low concentration (tissues) to produce its action. With time the drug will be inactivated (metabolized) by the tissue, and more doses of the drug may be administered, creating a continual concentration gradient from blood to tissue. Diffusion assumes that the chemical—in this case, the drug—is able to freely cross the plasma membrane. This is not the case for all drugs.

Large molecules, ionized drugs, and water-soluble agents have difficulty crossing plasma membranes by simple diffusion. These agents may require carrier, or transport, proteins to cross membranes. A drug that moves into a cell along its concentration gradient with help from a membrane carrier protein is using the process of facilitated diffusion. This process does not require energy expenditure from the cell, but it does require that a specific carrier protein be present on the plasma membrane. Transport proteins are selective and only carry molecules that have specific structures.

Some drugs cross membranes against their gradient, from low concentration to high concentration, through the process of active transport. This requires expenditure of energy on the part of the cell and a carrier protein. Carrier proteins that assist in active transport are sometimes called pumps.

Plasma membranes consist of a lipid bilayer, with proteins and other molecules interspersed in the membrane. This lipophilic membrane is relatively impermeable to large molecules, ions, and polar molecules. These physical characteristics have direct application to pharmacokinetics. For example, drug molecules that are small, nonionized, and lipid soluble will usually pass through plasma membranes by simple diffusion and more easily reach their target cells. Small water-soluble agents such as urea, alcohol, and water can enter through pores in the plasma membrane. However, large molecules, ionized drugs, and water-soluble agents will have more difficulty crossing plasma membranes. These agents may use other means to gain entry, such as carrier proteins or active transport. In some cases, the drug may not need to enter the cell to produce its effects: once bound to the plasma membrane, some drugs activate a second messenger within the cell, which produces the physiological change (see Chapter 4).

Absorption of Medications

3.3 Absorption is the process of moving a drug from the site of administration to the bloodstream. Absorption of a drug molecule depends on its size, lipid solubility, degree of ionization, and interactions with food or other medications.

Absorption is a process involving the movement of a substance from its site of administration, across body membranes, to circulating fluids. Absorption may occur across the skin and associated mucous membranes or across membranes that line the GI or respiratory tract. Most drugs, with the exception of many topical medications, intestinal anti-infectives, and some radiological contrast agents, must be absorbed to produce an effect.

Absorption is the primary pharmacokinetic factor determining the length of time it takes a drug to produce its effect. In general, the more rapid the absorption, the faster the onset of drug action. Drugs that are used in critical care are designed to be absorbed within seconds or minutes. At the other extreme are drugs, such as some hormones, that may be injected deep into tissue in order to absorb slowly over a few weeks or months.

NCLEX Success Tips

The IV route does not involve absorption as a step after IV administration because it bypasses absorption barriers and results in an immediate systemic response. The fastest route of absorption is the inhalation route.

The body must absorb drugs that are administered PO, IM, sub Q, intradermally, or by nebulizer (metered dose inhaler) before the system can respond.

Absorption is conditional on many factors. Drugs administered by IV have the most rapid onset of action. Drugs in elixir or syrup formulations are absorbed faster than those in tablets or capsules. Drugs administered in high doses are generally absorbed faster and have a more rapid onset of action than those given in low concentrations. Digestive motility, exposure to enzymes in the digestive tract, and blood flow to the site of drug administration also affect absorption.

The degree of ionization of a drug also affects its absorption. A drug's ability to become ionized depends on the surrounding pH, which is a measure of the acidity or basicity of a solution. Acetylsalicylic acid (ASA) provides an excellent example of the effects of ionization on absorption, as depicted in Figure 3.3. In the acid environment of the stomach, ASA is in its nonionized form and is thus readily absorbed and distributed by the bloodstream. As ASA enters the alkaline environment of the small intestine, however, it becomes ionized. In its ionized form, ASA is not as likely to be absorbed and distributed to target cells. Unlike acidic drugs, medications that are weakly basic are in their nonionized form in an alkaline environment; therefore, basic drugs are absorbed and distributed better in alkaline environments, such as in the small intestine. The pH of the local environment directly

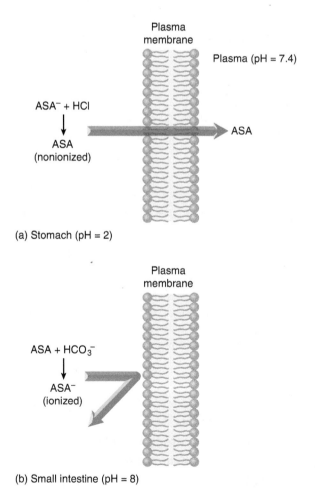

(a) Stomach (pH = 2)

(b) Small intestine (pH = 8)

Figure 3.3 Effect of pH on drug absorption: (a) a weak acid such as acetylsalicylic acid (ASA) is in a nonionized form in an acidic environment, and absorption occurs; (b) in a basic environment, ASA is mostly in an ionized form, and absorption is prevented.

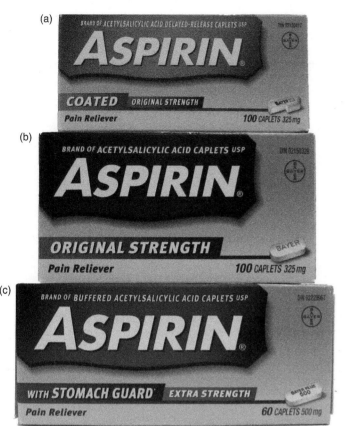

(a)

ASPIRIN®

BRAND OF ACETYLSALICYLIC ACID DELAYED-RELEASE CAPLETS USP

COATED   ORIGINAL STRENGTH

Pain Reliever   100 CAPLETS 325mg

(b)

ASPIRIN®

BRAND OF ACETYLSALICYLIC ACID CAPLETS USP

ORIGINAL STRENGTH

Pain Reliever   100 CAPLETS 325mg

(c)

ASPIRIN®

BRAND OF BUFFERED ACETYLSALICYLIC ACID CAPLETS USP

WITH STOMACH GUARD   EXTRA STRENGTH

Pain Reliever   60 CAPLETS 500mg

Figure 3.4   Drug products for oral use: (a) enteric-coated products are intended to absorb in the alkaline environment of the small intestine; (b) regular products dissolve and begin to absorb in the stomach; (c) buffered products contain ions that decrease gastric acidity and slow absorption.

Source: Shirley King.

influences drug absorption through ionization of the drug. In the simplest terms, it may help the student to remember that acids are absorbed in acids, and bases are absorbed in bases.

- Acids are absorbed in acids because they are nonionized. When acid is added to an acid, no chemical reaction will take place and hence no ions will be formed.

- Bases are absorbed in bases because they are nonionized. When an acid is added to a base, a chemical reaction leading to the formation of ions will take place.

Drug manufacturers deliberately alter the forms of some drugs to manage these factors, as depicted in the examples in Figure 3.4. Drug products for oral use may be in regular, buffered, or enteric-coated forms. Enteric-coated products are intended to absorb in the alkaline environment of the small intestine. Regular (uncoated) acidic products dissolve and absorb in the stomach. Buffered products contain ions that decrease gastric acidity and slow the absorption of acidic drugs.

Some clients, particularly children, have difficulty swallowing tablets and capsules. Crushing tablets or opening capsules and sprinkling the medication over food or mixing it with juice may make the drug more palatable and easier to swallow. The nurse should not crush tablets or open capsules, however, unless the manufacturer specifically states that this is permissible. In

general, the following types of drugs should not be chewed, crushed, or opened:

- **Extended-release formulations.** These drugs contain a high amount of medication that is intended to be released over an extended period. Opening the capsule or crushing the tablet will release the entire drug immediately, possibly resulting in a toxic effect. Sustained-release capsules should never be split open, crushed, or chewed because doing so may alter the drug's absorption rate, causing adverse reactions or subtherapeutic activity. The nurse should check with the pharmacist for alternative forms of the medication if it needs to be crushed or opened, such as when administering medications via nasogastric (NG) or percutaneous endoscopic gastrostomy (PEG) tube. Sustained-release capsules should be swallowed whole if the client has an intact swallowing reflex.

- **Enteric-coated drugs.** When crushed or opened, these drugs are exposed to stomach acid, which may destroy them. In addition, the drugs may irritate the stomach mucosa and cause nausea or vomiting.

- **Drugs with oral cavity effects.** Drugs that have a bitter taste are often coated with a thin layer of glucose or inert material to mask their taste. If crushed or opened, the bitter taste is experienced. Other drugs stain the teeth or cause an anesthetic-like effect on the tongue if crushed and exposed to the oral cavity. In addition, some drugs irritate the oral mucosa.

As an alternative to crushing, some drugs are available in liquid form for clients who have difficulty swallowing tablets or capsules. Liquid forms include elixirs, syrups, and suspensions. Liquid drugs are usually heavily flavoured and sweetened to mask their bitter taste.

In recent years, two alternatives to tablets, capsules, and liquids have been developed. Orally disintegrating tablets (ODTs) and oral soluble films are designed to dissolve in the oral cavity in less than 30 seconds, without the need to drink water. These dosage forms are convenient and especially appropriate for clients who have difficulty chewing or swallowing and clients who are mentally impaired, nauseated, or uncooperative. ODTs and soluble films are now available for dozens of medications.

Conventional tablets, liquids, and capsules have certain disadvantages. The client must be conscious and able to swallow properly. Certain types of drugs, including proteins such as insulin, are inactivated by the digestive enzymes in the stomach and small intestine. Furthermore, drugs absorbed from the stomach and small intestine first travel to the liver, where they may be inactivated before they ever reach their target organs—a process called **first-pass effect** (first-pass metabolism). There is also significant variation among clients in the motility of the GI tract and in its ability to absorb medications. In addition, children and some adults have an aversion to swallowing large tablets and capsules or to taking oral medications that taste bad.

Drug-drug or food-drug interactions may influence absorption. Many examples of these interactions have been discovered. For example, administering tetracyclines with food or drugs containing calcium, iron, or magnesium can significantly delay absorption of the antibiotic. High-fat meals can slow stomach motility significantly and delay the absorption of oral medications taken with the meal. The absorption of acidic drugs may be hastened by drinking citrus fruit juices that increase gastric acidity. Consuming alkaline substances with enteric-coated drugs may cause the coating to begin to break down prematurely, before it reaches the intended alkaline environment of the small intestine. Dietary supplements may also affect absorption. Common ingredients in herbal weight loss products, such as aloe leaf, guar gum, senna, and yellow dock, exert a laxative effect that may decrease intestinal transit time and reduce drug absorption (Scott & Elmer, 2002). Dietary intake can alter the effectiveness of some drugs; for example, dairy products bind certain antibiotics and make them ineffective. There is a food-drug interaction between repaglinide (GlucoNorm) and grapefruit juice that may inhibit metabolism of repaglinide. A client who is taking phenelzine (Nardil), a monoamine oxidase inhibitor, needs to avoid foods that are rich in tyramine because this food-drug combination can cause hypertensive crisis. The client should be given a list of foods to avoid and should report headaches, palpitations, and a stiff neck to the nurse.

Grapefruit juice, but not orange juice, inhibits the activity of an enzyme (cytochrome P450 3A4) in the intestinal wall. Even when taken in small quantities, grapefruit juice can significantly increase the absorption of some drugs, such as nifedipine (Adalat). The nurse must be aware of drug interactions and advise clients to avoid known combinations of foods and medications that significantly affect drug absorption and action.

Distribution of Medications

3.4 Distribution represents how drugs are transported throughout the body. Distribution depends on the formation of drug-protein complexes and special barriers such as the fetal-placental and blood-brain barriers.

Distribution describes how pharmacological agents are transported throughout the body. The simplest factor determining distribution is the amount of blood flow to body tissues. The heart, liver, kidneys, and brain receive the most blood supply. Skin, bone, and adipose tissue receive a lower blood flow; therefore, it is more difficult to deliver high concentrations of drugs to these areas.

The physical properties of a drug greatly influence how it moves throughout the body after administration. Lipid solubility is an important characteristic because this determines how quickly a drug is absorbed, mixes within the bloodstream, crosses membranes, and becomes localized in body tissues. Lipid-soluble agents are not limited by the barriers that normally stop water-soluble drugs; therefore, they are more completely distributed to body tissues.

Some tissues have the ability to accumulate and store drugs after absorption. The bone marrow, teeth, eyes, and adipose tissue have an especially high **affinity**, or attraction, for certain medications. Examples of agents that are attracted to adipose tissue are diazepam (Valium) and lipid-soluble vitamins. Tetracycline binds to calcium salts and accumulates in the bones and teeth. Once stored in tissues, drugs may remain in the body for many months and be released very slowly back into circulation. For example, the therapeutic effects of alendronate (Fosamax), a

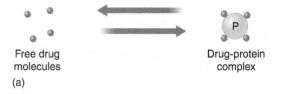

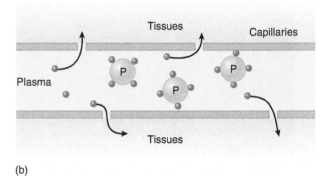

Figure 3.5   Plasma protein binding and drug availability: (a) the drug exists in a free state or bound to plasma protein; (b) drug-protein complexes are too large to cross membranes.

drug for osteoporosis, continue for many months after the drug is discontinued.

Not all drug molecules in the plasma will reach their target cells because many drugs bind reversibly to plasma proteins, particularly albumin, to form **drug-protein complexes**. Drug-protein complexes are too large to cross capillary membranes; therefore, the drug is not available for distribution to body tissues. Drugs bound to proteins circulate in the plasma until they are released or displaced from the drug-protein complex. Only unbound (free) drugs can reach their target cells. This concept is illustrated in Figure 3.5.

Drugs and other chemicals compete with each other for plasma protein binding sites, and some agents have a greater affinity for these binding sites than others. Drug-drug and food-drug interactions may occur when one agent displaces another from plasma proteins. The displaced medication can immediately reach high levels in the blood and produce adverse effects. An example is the anticoagulant warfarin (Coumadin). After administration, 99% of warfarin molecules are bound to plasma proteins. Drugs such as ASA or cimetidine (Tagamet) displace warfarin from the drug-protein complex, thus raising blood levels of free warfarin and dramatically enhancing the risk for hemorrhage. Most drug guides indicate the percentage of medication bound to plasma proteins; when giving multiple drugs that are highly bound, the nurse should monitor the client closely for adverse effects.

The brain and placenta possess special anatomical barriers that inhibit many chemicals and medications from entering. These barriers are referred to as the **blood-brain barrier** and **fetal-placental barrier**, respectively. Some medications, such as sedatives, antianxiety agents, and anticonvulsants, readily cross the blood-brain barrier to produce their actions on the central nervous system (CNS). On the other hand, most antitumour medications cannot cross this barrier, making brain cancers difficult to treat with chemotherapy.

The fetal-placental barrier serves an important protective function because it prevents potentially harmful substances from passing from the mother's bloodstream to the fetus. However, substances such as alcohol, cocaine, caffeine, and certain prescription medications easily cross the fetal-placental barrier and could potentially harm the fetus. Because of this, no prescription medication, over-the-counter (OTC) drug, or herbal therapy should be taken by a client who is pregnant without first consulting a healthcare provider. Healthcare providers should always question female clients in the childbearing years about their pregnancy status before prescribing a drug. Chapter 6 presents a list of drug pregnancy categories to assess fetal risk.

Metabolism of Medications

3.5 Metabolism is a process that changes a drug's form and makes it more likely to be excreted. Changes in hepatic metabolism can significantly affect drug action.

Metabolism, also called **biotransformation**, is the process of chemically converting a drug to a form that is usually removed from the body more easily. The rate and ability of the liver to metabolize medications will be altered in a client with liver disease. Therefore, it is essential to understand how each medication is metabolized. The dose of the administered drug has to be adjusted, usually lowered if the drug is metabolized in the liver. The nurse can expect prolonged or exaggerated action of the medication administered in a client with liver disease.

Metabolism involves a study of the complex biochemical pathways and reactions that alter drugs, nutrients, vitamins, and minerals. The liver is the primary site of drug metabolism, although the kidneys and cells of the intestinal tract also have high metabolic rates. Many types of biochemical reactions to medications, including hydrolysis, oxidation, and reduction, occur during phase I metabolism as the medications pass through the liver. Some drugs undergo phase II metabolism, during which the addition of side chains, known as **conjugates**, makes drugs more water soluble and more easily excreted by the kidneys.

In most cases, metabolic reactions change the structure of a drug so that it can be excreted by the body more easily. This often changes the drug from lipid soluble (easily absorbed and distributed) to water soluble, which is more easily excreted by the kidneys. In addition, once the molecule has been changed to water soluble, it is less able to enter tissues. The products of drug metabolism, or metabolites, usually have less pharmacological activity than the original molecule. In this way, metabolism provides an essential detoxifying effect for drugs and other substances entering the body.

On some occasions a metabolite may exhibit a *greater* therapeutic action than the original drug. This is the case for codeine. Although 90% of codeine is changed to inactive metabolites by the liver, 10% is converted to morphine, which has significantly greater ability to relieve severe pain. In a few cases the metabolite has greater toxicity than the original drug. Probably the most common example of this is acetaminophen (Tylenol), which is converted to a metabolite that is highly toxic to the liver.

Most metabolism in the liver is accomplished by the **hepatic microsomal enzyme system**. This enzyme complex is sometimes called the P450 system, named after cytochrome P450 (CYP), which is a key component of the system. As it relates to pharmacotherapy, the primary actions of the hepatic microsomal enzymes are to inactivate drugs and accelerate their excretion. In fact, some agents, known as **prodrugs**, have no pharmacological activity unless they are first metabolized to their active form by the body. Examples of prodrugs include benazepril (Lotensin) and losartan (Cozaar).

Changes in the function of the hepatic microsomal enzymes can significantly affect drug metabolism. A few drugs have the ability to increase metabolic activity in the liver, a process called **enzyme induction**. For example, phenobarbital (Phenobarb) causes the liver to synthesize more microsomal enzymes. By doing so, phenobarbital increases the rate of its own metabolism, as well as that of other drugs metabolized in the liver. Clients who are receiving phenobarbital require higher doses to achieve therapeutic effect.

Certain clients have decreased hepatic metabolic activity, which may alter drug action. In older clients, diminished hepatic and renal function commonly reduces drug metabolism and excretion. The nurse needs to check the client's most recent laboratory values such as creatinine and liver function tests to assess the functions of the kidneys and liver, respectively. The nurse also needs to keep in mind the importance of checking the blood levels for drugs, especially those with a narrow therapeutic index. Because adverse reactions are frequently related to drug blood level, the client may benefit from reduced drug dosages.

Hepatic enzyme activity is generally reduced in infants and older clients; therefore, pediatric and geriatric clients are more sensitive to drug therapy than are middle-aged clients. Clients with severe liver damage, such as that caused by cirrhosis, will require reductions in drug dosage because of their decreased metabolic activity. Genetic polymorphisms among ethnically diverse populations may result in differences in metabolic function (see Chapter 7). Certain genetic disorders in which clients lack specific metabolic enzymes have been recognized. Drug dosages in these clients must be adjusted accordingly, or an alternate drug may be prescribed. The nurse should assess patterns in a client's responses to previous medications for evidence of possible altered metabolism and pay careful attention to laboratory values that may indicate liver disease so that doses may be adjusted accordingly.

Metabolism has a number of additional therapeutic consequences. As illustrated in Figure 3.6, drugs absorbed after oral administration cross directly from the small intestine into the hepatic portal circulation, which carries blood to the liver before it is distributed to other body tissues. As blood passes through the liver circulation, some drugs can be completely metabolized to an inactive form before they ever reach the general circulation. This first-pass effect is an important mechanism, since a large number of oral drugs are rendered inactive by hepatic metabolic reactions. Alternate routes of delivery that bypass the first-pass effect (e.g., topical, sublingual, rectal, or parenteral routes) may need to be considered for these drugs.

The baseline level of hepatic microsomal enzyme function is genetically determined. Genetic differences in the function of CYP enzymes may cause people to metabolize drugs at widely

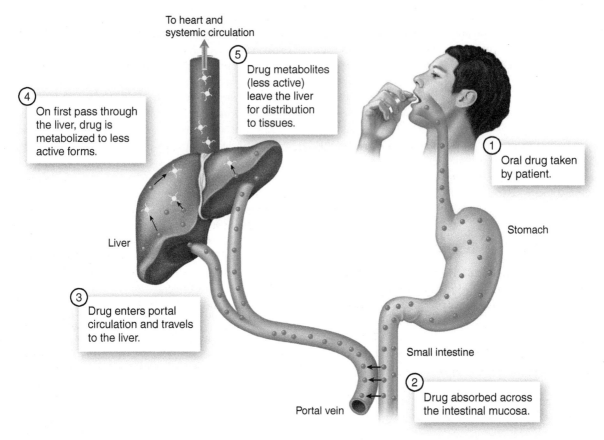

To heart and systemic circulation

⑤ Drug metabolites (less active) leave the liver for distribution to tissues.

④ On first pass through the liver, drug is metabolized to less active forms.

① Oral drug taken by patient.

Stomach

Liver

③ Drug enters portal circulation and travels to the liver.

Small intestine

② Drug absorbed across the intestinal mucosa.

Portal vein

Figure 3.6 First-pass effect: an oral drug is metabolized to an inactive form before it reaches target cells.

different rates. Some individuals metabolize at a faster rate, others at a slower rate. In these "slow metabolizers," normal drug doses may cause toxicity.

Certain lifestyle factors also affect CYP enzyme activity and thus may influence response to medications. Chronic alcohol consumption and tobacco use induce certain CYP enzymes. St. John's wort, a popular herbal remedy for depression, is an enzyme inducer and can affect the therapeutic response to certain medications. On the other hand, grapefruit juice is an inhibitor of cytochrome P450 3A4 activity. These examples underscore the importance of obtaining a thorough client history prior to initiating drug therapy.

Excretion of Medications

3.6 Excretion processes remove drugs from the body. Drugs are primarily excreted by the kidneys but may be excreted by the lung or glands, or into bile.

Drugs will continue to act on the body until they are either metabolized to an inactive form or removed from the body by **excretion**. The rate at which medications are excreted determines their concentration in the bloodstream and tissues. This is important because the concentration of drugs in the bloodstream determines their duration of action. Pathological states, such as liver disease or renal failure, often increase the duration of drug

action in the body because they interfere with natural excretion mechanisms. Dosing regimens must be carefully adjusted in clients with these pathological states.

Although drugs are removed from the body by numerous organs and tissues, the primary site of excretion is the kidney. In an average-sized person, approximately 180 L of blood are filtered by the kidneys each day. Free drugs, water-soluble agents, electrolytes, and small molecules are easily filtered by the glomerulus. Proteins, blood cells, conjugates, and drug-protein complexes are not filtered because of their large size.

Upon filtration, chemicals and drugs are subjected to the process of reabsorption in the renal tubule. Mechanisms of reabsorption are the same as for absorption elsewhere in the body. Nonionized and lipid-soluble drugs cross renal tubular membranes easily and return to the circulation; ionized and water-soluble drugs generally remain in the filtrate for excretion.

Drug-protein complexes and substances too large to be filtered by the glomerulus are sometimes secreted into the distal tubule of the nephron. For example, only 10% of a dose of penicillin G is filtered by the glomerulus; 90% is secreted into the renal tubule. As with metabolic enzyme activity, secretion mechanisms are less active in infants and older adults.

Certain drugs may be excreted more quickly if the pH of the filtrate changes. Weak acids such as ASA are excreted faster when the filtrate is slightly alkaline because ASA is ionized in an alkaline environment and the drug will remain in the filtrate and be excreted in the urine. Weakly basic drugs such as diazepam are excreted faster with a slightly acidic filtrate because they are ionized in this environment. Nurses should be aware of common foods that alter the pH of urine, since these may affect the excretion and duration of action of medications. Foods that acidify urine include cranberries, cheese, eggs, lentils, pasta, grains, plums, and prunes. Foods that alkalinize urine include milk, vegetables (except for corn), and fruits (except for cranberries, prunes, and plums). The relationship between pH and drug excretion can be especially important in critical care situations. To speed the renal excretion of acidic drugs such as ASA in an overdosed client, nurses can administer sodium bicarbonate. Sodium bicarbonate will make the urine more basic, which ionizes more ASA, causing it to be excreted more readily. The excretion of diazepam, on the other hand, can be enhanced by giving ammonium chloride, to acidify the filtrate.

Alteration of kidney function can dramatically affect pharmacokinetics. Clients with renal failure will have diminished ability to excrete medications and may retain drugs for an extended time. Doses for these clients must be reduced, to avoid drug toxicity. Because small to moderate changes in renal status can cause rapid increases in serum drug levels, the nurse must constantly monitor kidney function in clients receiving drugs that may be nephrotoxic or have a narrow margin of safety.

Other organs can serve as important sites of excretion. Drugs that can easily be changed into a gaseous form are especially suited for excretion by the respiratory system. The rate of respiratory excretion is dependent on factors that affect gas exchange, including diffusion, gas solubility, and pulmonary blood flow. The elimination of volatile anesthetics following surgery is primarily dependent on respiratory activity. The faster the breathing rate, the greater the excretion. Conversely, the respiratory removal of water-soluble agents such as alcohol is more dependent on blood flow to the lungs. The greater the blood flow into lung capillaries, the greater the excretion. In contrast to other methods of excretion, the lungs excrete most drugs in their original unmetabolized form.

Glandular activity is another elimination mechanism. Water-soluble drugs may be secreted into the saliva, sweat, or breast milk. The "funny taste" that clients sometimes experience when given IV drugs is due to the agent being secreted into the saliva. Another example of glandular excretion is the garlic smell that can be detected when standing next to a perspiring person who has recently eaten garlic. Excretion into breast milk is of considerable importance for basic drugs such as morphine and codeine, as these can achieve high concentrations and potentially affect the nursing infant. Nursing mothers should always check with their healthcare provider before taking any prescription medication, OTC drug, or herbal supplement. Pharmacology for the pregnant or breastfeeding client is discussed in Chapter 6.

Certain oral drugs travel through the GI tract without being absorbed and are excreted in the feces. Examples include mebendazole (Vermox), a drug used to kill intestinal worms, and barium sulphate, a radiological contrast agent. Some drugs are secreted in the bile, a process known as biliary excretion. In many cases, drugs secreted into the bile will enter the duodenum and eventually leave the body in the feces. However, most bile is circulated back to the liver by **enterohepatic recirculation**, as illustrated in Figure 3.7. A percentage of the drug may be recirculated numerous times with the bile. Biliary reabsorption

CONNECTIONS ◖ Lifespan Considerations

◖ Adverse Drug Effects and the Elderly

Adverse drug effects are more commonly recorded in elderly clients than in young adults or middle-aged clients because the geriatric population takes more drugs simultaneously (an average of seven) than do other age groups. In addition, chronic diseases that affect pharmacokinetics are present more often in the elderly. A recent report by the Canadian Institute for Health Information (CIHI, 2011) concluded that unintended, harmful reactions to drugs are a major problem in Canada and cause thousands of deaths and hospital admissions each year. According to CIHI, 1 in 200 Canadian seniors, compared to 1 in 1000 Canadians in other age groups, were admitted to hospital between 2010 and 2011 for drug side effects.

Blood thinners, often used to prevent heart attack and stroke, were the drug class most commonly associated with hospitalizations related to adverse drug reactions among seniors (12.6%). This was followed by chemotherapy drugs (12.1%) and opioids, a class of strong painkillers (7.4%). In older clients, diminished hepatic and renal function commonly reduces drug metabolism and excretion. Noncompliance or lack of adherence to drug regimen is often related to medication side effects in this age group. When developing a drug therapy regimen that will not interfere with a client's lifestyle, the nurse must consider the drug's adverse effects, because these may result in noncompliance.

is extremely influential in prolonging the activity of cardiac glycosides, certain antibiotics, and phenothiazines. Recirculated drugs are ultimately metabolized by the liver and excreted by the kidneys. Recirculation and elimination of drugs through biliary excretion may continue for several weeks after therapy has been discontinued.

Drug Plasma Concentration and Therapeutic Response

3.7 The therapeutic response of most drugs depends on their concentration in the plasma. The difference between the minimum effective concentration and the toxic concentration is called the therapeutic range.

The therapeutic response of most drugs is directly related to their level in the plasma. Although the concentration of the medication at its *target tissue* is more predictive of drug action, this quantity is impossible to measure in most cases. For example, it is possible to conduct a laboratory test that measures the serum level of lithium, a drug used for bipolar disorder, by taking a blood sample; it is a far different matter to measure the quantity of this drug in neurons within the CNS. It is common practice to monitor the plasma levels of drugs that have a low safety margin and to use these data to predict drug action or toxicity. Results of **therapeutic drug monitoring** are used by the healthcare provider to keep the drug dose within a predetermined therapeutic range. For example, the therapeutic range for the antibiotic vancomycin

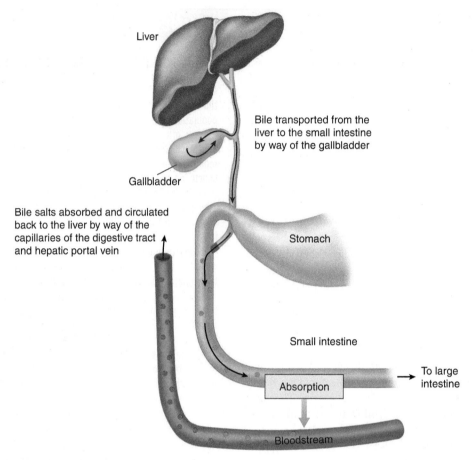

Figure 3.7   Enterohepatic recirculation.

(Vancocin) is 20 to 40 µg/mL, and the toxic level is considered to be greater than 80 µg/mL. For clients with severe infections, the nurse would carefully monitor the laboratory results for vancomycin to be certain that serum levels fall within the therapeutic range. Dosages would be adjusted upward or downward based on therapeutic drug monitoring and the client's responses. The nurse should always remember, however, that individual responses to drugs are highly variable and clients may experience toxic effects (or no effects) even if the serum concentration of the drug lies in the normal range.

Several important pharmacokinetic principles can be illustrated by measuring the serum level of a drug following a single-dose administration. These pharmacokinetic values are shown graphically in Figure 3.8. This figure demonstrates two plasma drug levels. First is the **minimum effective concentration**, the amount of drug required to produce a therapeutic effect. Second is the **toxic concentration**, the level of drug that will result in serious adverse effects. The plasma drug concentration between the minimum effective concentration and the toxic concentration is called the **therapeutic range** of the drug. These values have great clinical significance. For example, if the client has a severe headache and is given half of an ASA tablet, the plasma level will remain below the minimum effective concentration, and the client will not experience pain relief. Two or three tablets will increase the plasma level of ASA into the therapeutic range, and the pain will subside. Taking six or more tablets may result in adverse effects, such as GI bleeding or tinnitus. For each drug administered, the nurse's goal is to keep its plasma

concentration in the therapeutic range. For some drugs, this therapeutic range is quite wide; for other medications, the difference between a minimum effective dose and a toxic dose can be dangerously narrow.

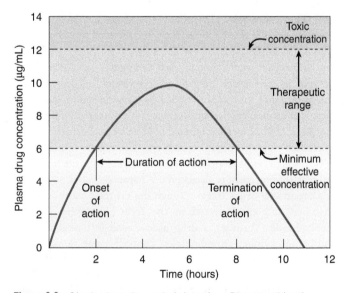

Figure 3.8   Single-dose drug administration. Pharmacokinetic values for this drug are as follows: onset of action, 2 hours; duration of action, 6 hours; termination of action, 8 hours after administration; peak plasma concentration, 10 µg/mL; time to peak drug effect, 5 hours; $t_{1/2}$, 4 hours.

Plasma Half-Life and Duration of Drug Action

3.8 Plasma half-life represents the duration of action for most drugs.

The most common description of a drug's duration of action is its **plasma half-life ($t_{1/2}$)**, defined as the length of time required for a medication to decrease concentration in the plasma by one-half after administration. Some drugs have a half-life of only a few minutes, while others have a half-life of several hours or days. The greater the half-life, the longer it takes a medication to be excreted. For example, a drug with a $t_{1/2}$ of 10 hours would take longer to be excreted and thus produce a longer effect in the body than a drug with a $t_{1/2}$ of 5 hours.

The plasma half-life of a drug is an essential pharmacokinetic variable that has important clinical applications. Drugs with relatively short half-lives, such as ASA ($t_{1/2}$ = 15 to 20 minutes), must be given every 3 to 4 hours. Drugs with longer half-lives, such as felodipine (Plendil) ($t_{1/2}$ = 11–16 hours), need only be given once a day.

Is it better to administer a drug with a short or long half-life? The answer depends on the client's condition and the treatment goal. Drugs with short half-lives are ideal for conditions and procedures that have a brief duration. For example, during a dental procedure, local anesthesia may be needed for only 15 to 20 minutes; therefore, procaine (Novocaine), with a half-life of 8 minutes, may be sufficient. Giving a drug with a long duration of action could cause adverse effects after the client leaves the office. As another example, a simple headache can be relieved with a short-acting drug such as aspirin ($t_{1/2}$ = 15 to 20 minutes) rather than a drug with a 10- or 12-hour duration. Because short-acting drugs are excreted rapidly, the risk for long-term adverse effects is reduced.

Long-duration drugs do have certain advantages. In the preceding example, procaine would not be suitable for a dental procedure that lasts 2 hours because multiple injections would be necessary. Long-duration drugs are beneficial in treating chronic conditions, such as heart failure or hypertension, and for the prevention of conditions such as migraine headaches, seizures, or pregnancy. As drugs stay in the body for prolonged periods, however, the risk for long-term adverse effects increases. This can become particularly serious for clients with significant renal or hepatic impairment; diminished metabolism and excretion will cause the plasma half-life of a drug to increase, and the concentration may reach toxic levels. In these clients, medications must be given less frequently, or the dosages must be reduced.

As a rule of thumb, when a drug is discontinued it takes approximately four half-lives before the agent is considered "functionally" eliminated. After four half-lives, 94% of the drug has been eliminated. In the case of procaine, which has a half-life of only 8 minutes, the drug is considered eliminated in 32 minutes. Although some drug remains, the amount is too small to produce any beneficial or toxic effect. Note, however, that this "rule of thumb" does not apply to all drugs; it certainly does not apply to medications administered to clients with renal or hepatic impairment.

Loading Doses and Maintenance Doses

3.9 Repeated dosing allows a plateau drug plasma level to be reached. Loading doses allow a therapeutic drug level to be reached rapidly.

Few drugs are administered as a single dose. Repeated doses result in an accumulation of drug in the bloodstream, as shown in Figure 3.9. Eventually, a plateau will be reached where the level of drug in the plasma is maintained continuously within the therapeutic range. At this level, the amount of drug administered has reached equilibrium with the amount of drug being eliminated, resulting in a continuous therapeutic level of drug being distributed to body tissues. Theoretically, it takes approximately four half-lives to reach this equilibrium. If the medication is given as a continuous infusion, the plateau can be reached quickly and be maintained with little or no fluctuation in drug plasma levels.

The plateau may be reached faster by the administration of loading doses followed by regular maintenance doses. A **loading dose** is a higher amount of drug, often given only once or twice, that is administered to "prime" the bloodstream with a level sufficient to quickly induce a therapeutic response. Before plasma levels can drop back toward zero, intermittent **maintenance doses** are given to keep the plasma drug concentration in the therapeutic range. Although blood levels of the drug fluctuate with this approach, the equilibrium state can be reached almost as rapidly as with a continuous infusion. Loading doses are particularly important for drugs with prolonged half-lives and for situations in which it is critical to raise drug plasma levels quickly, as might be the case when administering an antibiotic for a severe infection. In Figure 3.9, notice that it takes almost five doses (48 hours) before a therapeutic level is reached using a routine dosing schedule. With a loading dose, a therapeutic level is reached within 12 hours.

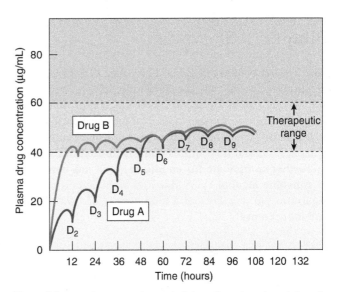

Figure 3.9 Multiple-dose drug administration: drug A and drug B are administered every 12 hours; drug B reaches the therapeutic range faster because the first dose is a loading dose.

CHAPTER

3 Understanding the Chapter

Key Concepts Summary

The numbered key concepts provide a succinct summary of the important points from the corresponding numbered section within the chapter. If any of these points are not clear, refer to the numbered section within the chapter for review.

3.1 Pharmacokinetics focuses on the movement of drugs throughout the body after they are administered. The four processes of pharmacokinetics are absorption, metabolism, distribution, and excretion.

3.2 The physiological properties of plasma membranes determine movement of drugs throughout the body.

3.3 Absorption is the process of moving a drug from the site of administration to the bloodstream. Absorption of a drug molecule depends on its size, lipid solubility, degree of ionization, and interactions with food or other medications.

3.4 Distribution represents how drugs are transported throughout the body. Distribution depends on the formation of drug-protein complexes and special

barriers such as the fetal-placental and blood-brain barriers.

3.5 Metabolism is a process that changes a drug's form and makes it more likely to be excreted. Changes in hepatic metabolism can significantly affect drug action.

3.6 Excretion processes remove drugs from the body. Drugs are primarily excreted by the kidneys but may be excreted by the lung or glands, or into bile.

3.7 The therapeutic response of most drugs depends on their concentration in the plasma. The difference between the minimum effective concentration and the toxic concentration is called the therapeutic range.

3.8 Plasma half-life represents the duration of action for most drugs.

3.9 Repeated dosing allows a plateau drug plasma level to be reached. Loading doses allow a therapeutic drug level to be reached rapidly.

Chapter 3 Scenario

John Kessler is 84 years old and has been ill with multiple debilitating chronic diseases for a long time; his prognosis is poor. He has had uncontrolled diabetes for more than 20 years and has experienced many complications due to this condition. Three years ago, he developed chronic renal failure, and he requires dialysis three times a week. To further complicate his condition, John has continued to consume alcohol every day and smokes one pack of cigarettes per day. He has a long history of both alcohol and tobacco use.

Five days ago, John's daughter noticed that he was becoming increasingly weak and lethargic. Last night, when his temperature reached 38.8°C and he became confused, John's daughter took him to the emergency department, and he was admitted to the medical unit. A chest x-ray this morning revealed bilateral pneumonia. John is

receiving multiple medications through both the intravenous (IV) and inhalation routes.

Critical Thinking Questions

1. What factors may influence drug metabolism or excretion in this client?

2. Discuss why drug elimination for this client may complicate the pharmacotherapy.

3. How will the IV or inhalation drug therapy affect the absorption of his medications?

4. John will receive a loading dose of IV antibiotic and then be placed on maintenance doses every 6 hours. What is the purpose of this regimen? Why would this client be a candidate for a loading dose?

See Answers to Critical Thinking Questions in Appendix B.

NCLEX Practice Questions

1 A nurse is teaching a client about a newly prescribed medication. Which statement by the client would indicate the need for further medication education?

   a. "The liquid form of the drug will be absorbed faster than the tablets."

   b. "If I take more, I'll have a better response."

   c. "Taking this drug with food will decrease how much of it gets in my system."

   d. "I can consult my healthcare provider if I experience unexpected adverse effects."

2 A nurse is caring for several clients. Which client will the nurse anticipate to be most likely to experience an alteration in drug metabolism?

   a. A 3-day-old premature infant

   b. A 22-year-old pregnant female

   c. A 32-year-old man with kidney stones

   d. A 50-year-old executive with hypertension

3 A client is receiving multiple medications, including one drug specifically used to stimulate gastric peristalsis. What influence could this drug have on additional oral medications?

   a. Increased absorption

   b. Reduced excretion

   c. Decreased absorption

   d. Enhanced distribution

4 A client is being discharged from the hospital with a nebulizer for self-administration of inhalation medication. Which statement by the client would indicate to the nurse that client education has been successful?

   a. "Inhaled medications should only be taken in the morning."

   b. "Doses for inhaled medication are larger than for oral medication."

   c. "Medicines taken by inhalation produce a very rapid response."

   d. "Inhaled drugs are often rendered inactive by hepatic metabolic reactions."

5 A nurse is caring for a client with hepatitis and resulting hepatic impairment. The nurse would expect the duration of action of most of the client's medications to

   a. Decrease

   b. Improve

   c. Be unaffected

   d. Increase

See Answers to NCLEX Practice Questions in Appendix A.

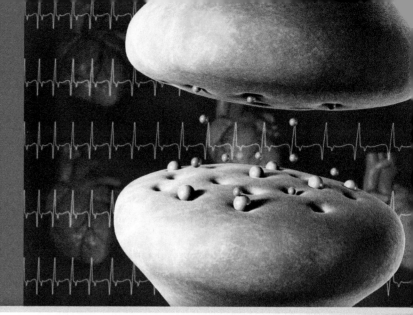

David Mack/Science Source

CHAPTER
4
Pharmacodynamics

LEARNING OUTCOMES

After reading this chapter, the student should be able to:

1. Apply principles of pharmacodynamics to clinical practice.
2. Discuss how frequency response curves may be used to explain how clients respond differently to medications.
3. Explain the importance of the median effective dose (ED_{50}) to clinical practice.
4. Compare and contrast median lethal dose (LD_{50}) and median toxicity dose (TD_{50}).
5. Correlate a drug's therapeutic index to its margin of safety.
6. Identify the significance of the graded dose-response relationship to clinical practice.
7. Compare and contrast the terms *potency* and *efficacy*.
8. Distinguish between an agonist, partial agonist, and antagonist.
9. Explain the relationship between receptors and drug action.
10. Explain possible future developments in the field of pharmacogenetics.

CHAPTER OUTLINE

▸ Pharmacodynamics and Inter-Individual Variability

▸ Therapeutic Index Describes a Drug's Margin of Safety

▸ The Graded Dose-Response Relationship and Therapeutic Response

▸ Potency and Efficacy

▸ Cellular Receptors and Drug Action

▸ Types of Drug-Receptor Interactions

▸ Pharmacology of the Future: Customizing Drug Therapy

In clinical practice, nurses quickly learn that medications do not affect all clients in the same way: a dose that produces a dramatic response in one client may have no effect on another. In some cases, the differences among clients are predictable, based on the pharmacokinetic principles discussed in Chapter 3. In other cases, the differences in response are not easily explained. Despite this client variability, healthcare providers must choose optimal doses while avoiding unnecessary adverse effects. This is not an easy task given the wide variation of client responses within a population. This chapter examines the mechanisms by which drugs affect clients and how the nurse can apply these principles to clinical practice.

Pharmacodynamics and Inter-Individual Variability

4.1 Pharmacodynamics is the area of pharmacology concerned with how drugs produce *change* in clients and the differences in client responses to medications.

The term **pharmacodynamics** is composed of the root words *pharmaco*, which means "medicine," and *dynamics*, which means "change." In simplest terms, pharmacodynamics refers to how a drug *changes* the body. A more complete definition explains pharmacodynamics as the branch of pharmacology concerned with the mechanisms of drug action and the relationships between drug concentration and responses in the body.

Pharmacodynamics has important clinical applications. Healthcare providers must be able to predict whether a drug will produce a significant change in clients. Although clinicians usually begin therapy with average doses taken from a drug guide, intuitive experience often becomes the practical method for determining which doses of medications will be effective in a given client. Knowledge of therapeutic indexes, dose-response relationships, and drug-receptor interactions will help the nurse to provide safe and effective treatment.

Inter-individual variability in responses to drugs can best be understood by examining a frequency distribution curve. A **frequency distribution curve**, shown in Figure 4.1, is a graphical representation of the number of individuals who respond to a drug at different doses. On the horizontal axis, notice the wide range of doses that produced the responses shown in the curve. A few individuals responded to the drug at very low doses (10 to 20 mg). As the dose was increased, more and more individuals responded. Some required very high doses to elicit the desired

response. The peak of the curve (50 mg) indicates the largest number of individuals responding to the drug. The curve does not show the *magnitude* of response, only whether a measurable response occurred. As an example, think of the given response to an antihypertensive drug as being a reduction of 20 mm Hg in systolic blood pressure. A few individuals experience the desired 20 mm Hg reduction at a dose of only 10 mg of drug. A 50-mg dose produces the largest number of individuals with a 20 mm Hg reduction in blood pressure; however, a few individuals need as much as 90 mg of drug to produce the same 20 mm Hg reduction.

The dose in the middle of the frequency distribution curve represents the drug's **median effective dose (ED_{50})**. The ED_{50} is the dose required to produce a specific therapeutic response in 50% of a group of clients. Drug guides sometimes report the ED_{50} as the average or standard dose.

The inter-individual variability shown in Figure 4.1 has important clinical implications. First, the nurse should realize that the standard or average dose predicts a satisfactory therapeutic response for only *half* of the population. In other words, many clients will require more or less than the average dose for optimum pharmacotherapy. Using the systolic blood pressure example, assume that a large group of clients is given the average dose

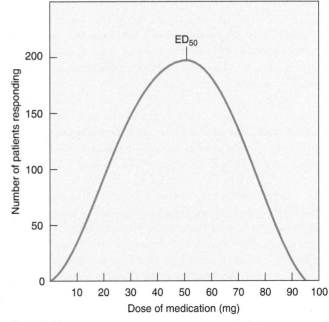

Figure 4.1 Frequency distribution curve: inter-individual variability in drug response.

of 50 mg. Some of these clients will experience toxicity at this level because they only needed 10 mg to achieve blood pressure reduction. Other clients in this group will probably have no reduction in blood pressure. By observing the client, taking vital signs, and monitoring associated laboratory data, the skill of the nurse is critical in determining whether the average dose is effective for the client. It is not enough to simply memorize an average dose for a drug; the nurse must know when and how to adjust this dose to obtain the optimum therapeutic response.

Therapeutic Index Describes a Drug's Margin of Safety

4.2 The therapeutic index, expressed mathematically as $TD_{50} \div ED_{50}$, is a value representing the margin of safety of a drug. The higher the therapeutic index, the safer the drug.

Administering a dose that produces an optimum therapeutic response for each individual client is only one component of effective pharmacotherapy. The nurse must also be able to predict whether the dose being given is safe for the client.

Frequency distribution curves can also be used to represent the safety of a drug. For example, the **median lethal dose (LD_{50})** is often determined in preclinical trials as part of the drug development process discussed in Chapter 1. The LD_{50} is the dose of drug that will be lethal in 50% of a group of animals. As with ED_{50}, a group of animals will exhibit considerable variability in the lethal dose; what may be a non-toxic dose for one animal may be lethal for another.

To examine the safety of a particular drug, the LD_{50} can be compared to the ED_{50}, as shown in Figure 4.2. In the top example, 10 mg of drug X is the average *effective* dose, and 40 mg is the average *lethal* dose. The ED_{50} and LD_{50} are used to calculate an important value in pharmacology, the **therapeutic index (TI)**, which is the ratio of a drug's LD_{50} to its ED_{50}.

The larger the difference between the two doses, the greater the therapeutic index. In Figure 4.2(a), the therapeutic index is 4 (40 mg ÷ 10 mg). Essentially, this means that it would take an error in magnitude of *approximately* 4 times the average dose to be lethal to a client. In terms of dosage, this is a relatively safe drug, and small to moderate medication errors or changes in the drug's bioavailability would likely not be fatal. Thus, the TI is a measure of a drug's safety margin: the higher the value, the safer the medication. Drugs exhibit a wide range of TIs, from 1 to 2 to greater than 100. As another example, the therapeutic index of a second drug is shown in Figure 4.2(b). Drug Z has the same ED_{50} as drug X, but shows a different LD_{50}. The TI for drug Z is only 2 (20 mg ÷ 10 mg). The difference between an effective dose and a lethal dose is very small for drug Z; therefore, the drug has a narrow safety margin. The therapeutic index offers the nurse practical information on the safety of a drug and a means to compare one drug to another.

Because the LD_{50} cannot be determined experimentally in humans, the **median toxicity dose (TD_{50})** is a more practical value in the clinical setting. The TD_{50} is the dose that will produce a given toxicity in 50% of a group of clients. The TD_{50} value may be extrapolated from animal data or based on adverse effects recorded in clinical trials.

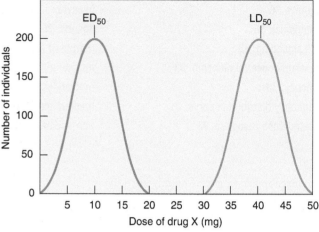

(a) Drug X : TI = $\dfrac{LD_{50}}{ED_{50}} = \dfrac{40}{10} = 4$

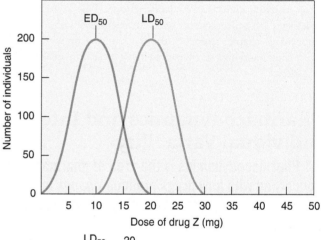

(b) Drug Z : TI = $\dfrac{LD_{50}}{ED_{50}} = \dfrac{20}{10} = 2$

Figure 4.2 Therapeutic index: (a) drug X has a therapeutic index (TI) of 4; (b) drug Z has a therapeutic index of 2.

The **margin of safety (MOS)** is another index of a drug's effectiveness and safety. The MOS is calculated as the amount of drug that is lethal to 1% of animals (LD_1) divided by the amount of drug that produces a therapeutic effect in 99% of animals (ED_{99}). In general, the higher the MOS value, the safer the medication. Of course, this considers only the lethality of the drug and does not account for non-lethal, though serious, adverse effects that may occur at lower doses.

NCLEX Success Tips

The nurse should keep in mind that clients with decreased renal function and decreased creatinine clearance will require a change in their medication dosages to avoid toxicity.

The nurse should arrange to get blood levels for medication with narrow therapeutic index on a scheduled basis.

The nurse should collaborate with the dietitian to ensure that food-drug interactions are kept to a minimum to avoid drug toxicity while clients are receiving medication with narrow therapeutic index.

The Graded Dose-Response Relationship and Therapeutic Response

4.3 The graded dose-response relationship describes how the therapeutic response to a drug changes as the medication dose is increased.

In the previous examples, frequency distribution curves were used to graphically visualize client differences in responses to medications in a *population*. It is also useful to visualize the variability in responses observed within a *single client*. A dose-response curve plots the drug dose administered to the client versus the intensity or degree of response obtained.

How does a client respond to varying doses of a drug? Common sense suggests that a larger dose would produce more drug effect. For example, an antibiotic would kill more bacteria if the dose was increased from 10 mg to 20 mg. An antihypertensive drug would cause a greater reduction in blood pressure if the dose was increased from 50 mg to 100 mg. These simple examples describe the **dose-response relationship**, one of the most fundamental concepts in pharmacology. The graphical representation of this relationship is called a dose-response curve, as illustrated in Figure 4.3. By observing and measuring an individual's response at different doses of the drug, one can explain several important clinical relationships.

The three distinct phases of a dose-response curve indicate essential pharmacodynamic principles that have relevance to clinical practice. Phase 1 occurs at the lowest doses. The flatness of this portion of the curve indicates that few target cells have yet been affected by the drug. Phase 2 is the straight-line portion of the curve. This portion often shows a linear relationship between the amount of drug administered and the degree of response obtained. For example, if the dose is doubled, the response is

twice as great. This is the most desirable range of doses for pharmacotherapeutics since giving more drug results in proportionately more effect; a lower drug dose produces less effect. In phase 3, a plateau is reached in which increasing the drug dose produces no additional therapeutic response. This may occur for a number of reasons. One explanation is that all receptors for the drug are occupied. It could also mean that the drug has brought 100% relief, such as when a migraine headache has been terminated; giving higher doses produces no additional relief. In phase 3, although increasing the dose does not result in more therapeutic effect, the nurse should be mindful that increasing the dose may produce adverse effects.

The dose-response curve in Figure 4.3 is smooth and continuous; therefore, it is sometimes called a **graded dose-response** curve. This is important to pharmacotherapeutics because by adjusting the dose in small increments at a time, the prescriber is able to attain virtually any degree of therapeutic response (0% to 100%) within the linear range of drug doses. This is especially true when using the intravenous (IV) route, during which the nurse can adjust the infusion rate in very small increments.

Potency and Efficacy

4.4 Potency, the dose of medication required to produce a particular response, and efficacy, the magnitude of maximum response to a drug, are means of comparing medications.

Within a pharmacological class, not all drugs are equally effective at treating a disorder. For example, some antineoplastic drugs kill more cancer cells than others, some antihypertensive agents lower blood pressure to a greater degree than others, and some analgesics relieve severe pain better than others in the same class. Furthermore, drugs in the same class are effective at different doses; one antibiotic may be effective at a dose of 1 mg/kg, whereas another is most effective at 100 mg/kg. Nurses need a method to compare one drug to another so that they can administer treatment effectively.

There are two fundamental ways to compare medications within therapeutic and pharmacological classes. First is the concept of **potency**. A drug that is more potent will produce a therapeutic effect at a lower dose compared with another drug in the same class. Consider two agents, drug X and drug Y, which both produce a 20 mm Hg drop in blood pressure. If drug X produced this effect at a dose of 10 mg and drug Y produced this effect at 60 mg, drug X is said to be more potent. Thus, potency is a way to compare the doses of two independently administered drugs in terms of how much is needed to produce a particular response. A useful way to visualize the concept of potency is by examining dose-response curves. Compare the two drugs shown in Figure 4.4(a). In this example, drug A is more potent because it requires a lower dose to produce the same response.

The second method used to compare drugs is **efficacy**, which is the magnitude of maximum response that can be produced from a particular drug. In the example shown in Figure 4.4(b), drug A is more efficacious because it produces a higher maximum response.

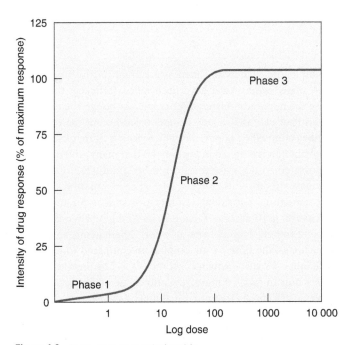

Figure 4.3 Dose-response relationship.

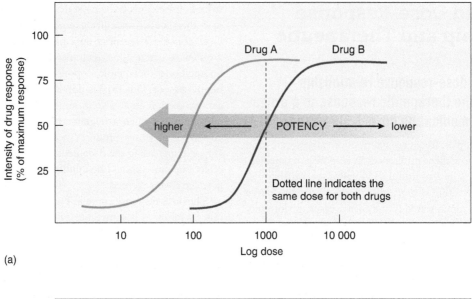

(a)

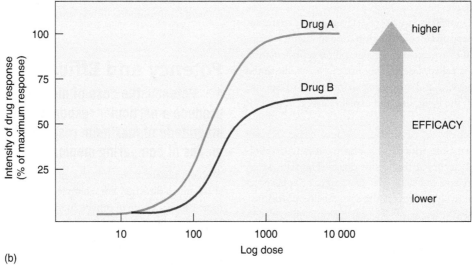

(b)

Figure 4.4 Potency and efficacy: (a) drug A has greater potency than drug B; (b) drug A has greater efficacy than drug B.

Which is more important to the success of pharmacotherapy, potency or efficacy? Perhaps the best way to understand these concepts is to use the specific example of headache pain. Two common over-the-counter (OTC) analgesics are ibuprofen (Advil, Motrin; 200 mg) and acetylsalicylic acid (Aspirin; 650 mg). The fact that ibuprofen relieves pain at a lower dose indicates that this agent is *more potent* than acetylsalicylic acid. At recommended doses, however, both are equally effective at relieving headache pain, thus they have the *same efficacy*. However, if the client is experiencing severe pain, neither acetylsalicylic acid nor ibuprofen has sufficient efficacy to bring relief. Narcotic analgesics such as morphine have greater efficacy than acetylsalicylic acid and ibuprofen and could effectively treat this type of pain. From a pharmacotherapeutic perspective, efficacy is almost always more important than potency. In the headache pain example, the average dose is unimportant to the client, but headache relief is essential. As another example, the client with cancer is much more concerned about how many cancer cells have been killed (efficacy) than what dose the nurse administered (potency). Although the nurse will often hear claims that one drug is more potent than another, a more compelling concern is which drug is more efficacious.

Although it is stated in Section 4.3 that many adverse effects are related to dose—that higher doses produce more intense adverse effects—this is true only when comparing doses of the same drug. For example, a therapeutic dose for amlodipine (Norvasc) is 10 mg/day. Giving 20 or 30 mg of amlodipine will most certainly increase the risk for experiencing an adverse effect. Can the dose of amlodipine be compared to a dose of nifedipine (Adalat), which is 60 mg/day? The answer is absolutely not. In fact, 10 mg of amlodipine gives the same risk of adverse effects as 60 mg of nifedipine. *The point is that when two different drugs are compared, one cannot assume that the drug with the lower dose gives fewer adverse effects.*

Cellular Receptors and Drug Action

4.5 Drug receptor theory is used to explain the mechanism of action of many medications.

Most drugs produce their actions by activating or inhibiting specific cellular receptors. Drugs rarely create new actions in the body; instead, they enhance or inhibit existing physiological and biochemical processes. **Cell signalling** is part of a complex system of communication that enables cells to perceive and correctly respond to their environment and carry out basic cellular activities. Errors in cellular information processing are responsible for diseases such as diabetes, cancer, and autoimmune disorders. Cells receive information from their environment through a class of molecules known as **receptors**. A receptor is a molecule to which a medication binds to initiate its effect. While many receptors are cell surface proteins, some are found inside cells. Molecules that activate (or in some cases inhibit) receptors are called receptor **ligands**. These ligands can be classified as hormones, neurotransmitters, cytokines, or growth factors. The information that cells receive is then processed through signalling pathways. Activation of specific target proteins causes a particular cell response. Different types of cells may have the same receptor and receive the same signal but have different target proteins that produce different responses when activated.

Drugs act by modulating or changing existing physiological and biochemical processes. To effect such changes requires that the drug interact with specific molecules and chemicals normally found in the body. The concept of a drug binding to a receptor to cause a change in body chemistry or physiology is a fundamental theory in pharmacology. Receptor theory explains the mechanisms by which most drugs produce their effects. However, it is important to understand that these receptors do not exist in the body solely to bind drugs. Their normal function is to bind endogenous molecules such as hormones, neurotransmitters, and growth factors.

NCLEX Success Tips

The nurse should keep in mind that receptors are either stimulated using agonists or inhibited using antagonists. The decision to inhibit or to stimulate a certain receptor depends on the desired therapeutic indication. However, it is worth noting that drugs are not completely organ-specific when they inhibit or stimulate a receptor on a specific organ; they tend to work the same way on other organs, leading to unwarranted side effects.

Beta receptors have two types (B1 and B2). The beta receptors in the heart and lungs are often targeted by different medications. An easy way to remember which type of receptor is located in which organ is to recall that you have one heart (hence B1) and two lungs (hence B2). Students should understand the function that results from stimulation or inhibition of these receptors in order to understand the mechanism of action and the side effects of drugs that work on these receptors.

Although a drug receptor can be any type of macromolecule, the vast majority are proteins. As shown in Figure 4.5, a receptor may be depicted as a three-dimensional protein associated with a cellular plasma membrane. The extracellular structural component of a receptor often consists of several protein subunits arranged around a central canal or channel. Other receptors consist of many membrane-spanning segments inserted across the plasma membrane.

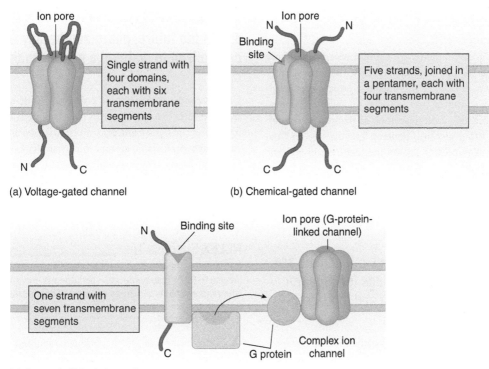

(a) Voltage-gated channel

(b) Chemical-gated channel

(c) G-protein-linked channel

Figure 4.5 Cellular receptors.

A drug attaches to its receptor in a specific manner, much like a lock and key. Small changes to the structure of a drug, or its receptor, may weaken or even eliminate binding between the two molecules. Once bound, drugs may trigger a series of **second messenger** events within the cell, such as the conversion of adenosine triphosphate (ATP) to cyclic adenosine monophosphate (cyclic AMP), the release of intracellular calcium, or the activation of specific G proteins and associated enzymes. These biochemical cascades initiate the drug's action by either stimulating or inhibiting a normal activity of the cell.

Not all receptors are bound to plasma membranes; some are intracellular molecules such as DNA or enzymes in the cytoplasm. By interacting with these types of receptors, medications are able to inhibit protein synthesis or regulate events such as cell replication and metabolism. Examples of agents that bind intracellular components include steroid medications, vitamins, and hormones.

Receptors and their associated drug mechanisms are extremely important in therapeutics. Receptor subtypes are being discovered and new medications are being developed at a faster rate than at any other time in history. These subtypes permit the "fine-tuning" of pharmacology. For example, the first medications affecting the autonomic nervous system affected all autonomic receptors. It was discovered that two basic receptor types existed in the body, alpha and beta, and drugs were then developed that affected only one type. The result was more specific drug action, with fewer adverse effects. Still later, several subtypes of alpha and beta receptors, including alpha-1, alpha-2, beta-1, and beta-2, were discovered that allowed even more specificity in pharmacotherapy. In recent years, researchers have further divided and refined these subtypes and discovered other receptors such as beta-3. It is likely that receptor research will continue to result in the development of new medications that activate very specific receptors and thus direct drug action that avoids unnecessary adverse effects.

Some drugs act independently of cellular receptors. These agents are associated with other mechanisms, such as changing the permeability of cellular membranes, depressing membrane excitability, or altering the activity of cellular pumps. Actions such as these are often described as **non-specific cellular responses**. Ethyl alcohol, general anesthetics, and osmotic diuretics are examples of agents that act by non-specific mechanisms.

Types of Drug-Receptor Interactions

4.6 Agonists, partial agonists, and antagonists are substances that compete with drugs for receptor binding and can cause drug-drug and food-drug interactions.

When a drug binds to a receptor, several therapeutic consequences can result. In simplest terms, a specific activity of the cell is either enhanced or inhibited. The actual biochemical mechanism underlying the therapeutic effect, however, may be extremely complex. In some cases, the mechanism of action is not known.

When a drug binds to its receptor, it may produce a response that *mimics* the effect of the endogenous regulatory molecule. For example, when the drug bethanechol is administered, it binds to acetylcholine receptors in the autonomic nervous system and produces the same actions as acetylcholine. A drug that produces the same type of response as the endogenous substance is called an **agonist**. Agonists sometimes produce a greater maximum response than the endogenous chemical. The term **partial agonist** describes a medication that produces a weaker, or less efficacious, response than an agonist.

A second possibility is that a drug will occupy a receptor and *prevent* the endogenous chemical from acting. This drug is called an **antagonist**. For example, protamine sulfate acts as "antidote" to heparin, and in its presence the body loses the anticoagulant action expected from heparin. Naloxone (Narcan) is an opioid antagonist that is used as an antidote for opioids.

Antagonists often compete with agonists for the receptor binding sites. For example, the drug atropine competes with acetylcholine for specific receptors in the autonomic nervous system. If the dose is high enough, atropine will inhibit the effects of acetylcholine because acetylcholine cannot bind to its receptors.

Not all antagonism is associated with receptors. *Functional* antagonists inhibit the effects of an agonist, not by competing for a receptor but by changing pharmacokinetic factors. For example, antagonists may slow the absorption of a drug. By speeding up metabolism or excretion, an antagonist can enhance the removal of a drug from the body. The relationships that occur between agonists and antagonists explain many of the drug-drug and food-drug interactions that occur in the body.

Pharmacology of the Future: Customizing Drug Therapy

4.7 In the future, pharmacotherapy will likely be customized to match the genetic makeup of each client.

Until recently, it was thought that single drugs should provide safe and effective treatment to every client in the same way. Unfortunately, a significant portion of the population either develops unacceptable side effects to certain drugs or is unresponsive to them. Many scientists and clinicians are now discarding the one-size-fits-all approach to drug therapy, which was designed to treat an entire population without addressing important inter-individual variation.

NCLEX Success Tip

Red blood cells with decreased levels of glucose-6-phosphate dehydrogenase (G6PD) may hemolyze—and anemia and jaundice may occur—when exposed to certain drugs, such as sulfonamides, acetylsalicylic acid, thiazide diuretics, and vitamin K.

With the advent of the Human Genome Project and other advances in medicine, researchers are hopeful that future drugs can be customized for clients with specific genetic similarities. In the past, unpredictable and unexplained drug reactions have been labelled **idiosyncratic responses**. For example, the most common

Special Considerations

◀ Enzyme Deficiency in Certain Ethnic Populations

Pharmacogenetics has identified a number of people who are deficient in the enzyme glucose-6-phosphate dehydrogenase (G6PD). This enzyme is essential in carbohydrate metabolism. Males of Mediterranean and African descent are more likely to express this deficiency. According to Carter (2012), G6PD deficiency is the most common enzyme deficiency worldwide. It is estimated to affect 400 million people worldwide. The disorder is caused by mutations in the DNA that encode for G6PD, resulting in one or more amino acid changes in the protein molecule. Following administration of certain drugs, such as primaquine, sulfonamides, and nitrofurantoin (Macrobid), an acute hemolysis of red blood cells occurs due to the breaking of chemical bonds in the hemoglobin molecule. Up to 50% of the circulating red blood cells may be destroyed. Genetic typing does not always predict toxicity; therefore, the nurse must observe clients carefully following the administration of these medications. Fortunately, there are good alternative choices for these medications.

Carter, S. M. (2012). *Glucose-6-phosphate dehydrogenase deficiency*. Retrieved from http://emedicine.medscape.com/article/200390-overview

adverse reaction to dantrolene (Dantrium) is muscle weakness. However, the drug may also depress liver function or cause idiosyncratic hepatitis. It is hoped that by performing a DNA test before administering a drug, these idiosyncratic side effects can someday be avoided.

Pharmacogenetics is the area of pharmacology that examines the role of genetic variation in drug response. The greatest advances in pharmacogenetics have been the identification of subtle genetic differences in drug-metabolizing enzymes. Genetic differences in these enzymes are responsible for a significant portion of drug-induced toxicity. It is hoped that the use of pharmacogenetic information may someday allow for customized drug therapy. Although therapies based on a client's genetically based response may not be cost effective at this time, pharmacogenetics may radically change the way pharmacotherapy will be practised in the future.

CHAPTER

4 Understanding the Chapter

Key Concepts Summary

The numbered key concepts provide a succinct summary of the important points from the corresponding numbered section within the chapter. If any of these points are not clear, refer to the numbered section within the chapter for review

4.1 Pharmacodynamics is the area of pharmacology concerned with how drugs produce *change* in clients and the differences in client responses to medications.

4.2 The therapeutic index, expressed mathematically as $TD_{50} \div ED_{50}$, is a value representing the margin of safety of a drug. The higher the therapeutic index, the safer the drug.

4.3 The graded dose-response relationship describes how the therapeutic response to a drug changes as the medication dose is increased.

4.4 Potency, the dose of medication required to produce a particular response, and efficacy, the magnitude of maximum response to a drug, are means of comparing medications.

4.5 Drug receptor theory is used to explain the mechanism of action of many medications.

4.6 Agonists, partial agonists, and antagonists are substances that compete with drugs for receptor binding and can cause drug-drug and food-drug interactions.

4.7 In the future, pharmacotherapy will likely be customized to match the genetic makeup of each client.

Chapter 4 Scenario

Katherine Hunter prides herself on being a wise consumer and cautiously examines the claims made by manufacturers for all of her purchases. She researches everything she buys, such as automobiles, household appliances, and medications. Recently, she has begun to seriously consider assertions made by the advertisements for various types of antacids. Most brands claim to be the most efficient in relieving the symptoms of indigestion. Others claim to be the most potent antacid available without a prescription. Some products claim that they not only relieve heartburn, but also supply the body with needed vitamins and minerals. When purchasing an OTC medication, all Katherine wants is something that will work quickly with few adverse effects.

Critical Thinking Questions

1. How would you teach Katherine the difference between potency and efficacy?
2. Which of the two concepts (potency and efficacy) would be most important for selecting a drug? Why?
3. What are the drawbacks of comparing two different medications?

See Answers to Critical Thinking Questions in Appendix B.

NCLEX Practice Questions

1 What parameters does a nurse use to determine whether the average dose of a medication is effective for a client? Select all that apply.
   a. Physical examination
   b. Vital signs
   c. Laboratory values
   d. Dosage time
   e. Efficacy

2 The nurse knows that a drug with a high therapeutic index is
   a. Probably safe
   b. Often dangerous
   c. Frequently risky
   d. Most likely effective

3 While reviewing a drug manufacturer's package insert, a nurse reads about the dose-response curve. The purpose of the dose-response curve is to illustrate the relationship between
   a. The amount of a drug administered and the degree of response it produces
   b. The prevalence of toxic effects in a given population
   c. The degree of response and the total duration of action of the drug
   d. The peak serum drug levels when half the dose is administered

4 A client with myasthenia gravis has been receiving neostigmine (Prostigmin), a cholinergic agonist, for the past 2 years. The nurse is ready to administer benztropine (Cogentin), a cholinergic antagonist. Which result will likely occur when these drugs are combined?
   a. Neostigmine will exhibit a greater effect.
   b. Neostigmine will exhibit a lesser effect.
   c. Neostigmine will not be affected by the administration of benztropine.
   d. Neostigmine will first exhibit a greater effect, followed by a lesser effect.

5 When considering pharmacodynamic principles for a client's drug therapy, the nurse is aware that affinity for a receptor is most closely associated with a drug's
   a. Potency
   b. Efficacy
   c. Metabolism
   d. First-pass effect

See Answers to NCLEX Practice Questions in Appendix A.

Pharmacology and the Nurse-Client Relationship

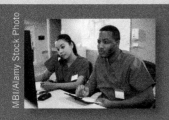

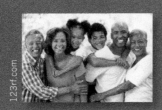

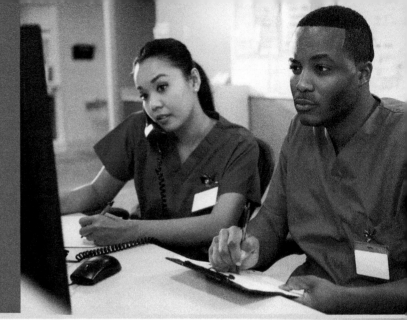
MBI/Alamy Stock Photo

CHAPTER

5

The Nursing Process in Pharmacology

LEARNING OUTCOMES

After reading this chapter, the student should be able to:

1. Explain the steps of the nursing process in relation to pharmacotherapeutics.
2. Identify assessment data to be gathered to ensure safe medication administration.
3. Develop appropriate nursing diagnoses for clients receiving medications.
4. Set realistic goals and outcomes during the planning stage for clients receiving medications.
5. Discuss key intervention strategies to be carried out for clients receiving medications.
6. Evaluate the outcomes of medication administration.
7. Apply the nursing process when giving medications, using the Nursing Process Focus flowcharts found in Chapters 13 through 63.

CHAPTER OUTLINE

▶ Review of the Nursing Process

▶ Assessing the Client in Relation to Drug Administration

▶ Diagnosing for the Client Receiving Medications

▶ Setting Goals and Outcomes for Drug Administration

▶ Key Interventions for Drug Administration

▶ Evaluating the Effects of Drug Administration

The nursing process, a systematic method of problem solving in nursing practice, forms the foundation of all nursing interventions. The use of the nursing process is particularly essential during medication administration. By using the steps of the nursing process, nurses can ensure that the interdisciplinary practice of pharmacology results in safe, effective, and individualized medication administration and outcomes for all clients under their care.

Review of the Nursing Process

5.1 The nursing process is a systematic method of problem solving and consists of clearly defined steps: assessing; diagnosing client problems, strengths, and needs; planning care through the formulation of goals and outcomes; implementing interventions; and evaluating the care provided.

Most nursing students enter a pharmacology course after taking a course on the fundamentals of nursing, during which the steps of the **nursing process** are discussed in detail. This section presents a brief review of those steps before discussing in detail how they can be applied to pharmacotherapy. Students who are unfamiliar with the nursing process are encouraged to consult one of the many excellent fundamentals of nursing textbooks for a more detailed explanation. Although these steps have been described in a cyclical form, the nursing process is a dynamic process, with each step emanating from the previous steps and affecting future steps within the process.

Assessing, the first step in the nursing process, is an ongoing process that begins with the nurse's initial contact with the client and continues with every interaction thereafter. During the initial assessment, **baseline data** that will be compared to information obtained during later interactions are gathered. Assessing consists of gathering **subjective data**, which include what the client says or perceives, and **objective data**, which are gathered through physical assessment, laboratory tests, and other diagnostic sources.

NCLEX Success Tips

Assessment is a crucial step that, if done thoroughly and competently, can mitigate medication errors. Medication-specific assessment is a necessary step to ensure client safety and best practice.

If the nurse discovers a medication error, the initial step is client assessment. Reporting and documenting can wait while the nurse ensures the client's well-being. As such, the most immediate action should be to assess the client's condition and to report it to the physician.

During assessment, it is crucial for the nurse to listen to the client and respect his or her knowledge about the medication. The nurse must not dismiss the client's concerns nor suggest possible explanations without investigating the specific situation. If the nurse has the wrong medication, the client can prevent a medication error prior to the nurse's administering it.

Identifying patterns, or **diagnosing**, is the second step in the nursing process. This step begins once the initial assessment data are gathered. The nurse interprets, analyzes, and synthesizes data in order to identify patterns of problems, health and safety risks, related needs, and strengths. If gaps in the data are observed, the nurse collects the missing data. The judgments made by nurses in this step are commonly referred to as **nursing diagnoses** to differentiate them from medical diagnoses. Identifying patterns, or diagnosing, provides the basis for establishing goals and outcomes, planning interventions to meet those goals and outcomes, and evaluating the effectiveness of the care provided to the client.

Diagnosing is often the most challenging part of the nursing process. Sometimes the nurse identifies what is believed to be the client's problem, only to discover after further assessment that the planned goals, outcomes, and interventions have not "solved" the problem. Diagnosing is an ongoing reasoning process and focuses on the client's problems and needs. A nursing role in primary health care is to enable clients to become active participants in their own care. By verifying identified problems and their associated needs collaboratively with the client, the nurse encourages the client to take a more active role in resolving these problems.

Identifying patterns in health problems and needs is integral to the nursing process. Use of the term *diagnosing* to describe this activity is common to most nursing practice models. In this text, the terms *diagnosing* and *nursing diagnoses* are used generally and do not refer specifically to the structured list of nursing diagnoses approved by the North American Nursing Diagnosis Association (NANDA).

In **planning**, the third step of the nursing process, the nurse plans ways to assist the client to resolve problems and return to an optimum level of wellness. Short-term or long-term **goals** that focus on what the client will be able to do or achieve, not on what the nurse will do, are established. **Outcomes** are the objective measures of those goals. They specifically define what the client will do, under what circumstances, and within what time frame. Goals and outcomes are also verified with the client or caregiver and are prioritized according to the clients' preferences and to address immediate needs first.

Planning links strategies, or interventions, to the established goals and outcomes. It is the formal written process that communicates with all members of the healthcare team what the nurse will do to assist the client in meeting those goals. Each healthcare organization decides how this plan of care will be communicated, and the plan may be nurse centred or interdisciplinary.

Implementing, the fourth step in the nursing process, occurs when the nurse caries out the planned nursing interventions. Interventions are designed to meet the client's needs and to ensure safe, effective care. As the nurse provides care, reassessment is ongoing and new data are compared to earlier data. The nurse compares the data to established nursing diagnoses, goals, and outcomes and begins the process of **evaluating**, the fifth step in the nursing process. Established needs are reviewed while taking into consideration the client's response to care. More assessment data are gathered as needed, and goals and outcomes are considered as to whether they were met, partially met, or not met at all. The process comes full circle as new or modified needs are identified and diagnosed, goals and outcomes are redefined, and new interventions are planned and implemented.

Nursing has not always relied on such an organized approach to nursing care but has always been concerned with delivering safe and effective care. The administration of medications requires the use of the nursing process to ensure the best possible outcomes for the client. These steps will now be applied specifically to drug administration.

Assessing the Client in Relation to Drug Administration

5.2 Assessing the client who is receiving medications includes obtaining health history information, physical assessment data, laboratory values, and other measurable data and assessing medication effects, both therapeutic and side effects. It also includes assessment of the medication ordered in relation to the client's medical condition, culture, ethnicity, gender, age, and other factors.

A health history and physical assessment are usually completed during the initial meeting between a nurse and a client. Many pieces of data are gathered during this initial assessment, and they have specific implications for the process of drug administration. Ongoing assessments after this time provide additional data to help the nurse evaluate the outcomes of medication use. This section discusses pertinent assessment components and how they relate to drug administration.

The initial health history is tailored to the client's clinical condition. A complete history is the most detailed, but the appropriateness of this history must be considered given the client's condition. Often a problem-focused or "chief complaint" history is taken, focusing on the symptoms that led the client to seek care. In any history, key components that may affect the successful outcome of drug administration must be assessed. Essential questions to ask in the initial history relate to allergies; past medical history; medications used currently and in the recent past; responses to medications taken in the past; patterns of compliance with medications; personal and social history, such as the use of alcohol, tobacco, or caffeine; health risks, such as the use of street drugs or illicit substances; and reproductive health questions, such as the pregnancy status of women of childbearing age. Table 5.1 provides pertinent questions that may be asked during an initial health history to provide baseline data before the administration of medications. The health history is tailored to the client's condition, so all questions may not be appropriate during the initial assessment. Keep in mind that what is *not* being said may be as important, or more important, than what *is* said. For instance, a client may deny

or downplay any symptoms of pain while grimacing or guarding a certain area from being touched. Nurses must use their keen skills of observation during the history to gather such critical data.

NCLEX Success Tips

As a safety precaution, the nurse should discard any unlabelled syringes containing medication. The nurse must administer only the medication that he or she has prepared.

The most important question to ask prior to administering antibiotics is allergies.

Along with the health history, a physical assessment is completed to gather objective data on the client's condition. Vital signs, height and weight, a head-to-toe physical assessment, and laboratory specimens may be obtained. These values provide the baseline data used to compare with future assessments and to guide the healthcare provider in deciding which medications to prescribe. Many medications can affect the heart rate and blood pressure, and these vital signs should be noted. Baseline electrolyte values are important parameters to obtain because many medications affect electrolyte balance. Renal and hepatic function tests are essential for many clients, particularly older adults and those who are critically ill, as these will be used to determine the proper drug dosage.

In addition to assessing the client, the nurse must assess the prescribed medication. Is the order complete? Is the order current or has it expired? Are the drug, dose, route, and time of administration specified and appropriate for this client, considering factors such as the client's age, gender, weight, ethnicity, and medical diagnoses? Are there any contraindications to using this drug for this client? Does the drug require special assessments or client teaching?

Once pharmacotherapy is initiated, ongoing assessments are conducted to determine the effects of the medications. Assessment should first focus on determining whether the client is experiencing the expected therapeutic benefits from the medications. For example, if a drug is given for symptoms of pain, is the pain subsiding? If an antibiotic is given for an infection, are the signs of that infection—elevated temperature, redness or swelling, drainage from infected sites, etc.—improving over time? If a client is not experiencing the therapeutic effects of the medication, further assessment must be done to determine the reason. Dosages and the scheduling of medications are reviewed, and serum drug levels may be obtained.

Assessment during pharmacotherapy also focuses on any side or adverse effects the client may be experiencing. Often these effects are manifested in dermatological, cardiovascular, gastrointestinal, or neurological symptoms. Here again, baseline data are compared with the current assessment to determine what changes have occurred since the initiation of pharmacotherapy. The Nursing Process Focus flowcharts provided in Chapters 13 through 63 illustrate key assessment data to be gathered associated with specific medications or classes of drugs.

Finally, an assessment of the ability of the client to assume responsibility for his or her own drug administration is necessary. Will the client require assistance obtaining or affording the prescribed medications, or taking them safely? What kind of medication storage facilities exist and are they adequate to protect the

TABLE 5.1   Health History Assessment Questions Pertinent to Drug Administration

Health History Component	Pertinent Questions
Chief complaint	• How do you feel? (Describe.) • Are you having any pain? (Describe.) • Are you experiencing other symptoms? (Especially pertinent to medications are nausea, vomiting, headache, itching, dizziness, shortness of breath, nervousness or anxiousness, palpitations or heart "fluttering," weakness, and fatigue.)
Allergies	• Are you allergic to any medications? • Are you allergic to any foods, environmental substances (e.g., pollen or "seasonal" allergies), tape, soaps, or cleansers? • What specifically happens when you experience an allergy?
Past medical history	• Do you have a history of diabetes, heart or vascular conditions, respiratory conditions, or neurological conditions? • Do you have any dermatological conditions? • How have these conditions been treated in the past? How are they being treated currently?
Family history	• Has anyone in your family experienced difficulties with any medications? (Describe.) • Does anyone in your family have any significant medical problems?
Drug history	• What prescription medications are you currently taking? (List drug name, dosage, frequency of administration.) • What non-prescription/over-the-counter (OTC) medications are you taking? (List drug name, dosage, frequency.) • What drugs, prescription or OTC, have you taken within the past month or two? • Have you ever experienced any side effects or unusual symptoms with any medications? (Describe.) • What do you know, or what have you been taught, about these medications? • Do you use any herbal or homeopathic remedies? Any nutritional substances or vitamins?
Health management	• When was the last time you saw a healthcare provider? • What is your normal diet? • Do you have any trouble sleeping?
Reproductive history	• Is there any possibility you are pregnant? (Ask *every* woman of childbearing age.) • Are you breastfeeding?
Personal and social history	• Do you smoke? • What is your normal alcohol intake? • What is your normal caffeine intake? • Do you have any religious or cultural beliefs or practices concerning medications or your health that we should know about? • What is your occupation? What hours do you work? • Do you have any concerns regarding insurance or the ability to afford medications?
Health risk history	• Do you have any history of depression or other mental illness? • Do you use any street drugs or illicit substances?

client, others in the home, and the efficacy of the medication? Does the client understand the uses and effects of this medication and how it is properly taken? Would assessment data suggest that the use of this medication might present a problem, such as difficulty swallowing large capsules or an inability to administer medication when home anticoagulant therapy has been ordered parenterally?

Diagnosing for the Client Receiving Medications

5.3 Diagnosing occurs after an analysis of the assessment data and identifies the client's problems and needs in relation to drug administration. Nursing diagnoses are verified with the client or caregiver.

Assessment data are analyzed in order to identify patterns of problems, health and safety risks, related needs, and strengths. This process is referred to as diagnosing. The identified patterns are summarized in a list of nursing diagnoses. The nursing diagnoses are verified and prioritized in collaboration with the client. They are then used to set goals and plan care. This section discusses common nursing diagnoses related to medication administration, and the development of appropriate nursing diagnosis statements.

Diagnosing that focuses on drug administration is the same as for other client condition-specific responses. Nursing diagnoses may address actual problems, such as the treatment of pain; focus on potential problems, such as a risk for fluid volume imbalance; or concentrate on maintaining the client's current level of wellness. There are many problems and needs common to clients receiving medications. The nurse can manage some problems independently, whereas other problems are multidisciplinary and require collaboration with other members of the healthcare team. For any of the medications given to a client, there are often combinations of nursing-independent and collaborative diagnoses that can be established.

NCLEX Success Tip

The nurse can formulate nursing diagnoses only after completing the assessment or data collection step in the nursing process. Jumping to conclusions or making assumptions before analyzing essential assessment data and identifying specific signs/symptoms and probable cause could endanger the client and result in medication errors.

Two of the most common nursing diagnoses in medication administration are inadequate knowledge and nonadherence. Inadequate knowledge may occur because the client has been given a new prescription and has no previous experience with the medication. It may also occur when a client has not received adequate education about the drugs used in the treatment of his or her condition. When obtaining a medication history, the nurse should assess the client's knowledge of the drugs currently being taken and evaluate whether the drug education has been adequate. Sometimes a client refuses to take a drug that has been prescribed or refuses to follow the administration directions correctly. Non-adherence assumes that the client has been properly educated about the medication and has made an informed decision not to take it. Because labelling a client's response as non-compliant may have a negative impact on the nurse-client relationship, it is vital that the nurse assess all possible factors leading to the nonadherence *before* establishing this diagnosis. Does the client understand why the medication has been prescribed? Has dosing and scheduling information been explained? Are side effects causing the client to refuse the medication? Do social issues or cultural, religious, or health beliefs have an impact on the client taking the medication? Is the nonadherence related to inadequate resources, either financial or social? A thorough assessment of possible causes should be conducted before labelling the client's response as non-compliant.

Nursing diagnoses applicable to drug administration are often collaborative problems that require communication with other healthcare providers. For example, fluid volume deficit related to diuretic drugs may require additional interventions such as medical orders by the physician to ensure that electrolytes and intravascular fluid volume remain within normal limits. Independent of medical orders, nurses may assist the client with ambulation if weakness or postural hypotension occurs as a result of fluid volume deficit.

Setting Goals and Outcomes for Drug Administration

5.4 In planning, goals and outcomes are established from the nursing diagnoses. Goals focus on what the client should be able to achieve, and outcomes provide the specific, measurable criteria that will be used to measure goal attainment. Interventions are planned to meet the goals.

After the nurse has gathered client assessment data, identified patterns and needs, and established priorities, the goals and outcomes are developed to assist the nurse in planning care, carrying out interventions, and evaluating the effectiveness of that care. Before administering and monitoring the effects of medications, nurses should establish clear goals and outcomes so that planned interventions ensure safe and effective use of these agents.

Goals are somewhat different than outcomes. Goals focus on what the client should be able to achieve and do, based on the nursing diagnosis established from the assessment data. Outcomes provide the specific, measurable criteria that will be used to evaluate the degree to which the goal was met. For example, a goal may be that the client will learn to self-inject insulin. One outcome related to this goal may be that the client will demonstrate the correct technique for withdrawing insulin from a vial into a syringe without prompting. Both goals and outcomes are focused on what the client will achieve or do, are realistic, and are verified with the client or caregiver. Priorities are established based on the assessment data and nursing diagnoses, with high-priority needs addressed before low-priority items. Safe and effective administration of medications, with the best therapeutic outcome possible, is the overall goal of any nursing plan of care.

Goals may be focused on the short term or long term, depending on the setting and situation. In the acute care or ambulatory setting, short-term goals may be most appropriate, whereas in the rehabilitation setting, long-term goals may be more commonly identified. For a client with a thrombus in the lower extremity who has been placed on anticoagulant therapy, a short-term goal may be that the client will not experience an increase in clot size as evidenced by improving circulation to the lower extremity distal to the clot. A long-term goal might focus on teaching the client to effectively administer parenteral anticoagulant therapy at home. Like assessment data, goals should focus first on the therapeutic outcomes of medications, then on the limitation or treatment of side effects. For the client on pain medication, relief of pain is a priority established before treating the nausea, vomiting, or dizziness caused by the medication. The Nursing Process Focus flowcharts provided in Chapters 13 through 63 outline some of the common goals that might be developed with the client.

CONNECTIONS   **Special Considerations**

◀ Clients with Speaking, Visual, or Hearing Impairments

Speaking impairments may make obtaining responses from the client difficult. Communication may be facilitated by having the client write, demonstrate, or draw responses. Clarify by paraphrasing the response back to the client. Use gestures, body language, and yes or no questions if writing or drawing is difficult. Allow adequate time for responses. Be especially aware of nonverbal clues, such as grimacing, when performing interventions that may cause discomfort or pain.

Provide adequate lighting for clients with visual impairments and be aware of the phrasing of verbal communication and how phrasing affects the message conveyed. Remember that the nonverbal cues involved in communication may be missed by the client. Repeat and restate the client's responses to ensure that the message has been understood in the absence of nonverbal cues. Explain interventions in detail before implementing procedures or activities with the client.

Clients with hearing impairments benefit from communication that is spoken clearly and slowly in a low-pitched voice. Sit near the client and avoid speaking loudly or shouting, especially if hearing devices are used. Limit the amount of background noise when possible. Write or draw to clarify verbal communication and use nonverbal gestures and body language to aid communication. Allow adequate time for communication and responses. Alert other members of the healthcare team that the client has a hearing impairment and may not hear a verbal answer given over an intercom system after having pressed the call light.

Outcomes are the specific criteria used to measure attainment of the selected goals. They are written to include the subject (the client in most cases), the actions required by that subject, the circumstances under which the actions are to be carried out, the expected performance, and the specific time frame in which the performance will be accomplished. For the client who will be taught to self-administer anticoagulant therapy at home, an outcome may be written as follows: client will demonstrate the injection of enoxaparin (Lovenox) using the preloaded syringe provided, given subcutaneously into the anterior abdominal areas, in 2 days (1 day prior to discharge). This outcome includes the subject (client), actions (demonstrate the injection), circumstances (using a preloaded syringe), performance (subcutaneous injection into the abdomen), and time frame (2 days from now; 1 day before discharge home). Writing specific outcomes also gives the nurse a concrete time frame to work toward to assist the client to meet the goals.

After goals and outcomes are identified based on the nursing diagnoses, a plan of care is written. Each agency determines whether this plan will be communicated as nursing centred, interdisciplinary, or both. All plans should be client focused and verified with the client or caregiver. The goals and outcomes identified in the plan of care will assist the nurse, and other healthcare providers, in carrying out interventions and evaluating the effectiveness of that care.

Key Interventions for Drug Administration

5.5 Interventions are implemented in order to return the client to an optimum level of wellness. These include the safe and effective administration of medications. Key interventions required of the nurse include monitoring drug effects, documenting medications, promoting optimal responses to medications, preventing or limiting adverse effects, and client teaching.

After the plan of care has been written, explicitly stating any goals and outcomes based on established nursing diagnoses, the nurse implements this plan. Interventions are aimed at returning the client to an optimum level of wellness and limiting adverse effects related to the client's medical diagnosis or condition. The nurse plays a key role in promoting optimal responses to drugs and minimizing adverse effects. Chapter 9 discusses interventions specific to drug administration, such as the 10 rights of drug administration and the techniques of administering medications. This section focuses on other key intervention strategies that the nurse completes for a client receiving medications.

A thorough knowledge of pharmacokinetics and pharmacodynamics is essential for the safe and effective care of clients who are receiving medications. Not only medications, but almost every intervention that the nurse provides may influence biochemical and psychological responses in a client. For example, providing a warm blanket can affect endogenous stress hormone

levels differently than administering an intramuscular injection. This, in turn, can influence blood flow and other bodily processes that affect drug responses. Ways in which the nurse can influence pharmacokinetics through purposeful use of dietary modifications and other supportive therapies are presented in Chapter 3.

Monitoring drug effects is a primary intervention that nurses perform. A thorough knowledge of the actions of each medication is necessary to carry out this monitoring process. The nurse should first monitor for the identified therapeutic effect. A lack of sufficient therapeutic effect suggests the need to reassess pharmacotherapy and related interventions. Monitoring may require a reassessment of the client's physical condition, vital signs, body weight, laboratory values, and/or serum drug levels. The client's statements about pain relief, as well as objective data such as a change in blood pressure, are used to monitor the therapeutic outcomes of pharmacotherapy. The nurse also monitors for side and adverse effects and attempts to prevent or limit these effects when possible. Some side effects may be managed by the nurse independent of medical orders, whereas others require collaboration with physicians to alleviate client symptoms. For example, a client with nausea and vomiting after receiving a narcotic pain reliever may be comforted by the nurse, who provides small frequent meals, sips of carbonated beverages, or changes of linen. However, the physician may need to prescribe an antiemetic drug to control the side effect of intense nausea.

Documentation of both therapeutic and adverse effects is completed during the intervention phase. This includes appropriate documentation of the administration of the medication as well as the effects observed. Additional objective assessment data, such as vital signs, may be included in the documentation to provide more details about the specific drug effects. A client's statements can add subjective details to the documentation. Each healthcare facility determines where, when, and how to document the administration of medications and any follow-up assessment data that have been gathered. The nurse's role in reporting adverse drug reactions is presented in Chapter 8.

Client teaching is a vital component of the nurse's interventions for a client receiving medications. Knowledge deficit and even nonadherence are directly related to the type and quality of medication education that a client has received. Nurse practice standards and regulating bodies such as professional nursing associations consider teaching to be a primary role for nurses, giving it the weight of law and key importance in accreditation standards. Because the goal of pharmacotherapy is the safe administration of medications, with the best therapeutic outcomes possible, teaching is aimed at providing the client with the information necessary to ensure that this occurs. Every nurse-client interaction can present an opportunity for teaching. Small portions of education given over time are often more effective than large amounts of information given on only one occasion. Discussing medications each time they are administered is an effective way to increase the amount of education accomplished. Providing written material also assists the client to retain the information and review it later. Some medications come with a self-contained teaching program that includes videotapes. A word of caution on the use of audio and print material is necessary, however: The client must be able to read and understand the material provided. Pharmacies may dispense client education pamphlets that detail all of the effects of a medication and the monitoring required, but they are ineffective if the reading level is above what the client can understand or if they are in a language unfamiliar to the client. Having the client "teach" the nurse, or summarize key points after the teaching has been provided, is a safety check that may be used to verify that the client understands the information provided.

Elderly and pediatric clients often present special challenges to client teaching. Age-appropriate print or video materials and teaching that is repeated slowly and provided in small increments may assist the nurse in teaching these clients. It is often necessary to co-teach the client's caregiver.

NCLEX Success Tips

For questions about medication history, do not forget to ask about over-the-counter and herbal supplements in addition to prescription medications.

Double-check drug dosages and make sure the client's answers pass the common sense test (e.g., a subcutaneous dose should not be more than 1 mL for an adult).

Question any medication order that is not written clearly, is an unusual dose, or is not in keeping with treatment for the client's known health problems.

Accurately identify the client by asking him or her to state his or her name. If the client is nonverbal, the next best method is to check the client's administration bracelet. Be especially careful when there are two clients or more in a room. Use two unique identifiers as per agency policy.

If a client questions a medication or states that it is different from one taken at home, stop and recheck the medication order and the client history.

Table 5.2 summarizes key areas of teaching and provides sample questions the nurse might ask, or observations that can be made, to verify that teaching has been effective. The Nursing

Process Focus flowcharts in Chapters 13 through 63 also supply information on specific drugs and drug classes that is important to include in client teaching.

Evaluating the Effects of Drug Administration

5.6 Evaluating whether the medication is producing the desired effects is an important nursing responsibility. Evaluation begins a new cycle as new assessment data are gathered and analyzed, nursing diagnoses are reviewed, goals and outcomes are refined, and new interventions are carried out.

Evaluation is the final step of the nursing process. It considers the effectiveness of the interventions in meeting established goals and outcomes. The process comes full circle as the nurse reassesses the client, reviews the nursing diagnoses, makes necessary changes, reviews and rewrites goals and outcomes, and carries out further interventions to meet those goals and outcomes. When evaluating the effectiveness of drug administration, the nurse assesses for therapeutic effects and a minimal occurrence of side or adverse effects. For example, Advair Diskus is a combination of steroid and bronchodilator used in the treatment of chronic asthma and chronic obstructive airway disease. The medication is intended to be used daily. Evaluation of its effectiveness includes assessing improvement in respiratory status and in the client's ability to perform activities of daily living and quality of life activities such as walking and playing.

The nurse also evaluates the effectiveness of teaching provided and notes areas where further drug education is needed. Evaluation is not the end of the process, but the beginning of another cycle as the nurse continues to work to ensure safe and effective

TABLE 5.2 Important Areas of Teaching for Clients Receiving Medications	
Area of Teaching	**Important Questions and Observations**
Therapeutic use and outcomes	• Can you tell me the name of your medicine and what the medicine is used for? • What will you look for to know that the medication is effective? (How will you know that the medicine is working?)
Monitoring side and adverse effects	• Which side effects can you handle by yourself? (e.g., simple nausea, diarrhea) • Which side effects should you report to your healthcare provider? (e.g., extreme cases of nausea or vomiting, extreme dizziness, bleeding)
Medication administration	• Can you tell me how much of the medication you are to take? (mg, number of tablets, mL of liquid, etc.) • Can you tell me how often you are to take it? • What special requirements are necessary when you take this medication? (e.g., take with a full glass of water, take on an empty stomach and remain upright for 30 minutes) • Is there a specific order in which you are to take your medications? (e.g., bronchodilator before corticosteroid inhaler) • Can you show me how you will give yourself the medication? (e.g., eye drops, subcutaneous injections) • What special monitoring is required before you take this medication? (e.g., pulse rate) Can you demonstrate this for me? Based on that monitoring, when should you NOT take the medication? • Do you know how, or where, to store this medication? • What should you do if you miss a dose?
Other monitoring and special requirements	• Are there any special tests you should have related to this medication? (e.g., fingerstick glucose levels, therapeutic drug levels) • How often should these tests be done? • What other medications should you NOT take with this medication? • Are there any foods or beverages you must not have while taking this medication?

CONNECTIONS Cultural Considerations

◀ Non-English-Speaking and Culturally Diverse Clients

Nurses should know in advance what translation services and interpreters are available in their healthcare facility to assist with communication. The nurse should use an interpreter's services when available, validating with the interpreter that he or she is able to understand the client. Many dialects are similar but not the same, and knowing another language is not the same as understanding the culture. Can the interpreter understand the client's language and cultural expressions or nuances well enough for effective communication to occur? If a family member is interpreting, especially if a child is interpreting for a parent or relative, the nurse should ensure that the interpreter first understands and repeats the information back to the nurse before explaining it to the client in the client's own language. This is especially important if

the interpretation is a summary of what has been said rather than a line-by-line interpretation. Before an interpreter is available, or if one is unavailable, use pictures, simple drawings, nonverbal cues, and body language to communicate with the client.

In some cultures, time may not be important and compliance with dosage schedules may require greater emphasis. Be aware of culturally based nonverbal communication behaviours (e.g., use of personal space, eye contact, or lack of eye contact). Gender sensitivities related to culture (e.g., male nurse or physician for female clients) and the use of touch are often important issues. In Western cultures, an informal and personal style is often the norm. When working with older clients and clients of other cultures, adopting a more formal style may be more appropriate.

medication use and active client involvement in his or her care. It is a checkpoint at which the nurse considers the overall goal of safe and effective administration of medications, with the best therapeutic outcome possible, and takes the steps necessary to ensure success. The nursing process acts as the overall framework to work toward this success.

NCLEX Success Tip

Students can use the nursing process as a guide or map while answering NCLEX questions. For example, assessment is a step prior to intervention, so if the stem of the question is about assessment, any distractor that focuses on planning, diagnosing, or intervention can be eliminated.

CHAPTER 5

Understanding the Chapter

Key Concepts Summary

The numbered key concepts provide a succinct summary of the important points from the corresponding numbered section within the chapter. If any of these points are not clear, refer to the numbered section within the chapter for review.

5.1 The nursing process is a systematic method of problem solving and consists of clearly defined steps: assessing; diagnosing client problems, strengths, and needs; planning care through the formulation of goals and outcomes; implementing interventions; and evaluating the care provided.

5.2 Assessing the client who is receiving medications includes obtaining health history information, physical assessment data, laboratory values, and other measurable data and assessing medication effects, both therapeutic and side effects. It also includes assessment of the medication ordered in relation to the client's medical condition, culture, ethnicity, gender, age, and other factors.

5.3 Diagnosing occurs after an analysis of the assessment data and identifies the client's problems and needs in

relation to drug administration. Nursing diagnoses are verified with the client or caregiver.

5.4 In planning, goals and outcomes are established from the nursing diagnoses. Goals focus on what the client should be able to achieve, and outcomes provide the specific, measurable criteria that will be used to measure goal attainment. Interventions are planned to meet the goals.

5.5 Interventions are implemented in order to return the client to an optimum level of wellness. These include the safe and effective administration of medications. Key interventions required of the nurse include monitoring drug effects, documenting medications, promoting optimal responses to medications, preventing or limiting adverse effects, and client teaching.

5.6 Evaluating whether the medication is producing the desired effects is an important nursing responsibility. Evaluation begins a new cycle as new assessment data are gathered and analyzed, nursing diagnoses are reviewed, goals and outcomes are refined, and new interventions are carried out.

Critical Thinking Questions

1 A 13-year-old client who is a cheerleader and from a rural community has been diagnosed with type 1 diabetes. She is supported by a single mother who is frustrated with her daughter's eating habits. The client has lost weight since beginning her insulin regimen. The nurse notes that the client and her mother, who is very well dressed, are both extremely thin. Identify additional data that the nurse would need to obtain before making the nursing diagnosis of nonadherence.

2 Regarding the client in Question 1, her drug regimen is evaluated and the healthcare provider suggests a subcutaneous insulin pump to help control the client's fluctuating blood glucose levels. Identify three client needs related to this new therapy.

3 A nursing student is assigned to a licensed preceptor who is administering oral medications. The student notes that the preceptor administers the drugs safely but routinely fails to offer the client information about the drug being administered. Discuss this action in relation to the concept of safe drug administration.

See Answers to Critical Thinking Questions in Appendix B.

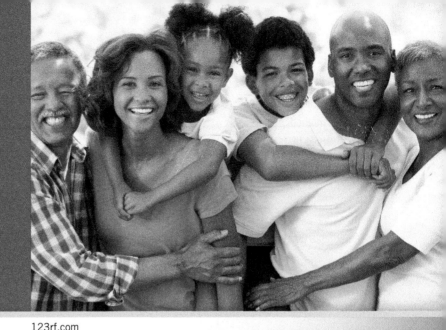
123rf.com

CHAPTER

6

Lifespan Considerations in Pharmacotherapy

LEARNING OUTCOMES

After reading this chapter, the student should be able to:

1. Discuss the basic concepts of human growth and development in relation to pharmacotherapeutics.

2. Explain how physical, cognitive, and psychomotor development influence pharmacotherapeutics.

3. Match the six pregnancy categories with their definitions.

4. Describe physiological changes during pregnancy that may affect the absorption, distribution, metabolism, and excretion of drugs.

5. Identify factors that influence the transfer of drugs into breast milk.

6. Outline important points in client and family education regarding drug use during pregnancy and lactation.

7. Identify the importance of teaching the breastfeeding mother about prescription and over-the-counter (OTC) drugs, as well as the use of herbal products.

8. Describe physiological and biochemical changes that occur in the older adult, and how these affect pharmacotherapy.

9. Discuss the nursing and pharmacological implications associated with each of the following developmental age groups: prenatal, infancy, toddlerhood, preschool, school age, adolescence, young adulthood, middle adulthood, and older adulthood.

CHAPTER OUTLINE

▶ Pharmacotherapy Across the Lifespan

▶ Pharmacotherapy During Pregnancy and Lactation

  ▶ Pharmacotherapy During Pregnancy

  ▶ Pharmacokinetics During Pregnancy

  ▶ Gestational Age and Pharmacotherapy

  ▶ Pregnancy Drug Categories

  ▶ Pharmacotherapy During Lactation

▶ Pharmacotherapy During Childhood

  ▶ Pharmacotherapy in the Pediatric Population

  ▶ Medication Safety for Pediatric Clients

  ▶ Calculating Drug Dosages for the Pediatric Client

  ▶ Adverse Drug Reactions in Children and Promoting Adherence

  ▶ Pharmacotherapy of Toddlers

Beginning with conception and continuing throughout the lifespan, the organs and systems within the body undergo predictable physiological alterations that influence the absorption, metabolism, distribution, and elimination of medications. Nurses must have knowledge of such changes to ensure that drugs are delivered in a safe and effective manner to clients of all ages. The purpose of this chapter is to examine how principles of developmental physiology and lifespan psychology apply to pharmacotherapeutics.

Pharmacotherapy Across the Lifespan

6.1 To contribute to safe and effective pharmacotherapy, it is essential for the nurse to comprehend and apply fundamental concepts of growth and development.

To collaborate effectively with the client, healthcare providers must consider the biophysical, psychosocial, ethnocultural, and spiritual characteristics that are unique to the client. To provide holistic and individualized care for the person receiving pharmacotherapy, nurses must understand *normal* growth and developmental patterns that occur throughout the lifespan. Growth characterizes the progressive increase in physical (body) size. Development refers to the functional evolution of the physical, psychomotor, and cognitive capabilities of a living being. It is from this benchmark that *deviations* from the norm can be recognized so that health pattern impairments can be addressed appropriately. The very nature of pharmacology requires that the specifics of age, growth, and development for each client be considered in relation to pharmacokinetics and pharmacodynamics.

PHARMACOTHERAPY DURING PREGNANCY AND LACTATION

The nurse caring for the pregnant or lactating woman faces the challenge of concurrently being responsible for the health and safety of two persons, knowing that most medications cross the placenta and are secreted in breast milk. Despite potential risks to the fetus, first-trimester use of prescription drugs has increased by more than 60% in the past 30 years (Mitchell et al., 2011). With the availability of the Internet, women may choose to search for drug information online, but Peters et al. (2013) found that even lists of "safe" drugs found in web-based information were inadequate and might provide false reassurance to women about the adverse effects posed by drugs taken during pregnancy.

The decision to initiate pharmacotherapy during pregnancy and lactation is made in collaboration with the pregnant client, with consideration of the risks and benefits for her and her fetus. Most drugs have not been tested in pregnant women and infants. When possible, drug therapy is postponed until after pregnancy and lactation, or safer alternatives are attempted. There are some conditions, however, that are severe enough to require pharmacotherapy in pregnant and lactating clients. These conditions include pre-existing illness, maternal illness unrelated to the pregnancy, and complications related to pregnancy. For example, if the client has epilepsy, hypertension, or a psychiatric disorder prior to the pregnancy, it could be unwise to discontinue therapy during pregnancy or lactation. Conditions such as gestational diabetes and gestational hypertension occur during pregnancy and must be treated for the safety of the growing fetus. In all cases, healthcare practitioners evaluate the therapeutic benefits of a given medication against its potential adverse effects and support the woman who may feel guilty for taking medically necessary drugs during pregnancy.

NCLEX Success Tips

During pregnancy, calorie needs increase by about 300 Cal/day; during lactation, they increase by 500 Cal/day.

The intake of a balanced diet is important for avoiding protein deficiency, which can alter drug distribution.

Adequate intake of folic acid is important for preventing neural tube defects.

Clients should avoid consuming non-nutritive substances (pica) that would replace essential nutrients and/or interfere with the absorption of supplemental vitamins during pregnancy.

Pharmacotherapy During Pregnancy

6.2 Pharmacotherapy during pregnancy should be conducted only when the benefits to the mother outweigh the potential risks to the unborn child.

The placenta is a semipermeable membrane through which some substances are passed to the fetus and by which others are blocked. The fetal membranes contain enzymes that detoxify certain substances as they cross the membrane. For example, insulin from the mother is inactivated by placental enzymes during the early stages of pregnancy, preventing it from reaching the fetus. In general, drugs that are water soluble, ionized, or bound to plasma proteins are less likely to cross the placenta.

NCLEX Success Tips

Chronically malnourished clients are at higher risk of drug toxicity due to decreased albumin (protein) levels. Having decreased albumin levels means that more free (active) drug is available in the blood. Liver disease can also influence protein levels and put clients at risk for drug toxicity or exaggerated action. Medications that are highly protein-bound are generally safe during pregnancy.

Constipation as a result of iron intake can be corrected by natural laxatives such as prunes and water rather than by medications that may be teratogenic.

Do not use agonist-antagonists for women with opioid dependence because antagonist activity could precipitate withdrawal (abstinence) symptoms in the mother and the neonate (irritability, hyperactive reflexes, tremors, seizures, yawning, sneezing, vomiting and diarrhea, and excessive crying by the neonate).

Pharmacokinetics During Pregnancy

6.3 During pregnancy, major physiological and anatomical changes occur that can alter the pharmacokinetics and pharmacodynamics of administered drugs.

During pregnancy, major physiological and anatomical changes occur in the endocrine, gastrointestinal (GI), cardiovascular, circulatory, and renal systems. Some of these changes alter the pharmacodynamics of drugs administered to the client and may affect the success of pharmacotherapy, as follows:

- Absorption: Hormonal changes as well as the pressure of the expanding uterus on the blood supply to abdominal organs affect the absorption of drugs. Gastric emptying is delayed, and transit time for food and drugs in the GI tract is slowed by progesterone, which allows a longer time for absorption of oral drugs. Gastric acidity is also decreased, which can affect the absorption of certain drugs. Changes in the respiratory system during pregnancy—increased tidal volume and pulmonary vasodilation—may cause inhaled drugs to be absorbed more quickly.

- Distribution and metabolism: Hemodynamic changes in the pregnant client increase cardiac output and plasma volume and change regional blood flow. The increased blood volume (up to 50%) in the woman's body causes dilution of drugs and decreases plasma protein concentrations, affecting drug distribution. Blood flow to the uterus, kidneys, and skin is increased, whereas flow to the skeletal muscles is diminished. Alterations in lipid levels may alter drug transport and distribution, especially during the third trimester. Drug metabolism is significantly altered during pregnancy (Isoherranen & Thummel, 2013) and increases for certain drugs, most notably anticonvulsants such as carbamazepine (Tegretol), phenytoin (Dilantin),

and valproic acid (Depakene, Epival), which may require higher doses during pregnancy.

- Excretion: By the third trimester of pregnancy, blood flow through the kidneys increases by 50% to 70%. This increase has a direct effect on renal plasma flow, glomerular filtration rate, and renal tubular absorption. Therefore, drug excretion rates may be increased, affecting dosage timing and onset of action.

Gestational Age and Pharmacotherapy

6.4 Gestational age must be considered when prescribing drugs to pregnant clients.

The **prenatal** stage is the time span from conception to birth. This stage is subdivided into the embryonic period (conception to 8 weeks) and the fetal period (8 to 40 weeks or birth). In terms of pharmacotherapy, this is a strategic stage because the health and welfare of both the pregnant client and the baby in utero are taken into consideration (Figure 6.1). Pharmacologically, the focus must be to eliminate potentially toxic agents that may harm the mother or unborn child. Agents that cause fetal malformations are termed **teratogens**. The baseline incidence of fetal malformations is approximately 3% of all pregnancies. Although causes of fetal malformations are difficult to confirm, Health Canada estimates that chemical and drug exposure, including alcohol and tobacco use, accounts for about 10% to 12% of these malformations.

NCLEX Success Tip

The nurse should remind the client that raw fish, including tuna, should be avoided during pregnancy due to the risk of the fish being contaminated with mercury and other potential teratogens.

The **placenta** is a temporary organ that allows for nutrition and gas exchange between the mother and the fetus. As much as 10% of the mother's cardiac output circulates through the placenta. Although the blood of the mother does not circulate through the fetus, capillary-like structures in the placenta allow an extensive exchange of substances. The placenta offers a degree of protective filtration of the maternal blood, preventing certain harmful substances from

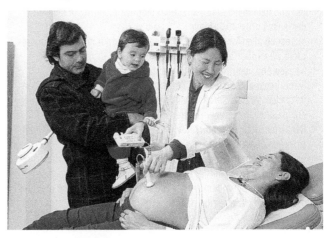

Figure 6.1 Pharmacotherapy of the pregnant client.
Source: © Jenny Thomas Photography.

reaching the fetus. Nutritional substances such as vitamins, fatty acids, glucose, and electrolytes freely pass from mother to fetus.

Most drugs cross the placenta and pass from mother to fetus by simple diffusion. A few drugs cross by way of active transport. The role the placenta plays in drug metabolism is under study. It is known that metabolic enzymes are present in the placenta and likely contribute to drug metabolism. What is not known with certainty is how a particular drug is metabolized through the placenta. Some drugs may be metabolized extensively and presumably have little or no effect on the developing fetus, whereas other drugs may be altered to become toxic metabolites capable of harm. It should be understood that drugs may cause fetal harm without crossing the placenta or entering the fetal blood. For example, certain drugs may cause constriction of placental blood vessels, impairing nutrient exchange. Other drugs can alter maternal physiology to such an extent that the fetus is affected.

Multiple factors affect the transfer of drugs across the placenta. These variables are the same as those that affect the movement of substances across other biological membranes, and they include:

- The plasma drug level in the mother
- Lipid solubility characteristic of the drug
- The drug's molecular size
- Drug protein binding capability
- Drug ionization
- Blood flow to the placenta

During the first trimester (conception to 3 months) of pregnancy, when the skeleton and major organs begin to develop, the fetus is at greatest risk for developmental anomalies. If teratogenic drugs are used by the mother, major fetal malformations may occur, or the drug may even precipitate a spontaneous abortion. Unfortunately, accidental exposure can occur because the mother may take a medication before she knows she is pregnant. Whenever possible, drug therapy should be delayed until after the first trimester of pregnancy.

CONNECTIONS Special Considerations

◀ **Altered Pharmacokinetics During Pregnancy**

- Increased progesterone levels can lead to delayed gastric emptying and decreased small intestinal motility, resulting in delayed or decreased drug *absorption*.
- Increased alveolar ventilation and cardiac output may lead to more rapid *absorption* of intramuscular and inhaled drugs.
- Nausea and vomiting may prevent drug *absorption*.
- Some hepatic enzymes are induced during pregnancy, resulting in increased *metabolism* of some drugs, whereas other hepatic enzymes are inhibited, resulting in decreased *metabolism* of other drugs.
- Renal blood flow is markedly increased, resulting in more rapid *excretion* of many drugs.
- Increased maternal blood volume may cause a decrease in serum concentration of the drug, thus decreasing *distribution*.
- Decreased serum albumin and protein levels may decrease plasma protein binding of some drugs, resulting in more free drug and increased drug *distribution*.

Based on Gibson, P. (2003). Baby safe: Which drugs are safe during pregnancy? *Canadian Journal of CME, 15*, 67–76.

During the second trimester (4 to 6 months) of pregnancy, the development of the major organs has progressed considerably; however, exposure to certain substances taken by the mother can still cause considerable harm to the fetus. The nurse-client relationship is vital during this time, especially in terms of teaching. A woman who is pregnant can mistakenly believe that her unborn infant is safe from anything she consumes because the "infant is fully formed and just needs time to grow." During prenatal visits, the nurse must be vigilant in assessing and evaluating each client so that any mistaken beliefs can be clarified.

During the third trimester (7 to 9 months) of pregnancy, blood flow to the placenta increases and placental vascular membranes become thinner. Such alterations allow the transfer of more substances from the maternal circulation to the fetal blood. As a result, the fetus will receive larger doses of medications and other substances taken by the mother. Because the fetus lacks mature metabolic enzymes and efficient excretion mechanisms, medications will have a prolonged duration of action in the unborn child.

Pregnancy Drug Categories

6.5 Pregnancy drug categories guide the healthcare provider in prescribing drugs for pregnant clients.

Health Canada uses the drug pregnancy categories developed by the United States Food and Drug Administration (FDA) to rate medications as to their risks during pregnancy. Table 6.1 shows the six pregnancy categories, which guide the healthcare team and the client in selecting drugs that are the least hazardous for the fetus. Nurses who routinely work with women who are pregnant must learn the pregnancy categories for medications commonly prescribed for their clients. Examples of category D or X drugs that have been associated with teratogenic effects include testosterone, estrogens, ergotamine (Ergomar), all angiotensin-converting enzyme (ACE) inhibitors, methotrexate, thalidomide (Thalomid), tetracycline, valproic acid, and warfarin (Coumadin). In addition, alcohol, nicotine, and illicit drugs such as cocaine also affect the unborn child.

A teratogen is any substance, organism, or physical agent that interferes with growth or development of the embryo or fetus and produces a permanent abnormality or death. Potential fetal consequences of drug use include intrauterine fetal death, physical malformations, growth impairment, behavioural abnormalities, and neonatal toxicity.

NCLEX Success Tips

Consumption of any amount or type of alcohol isn't recommended during pregnancy because it increases the risk of fetal alcohol syndrome or fetal alcohol effect.

Pregnant moms should engage in low-impact aerobics during pregnancy.

Eating frequent, small meals will help the client maintain her energy level by keeping her blood glucose level relatively constant.

Taking a multivitamin supplement daily and eating a balanced diet are recommended during pregnancy.

Folic acid supplementation is recommended to prevent neural tube defects and anemia in pregnancy. Deficiencies increase the risk of hemorrhage during delivery and of infection.

The recommended dose prior to pregnancy is 400 mcg/day; during pregnancy and breastfeeding, the recommended dose is 600 to 800 mcg/day.

TABLE 6.1 FDA Pregnancy Categories

Category	Definition
A	Adequate, well-controlled studies in pregnant women have not shown an increased risk of fetal abnormalities. Example drugs: levothyroxine and folic acid
B	Animal studies have revealed no evidence of harm to the fetus; however, there are no adequate, well-controlled studies in pregnant women. or Animal studies have shown an adverse effect, but adequate, well-controlled studies in pregnant women have failed to demonstrate a risk to the fetus. Example drugs: metformin and pantoprazole
C	Animal studies have shown an adverse effect and there are no adequate, well-controlled studies in pregnant women. or No animal studies have been conducted and there are no adequate, well-controlled studies in pregnant women. Example drugs: gabapentin and prednisone
D	Studies, adequate, well controlled, or observational, in pregnant women have demonstrated a risk to the fetus; however, the benefits of therapy may outweigh the potential risk. Example drugs: lisinopril and lorazepam
X	Studies, adequate, well controlled, or observational, in animals or pregnant women have demonstrated positive evidence of fetal abnormalities. The use of the product is contraindicated in women who are or may become pregnant. Example drugs: atorvastatin and warfarin
N	FDA has not yet classified the drug. Example drugs: aspirin and acetaminophen

U.S. Food and Drug Administration, 2015. United States Department of Health and Human Services

It is impossible to experimentally test drugs for teratogenicity in human subjects during clinical trials. Although drugs are tested in pregnant laboratory animals, the structure of the human placenta is unique. Drug pregnancy categories are extrapolated from these animal data and may be crude approximations of the actual risk to a human fetus. The actual risk to a human fetus may be much less, or magnitudes greater, than that predicted from animal data. No prescription drug, over-the-counter (OTC) medication, or herbal product should be taken during pregnancy unless the physician verifies that the therapeutic benefits to the mother clearly outweigh the potential risks to the fetus.

The current A, B, C, D, X, and N pregnancy labelling system is simplistic and gives no specific clinical information to help guide nurses or their clients as to whether a medication is truly safe. The system does not indicate how the dose should be adjusted during pregnancy or lactation. Most drugs are category C, as very high doses often produce teratogenic effects in animals. The FDA is in the process of updating these categories to provide more descriptive information on the risks and benefits of taking each medication. The new labels are expected to include pharmacokinetic and pharmacodynamic information that will suggest optimum doses for the childbearing client. To gather this information, the FDA is encouraging all pregnant women who are taking medication to join a pregnancy registry that will survey drug effects on both the

client and the fetus or newborn. Evaluation of a large number of pregnancies is needed to determine the effects of a medication on the fetus.

Pharmacotherapy During Lactation

6.6 Breastfeeding clients must be aware that drugs and other substances can appear in milk and affect the infant.

Breastfeeding is highly recommended as a means of providing nutrition, emotional bonding, and immune protection to the neonate. Many drugs, however, are able to enter breast milk in small amounts, and a few have been shown to be harmful. As with the placenta, drugs that are ionized, water soluble, or bound to plasma proteins are less likely to enter breast milk. Central nervous system (CNS) medications are very lipid soluble and thus are more likely to be present in higher concentrations in milk and can be expected to have a greater effect on an infant. Although concentrations of CNS drugs in breast milk are found in higher amounts, they often remain at subclinical levels. Regarding the role of protein binding, drugs that remain in the maternal plasma bound to albumin are not able to penetrate the mother's milk supply. For example, warfarin is strongly bound to plasma proteins and thus has a low level in breast milk.

It is important for the nurse to understand factors that influence the amount of drug secreted into breast milk. This allows the nurse to aid the client in making responsible choices regarding lactation and in reducing exposure of her newborn to potentially harmful substances. The amount of drug that passes to the infant during lactation depends on multiple factors:

- **Plasma drug level in the mother.** The higher the dose of drug taken by the mother, the more will be secreted into breast milk. It is therefore standard practice that if a drug must be prescribed for a lactating client, the lowest effective dose should be ordered.

- **Solubility of the drug.** Highly lipid-soluble drugs enter the milk at higher concentrations. Drugs that act on the CNS are usually lipophilic and have a tendency to penetrate milk at higher concentrations.

- **Molecular size and protein binding.** Some drugs, such as heparin and insulin, are simply too large to pass through membranes by passive diffusion. In addition, when drugs are highly protein bound, they are less likely to enter the milk than those that are free.

- **Drug ionization.** Milk is slightly more acidic than plasma; the pH of milk is 7.2 and of plasma is 7.4. This pH gradient allows weakly basic drugs to transfer more readily into breast milk and accumulate due to ion trapping.

- **Drug half-life.** Drugs with short half-lives will be metabolized and eliminated quickly by the mother. This results in smaller amounts being secreted into breast milk.

It is imperative to teach the mother that many prescription medications, OTC drugs, and herbal products may be excreted in breast milk and have the potential to affect her child (Figure 6.2).

The same guidelines for drug use apply during the breastfeeding period as during pregnancy: drugs should be taken only if the benefits to the mother clearly outweigh the potential risks to the infant. The nurse should explore the possibility of postponing pharmacotherapy until the baby is weaned or perhaps selecting a safer, non-pharmacological alternative therapy. If a drug is indicated, it is sometimes useful to administer it immediately after breastfeeding, or when the infant will be sleeping for an extended period, so that the longest possible time elapses before the next feeding. This will reduce the amount of active drug in the mother's milk when she does breastfeed her infant. The nurse can assist the mother in protecting the child's safety by teaching her to avoid illicit drugs, alcohol, and tobacco products during breastfeeding. Also, the mother should be advised to consult a healthcare provider before taking any OTC drugs or herbal products.

When considering the effects of drugs on the breastfeeding infant, the amount of drug that actually reaches the infant's tissues must be considered. Some medications are destroyed in the infant's GI system, are unable to be absorbed through the wall of the GI tract, or are rapidly metabolized by the liver. Therefore, although many drugs are found in breast milk, some are present in such small amounts that they cause no harm.

The last key factor in the effect of drugs on the infant relates to the infant's ability to metabolize small amounts of drugs. Premature, neonatal, and ill infants may be at greater risk for adverse effects because they lack drug metabolizing enzymes.

Health Canada's Food and Nutrition Branch provides guidance on which drugs should be avoided during breastfeeding to protect the infant's safety. Medications that pass into breast milk are indicated in drug guides. Nurses who work with women who are pregnant or breastfeeding should refer to this information. Table 6.2 shows selected drugs that are compatible with breastfeeding and those that should be avoided. Table 6.3 lists classes of medications that may cause serious problems in a baby after breastfeeding.

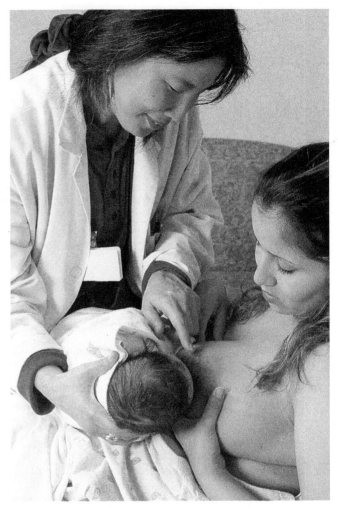

Figure 6.2   Pharmacotherapy of the breastfeeding client.
Source: © Jenny Thomas Photography.

TABLE 6.2   Selected Drugs Compatible with Breastfeeding

Class	Compatible Drugs	Drugs to Be Avoided
Analgesics (opioids)	Codeine and morphine in occasional doses	—
Analgesics (nonopioid)	Acetaminophen, aspirin, ibuprofen	—
Anti-infectives	Penicillins, trimethoprim, sulfisoxazole (over 1 month of age), macrolides, aminoglycosides, cephalosporins, isoniazid, fluconazole, acyclovir	Chloramphenicol, ciprofloxacin, tetracyclines, metronidazole
Antimigraine agents	Propranolol	Ergotamine
Antiseizure agents	Carbamazepine, diazepam (single dose), valproic acid, phenytoin	Ethosuximide
Cardiovascular agents	Iron salts, heparin, warfarin, verapamil, lidocaine, digoxin, prazosin, nifedipine, spironolactone, furosemide	Atenolol, ACE inhibitors, statins, hydrochlorothiazide
Central nervous system agents	Tricyclic antidepressants	Lithium carbonate
Cytotoxic agents and immunosuppressants	—	All drugs in this class should be avoided
Gastrointestinal agents	Aluminum hydroxide, magnesium hydroxide, promethazine (single dose)	Cimetidine, metoclopramide
Hormones	Prednisone, hydrocortisone (single dose), insulin, thyroid hormone, oxytocin (short term)	Oral contraceptives, estrogens, testosterone

Based on "Breastfeeding and Maternal Medication: Recommendations for Drugs in the Eleventh WHO Model List of Essential Drugs."
Copyright © 2002 World Health Organization. Retrieved from http://whqlibdoc.who.int/hq/2002/55732.pdf

TABLE 6.3 Classes of Medications That May Cause Serious Effects in a Baby Following Breastfeeding

Drug Class	Potential Adverse Effect
Antiepileptics (e.g. phenobarbitol, ethosuximide)	Sedation
Antineoplastics	Neutropenia
Beta-blockers	Lethargy, cyanosis, and bradycardia
Benzodiazepines	Sedation and weight loss
Ergot alkaloids	Vomiting and diarrhea
NSAIDs	Increased bleeding
Opioids	Sedation and withdrawal symptoms
Phenothiazines	Sedation
Pseudoephedrine	Inhibition of milk production

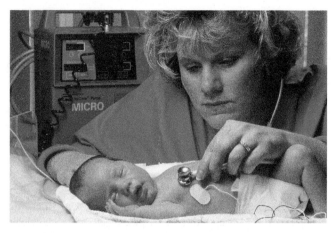

Figure 6.3 Pharmacotherapy of the infant.
Source: PearsonEducation/PH College.

NCLEX Success Tips

Neonates of women who smoked during pregnancy are small for their gestational age for two reasons: first, nicotine causes vasoconstriction, which reduces blood flow and, thus, nutrient transfer to the fetus; and second, smokers are at greater risk of poor nutrition.

Ask pregnant mothers to completely abstain from alcohol during pregnancy because a safe level of alcohol consumption during pregnancy has not yet been established. There is a lack of conclusive evidence surrounding the effects on the fetus of either social or moderate drinking.

PHARMACOTHERAPY DURING CHILDHOOD

Pharmacotherapy in the Pediatric Population

6.7 During infancy, pharmacotherapy is directed toward the safety of the child and teaching the parents how to properly administer medications and care for the infant.

Infancy is the period from birth to 12 months of age. During this time, nursing care and pharmacotherapy are directed toward safety of the infant, proper dosing of prescribed drugs, and teaching parents how to administer medications properly.

When an infant is ill, it is sometimes traumatic for the parents. By having knowledge of growth and development, the nurse can assist the parents in caring for the infant (Figure 6.3). The nurse should assess the infant's normal routines at home and attempt to follow these routines as closely as possible while the infant is hospitalized. Parents should be kept informed of specific orders for the infant, such as fluid restrictions. Encourage the parents to participate in the care of the infant as much as they are able. Medications administered at home to infants are often given via droppers into the eyes, ears, nose, or mouth. Infants with well-developed sucking reflexes may be willing to ingest oral drugs with a pleasant taste through a bottle nipple. Infant drops are given by placing the drops in the buccal pouch for the infant to swallow. Oral medications should be administered slowly to avoid aspiration. If rectal suppositories are administered,

the buttocks should be held together for 5 to 10 minutes to prevent expulsion of the drug before absorption has occurred.

Special considerations must be observed when administering intramuscular (IM) or intravenous (IV) injections to infants. Unlike adults, infants lack well-developed muscle masses, so the smallest needle appropriate for the drug—preferably a 1 cm (3/8-inch) needle—should be used. The vastus lateralis is the preferred site for IM injections because it has few nerves and is relatively well developed in infants. The gluteal site is usually contraindicated because of potential damage to the sciatic nerve, which may result in permanent disability. Because of the lack of choices for injection sites, the nurse must take care not to overuse a particular location, as inflammation and excessive pain may result. For IV sites, the feet and scalp often provide good venous access. After gaining IV access, it is important that the IV remain secured so that the infant does not dislodge it. It is also important to check the IV site frequently and assess for signs of inflammation or infiltration.

Medications for infants are often prescribed in milligrams per kilogram per day (mg/kg/24h) rather than according to the infant's age in weeks or months. An alternate method of calculating doses is to use the infant's body surface area (BSA). Because the liver and kidneys of infants are immature, drugs will have a greater impact due to their prolonged duration of action. For these reasons, it is important to consider age and size in determining safe dosages of medications for infants.

From early infancy, the natural immunity a child receives from the mother in utero slowly begins to decline. The child's developing immune system must then take over. Childhood diseases that were once damaging or fatal can now be controlled through routine immunizations. The nurse plays a key role in educating parents about the importance of keeping their child's immunizations current. Vaccinations are discussed in Chapter 41.

NCLEX Success Tips

The nurse should keep in mind that dosages of medications for infants are calculated according to infant weight. Note that an infant's weight doubles in the first 6 months and triples by 12 months.

Avoid giving infants cow's milk during the first year because it is deficient in essential fatty acids, iron, zinc, vitamin E, and vitamin C and ingestion in the first year could lead to anemia and, possibly, intestinal bleeding.

Medication Safety for Pediatric Clients

6.8 The nurse is a key member of the healthcare team in ensuring medication safety in pediatric clients.

The nurse is often responsible for administering medications to children. The importance of accurate drug dosage calculations, proper administration techniques, proper efforts to minimize adverse effects, and the need for overall safety cannot be overemphasized.

Principles of safe medication practice for pediatric clients are identical to those of adult clients. Medication safety is a team approach. Every level of responsibility is involved, including hospital-wide policies, prescriber actions, pharmacy guidelines, nursing interventions, and client and family adherence. Responsibility for preventing medication errors in pediatric clients is shared by every member of the team.

The safety and effectiveness of a medication regimen depends on proper procurement, storage, and administration of the drug. In the hospital setting, nurses are responsible for adherence to the basic rules of drug administration: right client, right drug, right route, right dose, at the right time. Younger pediatric clients may not be able to accurately identify themselves; therefore, it is imperative that the nurse use precautions to ensure that the right child receives the prescribed medication. The nurse must check the child's identification band against the medication record. Most hospitals' policies require that drugs such as digoxin (Lanoxin, Toloxin), heparin, insulin, chemotherapeutic agents, opioid analgesics, and barbiturates be double-checked with another nurse prior to administration. If the nurse suspects that a dose of medication ordered by the prescriber is outside the normal range, it is the nurse's responsibility to question the order because some drugs can be lethal to pediatric clients. The nurse should regularly check reputable online drug information sources for the most recent information on pediatric drugs and their adverse effects and can consult with the pharmacist as an additional resource.

Nursing Actions and Guidelines

- Check medication calculations with another professional member of the healthcare team.
- Confirm client identity before administration of each dose.
- Be familiar with medication ordering and dispensing systems.
- Verify drug orders before medication administration.
- Verify unusually large or small volumes or dosage units for a single client dose.
- When a client, parent, or caregiver questions whether a drug should be administered, listen attentively, answer questions, and double-check the medication order.
- Remain familiar with the operation of medication administration devices and the potential for errors with such devices, particularly patient-controlled analgesia (PCA) or infusion pumps.

Nursing Education and Communication

- Develop and maintain continuous education programs for nursing competencies in devices used for pediatric medication administration, particularly PCA and infusion pumps.
- Develop and maintain a pediatric medications knowledge base.
- Discuss medication orders with the prescriber whenever possible.
- Integrate and provide education for the client and caregiver regarding the medication regimen.
- Record and verify client identity, weight, allergies, and previous medication use.
- Be aware of and be involved in ongoing error-tracking systems and pharmacy programs. Encourage blame-free error reporting. Ensure that all staff members understand the method of reporting and are knowledgeable about the healthcare agency's system for reporting errors.

Calculating Drug Dosages for the Pediatric Client

6.9 The nurse must be accurate when calculating drug dosages for pediatric clients.

Nurses must consistently update their skills in calculating pediatric doses because errors in drug administration may have serious consequences. Drug dosage calculation for pediatric clients should be individualized, and nurses should take into consideration the child's age, height, weight, maturational state, and body surface area. All drug calculations for pediatric clients in critical care settings should be double-checked by the pharmacist and another nurse prior to administration.

Two common procedures for calculating pediatric dosages are the body weight method and the body surface area method. Use of the **body weight method** requires a calculation of the number of milligrams of drug, based on the child's weight in kilograms (mg/kg). A unit of time is usually included; for example, gentamicin (Garamycin) 5 mg/kg/24h. The body weight method is simple, and a dose can be calculated quickly. However, the serum concentrations of many drugs are not proportional to body weight, and body weight does not take into consideration pharmacokinetic variables such as changes in metabolism and elimination rates, as discussed in Chapter 3.

The **body surface area (BSA) method** uses an estimate of the child's BSA. This method is believed to be the most valid basis for dosage because it is related to certain physiological functions that account for the pharmacokinetic differences in pediatric clients. The BSA method better estimates blood volume, metabolism, and the effects of drugs. Measurements of the fluid volume compartment and the serum concentrations of drugs also correlate well with the BSA.

Using the BSA method, the child's height and weight are plotted on a **nomogram** (Figure 6.4), and a line is drawn between the two points. The point at which the line intersects the surface area (SA) line is the child's BSA. The dose is calculated as BSA ÷ 1.73 × Adult dose × Pediatric dose.

Other methods, including electronic calculators, are used to estimate pediatric doses. Each method has specific advantages and disadvantages. The student should refer to a medication mathematics text for practice calculation examples.

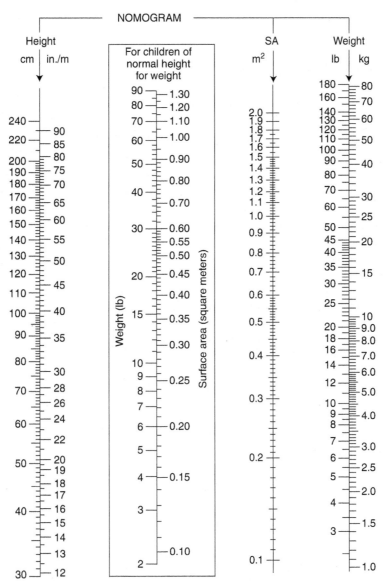

Figure 6.4   West nomogram for estimation of surface areas.

"Figure 715.1" from *Nelson Textbook of Pediatrics,* 18E by R. M. Kliegman, R. E. Behrman, H. B. Jenson, and B. M. D. Stanton. Copyright © 2007 by Saunders, an imprint of Elsevier Inc. Used by permission of Elsevier, Inc.

Adverse Drug Reactions in Children and Promoting Adherence

6.10 Pediatric clients are more susceptible than adults to adverse drug effects.

Because of their smaller size and immature or developing organ systems, pediatric clients are more susceptible to adverse effects. The nurse may find it challenging to identify adverse effects because infants and young children often do not have the maturity or verbal skills to accurately describe their feelings following medication administration. Identifying pediatric adverse effects will depend on the skill and ability of the nurse in assessing subtle changes in a client's response. For example, a child on diuretics

should have strict intake and output measurements to help determine whether the drug is working properly. Excessive weight gain could be caused by edema resulting from poor kidney excretion, or weight loss might be due to excessive diuresis. Signs of ototoxicity may go unnoticed for a long time unless someone checks that the child no longer responds to verbal commands. It may be necessary to consult a psychologist to identify signs of suicidal ideation from antidepressant use in adolescents.

Most types of adverse effects that occur in children age 1 or older are the same as those seen in adults. As with adults, the majority of adverse effects are dose related; therefore, the nurse must pay close attention to the proper dose and frequency of drug administration. Knowing specific drugs and their adverse effects in the adult population will help the nurse to quickly identify signs and symptoms of adverse effects in pediatric clients. For example, antibiotics such as amoxicillin (Amoxil) frequently result in diarrhea in both adults and children. Antianxiety agents, antidepressants, and antipsychotic drugs that cause CNS depression will likely cause drowsiness in both adults and children.

A few types of adverse effects are specific to children due to their immature or developing organs and tissues. For example, tetracycline must be avoided in the neonate because of the potential for permanent staining of the teeth. Sulfonamides can cause jaundice in neonates, and aspirin is contraindicated in children with fever due to the potential for Reye's syndrome. Glucocorticoids can inhibit growth.

Like adults, children may also experience drug interactions. Drugs that are most likely to contribute to drug interactions in pediatric clients are those with high potency, narrow therapeutic index, and extensive protein binding, and those that affect vital organ functions or hepatic metabolism.

Often parents' first response to their child's illness is to provide home remedies. OTC and herbal treatments are extremely common in some households, and research suggests that their use is on the rise among a large segment of the population. The nurse must become aware of commonly used OTC and herbal remedies in order to advise the families about their pros and cons. Parents must understand that OTC and herbal therapies may have adverse effects of their own and may interact with prescription medications. Herbal remedies commonly used in homes include St. John's wort, Echinacea, ginseng, licorice, and sassafras.

A drug will fail to achieve optimum therapeutic outcomes if it is not taken properly. Adherence, also called compliance, is taking the drug according to the instructions on the label or those provided by the prescriber. Maximizing adherence to the medication regimen is a major goal of the pediatric nurse. The nurse must assess the client and family to determine factors that could affect the family's ability to assist the child with the medication regimen and to develop strategies that will enhance medication adherence. The more complex, expensive, and inconvenient the medication regimen, the less likely the child and family will adhere. Children are most likely to adhere to their medication regimen if the following conditions exist:

- High expectations of successful outcome of the therapy
- Supportive family members who are able to communicate with the prescriber
- Positive interactions with the nurse and caregivers
- Minimal adverse effects from the medications
- Simple, short-term, inexpensive regimen with minimum disruption to daily routine

The nurse works with the child and family to enhance adherence by applying direct measures. The child and family should be asked directly whether they have doubts about their ability to adhere to the regimen. If there is doubt, the nurse should explore the areas of concerns with the family and start by teaching the importance of the drug, route of administration, expected outcomes, and possible adverse effects. For long-term drug therapy, the nurse may have to arrange follow-up appointments to assess drug responses or to administer the oral drug to the child and observe the drug being swallowed. This technique is known as **directly observed therapy (DOT)**. In extreme cases when the child does not appear to be responding appropriately to the prescribed regimen, periodic measurement of plasma drug levels can help to determine the amount of drug ingested and whether it has been taken as prescribed.

Pharmacotherapy of Toddlers

6.11 Medication administration to toddlers can be challenging; short, concrete explanations followed by immediate medication administration are usually best for the toddler.

Toddlerhood is the age from 1 to 3 years. During this period a toddler displays a tremendous sense of curiosity. The child begins to explore, wants to try new things, and tends to place everything in the mouth. This becomes a major concern for medication and household product safety. The nurse must be instrumental in teaching parents that poisons come in all shapes, sizes, and forms and include medicines, cosmetics, cleaning supplies, arts and crafts materials, plants, and food products that are improperly stored. Parents should be instructed to request child-resistant containers from the pharmacist and to store all medications in secure cabinets.

Toddlers can swallow liquids and may be able to chew solid medications. When prescription drugs are supplied as flavoured elixirs, it is important to stress that the child not be given access to the medication. Drugs must never be left at the bedside or within easy reach of the child. For a child who has access to a bottle of cherry-flavoured acetaminophen, the tasty liquid may produce a fatal overdose. About half of all poisonings reported to poison control centres occur in children younger than 6 years old. Nurses should educate parents about the following means to protect their children from poisoning:

- Read and carefully follow directions on the label before using drugs and household products.
- Ask a healthcare provider (e.g., pharmacist, nurse, physician) if unsure of correct dosing.
- Store all drugs and harmful agents out of the reach of children and in locked cabinets.
- Keep all household products and drugs in their original containers. Never put chemicals in empty food or drink containers.
- Always ask for medication to be placed in child-resistant containers.
- Never tell children that medicine is candy.
- Keep a bottle of syrup of ipecac in the home to induce vomiting. **Do not give this medication unless instructed to do so by a healthcare provider.**
- Keep the number for the poison control centre near phones, and call immediately on suspicion of a poisoning.
- Never leave medication unattended in a child's room or in areas where the child plays.

Administration of medications to toddlers can be challenging for the nurse. At this stage, the child is rapidly developing increased motor ability and learning to assert independence but has extremely limited ability to reason or understand the relationship of medicines to health. Giving long, detailed explanations to the toddler will prolong the procedure and create additional anxiety.

Short, concrete explanations followed by immediate drug administration are best for this age group. Physical comfort in the form of touching, hugging, or verbal praise after medication administration is important.

Oral medications that taste bad should be mixed with a vehicle such as jam, syrup, or fruit puree, if possible. The medication may be followed with a carbonated beverage or mint-flavoured candy. Nurses should teach parents to avoid placing medicine in milk, orange juice, or cereals because the child may associate these healthy foods with bad-tasting medications. Pharmaceutical companies often formulate pediatric medicines in sweet syrups to increase the ease of medication administration.

IM injections for toddlers may be given into the vastus lateralis muscle. IV injections may use scalp or feet veins; additional peripheral site options become available in late toddlerhood. Suppositories may be difficult to administer due to the resistance of the child. For any of these invasive administration procedures, having a parent in close proximity will usually reduce the toddler's anxiety and increase cooperation. Ask the parent prior to the procedure if he or she would like to assist. The nurse should take at least one helper into the room to assist in restraining the toddler, if necessary.

CONNECTIONS ◖ Special Considerations

◄ Pediatric Drug Research and Labelling

An estimated 75% of the medications prescribed for children contain no specific dosing information for pediatric clients. Without specific labelling information, healthcare providers have largely based their doses on the smaller weight of the child. Children, however, are not merely small adults; they have unique differences in physiology and biochemistry that may place them at risk for effects of drug therapy.

Inclusion of children in clinical trials is an expensive and potentially risky process. Large numbers of children in different age groups are needed for adequate drug testing. Manufacturers also face liability and malpractice issues associated with testing new medications in children. The United States Food and Drug Administration provided financial incentives for pharmaceutical manufacturers to test drugs in children. As a result, more than 28 drugs have been investigated in children, and 18 drug labels have been changed to incorporate the results of the research findings. Drugs that now have more specific pediatric labelling include ibuprofen (Advil, Motrin), ranitidine (Zantac), fluvoxamine (Luvox), and midazolam (Versed).

Pharmacotherapy of Preschoolers and School-Aged Children

6.12 Preschool and younger school-aged children can begin to assist with medication administration.

The **preschool child** ranges in age from 3 to 5 years. During this period, the child begins to refine gross and fine motor skills and develop language abilities. The child initiates new activities and becomes more socially involved with other children.

Preschoolers can sometimes comprehend the difference between health and illness and that medications are administered to help them feel better. Nonetheless, medications and other potentially dangerous products must still be safely stowed out of the child's reach.

In general, principles of medication administration that pertain to the toddler also apply to this age group. Preschoolers cooperate in taking oral medications if they are crushed or mixed with food or flavoured beverages. After a child has been walking for about a year, the ventrogluteal site may be used for IM injections, as it causes less pain than the vastus lateralis site. The scalp veins can no longer be used for IV access; peripheral veins are used for IV injections.

Like the toddler, preschoolers often physically resist medication administration and a long, detailed explanation of the procedure will promote anxiety. A brief explanation followed quickly by medication administration is usually the best method. Uncooperative children may need to be restrained, and clients over 4 years of age may require two adults to administer the medication. Before and after medication procedures, the child may benefit from opportunities to play-act troubling experiences with dolls. When the child plays the role of doctor or nurse by giving a "sick" doll a pill or injection, comforting the doll, and explaining that the doll will

now feel better, the little actor feels safer and more in control of the situation.

The **school-aged child** is between 6 and 12 years of age. Some refer to this period as the middle childhood years. This is the time in a child's life when there is progression away from the family-centred environment to the larger peer relationship environment. Rapid physical, mental, and social development occur and early ethical-moral development begins to take shape. Thinking processes become progressively logical and more consistent.

During this time, most children remain relatively healthy, with immune system development well under way. Respiratory infections and GI upsets are the most common complaints. Because the child feels well most of the time, there is little concept of illness or the risks involved with ingesting a harmful substance offered to the child by a peer or older person.

The nurse is usually able to gain considerable cooperation from school-aged children. Longer, more detailed explanations may be of value because the child has developed some reasoning ability and can understand the relationship between the medicine and feeling better. When children are old enough to welcome choices, they can be offered limited dosing alternatives to provide a sense of control and encourage cooperation. The option of taking one medication before another or the chance to choose which drink will follow a chewable tablet helps to distract children from the issue of whether they will take the medication at all. It also makes an otherwise strange or unpleasant experience a little more enjoyable. Making children feel that they are willing participants in medication administration, rather than victims, is an important foundation for compliance. Praise for cooperation is appropriate for any pediatric client and will set the stage for successful medication administration in the future.

School-aged children can take chewable tablets and may be able to swallow tablets or capsules. Many still resist injections;

however, an experienced pediatric nurse can usually administer parenteral medications quickly and compassionately, without the need to restrain the child. The ventrogluteal site is preferred for IM injections, although the muscles of older children are developed enough for the nurse to use other sites.

Pharmacotherapy of Adolescents

6.13 Pharmacological compliance in the adolescent is dependent on understanding and respecting the uniqueness of the person in this stage of growth and development.

Adolescence is the time between ages 13 and 18 years. A person in this age group is able to think in abstract terms and come to logical conclusions based on a given set of observations. Rapid physical growth and psychological maturation have a great impact on personality development. The adolescent relates strongly to peers, wanting and needing their support, approval, and presence. Physical appearance and conformity with peers in terms of behaviour, dress, and social interactions is important.

The most common needs for pharmacotherapy in this age group are skin problems, headaches, menstrual symptoms, and sports-related injuries. There is an increased need for contraceptive information and counselling about sexually related health problems. Since bulimia occurs in this population, the nurse should carefully question adolescents about their eating habits and their use of OTC appetite suppressants or laxatives. Tobacco use and illicit drug experimentation may be prevalent in this population. Teenage athletes may use amphetamines to delay the onset of fatigue, as well as anabolic steroids to increase muscle strength and endurance. The nurse assumes a key role in educating adolescent clients about the hazards of tobacco use and illicit drugs.

The adolescent has a need for privacy and control in drug administration. The nurse should seek complete cooperation and communicate with the teen more in the manner of an adult than a child. Teens usually appreciate thorough explanations of their treatment, and ample time should be allowed for them to ask questions. Adolescents are often reluctant to admit their lack of knowledge, so the nurse should carefully explain important information about their medications and expected side effects, even if the client claims to understand. Teens are easily embarrassed, and the nurse should be sensitive to their need for self-expression, privacy, and individuality, particularly when parents, siblings, or friends are present.

PHARMACOTHERAPY IN ADULTHOOD

When considering adult health, it is customary to divide this period of life into three stages: **young adulthood** (18 to 40 years), **middle adulthood** (40 to 65 years), and **older adulthood** (older than 65 years). Within each of these divisions are similar biophysical, psychosocial, and spiritual characteristics that affect nursing and pharmacotherapy.

Pharmacotherapy of Young and Middle-Aged Adults

6.14 Young adults comprise the healthiest age group and generally need few prescription medications. Middle-aged adults begin to suffer from lifestyle-related illnesses such as hypertension.

The health status of younger adults is generally good; absorption, metabolic, and excretion mechanisms are at their peak. There is minimal need for prescription drugs unless chronic diseases such as diabetes or immune-related conditions exist. The use of vitamins, minerals, and herbal remedies is prevalent in young adulthood. Prescription drugs are usually related to contraception or agents needed during pregnancy and delivery. Medication compliance is positive within this age range, as there is clear comprehension of benefit in terms of longevity and feeling well.

Substance abuse is a cause for concern in the 18 to 24 age group, with alcohol, tobacco products, amphetamines, and illicit drugs (marijuana and cocaine) being a problem. For young adults who are sexually active with multiple partners, prescription medications for the treatment of herpes, gonorrhea, syphilis, and human immunodeficiency virus (HIV) infection may be necessary.

The physical status of the middle-aged adult is on par with the young adult until about 45 years of age. During this period of life, numerous transitions occur that often result in excessive stress. Middle-aged adults are sometimes referred to as the "sandwich generation" because they are often caring for aging parents as well as children and grandchildren. Because of the pressures of work and family, they often take medication to control health alterations that could best be treated with positive lifestyle modifications. The nurse must emphasize the importance of lifestyle choices, such as limiting lipid intake, maintaining optimum weight, and exercising, to overall health.

Health impairments related to cardiovascular disease, hypertension, obesity, arthritis, cancer, and anxiety begin to surface in

---

CONNECTIONS **Special Considerations**

◀ Gender-Related Differences in Pharmacokinetics

- Oral contraceptives and sex hormone replacement therapies for women can affect hepatic *metabolism* and other metabolism of drugs.
- The *metabolism* of alcohol is slower in women.
- Renal function is greater in men, resulting in more efficient drug *excretion*.
- Hormonal fluctuations in women across the menstrual cycle and the lifespan may affect all phases of pharmacokinetics; research is needed to assess the effects.
- Body size and surface area, which are usually greater in men, can affect drug *distribution*.
- Adipose tissue, which is usually greater in women, can affect drug storage.

middle age. Gender-related differences in pharmacokinetics and disease comorbidity may influence pharmacotherapy. The use of drugs to treat hypertension, hyperlipidemia, digestive disorders, erectile dysfunction, and arthritis is becoming more common. Respiratory disorders related to lifelong tobacco use or exposure to secondhand smoke and environmental toxins may develop that require drug therapies. Adult onset diabetes mellitus often emerges during this time of life. The use of antidepressants and antianxiety agents is prominent in the over-50 population.

Pharmacotherapy of Older Adults

6.15 Older adults take more medications and experience more adverse drug events than any other age group. For drug therapy to be successful, the nurse must make accommodations for age-related changes in physiological and biochemical functions.

During the 20th century, an improved quality of life and the ability to effectively treat many diseases contributed to increased longevity. The risk of chronic health disorders is greater in older adults, and they are more likely to be prescribed drugs to treat them. The taking of multiple drugs concurrently, known as **polypharmacy**, has become commonplace among many older adults. Polypharmacy dramatically increases the risk of drug interactions and side effects.

Although predictable physiological and psychosocial changes occur with aging, significant variability exists among clients. Cognitive decline and memory loss may occur in older adults. However, many older adults are healthy and live independently. The nurse should avoid preconceived notions that elderly clients will have physical or cognitive impairment simply because they have reached a certain age. Careful assessment is always necessary (Figure 6.5).

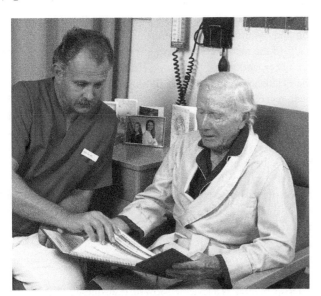

Figure 6.5 Pharmacotherapy of the older adult.
Source: PearsonEducation/PH College.

When administering medications to older adults, offer the client the same degree of independence and dignity that would be afforded middle-aged adults, unless otherwise indicated. Like their younger counterparts, older clients have a need to understand why they are receiving a drug and what outcomes are expected. Accommodations must be made for older adults who have certain impairments. Visual and auditory changes make it important for the nurse to provide drug instructions in large type and to obtain client feedback to be certain that medication instructions have been understood. Elderly clients with cognitive decline and memory loss can benefit from aids such as alarmed pill containers, medicine management boxes, and clearly written instructions. During assessment, the nurse should determine if the client is capable of self-administering medications or whether the assistance of a caregiver will be required. As long as small children are not present in the household, older clients with arthritis should be encouraged to ask the pharmacist for medication bottles with caps specially designed for ease of opening.

Older clients experience more adverse effects from drug therapy than any other age group. Although some of these effects are due to polypharmacy, many of the adverse events are predictable, based on normal physiological and biochemical processes that may occur during aging. The principal complications of drug therapy in the older adult population are degeneration of organ systems, multiple and severe illnesses, multiple drug therapy, and unreliable compliance. By understanding these changes, the nurse can avoid

CONNECTIONS ❙ Special Considerations

◀ Altered Pharmacokinetics During Older Adulthood

- Increased gastric pH, delayed gastric emptying, and decreased peristaltic rate may affect medication *absorption*. Often, when laxatives are used to compensate for slower peristalsis, medications may be rapidly *excreted* from the body before they can provide their full therapeutic benefit.
- The liver's production of enzymes decreases, thus decreasing hepatic drug metabolism and resulting in increased serum drug concentration; more drug is available for *distribution* and the effects of some drugs are prolonged.
- The aging liver produces less albumin, resulting in decreased plasma protein binding and increased levels of free drug in the bloodstream; *distribution*, drug effects, and the potential for drug-drug interactions are increased.
- The ratio of body fat to water increases, affecting *distribution* and storage of fat-soluble drugs and vitamins. The ratio of fat to muscle increases, slowing *metabolism*.
- The aging cardiovascular system causes decreased cardiac output and less efficient blood circulation, which slow drug *distribution*. This makes it important to initiate pharmacotherapy with smaller dosages and slowly increase the amount to a safe, effective level.
- The percentage of body water decreases, contributing to dehydration and changes in drug concentration and *distribution*. The risk of drug toxicity is increased by fluid deficit.
- Blood flow to the kidney decreases, resulting in a decrease in the amount of drug being delivered to the kidney for *excretion*.

many adverse drug effects in older clients. In older clients, the functioning of all major organ systems slowly declines. For this reason, all phases of pharmacokinetics are affected, and appropriate adjustments in therapy need to be implemented. Although most of the pharmacokinetic changes are due to reduced hepatic and renal drug elimination, other systems may also show a variety of changes. For example, immune system function diminishes with aging, so autoimmune diseases and infections occur more frequently in elderly clients. Therefore, there is an increased need for influenza and pneumonia vaccinations. Normal physiological changes that affect pharmacotherapy of the older adult are summarized as follows:

- Absorption: In general, absorption of drugs is slower in the older adult because of diminished gastric motility and decreased blood flow to digestive organs. Increased gastric pH can delay absorption of medications that require high acidity to dissolve.

- Distribution: Increased body fat in the older adult provides a larger storage compartment for lipid-soluble drugs and vitamins. Plasma levels are reduced, and the therapeutic response is diminished. Older adults have less body water, making the effects of dehydration more dramatic and increasing the risk for drug toxicity. For example, elderly clients who have reduced body fluid experience more orthostatic hypotension. The decline in lean body mass and total body water leads to an increased concentration of water-soluble drugs because the drug is distributed in a smaller volume of water. The aging liver produces less albumin, resulting in decreased plasma protein binding ability and increased levels of free drug in the bloodstream, thereby increasing the potential for drug-drug interactions. The aging cardiovascular system has decreased cardiac output and less efficient blood circulation, which slow drug distribution. This makes it important to initiate pharmacotherapy with smaller dosages and slowly increase the amount to a safe, effective level.

- Metabolism: The liver's production of enzymes decreases, liver mass decreases, and the visceral blood flow is diminished, resulting in reduced hepatic drug metabolism. This change leads to an increase in the half-life of many drugs, which prolongs and intensifies the drug response. The decline in hepatic function reduces first-pass metabolism. (Recall that first-pass metabolism relates to the amount of a drug that is metabolized during the first circulation through the liver after the drug has been absorbed by the intestinal tract.) Therefore, plasma levels are elevated, and tissue concentrations are increased for the particular drug. This change alters the standard dosage, the interval between doses, and the duration of side effects.

- Excretion: Older adults have reductions in renal blood flow, glomerular filtration rate, active tubular secretion, and nephron function. This decreases excretion for drugs that are eliminated by the kidneys. When excretion is reduced, serum drug levels and the potential for toxicity markedly increase. Administration schedules and dosage amounts may need to be altered in many older adults because of these changes in kidney function. Keep in mind that the most common cause of adverse drug reactions in older adults is the accumulation of toxic amounts of drugs secondary to impaired renal excretion.

Adherence to the Therapeutic Regimen

6.16 Adherence to the therapeutic regimen is a major challenge for many older adults.

Drug adherence or compliance is the willingness and ability to take medications as instructed on the label or by the healthcare provider. Healthcare providers often assume that clients leaving the clinic or hospital will be adherent, fill their prescriptions, and take their medications as directed. It may be surprising to learn that more than a third of clients report that they are often nonadherent with drug therapy. Reasons for nonadherence are many and varied but include the following client responses (Martin et al., 2010):

- Did not have the medicine on hand when it was time to take the dose (31%)
- Ran out of medicine (29.5%)
- Bothered by side effects (22.4%)
- Change in daily routine (21.4%)
- Felt better (16.4%)

Although nonadherence is not unique to older adults, this population is especially vulnerable. Older adult clients are more likely to have visual impairment, functional disabilities, and cognitive dysfunction that may be sources of medication errors and nonadherence. Functional hearing loss can prevent older adults from understanding the verbal instructions given by the healthcare provider. The large number of drugs taken by some older adults makes for a complicated dosing schedule that can be confusing for clients of any age.

Successful management of medical problems depends on a client's adherence to the regimen. One of the main responsibilities of the nurse is to assess barriers to medication adherence in the older adult. Studies suggest that nonadherence is affected by three factors: the individual client, the healthcare provider, and the client's social support network.

Adherence at the client level requires the client's comprehension and commitment to the treatment. The client must be able to afford the medication, believe in its efficacy, appropriately self-administer, and adjust to lifestyle changes that may be required. The healthcare provider must be able to effectively instruct the client regarding a medication's efficacy, prescribe cost-effective medication, decrease the complexity of the regimen, and provide manageable and understandable instructions. Nurses play a key role in assessing the client's understanding of the medications that have been ordered and assessing client concerns about cost or adverse effects.

The nurse should provide the older adult's spouse or caregiver with adequate information about the client's medication regimen, expected lifestyle changes, and the need for emotional support and monitoring. Table 6.4 lists reasons that clients give for nonadherence and provides suggestions for the nurse to promote adherence.

Drug misuse is a specific form of nonadherence that is common among older adults. Misuse includes overuse, underuse, or in some cases, erratic use. This misuse may be accidental or

TABLE 6.4 Promoting Adherence in the Older Adult Client

Reasons for nonadherence	• Unpleasant adverse effects • Forgetfulness • Cognitive or physical impairment • Poor or misunderstood instructions • Complicated regimens • Inability or refusal to purchase the medication • Health beliefs about medications
Ways the nurse can promote adherence	• Assist the older adult in comprehending and committing to the drug treatment regimen. • Communicate the instructions in such a manner that the older patient fully understands the purpose of the treatment. • Provide the older patient with social support services to obtain the medications. • Work with a pharmacist to ensure that the medication is dispensed in containers that are easily opened and in formulations that are easily taken. • Make sure all drugs are clearly labelled with instructions. • Simplify the regimen to reduce the number of drugs and doses per day. • Suggest that the older patient use a daily or weekly pill counter. • Provide the patient with a check-off calendar to document each time a medication is taken. • Engage family members or friends in supporting the older patient in efforts to comply. • Encourage the older patient to report signs of adverse effects. • Schedule periodic tests to determine plasma drug levels. • Place follow-up calls to high-risk patients.

deliberate. Self-adjusting the medication dose is a common practice: clients change their dose level depending on how they feel. Some believe that taking extra doses will speed their recovery. Clients rarely report such practices to their healthcare provider. Drug misuse may have serious consequences: many older adult visits to emergency departments are drug related, with nonadherence accounting for a substantial percentage.

CHAPTER

6 Understanding the Chapter

Key Concepts Summary

6.1 To contribute to safe and effective pharmacotherapy, it is essential for the nurse to comprehend and apply fundamental concepts of growth and development.

6.2 Pharmacotherapy during pregnancy should be conducted only when the benefits to the mother outweigh the potential risks to the unborn child.

6.3 During pregnancy, major physiological and anatomical changes occur that can alter the pharmacokinetics and pharmacodynamics of administered drugs.

6.4 Gestational age must be considered when prescribing drugs to pregnant clients.

6.5 Pregnancy drug categories guide the healthcare provider in prescribing drugs for pregnant clients.

6.6 Breastfeeding clients must be aware that drugs and other substances can appear in milk and affect the infant.

6.7 During infancy, pharmacotherapy is directed toward the safety of the child and teaching the parents how to properly administer medications and care for the infant.

6.8 The nurse is a key member of the healthcare team in ensuring medication safety in pediatric clients.

6.9 The nurse must be accurate when calculating drug dosages for pediatric clients.

6.10 Pediatric clients are more susceptible than adults to adverse drug effects.

6.11 Medication administration to toddlers can be challenging; short, concrete explanations followed by immediate medication administration are usually best for the toddler.

6.12 Preschool and younger school-aged children can begin to assist with medication administration.

6.13 Pharmacological compliance in the adolescent is dependent on understanding and respecting the uniqueness of the person in this stage of growth and development.

6.14 Young adults comprise the healthiest age group and generally need few prescription medications. Middle-aged adults begin to suffer from lifestyle-related illnesses such as hypertension.

6.15 Older adults take more medications and experience more adverse drug events than any other age group. For drug therapy to be successful, the nurse must make accommodations for age-related changes in physiological and biochemical functions.

6.16 Adherence to the therapeutic regimen is a major challenge for many older adults.

Chapter 6 Scenario

May David, a 22-year-old woman, comes to the clinic to obtain a pregnancy test. She has not had her menstrual period for the past 6 weeks but claims that infrequent menses are not unusual for her. She feels nauseous in the mornings, but the feeling is only temporary. You ask May, "Is it possible that you might be pregnant?" May's response is "I doubt it, since we have always used a condom during intercourse." She goes on to explain that she has been taking an antiseizure medication for several years to control her epilepsy and is taking some herbal medicines to promote a feeling of well-being.

May's vital signs are as follows: temperature, 36.7°C; pulse, 68 beats/minute; respiration, 18 breaths/minute; and blood pressure, 110/70 mm Hg. She is 1.7 m tall and is surprised that she has gained 2.3 kg in the past 4 weeks, bringing her weight to 65.8 kg. A urine specimen is sent to the laboratory to test for human chorionic gonadotropin (HCG). A complete physical examination is performed, followed by a vaginal examination via speculum. All physical findings are within normal limits except for the urine qualitative HCG, which is positive and quantitative (HCG = 550), indicating pregnancy. May smokes approximately half a pack of cigarettes per day.

Critical Thinking Questions

1. What are some key points the nurse will discuss with May regarding her condition and the medication she is taking?

2. What education should the nurse provide for May regarding the use of medication during pregnancy?

3. While caring for May, the nurse must consider pregnancy drug categories. In your own words, explain these categories.

4. What effect does May's tobacco use possibly have on her unborn baby?

See Answers to Critical Thinking Questions in Appendix B.

NCLEX Practice Questions

1 A client in her first trimester of pregnancy asks the nurse which medications to avoid during pregnancy. The nurse's response is based on the knowledge that during pregnancy,

   a. Most over-the-counter medications are safe.

   b. When possible, drug therapy is postponed until after pregnancy and lactation.

   c. It is wise to discontinue all drugs used to treat medical conditions.

   d. The decision of whether or not to take medication is the responsibility of the woman.

2 A nurse is preparing to discuss drug use during pregnancy with a group of nursing students. The main topic is FDA drug classifications. Which of the following drugs should the nurse explain to be most detrimental to the fetus?

   a. Category A

   b. Category B

   c. Category C

   d. Category X

3 A pregnant client asks the nurse what factors determine whether a drug will cross the placenta. The nurse's response will be based on which of the following principles?

   a. Highly lipid-soluble drugs cross the placental membrane more easily than do drugs with low lipid solubility.

   b. The lower the lipid content, the more easily the drug crosses the placental membrane.

   c. Drugs with large molecular weights pass rapidly through the placental membrane.

   d. Highly protein bound drugs pass rapidly through the placental membrane.

4 A nurse is administering medication to a group of pregnant women. At which stage of fetal development is it *least* likely for congenital malformations to occur?

   a. 1 to 2 weeks

   b. 3 to 4 weeks

   c. 5 to 6 weeks

   d. 7 to 8 weeks

5 The community health nurse is visiting a postpartum mother who is breastfeeding her 3.2-kg (7-lb) infant daughter. Which of the following statements made by the mother would indicate that further teaching is necessary? Select all that apply.

a. "When using over-the-counter medications, I should take only the lowest effective dose."

b. "The higher the dose of medication, the more likely it is that it will be secreted into the breast milk."

c. "I shouldn't take any drugs while I'm breastfeeding, not even prescription drugs."

d. "Medication in liquid form should be avoided since it more readily enters the breast milk."

e. "Now that I'm no longer pregnant, I don't need to worry about the medicines I take affecting my baby."

See Answers to NCLEX Practice Questions in Appendix A.

UNIT

3

Professional, Personal, and Cultural Influences on Pharmacotherapy

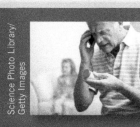

Science Photo Library/ Getty Images

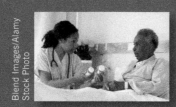

Blend Images/Alamy Stock Photo

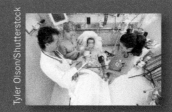

Tyler Olson/Shutterstock

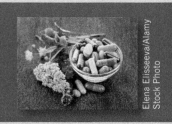

Elena Elisseeva/Alamy Stock Photo

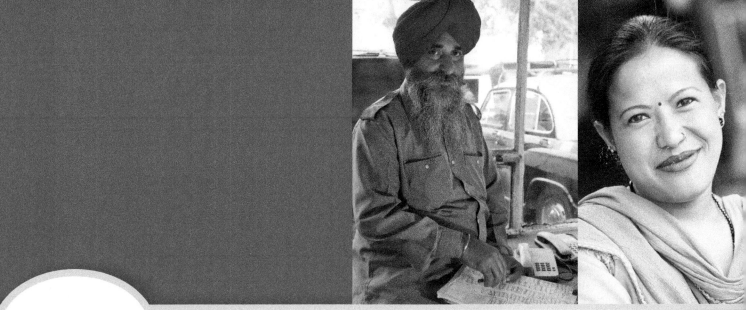

Indiapicture/Alamy Stock Photo   Kadmy/Fotolia

CHAPTER

7 Individual, Psychosocial, and Cultural Influences on Drug Responses

LEARNING OUTCOMES

After reading this chapter, the student should be able to:

1. Describe fundamental concepts underlying a holistic approach to pharmacotherapy.

2. Describe the components of the human integration pyramid model.

3. Identify psychosocial and spiritual factors that can affect pharmacotherapeutics.

4. Explain how ethnicity can affect pharmacotherapeutic outcomes.

5. Identify examples of how cultural values, beliefs, and practices can influence pharmacotherapeutic outcomes.

6. Explain how community and environmental factors can affect pharmacotherapeutic outcomes.

7. Convey how genetic polymorphisms can influence pharmacotherapy.

8. Relate the implications of gender to the actions of certain drugs.

9. Explain how pharmacogenomics may lead to customized drug therapy.

CHAPTER OUTLINE

▸ The Concept of Holistic Pharmacotherapy

▸ Psychosocial Influences on Pharmacotherapy

▸ Cultural and Ethnic Influences on Pharmacotherapy

▸ Community and Environmental Influences on Pharmacotherapy

▸ Genetic Polymorphisms and Their Influence on Pharmacotherapy

▸ Gender Influences on Pharmacotherapy

It is convenient for a nurse to learn an average drug dose, administer the medication, and expect all clients to achieve the same outcomes. Unfortunately, this rarely occurs. For example, the same dose of an antihypertensive drug can result in a desired therapeutic effect in one client and produce no effect or profound hypotension in other clients. For pharmacotherapy to be successful, the needs of each individual client must be assessed and evaluated. In Chapter 3, variables such as absorption, metabolism, plasma protein binding, and excretion were examined in an attempt to explain how these modify client responses to drugs. In Chapter 4, variability among client responses was explained in terms of differences in drug-receptor interactions. This chapter examines additional psychological, social, and biological variables that must be considered for optimum pharmacotherapy.

The Concept of Holistic Pharmacotherapy

7.1 To deliver holistic treatment, the nurse must consider the client's psychosocial and spiritual needs in a social context.

To deliver the highest quality of care, the nurse must fully recognize the individuality and totality of the client. Each person must be viewed holistically as an integrated biological, psychosocial, cultural, spiritual, communicating whole, existing and functioning within the environment. This approach helps to better understand how risk factors such as age, genetics, biological characteristics, personal habits, lifestyle, and environment increase a person's likelihood of acquiring specific diseases and influence pharmacotherapeutic outcomes.

The human integration pyramid, shown in Figure 7.1, is a model of six categories that compartmentalizes the functional environment in which human beings exist while maintaining an interrelated connection between them. This representation provides a useful approach to addressing the nursing and pharmacological needs of clients within the collaborative practices of healthcare delivery. Where appropriate, concepts illustrated in the pyramid are presented throughout this text as they relate to the various drug categories. All levels of the pyramid are important and connected: some are specific to certain drug classes and nursing activities, whereas others apply more diversely across the nursing-pharmacology spectrum.

By its very nature, modern (Western) medicine as it is practised in Canada is seemingly incompatible with **holistic** medicine. Western medicine focuses on specific diseases, their causes, and treatments. Disease is viewed as a malfunction of a specific organ or system. Sometimes the disease is viewed even more specifically and is categorized as a change in DNA structure or a malfunction of one enzyme. Sophisticated technology is used to image and classify the specific structural or functional abnormality. Somehow,

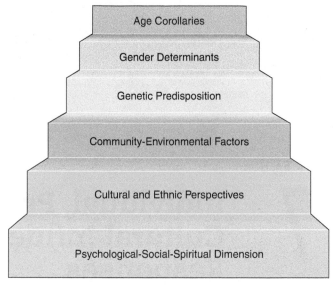

Figure 7.1 The human integration pyramid care model.

the total client is lost in this focus on categorizing disease. Too often it does not matter how or why the client developed cancer, diabetes, or hypertension, or how the client feels about it; the psychosocial and cultural dimensions are lost. Yet these dimensions can have a profound impact on the success of pharmacotherapy. The nurse must consciously direct care toward a holistic treatment of each individual client, in his or her psychosocial, spiritual, and social context.

Psychosocial Influences on Pharmacotherapy

7.2 The psychosocial domain must be considered when taking clients' medical histories. Positive attitudes and high expectations about therapeutic outcomes in the client may increase the success of pharmacotherapy.

Whereas science and medicine are founded on objective, logical, critical deliberation, psychology and sociology are based more on intuitive and subjective considerations. **Psychology** is the science that deals with normal and abnormal mental processes and their impact on behaviour. **Sociology** studies human behaviour within the context of groups and societies. **Spirituality** incorporates the capacity to love, to convey compassion and empathy, to give and forgive, to enjoy life, and to find peace of mind and fulfillment in living. The spiritual life overlaps with components of the emotional, mental, physical, and social aspects of living.

From a healthcare perspective, every human being should be considered an integrated psychological, social, and spiritual being.

Health impairments related to an individual's psychosocial situation often require a blending of individualized nursing care and therapeutic drugs, in conjunction with psychotherapeutic counselling. The term *psycho-social-spiritual* is appearing more frequently in nursing literature. It is now acknowledged that when clients have strong spiritual or religious beliefs, these may greatly influence their perceptions of illness and their preferred modes of treatment. In many situations, these beliefs have a strong bearing on pharmacotherapy. When illness imposes threats to health, the client commonly presents with psychological, social, and spiritual issues along with physical symptoms. Clients face concerns related to ill health, suffering, loneliness, despair, and death, and at the same time look for meaning, value, and hope in their situation. Such issues can have a great impact on wellness and preferred methods of medical treatment, nursing care, and pharmacotherapy.

The client's psychosocial history is an essential component of the initial client interview and assessment. This history delves into the personal life of the client, with inquiries directed toward lifestyle preferences, religious beliefs, sexual practices, alcohol intake, and tobacco and non-prescription drug use. For example, a highly stressed, middle-aged client who is struggling with a new business might find it difficult to focus on wellness goals such as maintaining normal blood pressure and cholesterol levels. The nurse must show extreme sensitivity when gathering psychosocial data. If a trusting nurse-client relationship is not established quickly, the client will be reluctant to share important personal data that could affect nursing care.

The psychological dimension can exert a strong influence on pharmacotherapy. Clients who are convinced that their treatment is important and beneficial to their well-being will demonstrate better compliance with drug therapy. The nurse must ascertain the client's goals in seeking treatment and determine whether drug therapy is compatible with those goals. Past experiences with health care may lead a client to distrust medications. Drugs may not be acceptable for the social environment of the client. For example, having to take drugs at school or in the workplace may cause embarrassment; clients may fear that they will be viewed as weak, unhealthy, or dependent.

In some cases, the client assessment may indicate a need to address psychosocial interventions before pharmacotherapy begins. Behavioural or cognitive therapies may be employed to reduce negative thoughts and behaviours that could affect therapy. In children or adolescents, attempts at psychosocial therapies may be a prerequisite to initiating pharmacotherapy for conditions such as attention-deficit disorder, major depressive disorder, or bipolar disorder. The integrated use of pharmacological and psychosocial therapies is believed to increase therapeutic success in addiction treatment.

NCLEX Success Tips

The development of alcoholism is influenced by biological, sociocultural, and environmental factors. The biological theories of alcoholism explicitly implicate genetic factors as having a major impact on the development of alcoholism in some people.

The disease concept of alcoholism allows the person with the disease not to feel guilty about having caused the illness. The nurse should stress that the one with the disease is still responsible for using alcohol; he or she alone decides whether or not to take that drink.

Using the disease of alcoholism as an excuse to drink and to avoid taking responsibility reflects ongoing denial about the disease.

Children of alcoholic parents are more likely to become alcoholics—even if they are raised in an alcohol-free environment—than are the children of nonalcoholic parents.

The nurse can inquire about the client's attitudes regarding the intake of alcohol whenever necessary, as long as this is done while respecting the client's religious beliefs, which is important in providing holistic client care. For example, nurses should not assume that all Muslims abstain from eating pork and drinking alcohol.

Asking about the client's preference is the best and safest way to ensure culturally competent care. The nurse can ask whether the client identifies with a cultural, ethnic, or religious group, and explain that he or she is asking so to ensure that the client's beliefs, practices, and values are incorporated into the care plan. This will promote client-focused care.

Alcohol can be part of nursing intervention. For example, prior to administering subcutaneous (SC) or intramuscular (IM) injections, some clients may refuse to have alcohol in contact with their skin for religious reasons. The nurse should respect their decision and find an alternative antiseptic solution to clean the skin before injection.

Clients who display positive attitudes about their personal health and have high expectations regarding the results of their pharmacotherapy are more likely to achieve positive outcomes. The nurse plays a pivotal role in encouraging the client's positive expectations. The nurse must always be forthright in explaining drug actions and potential side effects. Trivializing the limitations of pharmacotherapy or minimizing potential adverse effects can cause the client to have unrealistic expectations about treatment. The nurse-client relationship may be jeopardized, and the client may acquire an attitude of distrust.

Cultural and Ethnic Influences on Pharmacotherapy

7.3 Culture and ethnicity are two interconnected factors that can affect nursing care and pharmacotherapy. Differences in diet, use of alternative therapies, perceptions of wellness, and genetic makeup can influence a client's drug response.

Despite the apparent diverse cultural and ethnic differences among humans, we are indeed one species. It has been estimated that all humans share 99.8% of the same DNA sequences. The remaining

CONNECTIONS Special Considerations

◄ Alcoholism: Cultural and Environmental Influences

Alcoholism is considered a disease with both social and biological components. It clearly has a genetic basis that sensitizes some individuals to the action of ethanol. It also is known to develop in individuals who are exposed, from an early age, to situations in which drinking is considered socially acceptable. It is supported by cultural customs, poverty, traumatic experiences, and other environmental factors. The nurse is often the key healthcare professional who is trained to identify these factors during client assessment and to refer the client to the proper health or social agency for assistance. The condition must be considered and treated in a holistic and compassionate manner if the problem is to be controlled.

◀ Religious Affiliation and Disease Incidence

Religious affiliation is correlated with a reduction in the incidence of some diseases such as cancer and coronary artery disease. Religious and spiritual factors often figure into important decisions for clients who are facing terminal illness and death—for example, the decision to create advance directives such as a living will and a durable power of attorney for health care. Considerations of the meaning, purpose, and value of human life are used to make choices about the desirability of cardiopulmonary resuscitation and aggressive life support and whether and when to forgo life support and accept death as appropriate and natural under the circumstances.

0.2% of the sequences that differ are shared among peoples with similar historical and geographical heritage.

NCLEX Success Tip

Avoid generalizing and stereotyping (expecting that all people within an ethnic or cultural group are alike and share the same beliefs and attitudes).

An **ethnic** group is a community of people who have a common history and similar genetic heritage. Members of an ethnic group share distinctive social and cultural traditions, which are maintained from generation to generation. These beliefs include a shared perception of health and illness.

Culture is a set of beliefs, values, religious rituals, and customs shared by a group of people. In some respects, culture and ethnicity are similar, and many people use the words interchangeably. Ethnicity more often is used to refer to biological and genetic similarities. For example, many African Canadians have adopted the cultural norms of European Canadians. Others have kept some of the African cultural traditions and beliefs that have been passed on from generation to generation. As a group, however, all African Canadians share genetic similarities with people who live in Africa today and thus are considered to belong to the same ethnic group.

Culture can be a dominant force that influences the relationship between the client and the nurse. The practitioner-client relationship is a cross-cultural encounter, with the client bringing to the relationship religious and ideological beliefs that may challenge or conflict with what the healthcare provider believes to be in the best interest of the client. The client's definition of illness is, in fact, often based on cultural beliefs and values. It is also important to remember that diversity exists not only *between* different cultures but also *within* individual cultures. Examples include differences between age groups or between genders within a given culture.

Cultural sensitivity must be demonstrated by the nurse during the initial phase of the nursing process, when the nurse and the client first meet and culturally specific information is obtained during the medical history. Cultural competence requires knowledge of the values, beliefs, and practices of various peoples, along with an attitude of awareness, openness, and sensitivity. Understanding and respecting the beliefs of the client are key to establishing and maintaining a positive therapeutic relationship that culminates in culturally sensitive nursing care. Therapeutic communication mandates that all healthcare providers bear in mind the cultural, racial, and social factors that make up each person and how these affect behaviour. Failure to take these beliefs seriously can undermine the client's ability to trust the nurse and may even persuade some clients to avoid seeking medical care when it is needed.

Culture and ethnicity can affect pharmacotherapy in many ways. The nurse must keep in mind the following variables when treating clients in different ethnic groups:

- Diet: Every culture has a unique set of foods and spices, which have the potential to affect pharmacotherapy. For example, some Asian diets tend to be high in carbohydrates and lower in protein and fat. African Canadian diets tend to be higher in lipid content.

- Alternative therapies: Many cultural groups believe in using herbs and other alternative therapies either along with or in place of modern medicines. Some of these folk remedies and traditional treatments have existed for thousands of years and helped to form the foundation for modern medical practice. Some Chinese clients may go to herbalists to treat their illnesses. Aboriginal peoples often take great care in collecting, storing, and using herbs to treat and prevent disease. Certain cultures use spices and herbs to maintain a balance of hot and cold, which is thought to promote wellness. Therapeutic massage, heat, and tea infusions are used by many cultures. The nurse needs to interpret how these herbal and alternative therapies will affect the desired pharmacotherapeutic outcomes.

NCLEX Success Tips

Herbs are not intended for acute illness episodes or long-term therapy.

Their therapeutic effectiveness is slower than that of prescription medications; it may take as long as several weeks, depending on the herb.

Safe use of herbs in pregnancy and lactation is either contraindicated or unknown. They may dry up breast milk during lactation, although ginger may be an exception.

Explain that clients should start with one herb at a time, at a lower than recommended dose, and closely monitor their response.

Herbs may cause allergic reactions and adverse effects. If this occurs, discontinue using the herb and report the symptoms to the healthcare provider.

- Beliefs about health and disease: Each culture has distinct ways of viewing sickness and health. Some individuals seek the assistance of people in their community who they believe are blessed with healing powers. First Nations people may seek help from a tribal medicine man. Some African Canadians may know of neighbours who have gifts of healing through the laying on of hands. Clients may place great trust in these alternative healers. Culturally sensitive care respects the local knowledge, values, and wisdom of ethnic groups.

- Genetic differences: With the advent of DNA sequencing, hundreds of structural variants in metabolic enzymes have been discovered. Some of these appear more frequently in certain ethnic groups and have an impact on pharmacotherapeutics, as discussed in Section 7.5.

Community and Environmental Influences on Pharmacotherapy

7.4 Community and environmental factors affect health and the public's access to health care and pharmacotherapy. Inadequate access to healthcare resources and an inability to read or understand instructions may have a negative impact on treatment outcomes.

A number of community and environmental factors that influence disease and its subsequent treatment have been identified. Population growth, complex technological advances, and evolving globalization patterns have all affected health care. Communities vary significantly with regard to urbanization, age distribution, socioeconomic status, occupational pattern, and industrial growth. All of these have the potential to affect health and access to pharmacotherapy.

Access to health care is perhaps the most obvious community-related influence on pharmacotherapy. There are many potential obstacles to obtaining appropriate health care. Without an adequate prescription drug plan, some people on limited incomes are reluctant to seek health care for fear that the cost of prescription drugs may be too high. Older adults may fear losing their retirement savings or being placed in a nursing home for the remainder of their lives. Families living in rural areas may have to travel great distances to obtain necessary treatment. The nurse must be aware of these variables and have knowledge of agencies in the local community that can assist in improving healthcare access.

Literacy is another community-related variable that can affect health care. The 2003 Adult Literacy and Life Skills Survey (ALL Survey) measured the literacy skills of adults in seven countries, including Canada, and found that 4 in 10 Canadian adults lack the literacy skills that are desired for a knowledge-based economy. Canada's Aboriginal population has even lower literacy rates, and 22% of adult Canadians have serious problems dealing with printed materials. People who do not have access to computers also have significantly lower literacy skills than computer users. The functional illiteracy rate is higher in non-English-speaking individuals and older adults. The nurse must be aware that these clients may not be able to read drug labels, understand written treatment instructions, or read brochures describing their disease or therapy. Functional illiteracy can result in a lack of understanding about the importance of pharmacotherapy and lead to poor compliance. The nurse must attempt to identify clients with low literacy and provide them with brochures, instructions, and educational materials that can be understood. For non-English-speaking clients or those for whom English is their second language, the nurse should have proper materials in the client's primary language or should provide an interpreter who can help with accurate interpretation. The nurse should ask the client to repeat important instructions, to ensure comprehension. The use of more graphical materials is appropriate for certain therapies.

For many clients, belief in a higher spiritual being is important to wellness, and prayer may be an essential component of daily life. When serious illness occurs, or when death is imminent, clients may find comfort in and support from religious rituals and artifacts. The nurse should provide proper spiritual support for these clients. The nurse may want to provide information on local ministers, priests, or rabbis who visit the hospital on a regular basis. Spiritual guidance may provide clients with positive expectations regarding their health and may improve compliance with pharmacotherapy.

Genetic Polymorphisms and Their Influence on Pharmacotherapy

7.5 Genetic differences in metabolic enzymes that occur among different ethnic groups must be considered for effective pharmacotherapy. Small differences in the structure of enzymes can result in profound changes in drug metabolism.

Although humans are 99.8% alike in their DNA sequences, the remaining 0.2% may result in significant differences in clients' ability to metabolize medications. These differences are created when a mutation occurs in the gene (a portion of DNA) responsible for encoding a certain metabolic enzyme. A single base mutation in DNA may result in an amino acid change in the enzyme, which changes its function. Hundreds of such mutations have been identified. These changes in enzyme structure and function are called **genetic polymorphisms**. The change may result in either increased or decreased drug metabolism depending on the exact type of genetic polymorphism. The study of these polymorphisms is called pharmacogenetics.

Genetic polymorphisms are most often identified in specific ethnic groups because people of an ethnic group have been located in the same geographical area and have married others within the same ethnic group for many generations. This allows the genetic polymorphism to be amplified within that population.

The relationship between genetic factors and drug response has been documented for decades. The first polymorphism was discovered in the enzyme acetyltransferase, which metabolizes isoniazid (Isotamine). The metabolic process, known as acetylation, occurs slowly in certain Caucasians. The slow clearance can cause the drug to build up to toxic levels in these clients, who are known as slow acetylators. The opposite effect, fast acetylation, is found in many Japanese people.

In recent years, several other enzyme polymorphisms have been identified. People of Asian descent are less likely to be able to metabolically convert codeine to morphine due to an inherent absence of the enzyme debrisoquine hydroxylase, a defect that interferes with the analgesic properties of codeine. As another example, some persons of African descent receive decreased effects from beta-adrenergic antagonist drugs such as propranolol (Inderal) due to genetically influenced variances in plasma renin levels. A set of oxidation enzyme polymorphisms that alter the response to warfarin (Coumadin), diazepam (Valium), and several other medications has been found. Table 7.1 summarizes the three most common enzyme polymorphisms.

TABLE 7.1 Enzyme Polymorphisms of Importance to Pharmacotherapy

Enzyme	Result of Polymorphism	Drugs Using This Metabolic Enzyme/ Pathway
Acetyltransferase	Slow acetylation in Scandinavians, Jews, North African Caucasians; fast acetylation in Japanese	Isoniazid, chlordiazepam, hydralazine, procainamide, caffeine
Debrisoquine hydroxylase	Poor metabolization in Asians and Africans	Imipramine, perphenazine, haloperidol, propranolol, metoprolol, codeine, morphine
Mephenytoin hydroxylase	Poor metabolization in Asians and Africans	Diazepam, imipramine, barbiturates, warfarin

Pharmacogenetics is the study of specific genetic variations that alter a client's responses to medications. *Pharmacogenomics* is a related term that is more general in scope, referring to the network of genes that govern a person's response to drug therapy. Both pharmacogenetics and pharmacogenomics attempt to identify genetic differences in metabolism or receptor targets that affect individual drug responses, with the ultimate goal of improving the safety and effectiveness of drug therapy through the use of genetically guided treatment. It is expected that these fields will reveal data that will someday allow drug therapy to be customized for each individual client based on his or her genetic profile.

Gender Influences on Pharmacotherapy

7.6 Gender can influence many aspects of health maintenance, promotion, and treatment, as well as medication response.

A person's gender influences many aspects of health maintenance, promotion, and treatment, as well as drug response. It is a substantiated fact, for example, that women pay more attention to changes in health patterns and seek health care earlier than their male counterparts. Conversely, many women do not seek medical attention for potential cardiac problems because heart disease is considered to be a "man's disease." Alzheimer's disease affects both men and women, but studies in various populations have shown that between 1.5 and 3 times as many women as men suffer from the disease. Alzheimer's disease is becoming recognized as a major "women's health issue," comparable to osteoporosis, breast cancer, and fertility disorders.

Acceptance or rejection of the use of particular categories of medication may be gender based. Because of the side effects associated with certain medications, some clients do not take them appropriately—or take them at all. A common example is the use of certain antihypertensive agents in men. These may cause, as a common side effect, male impotence. In certain instances, male clients have suffered a stroke because they abruptly stopped taking the drug and did not communicate this fact to their healthcare provider. With open communication, dilemmas regarding drug problems and side effects can be discussed so that alternative drug therapies can be considered. As with so many areas of health care, appropriate client teaching by the nurse is a key aspect in preventing or alleviating pharmacology-related health problems.

Research has found many examples of differences in drug response between men and women. If males and females contain nearly all of the same genes, how can these differences be explained? Although they may have identical genes, the "expression" of the genes differs greatly. For example, both males and females possess the same genes for hepatic metabolic enzymes, but one gender may produce more of a certain enzyme, thus producing a different degree of drug action. An example of a gender difference in pharmacological outcome is aspirin, which is more effective at preventing heart attacks in men than in women.

Local and systemic responses to some medications can differ between genders. These response differences may be based on differences in body composition, such as the fat-to-muscle ratio. In addition, cerebral blood flow variances between males and females may alter the response to certain analgesics. Some of the benzodiazepines used for anxiety have slower elimination rates in women, and this difference becomes even more significant if the woman is taking oral contraceptives concurrently. There are numerous gender-related situations that the nurse must understand in order to monitor drug actions and effects appropriately.

Until recently, the vast majority of drug research studies were conducted using only male subjects. It was wrongly assumed that the conclusions of these studies applied in the same manner to females. In the late 1990s, Health Canada formalized policies that require the inclusion of subjects of both genders during development of drugs intended for use by both genders. These policies include analyses of clinical data by gender, assessment of potential pharmacokinetic and pharmacodynamic differences between genders, and where appropriate, conducting additional studies specific to women's health.

CHAPTER

7

Understanding the Chapter

Key Concepts Summary

The numbered key concepts provide a succinct summary of the important points from the corresponding numbered section within the chapter. If any of these points are not clear, refer to the numbered section within the chapter for review.

7.1 To deliver holistic treatment, the nurse must consider the client's psychosocial and spiritual needs in a social context.

7.2 The psychosocial domain must be considered when taking clients' medical histories. Positive attitudes and high expectations about therapeutic outcomes in the client may increase the success of pharmacotherapy.

7.3 Culture and ethnicity are two interconnected factors that can affect nursing care and pharmacotherapy. Differences in diet, use of alternative therapies, perceptions of

wellness, and genetic makeup can influence a client's drug response.

7.4 Community and environmental factors affect health and the public's access to health care and pharmacotherapy. Inadequate access to healthcare resources and an inability to read or understand instructions may have a negative impact on treatment outcomes.

7.5 Genetic differences in metabolic enzymes that occur among different ethnic groups must be considered for effective pharmacotherapy. Small differences in the structure of enzymes can result in profound changes in drug metabolism.

7.6 Gender can influence many aspects of health maintenance, promotion, and treatment, as well as medication response.

Chapter 7 Scenario

While travelling out of province with her husband to visit her children and grandchildren, Aponi Nampeyo became ill and was hospitalized. After being examined in the emergency department, she was diagnosed with appendicitis and underwent an emergency appendectomy. Aponi is Aboriginal and has lived most of her life on a reserve. She is well educated but not overly talkative, and she is comfortable with silence.

Aponi willingly accepts Western medical treatments. However, she also relies on traditional herbs and remedies from her youth. As the nurse caring for this client, you are curious about her culture and health practices. However, you do not want to appear nosy or intrusive.

Critical Thinking Questions

1. Should nurses discuss cultural beliefs with clients? Explain your answer.

2. Describe how the nurse could learn about Mrs. Nampeyo's culture.

3. Are most healthcare workers culturally competent? Why or why not?

See Answers to Critical Thinking Questions in Appendix B.

NCLEX Practice Questions

1 In initiating holistic care with a client who has chronic headaches, which action would the nurse take?

a. Tell the client to take Tylenol as directed on the label.

b. Ask the client what he or she believes may be contributing to the problem.

c. Monitor the client's pupil response to light.

d. Refer the client to an ophthalmologist for an eye exam.

2 Various psychosocial variables may influence nonadherence to pharmacotherapy. An example of this is when a client reports that a prescribed drug

a. Produces an unpleasant aftertaste

b. Is a very large tablet and difficult to swallow

c. Is too expensive for the client to afford

d. Potentially causes hepatotoxicity

3 An Aboriginal client states, "I will take only medications that are approved by the shaman." The nurse understands that this statement reflects the client's

a. Ethnicity

b. Cultural belief

c. Genetic polymorphisms

d. Health-related bias

4 Which of the following is considered a gender factor that may influence effective pharmacotherapy? Select all that apply.

a. Fat-to-muscle ratio

b. Cerebral blood flow

c. Limited drug research on females

d. Health beliefs

e. Dietary considerations

5 Which is the most effective method for a nurse to recognize client-specific genetic influences?

a. Ask the client if there have been drug dose–related problems in the past.

b. Consult reference books and the Internet for information.

c. Observe the effects in other clients of a similar racial-ethnic background.

d. Be cautious with all drugs and observe individual client responses.

See Answers to NCLEX Practice Questions in Appendix A.

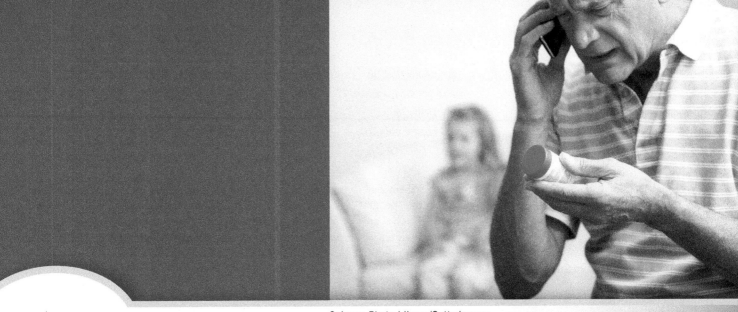

CHAPTER

8

Drug Effects, Adverse Reactions, and Interactions

LEARNING OUTCOMES

After reading this chapter, the student should be able to:

1. Differentiate between adverse effects and side effects.

2. Create a plan to minimize or prevent adverse drug events in clients.

3. Describe the incidence and characteristics of drug allergies.

4. Explain how idiosyncratic reactions differ from other types of adverse effects.

5. Explain why certain drugs with carcinogenic or teratogenic potential are used in pharmacotherapy.

6. Report the characteristic signs, symptoms, and treatment for each of the following organ-specific adverse events: nephrotoxicity, neurotoxicity, hepatotoxicity, dermatological toxicity, bone marrow toxicity, cardiotoxicity, and skeletal muscle and tendon toxicity.

7. Use examples to explain the importance of drug interactions to pharmacotherapy.

8. Describe the mechanisms of drug interactions that alter absorption, distribution, metabolism, or excretion.

9. Differentiate among additive, synergistic, and antagonistic drug interactions.

10. Identify examples of food-drug interactions that may affect pharmacotherapeutic outcomes.

CHAPTER OUTLINE

▸ The Nurse's Role in Preventing and Managing Adverse Drug Effects

▸ The Canadian Adverse Drug Reaction Information System

▸ Allergic Reactions

▸ Idiosyncratic Reactions

▸ Drugs That Have the Ability to Induce Cancer or Cause Birth Defects

▸ Drug Toxicity

▸ Drug Interactions

▸ Pharmacokinetic Drug Interactions

▸ Pharmacodynamic Drug Interactions

▸ Food, Nutrient, and Dietary Supplement Interactions

KEY TERMS

additive effect, 83	drug interaction, 80	side effects, 76
adverse drug effect, 76	idiosyncratic response, 77	synergistic effect, 83
antagonistic effect, 83	ototoxicity, 79	teratogens, 78
drug allergies, 77	risk–benefit ratio, 78	

Drugs are administered with the goal of producing a therapeutic effect. However, all drugs produce both intended therapeutic effects and unintended effects. An **adverse drug effect** is an undesirable and potentially harmful action caused by the administration of medication. Adverse effects, also called adverse events, are a significant component of pharmacotherapy and, when severe, may cause treatment to be discontinued or result in permanent harm to the client. The purpose of this chapter is to examine the different types of adverse effects and drug interactions, so that the nurse can minimize their impact on treatment outcomes.

The Nurse's Role in Preventing and Managing Adverse Drug Effects

8.1 The nurse plays a key role in preventing and managing adverse drug effects.

Although every drug has the *potential* to produce adverse events, most pharmacotherapy can be conducted without significant undesirable effects. Indeed, drugs that produce serious adverse effects are screened and removed from consideration during the drug development and approval process or are restricted for treating only serious health conditions such as cancer. Clients expect that their drugs, including over-the-counter (OTC) medications, herbal products, and dietary supplements, will be free from serious adverse effects when taken as directed. Although the majority of drugs are very safe, adverse effects cannot be avoided entirely.

Side effects are types of drug effects that are predictable and that may occur even at therapeutic doses. Side effects are less serious than adverse effects. Clients are often willing to tolerate annoying side effects if they believe that the drug will improve their condition or prevent a disease. The distinction between an adverse effect and a side effect, however, is often unclear. For example, is headache a side effect or an adverse effect? What about nausea? The answer lies in the severity of the symptoms. Headache or nausea may be minor (side effects), or they may become intense and disabling (adverse effects).

Adverse drug events may be specific to a single type of tissue or affect multiple organ systems. The most common adverse events are nausea and vomiting, which may occur when drugs are administered by any route. Headache and changes in blood pressure are also very common adverse drug events. Some adverse effects, although rare, are serious enough to warrant regular or continuous monitoring. Many adverse effects are extensions of a drug's pharmacological actions. These types of events are considered dose dependent: as the drug dose increases, the risk for adverse effects also increases. For example, antihypertensive drugs are given to lower blood pressure, but high doses cause hypotension, which may manifest as dizziness or fainting. Drugs for treating insomnia or anxiety may depress brain activity too much at higher doses, resulting in drowsiness or daytime sedation. Knowing the therapeutic actions of the drug enables the nurse to predict the signs and symptoms of many of the adverse effects that occur during treatment. It is important for nurses and their clients to understand that the difference between a drug being a beneficial medication or a toxic substance is often simply a matter of dose.

Can adverse effects be prevented? Although nurses play a key role in minimizing the number and severity of adverse events in their clients, some adverse effects simply cannot be predicted or prevented. However, skilled healthcare providers, including nurses, have multiple ways to minimize or prevent adverse effects, from having expert knowledge of how a drug acts to obtaining a comprehensive medical history from their clients. The following are means that healthcare providers use to minimize or prevent adverse drug events in their clients:

- **Obtain a thorough medical history.** The medical history of the client may reveal drug allergies or conditions that contraindicate the use of certain drugs. The history may also identify prescription drugs, OTC drugs, dietary supplements, and herbal products taken by the client that could negatively interact with the prescribed medication.

- **Thoroughly assess the client and all diagnostic data.** Assessment may reveal underlying hepatic or renal impairment that will affect the way the drug is handled by the body. The very young and the elderly are most susceptible to drug reactions because metabolism and excretion of drugs in these populations are less predictable. To prevent adverse effects, average drug doses should be adjusted based on careful client assessment.

- **Prevent medication errors.** Administering the incorrect dose or giving the drug to the wrong client may cause unnecessary adverse effects. Methods of preventing medication errors are described in detail in Chapter 10.

- **Monitor pharmacotherapy carefully.** Monitor client signs and symptoms regularly after initial drug doses or when doses are increased. This is especially critical when caring for clients who are very ill or when giving parenteral agents. Clients who are receiving drugs that have frequent or potentially severe adverse effects should be monitored continuously until the baseline effects of the drug have been established.

- **Know the drugs.** It is essential for nurses to know the most frequent and most serious adverse effects for every drug administered. A comprehensive knowledge of the drugs, herbal products, and supplements taken by their clients helps nurses to monitor for and identify adverse effects and provide the necessary interventions before they become serious.

- **Be prepared for the unusual.** Anaphylaxis may occur immediately and unpredictably, and other adverse effects may be delayed, occurring days, weeks, or months after therapy is initiated. Some drugs produce actions opposite to those expected. Clients may be reluctant to report certain adverse effects (such as impotence) without prompting by the nurse.

- **Question unusual orders.** If the nurse suspects that the wrong dose has been ordered or the pharmacy has filled the order incorrectly, the drug should not be administered until the prescriber or the pharmacy has been contacted.

- **Teach clients about adverse effects.** The client is the nurse's ally in identifying and preventing adverse effects. Teaching clients what therapeutic and adverse effects to expect from the drug and which types of symptoms to report to their healthcare providers is important in self-management and preventing serious adverse events. Furthermore, inadequate teaching may result in poor client adherence to the drug regimen and suboptimal treatment outcomes.

The Canadian Adverse Drug Reaction Information System

8.2 Health Canada continues to monitor for new adverse events after a drug is approved and marketed.

The Canadian Adverse Drug Reaction Information System (CADRIS) is a database of suspected adverse reactions to drugs, biologics, and natural health products reported to Health Canada's Canadian Adverse Drug Reaction Monitoring Program (CADRMP). These reports are submitted voluntarily by health professionals and consumers. Reports are monitored and may result in warnings to consumers about the safety of a drug or in a drug being pulled from pharmacy shelves.

Allergic Reactions

8.3 Allergic reactions are caused by a hyperresponse of the immune system.

Drug allergies are common events, comprising 6% to 10% of all adverse drug effects. Although drug allergies may elicit a diverse range of client symptoms, all are caused by a hyperresponse of body defences. Depending on the type of allergic response, basophils, mast cells, eosinophils, or lymphocytes secrete chemical mediators that trigger the allergic response. Specific chemical mediators of allergy include histamine, serotonin, leukotrienes, prostaglandins, and complements.

Several characteristics define a drug allergy. Allergies typically occur with very small amounts of drug; the severity of allergy symptoms is usually not proportional to the dose. The symptoms of allergy are unrelated to the pharmacological actions of the drug; anaphylaxis has the same symptoms regardless of the drug that induces it. Clients often exhibit cross-allergy, an allergic reaction to drugs with a similar structure, such as those from the same pharmacological class. Drug allergies require a previous exposure to the drug (or a very similar drug). This sensitizes the client to subsequent exposures, during which a hyperresponse of body defences is rapidly mounted upon re-exposure to the drug.

The signs and symptoms of drug allergy are variable and range from minor to life threatening. Symptoms may appear within minutes after the drug is administered, or they may develop after prolonged pharmacotherapy. Because the signs and symptoms of drug allergy are nonspecific, it is sometimes difficult to attribute an allergy symptom to any given drug, especially in clients who are receiving multiple drugs. Complicating an accurate diagnosis is that symptoms of drug allergy are the same as those of allergy to other substances, such as certain foods, or environmental triggers, such as insect stings, animal dander, or dust mites. It is important to determine the source of the allergy, especially in clients with severe reactions, so that the offending drug or environmental substance can be avoided in the future. The pharmacological treatment of allergy is discussed in Chapter 42.

Although allergic reactions are possible with most drugs, some medications exhibit a relatively higher incidence. The drugs or drug classes most likely to cause allergic reactions include penicillins and related antibiotics (monobactams and cephalosporins); radiological contrast media containing iodine; insulin; nonsteroidal anti-inflammatory drugs (NSAIDs), including aspirin; sulfonamides; cancer chemotherapy agents; preservatives (sulphites and paraben); and certain antiseizure drugs.

Clients are usually unaware of the true definition of allergy and often report any adverse effect they experience as a drug allergy. For example, many clients experience acute nausea and vomiting with narcotic analgesics such as codeine and will report that they have an allergy to codeine during a drug history. In fact, these symptoms are not caused by an overactive immune response and thus do not constitute a true allergy. Inaccurate reporting of allergies may lead to the healthcare provider avoiding the use of entire drug classes and prescribing more expensive second-line medications that could be less effective or produce more adverse effects.

Idiosyncratic Reactions

8.4 Idiosyncratic reactions are unusual drug responses often caused by genetic differences among clients.

Idiosyncratic response is an adverse drug effect that produces unusual and unexpected symptoms that are not related to the pharmacological action of the drug. Idiosyncratic reactions are not classified as allergies because they are not immune related. They are rare and unpredictable and vary from client to client.

Many, though not all, idiosyncratic reactions are due to unique, individual genetic differences among clients. For example, mutations involving specific metabolic enzymes may cause certain clients to be extremely sensitive to the effects of a drug or to be resistant to it. The drug may be handled by a different metabolic pathway, resulting in the accumulation of a metabolite that gives a different and unexpected response from the original drug.

Historically, the term *idiosyncratic* has been used to denote any drug effect that could not be explained. With advances in the understanding of drug mechanisms, more and more drug responses are now understood. With improved reporting of adverse drug events, rare and "unexpected" events are now documented and may be "expected." Therefore, use of the term *idiosyncratic*, although still common in clinical practice, will likely diminish with time.

Drugs That Have the Ability to Induce Cancer or Cause Birth Defects

8.5 Some drugs have the ability to induce cancer or cause birth defects.

Most adverse effects occur within minutes or hours after a drug is administered; some develop after several days or weeks of pharmacotherapy. In a few instances, the adverse effect may occur years or even decades after the drug was administered. Such is the case with drug-induced cancer.

Why would a drug be approved and given to clients if it was known to cause cancer in humans? The answer lies in the **risk–benefit ratio**. If a client has a condition that is likely to cause premature death if left untreated, the benefits of taking a drug with carcinogenic potential may outweigh the long-term risks. This assumes, of course, that effective, safer alternatives are not available.

Of the thousands of drugs and drug combinations approved for pharmacotherapy, only a few increase the risk of acquiring cancer. Most of these drugs, shown in Table 8.1, fall into three primary classes: antineoplastics, immunosuppressants, and hormonal agents.

Some antineoplastics are known chemical carcinogens. With the goal of eliminating cancer cells, some of these drugs cause molecular damage or mutations in DNA. Although much of the DNA damage in normal cells is repaired by enzymes, some mutations persist and accumulate in cells as a person ages, increasing cancer risk. The initial damage done by the drug may take decades to manifest as cancer. Leukemia is the type of cancer with the greatest cancer risk from antineoplastic therapy. However, the client may never develop cancer as a result of these medications; indeed, the majority of clients who receive antineoplastic drugs do not develop the disease. Because pharmacotherapy combined with surgery and radiation therapy can result in a total cure for some clients, the benefit of drug therapy outweighs the small risk of developing cancer later in life.

The second class of drugs that can induce cancer is the immunosuppressants. These medications are administered to dampen the immune system of clients who are receiving transplanted tissues or who have serious inflammatory disorders. Because a natural function of the immune system is to remove cancer cells that form in the body, any drug that inhibits this system would be expected to have some degree of cancer risk. Lymphoma is the most frequent type of cancer resulting from immunosuppressant use. Again, the risk is small compared to the benefits provided by these drugs.

The third group that may cause cancer consists of hormones or hormone antagonists. Little is known about the mechanisms by which hormone imbalances lead to cancer, and the topic is a subject of ongoing research. In some cases, hormones protect the client from cancer, or they may reduce the incidence of one type of cancer but increase the risk for another type. Probably the best studied of the hormone mechanisms is how estrogen binds to its intracellular receptors. About 70% of clients with breast cancer are estrogen receptor (ER)–positive: the hormone promotes tumour formation in the mammary gland. Cancers caused by hormones or hormone antagonists tend to affect reproductive organs, such as the vagina, uterus, or breast.

A similar question might be asked about drugs that cause birth defects, or **teratogens**. Why would a drug be approved if it was shown to produce birth defects in laboratory animals during the preclinical stage of drug testing? The answer to this question is very different from that for cancer-inducing drugs.

Teratogens affect a small percentage of the overall population: those who are pregnant. In most cases, these drugs are safe to use in males and in adults outside their childbearing years. Therefore, known teratogens may be approved for indications in clients who do not have the potential to become pregnant. When approved for females with reproductive potential, however, these drugs have increased risks. Although a pregnancy test may be performed prior to pharmacotherapy and the nurse may warn the client to discontinue the drug if pregnancy is suspected, the potential still remains for exposing an embryo or fetus to a toxic agent. In females with reproductive potential, teratogenic drugs are not used unless they have clear benefits that outweigh the possible risk of birth defects. All healthcare providers must carefully assess client compliance with instructions against this potential risk.

The nurse should remember that drugs are not tested in pregnant humans before Health Canada approval and that animal testing cannot predict with great accuracy the drug's effects on a human fetus. In some cases, the risks to a human embryo or fetus have been determined after a drug has been approved. The U.S. Food and Drug Administration (FDA) has established pregnancy drug categories, which gauge the risk of a drug causing birth defects (see Chapter 6). All drug use should be assumed dangerous during pregnancy, unless data have otherwise demonstrated the drug to be safe. No woman should take a drug, herbal product, or dietary supplement during pregnancy unless it is approved by the client's healthcare provider.

TABLE 8.1 Selected Drugs Suspected of Causing Cancer in Humans

Class	Drug	Type of Cancer
Antineoplastic	Adriamycin Chlorambucil Cisplatin Cyclophosphamide Dacarbazine Doxorubicin Etoposide Metronidazole Nitrosoureas Phenytoin Propylthiouracil Teniposide	Leukemia, urinary bladder
Hormones and hormone antagonists	Anabolic steroids Estrogen replacement therapy and oral contraceptives Progesterone Tamoxifen	Uterus, breast, hepatic
Immunosuppressants	Azathioprine Cyclosporine	Lymphoma, skin

Drug Toxicity

8.6 Drug toxicity may be specific to particular organs.

Very few drugs produce adverse effects in every organ system; these agents would be too toxic for safe pharmacotherapy. Instead, adverse effects are often organ specific, targeting one or a few organs. It is important for the nurse to learn these specific toxicities so that appropriate signs, symptoms, and diagnostic tests can be carefully monitored. Selected organ-specific toxicities are summarized in Table 8.2.

Nephrotoxicity

The kidneys are one of the most common organs affected by drugs. This is because these organs filter large volumes of blood, and most drugs are excreted by the renal route. Some drugs are reabsorbed or secreted by the kidney, exposing renal tubule cells to high concentrations of these agents. A few obstruct the urinary system by causing crystalluria in the urinary tract. Drug nephrotoxicity may manifest as acute symptoms that appear after one or several doses or as chronic symptoms that appear after several months of pharmacotherapy.

NCLEX Success Tips

Intrinsic renal failure results from damage to the kidney, such as from nephrotoxic injury caused by contrast media, antibiotics, corticosteroids, or bacterial toxins.

A client who is taking potentially nephrotoxic antibiotics should notify the nurse if his or her urine is cloudy, smoky, or pink; early signs of nephrotoxicity are manifested by changes in urine colour.

TABLE 8.2   Organ-Specific Toxicity

Toxicity	Example Drugs and Classes
Bone marrow	ACE inhibitors, antimalarials, antineoplastics, antiseizure drugs (carbamazepine, phenytoin), antithyroid drugs, cephalosporins, chloramphenicol, chlorpromazine, chlorpropamide, cimetidine, loop diuretics, methyldopa, NSAIDs, phenylbutazone, sulfonamides
Cardiotoxicity	Anthracycline antineoplastics (daunorubicin, doxorubicin, epirubicin, idarubicin, mitoxantrone)
Dermatological	Antiseizure drugs (carbamazepine, phenobarbital, phenytoin), cephalosporins, erythromycin, NSAIDs, penicillin, radiological contrast media, sulfonamides, tetracyclines
Hepatotoxicity	Carbamazepine, chlorpromazine, statins (HMG CoA reductase inhibitors)
Nephrotoxicity	ACE inhibitors, acyclovir, aminoglycosides, amphotericin B, cisplatin and other platinum-based antineoplastics, cocaine, cyclosporine, NSAIDs, radiological contrast media, sulfonamides, tacrolimus
Neurotoxicity	Aminoglycosides, cisplatin, ethanol, loop diuretics, methyldopa, salicylates, vincristine
Skeletal muscle and tendon toxicity	Fluoroquinolone antibiotics, statins

It is critical for the healthcare provider to identify at-risk clients and attempt to prevent drug-induced nephrotoxicity. Means for prevention include providing proper hydration, monitoring urinary laboratory values, and adjusting doses appropriately for clients with renal impairment. Clients with serious renal impairment should not receive nephrotoxic drugs unless other therapeutic options have been exhausted.

Neurotoxicity

Although the blood-brain barrier prevents many drugs from reaching the brain, neurotoxicity is a relatively common adverse effect of certain drug classes. This is because the brain receives a large percentage of the blood supply and is especially sensitive to small amounts of toxic substances. For sedatives, antidepressants, antianxiety drugs, antiseizure drugs, and antipsychotics, the difference between a therapeutic dose and one that produces adverse effects may be very small. Indeed, drowsiness is seen in a majority of clients who are receiving these drugs when therapy is initiated. Signs and symptoms of toxicity in the central nervous system (CNS) include depression, mania, sedation, behavioural changes, suicidal feelings, hallucinations, and seizures. The special senses may be affected, including visual changes, loss of balance, and hearing impairment. Hearing impairment, or **ototoxicity**, can result from drug-induced damage to the eighth cranial nerve.

Effective teaching is essential when clients are beginning therapy with potentially neurotoxic drugs. The nurse should warn clients not to drive vehicles or perform other hazardous tasks until they are familiar with the effects of these drugs. Caregivers should be taught to report changes in client behaviour because the person receiving the medication may have difficulty recognizing these signs. The nurse should be aware that neurotoxic drugs can significantly worsen pre-existing mental health disorders. Serious symptoms such as seizures, delirium, suicidal ideation, or significant visual or hearing impairment should be immediately reported to the prescriber.

NCLEX Success Tips

Neurotoxicity, the primary adverse effect of vincristine, may be manifested as blindness. Clients must report this promptly.

Neurotoxicity may also cause peripheral neuropathy.

Hepatotoxicity

The liver receives all drugs absorbed in the stomach and intestinal mucosa via the hepatic portal veins. A major function of the liver is to metabolize and detoxify drugs and other chemicals that enter the body; therefore, it should not be surprising that hepatotoxicity is one of the most common adverse drug effects. Effects of hepatotoxic drugs range from minor, transient increases in liver enzyme values to fatal hepatitis.

The nurse should regularly monitor liver enzyme tests when administering hepatotoxic drugs because changes in these laboratory values are early signs of liver toxicity. Symptoms of liver impairment are vague and nonspecific and include right upper quadrant pain, anorexia, bloating, fatigue, and nausea or vomiting. During chronic hepatotoxicity, jaundice, itching, and easy bruising are evident. In serious cases, the liver will be unable to metabolize other drugs, resulting in high serum drug levels. Extreme care must be taken when administering potentially hepatotoxic drugs to clients with pre-existing liver disease.

Dermatological Toxicity

Drug reactions affecting the skin are some of the most common types of adverse effects. These reactions may be caused by a hypersensitivity response or by nonimmune-type responses. Rash, the most common cutaneous drug reaction, usually occurs within 1 to 2 weeks of initiation of drug therapy and resolves without serious complications. Drug-induced rash is sometimes accompanied by itching (pruritus). Although almost any drug can cause rash, antibiotics are the most frequent drug class causing this condition. Urticaria (hives) are raised welts that are often accompanied by intense pruritus and, although less common than rash, are a symptom of a potential allergic reaction that could lead to anaphylaxis.

NCLEX Success Tip

A client who is receiving a blood product requires assessment for signs and symptoms of allergic reaction and anaphylaxis, including pruritus (itching), urticaria (hives), facial or glottal edema, and shortness of breath. If such a reaction occurs, the nurse should stop the transfusion immediately—but leave the intravenous line intact—and notify the physician. Usually, an antihistamine such as diphenhydramine hydrochloride is administered. Epinephrine and corticosteroids may be administered for severe reactions.

Serious and even fatal dermatological toxicity can occur. In angioedema, swelling occurs in the dermis, periorbital region, and around the mouth and throat. Angioedema is a severe drug reaction because the swelling may impair breathing and may be fatal. Phototoxicity is a type of drug-induced dermatological toxicity in which certain drugs cause the skin to absorb excess ultraviolet radiation from the sun or heat lamps. Symptoms resemble sunburn and are best prevented by advising clients to avoid direct sunlight. Phototoxicity resolves when the drug is discontinued.

Most types of drug-induced dermatological toxicity do not require pharmacological treatment. If pruritus is prominent, an antihistamine or a corticosteroid may be administered. In all cases of serious drug-induced hypersensitivity, the nurse should discontinue the drug until the cause of the skin condition can be diagnosed.

Bone Marrow Toxicity

Drugs that affect the bone marrow are of great concern because of the possibility of serious and perhaps fatal outcomes. The bone marrow serves as a nursery for the production of red blood cells, white blood cells, and platelets. Drugs may affect only one of these types of cells or all three. When all three groups are affected, drug-induced pancytopenia or aplastic anemia occurs, and the client is at great risk for serious illness. Loss of white blood cells may cause agranulocytosis or neutropenia, which places the client at risk for serious infections. The drug class most likely to cause bone marrow toxicity is the antineoplastics. Bone marrow toxicity is the dose-limiting factor with these drugs (see Chapter 60).

NCLEX Success Tips

Chemotherapeutic agents produce bone marrow depression, resulting in reduced red blood cell counts (anemia), reduced white blood cell counts (leukopenia), and reduced platelet counts (thrombocytopenia); this is collectively known as pancytopenia.

Neutropenia is the presence of a reduced number of neutrophils in the blood and is caused by bone marrow depression induced by chemotherapeutic agents.

Risk for infection takes priority in clients with severe bone marrow depression. This is because they have a decrease in white blood cells, which are the cells that fight infection. Therefore, the nurse should monitor temperature and blood cell count.

The role of the nurse in preventing bone marrow toxicity is to carefully monitor laboratory data and recognize changes that suggest impending toxicity, such as decreases in red blood cells, white blood cells, or platelets. In many cases, bone marrow toxicity can be quickly reversed if the condition is recognized early and the drug is discontinued. Furthermore, the nurse should carefully monitor the therapeutic regimen of clients who have pre-existing blood cell disorders because adding a drug with bone marrow toxicity may worsen these conditions.

Cardiotoxicity

Some drugs damage cardiac muscle cells, affecting the ability of the heart to effectively pump blood to the tissues. The most common cardiotoxic drugs are all antineoplastic medications. The cardiotoxicity of these drugs can be severe and lead to bradycardia, tachycardia, heart failure, and acute left ventricular failure. The nurse administering cardiotoxic drugs must be vigilant in observing for signs of cardiotoxicity such as excessive fatigue, cough, shortness of breath (especially when recumbent), weight gain, or peripheral edema.

NCLEX Success Tip

Imipramine, a tricyclic antidepressant, is a cardiotoxic medication for which routine electrocardiograms are needed.

Skeletal Muscle and Tendon Toxicity

Skeletal muscle is relatively resistant to the effects of drugs, despite its extensive blood supply. In skeletal muscle, the incidence of drug-induced myopathy is low, but it may be serious when it does occur. The most severe myopathy is rhabdomyolysis, a syndrome characterized by extensive muscle necrosis with the release of muscle enzymes and other constituents into the circulation. Rhabdomyolysis is a rare though serious adverse effect of statins, common medications used to treat excessive lipid levels in the blood.

To prevent skeletal muscle or tendon toxicity, the nurse should assess for unexplained muscle or joint soreness or pain during therapy. Laboratory tests such as creatine kinase should be evaluated regularly during therapy with drugs that have muscle toxicity.

Drug Interactions

8.7 Drug interactions may significantly affect pharmacotherapeutic outcomes.

A **drug interaction** occurs when a substance increases or decreases a drug's actions. The substance causing the interaction may be another drug, a dietary supplement, an herbal product, or a food. The substance participating in the drug interaction must be external to the body and is usually taken concurrently with the medication. Although substances that are naturally found in the body (endogenous substances) routinely interact with drugs, these are not considered drug interactions because they are part of the body's normal response to the drug.

Because clients often take multiple drugs concurrently, drug interactions occur continually. Even if only one drug is taken, the potential for a food-drug interaction still exists. Although drug interactions are impossible to eliminate entirely, most interactions go unnoticed and treatment outcomes are rarely affected. Indeed, it is likely that most drug interactions have yet to be documented or researched because they do not cause clinically noticeable effects or harm to the client.

Some drug interactions are important to pharmacology because they are known to cause adverse effects or otherwise affect treatment outcomes. By studying the mechanisms of potential drug interactions, the nurse can prevent certain adverse effects and optimize treatment outcomes. For example, if the client is receiving gentamicin (Garamycin), the nurse should use caution when administering acyclovir (Zovirax), because the drug combination can cause higher than normal levels of acyclovir in the blood. The prescriber should reduce the dose of acyclovir or substitute a different drug. *Understanding drug interactions can directly affect the success of pharmacotherapy.*

Drug interactions occur by dozens of different mechanisms. To simplify their study, it may be helpful to remember that drug interactions can have three basic effects on the action of a drug:

- The actions of the drug can be *inhibited*, resulting in less therapeutic action. For example, milk interferes with the absorption of tetracycline, causing a lower serum level of antibiotic, thus diminishing its therapeutic effects.

- The actions of the drug may be *enhanced*, causing a greater therapeutic response. For example, co-administration of the two antiviral drugs lopinavir and ritonavir (Kaletra) causes a greater reduction in levels of human immunodeficiency virus (HIV) than occurs when either drug is used alone.

- The drug interaction may produce a totally *new and different response*. For example, when used alone disulfiram (Antabuse) has no pharmacological effects. When taken with alcohol, however, the combination produces dramatic new actions such as severe headache, flushing, dyspnea, palpitations, and blurred vision.

Pharmacokinetic Drug Interactions

8.8 Pharmacokinetic drug interactions include changes in the absorption, distribution, metabolism, or excretion of medications.

Recall from Chapter 3 that pharmacokinetics is the branch of pharmacology that deals with how the body acts on a drug after it is administered. Many drug interactions involve some aspect of the pharmacokinetics of the medication. When studying drug interactions, it is convenient to use the same categories for pharmacokinetics that are presented in Chapter 3. The general types of pharmacokinetic interactions are illustrated in Figure 8.1.

Absorption

Most drugs need to be absorbed to produce their actions. Any substance that affects absorption has the potential to influence drug response. In fact, this is one of the most common mechanisms of drug interactions. By interfering with normal absorption, drug action may be inhibited or enhanced. Increasing absorption will raise drug serum levels and produce an enhanced effect; substances that inhibit absorption have the opposite effect.

The simplest way to affect absorption is to change the speed of substances moving through the gastrointestinal (GI) tract. Opioids such as morphine (Kadian, M-Eslon, MS Contin, MS-IR, Statex) or heroin will slow peristalsis, giving drugs additional time for absorption. Laxatives and drugs that stimulate the parasympathetic nervous system will speed substances through the GI tract, diminishing the absorption time of other drugs. The bile acid resins such as cholestyramine (Questran) bind other drugs and prevent their absorption.

Many drug-drug interactions caused by changes in absorption may be prevented by taking the two drugs at least 2 to 3 hours apart. In the case of food-drug interactions, the interacting food should be avoided, or the drug may be taken on an empty stomach. Taking drugs on an empty stomach, however, may increase the incidence of nausea or vomiting, which could result in loss of the drug before complete absorption occurs. The nurse must teach clients with drug-induced nausea not to take drugs with antacids or milk unless approved by the prescriber. Antacids are alkaline (basic) substances that raise the pH of the GI contents and have the potential to change the percentage of ionized drug. Ionized forms of drugs are less able to cross the intestinal mucosa than nonionized forms.

Distribution

Distribution is the movement of a drug from its site of absorption to its site of action. Many drugs travel through the blood bound to plasma proteins; when bound, the drug is unable to leave the blood to reach its target. Drugs may compete for available binding sites on plasma proteins; one drug may prevent another from binding to plasma proteins or may displace a drug from its binding sites. If this occurs, the amount of unbound or free drug increases, potentially raising the drug serum concentration to toxic levels. For example, diazepam (Valium) displaces phenytoin (Dilantin) from plasma proteins, causing a rapid increase in the plasma concentration of free phenytoin and an increased risk for adverse effects. Drugs that have a high potential for displacing other drugs from protein binding sites include aspirin and other NSAIDs, phenylbutazone, and sulfonamides.

A second potential drug-drug interaction involving distribution can occur if the pH of the plasma is altered by a drug. For example, when an alkaline substance such as sodium bicarbonate is infused, the pH of plasma increases, causing acidic drugs to become ionized. The ionized acidic drugs are less able to cross membranes and they accumulate in the extracellular spaces, creating an ionization (pH) gradient. The pH gradient moves acidic drugs from inside cells to the extracellular spaces, thus altering distribution.

Metabolism

A large number of drugs are metabolized by hepatic enzymes. Drug metabolites generally have less activity than the original drug

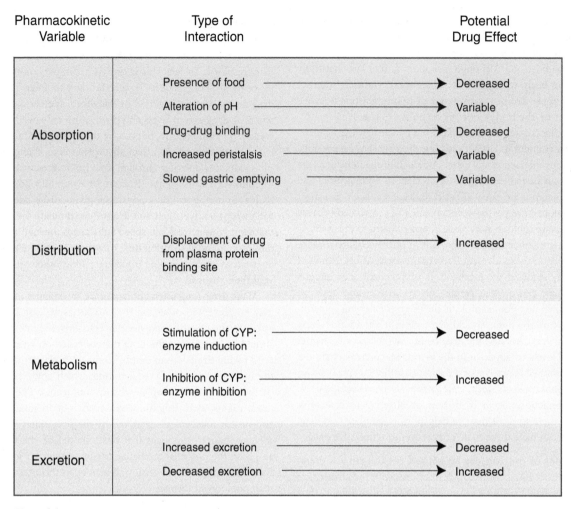

Figure 8.1   Types of pharmacokinetic drug-drug interactions.

and are more readily excreted by the kidneys. Any drug-induced change in the activity of hepatic enzymes has the potential to cause drug-drug interactions.

Certain drugs have the ability to increase (induce) or decrease (inhibit) hepatic enzyme activity. Inducers such as phenobarbital (Phenobarb) will increase drug metabolism, thus promoting the inactivation and excretion of other drugs. Clinically, this will be observed as diminished drug effectiveness. For example, if phenobarbital is administered concurrently with the antihypertensive drug nifedipine (Adalat), less blood pressure reduction will result. The dose of nifedipine will need to be increased to produce an optimal therapeutic effect. However, care must be taken if the inducer is discontinued because hepatic enzyme activity will return to baseline levels in a few days or weeks. Once hepatic enzymes return to normal, the dose of nifedipine will have to be adjusted downward to avoid toxicity. Also, remember that a few drugs (prodrugs) are *activated* by metabolism. Increasing the metabolism of prodrugs will cause an increase, rather than a decrease, in therapeutic response.

Drug interactions involving hepatic metabolism are some of the most complex in pharmacology. Although many of these interactions are not clinically significant, others clearly have the potential to affect therapeutic outcomes. The nurse will need to remember which drugs are inducers, inhibitors, and substrates of

CYP enzymes to optimize pharmacotherapeutic outcomes and minimize adverse effects.

Excretion

Most drugs are eliminated from the body through renal excretion. A drug interaction may occur if a substance changes the glomerular filtration rate (GFR), the amount of fluid (in mL) filtered by the kidney per minute. The higher the GFR, the more rapid will be the excretion of other drugs.

A second type of excretion-related interaction may occur if one drug changes the secretion or reabsorption of another drug in the renal tubule. For example, methotrexate competes with NSAIDs for the same secretion mechanism. If taken concurrently, NSAIDs will block the secretion of methotrexate, thus raising drug serum levels and increasing the potential for methotrexate toxicity.

Renal elimination may also be affected by drugs that change the pH of the filtrate in the renal tubules. Changing the pH causes drugs to become more (or less) ionized. The excretion of weak acids can be significantly increased by alkalinizing the urine through the administration of sodium bicarbonate. This drug interaction may be used therapeutically to promote more rapid excretion of acidic drugs such as aspirin during overdose situations. Similarly, excretion of weak bases can be increased by acidifying the urine through the administration of ammonium chloride.

Not all excretion-related drug interactions involve the kidneys. Some drugs are extensively excreted by the biliary system, and two drugs excreted in this way may interact through this mechanism. For example, pravastatin (Pravachol) and cyclosporine (Sandimmune, Neoral) use the same carrier protein to move drug molecules from the liver to bile. Giving the two drugs concurrently will slow the biliary excretion of pravastatin and raise its serum concentration to potentially toxic levels. Because biliary excretion is not the dominant form of elimination for most drugs, this type of drug-drug excretion interaction is far less common than those involving the kidneys.

Pharmacodynamic Drug Interactions

8.9 Pharmacodynamic drug interactions include additive, synergistic, or antagonistic effects.

Recall from Chapter 4 that pharmacodynamics is the branch of pharmacology that examines the mechanisms of drug action, meaning how a drug changes the body. Many drugs produce their actions by binding to specific receptors. When two drugs compete for the same receptor or activate receptors that produce opposite effects, drug interactions are possible. Many common interactions encountered in clinical practice are pharmacodynamic in nature.

During a pharmacodynamic drug interaction, drug action may be either enhanced or inhibited. The result of the interaction may be desirable (increased therapeutic response, decreased adverse effect) or undesirable (decreased therapeutic response, increased adverse effect).

The pharmacodynamic drug interaction that is easiest to visualize is the **additive effect**. In this interaction, two drugs from a similar therapeutic class produce a combined summation response. This is used extensively in treating hypertension. For example, a diuretic may be used to lower systolic blood pressure by 10 mm Hg, and a beta blocker may be added to the regimen to produce another 15 mm Hg reduction. Combined, the two drugs produce a 25 mm Hg reduction. Why would two drugs (with more expense to the client), rather than a single drug, be prescribed? There are two rationales. First, to produce a 25 mm Hg reduction using only the diuretic, the dose would have to be increased. Keeping the doses of both the diuretic and the beta blocker low and taking advantage of their additive effect reduces the potential for adverse drug events caused by high doses of medication. Second, some drugs have low efficacy, and it may not be possible to achieve a 25 mm Hg reduction with a single drug. The maximum effect from the diuretic may have been a 10 mm Hg reduction, so another drug would need to be added to the regimen to achieve a greater response. In this example, the two drugs act at very different types of receptors to produce the additive therapeutic response: beta blockers in cardiac muscle and diuretics in the renal tubules.

It should be remembered that additive effects also apply to adverse effects. This is seen frequently in drugs that affect the CNS. For example, narcotic analgesics, antidepressants, antiseizure drugs, and antianxiety drugs all may cause sedation as a side effect. When taken concurrently, drugs from these classes can cause additive sedation that could profoundly affect the ability to safely operate a vehicle, for example. Caution must always be used when administering multiple medications that have similar adverse effects such as nephrotoxicity, hepatotoxicity, or bone marrow toxicity.

Another pharmacodynamic drug interaction that produces an enhanced response is a **synergistic effect**. In this interaction, the effect of the two drugs is greater than would be expected from simply adding the two individual drugs' responses. This type of interaction is used extensively in treating infections. For example, Synercid is a combination drug that contains quinupristin and dalfopristin, two antibiotics that are effective against resistant *Staphylococcus* infections. Both drugs bind to the bacterial ribosome and produce greater killing than would be predicted from adding the two individual drugs' effects. Another example is the combination antibiotic Bactrim, which combines trimethoprim and sulfamethoxazole to produce a synergistic effect on bacterial cell killing.

A third type of pharmacodynamic interaction occurs when adding a second drug results in a diminished pharmacological response. This **antagonistic effect** can result in drug actions being "cancelled." For example, drugs that activate the sympathetic nervous system, such as epinephrine, will increase the heart rate and dilate the bronchi. A drug such as carvedilol (Coreg) will have the opposite effects: slowed heart rate and bronchoconstriction. Therefore, carvedilol is considered an antagonist to epinephrine and may cancel its actions, depending on the doses of the two drugs. Why would a nurse administer drugs with opposite actions? This is generally done to reduce the adverse effects of a drug.

In some cases, antagonists are used to treat symptoms of drug overdose. For example, clients who take an overdose of narcotics such as morphine or heroin experience coma and life-threatening CNS depression. The administration of naloxone (Narcan), a specific narcotic antagonist, can quickly reverse some of the serious adverse effects of morphine.

Pharmacodynamic interactions can be indirect and complex. The well-documented drug interaction between digoxin (Lanoxin, Toloxin) and diuretics, such as furosemide (Lasix), is an excellent example of an indirect effect. Furosemide enhances the excretion of potassium ion (hypokalemia), which increases the cardiotoxicity of digoxin. This can be a life-threatening interaction. Another example is the inhibition of vitamin K production in the intestine caused by antibiotics. If the client is also taking warfarin (Coumadin), bleeding may occur because the liver is prevented from producing certain clotting factors. Again, the antibiotic did not directly interact with warfarin, yet the combination produced a serious adverse effect.

Food, Nutrient, and Dietary Supplement Interactions

8.10 Food, nutrients, and dietary supplements may interact with medications and affect their actions.

Historically, interactions between drugs and food, dietary supplements, and herbal products have been largely dismissed as clinically unimportant. Although a few interactions (such as tetracyclines with calcium products) have been documented for decades, only since the late 1980s have food-drug interactions been recognized as important to maximizing pharmacotherapeutic outcomes. The interaction that prompted the increased interest in this topic was that of a benign and healthy substance: grapefruit juice. The interaction was discovered by chance in a research study designed to examine the effects of alcohol on felodipine, a calcium channel blocker. The researchers used grapefruit juice incidentally to disguise the taste of the alcohol.

Clients often take medications with juice because it covers up the bitter taste of a drug and provides a plentiful source of vitamins and minerals. Unfortunately, grapefruit juice also contains substances that increase the absorption of certain oral drugs. This occurs because grapefruit juice inhibits the enzyme CYP3A4 in the wall of the intestinal tract. As drugs are absorbed, they are not inactivated by CYP3A4, and higher amounts reach the circulation. Surprisingly, the inhibition from grapefruit juice may last for up to 3 days after drinking the juice. The substances in the juice that inhibit CYP3A4 enzymes are called furanocoumarins. Fortunately, only a few drug classes interact with grapefruit juice. These include benzodiazepines, certain calcium channel blockers, and statins (HMG-CoA reductase inhibitors).

Most of the food-drug interactions discovered thus far act by either increasing or decreasing the absorption or bioavailability of the drug. Food-drug interactions are easily avoided by timing the drug dose appropriately with the food or supplement. In most cases, there should be a minimum 2-hour gap between ingestion of the food and the drug. In a few cases, the drug should be administered with food to increase its absorption.

Very few interactions of drugs with herbal products have been clearly documented. As more clients take these products, however, research is demonstrating that certain drug-herb combinations may significantly affect pharmacotherapy. Because clients view herbal products as natural, they do not usually mention them when recording their medication history; therefore, the healthcare provider must ask specific questions about their use.

Perhaps the most widely studied herb is St. John's wort, which is taken by clients as a complementary or alternative therapy for depression. The herb induces hepatic metabolic enzymes, which can reduce the effectiveness of certain prescription medications, including antidepressants, warfarin, and benzodiazepines. A second herb that has been extensively studied is ginkgo biloba, which is taken to improve circulation and memory. Ginkgo may produce additive anticoagulant effects when taken with warfarin or antiplatelet drugs. It can also antagonize the effects of antiseizure drugs, thus increasing the risk for seizures. Because both St. John's wort and ginkgo can significantly affect drug action, the nurse should assess for the use of these substances when obtaining the client's health history.

CHAPTER

8 Understanding the Chapter

Key Concepts Summary

The numbered key concepts provide a succinct summary of the important points from the corresponding numbered section within the chapter. If any of these points are not clear, refer to the numbered section within the chapter for review.

8.1 The nurse plays a key role in preventing and managing adverse drug effects.

8.2 Health Canada continues to monitor for new adverse events after a drug is approved and marketed.

8.3 Allergic reactions are caused by a hyperresponse of the immune system.

8.4 Idiosyncratic reactions are unusual drug responses often caused by genetic differences among clients.

8.5 Some drugs have the ability to induce cancer or cause birth defects.

8.6 Drug toxicity may be specific to particular organs.

8.7 Drug interactions may significantly affect pharmacotherapeutic outcomes.

8.8 Pharmacokinetic drug interactions include changes in the absorption, distribution, metabolism, or excretion of medications.

8.9 Pharmacodynamic drug interactions include additive, synergistic, or antagonistic effects.

8.10 Food, nutrients, and dietary supplements may interact with medications and affect their actions.

Chapter 8 Scenario

The more medication an individual takes, the more likely it is that an adverse reaction may occur. For Elizabeth Washington this is a real possibility, because she takes multiple medications for various physical problems. Elizabeth is a 77-year-old Canadian of African descent who has several chronic conditions that require pharmacotherapy, including diabetes, heart failure, arthritis, and depression. She has been wheelchair bound since her stroke 2 years ago and has lost functional ability of her left side.

Unfortunately, Elizabeth does not have a regular family physician and moves from clinic to clinic. Her medical record is extensive and includes her health history for the last 15 years. Because her medical history record is so lengthy, Elizabeth fears that new doctors will not take the time to read the entire file before prescribing the newest treatment or therapy.

Critical Thinking Questions

1. Identify ways that you can minimize or prevent adverse drug events in this client.

2. What existing conditions make Elizabeth more susceptible to a drug reaction?

3. Discuss how drug reactions can affect pharmacokinetics.

4. Differentiate among additive, synergistic, and antagonist drug effects.

See Answers to Critical Thinking Questions in Appendix B.

NCLEX Practice Questions

1 Prior to the administration of an antibiotic, the client informs the nurse of having experienced an allergic reaction 4 years ago. Based on this information, what should the nurse do first?

 a. Ask the client to describe the reaction further.

 b. Notify the healthcare provider on call about the client's statements.

 c. Administer the dose and observe the client for a reaction.

 d. Check the medical administration record for documented allergies.

2 A nurse is researching a new drug prior to administration. The drug handbook states that the adverse effects are "dose related," which means that

 a. As the dose increases, the risk of adverse effects also increases.

 b. Adverse effects should be expected after the first dose.

 c. Oral preparations will produce the most adverse effects.

 d. The timing of each dose should be correlated with the presence of adverse effects.

3 The client is receiving a medication that may cause nephrotoxicity. To decrease the risk of this adverse reaction, the nurse should encourage the client to

 a. Avoid sunbathing and exposure to direct sunlight.

 b. Increase the intake of potassium-enriched foods.

 c. Abstain from alcoholic beverages.

 d. Increase fluid intake to promote adequate hydration.

4 When observing a client for bone marrow toxicity, the nurse will monitor for

 a. Increased complaints of muscle and bone pain in the lower extremities

 b. A decrease in red blood cells, white blood cells, and platelets

 c. A decrease in the range of motion of the upper and lower extremities

 d. An increase in hepatic enzymes

5 The client is receiving a medication that causes hepatotoxicity. Which symptoms would alert the nurse that this drug-related toxicity has occurred?

 a. Black furry tongue and vaginal yeast infection

 b. Sudden reduction in blood pressure on rising

 c. Right upper quadrant pain, anorexia, and jaundice

 d. Uncontrollable movements in the face, arms, and legs

See Answers to NCLEX Practice Questions in Appendix A.

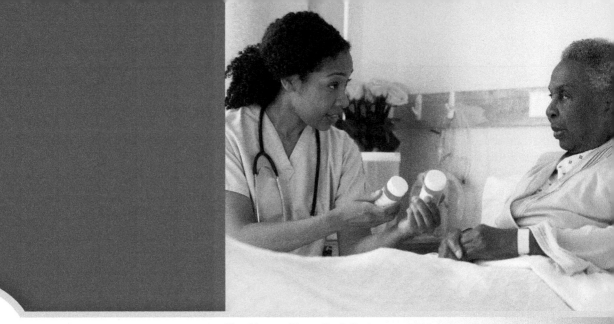

Blend Images/Alamy Stock Photo

CHAPTER

9

Principles of Drug Administration

LEARNING OUTCOMES

After reading this chapter, the student should be able to:

1. Discuss drug administration as a component of safe, effective nursing care, using the nursing process.

2. Describe the roles and responsibilities of the nurse regarding drug administration.

3. Explain how the 10 rights of drug administration affect client safety.

4. Give specific examples of how the nurse can increase client adherence in taking medications.

5. Interpret drug orders that contain abbreviations.

6. Compare and contrast the three systems of measurement used in pharmacology.

7. Explain the proper methods to administer enteral, topical, and parenteral drugs.

8. Compare and contrast the advantages and disadvantages of each route of drug administration.

CHAPTER OUTLINE

▶ Nursing Management of Drug Administration

  ▸ Medication Knowledge, Understanding, and Responsibilities of the Nurse

  ▸ The Rights of Drug Administration

  ▸ Client Adherence and Successful Pharmacotherapy

  ▸ Drug Orders and Time Schedules

  ▸ Systems of Measurement

▶ Routes of Drug Administration

  ▸ Enteral Drug Administration

  ▸ Topical Drug Administration

  ▸ Parenteral Drug Administration

The primary role of the nurse in drug administration is to ensure that prescribed medications are delivered in a safe manner. Drug administration is an important component of providing comprehensive nursing care that incorporates all aspects of the nursing process. In the course of drug administration, nurses collaborate closely with physicians, pharmacists, and, of course, their clients. The purpose of this chapter is to introduce the roles and responsibilities of the nurse in delivering medications safely and effectively.

NURSING MANAGEMENT OF DRUG ADMINISTRATION

Medication Knowledge, Understanding, and Responsibilities of the Nurse

9.1 The nurse must have comprehensive knowledge of the actions and side effects of drugs before they are administered to limit the number and severity of adverse drugs reactions.

Whether administering drugs or supervising drug use, the nurse is expected to understand the pharmacotherapeutic principles for all medications received by each client. Given the large number of different drugs and the potential consequences of medication errors, this is indeed an enormous task. The nurse's responsibilities include knowledge and understanding of the following:

- What drug is ordered
- Drug name (generic and trade) and classification
- Intended or proposed use
- Effects on the body
- Contraindications
- Special considerations (i.e., how age, gender, weight, body fat distribution, diet, genetics, and individual pathophysiological states affect pharmacokinetics, pharmacodynamics, and overall pharmacotherapeutic response)
- Side effects
- Why the medication has been prescribed for this particular client

- How the medication is to be administered, including dosage ranges
- What nursing process considerations related to the medication apply to this client

Before any drug is administered, the nurse must obtain and process pertinent information regarding the client's medical history, physical assessment, disease processes, and learning needs and capabilities. Growth and developmental factors must always be considered. It is important to remember that a large number of variables influence a client's response to medications. Having a firm understanding of these variables can increase the success of pharmacotherapy.

A major role of the nurse in pharmacotherapy is to promote optimal responses to the medication and to prevent or limit the number and severity of adverse drug events. Many adverse drug reactions (ADRs) are preventable. Professional nurses can routinely prevent many serious adverse drug reactions in their clients by applying their experience and knowledge of pharmacotherapeutics to clinical practice. Some ADRs, however, are not preventable. It is vital that the nurse be prepared to recognize and respond to potential adverse effects of medications. Professional responsibilities in reporting ADRs are discussed in Chapter 10.

Allergic and anaphylactic reactions are particularly serious ADRs that must be carefully monitored and prevented when possible. An **allergic reaction** is an acquired hyperresponse of body defences to a foreign substance (allergen). Signs of allergic reactions vary in severity and include skin rash with or without itching, edema, nausea, diarrhea, runny nose, and reddened eyes with tearing. Upon discovering that the client is allergic to a product, it is the nurse's responsibility to alert all personnel by documenting the allergy in the medical record and by applying labels to the chart and **medication administration record (MAR)**. An appropriate, agency-approved bracelet should be placed on the client next to the identification bracelet to alert all caregivers of the specific drug allergy. It is good practice to verify allergy information on the bracelet with the client. Stress at the time of hospitalization may cause the client to forget to mention a significant allergy. Information related to drug allergy must be communicated to the physician and pharmacist so that the medication regimen can be evaluated for cross-sensitivity between various pharmacological products.

The Rights of Drug Administration

9.2 The 10 rights and 3 checks are guidelines to safe drug administration, which is a collaborative effort among nurses, physicians, and other healthcare professionals.

The **10 rights of drug administration** form the operational basis for the safe delivery of medications. The 10 rights offer simple and practical guidance for the nurse during drug preparation, delivery, administration, and documentation. If followed consistently, the chance of a medication error is greatly reduced. The 10 rights are as follows:

1. Right drug
2. Right client
3. Right dose
4. Right route of administration
5. Right time of delivery and frequency
6. Right documentation
7. Right history and assessment
8. Drug approach and right to refuse
9. Right drug-drug interaction and evaluation
10. Right education and information

The 10 rights require that the nurse complete the assessment of the client and research the prescribed drug, as discussed in Chapter 5. Once the nurse determines that the drug as prescribed is appropriate and safe for this client at this time, the drug is prepared adhering to the "rights" and administered in accordance with the guidelines for safe drug administration presented in Table 9.1.

The **three checks of drug administration** that nurses use in conjunction with the 10 rights help to ascertain client safety and drug effectiveness. Traditionally, these checks incorporate checking the drug against the MAR or the medication information system at the following times:

1. When removing the drug from the medication drawer, refrigerator, or controlled substance locker
2. When preparing the drug, pouring it, taking it out of the unit dose container, or connecting the intravenous (IV) tubing to the bag
3. Immediately before administering the drug to the client

Despite all attempts to provide safe drug delivery, errors continue to occur, some of which are fatal. Although the nurse is held accountable for preparing and administering medications, safe drug practices are a result of multidisciplinary endeavours. Responsibility for accurate drug administration lies with multiple individuals, including physicians, pharmacists, and other healthcare professionals. Factors that contribute to medication errors and strategies to prevent medication errors are presented in Chapter 10. The student should review the guidelines for safe drug administration in Table 9.1 before proceeding to subsequent sections.

Client Adherence and Successful Pharmacotherapy

9.3 For pharmacological adherence, the client must understand and personally accept the value associated with the prescribed drug regimen. Understanding the reasons for nonadherence can help the nurse to increase the success of pharmacotherapy.

Adherence is a major factor that affects pharmacotherapeutic success. As it relates to pharmacology, **adherence** is taking a medication in the manner prescribed by the practitioner or, in the case of over-the-counter (OTC) drugs, following the instructions on the label. Client nonadherence ranges from not taking the medication at all to taking it at the wrong time or in the wrong manner.

TABLE 9.1   Guidelines for Safe Drug Administration

Certain protocols and techniques are common to all methods of drug administration:
- Know and apply the medication policies of the hospital or agency.
- Review the medication order and check for drug allergies.
- Wash hands and apply gloves, if indicated.
- Use aseptic technique when preparing and administering parenteral medications.
- Identify the client by asking the person to state his or her full name (or by asking the parent or guardian), checking the identification band, and comparing this information with the MAR.
- Ask the client about known allergies.
- Inform the client of the drug name, intended effect, and method of administration.
- Position the client for the appropriate route of administration.
- For enteral drugs, assist the client to a sitting position.
- If the drug is pre-packaged (unit dose), remove it from its packaging at the bedside, when possible. This enables the nurse to check the package label directly, provides a safe way to preserve the medication if the client is unable to receive the drug at the last moment (e.g., vomits), and provides an opportunity for the nurse to demonstrate checking the label for the "right drug" for able clients.
- Unless specifically instructed to do so in the orders, do not leave drugs at the bedside. Remain with the client until all medication has been swallowed.
- When giving more than one medication to a client, the following chronological order is recommended: give tablets and capsules followed by water or other liquid; then give liquids diluted with water as required. Cough medicine is given undiluted and is not followed by liquids. Sublingual and buccal tablets are given last.
- Document the medication administration and any pertinent client responses on the MAR. Documenting immediately after administration decreases the chance that another dose of the drug will be given by another caregiver.

Although the nurse may be extremely conscientious in applying all of the principles of effective drug administration, these strategies are of little value unless the client agrees that the prescribed drug regimen is personally worthwhile. Before administering the drug, the nurse should use the nursing process to formulate a personalized care plan that will best enable the client to become an active participant in his or her care (see Chapter 5). This allows the client to accept or reject the pharmacological therapy based on accurate information that is presented in a manner that addresses individual learning styles. It is imperative to remember that a responsible, well-informed adult always has the legal option of refusing to take any medication.

In the plan of care, it is important to address essential information that the client must know regarding the prescribed medications. This includes factors such as the name of the drug; why it has been ordered; expected drug actions; associated side effects; and potential interactions with other medications, foods, herbal supplements, or alcohol. Clients need to be reminded that they share an active role in ensuring their own medication effectiveness and safety.

Many factors can influence whether clients comply with pharmacotherapy. The drug may be too expensive or not approved by the client's health insurance plan. Clients sometimes forget doses of medications, especially when they must be taken three or four times per day. Clients often discontinue the use of drugs that have annoying side effects or those that impair major lifestyle choices. Adverse effects that often prompt nonadherence are headache, dizziness, nausea, diarrhea, and impotence.

Clients often take medications in an unexpected manner, sometimes self-adjusting their doses. Some clients believe that if one tablet is good, two must be better. Others believe that they will become dependent on the medication if it is taken as prescribed; therefore, they take only half the required dose. Clients are usually reluctant to admit or report nonadherence to the nurse for fear of being reprimanded or feeling embarrassed. Because the reasons for nonadherence are many and varied, the nurse must be vigilant in questioning clients about their medications. When pharmacotherapy fails to produce the expected outcomes, nonadherence should be considered a possible explanation.

Drug Orders and Time Schedules

9.4 There are established orders and time schedules by which medications are routinely administered. Documentation of drug administration and reported side effects are important responsibilities of the nurse.

Healthcare providers use accepted abbreviations to communicate the directions and times for drug administration, although for safety reasons abbreviations must be used minimally. Table 9.2 lists common abbreviations.

TABLE 9.2	Drug Administration Abbreviations		
Abbreviation	**Meaning**	**Abbreviation**	**Meaning**
ac	before meals	qd	every day*
ad lib	as desired/directed	qh	every hour
AM	morning	qhs	bedtime (every night)*
bid	twice per day	qid	four times per day
cap	capsule	qod	every other day*
/d	per day	q2h	every 2 hours (even)
gtt	drop	q4h	every 4 hours (even)
h or hr	hour	q6h	every 6 hours (even)
hs	hour of sleep/ bedtime	q8h	every 8 hours (even)
no	number	q12h	every 12 hours
pc	after meals; after eating	Rx	take
PM	afternoon	STAT	immediately; at once
PO	by mouth; orally	tab	tablet
PRN or prn	when needed/ necessary	tid	three times per day
q	every		

*The Institute for Safe Medication Practices recommends the following changes to avoid medication errors: for qd, use "daily" or "every day"; for qhs, use "nightly"; for qod, use "every other day."

A **STAT order** refers to any medication that is needed immediately and is to be given only once. It is often associated with emergency medications that are needed for life-threatening situations. The term *STAT* comes from *statim*, the Latin word meaning "immediately." The physician normally notifies the nurse of any STAT order, so that the medication can be obtained from the pharmacy and administered immediately. The time frame between writing the order and administering the drug should be 5 minutes or less. Although not as urgent, an **ASAP order** (as soon as possible order) should be available for administration to the client within 30 minutes of the written order.

The **single order** is for a drug that is to be given only once and at a specific time, such as a preoperative order. A **PRN order**, from the Latin *pro re nata*, is administered *as required* by the client's condition. The nurse makes the judgment, based on client assessment, as to when such a medication is to be administered. A **continuing order** is for a drug that is to be given on an ongoing basis for a specific number of doses or days. An example is "ampicillin 250 mg PO qid for 5 days." Continuing orders usually are initiated within 2 hours of the time the order is written by the physician. Sometimes a **standing order** is written in advance of a routine situation and is to be carried out under specific circumstances. An example is a set of postoperative PRN prescriptions that are written for all clients who have undergone a specific surgical procedure. "Acetaminophen elixir 325 mg PO q4h PRN sore throat" may be ordered for all clients who have undergone a tonsillectomy. The nurse must then assess the safety of implementing the order for a particular client. Because of the legal implications of putting all clients into a single treatment category, such orders are not permitted in some facilities. It is important to be aware that agencies differ in the way they define the terms *continuing order* and *standing order* and to clarify how the term is defined in a particular agency.

Agency policies dictate that drug orders be reviewed by the attending physician within specific time frames. Prescriptions for narcotics and other scheduled drugs are often automatically discontinued after specific time frames depending on practice environment, unless specifically reordered by the physician. Automatic stop orders do not generally apply when the number of doses, or an exact period of time, is specified.

Some medications must be taken at specific times. If a drug causes stomach upset, it is usually administered with meals to prevent epigastric pain, nausea, and vomiting. Other medications should be administered between meals because food interferes with absorption. Some central nervous system (CNS) drugs and antihypertensives are best administered at bedtime because they may cause drowsiness. Sildenafil (Viagra) is unique in that it should be taken 30 to 60 minutes prior to expected sexual intercourse to achieve an effective erection. The nurse must pay careful attention to educating clients about the timing of their medications to enhance adherence and to increase the potential for therapeutic success.

Once medications are administered, the nurse must correctly document that they have been given to the client. It is necessary to include the drug name, dosage, time administered, any assessments, and the nurse's signature. If a medication is refused or omitted, this fact must be recorded on the appropriate form within the medical record. It is customary to document the reason, when possible. Should the client voice any concerns or complaints about the medication, these are also included.

Systems of Measurement

9.5 Systems of measurement used in pharmacology include the metric, apothecary, and household systems. Although the metric system is most commonly used, the nurse must be able to convert dosages among the three systems of measurement.

Dosages are labelled and dispensed according to their weight, quantity, or volume. Three systems of measurement are used in pharmacology: metric, apothecary, and household.

The **International System of Units (SI)**, the modern **metric system**, is the most common system of drug measurement. The volume of a drug is expressed in terms of the litre (L) or millilitre (mL). The cubic centimetre (cc) is a common measurement of volume that is equivalent to 1 mL of fluid. The metric weight of a drug is stated in terms of kilograms (kg), grams (g), milligrams (mg), or micrograms (mcg or μg). A **unit (U)** is a particular quantity. Insulin is an example of a drug that is prescribed in units.

The **apothecary system** and **household system of measurement** are older systems of measurement. Although most physicians and pharmacies use the metric system, these older systems are still encountered. Approximate equivalents between metric, apothecary, and household units of volume and weight are listed in Table 9.3.

Because Canadians are very familiar with the teaspoon, tablespoon, and cup, it is important for the nurse to be able to convert between the household and metric systems of measurement. In the hospital, a glass of fluid is measured in millilitres or cubic centimetres: an 8-ounce glass of water is recorded as 240 mL. If a client being discharged is ordered to drink 2400 mL of fluid per day, the nurse may instruct the client to drink ten 8-ounce glasses, or 10 cups, of fluid per day. Likewise, when a child is to be given a drug that is administered in elixir form, the nurse should explain that 5 mL of the drug is the same as 1 teaspoon. The nurse

TABLE 9.3 Approximate Metric, Apothecary, and Household Measurement Equivalents

Metric	Apothecary	Household
1 mL	15 minims	15 drops
5 mL	1 fluidram	1 teaspoon or 75 drops
15 mL	4 fluidrams	1 tablespoon or 3 teaspoons
30 mL	8 fluidrams or 1 fluid ounce	2 tablespoons
240–250 mL	8 fluid ounces (1/2 pint)	1 glass or cup
500 mL	1 pint	2 glasses or 2 cups
1 L	32 fluid ounces or 1 quart	4 glasses or 4 cups or 1 quart
1 mg	1/60 grain	—
60–64 mg	1 grain	—
300–325 mg	5 grains	—
1 g	15–16 grains	—
1 kg	—	2.2 pounds

To convert grains to grams: divide grains by 15 or 16.

To convert grams to grains: multiply grams by 15 or 16.

To convert minims to millilitres: divide minims by 15.

should encourage the use of accurate medical dosing devices at home, such as oral dosing syringes, oral droppers, cylindrical spoons, and medication cups. These are preferred over the traditional household measuring spoon because they are more accurate. Eating utensils that are commonly referred to as teaspoons or tablespoons often do not hold the volume that their names imply.

ROUTES OF DRUG ADMINISTRATION

The three broad categories of routes of drug administration are enteral, topical, and parenteral, with subsets within each category. Each route has both advantages and disadvantages. While some drugs are formulated to be given by several routes, others are specific to only one route. Pharmacokinetic considerations, such as how the route of administration affects drug absorption and distribution, are discussed in Chapter 3.

Enteral Drug Administration

9.6 The enteral route includes drugs given orally and those administered through nasogastric or gastrostomy tubes. This is the most common route of drug administration.

The **enteral route** of drug administration includes drugs given orally and those administered through nasogastric or gastrostomy tubes. Oral drug administration is the most common, the most convenient, and usually the least costly of all routes. It is also considered the safest route because the skin barrier is not compromised and, in cases of overdose or error, medications remaining in the stomach can be retrieved. Oral preparations are available in tablet, capsule, and liquid forms. Medications administered by the enteral route take advantage of the vast absorptive surfaces of the oral mucosa, stomach, or small intestine.

Tablets and Capsules

Tablets and capsules are the most common forms of drugs. Clients prefer tablets or capsules over other routes and forms because of their ease of use. In some cases, tablets may be scored for more individualized dosing. Clients should be instructed to take tablets and capsules with a full glass of water and then to sit up for 15 minutes.

Some clients, particularly children, have difficulty swallowing tablets and capsules. Although crushing tablets or opening capsules and sprinkling the drug over food or mixing it with juice could make it more palatable and easier to swallow, this should be avoided in many situations. Do *not* crush tablets or open capsules unless the manufacturer specifically states that this is permissible. Some drugs are inactivated by crushing or opening, while others severely irritate the stomach mucosa and cause nausea or vomiting. Occasionally, drugs should not be crushed because they irritate the oral mucosa, are extremely bitter, or contain dyes that stain the teeth. Most drug guides provide lists of drugs that may not be crushed. Another reason not to mix medicine with food is that children may become less willing to eat the food. Guidelines for administering tablets and capsules are given in Table 9.4.

NCLEX Success Tips

Do not break or crush enteric-coated medications, which are designed for release and absorption in the small intestine.

As a rule, do not break or crush extended-release medications. Some scored formulations can be broken without affecting the release mechanism, and some mixed-release capsules can be opened and their contents sprinkled on food. Read product literature carefully.

The strongly acidic contents within the stomach can present a destructive obstacle to the absorption of some medications. To overcome this barrier, tablets may have a hard, waxy coating that enables them to resist the acidity. These **enteric-coated** tablets are designed to dissolve in the alkaline environment of the small intestine. It is important that the nurse not crush enteric-coated tablets, as the medication would then be directly exposed to the stomach environment.

Studies have clearly demonstrated that adherence declines as the number of doses per day increases. With this in mind, pharmacologists have attempted to design new drugs so that they may be administered only once or twice daily. **Sustained-release** tablets or capsules are designed to dissolve very slowly. This releases the medication over an extended time and results in a longer duration of action for the medication. Also called extended-release (XR), long-acting (LA), or slow-release (SR) medications, these forms allow for the convenience of once- or twice-daily dosing. Extended-release medications must not be crushed or opened.

Giving medications by the oral route has certain disadvantages. The client must be conscious and able to swallow properly. Certain types of drugs, including proteins, are inactivated by digestive enzymes in the stomach and small intestine. Medications absorbed from the stomach and small intestine first travel to the liver, where they may be inactivated before they ever reach their target organs. This process, called first-pass metabolism, is discussed in Chapter 4. The significant variation in the motility of the gastrointestinal (GI) tract and in its ability to absorb medications can create differences in bioavailability. In addition, children and some adults have an aversion to swallowing large tablets and capsules or to taking oral medications that are distasteful.

Sublingual and Buccal Drug Administration

For sublingual and buccal administration, the tablet is not swallowed but kept in the mouth. The mucosa of the oral cavity contains a rich blood supply that provides an excellent absorptive surface for certain drugs. Medications given by this route are not subjected to destructive digestive enzymes and do not undergo hepatic first-pass metabolism.

For the **sublingual (SL)** route, the medication is placed under the tongue and allowed to dissolve slowly, as shown in Figure 9.1(a). Because of the rich blood supply in this region, the sublingual route results in a rapid onset of action. Sublingual dosage forms are most often formulated as rapidly disintegrating tablets or soft gelatin capsules filled with liquid drug.

When multiple drugs have been ordered, the sublingual preparations should be administered after oral medications have been swallowed. The client should be instructed not to move the drug with the tongue and not to eat or drink anything until the medication has dissolved completely. The sublingual mucosa is not suitable for

TABLE 9.4 Enteral Drug Administration

Drug Form	Administration Guidelines
Tablet, capsule, and liquid	1. Assess that the client is alert and has the ability to swallow.
	2. Place tablets or capsules into medication cup. (A tablet in a single dose packet may be torn at the top, ready to hand to the client.)
	3. If liquid, shake the bottle to mix the agent (if it is a suspension) and measure the dose into the cup at eye level.
	4. Hand the client the medication cup.
	5. Offer a glass of water to facilitate swallowing the medication. Milk or juice may be offered if not contraindicated.
	6. Remain with the client until all medication is swallowed.
Sublingual	1. Assess that the client is alert and has the ability to hold medication under the tongue.
	2. Place sublingual tablet under the client's tongue.
	3. Instruct the client not to chew or swallow the tablet or move the tablet around with the tongue.
	4. Instruct the client to allow tablet to dissolve completely before swallowing saliva.
	5. Remain with the client to determine that all of the medication has dissolved.
	6. Offer a glass of water, if the client desires.
Buccal	1. Assess that the client is alert and has the ability to hold medication between the gums and the cheek.
	2. Place the buccal tablet between the gum line and the cheek.
	3. Instruct the client not to chew or swallow the tablet or move the tablet around with the tongue.
	4. Instruct the client to allow the tablet to dissolve completely before swallowing saliva.
	5. Remain with the client to determine that all of the medication has dissolved.
	6. Offer a glass of water, if the client desires.
Nasogastric and gastrostomy	1. Administer liquid forms when possible to avoid clogging the tube.
	2. If solid, crush finely into powder and mix thoroughly with at least 30 mL of warm water until dissolved.
	3. Assess and verify tube placement.
	4. Turn off feeding, if applicable to the client.
	5. Aspirate stomach contents and measure the residual volume. If greater than 100 mL for an adult, check agency policy.
	6. Return residual via gravity and flush with water.
	7. Pour medication into syringe barrel and allow it to flow into the tube by gravity. Give each medication separately, flushing between with water.
	8. Keep head of bed elevated for 1 hour to prevent aspiration.
	9. Re-establish continual feeding, as scheduled. Keep head of bed elevated 45 degrees to prevent aspiration.

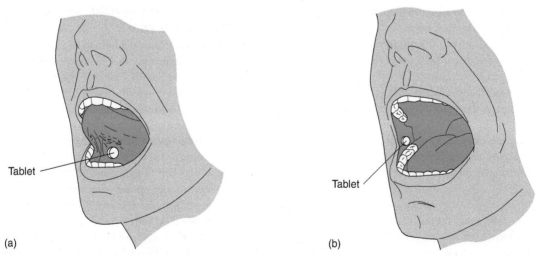

Tablet

(a)

Tablet

(b)

Figure 9.1 (a) Sublingual drug administration; (b) buccal drug administration.

extended-release formulations because it is a relatively small area and is constantly being bathed by a substantial amount of saliva. Table 9.4 presents important points regarding sublingual drug administration.

To administer by the **buccal route**, the tablet or capsule is placed in the oral cavity between the gum and the cheek, as shown in Figure 9.1(b). The client must be instructed not to manipulate the medication with the tongue; otherwise it could get displaced to the sublingual area, where it would be absorbed more rapidly, or to the back of the throat, where it could be swallowed. The buccal mucosa is less permeable to most medications than the sublingual area, providing for slower absorption. The buccal route is preferred over the sublingual route for sustained-release delivery because of its greater mucosal surface area. Drugs formulated for buccal administration generally do not cause irritation and are small enough to not cause discomfort to the client. Like the sublingual route, the buccal route avoids first-pass metabolism by the liver and the enzymatic processes of the stomach and small intestine. Table 9.4 provides important guidelines for buccal drug administration.

Elixirs, Syrups, and Suspensions

Liquids come in three forms. Elixirs contain drugs that are in a solution of water and alcohol. Cough medicines are often available as elixirs. A syrup contains the drug in a sugary, sticky solution. Acetaminophen is available as a syrup, for example. A suspension contains finely divided drug particles dispersed in a liquid. A suspension must always be shaken to ensure that the drug is dispersed evenly throughout the liquid before it is poured. Failure to shake the bottle every time it is used allows the drug to settle to the bottom, so the last dose poured would contain the largest dose of drug. Some antibiotics are available in suspensions.

Nasogastric and Gastrostomy Drug Administration

Clients with a nasogastric tube or enteral feeding mechanism such as a gastrostomy tube may have their medications administered through these devices. A nasogastric (NG) tube is a soft, flexible tube inserted by way of the nasopharynx with the tip lying in the stomach. A gastrostomy (G) tube is surgically placed directly into the client's stomach. Generally, the NG tube is used for short-term treatment, whereas the G tube is inserted for clients who require long-term care. Drugs administered through these tubes are usually in liquid form. Although solid drugs can be crushed or dissolved, they tend to cause clogging of the tubes. Sustained-release drugs should not be crushed and administered through NG or G tubes. Drugs administered by this route are exposed to the same physiological processes as those given orally. Table 9.4 lists important guidelines for administering drugs through NG and G tubes.

NCLEX Success Tips

If the client is receiving enteral feeding, ensure the compatibility of medication and feeding; if they are not compatible, turn off tube feeding for 30 to 60 minutes before and after medication administration.

Flush the enteral tube with approximately 30 mL of water following each medication.

If the enteral tube is connected to suction, disconnect it from suction for at least 30 minutes after administering medication.

Maintain the client in semi-Fowler's position for at least 30 minutes following administration of medication.

Topical Drug Administration

9.7 Topical drugs are applied locally to the skin or membranous linings of the eye, ear, nose, respiratory tract, urinary tract, vagina, and rectum.

Topical drugs are those applied locally to the skin or the membranous linings of the eye, ear, nose, respiratory tract, urinary tract, vagina, and rectum. These applications include the following:

- Dermatological preparations: Drugs are applied to the skin; this is the topical route most commonly used. Formulations include creams, lotions, gels, powders, and sprays.

- Instillations and irrigations: Drugs are applied into body cavities or orifices. These include the eyes, ears, nose, urinary bladder, rectum, and vagina.

- Inhalations: Drugs are applied to the respiratory tract by inhalers, nebulizers, or positive pressure breathing apparatuses. The most common indication for inhaled drugs is bronchoconstriction due to bronchitis or asthma; however, a number of illegal, abused drugs are taken by this route because it provides a very rapid onset of drug action.

NCLEX Success Tips

After performing hand hygiene, apply gloves to prevent drug absorption through the fingertips.

Alternate application areas to prevent skin irritation and apply to clean, dry, intact, and hairless skin.

Many drugs are applied topically to produce a *local* effect. For example, antibiotics may be applied to the skin to treat skin infections. Antineoplastic agents may be instilled into the urinary bladder via a catheter to treat tumours of the bladder mucosa. Corticosteroids are sprayed into the nostrils to reduce inflammation of the nasal mucosa due to allergic rhinitis. Local, topical delivery produces fewer side effects compared with the same drug given orally or parenterally. This is because, when given topically, these drugs are absorbed very slowly and the amounts that reach the general circulation are minimal.

Some drugs are given topically to provide for slow release and absorption of the drug to the general circulation. These agents are given for their *systemic* effects. For example, a nitroglycerin patch is not applied to the skin to treat a local skin condition but to treat a systemic condition—coronary artery disease. Likewise, prochlorperazine suppositories are inserted rectally not to treat a disease of the rectum but to alleviate nausea.

The distinction between topical drugs given for local effects and those given for systemic effects is an important one for the nurse. In the case of local drugs, absorption is undesirable and may cause side effects. For systemic drugs, absorption is essential for the therapeutic action of the drug. With either type of topical agent, drugs should not be applied to abraded or denuded skin, unless this is ordered by a physician.

Transdermal Delivery System

The use of transdermal patches provides an effective means of delivering certain medications. Examples include nitroglycerin for angina pectoris and scopolamine (Buscopan, Transderm-V) for motion sickness. Although transdermal patches contain a specific amount of drug, the rate of delivery and the actual dose received may be variable. Patches are changed on a regular basis, using a site rotation routine, which should be documented in the MAR. Before applying a transdermal patch, the nurse should verify that the previous patch has been removed and disposed of appropriately. Drugs to be administered by this route avoid the first-pass effect in the liver and bypass digestive enzymes. Table 9.5 and Figure 9.2 explain the major points of transdermal drug delivery.

TABLE 9.5   Topical Drug Administration

Drug Form	Administration Guidelines
Transdermal	1. Obtain transdermal patch and read manufacturer's guidelines. Application site and frequency of changing differ according to medication. 2. Apply gloves before handling to avoid absorption of the agent by the nurse. 3. Remove previous medication or patch and cleanse area. 4. If using a transdermal ointment, apply the ordered amount of medication in an even line directly on the pre-measured paper that accompanies the medication tube. 5. Press patch or apply medicated paper to clean, dry, and hairless skin. 6. Rotate sites to prevent skin irritation. 7. Label patch with date, time, and initials.
Ophthalmic	1. Instruct the client to lie supine or to sit with head slightly tilted back. 2. With non-dominant hand, pull the client's lower lid down gently to expose the conjunctival sac, creating a pocket. 3. Ask the client to look upward. 4. Hold eyedropper 0.5 cm above the conjunctival sac. Do not hold dropper over eye, as this may stimulate the blink reflex. 5. Instill prescribed number of drops into the centre of the pocket. Avoid touching eye or conjunctival sac with tip of eyedropper. 6. If applying ointment, apply a thin line of ointment evenly along inner edge of lower lid margin, from inner to outer canthus. 7. Instruct the client to close eye gently. Apply gentle pressure with finger to the nasolacrimal duct at the inner canthus for 1–2 minutes to avoid overflow drainage into nose and throat, thus minimizing risk of absorption into the systemic circulation. 8. With tissue, remove excess medication around eye. 9. Replace dropper. Do not rinse eyedropper.
Otic	1. Instruct the client to lie on side or to sit with head tilted so that affected ear is facing up. 2. If necessary, clean the pinna of the ear and the meatus with a clean washcloth to prevent any discharge from being washed into the ear canal during instillation of the drops. 3. Position pinna backward and upward for an adult (see Figure 9.4, p. 96). Position pinna backward and slightly downward for a child (see Figure 9.5, p. 96). This straightens the ear canal. 4. Hold dropper 0.5 cm above ear canal and instill prescribed number of drops into the side of the ear canal, allowing drops to flow downward. Avoid placing drops directly on the tympanic membrane. 5. Gently apply intermittent pressure to the tragus of the ear three or four times. 6. Instruct the client to remain on side for up to 10 minutes to prevent loss of medication. 7. If cotton ball is ordered, pre-soak with medication and insert it into the outermost part of ear canal. 8. Wipe any solution that may have dripped from the ear canal with a tissue.
Nasal drops or sprays	1. Ask the client to blow the nose to clear nasal passages. 2. Instruct the client to lie or sit with head tilted back and slightly toward the side of the target nostril/sinus (head tilted slightly to the left for the left nostril/sinus; head tilted slightly to the right for the right nostril/sinus). 3. Draw up correct volume of drug into dropper if a drop. 4. Instruct the client to open and breathe through the mouth. 5. Hold tip of the dropper or spray just above the nostril and pointing toward the ear and, without touching nose with the dropper, direct the solution laterally toward the midline of the superior concha of the ethmoid bone—not the base of the nasal cavity, where it will run down the throat and into the eustachian tube. 6. Ask the client to remain in position for 5 minutes. 7. Discard any remaining solution that is in the dropper.
Vaginal	1. Instruct the client to assume a supine position with knees bent and separated. 2. Place water-soluble lubricant into medicine cup.

TABLE 9.5 Topical Drug Administration (*continued*)

Drug Form	Administration Guidelines
	3. Apply gloves; open suppository and lubricate the rounded end.
	4. Expose the vaginal orifice by separating the labia with non-dominant hand.
	5. Insert rounded end of the suppository about 8–10 cm along the posterior wall of the vagina, or as far as it will pass.
	6. If using a cream, jelly, or foam, gently insert applicator 5 cm along the posterior vaginal wall and slowly push the plunger until empty. Remove applicator and place on a paper towel.
	7. Ask the client to lower legs and remain lying in the supine or side-lying position for 5–10 minutes following insertion.
Rectal suppositories	1. Instruct the client to lie on left side (Sims' position).
	2. Apply gloves; open suppository and lubricate the rounded end.
	3. Lubricate the gloved forefinger of the dominant hand with water-soluble lubricant.
	4. Inform the client when the suppository is to be inserted; instruct the client to take slow, deep breaths and deeply exhale during insertion to relax the anal sphincter.
	5. Gently insert the lubricated end of suppository into the rectum, beyond the anal-rectal ridge to ensure retention.
	6. Instruct the client to remain in Sims' position or to lie supine to prevent expulsion of the suppository.
	7. Instruct the client to retain the suppository for at least 30 minutes to allow absorption to occur, unless the suppository is administered to stimulate defecation.

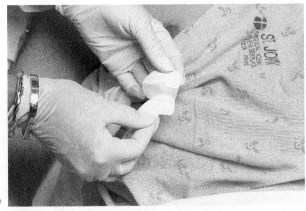
(a)

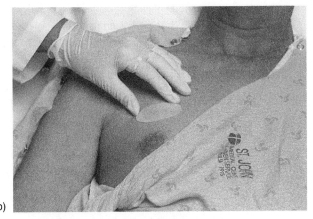
(b)

Figure 9.2 Transdermal patch administration: (a) protective coating is removed from the patch; (b) patch immediately applied to clean, dry, hairless skin and labelled with date, time, and initials.
Source: Pearson Education/PH College.

NCLEX Success Tip

Drop the prescribed number of drops into the lower subconjunctival sac while applying pressure to the inner canthus to reduce systemic absorption of the medication. Apply ointment along the inside edge of the entire lower eyelid, from the inner canthus to the outer canthus.

Ophthalmic Administration

The ophthalmic route is used to treat local conditions of the eye and surrounding structures. Common indications include excessive dryness, infections, glaucoma, and dilation of the pupil during eye examinations. Ophthalmic drugs are available in the form of eye irrigations, drops, ointments, and medicated discs. Table 9.5 and Figure 9.3 give guidelines for adult administration. Although the procedure is the same with a child, it is advisable to enlist the help of an adult caregiver. In some cases, the infant or toddler may need to be immobilized with arms wrapped to prevent accidental injury to the eye during administration.

For the young child, demonstrating the procedure using a doll facilitates cooperation and decreases anxiety.

NCLEX Success Tip

Straighten out the ear canal. For an infant or young child, pull pinna of the ear gently downward and backward. For an adult, pull pinna gently upward and backward.

Otic Administration

The otic route is used to treat local conditions of the ear, including infections and soft blockages of the auditory canal. Otic medications include eardrops and irrigations, which are usually ordered for cleaning purposes. Figure 9.4 illustrates the procedure for otic administration in adults. Administration to infants and young children must be performed carefully to avoid injury to sensitive structures of the ear, as shown in Figure 9.5. Table 9.5 presents key points in administering otic medications.

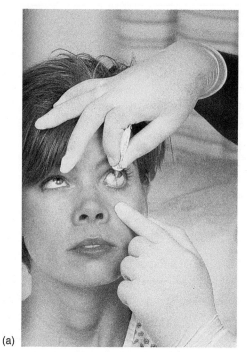

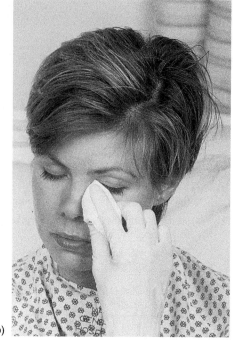

(a)

(b)

Figure 9.3   Ophthalmic administration: (a) instilling an eye ointment into the lower conjunctival sac; (b) pressing on the nasolacrimal duct.

Source: © Jenny Thomas Photography.

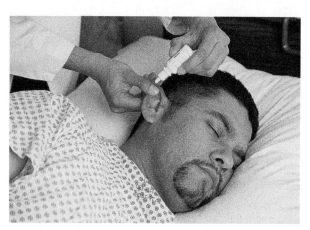

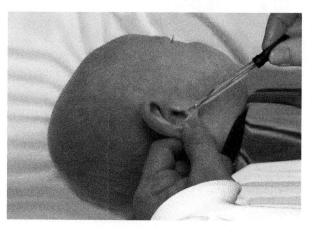

Figure 9.4   Position the pinna backward and upward when instilling eardrops in adults.

Source: © Elena Dorfman.

Figure 9.5   Position the pinna backward and slightly downward when instilling eardrops in children.

Source: Shirley King.

NCLEX Success Tip

Instruct the client not to sneeze or blow his or her nose and to keep the head tilted back for 5 minutes until the medication is absorbed.

Nasal Administration

The nasal route is used for both local and systemic drug administration. The nasal mucosa provides an excellent absorptive surface for certain medications. Advantages of this route include ease of use and avoidance of the first-pass effect and digestive enzymes. Nasal spray formulations of corticosteroids have revolutionized

the treatment of allergic rhinitis due to their high safety margin when administered by this route.

Although the nasal mucosa provides an excellent surface for drug delivery, there is the potential for damage to the cilia within the nasal cavity, and mucosal irritation is common. In addition, unpredictable mucous secretion among some individuals may affect drug absorption from this site.

Drops or sprays are often used for their local **astringent effect**, which is to shrink swollen mucous membranes or to loosen secretions and facilitate drainage. This brings immediate relief from the nasal congestion caused by the common cold. The nose also provides the route to reach the nasal sinuses

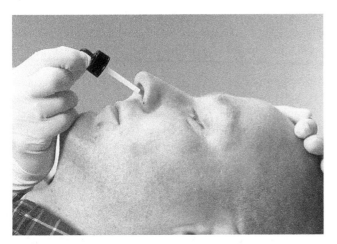

Figure 9.6 Nasal drug administration.
Source: Pearson Education/PH College.

and the eustachian tube. Proper positioning of the client prior to instilling nose drops for sinus disorders depends on which sinuses are being treated. The same holds true for treatment of the eustachian tube. Table 9.5 and Figure 9.6 illustrate important points related to nasal drug administration.

Vaginal Administration

The vaginal route is used to deliver medications for treating local infections and to relieve vaginal pain and itching. Vaginal medications are inserted as suppositories, creams, jellies, or foams. It is important that the nurse explain the purpose of treatment and provide for privacy and client dignity. Before inserting vaginal drugs, the nurse should instruct the client to empty her bladder to lessen both the discomfort during treatment and the possibility of irritating or injuring the vaginal lining. The client should be offered a perineal pad following administration. Figure 9.7 illustrates administration of a vaginal suppository and cream. Table 9.5 provides guidelines regarding vaginal drug administration.

Rectal Administration

The rectal route may be used for either local or systemic drug administration. It is a safe and effective means of delivering drugs to clients who are comatose or who are experiencing nausea and vomiting. Rectal drugs are normally in suppository form, although a few laxatives and diagnostic agents are given via enema. Although absorption is slower than by other routes, it is steady and reliable provided the medication can be retained by the client. Venous blood from the lower rectum is not transported by way of the liver; therefore, the first-pass effect is avoided, as are the digestive enzymes of the upper GI tract. Table 9.5 gives details regarding rectal suppository administration.

Parenteral Drug Administration

9.8 Parenteral administration is the dispensing of medications via a needle, usually into the skin layers (intradermal), subcutaneous tissue (subcutaneous), muscles (intramuscular), or veins (intravenous).

Parenteral administration refers to the dispensing of medications by routes other than oral or topical. The **parenteral route** delivers drugs via a needle into the skin layers, subcutaneous tissue, muscles, or veins. More advanced parenteral delivery includes administration into arteries, body cavities (such as intrathecal), and organs (such as intracardiac). Parenteral drug administration is much more invasive than topical or enteral administration. Because of the potential for introducing pathogenic microbes directly into the blood or body tissues, aseptic techniques must be strictly applied. The nurse is expected to identify and use appropriate materials for parenteral drug delivery, including specialized equipment and techniques involved in the preparation and administration of injectable products. The nurse must know the correct anatomical locations for parenteral administration and the safety procedures regarding hazardous equipment disposal.

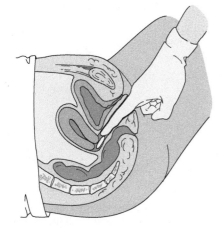

(a)

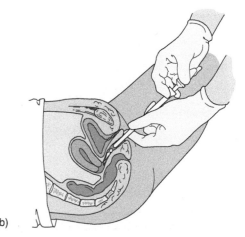

(b)

Figure 9.7 Vaginal drug administration: (a) instilling a vaginal suppository; (b) using an applicator to instill a vaginal cream.
Pearson Education

NCLEX Success Tip

Ensure the compatibility of a piggyback medication with the currently infusing IV solution and ingredients (such as potassium) or medications. If they are compatible, discontinue the primary infusion temporarily if it's safe to do so, or start a second IV line. Set up the secondary set, following the procedure for setting up an IV.

Intradermal and Subcutaneous Administration

Injection into the skin delivers drugs to the blood vessels that supply the various layers of the skin. Drugs may be injected either intradermally or subcutaneously. The major difference between these methods is the depth of injection. An advantage of both methods is that they offer a means of administering drugs to clients who are unable to take them orally. Drugs administered by these routes avoid the hepatic first-pass effect and digestive enzymes. Disadvantages are that only small volumes can be administered, and injections can cause pain and swelling at the injection site.

An **intradermal (ID)** injection is administered into the dermis layer of the skin, as illustrated in Figure 9.8. Because the dermis contains more blood vessels than the deeper subcutaneous layer, drugs are more easily absorbed. This method is usually employed for allergy and disease screening (Mantoux test) or for local anesthetic delivery prior to venous cannulation. Intradermal injections are limited to very small volumes of drug, usually only

0.1 to 0.2 mL. The usual sites for ID injections are the non-hairy skin surfaces of the upper back, over the scapulae, the high upper chest, and the inner forearm. Guidelines for intradermal injections are provided in Table 9.6.

A **subcutaneous (SC)** injection is delivered to the subcutaneous (fatty) tissue. Insulin, heparin, vitamins, some vaccines, and other medications are given in this tissue because it is easily accessible and contains no large blood vessels. Body sites that are ideal for SC injections include the following:

- Outer aspect of the upper arms, in the area above the triceps muscle
- Middle two-thirds of the anterior thigh area
- Subscapular areas of the upper back
- Upper dorsogluteal and ventrogluteal areas
- Abdominal areas, above the iliac crest and below the diaphragm, 4 to 5 cm out from the umbilicus

Subcutaneous doses are small in volume, usually ranging from 1.5 to 2 mL. The needle size varies with the client's quantity of body fat. The length is usually one-half the size of a pinched or bunched skin fold that can be grasped between the thumb and forefinger. It is important to rotate injection sites in an orderly and documented manner to promote absorption, minimize tissue damage, and alleviate discomfort. For insulin, however, rotation should be within an anatomical area to promote reliable absorption and maintain consistent blood glucose levels.

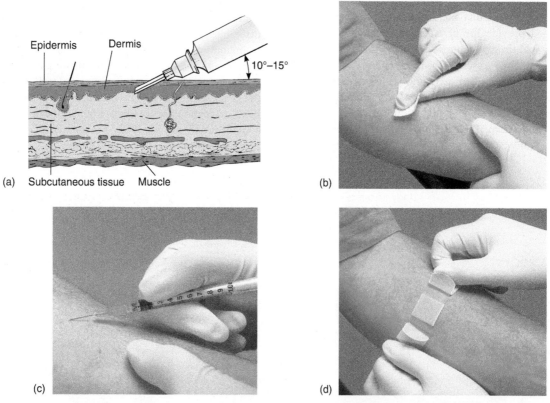

Figure 9.8 Intradermal drug administration: (a) cross-section of skin showing depth of needle insertion; (b) the administration site is prepared; (c) the needle is inserted, bevel up, at a 10- to 15-degree angle; (d) the needle is removed and the puncture site is covered with an adhesive bandage.

Pearson Education

TABLE 9.6 Parenteral Drug Administration

Drug Form	Administration Guidelines
Intradermal (ID)	1. Prepare medication in a tuberculin or 1-mL syringe, using a 25- to 27-gauge, 1.0- to 1.6-cm (3/8- to 5/8-inch) needle. 2. Apply gloves and cleanse injection site with antiseptic swab in a circular motion. Allow to air-dry. 3. With thumb and index finger of non-dominant hand, spread skin taut. 4. Insert needle, with bevel facing upward, at angle of 10–15 degrees. 5. Advance needle until entire bevel is under skin; do not aspirate. 6. Slowly inject medication to form small wheal or bleb. 7. Withdraw needle quickly, and pat site gently with sterile 5 × 5 cm (2 × 2 inch) gauze pad. Do not massage area. 8. Instruct the client not to rub or scratch area.
Subcutaneous (SC)	1. Prepare medication in a 1- to 3-mL syringe using a 23- to 25-gauge, 1.3- to 1.6-cm (1/2- to 5/8-inch) needle. For heparin and insulin, the recommended needle is 1 cm (3/8 inch) and 25–27 gauge. Insulin syringes are marked in units and usually have needles already attached. 2. Choose site, avoiding areas of bony prominence, major nerves, and blood vessels. For heparin, check agency policy for the preferred injection sites. 3. Check previous rotation sites and select a new area for injection. (Selection of sites for insulin is discussed in Chapter 28.) 4. Apply gloves and cleanse injection site with antiseptic swab in a circular motion. Allow to air-dry. 5. Bunch the skin between thumb and index finger of non-dominant hand or spread taut if there is substantial SC tissue. 6. Insert needle at 45- or 90-degree angle depending on body size and depth of SC tissue: 90 degrees if obese or average; 45 degrees if underweight. If the client is very thin, gather skin at area of needle insertion and administer at 90-degree angle. 7. Aspiration is usually not required for SC injections. If agency policy requires aspiration for non-heparin injections, aspirate by pulling back on plunger. If blood appears, withdraw the needle, discard the syringe, and prepare a new injection. For heparin, do not aspirate, as this can damage surrounding tissues and cause bruising. 8. Inject medication slowly. 9. Remove needle quickly, and gently pat site with antiseptic swab or gauze. For heparin, do not massage the site, as this may cause bruising or bleeding.
Intramuscular (IM): ventrogluteal site	1. Prepare medication using a 20- to 23-gauge, 3.8-cm (1.5-inch) needle. 2. Apply gloves and cleanse ventrogluteal injection site with antiseptic swab in a circular motion. Allow to air-dry. 3. Locate site by placing the non-dominant hand with heel on the greater trochanter and thumb toward umbilicus. Point to the anterior iliac spine with the index finger, spreading the middle finger to point toward the iliac crest (forming a V). Injection of medication is given within the V-shaped area of the index and third finger. 4. Insert needle with smooth, dart-like movement at a 90-degree angle within V-shaped area. 5. Aspirate, and observe for blood. If blood appears, withdraw the needle, discard the syringe, and prepare a new injection. 6. Inject medication slowly with smooth, even pressure on the plunger. 7. Remove needle quickly. 8. Apply pressure to site with a dry, sterile 5 × 5 cm (2 × 2 inch) gauze and massage vigorously to create warmth and promote absorption of the medication into the muscle.
Intravenous (IV)	1. To add drug to an IV fluid container: 　a. Verify order and compatibility of drug with IV fluid. 　b. Prepare medication in a 5- to 20-mL syringe using a 2.5- to 3.8-cm (1- to 1.5-inch), 19- to 21-gauge needle. 　c. Locate medication port on IV fluid container and cleanse with antiseptic swab. 　d. Carefully insert needle or access device into port and inject medication. 　e. Withdraw needle and mix solution by rotating container end to end. 　f. Apply gloves and assess injection site for signs and symptoms of inflammation or extravasation. 　g. Hang container and check infusion rate. 2. To add drug to an IV bolus (IV push) using existing IV line or IV lock (reseal): 　a. Verify order and compatibility of drug with IV fluid. 　b. Determine the correct rate of infusion. 　c. Determine if IV fluids are infusing at proper rate (IV line) and that IV site is adequate. 　d. Prepare drug in a syringe with 25- to 26-gauge needle.

(continued)

TABLE 9.6 Parenteral Drug Administration (*continued*)

Drug Form	Administration Guidelines
	e. Apply gloves and assess injection site for signs and symptoms of inflammation or extravasation.
	f. Select injection port, on tubing, closest to insertion site (IV line).
	g. Cleanse tubing or lock port with antiseptic swab and insert needle into port.
	h. If administering medication through an existing IV line, occlude tubing by pinching just above the injection port.
	i. Slowly inject medication over designated time, not usually faster than 1 mL/min, unless specified.
	j. Withdraw syringe. Release tubing and ensure proper IV infusion if using an existing IV line.
	k. If using an IV lock, check agency policy for use of saline flush before and after injecting medications.

Movement from one anatomical area to another should occur in a systematic order in accordance with agency and regional policies. Movement to a new anatomical area will allow previous areas time to rejuvenate.

Site preparation should be in accordance with agency policy. Alcohol preparation may be preferred for hygienic reasons in some situations. However, alcohol swabs can be drying and toxic to cells with repeated application, and some clients prefer to cleanse the site with soapy water and rinse with plain water prior to injection. Soap and water and proper site rotation may help to reduce **lipoatrophy**, the damage and scarring of subcutaneous tissue, in diabetic clients. When performing SC injections, it is not necessary to aspirate prior to the injection. Note that tuberculin syringes and insulin syringes are not

interchangeable, so the nurse should not substitute one for the other. Table 9.6 and Figure 9.9 provide important information regarding SC drug administration.

Intramuscular Administration

An **intramuscular (IM)** injection delivers medication into specific muscles. Because muscle tissue has a rich blood supply, medication moves quickly into blood vessels to produce a more rapid onset of action than with oral, ID, or SC administration. The anatomical structure of muscle permits this tissue to receive a larger volume of medication than the subcutaneous region. An adult with well-developed muscles can safely tolerate up to 5 mL of medication in a large muscle, although only 2 to 3 mL

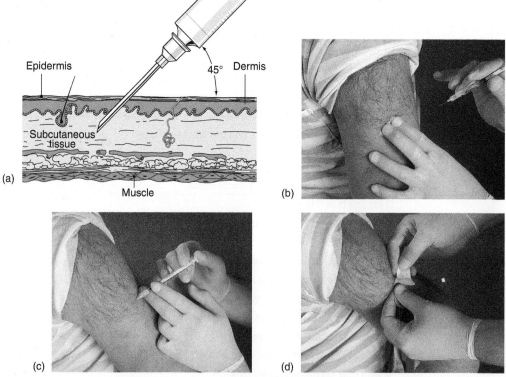

Figure 9.9 Subcutaneous drug administration: (a) cross-section of skin showing depth of needle insertion; (b) the administration site is prepared; (c) the needle is inserted, bevel up, at a 45-degree angle; (d) the needle is removed and the puncture site is covered with an adhesive bandage.
Pearson Education

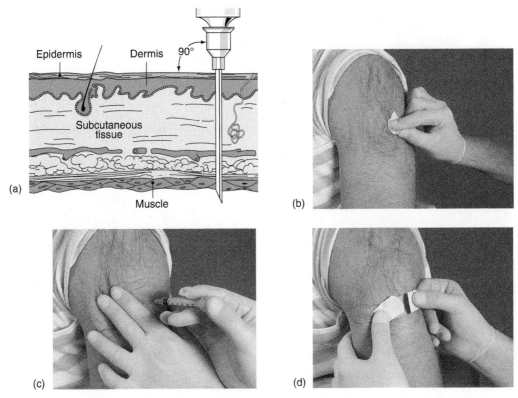

Figure 9.10 Intramuscular drug administration: (a) cross-section of skin showing depth of needle insertion; (b) the administration site is prepared; (c) the needle is inserted at a 90-degree angle; (d) the needle is removed and the puncture site is covered with an adhesive bandage.

Pearson Education

is recommended. The deltoid and triceps muscles should receive a maximum of 1 mL.

A major consideration for the nurse regarding IM drug administration is the selection of an appropriate injection site. Injection sites must be located away from bone, large blood vessels, and nerves. The size and length of needle are determined by body size and muscle mass, the type of drug to be administered, the amount of adipose tissue overlying the muscle, and the age of the client. Information regarding IM injections is given in Table 9.6 and Figure 9.10. The four common sites for intramuscular injections are as follows:

- Ventrogluteal: This is the preferred site for IM injections. This area provides the greatest thickness of gluteal muscles, contains no large blood vessels or nerves, is sealed off by bone, and contains less fat than the buttock area, thus eliminating the need to determine the depth of subcutaneous fat. It is a suitable site for children and infants over 7 months of age.
- Deltoid: This site is used in adults and well-developed teens for volumes of medication not to exceed 1 mL. Because the radial nerve lies in close proximity, the deltoid is not generally used except for small-volume vaccines, such as hepatitis B in adults.
- Dorsogluteal: This site is used for adults and for children who have been walking for at least 6 months. The site is safe as

long as the nurse appropriately locates the injection landmarks to avoid puncture or irritation of the sciatic nerve and blood vessels.

- Vastus lateralis: Usually thick and well developed in both adults and children, the middle third of the muscle is the site for IM injections.

Intravenous Administration

Intravenous (IV) medications and fluids are administered directly into the bloodstream and are immediately available for use by the body. The IV route is used when a very rapid onset of action is desired. Like other parenteral routes, IV medications bypass the enzymatic process of the digestive system and the first-pass effect of the liver. The three basic types of IV administration are as follows:

- Large-volume infusion: This is used for fluid maintenance, replacement, or supplementation. Compatible drugs may be mixed into a large-volume IV container with fluids such as normal saline or Ringer's lactate. Table 9.6 and Figure 9.11 describe and illustrate this technique. Do not add a drug to an IV bag that is already connected to the client and infusing, because concentrated drug may be drawn into the infusion line before being distributed in the solution bag. An IV drug should be added to a full bag of solution, rotated to promote even distribution, and then connected to the client.

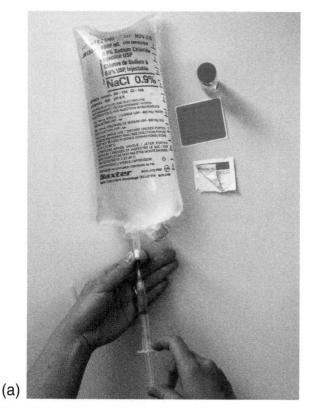

(a)

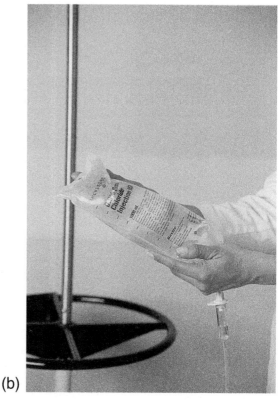

(b)

Figure 9.11 Adding a drug to an IV solution bag: (a) inserting the drug through the injection port of the IV bag; (b) rotating the IV bag to distribute the drug.

Sources: (a) Shirley L. King; (b) © Elena Dorfman.

- Intermittent infusion: This is a small amount of IV solution that is arranged tandem or piggybacked to the primary large-volume infusion. It is used to instill adjunct medications, such as antibiotics or analgesics, over a short time period. This is illustrated in Figure 9.12.

- IV bolus (push): A concentrated dose is delivered directly to the circulation via syringe. This is used to administer single-dose medications. Bolus injections may be given through an intermittent injection port or by direct IV push. Details on the bolus administration technique are given in Table 9.6 and Figure 9.13.

Although the IV route offers the fastest onset of drug action, it is also the most dangerous. Once injected, the medication cannot be retrieved. If the drug solution or the needle is contaminated, pathogens have a direct route to the bloodstream and body tissues. Clients who are receiving IV injections must be closely monitored for adverse reactions. Some adverse reactions occur immediately after injection; others may take hours or days to appear. Antidotes for drugs that can cause potentially dangerous or fatal reactions must always be readily available.

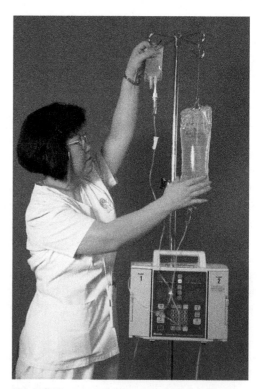

Figure 9.12 An intermittent IV infusion given piggyback to the primary infusion.

Source: Pearson Education/PH College.

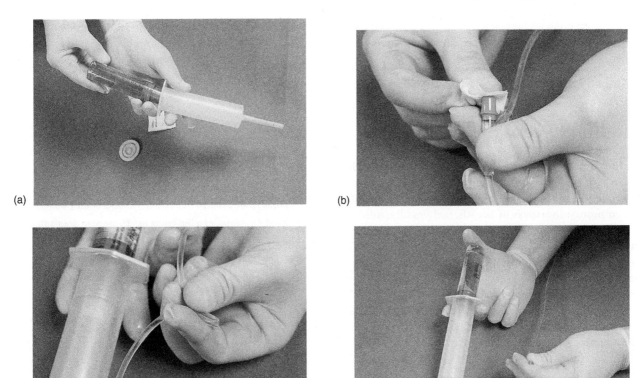

Figure 9.13 Intravenous bolus administration: (a) drug is prepared; (b) administration port is cleaned; (c) line is pinched; (d) drug is administered.

Source: Pearson Education/PH College.

CHAPTER
9   Understanding the Chapter

Key Concepts Summary

The numbered key concepts provide a succinct summary of the important points from the corresponding numbered section within the chapter. If any of these points are not clear, refer to the numbered section within the chapter for review.

9.1 The nurse must have comprehensive knowledge of the actions and side effects of drugs before they are administered to limit the number and severity of adverse drugs reactions.

9.2 The 10 rights and 3 checks are guidelines to safe drug administration, which is a collaborative effort among nurses, physicians, and other healthcare professionals.

9.3 For pharmacological adherence, the client must understand and personally accept the value associated with the prescribed drug regimen. Understanding the reasons for

nonadherence can help the nurse to increase the success of pharmacotherapy.

9.4 There are established orders and time schedules by which medications are routinely administered. Documentation of drug administration and reported side effects are important responsibilities of the nurse.

9.5 Systems of measurement used in pharmacology include the metric, apothecary, and household systems. Although the metric system is most commonly used, the nurse must be able to convert dosages among the three systems of measurement.

9.6 The enteral route includes drugs given orally and those administered through nasogastric or gastrostomy tubes. This is the most common route of drug administration.

9.7   Topical drugs are applied locally to the skin or membranous linings of the eye, ear, nose, respiratory tract, urinary tract, vagina, and rectum.

9.8   Parenteral administration is the dispensing of medications via a needle, usually into the skin layers (intradermal), subcutaneous tissue (subcutaneous), muscles (intramuscular), or veins (intravenous).

Chapter 9 Scenario

Mr. Jim is a 75-year-old patient on a cardiac unit. He is known to have hypertension and diabetes mellitus type 2. He arrived at the emergency department with the following symptoms: shortness of breath, tachycardia, mild confusion, and slight chest pain. Mr. Jim was stabilized and admitted for further investigation. During the a.m. shift, while the nurse is administering Mr. Jim's medication, the client claims that the colours of the hypertension and diabetes tablets that the nurse wants him to take are different from the colours of the drugs he receives at home. Because of this difference in colours, Mr. Jim refuses to take the medications.

Critical Thinking Questions

1. Why is it that errors continue to occur despite the fact that the nurse follows the 10 rights and 3 checks of drug administration?

2. What strategies can the nurse use to promote drug adherence for a client who is refusing to take his or her medication?

3. Compare the oral, topical, IM, SC, and IV routes. Which has the fastest onset of drug action? Which routes avoid the hepatic first-pass effect? Which require strict aseptic technique?

See Answers to Critical Thinking Questions in Appendix B.

NCLEX Practice Questions

1 For safety reasons, if a client is at risk of not being able to swallow safely and might aspirate, the best nursing action is to

   a. Reposition the patient

   b. Change the medication to a liquid form and try again

   c. Withhold the medication and contact the person who prescribed it

   d. Crush the medication, as this decreases the chance of choking or aspirating

2 When administering a sublingual medication, which of the following instructions should the nurse provide to the client?

   a. Do not chew or swallow the tablet.

   b. Keep the head of the bed elevated for at least 1 hour.

   c. Keep the tablet between the gums and cheek.

   d. Drink a lot of water to ensure that the tablet is dissolved.

3 A one-time (single) order indicates that

   a. The client can choose when he or she will use it

   b. A medication is to be given immediately

   c. The medication is to be given only once at a specified time

   d. One additional dose can be administered after a routine medication order has been discontinued

4 When administering all medications, they should be kept as clean as possible. Which of the following types of medication must be kept sterile when administering them?

   a. Oral solutions

   b. Vaginal irrigations

   c. Ophthalmic solutions

   d. Nasal instillations

5 Your client has two eye medications ordered for 1000. The nurse will

   a. Apply the second medication immediately after the first to avoid repeated irritation

   b. Contact the healthcare provider to change the scheduled times

   c. Wait 5 minutes between medications

   d. Wait 2 hours between medications

See Answers to NCLEX Practice Questions in Appendix A.

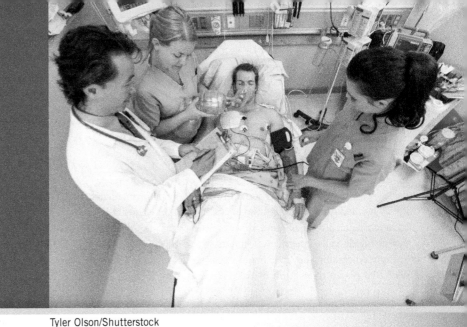

Tyler Olson/Shutterstock

10 Medication Incidents and Risk Reduction

LEARNING OUTCOMES

After reading this chapter, the student should be able to:

1. Explain how the ethical principles contained in the Code of Ethics for Registered Nurses by the Canadian Nurses Association (CNA) are used to guide nurses in their practice.

2. Apply general moral principles to the effective administration of medications.

3. Discuss the standards of care in the application of the nursing process.

4. Explain the importance of documentation in the administration of medications.

5. Discuss factors that contribute to medication incidents.

6. Identify the process in reporting and managing medication incidents.

7. Describe strategies that the nurse may implement to prevent medication incidents.

8. Describe the role of the nurse in reporting adverse drug reactions (ADRs).

9. Discuss client education that is important for safe medication usage.

CHAPTER OUTLINE

▶ Medication Incidents

▶ National Programs for Monitoring Medication Incidents and Reducing Risk

▶ Ethics and Standards of Nursing Practice

▶ Factors Contributing to Medication Incidents

▶ Drug Names and Medication Errors

▶ The Impact of Medication Incidents

▶ Documenting and Reporting Medication Incidents

▶ Strategies for Preventing Medication Incidents

▶ Providing Client Education for Safe Medication Usage

In their clinical practice, nurses are sensitive to the complexities of medication administration and the potential for incidents involving medications. Medication incidents that put clients at risk include medication errors and adverse drug reactions. Although nurses highly value proficiency and strive for 100% accuracy in giving medications, they may inadvertently be involved in an incident that places their client at risk for injury. Doing harm to a client is every nurse's greatest fear. "To do no harm" is the ethical principle of **non-maleficence**, and **beneficence** is the obligation to seek interventions that are beneficial for the client. These two principles guide nursing care in both theory and practice.

Medication Incidents

10.1 Medication incidents that put clients at risk include medication errors and adverse drug reactions. Medication incidents impede pharmacotherapeutic outcomes, increase hospitalization costs, and can result in serious illness or death.

Medication incidents that put clients at risk include medication errors and adverse drug reactions. Medication incidents impede pharmacotherapeutic outcomes, increase hospitalization costs, and can result in serious illness or death. An **adverse drug reaction (ADR)** is an undesired and unexpected client response to an administered medication. ADRs can range from rashes to anaphylaxis and death. **Medication errors** are situations where the wrong drug or medication is prescribed or given, the medication is improperly administered, or an incorrect dosage or protocol is used. According to Health Canada, medication errors are the most common single preventable cause of client injury. Medication incidents may lead to litigation against the nurse, physician, pharmacist, or healthcare agency. Medication errors occur even among the most conscientious healthcare professionals.

National Programs for Monitoring Medication Incidents and Reducing Risk

10.2 Health Canada has two programs aimed at monitoring and reducing the risk for medication incidents. Medication errors should be reported to the Canadian Medication Incident Reporting and Prevention System (CMIRPS). Adverse drug reactions should be reported to MedEffect. Both programs provide easy online reporting.

Health Canada is concerned with medication incidents at the national level. The Canadian Medication Incident Reporting and Prevention System (CMIRPS), funded by Health Canada, is a new national medication incident reporting and prevention system. A number of healthcare and client safety organizations, including the Canadian Patient Safety Institute (CPSI), Institute for Safe Medication Practices Canada (ISMP Canada), Canadian Institute for Health Information (CIHI), Canadian Nurses Association (CNA), Canadian Medical Association (CMA), and Canadian Pharmacists Association (CPhA), helped to develop the system. CMIRPS is aimed at promoting an open, "blame-free," non-punitive system that encourages healthcare practitioners to voluntarily report medication incidents.

CMIRPS categorizes errors using the algorithm (a step-by-step process) shown in Figure 10.1. This algorithm was developed by the National Coordinating Council for Medication Error Reporting and Prevention (NCC MERP) in the United States. Analysis focuses on the extent of harm that an error can cause, as shown in Figure 10.2, and is used to plan strategies to promote safe medication practices and prevent medication errors.

Health Canada's Marketed Health Products Directorate (MHPD) developed the MedEffect program to provide easy, centralized access to current, relevant, and reliable health product safety information. This includes access to Health Canada's advisories, warnings, and recalls; the *Canadian Adverse Reaction Newsletter* (CARN); and the Canadian Adverse Drug Reaction Monitoring Program (CADRMP).

The MedEffect program aims to increase awareness about the importance of reporting adverse drug reactions to Health Canada and to make it as simple as possible for health professionals and consumers to complete and file ADR reports via the Web, phone, fax, or mail. *It is the responsibility of the nurse to become familiar with this program and know how to file an ADR report in the event of an occurrence.* An ADR report should be filed whenever an ADR is suspected; confirmation of the ADR is not required. The accuracy of available drug information on potentially harmful effects depends on reporting. Sometimes ADR reports result in drugs being removed from the market to protect client safety.

Ethics and Standards of Nursing Practice

10.3 Standards of nursing practice include definition of roles, responsibilities, and practices relating to the safe delivery of medications.

Drug administration is one of the most important responsibilities of the nurse, and one that has obvious ethical and legal connections to nursing practice. Knowledge of applicable codes of **ethics** and standards of practice is essential to provide for client safety.

The CNA published the Code of Ethics for Registered Nurses to provide guidance for decision making concerning ethical matters and a basis for evaluating ethical nursing practice. The code

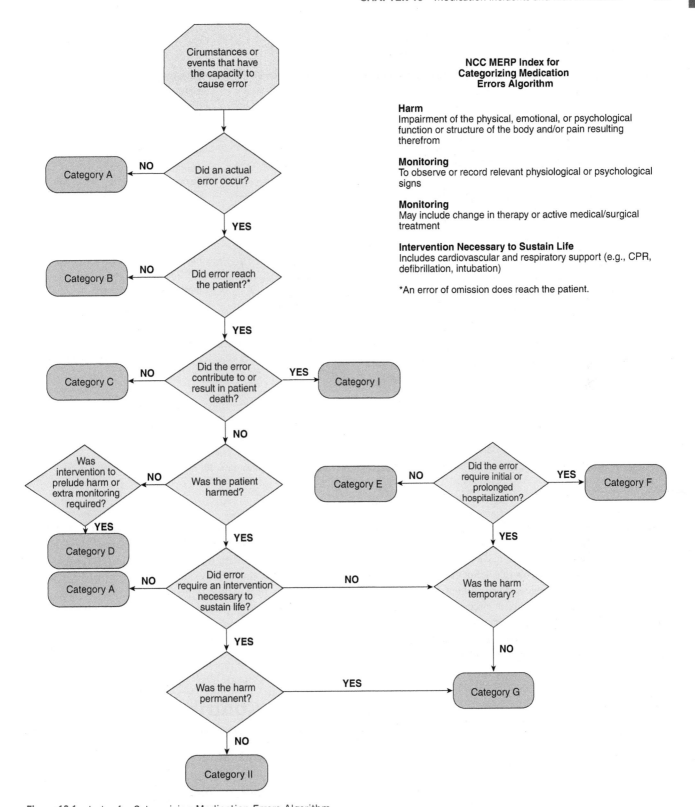

Figure 10.1 Index for Categorizing Medication Errors Algorithm.

informs nurses, other healthcare professionals, and members of the public about the ethical responsibilities and moral commitments expected of nurses. Because the registered nurse and nursing student are required to practise and administer medications in accordance with the code, they should obtain a current copy of the complete code from the CNA website.

Standards of professional practice specify the skills and learning that are expected to be possessed by members of a profession. Standards of professional practice demonstrate to the public, government, and other stakeholders that a profession is dedicated to maintaining public trust and upholding the criteria of its legal scope of practice.

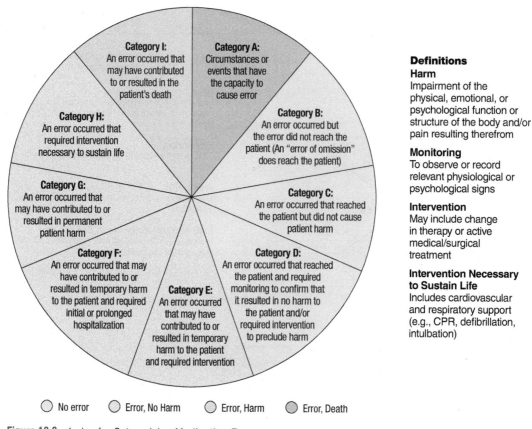

Definitions

Harm
Impairment of the physical, emotional, or psychological function or structure of the body and/or pain resulting therefrom

Monitoring
To observe or record relevant physiological or psychological signs

Intervention
May include change in therapy or active medical/surgical treatment

Intervention Necessary to Sustain Life
Includes cardiovascular and respiratory support (e.g., CPR, defibrillation, intulbation)

Category I:
An error occurred that may have contributed to or resulted in the patient's death

Category A:
Circumstances or events that have the capacity to cause error

Category H:
An error occurred that required intervention necessary to sustain life

Category B:
An error occurred but the error did not reach the patient (An "error of omission" does reach the patient)

Category G:
An error occurred that may have contributed to or resulted in permanent patient harm

Category C:
An error occurred that reached the patient but did not cause patient harm

Category F:
An error occurred that may have contributed to or resulted in temporary harm to the patient and required initial or prolonged hospitalization

Category E:
An error occurred that may have contributed to or resulted in temporary harm to the patient and required intervention

Category D:
An error occurred that reached the patient and required monitoring to confirm that it resulted in no harm to the patient and/or required intervention to preclude harm

○ No error   ○ Error, No Harm   ○ Error, Harm   ○ Error, Death

Figure 10.2 Index for Categorizing Medication Errors

In nursing, standards of practice are defined and enforced by provincial or territorial regulatory bodies (professional nursing associations). The rule of reasonable and prudent action also defines **standards of care**. This rule defines the standard of care as the actions that a reasonable and prudent nurse with equivalent preparation would do under similar circumstances. The nurse's actions would be legally judged by whether he or she acted within the standards of practice and whether the actions were what a reasonable and prudent nurse would have done when faced with a similar dilemma.

Standards of nursing practice include definition of roles, responsibilities, and practices, part of which includes the safe delivery of medications. Each province and territory has a professional nursing association or regulatory body that establishes, monitors, and enforces standards of professional practice. The professional nurse must be qualified to administer medications as specified in the standards for the particular province or territory in which he or she is working.

Every nurse and student nurse is responsible for consulting their provincial or territorial practice standards prior to implementing care to clients. Nurses are also responsible for regularly reviewing their nursing practice standards for amendments and updates.

Nurses who practise in clinical agencies need to understand and follow the policies and procedures governing medication administration of the organization in which they practise. These policies and procedures establish the standards of care

for that particular hospital or organization, and it is important that nurses adhere to those established policies and procedures. Common errors relate to failing to administer a medication at the prescribed time. For example, an agency policy may identify that it is permissible to give a medication 30 minutes early or 30 minutes late for medications taken four times a day. The standards of care and the agency's policy manual are designed to help the nurse prevent medication incidents and maintain client safety.

Factors Contributing to Medication Incidents

10.4 Numerous factors contribute to medication errors, including failing to adhere to the 10 rights of drug administration, failing to follow agency procedures or consider client variables, giving medications based on verbal orders, not confirming orders that are illegible or incomplete, and working under stressful conditions.

Safe medication administration involves collaboration between the nurse and the client and between the nurse and other members of the healthcare team. Factors that contribute to medication incidents include, but are not limited to, the following:

- Omitting one of the 10 rights of drug administration (see Chapter 9). Common errors include giving an incorrect dose, not giving an ordered dose, and giving an unordered drug.
- Failing to perform an agency system check. Both pharmacists and nurses must collaborate on checking the accuracy and appropriateness of drug orders prior to administering drugs to clients.
- Failing to account for client variables such as age, body size, and renal or hepatic function. Nurses should always review recent laboratory data and other information in the client's chart before administering medications, especially those drugs that have a narrow margin of safety.
- Giving medications based on verbal orders or phone orders, which may be misinterpreted or go undocumented. Nurses should remind the prescribing healthcare practitioner that medication orders must be in writing before the drug can be administered.
- Giving medications based on an incomplete order or an illegible order, when the nurse is unsure of the correct drug, dosage, or administration method. Incomplete orders should be clarified with the healthcare provider before the medication is administered. Characteristics of orders that improve safety include avoidance of certain abbreviations (Table 10.1) and inclusion of the following:
  - A brief notation of purpose (e.g., for pain)
  - Metric system measurements, except for therapies that use standard units (e.g., insulin or vitamins)
  - Client age and, when appropriate, weight
  - Drug name, exact metric weight or concentration, and dosage form
  - A leading zero preceding a decimal number less than one (e.g., 0.5 mg)
  - Avoidance of abbreviations for drug names (e.g., MOM, HCTZ) and avoidance of Latin directions for use
- Practising under stressful work conditions. The rate of medication errors increases when nurses have high stress levels and when individual nurses are assigned to clients who are the most acutely ill.

Clients, or their home caregivers, may also contribute to medication incidents by doing the following:

- Taking drugs prescribed by several healthcare practitioners without informing those providers about all prescribed medications
- Getting their prescriptions filled at more than one pharmacy
- Not filling or refilling their prescriptions
- Taking medications incorrectly
- Taking medications that may have been left over from a previous illness or prescribed for something else

NCLEX Success Tips

The nurse should be knowledgeable about drug dosages and possible interactions when administering medications.

The nurse must follow appropriate policies to correct dosage errors or to prevent potential interactions.

The nurse is responsible for questioning unclear or ambiguous physician orders.

The nurse must never carry out an order with which he or she is uncomfortable.

TABLE 10.1 Abbreviations to Avoid in Medication Administration

Abbreviation	Intended Meaning	Common Error
U	units	Mistaken as a zero or a four (4), resulting in overdose. Also mistaken for "cc" (cubic centimetres) when poorly written.
µg	micrograms	Mistaken for "mg" (milligrams), resulting in an overdose.
q.d.	Latin abbreviation for every day	The period after the "q" has sometimes been mistaken for an "I," and the drug has been given "qid" (four times daily) rather than daily.
q.o.d.	Latin abbreviation for every other day	Misinterpreted as "qd" (daily) or "qid" (four times daily). If the "O" is poorly written, it looks like a period or "I."
SC	subcutaneous	Mistaken as "SL" (sublingual) when poorly written.
t i w	three times a week	Misinterpreted as "three times a day" or "twice a week."
D/C	discharge; also discontinue	Medications have been prematurely discontinued when D/C (intended to mean "discharge") was misinterpreted as "discontinue," because it was followed by a list of drugs.
hs	half strength	Mistaken as the Latin abbreviation "hs" (hour of sleep).
cc	cubic centimetres	Mistaken as "U" (units) when poorly written.
AU, AS, AD	Latin abbreviation for both ears, left ear, right ear	Misinterpreted as the Latin abbreviation "OU" (both eyes), "OS" (left eye), "OD" (right eye).
IU	international unit	Mistaken as IV (intravenous) or 10 (ten).
MS, MS04, MgS04	Can mean morphine sulfate or magnesium sulfate	Confused for one another.

Drug Names and Medication Errors

10.5 Certain drugs have higher rates of medication errors.

Certain drugs have higher rates of medication errors. Some types of medication errors are independent of the drug being administered. For example, failure to perform adequate medication order checks, forgetting to give a dose, or administering the medication to the wrong client can occur with any medication. Some drugs, however, have higher error rates than others. Furthermore, when an error does occur, certain medications have greater potential to cause harm. Learning which drugs have the highest error rates and produce the most serious consequences can help the nurse to be more vigilant when administering these agents.

NCLEX Success Tips

Misinterpretation of handwriting remains a leading cause of medication errors in healthcare settings without computerized medical records or computer prescribing. The nurse must clarify prescriptions with the admitting physician to ensure medication accuracy and client safety.

It is not safe practice for the nurse to question the client regarding a diagnosis, nor to assume the medication has been correctly prescribed.

With thousands of generic and brand names for drugs, it is inevitable that some will look or sound similar; for example, *hydroxyzine* (Atarax) and *hydralazine* (Apresoline) or *Novolin* (Humulin) and *NovoLog* (NovoRapid). It is easy to understand how a verbal order given in a hurry over a cellphone could result in the wrong drug. It is likely that hundreds of medication errors occur each year because of look-alike or sound-alike drugs. This is a primary reason why verbal drug orders should always be confirmed in writing before being administered.

NCLEX Success Tip

Drugs that are similar in name—sometimes referred to as SALADs (sound-alike, look-alike drugs)—increase the risk of medication errors. The pharmacy should be consulted to help determine how to label each medication in such a way that draws attention to the name of the medication.

Drugs that have a narrow therapeutic index are more likely to cause serious consequences should a medication error occur. These drugs are not necessarily more error prone than others, but the nurse should give extra care when administering them due to their toxicity. The ISMP maintains lists of **high-alert medications** and defines these as "drugs that bear a heightened risk of causing significant patient harm when used in error." There are lists for both institutional and inpatient settings as well as for community and ambulatory agencies. Healthcare agencies may build in additional safeguards, such as independent double-checks or automated alerts, for these medications. Each client care unit may include its own additional list of high-alert medications. For example, high-alert drugs on a cancer unit or pediatric unit may differ from those on a medical-surgical unit.

NCLEX Success Tip

An example of a drug with narrow therapeutic index is digoxin (Lanoxin, Toloxin).

The Impact of Medication Incidents

10.6 Medication errors affect client morbidity, mortality, and length of hospital stay. Nurses must be vigilant to prevent errors and protect clients.

Medication incidents are the most common cause of morbidity and preventable death within hospitals. When a medication error occurs, the repercussions can be emotionally devastating for the nurse and extend beyond the particular nurse and client involved. A medication error can increase the client's length of stay in the hospital, which increases costs and the time that a client is separated from his or her family. The nurse who makes the medication error may suffer self-doubt and embarrassment. If a high error rate occurs within a particular unit, the nursing unit may develop a poor reputation within the facility. If frequent medication errors or serious errors are publicized, the reputation of the facility may suffer because it may be perceived as unsafe.

The goal of every healthcare organization should be to improve medication administration systems to prevent harm to clients caused by medication incidents. All errors, whether or not they affect the client, should be investigated with the goal of identifying ways to improve the medication administration process to prevent future errors. The investigation should occur in a non-punitive manner that will encourage staff to report errors, thereby building a culture of safety within an organization. An error can alert nurses and healthcare administrators to the fact that a new policy or procedure needs to be implemented to reduce or eliminate medication incidents.

Documenting and Reporting Medication Incidents

10.7 Nurses are legally and ethically responsible for reporting medication errors—whether or not they cause harm to a client—to the physician and for documenting them in the client's medical record and the incident report.

It is the nurse's legal and ethical responsibility to document and report all incidents involving medications. The nurse in charge and, in most cases, the physician are notified immediately about a medication incident. In some cases, serious adverse reactions caused by medication errors may require the immediate initiation of life-saving interventions for the client. Following such incidents, intense monitoring and additional medical treatments may be required.

Documenting in the Client's Medical Record

Agency policies and procedures provide guidance on reporting medication incidents. Documentation of the incident should occur in a factual manner: the nurse should avoid blaming or making judgments. Documentation in the medical record must include specific nursing interventions that were implemented following the incident to protect client safety, such as monitoring vital signs and assessing the client for possible complications. Documentation does not simply record that a medical incident occurred. Failure to document nursing actions implies either negligence or failure to acknowledge that the incident occurred. The nurse should also document all individuals who were notified of the incident. Incidents that involve a medication that was given in error or that was omitted should also be recorded on the medication administration record (MAR).

NCLEX Success Tip

Abbreviations can be misinterpreted. All healthcare professionals should avoid the use of easily misunderstood abbreviations.

Completing a Written Incident Report

In addition to documenting in the client's medical record, the nurse who made or discovered the incident should complete a written incident report. The specific details of the incident should be recorded in a factual and objective manner. The incident report provides the nurse with an opportunity to identify factors that contributed to the incident. Agency policy specifies whether a copy of the incident report is to be included in the client's medical record.

Accurate documentation in the medical record and the incident report is essential for legal reasons. These documents verify that the client's safety was protected and serve as tools to improve medication administration processes. Legal situations may worsen if there is an attempt to hide a mistake or delay corrective action, or if the nurse forgets to document interventions in the client's chart.

Hospitals and agencies monitor medication incidents through quality improvement programs. The results of quality improvement programs alert staff and administrative personnel about trends within particular units. Through data analyses, specific strategies can be developed to prevent such incidents.

Reporting at the National Level

Health Canada requests that nurses and other healthcare providers report medication incidents in order to build an up-to-date database that can be used to develop national strategies to improve medication safety. Medication errors, or situations that can lead to errors, may be reported in confidence directly to Health Canada through CMIRPS or ISMP Canada. Adverse drug reactions can be reported to Health Canada through MedEffect.

Strategies for Preventing Medication Incidents

10.8 Nurses can reduce medication incidents by adhering to the steps of the nursing process, knowing common types of medication errors and strategies for their prevention, and keeping up to date on pharmacotherapeutics.

What can the nurse do in the clinical setting to prevent medication incidents? The nurse can begin by using the four steps of the nursing process:

1. **Assessment:** Ask the client about allergies to food or medications, current health concerns, and use of over-the-counter (OTC) medications and herbal supplements. Ensure that the client is receiving the right dose, at the right time, and by the right route. Assess renal and liver function and check for impairments of other body systems that may affect pharmacotherapy. Identify areas of needed client education with regard to medications.

2. **Planning:** Minimize factors that contribute to medication errors. Avoid using abbreviations that can be misunderstood, question unclear orders, accept verbal orders only when the agency policy allows for it and make sure to repeat back verbal orders for confirmation, and follow specific facility policies and procedures related to medication administration. Have the client restate dosing directions, including the correct dose of medication and the right time to take it. Ask the client to demonstrate an understanding of the goals of therapy.

3. **Implementation:** Avoid distractions during medication administration if at all possible. When engaged in a medication-related task, focus entirely on the task. Noise, other events, and talking co-workers can distract the nurse's attention and result in a medication error. Practise the rights of medication administration: right client, right time and frequency of administration, right dose, right route of administration, right drug, and right documentation. Keep the following steps in mind as well:

   - Positively verify the identity of each client using two means (i.e., name and birthdate) before administering the medication, according to facility policy and procedures.

   - Use the correct procedures and techniques for all routes of administration. Use sterile materials and aseptic techniques when administering parenteral or eye medications.

   - Calculate medication doses correctly and measure liquid drugs carefully. Some medications, such as heparin, have a narrow safety margin for producing serious adverse effects. When giving these medications, ask a colleague to check the calculations to make certain the dosage is correct. Always double-check pediatric calculations prior to administration.

   - Open medications immediately prior to administering the medications and in the presence of the client.

   - Record the medication on the MAR immediately after administration.

   - Always confirm that the client has swallowed the medication. Never leave the medication at the bedside unless there is a specific order that medications may be left there.

   - Be alert for long-acting oral dosage forms with indicators such as LA, XL, and XR. These tablets or capsules must remain intact for the extended-release feature to be effective. Instruct the client not to crush, chew, or break the medication in half because doing so could cause an overdose.

   - Recheck any medications that the client states "look different" (e.g., different colour, larger pill).

4. **Evaluation:** Assess the client for expected outcomes and determine if any adverse effects have occurred.

Nurses must be zealous in keeping up to date on pharmacotherapeutics and should never administer a medication until they are familiar with its uses, contraindications, interactions, and side effects. There are many venues by which the nurse can obtain updated medication information. Each nursing unit should have current drug references available. Nurses can also call the pharmacy to obtain information about the drug or, if available, look it up on the Internet using reliable sources. Many nurses are now relying on personal digital assistants (PDAs) to provide current information. These devices can be updated daily or weekly by downloading information, so the information is always current. PDAs have the advantage of being portable for easy access right at the bedside or point of care. Nurses need to familiarize themselves with research on preventing medication errors to maintain evidence-based practice skills.

NCLEX Success Tips

If the nurse forgets his or her password, he or she should have computer support reset it. The nurse should never try to override the machine to get it to dispense the medication; doing so would be unsafe and could cause other medication errors.

The nurse should never give anyone the password nor delegate medication administration to a nursing assistant.

Nurses have a collaborative role to play in improving systems for managing medications in their practice settings. For example, nurses may make recommendations for improving lighting in a medication preparation area or for stocking and storing medications. Modifications to policies and procedures may be recommended. Nurses may advocate for use of modern technologies

CONNECTIONS   Lifespan Considerations

◀ Issues in Medication Safety and Risk Reduction

Children

Children are vulnerable to medication incidents because they receive medication dosages based on weight (which increases the possibility of dosage miscalculations) and the therapeutic dosages are much smaller.

- Always double-check calculations for pediatric clients with another nurse.
- Medications may need to be crushed or administered in a liquid form.
- Medications can have idiosyncratic effects on pediatric clients.
- Keep medications out of reach and use child-safe tops on medication containers.

Older Adults

Almost half of fatal medication errors occur in clients older than 60 years. There is an increase in the risk for errors in older adults because they often take multiple medications, have numerous healthcare providers, and may have normal age-related changes in pharmacokinetics.

- Be alert for individual responses to pharmacotherapy and assess laboratory reports.
- Complete a thorough medication history on admission.
- Provide written and oral instructions on discharge.

that could improve client safety, such as the use of automated, computerized, locked cabinets for medication storage; in this system, each nurse on the unit has a code for accessing the cabinet and removing a medication dose. These automated systems maintain an inventory of drug supplies. In addition, nurses may seek opportunities to become involved in committees that focus on examining and reducing the risk for medication incidents.

Providing Client Education for Safe Medication Usage

10.9 Adequate client education and adherence are essential strategies for safe medication usage. Client teaching includes providing age-appropriate medication handouts and encouraging clients to keep a list of all prescribed medications, OTC drugs, herbal therapies, and vitamins they are taking and to report them to all healthcare providers.

In the hospital setting, the physician, nurse, and pharmacist are largely responsible for preventing medication errors, and they collaborate to ensure that the client is receiving the correct drug in the manner designated by the prescriber. In the home setting, this responsibility relies on proper client adherence to drug therapy. For prescription drugs, healthcare providers provide the clients with verbal and written instructions on how and when to take the medication. Labels for OTC medications, herbal products, and dietary supplements indicate the correct method of taking the agent; however, clients do not always read or understand the information given.

Adherence is a major factor that affects pharmacotherapeutic outcomes and the risk for medication errors. As it relates to pharmacotherapy, **adherence**, or *compliance*, is defined as taking medications in the manner prescribed by the healthcare provider. In the case of OTC products, adherence means correctly following the instructions on the label. Client nonadherence (non-compliance) ranges from not taking the medication at all to taking it at the wrong time or at the wrong dose. It is estimated that approximately 50% of clients with chronic illnesses do not take their medications as prescribed, leading to increased complications, death, and additional costs.

Many factors can influence client adherence with pharmacotherapy. One of the most common sources of nonadherence is simply forgetting a dose of medication. This occurs frequently when the drug must be taken more than twice daily. Another source of nonadherence is that the drug may be too expensive or not approved by the client's health insurance plan. Clients often discontinue the use of drugs that have annoying adverse effects or that impair major lifestyle choices. Adverse effects that often prompt nonadherence are headache, dizziness, nausea, diarrhea, and impotence.

Clients often take medications in an unexpected manner, sometimes self-adjusting their doses. Some feel that if one tablet is good, two must be better. Others believe that they will become dependent on the medication if it is taken as prescribed; therefore, they take only half the necessary dose. Still others simply stop taking the medication when they start feeling better. Clients are usually reluctant to admit or report nonadherence to the nurse for fear of being reprimanded or feeling embarrassed.

Because reasons for nonadherence are many and varied, the nurse must be vigilant in questioning clients about taking their medications. When pharmacotherapy fails to produce the expected treatment outcomes, nonadherence should always be considered as a possible explanation. There are steps that the nurse can take to increase the potential for client adherence to the therapeutic regimen. All of these steps focus on effective teaching. Knowing that clients often feel overwhelmed by the amount of information provided and perceive that they lack a voice in the decision-making process, the nurse can discuss the prescription routine with the client and ask questions: Will the client be able to fill the prescription? How will it fit into the client's usual routine or with other medications? Listening for clues that suggest that the client is overwhelmed by the routines, the nurse then can ask further questions about what suggestions the client might have to make the routine workable. Clients may be reluctant to discuss these suggestions with their healthcare provider but may feel comfortable doing so with the nurse because of the nurse-client relationship.

In the plan of care, it is important to address essential information that the client must know regarding the prescribed medications. This includes factors such as the name of the medication, why it has been ordered, expected drug actions, associated adverse effects, and information on interactions with other medications, foods, herbal supplements, or alcohol. Clients should be encouraged to take an active role in ensuring the effectiveness of their medications and their own safety. It is important to remember that, unless diagnosed as mentally incompetent, a well-informed adult always has the legal option of refusing to take any medication. It is the nurse's responsibility, however, to ensure that the client has all of the necessary information to make an informed decision.

For clients who are receiving outpatient therapy or being released from a hospital, the nurse must carefully assess their ability to take their medications in a safe and effective manner. If the nurse believes that a client may have difficulty in properly administering the medications, caregivers should be consulted and other arrangements made to ensure that the client receives the correct drugs using the proper dosing schedule. At each successive healthcare visit, the nurse can review the medication history, asking questions about the prescribed medications. Being alert to reports that the client is not taking, or not correctly taking, the prescribed drugs may suggest an overwhelming, complex medication routine that needs to be reassessed if it is to be successful. Economic conditions sometimes result in difficult choices for clients between obtaining medications and other required necessities. Nurses provide medication education and follow-up that will result in positive health outcomes and the prevention of negative health effects and even larger expenditures as a result of poor medication adherence.

An essential strategy for avoiding medication errors is to educate the client. Provide age-appropriate handouts and audiovisual teaching aids about the medication, and provide contact information about whom to notify in the event of an adverse reaction. Teach clients to do the following:

- Keep a lifetime record of all medications and natural health products taken.
- Carry a list of all medications they are currently taking, including prescribed drugs, OTC drugs, dietary supplements, and herbals.
- Know the names of all medications they are currently taking, their uses, when they should be taken, and the doses.
- Know what side effects need to be reported immediately.
- Read the label prior to each drug administration.
- Use the measuring device that comes with liquid medications rather than using household measuring spoons.
- Do not use expired medications.
- Wear a MedicAlert bracelet for allergies and health conditions.
- Use one pharmacy for all prescriptions because the pharmacist is able to identify interactions and provide information about scheduling doses.
- Keep contact information for the nearest poison control centre accessible.
- Ask questions. Healthcare providers want to be partners in maintaining client safety with respect to medications.

CHAPTER 10

Understanding the Chapter

Key Concepts Summary

The numbered key concepts provide a succinct summary of the important points from the corresponding numbered section within the chapter. If any of these points are not clear, refer to the numbered section within the chapter for review.

10.1 Medication incidents that put clients at risk include medication errors and adverse drug reactions. Medication incidents impede pharmacotherapeutic outcomes, increase hospitalization costs, and can result in serious illness or death.

10.2 Health Canada has two programs aimed at monitoring and reducing the risk for medication incidents. Medication errors should be reported to the Canadian Medication Incident Reporting and Prevention System (CMIRPS). Adverse drug reactions should be reported to MedEffect. Both programs provide easy online reporting.

10.3 Standards of nursing practice include definition of roles, responsibilities, and practices relating to the safe delivery of medications.

10.4 Numerous factors contribute to medication errors, including failing to adhere to the 10 rights of drug administration, failing to follow agency procedures or consider client variables, giving medications based on verbal orders, not confirming orders that are illegible or incomplete, and working under stressful conditions.

10.5 Certain drugs have higher rates of medication errors.

10.6 Medication errors affect client morbidity, mortality, and length of hospital stay. Nurses must be vigilant to prevent errors and protect clients.

10.7 Nurses are legally and ethically responsible for reporting medication errors—whether or not they cause harm to a client—to the physician and for documenting them in the client's medical record and the incident report.

10.8 Nurses can reduce medication incidents by adhering to the steps of the nursing process, knowing common types of medication errors and strategies for their prevention, and keeping up to date on pharmacotherapeutics.

10.9 Adequate client education and adherence are essential strategies for safe medication usage. Client teaching includes providing age-appropriate medication handouts and encouraging clients to keep a list of all prescribed medications, OTC drugs, herbal therapies, and vitamins they are taking and to report them to all healthcare providers.

Chapter 10 Scenario

What happened to Ross Holland was truly a tragedy. He entered the hospital for simple sinus surgery and never recovered. Ironically, Ross was a vigilant man. As a veteran, he had seen the worst of combat for 4 years. During the last 6 months of the conflict, he survived in a prisoner-of-war camp. When he returned home, he took a job as a safety inspector in the automobile industry.

From a previous physical examination, Ross knew that he had a slightly irregular heartbeat, but he never really took it seriously. In fact, he did not mention it when the nurse was admitting him to the hospital. However, the condition became a problem soon after surgery. The nurse caring for Ross noticed a series of cardiac irregularities on the monitor and contacted the healthcare provider. The healthcare provider ordered Ross to receive a cardiac medicine immediately to correct the problem. In haste, the nurse failed to clarify the route by which the medication was to be given. In addition, the nurse was not familiar with the

medication's usual dose or any precautions that needed to be taken. As a result, the medication was given by direct intravenous administration without being diluted as directed on the medication bottle. Ross was given 100 times the normal dose. Consequently, he experienced seizure activity that lasted for 5 minutes followed by respiratory arrest. All efforts to resuscitate him were unsuccessful.

Critical Thinking Questions

1. Ultimately, who was responsible for this medication error: Ross? The healthcare provider? The nurse? Explain why.
2. Identify the contributing factors that resulted in the error.
3. What strategies should a nurse use to prevent medication errors?
4. What policy could healthcare facilities implement to avoid medication errors?

See Answers to Critical Thinking Questions in Appendix B.

NCLEX Practice Questions

1 It is 2:45 a.m. and a nurse has telephoned the prescriber to report that the client is experiencing an acute episode of postoperative pain. How can the nurse avoid medication errors when receiving a telephone order from a prescriber?

a. Decline to accept the telephone order.

b. Refuse to call the prescriber but attempt to comfort the client.

c. Instruct the client's family to call the prescriber.

d. Repeat the order back verbally to ensure accuracy.

2 A nurse cannot read the number of milligrams (mg) to be administered in a drug order written by the healthcare provider. It is questionable as to whether 125 mg, 1.25 mg, or 12.5 mg should be administered. What action would be most appropriate in preventing a medication error?

a. Telephone the healthcare provider about the illegible medication order.

b. Ask another nurse to read the questionable medication order.

c. Contact the pharmacist about the medication order.

d. Consult a drug handbook and administer the normal dose.

3 A nurse is counselling a client on a medication taken daily. Which strategy should the nurse include in this teaching session to prevent a medication error?

a. Insist on brand name drugs rather than generic drugs.

b. Have all prescriptions filled at one pharmacy.

c. Request that all prescriptions be placed in easily opened containers.

d. Consult the Internet about possible adverse effects.

4 When given a medication, a client tells the nurse, "I've never seen this pill before. It's not like the others I take." Which would be the most appropriate action for the nurse to take?

a. Instruct the client that different brands are frequently used.

b. Administer the medication in its existing form.

c. Verify the order and double-check the drug label.

d. Advise the client to talk with the healthcare provider, then administer the drug.

5 As a nurse enters a room to administer medication, the client states, "I'm in the bathroom. Please leave the medication on my bedside table, and I'll take it when I come out." Which would be the appropriate response?

a. "I will leave the medication and follow up with you in 30 minutes."

b. "You must take the medication now or refuse the dose."

c. "Let me know when you are ready, and I will return with your medicine."

d. "I've given the drug to your visitors. Take it when you come out of the bathroom."

See Answers to NCLEX Practice Questions in Appendix A.

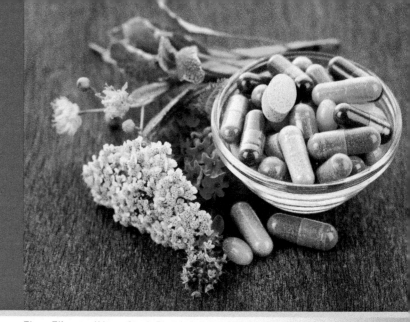

CHAPTER

11

Complementary and Alternative Therapies and Their Roles in Pharmacotherapy in Canada

LEARNING OUTCOMES

After reading this chapter, the student should be able to:

1. Explain the role of complementary and alternative medicine in client wellness.

2. Discuss reasons why herbal and dietary supplements have increased in popularity.

3. Identify the parts of an herb that may contain active ingredients and the types of formulations made from these parts.

4. Discuss the regulatory process for natural health products licensed for sale in Canada.

5. Describe some adverse effects that may be caused by herbal preparations.

6. Discuss the role of the nurse in teaching clients about complementary and alternative therapies.

7. Identify common herb-drug interactions.

CHAPTER OUTLINE

▶ Complementary and Alternative Therapies

▶ Brief History of Natural Health Products

▶ Regulation of Natural Health Products (NHPs)

▶ Herbal Product Formulations

▶ Herb-Drug Interactions: The Pharmacological Actions and Safety of Natural Products

▶ Specialty Supplements Used to Promote Wellness

KEY TERMS

botanical, 118	herb, 118	specialty supplements, 123
complementary and alternative medicine (CAM), 117	natural health products (NHPs), 119	

Natural therapies, including herbal products and other complementary therapies, are increasingly used by Canadians. Despite the fact that these therapies have not been subjected to the same scientific scrutiny as prescription medications, consumers have turned to these treatments for a variety of reasons. Many people have the impression that natural substances have more healing power than synthetic medications. This impression and the ready availability of herbal products at a reasonable cost have convinced many consumers to try them. This chapter examines the role of complementary and alternative therapies in the prevention and treatment of disease.

Complementary and Alternative Therapies

11.1 Complementary and alternative medicine (CAM) is a set of diverse therapies and healing systems used by many people for disease prevention and self-healing.

Complementary and alternative medicine (CAM) comprises an extremely diverse set of therapies and healing systems that are considered to be outside mainstream health care. Although diverse, the major CAM systems have the following common characteristics:

- Focus on treating each person as an individual
- Consider the health of the whole person
- Integrate mind and body
- Promote disease prevention, self-care, and self-healing
- Acknowledge the role of spirituality in health and healing

Because of its popularity, considerable attention is now being focused on the effectiveness, or lack of effectiveness, of CAM. Although research into these alternative systems is beginning to appear worldwide, few CAM therapies have been subjected to rigorous clinical and scientific study. It is likely that some of these therapies will be found to be ineffective, and others will become mainstream treatments. The line between what is defined as an alternative therapy and what is considered mainstream is constantly changing. Increasing numbers of healthcare providers are now accepting CAM therapies and recommending them to their clients. Table 11.1 lists many of these therapies.

Nurses have long known the value of CAM therapies in preventing and treating disease. Prayer, meditation, massage, and yoga, for example, have been used to treat both body and mind for centuries. From a pharmacotherapeutic perspective, the value of CAM therapies lies in their ability to reduce the need

TABLE 11.1 Complementary and Alternative Therapies

Healing Method	Examples
Biological-based therapies	Herbal therapies
	Nutritional supplements
	Special diets
Alternate healthcare systems	Naturopathy
	Homeopathy
	Chiropractic
	Aboriginal medicine (e.g., sweat lodges, medicine wheel)
	Chinese traditional medicine (e.g., acupuncture, Chinese herbs)
Manual healing	Massage
	Pressure point therapies
	Hand-mediated biofield therapies
Mind-body interventions	Yoga
	Meditation
	Hypnotherapy
	Guided imagery
	Biofeedback
	Movement-oriented therapies (e.g., music, dance)
Spiritual	Shamans
	Faith and prayer
Others	Bioelectromagnetics
	Detoxifying therapies
	Animal-assisted therapy

for medications. For example, if a client can find anxiety relief through herbal products, massage, or biofeedback therapy, the use of anxiolytic drugs may be reduced or eliminated. Reduction of traditional drug doses leads to fewer adverse effects.

The nurse should be sensitive to the client's need for alternative treatment and not be judgmental. Both advantages and limitations must be presented to clients so that they may make rational and informed decisions on their treatment. Pharmacotherapy and alternative therapies can serve complementary and essential roles in the healing of the total client.

Brief History of Natural Health Products

11.2 Natural products obtained from plants have been used as medicines for thousands of years.

An **herb** is technically a **botanical** without woody tissue such as stems or bark. Over time, the terms *botanical* and *herb* have come to be used interchangeably to refer to any plant product with some useful application either as a food enhancer, such as flavouring, or as a medicine.

The use of botanicals has been documented for thousands of years. One of the earliest recorded uses of plant products was a prescription for garlic in 3000 BCE. Eastern and Western medicine have recorded thousands of herbs and herb combinations reputed to have therapeutic value. Some of the most popular herbal supplements and their primary uses are shown in Table 11.2.

NCLEX Success Tip

Before surgery, nurses should keep in mind that some patients use garlic to help in controlling their blood pressure. The nurse must obtain a history of the approximate amount of garlic the client received prior to surgery. Garlic has anticoagulant properties and may cause bleeding if enough has been taken too close to surgery.

With the birth of the pharmaceutical industry in the late 1800s, interest in herbal medicines began to wane. Synthetic drugs could

TABLE 11.2   Popular Herbal Supplements

Herb	Medicinal Part	Primary Use(s)	Herb Feature (Chapter)
Acai	Berries	Vitamin and mineral supplement, antioxidant, possible weight loss	—
Aloe vera	Leaves	Topical application for minor skin irritations and burns	73
Bilberry	Berries and leaves	Terminate diarrhea, improve and protect vision, antioxidant	74
Black cohosh	Roots	Relief of menopausal symptoms	70
Chlorophyll/chlorella	Leaves	Improve digestion, vitamin and mineral supplement	—
Cranberry	Berries/juice	Prevent urinary tract infection	50
Echinacea	Entire plant	Enhance immune system, treat the common cold	42
Elderberry	Berries and flowers	Congestion in respiratory system due to colds and flu	—
Evening primrose	Oil extracted from seeds	Source of essential fatty acids, relief of premenstrual or menopausal symptoms, relief of rheumatoid arthritis and other inflammatory symptoms	—
Flaxseed (ground) and/or oil	Seeds and oil	Reduce blood cholesterol, laxative	35
Garlic	Bulbs	Reduce blood cholesterol, reduce blood pressure, anticoagulation	38
Ginger	Root	Antiemetic, antithrombotic, diuretic, promote gastric secretions, anti-inflammatory, increase blood glucose, stimulation of peripheral circulation	59
Ginkgo	Leaves and seeds	Improve memory, reduce dizziness	21
Ginseng	Root	Relieve stress, enhance immune system, decrease fatigue	—
Grape seed	Seeds/oil	Source of essential fatty acids, antioxidant, restore microcirculation to tissues	34
Green tea	Leaves	Antioxidant; lower LDL cholesterol; prevent cancer; relieve stomach problems, nausea, vomiting	63
Horny goat weed	Leaves and roots	Enhance sexual function	—
Milk thistle	Seeds	Antitoxin, protection against liver disease	—
Red rice yeast extract	Dried in capsules	Reduce blood cholesterol	—
Saw palmetto	Berries	Treatment of benign prostatic hyperplasia	71
Soy	Beans	Source of protein, vitamins, and minerals; relief of menopausal symptoms, prevent cardiovascular disease, anticancer	69
Stevia	Leaves	Natural sweetener	—
St. John's wort	Flowers, leaves, stems	Reduce depression, reduce anxiety, anti-inflammatory	19
Valerian	Roots	Relieve stress, promote sleep	—
Wheat or barley grass	Leaves	Improve digestion, vitamin and mineral supplement	—

be standardized and produced more cheaply than natural herbal products. Regulatory agencies required that products be safe and effective. The focus of health care was on diagnosing and treating specific diseases rather than on promoting wellness and holistic care. Most alternative therapies were no longer taught in medical or nursing schools; these healing techniques were criticized as being unscientific relics of the past.

Beginning in the 1970s and continuing to the present, alternative therapies and herbal medicines have experienced a remarkable resurgence, such that the majority of adults in Canada are currently using CAM therapies. These therapies now represent a multibillion-dollar industry. This increase in popularity is a result of a number of factors:

* Herbal products and dietary supplements were once available only in specialty health food stores but can now be purchased in virtually all supermarkets and pharmacies.

* Complementary therapies are aggressively marketed by the supplement industry as viable and natural alternatives to conventional medicine. The increased availability of the Internet as a marketing tool has led to websites with misleading information about the effectiveness of herbal and dietary supplements.

* The baby boomer generation has demonstrated a renewed interest in natural alternatives and preventive medicine.

* The gradual aging of the population has led people to seek therapeutic alternatives for chronic conditions such as pain, arthritis, anxiety, depression, hormone replacement therapy, and prostate difficulties.

* People have the impression that natural substances are safer than synthetic pharmaceuticals.

* The high cost of prescription medicines has driven people to seek less expensive alternatives.

* Nurses and other healthcare providers have been more proactive in promoting self-care and recommending CAM for their clients.

Regulation of Natural Health Products (NHPs)

11.3 Natural health products are regulated by the Natural Health Products Regulations of the Food and Drugs Act in Canada.

Internationally, the regulation of natural products varies. Generally, they are regulated as drugs in the European Union. In Australia, many products are classified as "complementary medicines." In the United States, many products are regulated as "dietary supplements," a category that does not require pre-market review or proof of safety or efficacy.

In Canada, vitamins and minerals, herbal products, homeopathic medicines, and other such products with health claims are classified as **natural health products (NHPs)**. A recent survey shows that 71% of Canadians regularly take vitamins and minerals and other NHPs. Since 2004, NHPs, also referred to as *complementary medicines* or *traditional remedies*, have been subject to the Natural Health Products Regulations of the Food and Drugs Act in Canada. The Natural and Non-prescription Health Products

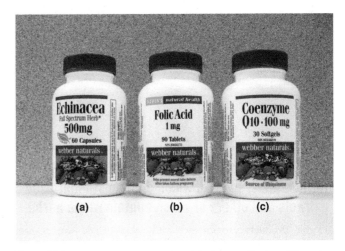

Figure 11.1 Natural health product labels may display different numbering systems: (a) no number, indicating that no health claims are made and the product has not been evaluated by Health Canada; (b) Natural Product Number (NPN), indicating that the product has been approved for sale by the NNHPD of Health Canada; (c) Drug Identification Number (DIN), indicating that the product has been evaluated by the Therapeutic Products Directorate of Health Canada and approved for sale in Canada.

Source: Shirley King.

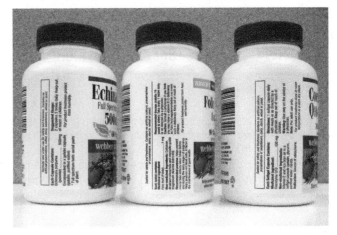

Figure 11.2 Labels on natural health products vary: some labels suggest a use for the product, some display warnings, but all recommend a dosage.

Source: Shirley King.

Directorate (NNHPD) is responsible for defining NHPs and determining licensing requirements, labelling standards, manufacturing practices, adverse event reporting, quality control, and more. Because the NNHPD was established recently, labels may differ among products. NHPs may display different numbering systems, as shown in Figure 11.1. Information about ingredients, indications, and cautions on the labels of NHPs may vary in completeness, as shown in Figure 11.2. To be licensed, an NHP must have at least some efficacy and be relatively safe at the recommended dosage. The NNHPD establishes tolerance levels for impurities in NHPs. Canadians want NHPs that are as free of contaminants as possible for a product that is natural. Potential contaminants include heavy metals, microorganisms, foreign matter, pesticides and herbicides, radioactive elements, and parts of other plants. The inclusion of unintended or undeclared botanicals in a product represents a serious problem, as it is one of the most common causes of adverse effects. For most botanicals, the biologically active ingredients that produce the desired therapeutic effect have not been conclusively identified. The nurse should access Health Canada's MedEffect website to monitor product safety concerns and recalls.

Herbal Product Formulations

11.4 Herbal products are available in a variety of formulations, some of which contain standardized extracts and others of which contain whole herbs.

Herbal products can interact with other drugs. Nurses need to have knowledge of products that can interact with prescription medications and affect health. The pharmacologically active chemicals in an herbal product may be present in only one specific part of the plant or in all parts. For example, the active chemicals in chamomile are in the above-ground portion that includes the leaves, stems, and flowers. For other herbs, such as ginger, the underground rhizomes and roots are used for their healing properties. If collecting herbs for home use, it is essential to know which portion of the plant contains the active chemicals.

Most traditional drugs contain only one active chemical. This chemical can be standardized and measured, and the amount of

---

CONNECTIONS   Special Considerations

◀ Herbal Products

- Because an herbal product comes from plants and is labelled "natural," this does not mean it is safe. Many plants are poisonous and are harmful to human bodies.
- Herbals can act in the same way as drugs and can cause side effects and health problems if not used correctly or if taken in large amounts.
- The active ingredients in many herbs and herbal products are not known. There may be dozens of active compounds in one herbal product.
- Research is needed to identify the active ingredients in herbals and determine how they work in the body.
- Actual contents of herbal products may differ from batch to batch depending on growing conditions and manufacturing processes. "Standardization" may not guarantee uniformity.
- Some herbal products have been found to be contaminated with lead, pesticides, microorganisms, and other substances.
- Women who are pregnant or nursing and children should be especially cautious about using herbal products.
- Clients who are taking prescription medications should be advised to consult their healthcare provider before using an herbal product. Some herbals are known to interact with medications in ways that cause health problems.
- Advertisements should be evaluated for accuracy since some may provide information that is unclear or misleading.
- Adverse effects of herbal products should be reported as for prescription medicines (see Chapter 10).

Based on Natural Health Products Directorate (NHPD), www.hc-sc.gc.ca. National Center for Complementary and Alternative Medicine (NCCAM), http://nccam.nih.gov/ Data modified from www.prenhall.com/drugguides

---

CONNECTIONS   Lifespan Considerations

◀ Dietary Supplements and the Older Adult

Can dietary supplements improve the health of older adults? A growing body of evidence is showing that the use of supplements can positively influence seniors' health. Dietary supplements have been successfully used to enhance older adults' immune systems, reduce short-term memory loss, lessen the risks of Alzheimer's disease, and improve overall health. Nutritional deficiencies greatly increase with age, and supplements help to prevent or eliminate these deficiencies in older adults. In addition, some research has shown that older adults who have low levels of folate and vitamin B_{12} have an increased risk for developing Alzheimer's disease. The nurse should assess the need for such supplements in all older adults. However, the nurse should be aware that herbal and dietary supplements can be expensive; therefore, supplements should not automatically be included in treatment plans. In addition, older adults should be educated as to the risks of megavitamin therapy.

---

drug received by the client is precisely known. It is a common misunderstanding that herbs also contain one active ingredient, which can be extracted and delivered to clients in precise doses, like drugs. Herbs may contain dozens of active chemicals, many of which have not yet been isolated, studied, or even identified. It is possible that some of these substances work together synergistically and may not have the same activity in isolation. Furthermore, the strength of an herbal preparation may vary depending on where the herb was grown and how it was collected and stored.

Some attempts have been made to standardize herbal extracts using a marker substance such as the percent of flavones in ginkgo or the percent of lactones in kava kava. Some of these standardizations are shown in Table 11.3. Until science can better characterize these substances, however, it is best to conceptualize the active ingredient of an herb as being the herb itself.

The two basic formulations of herbal products are solid and liquid. Solid products include pills, tablets, and capsules made from dried herbs (see Figure 11.1). Other solid products are salves and ointments that are administered topically. Liquid formulations are made by extracting the active chemicals from the plant using solvents such as water, alcohol, or glycerol. The liquids are then concentrated in various strengths and ingested. The various liquid formulations of herbal preparations are described in Table 11.4. Figure 11.3 illustrates formulations of the popular herbal *Ginkgo biloba*.

Herb-Drug Interactions: The Pharmacological Actions and Safety of Natural Products

11.5 Natural health products may have pharmacological actions and result in adverse effects, including significant interactions with prescription medications.

A key concept to remember when dealing with alternative therapies is that "natural" is not synonymous with "better" or "safe."

TABLE 11.3 Standardization of Select Herb Extracts

Herb	Standardization	Percent
Black cohosh rhizome	Triterpene glycosides	2.5
Cascara sagrada bark	Hydroxyanthracenic heterosides	20
Echinacea purpurea herb	Phenolics	4
Ginger rhizome	Pungent compounds	>10
Ginkgo leaf	Flavone glycosides	24–25
	Lactones	6
Ginseng root	Ginsenosides	20–30
Kava kava rhizome	Kavalactones	40–45
Milk thistle root	Silymarin	80
St. John's wort herb	Hypericins	0.3–0.5
	Hyperforin	3–5
Saw palmetto fruit	Total fatty acids	80–90

TABLE 11.4 Liquid Formulations of Herbal Products

Product	Description
Tea	Fresh or dried herbs are soaked in hot water for 5–10 minutes before ingestion; convenient
Infusion	Fresh or dried herbs are soaked in hot water for long periods, at least 15 minutes; stronger than teas
Decoction	Fresh or dried herbs are boiled in water for 30–60 minutes until much of the liquid has boiled off; very concentrated
Tincture	Extraction of active ingredients by soaking the herb in alcohol; alcohol remains as part of the liquid
Extract	Extraction of active ingredients using organic solvents to form a highly concentrated liquid or solid form; solvent may be removed or be part of the final product

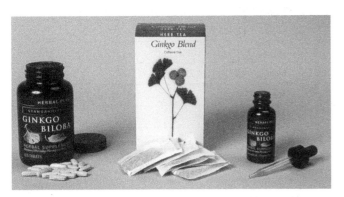

Figure 11.3 Three different ginkgo formulations: tablets, tea bags, and liquid extract.

Source: Shirley King.

There is no question that some botanicals contain powerful active chemicals that perhaps are more effective than currently approved medications. Thousands of years of experience, combined with current scientific research, have shown that some herbal remedies have therapeutic actions. However, the fact that a substance comes from a natural product does not make it safe or effective. For example, poison ivy is natural, but it certainly is not safe or therapeutic. Natural products may not offer an improvement over conventional therapy in treating certain disorders and, indeed, may be of no value whatsoever. Furthermore, a client who substitutes an unproven alternative therapy for an established, effective medical treatment may delay healing and suffer irreparable harmful effects.

The true extent of herb-drug interactions is unknown. Most reports in the medical literature are anecdotal, often given as a case report on a single client. It is often impossible to know the exact amount of herb taken because there is such a wide variation in the quality of products on the market, or even to know what chemical within the herb (either active ingredients or contaminants) may have caused the reported interaction. Relatively few controlled scientific studies of herb-drug or dietary supplement–drug interactions have been conducted. The majority of the information on these interactions is theoretical rather than clinically based.

Some herbal products contain ingredients that may serve as agonists or antagonists to prescription drugs. When obtaining medical histories, nurses should include questions on dietary supplements. Clients who are taking medications with potentially serious herb-drug interactions, such as insulin, warfarin (Coumadin), or digoxin (Lanoxin, Toloxin), should be warned to never take any herbal product or dietary supplement without first discussing their needs with a physician. Drug interactions with select herbs are outlined in Table 11.5.

When using natural products, one must also be aware of allergic reactions. Most herbal products contain a mixture of ingredients, many of which have not been identified. It is not unusual to find dozens of different chemicals in teas and infusions made from the flowers, leaves, or roots of a plant. Clients who have known allergies to food products or medicines should seek medical advice before taking a new herbal product. It is always wise to take the smallest amount possible when starting herbal therapy, even less than the recommended dose, to see if allergies or other adverse effects occur.

Nurses have an obligation to seek the latest medical information on herbal products since their clients may be using them to supplement traditional medicines. Clients should be advised to be skeptical of claims on the labels of dietary supplements and to seek health information from reputable sources. Nurses should never judge or condemn a client's use of alternative medicines, but instead should be supportive and seek to understand the client's goals associated with taking the supplements. They should also gather information about the benefits that the clients claim to experience. The healthcare provider will often need to educate clients on the role of CAM therapies in the treatment of their disorder and discuss which treatment or combination of treatments will best meet their health goals.

TABLE 11.5   Common Herb-Drug Interactions

Common and Scientific Names	Drugs of Interaction	Comments
echinacea (*Echinacea purpurea*)	Amiodarone	Possible increased hepatotoxicity
	Anabolic steroids	Possible increased hepatotoxicity
	Ketoconazole	Possible increased hepatotoxicity
	Methotrexate	Possible increased hepatotoxicity
feverfew (*Tanacetum parthenium*)	Acetylsalicylic acid (ASA)	Increased bleeding potential
	Heparin	Increased bleeding potential
	Nonsteroidal anti-inflammartory drugs (NSAIDs)	Increased bleeding potential
	Warfarin	Increased bleeding potential
garlic (*Allium sativum*)	ASA	Increased bleeding potential
	Insulin	Additive hypoglycemic effects
	NSAIDs	Increased bleeding potential
	Oral hypoglycemic agents	Additive hypoglycemic effects
	Warfarin	Increased bleeding potential
ginger (*Zingiber officinale*)	ASA	Increased bleeding potential
	Heparin	Increased bleeding potential
	NSAIDs	Increased bleeding potential
	Warfarin	Increased bleeding potential
ginkgo (*Ginkgo biloba*)	Anticonvulsants	May decrease anticonvulsant effectiveness
	ASA	Increased bleeding potential
	Heparin	Increased bleeding potential
	NSAIDs	Increased bleeding potential
	Tricyclic antidepressants	May decrease seizure threshold
	Warfarin	Increased bleeding potential
ginseng (*Panax quinquefolius, Eleutherococcus senticosus*)	Central nervous system (CNS) depressants	Potentiate sedation
	Digoxin	Increased toxicity
	Diuretics	May attenuate diuretic effects
	Insulin	Increased hypoglycemic effects
	Monoamine oxidase (MAO) inhibitors	Hypertension, manic symptoms, headaches, nervousness
	Oral hypoglycemic agents	Increased hypoglycemic effects
	Warfarin	Decreased anticoagulant effects
goldenseal (*Hydrastis canadensis*)	Diuretics	May attenuate diuretic effects
kava kava (*Piper methysticum*)	Barbiturates	Potentiate sedation
	Benzodiazepines	Potentiate sedation
	CNS depressants	Potentiate sedation
	Levodopa/carbidopa	Worsening of Parkinson's disease symptoms
	Phenothiazines	Increased risk and severity of dystonic reactions
St. John's wort (*Hypericum perforatum*)	CNS depressants	Potentiate sedation
	Cyclosporine	May decrease cyclosporine levels

TABLE 11.5 Common Herb-Drug Interactions (*continued*)

	Efavirenz	Decreased antiretroviral activity
	MAO inhibitors	May cause hypertensive crisis
	Opiate analgesics	Increased sedation
	Protease inhibitors	Decreased antiretroviral activity of indinavir
	Reserpine	Antagonize hypotensive effects
	Selective serotonin reuptake inhibitors	May cause serotonin syndrome*
	Theophylline	Decreased theophylline efficacy
	Tricyclic antidepressants	May cause serotonin syndrome*
	Warfarin	Decreased anticoagulant effects
valerian (*Valeriana officinalis*)	Barbiturates	Potentiate sedation
	Benzodiazepines	Potentiate sedation
	CNS depressants	Potentiate sedation

*Serotonin syndrome: headache, dizziness, sweating, agitation.

Source: Data modified from www.prenhall.com/drugguides.

Specialty Supplements Used to Promote Wellness

11.6 Specialty supplements are non-herbal dietary products widely used to promote wellness.

Specialty supplements are non-herbal dietary products used to enhance a wide variety of body functions. These supplements form a diverse group of products obtained from plant and animal sources. They are more specific in their action than herbal products and are generally targeted for one condition or a smaller group of related conditions. The most popular specialty supplements are listed in Table 11.6.

In general, specialty supplements have a legitimate rationale for their use. For example, chondroitin and glucosamine are natural substances in the body that are necessary for cartilage growth and maintenance. Amino acids are natural building blocks of muscle protein. Flaxseed and fish oils contain omega fatty acids that have been shown to reduce the risk of heart disease in certain clients.

As with herbal products, the link between most specialty supplements and their claimed benefits is unclear. In most cases, the body already has sufficient quantities of the substance; thus taking additional amounts may be of no benefit. In other cases, the supplement is marketed for conditions for which the supplement has no proven effect. The good news is that these substances are generally not harmful unless taken in large amounts. The bad news, however, is that they can give clients false hopes of an easy cure for chronic conditions such as heart disease or the pain of arthritis. As with herbal products, the healthcare provider should advise clients to be skeptical about any health claims regarding the use of these supplements.

TABLE 11.6 Select Specialty Supplements

Name	Primary Uses	Supplement Feature (Chapter)
Amino acids	Build protein, muscle strength, and endurance	—
Carnitine	Enhance energy and sports performance, heart health, memory, immune function, and male fertility	36
Chromium	Treatment of diabetes; hyperglycemia	66
Coenzyme Q10	Prevent heart disease, provide anti-oxidant therapy	29
DHEA	Boost immune and memory functions	—
Fish oil	Reduce cholesterol levels, enhance brain function, and increase visual acuity	68
Glucosamine and chondroitin	Alleviate arthritis and other joint problems	72
Lactobacillus acidophilus	Maintain intestinal health	60
Melatonin	Reduce sleeplessness and jet-lag during travel	18
Methyl sulfonyl methane (MSM)	Reduce allergic reactions to pollen and foods, relieve pain and inflammation of arthritis	—
Selenium	Reduce the risk of certain types of cancer	—
Vitamin C	Prevent colds	45

CHAPTER

11

Understanding the Chapter

Key Concepts Summary

The numbered key concepts provide a succinct summary of the important points from the corresponding numbered section within the chapter. If any of these points are not clear, refer to the numbered section within the chapter for review.

11.1 Complementary and alternative medicine (CAM) is a set of diverse therapies and healing systems used by many people for disease prevention and self-healing.

11.2 Natural products obtained from plants have been used as medicines for thousands of years.

11.3 Natural health products are regulated by the Natural Health Products Regulations of the Food and Drugs Act in Canada.

11.4 Herbal products are available in a variety of formulations, some of which contain standardized extracts and others of which contain whole herbs.

11.5 Natural health products may have pharmacological actions and result in adverse effects, including significant interactions with prescription medications.

11.6 Specialty supplements are non-herbal dietary products widely used to promote wellness.

Chapter 11 Scenario

Larry Bunch, who is 69 years old, was not only frustrating his daughter, but also annoying himself because of his forgetfulness. Since the death of his wife 2 years ago, his forgetfulness seems to have worsened. To remedy the situation, Larry purchased a bottle of ginkgo biloba at the health food store and began taking the supplement about 6 months ago.

Larry was hospitalized 3 years ago for a cardiac condition (atrial fibrillation). When he was discharged from the hospital, he was placed on an anticoagulant therapy to prevent blood clots from forming in his heart. Today, Larry goes to his healthcare provider's office for a scheduled blood test to determine the effectiveness of the anticoagulant.

When the results from the blood test return, it is noted that Larry's coagulation time is abnormally high. Based on the test, Larry is at high risk for hemorrhaging. As the nurse, you note that his vital signs are within normal limits, and he states that he feels well. However, you also observe some large bruises on Larry's arms, which he cannot explain.

Critical Thinking Questions

1. What is the relationship between this client's use of ginkgo biloba and the laboratory results?
2. What instructions should this client receive about taking the supplement?
3. Discuss the hazards that clients face when using complementary and alternative therapies.
4. What should the healthcare provider do concerning Larry's forgetfulness?

See Answers to Critical Thinking Questions in Appendix B.

NCLEX Practice Questions

1 A client asks why all healthcare providers do not rely on complementary and alternative medicine. Talking to this patient, the nurse knows that many complementary and alternative therapies

a. Have not been subjected to rigorous clinical studies

b. Consist only of old wives' tales and fables

c. Only provide a placebo effect

d. Are costly and not worth the risk

2 Which health teaching concept should be included in the instructions for a patient taking echinacea?

a. Dosage can be doubled if symptoms fail to resolve in 48 hours.

b. Limit fluid intake while taking this supplement.

c. Take the smallest amount possible when starting herbal therapy.

d. Allergic reactions are not possible with natural supplements.

3 Which patient is most likely to experience drug toxicity while taking herbal supplements?

a. An 80-year-old female with cirrhosis

b. A 58-year-old male with cardiac irregularities

c. A 30-year-old female with pneumonia

d. An 18-year-old male with chronic acne

4 A patient asks the nurse, "Why are herbal supplements so popular?" The nurse's answer will be based upon which factors? Select all that apply.

a. Herbal supplements can now be purchased in virtually all supermarkets.

b. Herbal supplements are aggressively marketed by the supplement industry.

c. Herbal supplements cost less than prescription medicines.

d. Herbal supplements are safer than synthetic pharmaceuticals.

e. Herbal supplements appeal to the aging population.

5 Polypharmacy may be of concern in the older adult population. A pharmacokinetic factor for this concern is that older adults

a. Are more likely to have difficulty using herbal products correctly

b. May spend too much on herbal products rather than prescriptions

c. May hold unrealistic expectations for the outcomes of herbal therapy

d. May have age-related changes in liver or kidney function

See Answers to NCLEX Practice Questions in Appendix A.

Pharmacology of Alterations in the Autonomic Nervous System

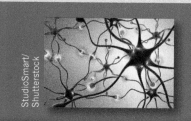

StudioSmart/
Shutterstock

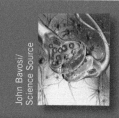

John Bavosi/
Science Source

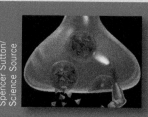

Spencer Sutton/
Science Source

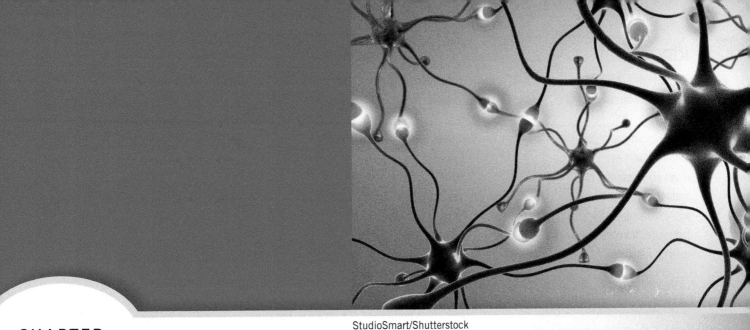

StudioSmart/Shutterstock

12 Brief Review of the Autonomic Nervous System and Neurotransmitters

LEARNING OUTCOMES

After reading this chapter, the student should be able to:

1. Distinguish between the functions of the central and peripheral nervous systems.

2. Discuss how drugs are classified according to their effects on each of the two fundamental divisions of the nervous system.

3. Compare and contrast the actions of the sympathetic and parasympathetic nervous systems.

4. Explain the process of synaptic transmission and the neurotransmitters that are important to the autonomic nervous system.

5. Discuss how drugs are used to modify functions of the autonomic nervous system.

6. Describe the actions of acetylcholine at cholinergic synapses.

7. Describe the actions of norepinephrine at adrenergic synapses.

8. Compare and contrast the types of responses that occur when a drug activates alpha$_1$-, alpha$_2$-, beta$_1$-, or beta$_2$-adrenergic receptors.

9. Compare the actions of the adrenal medulla with those of other sympathetic effector organs.

10. Explain how higher centres in the brain can influence autonomic functions.

CHAPTER OUTLINE

▸ The Nervous System

  ▸ The Two Major Subdivisions of the Nervous System

  ▸ The Peripheral Nervous System

  ▸ The Autonomic Nervous System: Sympathetic and Parasympathetic Branches

  ▸ Structure and Function of Synapses

  ▸ Acetylcholine and Cholinergic Transmission

  ▸ Norepinephrine and Adrenergic Transmission

▸ Autonomic Drugs

  ▸ Classification and Naming of Autonomic Drugs

acetylcholine (Ach), 132

acetylcholinesterase (AchE), 132

adrenergic, 133

adrenergic antagonists, 134

adrenergics, 134

alpha (α) receptors, 133

antiadrenergics, 134

anticholinergics, 134

autonomic nervous system (ANS), 128

beta (β) receptors, 133

catecholamines, 133

central nervous system (CNS), 128

cholinergic, 132

cholinergics, 134

fight-or-flight response, 129

ganglion, 131

monoamine oxidase (MAO), 133

muscarinic, 132

neurotransmitters, 131

nicotinic, 132

norepinephrine (NE), 132

parasympathetic nervous system, 129

peripheral nervous system, 128

postsynaptic neuron, 131

presynaptic neuron, 131

rest-and-digest response, 129

somatic nervous system, 128

sympathetic nervous system, 129

synapse, 130

synaptic transmission, 131

Neuropharmacology represents one of the largest, most complicated, and least understood branches of pharmacology. Nervous system drugs are used to treat a large and diverse set of conditions, including pain, anxiety, depression, schizophrenia, insomnia, and convulsions. By their action on nerves, medications are used to treat disorders that affect many body systems. Examples include abnormalities in heart rate and rhythm, hypertension, glaucoma, asthma, and even a runny nose.

The study of nervous system pharmacology extends over the next 13 chapters of this text. Traditionally, the study of neuropharmacology begins with the autonomic nervous system. A firm grasp of autonomic physiology is necessary to understand nervous, cardiovascular, and respiratory pharmacology. This chapter serves dual purposes. First, it is a comprehensive review of autonomic nervous system physiology, a subject that is often covered superficially in anatomy and physiology classes. Second, it introduces the four fundamental classes of autonomic medications discussed in Chapters 13 and 14.

THE NERVOUS SYSTEM

The Two Major Subdivisions of the Nervous System

12.1 The two major subdivisions of the nervous system are the central nervous system and the peripheral nervous system.

The nervous system is the master controller of most activities that occur within the body. Compared to the other major regulator, the endocrine system, the nervous system acts instantaneously to make adjustments that maintain vital functions.

The nervous system has two major divisions: the **central nervous system (CNS)** and the **peripheral nervous system**. The CNS consists of the brain and spinal cord. The peripheral nervous system consists of all nervous tissue outside the CNS, including sensory and motor neurons. The basic functions of the nervous system are as follows:

- Recognize changes in the internal and external environments

- Process and integrate the environmental changes that are perceived

- React to the environmental changes by producing an action or response

Figure 12.1 shows the functional divisions of the nervous system. In the peripheral nervous system, neurons either recognize changes to the environment (sensory division) or respond to these changes by moving muscles or secreting chemicals (motor division). The **somatic nervous system** consists of nerves that provide *voluntary* control over skeletal muscle. Nerves of the **autonomic nervous system (ANS)**, on the other hand, have *involuntary* control over the contraction of smooth muscle and cardiac muscle, and the secretion of glands. Organs and tissues regulated by neurons from the ANS include the heart, digestive tract, respiratory tract, reproductive tracts, arteries, salivary glands, and portions of the eye. Whereas only a few medications directly affect the somatic nervous system, a large number affect autonomic nerves.

The Peripheral Nervous System

12.2 The peripheral nervous system is divided into somatic and autonomic components.

With its immense potential and complexity, the human brain requires a continuous flow of information to accomplish its functions. In addition, the brain would be useless without a means to carry out its commands. The peripheral nervous system provides the brain with the means to communicate with and receive sensory messages from the outside world.

Neurons in the peripheral nervous system *recognize* changes to the environment (sensory division) and *respond* to those changes by moving muscles or secreting chemicals (motor division). The sensory division consists of specialized nerves that recognize touch, pain, heat, body position, light, or specific chemicals in body fluids. These sensory neurons send their messages to the spinal cord. Based on this information, the brain determines what messages are important, determines whether an action is needed, and plans an appropriate response.

The motor division is divided into two components. The somatic nervous system consists of nerves that provide for the voluntary control of skeletal muscle. The nerves of the autonomic nervous system (ANS) provide for the involuntary control of vital functions of the cardiovascular, digestive, respiratory, and genitourinary

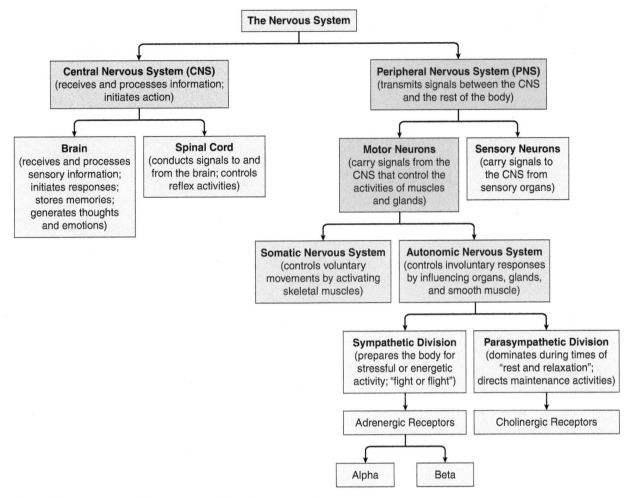

Figure 12.1 Functional divisions of the peripheral nervous system.

systems. The ANS controls vital life activities without people being aware of its functions. The three main activities of the ANS are:

- Contraction of smooth muscle of the bronchi, blood vessels, gastrointestinal (GI) tract, eye, and genitourinary tract
- Contraction of cardiac muscle
- Secretion of salivary, sweat, gastric, and bronchial glands

The ANS is particularly important to pharmacology because a large number of medications affect autonomic nerves. Some of these drug actions produce desirable, therapeutic effects, whereas others produce adverse effects. The remainder of this chapter reviews the structure and function of this complex system.

The Autonomic Nervous System: Sympathetic and Parasympathetic Branches

12.3 The autonomic nervous system is divided into two mostly opposing components: the sympathetic and parasympathetic branches.

The autonomic nervous system has two divisions: the sympathetic and the parasympathetic nervous systems. With a few exceptions,

organs and glands receive nerves from both branches of the autonomic nervous system. The ultimate action of the smooth muscle or gland depends on which branch is sending the most signals at a given time. The major actions of the two divisions are shown in Figure 12.2. It is essential that the student learn these actions early in the study of pharmacology because knowledge of autonomic effects is used to predict the actions and side effects of many drugs.

The **sympathetic nervous system** is activated under conditions of stress and produces a set of actions called the **fight-or-flight response**. Activation of this system will ready the body for an immediate response to a potential threat. The heart rate and blood pressure increase, and more blood is shunted to skeletal muscles. The liver immediately produces more glucose for energy. The bronchi dilate to allow more air into the lungs, and the pupils dilate for better vision.

Conversely, the **parasympathetic nervous system** is activated under non-stressful conditions and produces symptoms called the **rest-and-digest response**. Digestive processes are promoted, and heart rate and blood pressure decline. Not as much air is needed, so the bronchi constrict. Most of the actions of the parasympathetic division are opposite to those of the sympathetic division.

A proper balance of the two autonomic branches is required for internal homeostasis. Under most circumstances, the two branches

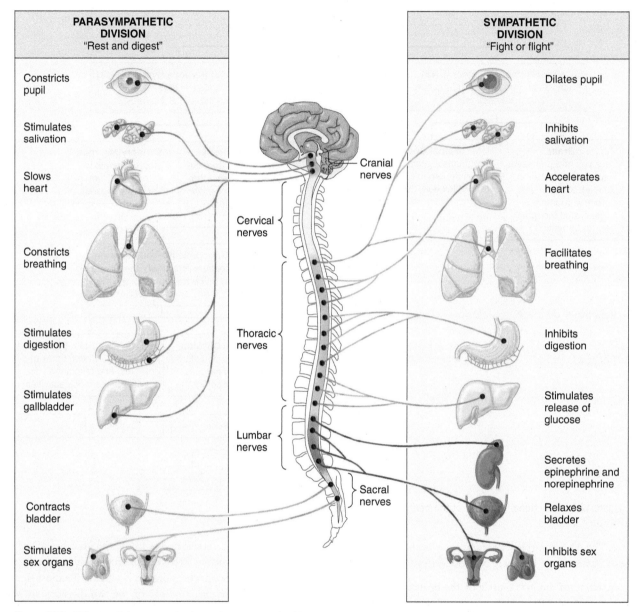

Figure 12.2 Effects of the sympathetic and parasympathetic nervous systems.
Source: Krogh, D. (2011). *Biology: A Guide to the Natural World* (5th ed., Fig. 27.8). Upper Saddle River, NJ: Prentice Hall. Reprinted by permission.

cooperate to achieve a balance of readiness and relaxation. Because they have mostly opposite effects, homeostasis may be achieved by changing one or both branches. For example, heart rate can be increased by either *increasing* the firing of sympathetic nerves or *decreasing* the firing of parasympathetic nerves. This allows the body a means of fine-tuning its essential organ systems.

The sympathetic and parasympathetic divisions are not always opposite in their effects. For example, the constriction of arterioles is controlled entirely by the sympathetic branch. Sympathetic stimulation causes constriction of arterioles, whereas lack of stimulation causes vasodilation. Sweat glands are controlled only by sympathetic nerves. In the male reproductive system, the roles are complementary. Erection of the penis is a function of the parasympathetic division, and ejaculation is controlled by the sympathetic branch.

Structure and Function of Synapses

12.4 Synaptic transmission allows information to be communicated between two nerves or from nerves to muscles or glands.

For information to be transmitted throughout the nervous system, neurons must communicate with each other and with muscles and glands. In the autonomic nervous system, this involves the connection of two neurons in series. As an action potential travels along the first nerve, it encounters a structure at the end called a **synapse**. The synapse contains a physical space called the synaptic cleft, which must be bridged for the impulse to reach the next nerve. The nerve carrying the original impulse is called

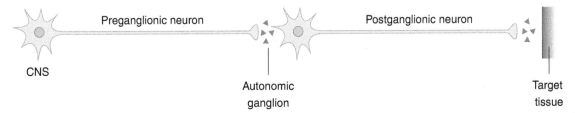

Figure 12.3 Basic structure of an autonomic pathway.

the **presynaptic neuron**. The nerve on the other side of the synapse, waiting to receive the impulse, is the **postsynaptic neuron**. If this connection occurs outside the CNS, it is called a **ganglion**. The basic structure of a synapse is shown in Figure 12.3.

The physical space of the synaptic cleft is bridged by **neurotransmitters**, which are released into the synaptic cleft when a nerve impulse reaches the end of the presynaptic neuron. The neurotransmitter diffuses across the synaptic cleft to reach receptors on the postsynaptic neuron, which results in the impulse being regenerated. Outside the CNS, the regenerated action potential travels along the postganglionic neuron until it reaches its target: a type of synapse called a neuroeffector junction, which is located on smooth muscle, cardiac muscle, or a gland. When released at the neuroeffector junction, the neurotransmitter induces the target tissue to elicit its characteristic response. Generally, the more neurotransmitter released into the synapse, the greater and longer lasting will be its effect. This process, called **synaptic transmission**, is illustrated in Figure 12.4. There are several different types of neurotransmitters located throughout the nervous system, and each is associated with particular functions.

A large number of drugs act by altering neurotransmitter activity in the ANS. Some medications are identical to endogenous neurotransmitters, or have a very similar chemical structure, and are able to directly activate a gland or muscle. Other drugs are used to stimulate or block the actions of natural neurotransmitters. A firm grasp of autonomic physiology is essential to understanding the actions and adverse effects of hundreds of drugs.

The two-neuron chain of the ANS allows multiple locations at which drugs can act. Some medications affect the outflow of nervous impulses at their source—the CNS. A second potential site for drug action is at the ganglia, the synapse where the preganglionic and postganglionic neurons meet. Yet a third possible site is at the end of the chain, at the neuroeffector junction of the target organs.

Although complex, actions of drugs that affect the ANS can be grouped into just a few categories. The five general mechanisms by which drugs affect synaptic transmission in the ANS are as follows:

- Medications may affect the *synthesis* of the neurotransmitter in the preganglionic nerve. Drugs that decrease neurotransmitter synthesis inhibit autonomic responses. Those that increase neurotransmitter synthesis have the opposite effect (enhance the autonomic response).

- Medications can prevent the *storage* of the neurotransmitter in vesicles within the preganglionic nerve. Prevention of neurotransmitter storage inhibits autonomic actions.

- Medications can influence the *release* of the neurotransmitter from the preganglionic nerve. Promoting neurotransmitter release stimulates autonomic responses, whereas preventing neurotransmitter release has the opposite effect (inhibit autonomic responses).

- Medications can *bind* to the neurotransmitter receptors on the postganglionic cell. Drugs that bind to receptors and stimulate the cell will increase autonomic responses. Those that attach to the postganglionic cell and prevent the natural neurotransmitter from reaching its receptors will inhibit autonomic actions.

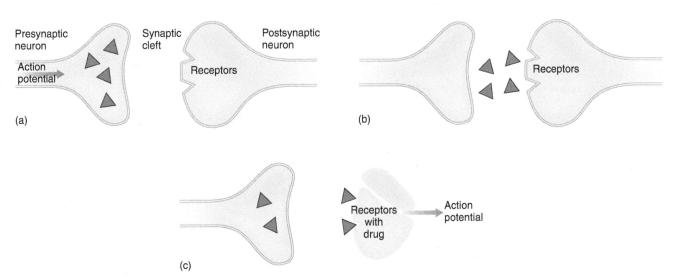

Figure 12.4 Synaptic transmission: (a) action potential reaches synapse; (b) neurotransmitter is released into synaptic cleft; (c) neurotransmitter reaches receptors to regenerate action potential.

• Medications can *prevent the destruction or reuptake* of the neurotransmitter. These drugs cause the neurotransmitter to remain in the synapse for a longer time and will stimulate autonomic actions.

It is important to understand that autonomic drugs are rarely given to correct physiological defects in the ANS itself. Compared to other body systems, the ANS has remarkably little disease. Rather, medications are used to stimulate or inhibit target organs or glands of the ANS, such as the heart, lungs, or digestive tract. With few exceptions, the disorder lies in the target organ, not the ANS. Thus when an autonomic drug is administered, the goal is not to treat an autonomic disease; it is to correct disorders of target organs through the drug's effects on autonomic nerves.

Acetylcholine and Cholinergic Transmission

12.5 Acetylcholine is the neurotransmitter released at cholinergic receptors, which may be nicotinic or muscarinic.

The two primary neurotransmitters of the autonomic nervous system are **norepinephrine (NE)**, also known as noradrenaline, and **acetylcholine (Ach)**. A detailed knowledge of the underlying physiology of these neurotransmitters is required for proper understanding of drug action. When reading the following sections, the student should refer to the sites of acetylcholine and norepinephrine action shown in Figure 12.5.

Nerves that release acetylcholine are called **cholinergic** nerves. There are two types of cholinergic receptors that bind acetylcholine; they are named after certain chemicals that bind to them:

• Nicotinic receptors: postganglionic neurons ending in ganglia in both the sympathetic and the parasympathetic nervous systems

• Muscarinic receptors: postganglionic neurons ending in neuroeffector target tissues in the parasympathetic nervous system

Early research on laboratory animals found that the actions of acetylcholine at the *ganglia* resemble those of nicotine, the active agent found in tobacco. Because of this similarity, receptors for acetylcholine in the ganglia are called **nicotinic** receptors. Nicotinic receptors are also present in skeletal muscle, which is controlled by the somatic nervous system. Because these receptors are present in so many locations, drugs that affect nicotinic receptors produce profound effects on both the autonomic and the somatic nervous systems. Activation of the nicotinic acetylcholine receptors causes tachycardia, hypertension, and increased tone and motility in the digestive tract. Although nicotinic receptor blockers were some of the first drugs used to treat hypertension, the only current therapeutic application of these agents, known as ganglionic blockers, is to produce muscle relaxation during surgical procedures. Activation of acetylcholine receptors at *postganglionic* nerve endings in the parasympathetic nervous system results in the classic symptoms of parasympathetic stimulation shown in Figure 12.2. Early research discovered that these actions closely resemble those produced when a client ingests the poisonous mushroom *Amanita muscaria*. Because of this similarity, these acetylcholine receptors were named **muscarinic** receptors. Unlike the nicotinic receptors that have few pharmacological applications, a number of medications affect muscarinic receptors, and these are discussed in subsequent sections of this chapter. The locations of nicotinic and muscarinic receptors are illustrated in Figure 12.5. Table 12.1 summarizes the actions produced by the two types of acetylcholine receptors.

The physiology of acetylcholine affords several mechanisms by which drugs may act. Acetylcholine is synthesized in the presynaptic nerve terminal from choline and acetyl coenzyme A. The enzyme that catalyzes this reaction is called **acetylcholinesterase (AchE)**, or simply cholinesterase. (Note that the suffix, *-erase*, can be thought of as wiping out the Ach.) Once synthesized,

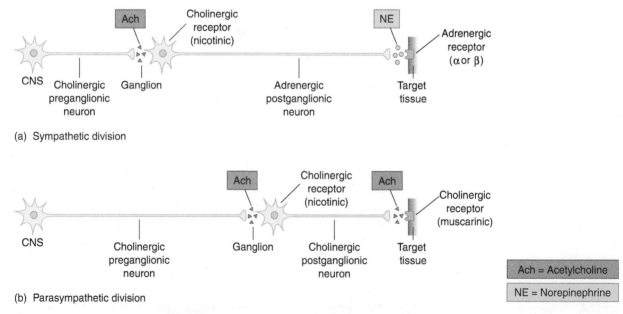

Figure 12.5   Receptors in the autonomic nervous system: (a) sympathetic division; (b) parasympathetic division.

TABLE 12.1 Types of Autonomic Receptors

Neurotransmitter	Receptor	Primary Locations	Responses
Acetylcholine (cholinergic)	Muscarinic	Parasympathetic target: organs other than the heart	Stimulation of smooth muscle and gland secretions
		Heart	Decreased heart rate and force of contraction
	Nicotinic	Postganglionic neurons and neuromuscular junctions of skeletal muscle	Stimulation of smooth muscle and gland secretions
Norepinephrine (adrenergic)	Alpha$_1$	All sympathetic target organs except the heart	Constricted blood vessels; dilated pupils
	Alpha$_2$	Presynaptic adrenergic nerve terminals	Inhibited release of norepinephrine
	Beta$_1$	Heart and kidneys	Increased heart rate and force of contraction; release of renin
	Beta$_2$	All sympathetic target organs except the heart	Inhibition of smooth muscle

acetylcholine is stored in vesicles in the presynaptic neuron. When an action potential reaches the nerve ending, acetylcholine is released into the synaptic cleft, where it diffuses across to find nicotinic or muscarinic receptors. Acetylcholine in the synaptic cleft is rapidly destroyed by acetylcholinesterase, and choline is reformed. The choline is taken up by the presynaptic neuron to make more acetylcholine, and the cycle is repeated. Drugs can affect the formation, release, receptor activation, or destruction of acetylcholine.

Some drugs (and poisons) can prevent the inactivation of Ach by blocking the acetylcholinesterase enzyme. These drugs will cause a prolonged action of Ach at the synapse. Other medications will prevent Ach from reaching its receptors, thus blocking its actions. Medications that interfere with the life cycle of Ach are presented in Chapter 13.

Pseudocholinesterase, also known as plasma cholinesterase, is another enzyme that destroys Ach. Found primarily in the liver, pseudocholinesterase rapidly inactivates Ach and drugs with a chemical structure similar to Ach as they circulate in the plasma. Some people are born with a genetic deficiency of this enzyme and are unable to inactivate succinylcholine (Quelicin), a surgical drug structurally similar to Ach. These clients are particularly sensitive to the effects of succinylcholine.

Norepinephrine and Adrenergic Transmission

12.6 Norepinephrine is the primary neurotransmitter released at adrenergic receptors, which may be alpha or beta.

In the sympathetic nervous system, norepinephrine is the neurotransmitter released at almost all postganglionic nerves. Norepinephrine belongs to a class of endogenous agents called **catecholamines**, all of which are involved in neurotransmission. Other catecholamines include epinephrine (adrenaline) and dopamine. The receptors at the ends of postganglionic sympathetic neurons are called **adrenergic**, which comes from the word *adrenaline*.

Adrenergic receptors are of two basic types: **alpha (α) receptors** and **beta (β) receptors**. These receptors are further divided into the subtypes alpha$_1$ and alpha$_2$ and beta$_1$, beta$_2$, and beta$_3$. Activation of each receptor subtype results in a characteristic set of physiological responses, which are summarized in Table 12.1.

The significance of these receptor subtypes to pharmacology cannot be overstated. Some drugs are selective and activate only one type of adrenergic receptor, whereas others affect all receptor subtypes. Furthermore, a drug may activate one type of receptor at low doses and begin to affect other receptor subtypes as the dose is increased. Committing the receptor types and their responses to memory is an essential step in learning autonomic pharmacology.

Norepinephrine is synthesized in the nerve terminal through a series of steps that require the amino acids phenylalanine and tyrosine. The final step of the synthesis involves the conversion of dopamine to norepinephrine. Norepinephrine is stored in vesicles until an action potential triggers its release into the synaptic cleft. It then diffuses across the cleft to alpha or beta receptors on the effector organ. The reuptake of norepinephrine back into the presynaptic neuron terminates its action. Once reuptake occurs, norepinephrine in the nerve terminal may be returned to vesicles for future use or destroyed enzymatically by **monoamine oxidase (MAO)**. The primary method for termination of norepinephrine action is through reuptake. Many drugs affect autonomic function by influencing the synthesis, storage, release, reuptake, or destruction of norepinephrine.

NCLEX Success Tips

A decreased acetylcholine level has been implicated as a cause of cognitive changes in healthy elderly clients and in the severity of dementia.

Choline acetyltransferase, an enzyme necessary for acetylcholine synthesis, has been found to be deficient in clients with dementia.

Norepinephrine is associated with aggression, sleep-wake patterns, and the regulation of physical responses to emotional stimuli, such as the increased heart and respiratory rates caused by panic.

The adrenal medulla is a tissue closely associated with the sympathetic nervous system that has a much different anatomical and physiological arrangement than the rest of the sympathetic branch. The preganglionic neuron from the spinal cord terminates in the adrenal medulla and releases the neurotransmitter epinephrine directly into the blood. Epinephrine travels to target organs, where it elicits the classic fight-or-flight symptoms. The action of epinephrine is terminated through hepatic metabolism rather than reuptake.

NCLEX Success Tips

A pheochromocytoma is a tumour of the adrenal medulla that secretes excessive catecholamine. Pheochromocytoma causes hypertension, tachycardia, hyperglycemia, hypermetabolism, and weight loss.

Excessive secretion of aldosterone in the adrenal cortex is also responsible for hypertension. This hormone acts on the renal tubule, where it promotes reabsorption of sodium and excretion of potassium and hydrogen ions.

Other types of adrenergic receptors exist. Beta$_3$ receptors are located in the central and autonomic nervous systems and may play a role in lipolysis. Although dopamine was once thought to function only as a chemical precursor to norepinephrine, research has determined that dopamine serves a larger role as neurotransmitter. Five dopaminergic receptors (D$_1$ through D$_5$) have been discovered in the CNS. Dopaminergic receptors in the CNS are important to the action of certain antipsychotic medicines (Chapter 19) and in the treatment of Parkinson's disease (Chapter 20). Dopamine receptors in the peripheral nervous system are located in the arterioles of the kidney and other viscera. These receptors likely have a role in autonomic function.

NCLEX Success Tips

Psychopharmacological therapy aims to restore the balance of neurotransmitters.

Cocaine blocks reuptake of norepinephrine, epinephrine, and dopamine, causing an excess of these neurotransmitters at postsynaptic receptor sites. Consequently, the drug is likely to cause tachyarrhythmias. As craving for the drug increases, a person addicted to cocaine typically experiences euphoria followed by depression.

Bupropion (Wellbutrin, Zyban) inhibits dopamine reuptake; it is an activating antidepressant and could cause agitation. Bupropion lowers the seizure threshold, especially at doses greater than 450 mg/day, and possible adverse effects are visual disturbances and increased libido. The nurse must closely monitor the client for suicidal feelings. As the client with major depression begins to feel better, he or she may have enough energy to carry out a suicide attempt.

Benztropine (Cogentin) is an anticholinergic administered to reduce extrapyramidal adverse effects in a client taking antipsychotic drugs. It works by restoring the equilibrium between the neurotransmitters acetylcholine and dopamine in the central nervous system (CNS).

Studies of the role of neurotransmitters in schizophrenia have shown that the disease results (in part) from an overactive dopamine system in the brain. Excessive dopamine activity may be responsible for such symptoms as hallucinations, agitation, delusional thinking, and grandiosity—forms of hyperactivity that have been linked to excessive dopamine activity.

Metoclopramide (Metonia) is a dopamine antagonist that stimulates motility of the upper gastrointestinal (GI) tract, increases lower esophageal sphincter tone, and blocks dopamine receptors at the chemoreceptor trigger zone. It may be used for delayed gastric emptying secondary to diabetic gastroparesis.

Levodopa-carbidopa (Sinemet), which is used to replace insufficient dopamine in a client with Parkinson's disease, may cause harmless darkening of the urine. Blurred vision is an expected adverse effect. The client should take levodopa-carbidopa shortly before meals, not at bedtime, and must continue to take it for life.

Extrapyramidal effects and antipsychotic-induced muscle rigidity are caused by a low level of dopamine. Dopamine receptor agonists reduce extrapyramidal symptoms such as bradyphrenia (slowed thought processes), akathisia (meaningless movements such as marching in place), or dystonia (abnormal muscle rigidity or movements).

Hallucinations, grandiosity, and delusional thinking are attributable to the effects of excessive dopamine activity.

Although it is often stated that control of the ANS is involuntary, this is an oversimplification. For example, strong emotions such as rage are seated in the brain, but they trigger the heart to race, the blood pressure to rise, and the respiration rate to increase. Mental depression can have the opposite effects. The smell of steak or chicken cooking on the grill can increase peristalsis, resulting in "grumbling" of the stomach and increased salivation. Clearly, autonomic actions can be modified by higher brain centres.

Drugs can affect the ANS by influencing these higher centres. For example, drugs that decrease anxiety or diminish the incidence of panic attacks can slow the heart rate and lower blood pressure through their ability to affect conscious thought. It is important to understand that these drugs do not necessarily act on autonomic receptors. Nor do clients consciously lower their blood pressure or heart rate. The autonomic effect is indirect, caused by a reduction of stress, and it is at a subconscious level. Controlling autonomic activity through conscious thought is the principle that underlies biofeedback therapy.

AUTONOMIC DRUGS

Classification and Naming of Autonomic Drugs

12.7 Given the opposite actions of the sympathetic and parasympathetic nervous systems, autonomic drugs are classified based on one of four possible actions.

Given the opposite actions of the sympathetic and parasympathetic nervous systems, autonomic drugs are classified based on one of four possible actions:

1. Stimulation of the sympathetic nervous system: These drugs are called **adrenergics**, sympathomimetics, or adrenergic agonists, and they produce the classic symptoms of the fight-or-flight response.

2. Stimulation of the parasympathetic nervous system: These drugs are called **cholinergics**, parasympathomimetics, or muscarinic agonists, and they produce the characteristic symptoms of the rest-and-digest response.

3. Inhibition of the sympathetic nervous system: These drugs are called **adrenergic antagonists**, **antiadrenergics**, or adrenergic blockers, and they produce actions *opposite* to those of the adrenergics.

4. Inhibition of the parasympathetic nervous system: These drugs are called **anticholinergics**, parasympatholytics, or muscarinic blockers, and they produce actions *opposite* to those of the cholinergics.

NCLEX Success Tip

Anticholinergic effects result from blockage of the parasympathetic nervous system and include urine retention, blurred vision, dry mouth, and constipation.

Students beginning their study of pharmacology often have difficulty understanding the terminology and actions of autonomic drugs. Upon examining the four drug classes, however, it is evident that only one group need be learned because the others are logical extensions of the first. If the fight-or-flight actions of the adrenergics are learned, the other three groups are either the same or opposite. For example, both the adrenergics and the anticholinergics increase heart rate and dilate the pupils. The other two groups, the cholinergics and the adrenergic antagonists, have the opposite effects of slowing heart rate and constricting the pupils. Although this is an oversimplification and exceptions do exist, it is a time-saving means of learning the basic actions and adverse effects of dozens of drugs that affect the autonomic nervous system. It should be emphasized again that mastering the actions and terminology of autonomic drugs early in the study of pharmacology will reap rewards later in the course when these drugs are applied to various systems.

CHAPTER 12

Understanding the Chapter

Key Concepts Summary

The numbered key concepts provide a succinct summary of the important points from the corresponding numbered section within the chapter. If any of these points are not clear, refer to the numbered section within the chapter for review.

12.1   The two major subdivisions of the nervous system are the central nervous system and the peripheral nervous system.

12.2   The peripheral nervous system is divided into somatic and autonomic components.

12.3   The autonomic nervous system is divided into two mostly opposing components: the sympathetic and parasympathetic branches.

12.4   Synaptic transmission allows information to be communicated between two nerves or from nerves to muscles or glands.

12.5   Acetylcholine is the neurotransmitter released at cholinergic receptors, which may be nicotinic or muscarinic.

12.6   Norepinephrine is the primary neurotransmitter released at adrenergic receptors, which may be alpha or beta.

12.7   Given the opposite actions of the sympathetic and parasympathetic nervous systems, autonomic drugs are classified based on one of four possible actions.

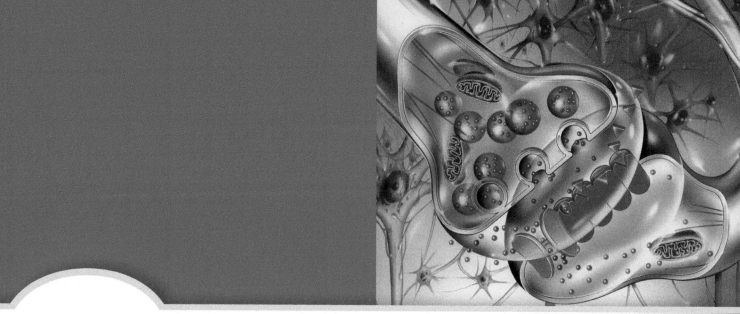
John Bavosi/Science Source

CHAPTER 13

Pharmacotherapy with Cholinergic Agonists and Antagonists

LEARNING OUTCOMES

After reading this chapter, the student should be able to:

1. Compare and contrast the mechanisms of action for direct- and indirect-acting cholinergic agonists.

2. Identify the actions of muscarinic agonists and their pharmacological uses.

3. Describe the pharmacotherapy of myasthenia gravis.

4. Explain the actions and pharmacological applications of nicotine.

5. For each of the drug classes listed in Protoype Drugs, identify the prototype and representative drugs and explain the mechanism(s) of drug action, primary indications, contraindications, significant drug interactions, pregnancy category, and important adverse effects.

6. Apply the nursing process to care for clients who are receiving pharmacotherapy with cholinergic agonists and antagonists.

7. Identify the physiological responses produced when a drug blocks cholinergic receptors.

8. Explain the actions of muscarinic antagonists and compare them with other cholinergic antagonists.

9. Explain how the therapeutic actions and adverse effects of the cholinergic antagonists can be explained by their blockade of muscarinic or nicotinic receptors.

CHAPTER OUTLINE

▸ Cholinergic Agonists

▸ Clinical Applications of Cholinergics

▸ Nicotinic Agonists (Nicotine)

▸ Anticholinergics

▸ Clinical Applications of Anticholinergics

PROTOTYPE DRUGS | Cholinergics

bethanechol (Duvoid)

NCLEX Success Tips

Bethanechol stimulates the smooth muscle of the bladder, causing it to release retained urine. Bethanechol doesn't act on the urinary sphincter, nor does it dilate the urethra. The bladder contains smooth muscle, not skeletal muscle.

Bethanechol will increase gastrointestinal (GI) motility, which may cause nausea, belching, vomiting, intestinal cramps, and diarrhea. Peristalsis is increased rather than decreased. With high doses of bethanechol, cardiovascular responses may include vasodilation, decreased cardiac rate, and decreased force of cardiac contraction, which may cause hypotension. Salivation or sweating may greatly increase.

Bethanechol, a cholinergic drug, may be used in gastroesophageal reflux disease (GERD) to increase lower esophageal sphincter pressure and facilitate gastric emptying. Cholinergic adverse effects may include urinary urgency, diarrhea, abdominal cramping, hypotension, and increased salivation. To avoid these adverse effects, the client should be closely monitored to establish the minimum effective dose.

ANTICHOLINERGICS

Atropine

NCLEX Success Tips

Atropine is an anticholinergic drug that decreases mucous secretions in the respiratory tract and dries the mucus membranes of the mouth, nose, pharynx, and bronchi. Moderate to large doses cause tachycardia and palpitations.

Atropine sulfate causes pupil dilation. This action is contraindicated for clients with glaucoma because it increases intraocular pressure.

The nurse should tell the client that, when used as preanesthesia medication, atropine and other cholinergic blocking agents reduce salivation and gastric secretions, thus helping to prevent aspiration of secretions during surgery. Atropine increases the heart rate and cardiac contractility, decreases bronchial secretions, and causes bronchodilation.

OTHER PROTOTYPES

Pr *benztropine (Cogentin)*

Pr *iptratopium (Atrovent)*

Cholinergic Agonists

13.1 Drugs can activate or suppress cholinergic receptors either directly or indirectly.

Recall from Chapter 12 that cholinergic receptors are located throughout the peripheral nervous system. To understand the effects of cholinergic drugs, it is important to review the locations of these receptors. In the autonomic nervous system, cholinergic

synapses are present at the neuroeffector junctions in the parasympathetic division and at the ganglia in both the parasympathetic and the sympathetic divisions. In the somatic nervous system, cholinergic synapses are present at the neuromuscular junctions, which result in skeletal muscle contraction. In addition, cholinergic synapses are present throughout the central nervous system (CNS).

The degree of activation at a cholinergic synapse is dependent on the amount of neurotransmitter, acetylcholine (Ach), interacting with its receptors. Drugs and other chemicals that increase the action of Ach at cholinergic receptors will promote rest-and-digest responses. These substances are called **cholinergic agonists**, or parasympathomimetics.

Also recall from Chapter 12 that there are two primary types of cholinergic receptors: muscarinic and nicotinic. Although Ach itself stimulates both types of receptors, drugs may be selective for only one type. For example, bethanechol (Duvoid) is selective for muscarinic receptors and thus it is called a **muscarinic agonist**. On the other hand, nicotine is selective for nicotinic receptors and therefore is classified as a **nicotinic agonist**. Note that both bethanechol and nicotine are considered cholinergic agonists; the terms *muscarinic* and *nicotinic* are used to specify which cholinergic synapses are activated. If the student has not yet learned the differences between muscarinic and nicotinic receptors, a summary of these differences is provided in Table 13.1.

Cholinergic agonists can activate cholinergic receptors directly or indirectly. Direct-acting drugs, such as bethanechol, enter the synaptic cleft and bind to Ach receptors to produce

TABLE 13.1 Types of Cholinergic Receptors and Their Actions

	Muscarinic	**Nicotinic**
Receptor location	Glands, smooth muscle, cardiac muscle	Skeletal muscle, autonomic ganglia, brain, adrenal gland*
General actions	Pupil constriction Decreased accommodation of the eye Increased GI motility Decreased heart rate Decreased blood pressure Increased glandular secretions (salivary, lacrimal, and sweat) Constriction of bronchial smooth muscle	Skeletal muscle contraction Initial stimulation of glandular secretion, followed by inhibition Increased heart rate Increased blood pressure
Antagonists	Atropine, scopolamine	Mecamylamine, succinylcholine, tubocurarine

*Some effects of nicotinic activation are caused by the release of epinephrine from the adrenal gland. The epinephrine subsequently activates the adrenergic receptors.

TABLE 13.2	Cholinergics	
Type	**Drug**	**Primary Use**
Direct acting (muscarinic agonists)	**Pr** bethanechol (Duvoid)	Increase urination
	pilocarpine (Salagen)	Glaucoma
Indirect acting (cholinesterase inhibitors)	edrophonium (Tensilon)	Diagnosis of myasthenia gravis
	galantamine (Reminyl)	Alzheimer's disease
	neostigmine (Prostigmin)	Myasthenia gravis, increase urination

typical rest-and-digest responses. Some of these direct-acting drugs cause the release of additional Ach into the synaptic cleft, thus enhancing the normal physiological responses caused by Ach. The direct-acting cholinergic agonists essentially act by the same mechanism as Ach itself.

Indirect-acting drugs inhibit acetylcholinesterase (AchE) (also called cholinesterase), the enzyme in cholinergic synapses that destroys Ach. By blocking the destruction of Ach, the neurotransmitter accumulates and remains in the synaptic cleft for a longer time to produce enhanced rest-and-digest responses. Some indirect drugs such as neostigmine (Prostigmin) bind only briefly to AchE and exhibit short durations of action. These drugs are called *reversible* cholinesterase inhibitors.

There are certain chemicals that bind *irreversibly* to AchE. For example, certain insecticides and nerve gas agents bind to AchE for prolonged periods and can cause significant mortality if ingested or absorbed. Because of the hazardous nature of these chemicals, irreversible cholinesterase inhibitors are not widely used in medicine.

Cholinergic agonists (parasympathomimetics) activate the parasympathetic nervous system and induce the rest-and-digest response. They are listed in Table 13.2. A few have clinical applications in the treatment of glaucoma, myasthenia gravis, and early Alzheimer's disease.

NCLEX Success Tip

A positive edrophonium test confirms the diagnosis of myasthenia gravis. After edrophonium administration, most clients with myasthenia gravis show markedly improved muscle tone within 30 to 60 seconds following administration, and muscle strength within 4 to 5 minutes (positive Tensilon test).

Clinical Applications of Cholinergics

13.2 Muscarinic agonists produce their effects by directly stimulating cholinergic receptors.

The classic cholinergic (parasympathomimetic) is acetylcholine (Ach), the endogenous neurotransmitter at cholinergic synapses

in the autonomic nervous system. Acetylcholine, however, has almost no therapeutic use because it is rapidly destroyed after administration and it produces many side effects. Recall that Ach is the neurotransmitter at the ganglia in both the parasympathetic and the sympathetic divisions and at the neuroeffector junctions in the parasympathetic nervous system, as well as in skeletal muscle. It is not surprising, then, that administration of Ach or drugs that mimic Ach will have widespread and varied effects on the body.

Cholinergics are divided into two subclasses, direct acting and indirect acting, based on their mechanism of action. Direct-acting agents bind to cholinergic receptors to produce the rest-and-digest response and increase smooth muscle tone. For example, bethanechol causes the detrusor muscle in the bladder wall to contract and expel urine. Because they are relatively resistant to the enzyme acetylcholinesterase, direct-acting agents have a longer duration of action than Ach. They are poorly absorbed across the gastrointestinal (GI) tract and generally do not cross the blood-brain barrier. They have little effect on Ach receptors in ganglia. Because they are moderately selective to muscarinic receptors when used at therapeutic doses, they are sometimes called muscarinic agonists.

The indirect-acting cholinergics, such as neostigmine (Prostigmin), inhibit the action of acetylcholinesterase. This inhibition allows endogenous Ach to avoid rapid destruction and remain on cholinergic receptors for a longer time, thus prolonging its action. These drugs are called cholinesterase inhibitors. Unlike the direct-acting agents, the cholinesterase inhibitors are non-selective and affect all Ach sites: autonomic ganglia, muscarinic receptors, skeletal muscle, and Ach sites in the CNS.

Physostigmine was one of the first indirect-acting cholinergics to be discovered. It was obtained from the dried ripe seeds of *Physostigma venenosum,* a plant found in West Africa. The bean of this plant was used in tribal rituals. During World War II, similar compounds were synthesized that produced potent neurological effects and could be used during chemical warfare. This class of agents now includes organophosphate insecticides, such as malathion and parathion, and toxic nerve gases such as sarin. Nurses who work in agricultural areas may become quite familiar with the symptoms of acute poisoning with organophosphates. Poisoning results in intense stimulation of the parasympathetic nervous system, which may result in death if untreated.

Because of their high potential for serious adverse effects, few cholinergics are widely used in pharmacotherapy. Some have clinical applications in ophthalmology because they reduce intraocular pressure in clients with glaucoma (Chapter 63). Others are used for their stimulatory effects on the smooth muscle of the bowel or urinary tract.

Several drugs in this class are used for their effects on Ach receptors in skeletal muscle or in the CNS, rather than for their parasympathetic action. **Myasthenia gravis** is a disease characterized by destruction of nicotinic receptors on skeletal muscle. Administration of neostigmine will stimulate skeletal muscle contraction and help to reverse the severe muscle weakness characteristic of this disease. Galantamine (Reminyl) is used to treat Alzheimer's disease because of its ability to inhibit cholinesterase and thus increase the amount of Ach at receptors in the CNS (Chapter 20).

PROTOTYPE DRUG | **Bethanechol (Duvoid)**

Actions and Uses: Bethanechol is a direct-acting cholinergic that interacts with muscarinic receptors to cause actions typical of parasympathetic stimulation. Its effects are most noted in the digestive and urinary tracts, where it will stimulate smooth muscle contraction. These actions are useful in increasing smooth muscle tone and muscular contractions in the GI tract following general anesthesia. In addition, it is used to treat non-obstructive urinary retention in clients with atony of the bladder.

Administration Alerts:

- Never administer by the intramuscular (IM) or intravenous (IV) route.
- Oral and subcutaneous (SC) doses are *not* interchangeable.
- Monitor blood pressure, pulse, and respirations before administration and for at least 1 hour after SC administration.
- Bethanechol is pregnancy category C.

Pharmacokinetics: Bethanechol is poorly absorbed from the GI tract, but it may still be administered orally (PO). It can be given by SC injection. Peak effect is 30 minutes SC and 60 minutes PO.

Adverse Effects and Interactions: The side effects of bethanechol are predicted from its parasympathetic actions. It should be used with extreme caution in clients with disorders that could be aggravated by increased contractions of the digestive tract, such as suspected obstruction, active ulcer, or inflammatory disease. The same caution should be exercised in clients with suspected urinary obstruction or chronic obstructive pulmonary disease (COPD). Side effects include increased salivation, sweating, abdominal cramping, and hypotension that could lead to fainting. It should not be given to clients with asthma.

Drug interactions with bethanechol include increased effects from cholinesterase inhibitors and decreased effects from procainamide (Procan), quinidine (Quinate), atropine, and epinephrine.

Nicotinic Agonists (Nicotine)

13.3 Nicotine acts by activating acetylcholine receptors at the ganglia.

Nicotinic agonists act by activating Ach receptors at the ganglia. Very few drugs are used for their effects on Ach nicotinic receptors located in the autonomic ganglia. These ganglia synapse with neurons that lead to skeletal muscles (nicotinic receptors) as well as with those that lead to effector organs (muscarinic receptors). Drugs that affect the ganglia have the potential to produce widespread, non-selective effects on the autonomic nervous system.

The only drug in widespread use that activates ganglionic receptors is nicotine. The most active component of tobacco smoke, nicotine, is well absorbed from the GI and respiratory mucosa as well as from the skin. Because nicotine acts at the ganglia, both parasympathetic and sympathetic responses are stimulated.

Stimulation of organ activity generally occurs with low doses, such as those acquired by cigarette smoking. Within seconds after smoking, activation of the CNS increases alertness. The heart rate and blood pressure increase, although these parameters may subsequently decrease due to the baroreceptor reflex. The emetic centre in the CNS is triggered, causing a feeling of nausea. As the level of nicotine in the blood falls, these same organ systems become depressed. Nicotine is pregnancy category D.

Nicotine is an extremely dangerous substance. Acute toxicity, which can occur due to the accidental ingestion of insecticides containing nicotine, may cause death due to paralysis of the respiratory muscles. The chronic effects of nicotine in tobacco smokers, such as lung cancer and emphysema, are well documented.

As a drug, nicotine is used as nicotine replacement therapy (NRT) in tobacco cessation programs. Delivery systems include chewing gum (Nicorette), transdermal patches (NicoDerm), and nasal spray (Nicotrol). Use of these products reduces the uncomfortable symptoms of nicotine withdrawal, such as difficulty sleeping, lack of concentration, depression, headaches, and food cravings. As tobacco use diminishes over an 8- to 12-week period, these products are gradually withdrawn.

The goal of NRT is to gradually reduce the client's physical dependence on nicotine. However, the nurse should remember that psychological dependence also occurs with nicotine and that most successful smoking cessation programs include behavioural modification therapy such as self-help groups. The consistent use of NRT roughly doubles a client's chances of quitting smoking, but a great deal of persistence and motivation is required.

Indirect-Acting Cholinergics

The indirect-acting cholinergic agonists inhibit the enzymatic destruction of Ach, allowing the neurotransmitter to remain on cholinergic receptors for a longer time. Like the direct-acting agonists, these drugs essentially prolong the actions of Ach. Unlike the direct-acting (muscarinic) agonists, however, the **acetylcholinesterase (AchE) inhibitors** are non-selective and affect Ach synapses located at the autonomic ganglia, muscarinic receptors, neuromuscular junctions, and Ach synapses in the CNS.

The muscarinic actions of the AchE inhibitors are identical to those described for the direct-acting drugs. As such, these drugs would be expected to increase peristalsis in the GI and urinary tracts, and some can decrease intraocular pressure.

Indirect-acting cholinergics are contraindicated for clients with mechanical obstruction of either the intestine or the urinary tract due to their ability to intensify smooth muscle contractions. Smooth muscle contractions can also occur in the bronchi, so extreme caution must be exercised when treating clients with asthma or COPD.

Because these medications can inhibit acetylcholinesterase at many locations, acetylcholine will accumulate at the muscarinic receptors and neuromuscular junctions and cause side effects such as increased salivation, increased muscle tone, urinary frequency, bronchoconstriction, and bradycardia. Monitor the client for drug-induced insomnia. Also assess pregnancy and breastfeeding status, as indirect-acting cholinergics are contraindicated in both situations.

Cholinergic crisis occurs when acetylcholine increases to toxic levels. Cholinergic crisis is characterized by excessive parasympathetic activity, including excessive salivation and profound muscle weakness. Atropine, an anticholinergic, should be available to counteract the increased levels of acetylcholine by providing selective blockage of muscarinic cholinergic receptors.

For clients with myasthenia gravis, it is important to perform a baseline physical assessment of neuromuscular and respiratory function. In myasthenia gravis, the nicotinic receptors on skeletal muscle are destroyed. As a result, the muscles of the respiratory tract and other muscle groups used for chewing, swallowing, and speaking are weakened. Therefore, it is important to assess the client's swallowing ability prior to administering an oral drug.

See Nursing Process Focus: Clients Receiving Cholinergic Therapy for specific points to include when teaching clients about indirect-acting cholinergics.

Direct-Acting Cholinergics

Because of the stimulation of the CNS by these agents, several additional nursing actions are required. These include assessment of past medical history for any of the following: angina pectoris, recent myocardial infarction, and dysrhythmias. Obtain history information on the possible use of lithium (Carbolith, Lithane) and adenosine (Adenocard) because both drugs are contraindicated due to their interaction with nicotine. Lithium is a CNS agent that can produce significant muscarinic blockade to atropine. Adenosine is an antidysrhythmic agent, and its effect with nicotine can cause an increased risk of heart block. For women who are breastfeeding, monitor their infant's respiratory patterns and any CNS changes prior to and after feedings. Monitor elderly clients for episodes of dizziness and sleep disturbances caused by CNS stimulation from the parasympathomimetic.

See Nursing Process Focus: Clients Receiving Cholinergic Therapy for specific points to include when teaching clients about direct-acting cholinergics.

NURSING PROCESS FOCUS

Clients Receiving Cholinergic Therapy

Assessment	Potential Nursing Diagnoses/Identified Patterns
Prior to administration: • Obtain complete health history, including vital signs, allergies, and drug history for possible drug interactions. • Assess reason for drug administration. • Assess for contraindications of drug administration. • Assess for urinary retention and urinary patterns initially and throughout therapy (direct acting). • Assess muscle strength, neuromuscular status, ptosis, diplopia, and chewing.	• Need for knowledge regarding drug therapy • Impaired physical mobility • Urinary incontinence • Risk for injury related to drug side effects

Planning: Client Goals and Expected Outcomes

The client will:

• Exhibit increased bowel/bladder function and tone by regaining normal pattern of elimination (direct acting)
• Exhibit a decrease in myasthenia gravis symptoms such as muscle weakness, ptosis, and diplopia (indirect acting)
• Demonstrate understanding of the drug by accurately describing the drug's purpose, action, side effects, and precautions

Implementation

Interventions (Rationales)	Client Education/Discharge Planning
All Cholinergics	
• Monitor for adverse effects such as abdominal cramping, diarrhea, excessive salivation, difficulty breathing, and muscle cramping. (These may indicate cholinergic crisis, which requires atropine.) • Monitor liver enzymes at initiation of therapy and weekly for 6 weeks (for possible hepatotoxicity). • Assess and monitor for appropriate self-care administration to prevent complications.	• Instruct client to report nausea, vomiting, diarrhea, rash, jaundice, change in colour of stool, or any other adverse reactions to the drug. • Instruct client to adhere to laboratory testing schedule for serum blood level tests of liver enzymes as directed. Instruct client to: • Take drug as directed on regular schedule to maintain serum levels and control symptoms • Not chew or crush sustained-release tablets • Take oral cholinergics on an empty stomach to lessen incidence of nausea and vomiting and to increase absorption

Direct Acting

- Monitor intake and output ratio. Palpate abdomen for bladder distention. (These drugs have an onset of action of 60 minutes due to binding of the drug to cholinergic receptors on the smooth muscle of the bladder, which contracts the bladder to stimulate urination.)
- Monitor for blurred vision (a cholinergic effect).
- Monitor for orthostatic hypotension.

- Advise client to be near bathroom facilities after taking drug.
- Advise client that blurred vision is a possible side effect and to take appropriate precautions.
- Instruct client not to drive or perform hazardous activities until effects of the drug are known.
- Instruct client to avoid abrupt changes in position and prolonged standing in one place.

Indirect Acting (Cholinesterase Inhibitors)

- Monitor muscle strength, neuromuscular status, ptosis, diplopia, and chewing to determine if the therapeutic effect is achieved.
- Schedule other medications around mealtimes unless contraindicated. (The indirect-acting cholinergic will aid in chewing and swallowing.)
- Schedule activities to avoid fatigue.
- Monitor for muscle weakness. (This symptom, depending on time onset, indicates cholinergic crisis—overdose—OR **myasthenic crisis**—underdose.)

- Instruct client to report difficulty with vision or swallowing.
- Instruct client to take indirect-acting cholinergic about 30 minutes before meal.
- Instruct client to plan activities according to muscle strength and fatigue.
- Instruct client to take frequent rest periods.

Instruct client to:

- Report any severe muscle weakness that occurs 1 hour after administration of medication
- Report any muscle weakness that occurs 3 or more hours after medication administration, as this is a major symptom of myasthenic crisis
- Not allow prescription to run out, especially if the medication is essential for breathing (respiratory muscle function)

Evaluation of Outcome Criteria

Evaluate effectiveness of drug therapy by confirming that client goals and expected outcomes have been met (see "Planning").

See Tables 13.2 and 13.3 for a list of drugs to which these nursing applications apply.

Anticholinergics

13.4 Anticholinergics act by blocking the effects of acetylcholine at muscarinic or nicotinic receptors.

Anticholinergics are drugs that inhibit parasympathetic impulses. By suppressing the parasympathetic division, symptoms of the fight-or-flight response are induced. The anticholinergics are listed in Table 13.3.

TABLE 13.3 Anticholinergics

Drug	Primary Use
Pr atropine	Increase heart rate, dilate pupils
benztropine (Cogentin)	Parkinson's disease
cyclopentolate (Cyclogyl)	Dilate pupils
dicyclomine (Bentylol)	Irritable bowel syndrome
glycopyrrolate	Produce a dry field prior to anesthesia, peptic ulcers
ipratropium (Atrovent)	Asthma
oxybutynin (Ditropan)	Incontinence
propantheline	Irritable bowel syndrome, peptic ulcer
scopolamine (Buscopan, Transderm-V)	Motion sickness, irritable bowel syndrome, adjunct to anesthesia
tiotropium (Spiriva)	COPD

Nursing Considerations

The role of the nurse in anticholinergic therapy involves careful monitoring of the client's condition and providing education as it relates to the prescribed drug treatment. Both direct-acting and indirect-acting cholinergics are contraindicated for clients with hypersensitivity. These drugs should not be used in clients with obstruction of the GI and urinary systems because they increase muscular tone and contraction.

Perform a thorough medical history, including medications the client is currently taking that could cause drug-drug interactions. Antihistamines, in particular, can lead to excessive muscarinic blockade. Check for a history of taking herbal supplements; some have atropine-like actions that potentiate the effects of the medication and can be harmful to the client. For example, aloe, senna, buckthorn, and cascara sagrada may increase atropine's effect, particularly with chronic use of these herbs.

This classification of drugs should not be used if the client has a history of acute angle-closure glaucoma. Anticholinergics block muscarinic receptors in the eye, creating paralysis of the iris sphincter, which can increase intraocular pressure. Safety has not been established for pregnancy and lactation. Anticholinergics may produce fetal tachycardia.

Anticholinergics are contraindicated in clients with heart disease and hypertension because blockade of cardiac muscarinic receptors prevents the parasympathetic nervous system from slowing the heart. This can result in an acceleration of heart rate that may exacerbate these conditions. Clients with hyperthyroidism should not be given these medications because in hyperthyroidism the heart rate is generally high, and administration of

◀ Impact of Anticholinergics on Male Sexual Function

A functioning autonomic nervous system is essential for normal male sexual health. The parasympathetic nervous system is necessary for erections, whereas the sympathetic division is responsible for the process of ejaculation. Anticholinergic drugs will block transmission of parasympathetic impulses and may interfere with normal erections. Adrenergic antagonists can interfere with the smooth muscle contractions in the seminal vesicles and penis, resulting in an inability to ejaculate.

For clients who are receiving autonomic nervous system medications, include questions about sexual activity during the assessment process. For male clients who are not sexually active, these side effects may be unimportant. For male clients who are sexually active, however, drug-induced sexual dysfunction may be a major cause of nonadherence. The client should be informed to expect such side effects and to report them to his healthcare provider immediately. In most cases, alternative medications that do not affect sexual function are available. Inform the client that supportive counselling is available.

◀ Valerian

Valerian root (*Valeriana officinalis*) is a perennial native to Europe and North America that is an herbal choice for nervous tension and anxiety. This natural product promotes rest without affecting rapid eye movement (REM) sleep and has a reputation for calming an individual without causing side effects or discomfort. Its name comes from the Latin *valere*, which means "to be well." One thing that is *not well*, however, is its pungent odour, although many users claim that the smell is well worth the benefits. Valerian also is purported to reduce pain and headaches without the worry of dependency. There is no drug hangover, as is sometimes experienced with tranquilizers and sedatives. It is available as a tincture (alcohol mixture), tea, or extract. Sometimes it is placed in juice and consumed immediately before taking a nap or going to bed.

anticholinergics can cause dysrhythmias due to norepinephrine release from sympathetic nerves that regulate heart rate.

The nurse should also assess for baseline bowel and bladder function. Renal conditions are contraindications to anticholinergic therapy because they impair the ability of the bladder to empty. Gastrointestinal conditions such as ulcerative colitis and ileus are contraindicated because blockade of muscarinic receptors in the intestine can decrease the tone and motility of intestinal smooth muscle, which can exacerbate intestinal conditions. Monitor clients with esophageal reflux and hiatal hernia because anticholinergics reduce GI motility. Clients with gastroesophageal reflux disease (GERD) and hiatal hernia experience decreased muscle tone in the lower esophageal sphincter and delayed stomach emptying. Anticholinergics exacerbate these symptoms, increasing the risk of esophageal injury and aspiration. Clients with Down syndrome may be more sensitive to the effects of atropine due to structural differences in the CNS caused by chromosomal abnormality (trisomy). Clients with Down syndrome also tend to have disorders such as GERD and heart disease, which may be adversely affected by anticholinergics.

Clinical Applications of Anticholinergics

13.5 Anticholinergics may be used to treat asthma, peptic ulcer, and Parkinson's disease, whereas acetylcholinesterase inhibitors may be used to treat Alzheimer's disease, glaucoma, and myasthenia gravis.

Agents that block the action of acetylcholine are known by a number of names, including anticholinergics, cholinergic blockers,

muscarinic antagonists, and parasympatholytics. Although the term *anticholinergic* is most commonly used, the most accurate term for this class of drug is **muscarinic antagonists** because at therapeutic doses, these drugs are selective for acetylcholine muscarinic receptors and thus have little effect on acetylcholine nicotinic receptors.

Anticholinergics act by competing with acetylcholine for binding of muscarinic receptors. When anticholinergics occupy these receptors, no response is generated at the neuroeffector organs. By suppressing the effects of acetylcholine, symptoms of sympathetic nervous system activation predominate. Most therapeutic uses of the anticholinergics are predictable extensions of their parasympathetic-blocking actions: dilation of the pupils, increase in heart rate, drying of secretions, and relaxation of the bronchi. Note that these are also symptoms of sympathetic activation (fight-or-flight response).

Therapeutic uses of anticholinergics include the following:

- GI disorders: Anticholinergics decrease the secretion of gastric acid in peptic ulcer disease (Chapter 34). They also slow intestinal motility and may be useful for reducing the cramping and diarrhea associated with irritable bowel syndrome (Chapter 35).
- Ophthalmic procedures: Anticholinergics may be used to cause mydriasis or cycloplegia during eye procedures (Chapter 63).
- Cardiac rhythm abnormalities: Anticholinergics can be used to accelerate the heart rate in clients experiencing bradycardia.
- Pre-anesthesia: Combined with other agents, anticholinergics can decrease excessive respiratory secretions and reverse the bradycardia caused by anesthetics (Chapter 24).
- Asthma: A few agents, such as ipratropium (Atrovent), are useful in treating asthma because of their ability to dilate the bronchi (Chapter 38).

The prototype drug atropine is used for several additional medical conditions because of its effective muscarinic receptor blockade. These applications include reversal of adverse muscarinic effects and treatment of muscarinic agonist poisoning, including that caused from overdose of bethanechol, cholinesterase inhibitors, or accidental ingestion of certain types of mushrooms or organophosphate pesticides.

Some of the anticholinergics are used for their effects on the CNS rather than their autonomic actions. Scopolamine (Buscopan, Transderm-V) is used for sedation and motion sickness, and benztropine (Cogentin) is prescribed to reduce the muscular tremor and rigidity associated with Parkinson's disease.

Anticholinergics exhibit a relatively high incidence of side effects. Important adverse effects that limit their usefulness include tachycardia, CNS stimulation, and the tendency to cause urinary retention in men with prostate disorders. Adverse effects such as dry mouth and dry eyes occur due to blockade of muscarinic receptors on salivary glands and lacrimal glands, respectively. Blockade of muscarinic receptors on sweat glands can inhibit sweating, which may lead to hyperthermia. Photophobia can occur due to the pupil being unable to constrict in response to bright light. Symptoms of overdose include fever, visual changes, difficulty swallowing, psychomotor agitation, and/or hallucinations. The development of safer, and sometimes more effective, drugs has greatly decreased the current use of anticholinergics. Exceptions include ipratropium (Atrovent) and tiotropium (Spiriva), which are a relatively new anticholinergics used for clients with COPD. Because they are delivered via aerosol spray, these agents produce more localized action with fewer systemic side effects than atropine.

PROTOTYPE DRUG | Atropine

Actions and Uses: By occupying muscarinic receptors, atropine blocks the parasympathetic actions of acetylcholine and induces symptoms of the fight-or-flight response. Most prominent are increased heart rate, bronchodilation, decreased motility in the GI tract, mydriasis, and decreased secretions from glands. At therapeutic doses, atropine has no effect on nicotinic receptors in ganglia or skeletal muscle.

Atropine is particularly important as an antidote to cholinergic toxicity. Atropine may also be used to suppress secretions during surgical procedures, to treat palliative care clients who have excess secretions, to increase the heart rate in clients with bradycardia,

and to dilate the pupil during eye examinations. Once widely used to cause bronchodilation in clients with asthma and to treat hypermotility diseases of the GI tract such as irritable bowel syndrome, atropine is now rarely prescribed for these disorders because of the development of drugs with less unpleasant side effects.

Pharmacokinetics: Atropine can be given by the IV, SC, IM, or PO route. Atropine is well absorbed. It is widely distributed, crosses the blood-brain barrier and placenta, and enters breast milk. It is mostly metabolized by the liver. About 40% is excreted unchanged by the kidneys. Its half-life is 4 to 5 hours in adults.

Administration Alerts:

- Atropine may be given by direct IV (push) or by infusion.
- It may cause initial paradoxical bradycardia, lasting up to 2 minutes, especially at lower doses.
- The drug may induce ventricular fibrillation in cardiac clients.
- Atropine is pregnancy category C.

Adverse Effects and Interactions: The side effects of atropine limit its therapeutic usefulness and are predictable extensions of its autonomic actions. Expected side effects include dry mouth, constipation, urinary retention, and an increased heart rate. Initial CNS excitement may progress to delirium and even coma. Atropine is usually contraindicated in clients with glaucoma because the drug may increase pressure within the eye. Accidental poisoning has occurred in children who eat the colourful, purple berries of the deadly nightshade, mistaking them for cherries. Symptoms of poisoning are those of intense parasympathetic stimulation.

Drug interactions with atropine include an increased effect with antihistamines, tricyclic antidepressants, quinidine, and procainamide. Atropine decreases effects of levodopa-carbidopa (Sinemet). Use with caution with herbal supplements, such as aloe, senna, buckthorn, and cascara sagrada, which may increase atropine's effect, particularly with chronic use of these herbs.

CHAPTER
13 Understanding the Chapter

Key Concepts Summary

The numbered key concepts provide a succinct summary of the important points from the corresponding numbered section within the chapter. If any of these points are not clear, refer to the numbered section within the chapter for review.

13.1 Drugs can activate or suppress cholinergic receptors either directly or indirectly.

13.2 Muscarinic agonists produce their effects by directly stimulating cholinergic receptors.

13.3 Nicotine acts by activating acetylcholine receptors at the ganglia.

13.4 Anticholinergics act by blocking the effects of acetylcholine at muscarinic or nicotinic receptors.

13.5 Anticholinergics may be used to treat asthma, peptic ulcer, and Parkinson's disease, whereas acetylcholinesterase inhibitors may be used to treat Alzheimer's disease, glaucoma, and myasthenia gravis.

Chapter 13 Scenario

Hilda Echoles is an 82-year-old client who lives alone in a two-storey house. Recently, she fell down the steps at her front door and fractured her right femur. She was taken to the nearest hospital and underwent a total hip replacement 2 weeks ago. Because she was nearing the time for her discharge, the urinary catheter, which was inserted during surgery, was removed. Since that time, Hilda has experienced urinary retention and required intermittent catheterization.

To aid in urinary elimination, her physician has ordered bethanechol (Duvoid) 20 mg three times per day. Because the medication has demonstrated some effectiveness in achieving bladder emptying, Hilda will be discharged on this medication until she sees her family doctor 2 weeks after discharge.

Critical Thinking Questions

1. As Hilda's nurse, you will be reviewing Hilda's discharge medications before she leaves the hospital. What pertinent information should she receive about bethanechol?

2. Hilda states, "Sometimes, my memory is not so good and I forget to take my medication." What should she do if she forgets a dose? List suggestions that you could provide to this client to help her remember her medication times and to ensure safe and effective administration.

3. What parameters would you use to determine the effectiveness of this drug therapy?

See Answers to Critical Thinking Questions in Appendix B.

NCLEX Practice Questions

1 A nurse discussing the adverse effects associated with a muscarinic agonist knows that reflex tachycardia may occur with this drug because

a. Baroreceptors acknowledge transient hypotension and signal the medulla to increase the heart rate.

b. This drug simulates the sinoatrial node in the right atrium.

c. Aortic receptors identify episodes of systolic hypertension and stimulate heart rhythms.

d. This drug stimulates bronchial smooth muscle contraction and a narrowing of the airway.

2 A nurse is discussing the therapeutic effects of bethanechol (Duvoid) with a patient who is receiving this drug for urinary retention. The nurse understands that bethanechol

a. Changes the diameter of the urethral opening

b. Increases the amount of urine made in the kidneys

c. Improves blood flow to the kidneys

d. Increases the contractions of the bladder and structures that promote urination

3 The nurse monitors the patient for which of the common adverse effects associated with bethanechol (Duvoid)? Select all that apply.

a. Abdominal discomfort

b. Sweating

c. Flushed skin

d. Constipation

e. Blurred vision

4 A healthcare provider has ordered neostigmine (Prostigmin) for each of the following patients. The nurse should question the order for which patient?

a. A patient with postoperative abdominal distention

b. A patient experiencing urinary retention

c. A patient with chronic obstructive pulmonary disease

d. A patient who has received nondepolarizing muscle relaxants

5 The provider orders neostigmine (Prostigmin) for a patient who has not urinated in the past 16 hours. The nurse collaborates with the prescriber about which action related to this drug therapy?

a. Heart rate less than 60 beats per minute

b. Change in pupillary size from 3 mm to 1 mm

c. Increased salivation

d. Respiratory rate of 16 breaths per minute

See Answers to NCLEX Practice Questions in Appendix A.

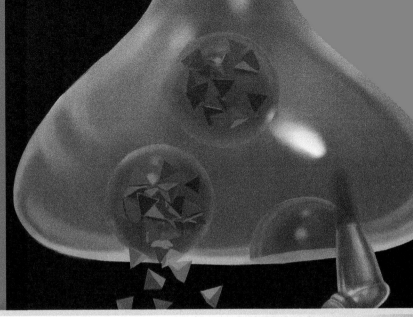

Spencer Sutton/Science Source

PROTOTYPE DRUGS

ADRENERGICS

Pr *phenylephrine (Neo-Synephrine)*

OTHER PROTOTYPES

Pr *norepinephrine (Levophed)*
Pr *dopamine*
Pr *epinephrine (Adrenalin)*

ANTIADRENERGICS

Pr *prazosin (Minipress)*

OTHER PROTOTYPES

Pr *atenolol (Tenormin)*
Pr *carvedilol (Coreg)*
Pr *doxazosin (Cardura)*
Pr *metoprolol (Lopresor)*
Pr *propranolol (Inderal)*
Pr *timolol*

CHAPTER 14

Pharmacotherapy with Adrenergic Agonists and Antagonists

LEARNING OUTCOMES

After reading this chapter, the student should be able to:

1. Identify the physiological responses produced when a drug activates adrenergic receptors.
2. Explain the direct and indirect mechanisms by which adrenergic agonists act.
3. Compare and contrast the characteristics of catecholamines and non-catecholamines.
4. Identify indications for pharmacotherapy with adrenergic agonists.
5. Apply the nursing process to care for clients who are receiving pharmacotherapy with adrenergic agonists.
6. Identify the physiological responses produced when a drug blocks adrenergic receptors.
7. Identify indications for pharmacotherapy with adrenergic antagonists.
8. Describe the first-dose phenomenon and how it may be prevented.
9. Explain the advantages of selective beta antagonists versus non-selective beta antagonists.
10. Explain why beta-adrenergic antagonists should never be abruptly discontinued.
11. Apply the nursing process to care for clients who are receiving pharmacotherapy with adrenergic antagonists.

CHAPTER OUTLINE

▸ Adrenergic Agonists and Antagonists

▸ Clinical Applications of Adrenergics

▸ Adrenergic Antagonists

▸ Clinical Applications of Adrenergic Antagonists

Adrenergic Agonists and Antagonists

14.1 Autonomic drugs are classified by which receptors they stimulate or block: adrenergic agonists stimulate adrenergic receptors of sympathetic nerves, whereas adrenergic antagonists inhibit the sympathetic division of the autonomic nervous system.

Adrenergics (sympathomimetics) stimulate adrenergic receptors, thereby activating the sympathetic nervous system and inducing symptoms characteristic of the fight-or-flight response. These drugs have clinical applications in the treatment of shock, hypotension, asthma, and the common cold. They are listed in Table 14.1.

NCLEX Success Tips

Clonidine (Catapres) is used as adjunctive therapy in opioid withdrawal. It is mainly used for the treatment of high blood pressure; however, when used along with treatment for opioid withdrawal (an off-labelled use), make a priority assessment for hypotension.

Clonidine is a central-acting adrenergic antagonist. It reduces sympathetic outflow from the central nervous system. Dry mouth, impotence, and sleep disturbances are possible adverse effects.

NCLEX Success Tips

Adverse effects of pseudoephedrine (Sudafed) are experienced primarily in the cardiovascular system and through sympathetic effects on the central nervous system (CNS). The most common CNS adverse effects include restlessness, dizziness, tension, anxiety, insomnia, and weakness. Common cardiovascular adverse effects include tachycardia, hypertension, palpitations, and arrhythmias.

Pseudoephedrine can increase blood pressure and increase urinary retention with an enlarged prostate and should be avoided.

Clinical Applications of Adrenergics

14.2 Adrenergics act directly by activating adrenergic receptors or indirectly by increasing the release of norepinephrine from nerve terminals. They are primarily used for their effects on the heart, bronchial tree, and nasal passages.

The adrenergics, also known as adrenergic agonists and sympathomimetics, produce many of the same responses as the anticholinergics. However, because the sympathetic nervous system has both alpha and beta subreceptors, the actions of many adrenergics are more specific and have wider therapeutic application (see Table 14.1).

TABLE 14.1	Adrenergics	
Drug	**Primary Receptor Subtype**	**Primary Use**
salbutamol (Ventolin)	Beta$_2$	Asthma
clonidine (Catapres)	Alpha$_2$ in central nervous system (CNS)	Hypertension
dobutamine (Dobutrex)	Beta$_1$	Cardiac stimulant
dopamine	Alpha$_1$ and beta$_1$	Shock
epinephrine (Adrenalin)	Alpha and beta	Cardiac arrest, asthma
formoterol (Foradil)	Beta$_2$	Asthma, chronic obstructive pulmonary disease
isoproterenol	Beta$_1$ and beta$_2$	Asthma, dysrhythmias, heart failure
methyldopa	Alpha$_2$ in CNS	Hypertension
norepinephrine (Levophed)	Alpha$_1$ and beta$_1$	Shock
Pr phenylephrine (Neo-Synephrine)	Alpha	Nasal congestion
pseudoephedrine (Sudafed)	Alpha and beta	Nasal congestion

Adrenergic agonists, also called **sympathomimetics**, are agents that activate adrenergic receptors in the sympathetic nervous system. Drugs in this class include naturally occurring (endogenous) substances such as norepinephrine (NE), epinephrine, and dopamine. NE is the major neurotransmitter in the sympathetic nervous system, whereas epinephrine is the primary hormone released by the adrenal medulla. Dopamine is the immediate biochemical precursor to NE and is a key neurotransmitter in certain regions of the central nervous system (CNS). In addition to their natural physiological roles in the body, NE, epinephrine, and dopamine are available as prescription drugs. A number of synthetic adrenergic agonists that mimic the effects of these natural neurotransmitters are also available. See Figure 14.1 for an illustration of the mechanisms of action of adrenergic agonists.

When administered as drugs, the adrenergic agonists induce symptoms of the fight-or-flight response. Their most important therapeutic actions are on the cardiovascular and respiratory systems. Activation of adrenergic receptors in the myocardium increases the heart rate (positive chronotropic effect) and the force of contraction (positive inotropic effect). Cardiac output increases. Constriction of vascular smooth muscle causes a rapid increase

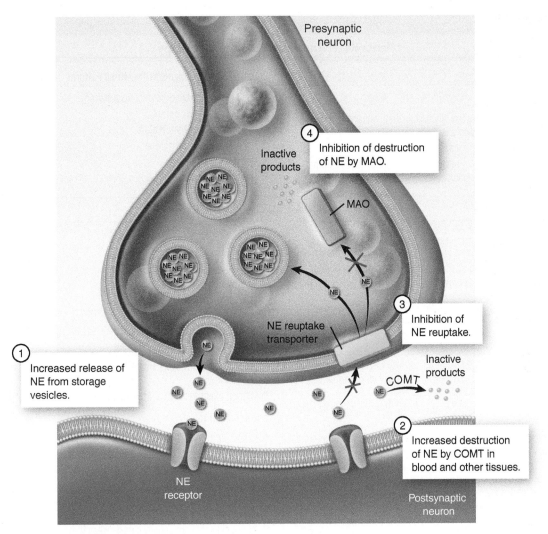

Figure 14.1 Mechanisms of action of adrenergic agonists: (1) stimulation of the release of norepinephrine (NE); (2) increased destruction of NE by catechol-O-methyltransferase (COMT); (3) inhibition of the reuptake of NE; (4) inhibition of the destruction of NE by monoamine oxidase (MAO).

in blood pressure. Administration by the parenteral or inhalation routes immediately relaxes bronchial smooth muscle, resulting in bronchodilation. Activation of adrenergic receptors in the smooth muscle of the gastrointestinal (GI) and urinary tracts slows peristalsis and may cause constipation and urine retention. Metabolic effects include increased oxygen consumption and increased blood glucose and lactate levels. Other adrenergic actions include reduction of glandular secretory activity and mydriasis.

It is important to remember that the symptoms of the fight-or-flight response elicited by the adrenergic agonists may be considered as therapeutic or adverse, depending on the condition of the client and the goals of pharmacotherapy. For example, if the client is in shock, increased blood pressure is a key therapeutic effect. However, if the client is taking an adrenergic agonist to treat nasal congestion, an increase in blood pressure is an adverse effect. Furthermore, a therapeutic effect may become an adverse effect if taken to extreme, such as raising blood pressure too much or causing excessive drying of the nasal or oral mucosa.

As discussed, actions produced by cholinergic (muscarinic) antagonists are similar to those of adrenergic agonists. This is

because blocking muscarinic receptors in the parasympathetic nervous system allows sympathetic nerve impulses to predominate. However, because the sympathetic nervous system has alpha and beta receptor subtypes, the actions of many adrenergic agonists are more specific, which allows for wider therapeutic applications due to a lower incidence of adverse effects.

Adrenergics may be classified as catecholamines or non-catecholamines. The catecholamines have a chemical structure similar to NE, have a short duration of action, and must be administered parenterally. The non-catecholamines can be taken orally and have longer durations of action because they are not rapidly destroyed by monoamine oxidase (MAO).

Most adrenergics act by directly binding to and activating adrenergic receptors. Examples include the three endogenous catecholamines: epinephrine, norepinephrine, and dopamine. Other medications in this class act indirectly by causing the release of NE from its vesicles on the presynaptic neuron or by inhibiting its reuptake or destruction. Those that act by indirect mechanisms, such as amphetamine and cocaine, are used for their central effects on the brain rather than their autonomic effects.

NURSING PROCESS FOCUS

Clients Receiving Anticholinergic Therapy

Assessment	Potential Nursing Diagnoses/Identified Patterns
Prior to administration: • Obtain complete health history, including drug history to determine possible drug interactions and allergies. • Assess reason for drug administration. • Assess heart rate, blood pressure, temperature, and elimination patterns (initially and throughout therapy).	• Need for knowledge regarding drug therapy • Decreased cardiac output • Changes in body temperature • Dry oral mucous membrane • Constipation • Urinary retention

Planning: Client Goals and Expected Outcomes

The client will:

• Exhibit a decrease in symptoms for which the medication is prescribed
• Demonstrate an understanding of the drug by accurately describing the drug's purpose, action, side effects, and precautions
• Verbalize techniques to avoid hazardous side effects associated with anticholinergic therapy

Implementation

Interventions (Rationales)	Client Education/Discharge Planning
• Monitor for signs of anticholinergic crisis resulting from overdosage: fever, tachycardia, difficulty swallowing, ataxia, reduced urine output, psychomotor agitation, confusion, hallucinations. • Report significant changes in heart rate, blood pressure, or the development of dysrhythmias. • Observe for side effects such as drowsiness, blurred vision, tachycardia, dry mouth, urinary hesitancy, and decreased sweating. • Provide comfort measures for dry mucous membranes, such as applying lubricant to moisten lips and oral mucosa, assisting in rinsing mouth, using artificial tears for dry eyes, as needed. • Minimize exposure to heat and cold and strenuous exercise. (Anticholinergics can inhibit sweat gland secretions due to direct blockade of the muscarinic receptors on the sweat glands. This can increase the risk for hyperthermia since sweating is necessary for clients to cool down.) • Monitor intake and output ratio. Palpate abdomen for bladder distention. • Monitor client for abdominal distention and auscultate for bowel sounds.	• Instruct client to report side effects related to therapy such as shortness of breath. • Instruct client to monitor vital signs. Instruct client to: • Report side effects. • Avoid driving and hazardous activities until effects of the drug are known. • Wear sunglasses to decrease the sensitivity to bright light. • Instruct client that oral rinses, sugarless gum or candy, and frequent oral hygiene may help to relieve dry mouth. Avoid alcohol-containing mouthwashes that can further dry oral tissue. • Advise client to limit activity outside when the temperature is hot. Strenuous activity in a hot environment may cause heat stroke. • Instruct client to notify healthcare provider if difficulty in voiding occurs. • Advise client to increase fluid and add bulk to the diet if constipation becomes a problem.

Evaluation of Outcome Criteria

Evaluate effectiveness of drug therapy by confirming that client goals and expected outcomes have been met (see "Planning").

See Table 14.1 for a list of drugs to which these nursing actions apply.

A few agents, such as ephedrine, act by both direct and indirect mechanisms.

Most effects of adrenergics are predictable based on their autonomic actions, depending on which adrenergic subreceptors are stimulated. Because the receptor responses are so different, the student will need to memorize the specific receptor subtypes activated by each adrenergic. Therapeutic applications of the different receptor subtype activations are as follows:

• Alpha$_1$ receptor agonists: Treatment of nasal congestion or hypotension; induction of mydriasis during ophthalmic examinations. Activation of alpha-adrenergic receptors causes a number of important physiological responses, most of which

relate to contraction of vascular smooth muscle. Like the non-selective adrenergic agonists, several of the selective alpha agonists are used to treat hypotension associated with shock and other critical care conditions. Alpha agonists may also be administered to treat clients who are susceptible to orthostatic hypotension.

A second application of alpha-adrenergic agonists is for the treatment of nasal congestion. During upper respiratory infections or allergic rhinitis, arterioles in the nose dilate and produce excess mucus. Alpha$_1$ agonists relieve nasal congestion by causing vasoconstriction of vessels that serve the nasal mucosa. Intranasal drugs such as phenylephrine (Neo-Synephrine) work within minutes and are highly effective at clearing the nasal passages. The intranasal route causes few systemic side effects because absorption is limited.

- Alpha$_2$ receptor agonists: Treatment of hypertension through non-autonomic (central-acting) mechanism. Activation of alpha$_2$-adrenergic receptors produces very different responses than alpha$_1$ activation. The most important responses to alpha$_2$ receptor agonists occur in the brain rather than in the peripheral nervous system. Unlike alpha$_1$ agonists, which increase sympathetic nervous system activity, alpha$_2$ agonists act in the CNS to *decrease* sympathetic activity. Methyldopa and clonidine (Catapres) are two drugs in this class. Because they decrease blood pressure, their primary therapeutic application is for the treatment of hypertension (see Chapter 51).

- Beta$_1$ receptor agonists: Treatment of cardiac arrest, heart failure, and shock. Pharmacologically, the most significant site that has beta$_1$ receptors is cardiac muscle. Activation of beta$_1$ receptors results in cardiac actions typical of the fight-or-flight response: increased heart rate (positive chronotropic effect), force of contraction (positive inotropic effect), and velocity of impulse conduction across the myocardium (positive dromotropic effect). These cardiac effects may be considered beneficial or adverse, depending on the condition of the client and the therapeutic goals.

  Drugs used for their beta$_1$-agonist actions are sometimes called **cardiotonic drugs** because they increase the force of contraction of the heart. In the treatment of heart failure or shock, they are administered to increase cardiac output. Another name applied to these drugs is **inotropic drugs** because they reverse the cardiac symptoms of shock by increasing the strength of myocardial contraction. The use of beta$_1$ agonists in treating heart failure is presented in Chapter 54.

- Beta$_2$ receptor agonists: Treatment of asthma and premature labour contractions. Beta$_2$-adrenergic receptors are more widely distributed than beta$_1$ receptors. Pharmacologically, the most important site is in the lung, where activation of beta$_2$ receptors leads to relaxation of bronchial smooth muscle. Beta$_2$-adrenergic agonists, commonly referred to as bronchodilators, are used extensively in the treatment of asthma and other pulmonary disorders. Autonomic drugs used as bronchodilators include non-selective adrenergic agonists as well as those that are selective for beta$_2$ receptors. Epinephrine is the best example of a non-selective drug that is an effective bronchodilator. Unfortunately, epinephrine exhibits a high incidence of adverse effects, such as hypertension and dysrhythmias, due to its stimulation of multiple receptor subtypes throughout the body.

Some adrenergics are non-selective, stimulating more than one type of adrenergic receptor. For example, epinephrine stimulates all four types of adrenergic receptors and is used for cardiac arrest and asthma. Pseudoephedrine (Sudafed) stimulates both alpha$_1$ and beta$_2$ receptors and is used as a nasal decongestant. Isoproterenol stimulates both beta$_1$ and beta$_2$ receptors and is used to increase the heart's rate and force of contraction and speed of electrical conduction, and occasionally is used to treat asthma. The non-selective drugs generally cause more autonomic-related side effects than the selective agents.

The side effects of the adrenergics are mostly extensions of their autonomic actions. Cardiovascular effects such as tachycardia, hypertension, and dysrhythmias are particularly troublesome and may limit therapy. Large doses can induce CNS excitement and seizures. Other adrenergic responses that may occur are dry mouth, nausea, and vomiting. Some of these agents cause anorexia, which has led to their historical use as appetite suppressants. Because of prominent cardiovascular side effects, adrenergics are now rarely used for this purpose.

Drugs in this class are presented as prototype drugs in many other chapters in this text: dopamine and norepinephrine in Chapter 17 and salmeterol in Chapter 38.

Nursing Considerations

Since the purposes and indications of drugs within this class vary greatly, the Nursing Process Focus applies to all clients who are receiving adrenergic drugs. For specific nursing considerations, contraindications, and precautions, see Chapters 17 and 38.

PROTOTYPE DRUG | **Phenylephrine (Neo-Synephrine)**

Actions and Uses: Phenylephrine is a selective alpha-adrenergic agonist that is available in several different formulations, including intranasal, ophthalmic, intramuscular (IM), subcutaneious (SC), and intravenous (IV). All of its actions and indications are extensions of its sympathetic stimulation. When applied intranasally by spray or drops, it reduces nasal congestion by constricting small blood vessels in the nasal mucosa. Applied topically to the eye during ophthalmic examinations, phenylephrine is used to dilate the pupil. The parenteral administration of phenylephrine can reverse acute hypotension caused by spinal anesthesia or vascular shock. Because it lacks beta-adrenergic agonist activity, it produces relatively few cardiac side effects at therapeutic doses. Its longer duration of activity and lack of significant cardiac effects give phenylephrine some advantages over epinephrine and norepinephrine in treating acute hypotension.

Administration Alerts:

- Do not use solution if it is brown or contains precipitate (particles).

- Parenteral administration can cause severe tissue injury with extravasation.

- Phenylephrine ophthalmic drops may damage soft contact lenses.

- Phenylephrine is pregnancy category C.

Pharmacokinetics: Phenylephrine is rapidly absorbed. It is metabolized in the liver and tissues by monoamine oxidase. Its half-life is unknown.

Adverse Effects and Interactions: When used topically or intranasally, side effects are uncommon. Intranasal use can cause burning of the mucosa and rebound congestion if used for prolonged periods (see Chapter 38). Ophthalmic preparations can cause narrow-angle glaucoma, secondary to their mydriatic effect. High doses can cause reflex bradycardia due to the elevation of blood pressure caused by stimulation of alpha$_1$ receptors. When administered parenterally, the drug should be used with caution in clients with advanced coronary artery disease or hypertension. Anxiety, restlessness, and tremor may occur due to the drug's stimulation effect on the CNS. Clients with hyperthyroidism may experience a severe increase in basal metabolic rate, resulting in increased blood pressure and tachycardia. Drug interactions may occur with MAO inhibitors, causing a hypertensive crisis. Increased effects may also occur with tricyclic antidepressants. This drug is incompatible with iron preparations (ferric salts).

Adrenergic Antagonists

14.3 Adrenergic antagonists inhibit the sympathetic division of the autonomic nervous system.

Adrenergic antagonists inhibit the sympathetic nervous system and produce many of the same rest-and-digest symptoms as the

---

NURSING PROCESS FOCUS

Clients Receiving Adrenergic Therapy

Assessment	Potential Nursing Diagnoses/Identified Patterns
Prior to administration: • Determine reason for drug administration. • Monitor vital signs, urinary output, and cardiac output (initially and throughout therapy). • For treatment of nasal congestion, assess the nasal mucosa for changes such as excoriation or bleeding. • Obtain complete health history, including allergies, drug history, and possible drug interactions.	• Need for knowledge regarding drug therapy • Adequate sleep • Nasal congestion • Risk for injury related to side effects of drug therapy • Decreased cardiac output • Risk for decreased tissue perfusion

Planning: Client Goals and Expected Outcomes

The client will:

• Exhibit a decrease in the symptoms for which the drug is being given
• Demonstrate understanding of the drug's action by accurately describing drug side effects and precautions
• Demonstrate proper nasal/ophthalmic drug instillation technique

Implementation

Interventions (Rationales)	Client Education/Discharge Planning
• Closely monitor IV insertion sites for extravasation with IV administration. Use an infusion pump to deliver the medication. • Use a tuberculin syringe when administering SC doses that are extremely small. • For metered dose inhalation, shake container well and wait at least 2 minutes between medications. It is important to use the correct number of sprays when using metered dose inhalers. • Instill only the prescribed number of drops when using ophthalmic solutions. • Monitor the client for side effects. (Side effects of adrenergics may be serious and limit therapy.) • Monitor breathing patterns and observe for shortness of breath and/or audible wheezing. • Observe the client's responsiveness to light. (Some adrenergics cause photosensitivity by affecting the pupillary light accommodation/response.) • Provide eye comfort by reducing exposure to bright light in the environment; shield the eyes with a rolled washcloth or eye bandages for severe photosensitivity. • For clients receiving nasal adrenergics, observe the nasal cavity. Monitor for rhinorrhea and epistaxis.	Instruct client to: • Use the drug strictly as prescribed, and not "double up" on doses. • Take medication early in the day to avoid insomnia. Instruct client to: • Immediately report shortness of breath, palpitations, dizziness, chest/arm pain or pressure, or other angina-like symptoms. • Consult healthcare provider before attempting to use adrenergics to treat nasal congestion or eye irritation. • Monitor blood pressure, pulse, and temperature to ensure proper use of home equipment. • Instruct client to immediately report any difficulty breathing. Instruct clients with a history of asthma to consult their healthcare provider before using over-the-counter (OTC) drugs to treat nasal congestion. • Instruct clients using ophthalmic adrenergics that transient stinging and blurred vision upon instillation is normal. Headache and/or brow pain may also occur. • Instruct client to avoid driving and other activities that require visual acuity until blurring subsides. Instruct client to: • Observe nasal cavity for signs of excoriation or bleeding (you are looking for signs of bleeding due to the potential of the adrenergic medication being absorbed systemically) before instilling nasal spray or drops; review procedure for safe instillation of nasal sprays or eye drops. • Limit OTC usage of adrenergics; inform client about rebound nasal congestion with prolonged use.

Evaluation of Outcome Criteria

Evaluate effectiveness of drug therapy by confirming that client goals and expected outcomes have been met (see "Planning").

See Table 14.1 for a list of drugs to which these nursing actions apply.

cholinergics. They compete with NE for adrenergic receptors; by blocking NE from reaching its receptors, symptoms of the fight-or-flight response are *prevented*. With reduced sympathetic activation, nerve impulses from the parasympathetic nervous system will predominate. In fact, most of the symptoms produced by adrenergic antagonists are those of parasympathetic activation. In other words, adrenergic antagonists and cholinergic agonists result in many of the same actions. They have wide therapeutic application in the treatment of hypertension. The adrenergic antagonists are listed in Table 14.2.

Clinical Applications of Adrenergic Antagonists

14.4 Adrenergic antagonists are primarily used for hypertension and are the most widely prescribed class of autonomic drug.

Adrenergic antagonists act by directly blocking adrenergic receptors. The actions of these agents are specific to either alpha or beta blockade. Medications in this class have great therapeutic application: they are the most widely prescribed class of autonomic drug.

Alpha-adrenergic antagonists, or simply alpha blockers, are used for their effects on vascular smooth muscle. By relaxing vascular smooth muscle in small arteries, alpha$_1$ blockers such as doxazosin cause vasodilation, which results in decreased blood pressure. They may be used either alone or in combination with other agents in the treatment of hypertension (Chapter 51). A second use is in the treatment of benign prostatic hyperplasia

due to their ability to increase urine flow (Chapter 32). The most common adverse effect of alpha blockers is **orthostatic hypotension**, which occurs when a client abruptly changes from a recumbent to an upright position. Reflex tachycardia, nasal congestion, and impotence are other important side effects that occur due to increased parasympathetic activity. Orthostatic hypotension is especially pronounced at the beginning of pharmacotherapy and when increasing the dose. This adverse effect is called the **first-dose phenomenon**. Because the first-dose phenomenon can cause syncope due to reduced blood flow to the brain, initial therapy begins with low doses, usually administered at bedtime.

Alpha$_1$ antagonists are occasionally used to treat pheochromocytoma and Raynaud's disease. **Pheochromocytoma** is a tumour, usually benign, arising from the adrenal medulla that is characterized by excessive secretion of catecholamines. A client with a pheochromocytoma will exhibit extreme hypertension, palpitations, dyspnea, anxiety, and profuse sweating. All are signs of excessive amounts of catecholamines. Although surgical removal is the usual treatment, alpha$_1$-receptor antagonists can be administered to block the peripheral vascular effects of natural (endogenous) catecholamines. This reduces the profound hypertension in clients who are high surgical risks.

NCLEX Success Tips

Excess catecholamine release occurs with pheochromocytoma and causes hypertension. The nurse should prepare to administer nitroprusside (a vasodilator) to control the hypertension until the client undergoes adrenalectomy to remove the tumour.

Pheochromocytoma causes excessive production of epinephrine and norepinephrine, natural catecholamines that raise blood pressure. Phentolamine—an alpha-adrenergic antagonist administered by IV bolus or drip—antagonizes the body's response to circulating epinephrine and norepinephrine, reducing blood pressure quickly and effectively. Although methyldopa is an antihypertensive agent available in parenteral form, it is not effective in treating hypertensive emergencies.

Felodipine, an antihypertensive agent, is available only in extended-release tablets and therefore does not reduce blood pressure quickly enough to correct hypertensive crisis.

In **Raynaud's disease**, vasospasms of vessels serving the fingers and toes can lead to intermittent pain and cyanosis of the digits. Emotional stress or cold temperatures usually exacerbate the disorder. The primary treatment is non-pharmacological: warming techniques and avoidance of cold. For those who require pharmacotherapy, administration of alpha$_1$ antagonists can diminish the vasospasm and bring symptomatic relief to clients. **Beta-adrenergic antagonists** may block beta$_1$ receptors, beta$_2$ receptors, or both. Regardless of their receptor specificity, the therapeutic applications of all beta blockers relate to their effects on the cardiovascular system. Beta blockers will decrease the rate and force of contraction of the heart and slow electrical conduction through the atrioventricular node. Drugs that selectively block beta$_1$ receptors, such as atenolol (Tenormin), are called cardioselective agents. Because they have little effect on non-cardiac tissue, they exert fewer side effects than non-selective agents such as propranolol (Inderal).

Drug	Primary Receptor Subtype	Primary Use
acebutolol (Rhotral, Sectral)	Beta$_1$	Hypertension, dysrhythmias, angina
atenolol (Tenormin)	Beta$_1$	Hypertension, angina
carvedilol (Coreg)	Alpha$_1$, beta$_1$, and beta$_2$	Hypertension
doxazosin (Cardura)	Alpha$_1$	Hypertension
metoprolol (Lopresor)	Beta$_1$	Hypertension
nadolol (Corgard)	Beta$_1$ and beta$_2$	Hypertension
phentolamine	Alpha	Severe hypertension
Pr prazosin (Minipress)	Alpha$_1$	Hypertension
propranolol (Inderal)	Beta$_1$ and beta$_2$	Hypertension, dysrhythmias, heart failure
sotalol (Rylosol)	Beta$_1$ and beta$_2$	Dysrhythmias
terazosin (Hytrin)	Alpha$_1$	Hypertension
timolol	Beta$_1$ and beta$_2$	Hypertension, angina, glaucoma

TABLE 14.2 Adrenergic Antagonists

The primary use of beta blockers is in the treatment of hypertension. Although the exact mechanism by which beta blockers reduce blood pressure is not completely understood, it is thought that the reduction may be due to the decreased cardiac output or suppression of renin release by the kidney. See Chapter 51 for a more comprehensive description of the use of beta blockers in hypertension management.

Beta-adrenergic antagonists have several other important therapeutic applications, discussions of which appear in many chapters in this text. By decreasing the cardiac workload, beta blockers can ease the symptoms of angina pectoris (Chapter 50). By slowing electrical conduction across the myocardium, beta blockers are able to treat certain types of dysrhythmias (Chapter 55). Other therapeutic uses include the treatment of heart failure (Chapter 54), myocardial infarction (Chapter 50), and narrow-angle glaucoma (Chapter 63).

Nursing Considerations

Because the purposes and indications of drugs within this class vary greatly, the Nursing Process Focus applies to all clients receiving adrenergic antagonist drugs. For specific nursing considerations, contraindications, and precautions, see Chapters 54 and 55 for more information about alpha- and beta-adrenergic blockers.

PROTOTYPE DRUG	Prazosin (Minipress)

Actions and Uses: Prazosin is a selective alpha$_1$-adrenergic antagonist that competes with norepinephrine at its receptors on vascular smooth muscle in arterioles and veins. Its major action is a rapid decrease in peripheral resistance that reduces blood pressure. It has little effect on cardiac output or heart rate, and it causes less reflex tachycardia than some other drugs in this class. Tolerance to prazosin's antihypertensive effects may occur. Its most common use is in combination with other agents, such as beta blockers or diuretics, in the pharmacotherapy of hypertension. Prazosin has a short half-life and is often taken two or three times per day.

Pharmacokinetics: Prazosin is 60% absorbed after oral administration. It is widely distributed and highly protein bound. It is extensively metabolized by the liver. Its half-life is 2 to 3 hours.

Administration Alerts:

- This drug increases urinary metabolites of vanillylmandelic acid (VMA) and norepinephrine, which are measured to screen for pheochromocytoma (adrenal tumour), so prazosin will cause false-positive results.
- Prazosin is pregnancy category C.

Adverse Effects and Interactions: Like other alpha blockers, prazosin has a tendency to cause orthostatic hypotension due to alpha$_1$ inhibition in vascular smooth muscle. In rare cases, this hypotension can be so severe as to cause unconsciousness about 30 minutes after the first dose. This is called the *first-dose phenomenon*. To avoid this situation, the first dose should be very low and given at bedtime. Dizziness, drowsiness, or lightheadedness may occur as a result of decreased blood flow to the brain due to the drug's hypotensive action. Reflex tachycardia may occur due to the rapid falls in blood pressure. The alpha blockade may also result in nasal congestion or inhibition of ejaculation.

Drug interactions include increased hypotensive effects with concurrent use of antihypertensives and diuretics.

NURSING PROCESS FOCUS

Clients Receiving Adrenergic Antagonist Therapy

Assessment	Potential Nursing Diagnoses/Identified Patterns
Prior to administration: • Assess vital signs, urinary output, and cardiac output (initially and throughout therapy). • Assess reason for drug administration. • Obtain complete health history, including allergies, drug history, and possible drug interactions.	• Need for knowledge regarding drug therapy • Impaired sensory perception • Risk for injury related to dizziness, syncope • Urinary retention • Sexual dysfunction

Planning: Client Goals and Expected Outcomes

The client will:

- Exhibit a decrease in blood pressure with no adverse effects
- Report a decrease in urinary symptoms such as hesitancy and difficulty voiding
- Demonstrate an understanding of the drug by accurately describing the drug's purpose, action, side effects, and precautions

Implementation

Interventions (Rationales)	Client Education/Discharge Planning
• For prostatic hypertrophy, monitor for urinary hesitancy/feeling of incomplete bladder emptying, interrupted urinary stream. • Monitor for syncope. (Alpha-adrenergic antagonists produce first-dose syncope phenomenon and may cause loss of consciousness.) • Monitor vital signs, level of consciousness, and mood. (Adrenergic antagonists can exacerbate existing mental depression.) • Monitor carefully for dizziness, drowsiness, or lightheadedness. (These are signs of decreased blood flow to the brain due to the drug's hypotensive action.) • Observe for side effects, which may include blurred vision, tinnitus, epistaxis, and edema. • Monitor liver function (due to increased risk for liver toxicity).	• Instruct client to report increased difficulty with urinary voiding to healthcare provider. Instruct client to: • Take this medication at bedtime, and to take the first dose *immediately* before getting into bed. • Avoid abrupt changes in position. • Warn client about the first-dose phenomenon; reassure that this effect diminishes with continued therapy. • Instruct client to immediately report any feelings of dysphoria. • Interview client regarding suicide potential; obtain a "no self-harm" verbal contract from the client. Instruct client: • To monitor vitals signs, especially blood pressure, ensuring proper use of home equipment • Regarding the normotensive range of blood pressure, instruct client to consult the nurse regarding "reportable" blood pressure readings • To report dizziness or syncope that persists beyond the first dose, as well as paresthesias and other neurological changes Instruct client: • That nasal congestion may be a side effect. • To report any adverse reactions to the healthcare provider. • Warn client about the potential danger of concomitant use of OTC nasal decongestants. Instruct client to: • Adhere to a regular schedule of laboratory testing for liver function as ordered by the healthcare provider • Report signs and symptoms of liver toxicity: nausea, vomiting, diarrhea, rash, jaundice, abdominal pain, tenderness or distention, or change in colour of stool Inform client of the importance of ongoing medication adherence and follow-up.

Evaluation of Outcome Criteria

Evaluate effectiveness of drug therapy by confirming that client goals and expected outcomes have been met (see "Planning").

See Table 14.2 for a list of drugs to which these nursing actions apply.

CHAPTER

14 Understanding the Chapter

Key Concepts Summary

The numbered key concepts provide a succinct summary of the important points from the corresponding numbered section within the chapter. If any of these points are not clear, refer to the numbered section within the chapter for review.

14.1 Autonomic drugs are classified by which receptors they stimulate or block: adrenergic agonists stimulate adrenergic receptors of sympathetic nerves, whereas adrenergic antagonists inhibit the sympathetic division of the autonomic nervous system.

14.2 Adrenergics act directly by activating adrenergic receptors or indirectly by increasing the release of norepinephrine from nerve terminals. They are primarily used for their effects on the heart, bronchial tree, and nasal passages.

14.3 Adrenergic antagonists inhibit the sympathetic division of the autonomic nervous system.

14.4 Adrenergic antagonists are primarily used for hypertension and are the most widely prescribed class of autonomic drug.

Chapter 14 Scenario

Alexia Howard is a 22-year-old woman with a history of asthma since childhood. She is presently a student at the local university, where she lives in the residence. Since the beginning of the semester, Alexia has experienced tremendous stress while trying to manage school and part-time employment. Her roommate, an animal lover, has brought stray dogs and cats into their room several times during the past few months until she could find good homes for them.

Today, Alexia arrives at the University Health Centre with tachypnea and acute shortness of breath with audible wheezing. She has not consistently taken her prescribed medications to avoid asthma attacks. A physical examination reveals a heart rate of 110 beats/minute and a respiratory rate of 40 breaths/minute with signs of accessory muscle use. Auscultation reveals decreased breath sounds with inspiratory and expiratory wheezing. She is coughing up small amounts of white sputum. Her saturated oxygen is 93% on room air.

An aerosol treatment with salbutamol (Ventolin) is ordered, using a small-volume nebulizer for 15 minutes. Peak flow measures after the treatment show marked improvement of airflow. On auscultation there is clearing of bilateral breath sounds. Alexia's respiratory rate at the time of discharge is 20 and her heart rate is 108. She verbalizes that she feels much better but a little nervous.

Alexia is discharged from the University Health Centre. She is given a prescription for inhaled steroids and instructed to resume her home medications and use them consistently.

Critical Thinking Questions

1. Discuss the mechanism of action associated with salbutamol (Ventolin).
2. Why is salbutamol being given to Alexia, and why is this route of administration being used?
3. What adverse effects is Alexia demonstrating as a result of the administration of salbutamol?

See Answers to Critical Thinking Questions in Appendix B.

NCLEX Practice Questions

1 A client who uses over-the-counter phenylephrine (Neo-Synephrine) nasal spray asks the nurse how the medication works. The nurse's response would be that

a. It helps to shrink the swelling in your nose by tightening the blood vessels there.

b. It works to locally destroy invading organisms that cause colds and flu.

c. It coats the nasal passages to reduce swelling.

d. It is absorbed after you swallow it to act as a decongestant.

2 A nurse is teaching a client about the use of an adrenergic agonist nasal spray at home. What client teaching is needed related to this medication? Select all that apply.

a. Do not share the nasal spray with another person.

b. Only use this drug for 3 to 5 days unless directed by a healthcare provider.

c. Symptoms of excessive use of this drug are lethargy and fatigue.

d. Infants and children should not use this medication unless directed by a healthcare provider.

e. This drug can be safely used by individuals with diabetes.

3 The healthcare provider prescribes epinephrine (adrenalin) to a client who was stung by several wasps 30 minutes ago. The nurse knows that the primary purpose of this medication for this client is to

a. Stop the systemic release of histamine produced by the mast cells.

b. Counteract the formation of antibodies in response to an invading antigen.

c. Increase the number of white blood cells produced to fight the primary invader.

d. Increase a declining blood pressure and dilate constricting bronchi associated with anaphylaxis.

4 A client takes a dose of salbutamol (Ventolin) prior to bedtime. Which effect would the nurse consider normal for this drug?

a. Insomnia

b. Sleepiness

c. Urticaria

d. Tinnitus

5 A beta-adrenergic agonist is prescribed for each of the following clients. For which client should the nurse question the order? Select all that apply.

a. A client with hyperthyroidism

b. A client with asthma

c. A client with shock

d. A client with dysrhythmias

e. A client with heart failure

See Answers to NCLEX Practice Questions in Appendix A.

UNIT

5

Pharmacology of Alterations in the Central Nervous System

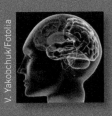

V. Yakobchuk/Fotolia

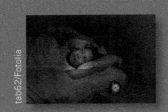

tab62/Fotolia

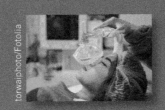

torwaiphoto/Fotolia

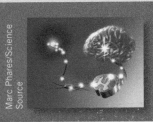

Marc Phares/Science Source

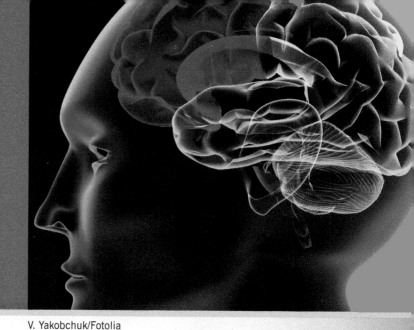
V. Yakobchuk/Fotolia

CHAPTER
15

Brief Review of the Central Nervous System

LEARNING OUTCOMES

After reading this chapter, the student should be able to:

1. Identify disorders for which central nervous system medications are prescribed.

2. Illustrate the major components of a synapse within the central nervous system.

3. Identify the major neurotransmitters in the central nervous system and their functions.

4. Describe the major structural regions of the brain and their primary functions.

5. Explain the major functional systems of the brain and their primary functions.

CHAPTER OUTLINE

▸ How Medications Affect the Central Nervous System

▸ Neurons and Neurotransmission

▸ Structural Divisions of the Central Nervous System

▸ Functional Systems of the Central Nervous System

KEY TERMS

basal nuclei, 161	glutamate, 159	serotonin, 159
dopamine, 158	limbic system, 161	synapses, 158
extrapyramidal system, 161	neuron, 157	
gamma-aminobutyric acid (GABA), 158	reticular activating system (RAS), 161	

Chapters 12 through 14 introduced the autonomic nervous system (ANS). The ANS is the system that provides involuntary control over vital functions of the cardiovascular, digestive, respiratory, and genitourinary systems. This chapter launches Unit 4, which examines the pharmacology of the central nervous system (CNS). The two components of the CNS, the brain and spinal cord, are collectively responsible for interpreting sensory information and formulating appropriate responses. Typical responses may include thinking (deciding if the sensory information is harmful or pleasurable), emotions (anger, depression, euphoria), or movement (running away, pounding a fist, hugging). The purpose of this chapter is to provide a brief review of concepts of CNS anatomy and physiology that are relevant to neuropharmacology.

How Medications Affect the Central Nervous System

15.1 Medications affect the central nervous system by stimulating or suppressing the firing of specific neurons.

Medications may be administered to treat specific neurological or psychiatric disorders of the CNS. Many drugs cause CNS adverse effects during pharmacotherapy, whereas some are self-administered to produce pleasurable psychoactive effects. At high doses, a large number of drugs affect the brain, and CNS toxicity is a dose-limiting factor in the pharmacotherapy of many diseases.

Of all divisions of pharmacology, CNS drug mechanisms are probably the least understood. For some medications, pharmacologists know only that the drug acts on the CNS and produces a therapeutic effect, and its mechanism of action remains largely unknown. There are two primary reasons for this lack of understanding about how CNS drugs produce their effects: the uniqueness of the human brain and the complexity of the disorders affecting it.

The human brain is truly unique, with no other species having the same complexity. It is not known if animals experience the same types of mental disorders as humans, and measurement of hallucinations, euphoria, or depression is difficult, if not impossible, in most species. Pharmacologists are certainly able to measure changes in brain activity or in the amounts of neurotransmitters in specific regions of the brain, but these do not adequately explain complex changes in thinking, mood, or behaviour. Without good animal models, pharmacologists must rely largely on empirical observations—evidence derived from giving the drugs to clients and determining what works rather than how it works.

Also complicating the study of CNS pharmacology is the fact that mental disorders themselves are incompletely understood. The physiological basis for disorders such as schizophrenia, major depression, bipolar disorder, panic attacks, or post-traumatic stress disorder is not well established. There is great client variability in symptoms and disease progression with these disorders, and social factors play important roles. Without a complete understanding of the etiology and pathophysiology of mental disorders, pharmacotherapy of these conditions and the development of new drug therapies for CNS disorders will remain challenging.

The next nine chapters present the major classes of drugs whose pharmacotherapeutic goal is to modify the activity of some portion of the CNS. A tenth chapter examines substances that are abused for their effects on the CNS. In a few cases, CNS drugs affect the function of very specific regions of the brain. Most CNS drugs, however, are nonspecific and affect multiple brain regions.

In the simplest terms, CNS drugs have two basic actions: they either stimulate (activate) or suppress (inhibit) the firing of neurons. In some cases, CNS drugs may have both actions: activation of some neurons and inhibition of others. The pharmacological effects of a CNS drug observed in a client are the result of precisely which neurons are changed, and how many are affected. As a result of neuron modification, the following beneficial effects of CNS drugs are observed and are studied in this unit:

- Reduction in anxiety
- Improved sleep patterns
- Elevated mood
- Management of psychotic symptoms
- Slowing of the progression of chronic degenerative diseases of the brain
- Termination and prevention of seizures
- Reduction in muscle spasms and spasticity
- Reduction of hyperactivity and mania
- Reduction in pain
- Induction of anesthesia

Neurons and Neurotransmission

15.2 Neurons in the central nervous system communicate with each other and with body tissues using neurotransmitters.

The **neuron** is the primary functional cell in all portions of the nervous system. The function of the neurons that make up the nervous system is to communicate messages through conduction of an action potential. In the CNS, the vast majority of neurons are communicating with other neurons. These neuronal pathways or circuits are extremely complex and provide the basis for the higher level functions of the brain such as thinking, memory, and intelligence.

Although a single neuron in the CNS serves no practical function, the interconnections among billions of neurons are a major part of what distinguishes the human brain from that of all other species.

Communication between neurons in the brain, as well as that between the brain and other organs, is provided through **synapses**. Synapses are junctions between two neurons, or between a neuron and a muscle or a gland. Synapses in the ANS are presented in detail in Chapter 12. The student should review that chapter before proceeding.

Synapses within the CNS operate by the same basic principles as those in the ANS. An action potential from the presynaptic neuron releases a neurotransmitter that moves across the synaptic cleft to activate receptors on the postsynaptic neuron. In some cases, the neuron may be excitatory, enhancing neural transmission. In other cases, the impulse inhibits a neurotransmitter from being released, or it causes the release of an inhibitory neurotransmitter that suppresses neuronal conduction. All interconnections in the CNS depend on transmission of the action potential from one neuron to another neuron, or to multiple neurons at synapses.

In the ANS only two neurotransmitters—acetylcholine (Ach) and norepinephrine (NE)—account for nearly all synaptic transmission. Although these two chemicals also are found in the CNS, more than 30 additional substances have been identified as neurotransmitters in the brain, making the study of neuronal communication in this organ very complex. Some neurotransmitters such as glutamate are primarily stimulatory, whereas others such as gamma-aminobutyric acid (GABA) inhibit neuronal activity. NE can activate or inhibit neuronal activity, depending on its location in the brain. A summary of relevant brain neurotransmitters is shown in Table 15.1.

Adrenergic synapses   Adrenergic synapses use NE as the neurotransmitter. Adrenergic synapses in the CNS are abundant in the hypothalamus, the limbic system, and the reticular activating system (RAS). NE activates parts of the brain to heighten alertness and is prominent during waking hours. Adrenergic neurons likely play a role in mood disorders such as depression and anxiety.

Drugs used to modify adrenergic synapses in the CNS include caffeine, amphetamines, and tricyclic antidepressants.

Cholinergic synapses   Cholinergic synapses use Ach as the neurotransmitter. In the brain, these synapses are most often stimulatory. Cholinergic synapses are abundant in the motor cortex and basal ganglia but are uncommon in other areas. Cholinergic synapses are especially important in the pathophysiology of Parkinson's disease and Alzheimer's disease. Ach is also a major neurotransmitter in the ANS.

Dopaminergic synapses   Dopaminergic synapses use dopamine as the neurotransmitter. **Dopamine** is a chemical precursor in the synthesis of NE and, like epinephrine and NE, is classified chemically as a catecholamine. Dopaminergic synapses are generally excitatory and affect arousal and wakefulness. However, two major receptor subtypes exist: D1 is stimulatory, and D2 is inhibitory. Cocaine and amphetamines produce their stimulatory actions by affecting dopamine receptors; marijuana is also thought to exert some of its psychoactive effects by increasing dopaminergic activity. Dopamine receptors are important in the pharmacotherapy of psychosis, Parkinson's disease, and depression.

Endorphins and enkephalins   Endorphins and enkephalins are small peptides secreted by neurons in the hypothalamus, pituitary, limbic system, and spinal cord. The receptor for these molecules is the opioid receptor, which is involved in pain transmission. Endorphins and enkephalins are sometimes called natural opiates because they produce effects very similar to those of morphine and other opioid drugs. Drugs used to modify the types of synapses in the CNS include opioids such as codeine and morphine.

Gamma-aminobutyric acid synapses   These synapses use **gamma-aminobutyric acid (GABA)** as the neurotransmitter. GABA synapses are the second most common type in the CNS, accounting for 30% to 40% of all brain synapses. GABA is the primary inhibitory neurotransmitter in the CNS and is found throughout the brain, with greatest abundance in the basal ganglia and hypothalamus. Several GABA receptor subtypes have been identified. GABA receptors are the primary site of action for

TABLE 15.1   Select Central Nervous System Neurotransmitters and Their Functions

Neurotransmitter	Abundance	Effect	Clinical Significance
Acetylcholine (Ach)	Widely distributed in the CNS; a major transmitter in the ANS	CNS: May be excitatory or inhibitory; controls voluntary skeletal muscle movement ANS: Activates the parasympathetic nervous system	Myasthenia gravis, Alzheimer's disease
Dopamine	Basal ganglia and limbic system	Usually excitatory; locomotion, attention, learning, and the reinforcing effects of abused drugs	Parkinson's disease; psychoses; motivation, pleasure
Endorphins and enkephalins	Widely distributed in the CNS and peripheral nervous system (PNS)	Usually inhibitory; reduction of pain	Opioids bind to endorphin receptors
Gamma aminobutyric acid (GABA)	Widely distributed in the CNS	Most common inhibitory CNS neurotransmitter	Seizure and anxiety disorders
Glutamate	Widely distributed in the CNS	Most common excitatory CNS neurotransmitter	Memory
Norepinephrine (NE)	Widely distributed in the CNS; a major transmitter in the ANS	CNS: May be excitatory or inhibitory ANS: Activates the sympathetic nervous system	Depression, memory, panic attacks
Serotonin	Common in the brainstem but also found in the limbic system, gastrointestinal tract, and platelets	Usually inhibitory	Anxiety, bipolar disorder, and depression

several classes of drugs, including the benzodiazepines and barbiturates, as well as other possible hypnotic agents (for example, zoplicone (Imovane)).

NCLEX Success Tips

Gabapentin (Neurontin) is structurally related to GABA but doesn't interact with GABA receptors, isn't converted into GABA or GABA agonist, doesn't inhibit GABA reuptake, and doesn't prevent degradation. Gabapentin may impair vision. Changes in vision, concentration, or coordination should be reported to the nurse. Gabapentin is an anticonvulsant used to treat several seizure disorders.

Gabapentin should not be stopped abruptly because of the potential for status epilepticus; this is a medication that must be tapered off.

It is to be stored at room temperature and out of direct light and should not be taken with antacids.

Glutamate synapses Glutamate synapses use the amino acid **glutamate** (glutamic acid) as the neurotransmitter. Glutamate is the most common neurotransmitter in the CNS, and its synapses are always excitatory in nature. It is found in nearly all regions of the brain. Several glutamate receptor subtypes have been identified, with the *N*-methyl-D-aspartate (NMDA) receptor being particularly important to memory and learning. In addition to glutamate, zinc, magnesium, glycine, and even phencyclidine (a hallucinogen) bind to the NMDA receptor, thus modulating neuronal activity. High amounts of glutamate can cause neuron death and may be the mechanism responsible for certain types of neurotoxicity.

Serotonergic synapses Serotonergic synapses use **serotonin**, also known as 5-hydroxytryptamine (5-HT), as the neurotransmitter. Although some serotonergic synapses are located in the CNS, 98% of the serotonergic receptors are found outside the CNS in platelets, mast cells, and other peripheral cells. Serotonergic receptors are found throughout the limbic (emotional) system of the brain, often in close association with adrenergic synapses. Serotonin is used by the body to synthesize the hormone melatonin in the pineal gland. Low serotonin levels in the CNS are associated with anxiety and impulsive behaviour, including suicidal ideation. Serotonergic receptors play an important role in the mechanism of action of antidepressant drugs.

NCLEX Success Tips

The nurse should pay special attention to medications that increase serotonin level in the CNS, such as monoamine oxidase inhibitors (MAOIs), selective serotonin reuptake inhibitors (SSRIs), serotonin–norepinephrine reuptake inhibitors (SNRIs), and many other CNS agents.

Clients taking an MAOI must wait 14 days after stopping the MAOI before starting an SSRI.

Structural Divisions of the Central Nervous System

15.3 The central nervous system is divided into several major structural components.

The brain consists of dozens of structural divisions that serve common functions. Identification of the many anatomical

components in the CNS is complex and beyond the scope of this text. This section focuses on regions of the CNS that have applications to neuropharmacology. For a more complete discussion of CNS anatomy, the student should consult anatomy and physiology textbooks. Basic brain structures are illustrated in Figure 15.1.

Cerebrum The cerebrum is the "thinking" part of the brain responsible for perception, speech, conscious motor movement, movement of skeletal muscles, memory, and smell. It is the largest part of the brain, by weight, and the most advanced. Portions of the cerebrum are organized for specialized functions. For example, the occipital lobe is associated with vision, and the frontal lobes are concerned with reasoning and planning. Other areas are specific to language, hearing, motor, or sensory functions.

Disorders of the cerebrum may be focal or generalized. Focal abnormalities, often the result of a stroke, occur in specific regions and may affect a single brain function such as vision, hearing, or movement of a particular limb. Generalized disorders of the cerebrum affect widespread areas or multiple regions and can produce drowsiness, coma, hallucinations, depression, or generalized anxiety.

Thalamus The thalamus is the major relay centre in the brain that sends sensory information such as sounds, sights, pain, touch, and temperature to the cerebral cortex for analysis. To reach the cerebrum, all sensory information must travel through the thalamus. Portions of the thalamus comprise the limbic system, an area that controls mood and motivation. Abnormalities of the thalamus have been associated with diverse mood disorders such as obsessive-compulsive disorder, bipolar disorder, anxiety, and panic disorder.

Hypothalamus The hypothalamus is the major visceral control centre in the body. Regulation of hunger, thirst, water balance, and body temperature are functions of this region. The hypothalamus is also part of the limbic system, which is associated with emotional balance. Some neurons in the hypothalamus connect to the brainstem to affect vital centres such as heart rate, respiratory rate, blood pressure, and pupil size. These responses are associated with the fight-or-flight response of the ANS. The many endocrine functions of the hypothalamus are discussed in Chapter 27. Disorders of the hypothalamus may affect some or all of these essential endocrine functions.

Cerebellum The cerebellum controls muscle movement, balance, posture, and tone. It is involved in learning fine motor skills that make muscular movements smooth and continuous. The cerebellum receives sensory information, including vision, position, equilibrium, and touch, and calculates the strength and extent of muscle movement needed to maintain posture and coordinate complex tasks such as walking, driving, or playing a musical instrument. Injury or disease in this region results in uncoordinated, jerky body movements.

Brainstem The brainstem, consisting of the medulla oblongata, pons, and midbrain, connects the spinal cord to the brain. Because of its critical location, it serves as the major relay centre for messages travelling to and from the brain. In addition, it

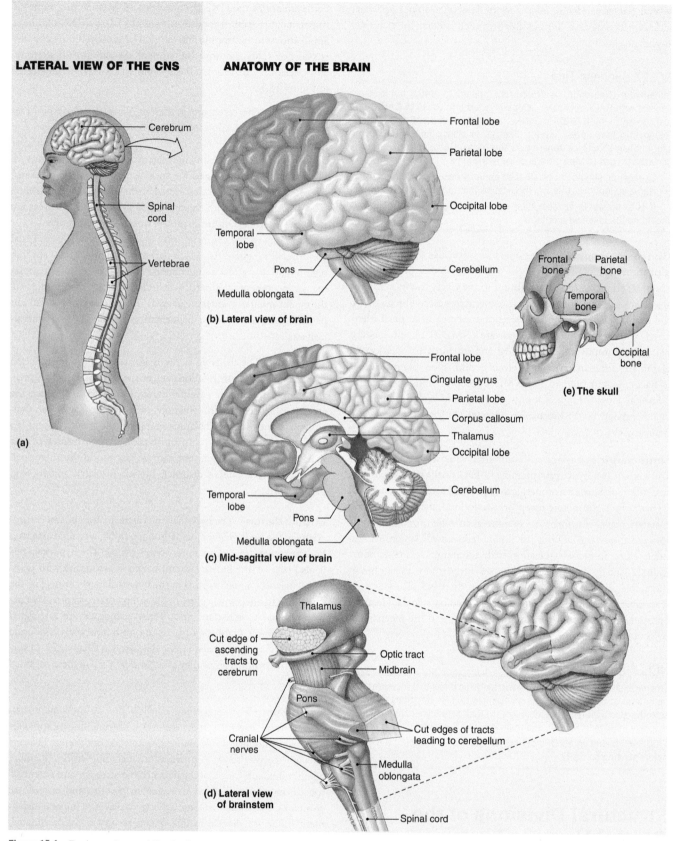

Figure 15.1   Basic anatomy of the brain.

Source: From *Human Physiology: An Integrated Approach* (2nd ed.) by D. U. Silverthorn, 2001. Reprinted and electronically reproduced by permission of Pearson Education, Inc., Upple Saddle River, NJ.

contains major reflex and control centres that involve breathing, heart rate, vision, swallowing, coughing, and vomiting. Injury to the brainstem can be fatal if vital centres are disrupted. The brainstem contains clusters of scattered neurons known as the reticular formation, which help to maintain alertness.

Spinal cord   The spinal cord is essentially a conduction pathway to and from the brain. Disruptions of these pathways will prevent transmission of nerve impulses and cause loss of sensory (paresthesia) or motor (paralysis) function.

Blood-brain barrier   The brain must receive a continuous supply of oxygen and glucose; interruptions for even brief periods may cause loss of consciousness. At the same time that it needs large quantities of nutrients, the brain must also protect itself from pathogens or toxins that may have entered the blood. Capillaries in most regions of the brain are not as porous as those in other organs; the endothelial cells form tight junctions, creating a seal or barrier to many substances. This is important to pharmacology because CNS drugs must be able to penetrate the blood-brain barrier to produce their effects.

Functional Systems of the Central Nervous System
15.4 Several functional divisions of the central nervous system are important to pharmacotherapy.

Functional brain systems are clusters of neurons that work together to perform a common function. These clusters may be located far apart from each other in the CNS, but they form a network that acts as a coordinated unit. Some CNS drugs produce their effects by modifying the functions of these systems.

Limbic system   The **limbic system** is a group of structures deep in the brain that are responsible for emotional expression, learning, and memory. Emotional states associated with this system include anxiety, fear, anger, aggression, remorse, depression, sexual drive, and euphoria. Signals routed through the limbic system ultimately connect with the hypothalamus. Through its connection with the hypothalamus, autonomic actions such as rapid heart rate, high blood pressure, or peptic ulcers are associated with intense emotional states. The limbic system also communicates with the cerebrum, which allows people to think and reflect on their emotional states. The connection to the cerebrum allows one to use logic to "override" emotional reactions that might be inappropriate or harmful. Parts of the limbic system also allow one to remember emotional responses.

Reticular activating system   Stimulation of the reticular formation causes heightened alertness and arousal of the brain as a whole. Inhibition causes general drowsiness and the induction of sleep.

The larger area in which the reticular formation is found is called the **reticular activating system (RAS)**. This structure projects from the brainstem to the thalamus. The RAS is responsible for sleeping and wakefulness and performs an alerting function for the cerebral cortex. It also acts as a filter, allowing one to ignore weak, repetitious, or unimportant sensory stimuli and to focus attention on individual tasks by transmitting information to higher brain centres. This is important in busy, noisy environments when a person must concentrate on a specific task, such as studying or reading. In any given situation, as much as 99% of all sensory information may be filtered and never reach consciousness.

The RAS has particular importance to pharmacology because many drugs act by decreasing neuronal activity in this system to cause drowsiness or sleep. Examples include alcohol and sedative-hypnotics. Lysergic acid diethylamide (LSD) interferes with portions of the RAS, causing unusual sensory experiences such as seeing odours or hearing colours.

Basal nuclei   The **basal nuclei**, also called basal ganglia, are a cluster of neurons in the brain that help to regulate the initiation and termination of skeletal muscle movement. They also help to initiate and terminate certain cognitive functions such as memory, learning, planning, and attention. Connections between the basal ganglia and the limbic system are thought to be associated with psychoses, attention deficit/hyperactivity disorder, and obsessive-compulsive disorder. Reduced dopaminergic transmission through the basal ganglia is the most common finding in Parkinson's disease.

Extrapyramidal system   Messages that control the voluntary movement of skeletal muscle originate in the cerebrum and travel down the CNS in tracts or pathways. The two motor pathways, travelling through the brain, brainstem, and spinal cord, are called pyramidal (direct) and extrapyramidal (indirect). The pyramidal tracts are voluntary tracts involved with the movement of skeletal muscles. The **extrapyramidal system** controls locomotion, complex muscular movements, and posture. The extrapyramidal system has particular importance to pharmacology because it is adversely affected by certain medications, especially the conventional antipsychotic agents. Adverse extrapyramidal symptoms include jerking motions; muscular spasms of the head, face, and neck; and akathisia, an inability to remain at rest. Some extrapyramidal symptoms resemble those of Parkinson's disease.

NCLEX Success Tip

Metoclopramide (Metonia), a prokinetic agent used as an antiemetic, has central antiemetic effects and antagonizes the action of dopamine, a catecholamine neurotransmitter. It can cause serious muscle problems called tardive dyskinesia (extrapyramidal effect) in which the client's muscles, especially of the face, move in unusual ways. Tardive dyskinesia may not be reversible.

CHAPTER

15

Understanding the Chapter

Key Concepts Summary

The numbered key concepts provide a succinct summary of the important points from the corresponding numbered section within the chapter. If any of these points are not clear, refer to the numbered section within the chapter for review.

15.1 Medications affect the central nervous system by stimulating or suppressing the firing of specific neurons.

15.2 Neurons in the central nervous system communicate with each other and with body tissues using neurotransmitters.

15.3 The central nervous system is divided into several major structural components.

15.4 Several functional divisions of the central nervous system are important to pharmacotherapy.

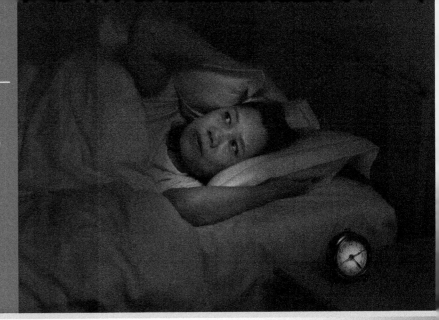

tab62/Fotolia

CHAPTER

16 Pharmacotherapy of Anxiety and Sleep Disorders

LEARNING OUTCOMES

After reading this chapter, the student should be able to:

1. Discuss factors contributing to anxiety and insomnia and explain some non-pharmacological therapies used to manage each of these disorders.

2. Identify drug classes used for treating anxiety and sleep disorders.

3. Explain the therapeutic action of drugs used to treat anxiety disorders and insomnia.

4. Describe the nurse's role in the pharmacological management of clients with anxiety disorders and insomnia.

5. For each of the drug classes listed in Prototype Drugs, identify a representative drug and explain its mechanism of action, therapeutic effects, and important adverse effects.

6. Describe and explain, based on pharmacological principles, the rationale for nursing assessment, planning, and interventions for clients with anxiety disorders and insomnia.

7. Use the nursing process to care for clients who are receiving drug therapy for anxiety and insomnia.

CHAPTER OUTLINE

▶ Anxiety Disorders

  ▶ Types of Anxiety Disorders

  ▶ Regions of the Brain Responsible for Anxiety and Wakefulness

  ▶ Sleep Disorders

  ▶ Anxiety Management Through Pharmacological and Non-Pharmacological Strategies

▶ Insomnia

  ▶ Insomnia and the Role of Melatonin

▶ Central Nervous System Depressants

  ▶ Treating Anxiety and Insomnia with CNS Depressants

▶ Benzodiazepines

  ▶ Treating Anxiety and Insomnia with Benzodiazepines

▶ Barbiturates

  ▶ Use of Barbiturates as Sedatives

  ▶ Other CNS Depressants for Anxiety and Sleep Disorders

Anxiety is a generalized feeling of worry, fear, or uneasiness about a perceived threat. This threat, such as an upcoming divorce or pharmacology test, may be clearly identifiable, or it may be an unfocused, general feeling of worry or dread. Anxiety is a normal, adaptive response to stress that prepares a person to deal with the perceived threat both physically and emotionally. However, when the anxiety is excessive or irrational, the client's quality of life may become seriously affected, and there will be an increased risk of developing chronic gastrointestinal (GI) and cardiovascular disorders. Anxiety disorders are the most common mental health illnesses encountered in clinical practice. This chapter discusses medications that treat anxiety, cause sedation, or help clients to sleep.

ANXIETY DISORDERS

According to the *International Classification of Diseases,* 10th edition (ICD-10), anxiety is a state of "apprehension, tension, or uneasiness that stems from the anticipation of danger, the source of which is largely unknown or unrecognized." Anxious individuals can often identify at least some factors that bring on their symptoms. Most state that their feelings of anxiety are disproportionate to any actual dangers.

Types of Anxiety Disorders

16.1 Generalized anxiety disorder is the most common type of anxiety; phobias, obsessive-compulsive disorder, panic attacks, and post-traumatic stress disorder are other important categories.

The anxiety experienced by people who are faced with a stressful environment is called **situational anxiety**. To a certain degree, situational anxiety is beneficial because it motivates people to accomplish tasks in a prompt manner—if for no other reason than to eliminate the source of nervousness. Situational stress may be intense, though clients often learn coping mechanisms to deal with the stress without seeking conventional medical intervention. From an early age, ego defence mechanisms begin to develop that serve as defences against anxiety.

Generalized anxiety disorder (GAD) is a difficult-to-control, excessive anxiety that lasts 6 months or more. It focuses on a variety of life events or activities and interferes with normal, day-to-day functions. It is by far the most common type of stress disorder, and the one most frequently encountered by the nurse. Symptoms include restlessness, fatigue, muscle tension, nervousness, inability to focus or concentrate, an overwhelming sense of dread, and sleep disturbances. Autonomic signs of sympathetic nervous system activation include blood pressure elevation, heart palpitations, varying degrees of respiratory change, dry mouth, and increased reflexes. Parasympathetic responses may consist of abdominal cramping, diarrhea, fatigue, urinary urgency, and numbness and tingling of the extremities. Females are slightly more likely to experience GAD, and its prevalence is highest in the 20 to 35 age group.

A second category of anxiety, called **panic disorder**, is characterized by intense feelings of immediate apprehension, fearfulness, terror, or impending doom that are accompanied by increased autonomic nervous system activity. Although panic attacks usually last less than 10 minutes, clients may describe them as seemingly endless. As much as 5% of the population will experience one or more panic attacks during their lifetime, with women being affected about twice as often as men.

Other categories of anxiety disorders include phobias, obsessive-compulsive disorder, and post-traumatic stress disorder. **Phobias** are fearful feelings attached to situations or objects. Common phobias include fear of snakes, spiders, crowds, or heights. Phobias compel a client to avoid the fearful stimulus. **Obsessive-compulsive disorder (OCD)** involves recurrent, intrusive thoughts or repetitive behaviours that interfere with normal activities or relationships. Common examples include fear of exposure to germs and repetitive handwashing. **Post-traumatic stress disorder (PTSD)** is a type of anxiety that develops in response to re-experiencing a previous life event. Traumatic life events such as war, physical or sexual abuse, natural disasters, or murder may lead to a sense of helplessness and re-experiencing of the traumatic event. In the aftermath of the terrorist attack on September 11, 2001, the incidence of PTSD increased considerably.

Regions of the Brain Responsible for Anxiety and Wakefulness

16.2 The limbic system and the reticular activating system are specific regions of the brain responsible for anxiety and wakefulness.

Neural systems associated with anxiety and restlessness include the limbic system and the reticular activating system. These are illustrated in Figure 16.1.

The **limbic system** is an area in the middle of the brain responsible for emotional expression, learning, and memory. Signals routed through the limbic system ultimately connect with the hypothalamus. Emotional states associated with this connection include anxiety, fear, anger, aggression, remorse, depression, sexual drive, and euphoria.

The hypothalamus is an important centre responsible for unconscious responses to extreme stress such as elevated blood pressure, elevated respiratory rate, and dilated pupils. These are responses associated with the fight-or-flight response of the autonomic nervous system, as discussed in Chapter 12.

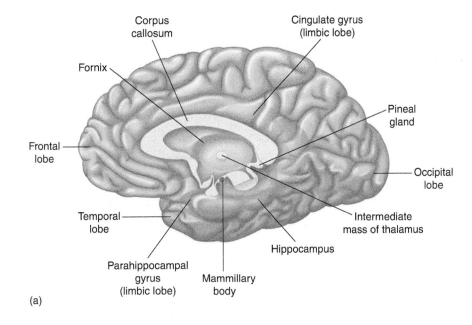

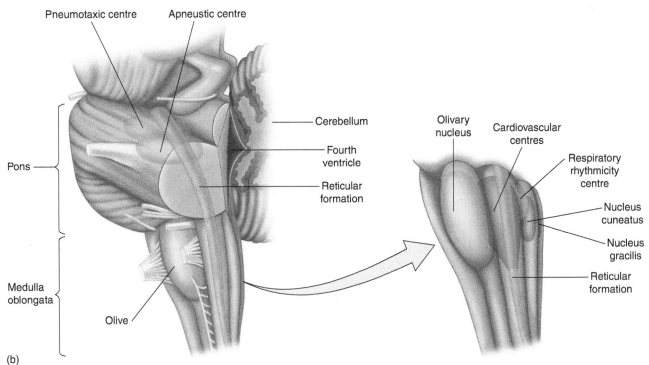

Figure 16.1 Brain regions strongly associated with anxiety, expressions of emotion, and a restless state: (a) the limbic system; (b) the reticular formation, a nucleus where nervous signals ascend to higher centres of the brain; this entire neural network is called the reticular activating system.

The many endocrine functions of the hypothalamus are discussed in Chapter 27.

The hypothalamus also connects with the **reticular formation**, a network of neurons found along the entire length of the brainstem, as shown in Figure 16.1(b). Stimulation of the reticular formation causes heightened alertness and arousal; inhibition causes general drowsiness and the induction of sleep.

The larger area in which the reticular formation is found is called the **reticular activating system (RAS)**. This structure projects from the brainstem to the thalamus. The RAS is responsible for sleeping and wakefulness and performs an alerting function for the cerebral cortex. It also helps a person to focus attention on individual tasks by transmitting information to higher brain centres.

If signals are prevented from passing through the RAS, no emotional signals are sent to the brain, resulting in a reduction in general brain activity. If signals coming from the hypothalamus are allowed to proceed, those signals are further routed through the RAS and on to higher brain centres. This is the neural mechanism thought to be responsible for emotions such as anxiety and fear. It is also the mechanism associated with restlessness and an interrupted sleeping pattern.

Sleep Disorders

16.3 Sleep occurs in distinct stages.

The process of sleep has been well studied. It has been established that all people need an adequate amount of sleep to function optimally, although the amounts change throughout the lifespan. For middle-aged adults, 7 to 8 hours of sleep appear to be adequate. Most older adults sleep less than 8 hours, and infants and babies require much more sleep. Although it is known that sleep is essential for wellness, scientists are unsure of its function or how much is needed to maintain optimum health. The following are some theories:

1. Inactivity during sleep gives the body time to repair itself.

2. Sleep is a function that evolved as a protective mechanism. Throughout history, nighttime was the safest time of day for resting.

3. Sleep involves "electrical" charging and discharging of the brain. The brain needs time to process and file new information collected throughout the day. When this is done without interference from the outside environment, these vast amounts of data can be retrieved later through memory.

Sleep occurs in two basic phases: rapid eye movement (REM) sleep and non–rapid eye movement (NREM) sleep. NREM sleep is further subdivided into four distinct stages based on the depth of sleep (see Table 16.1 for details). Drugs may affect the length of time spent in the different stages of sleep. Decreases in the neurotransmitters acetylcholine, norepinephrine, and serotonin signal the change from wakefulness to **non–rapid eye movement (NREM) sleep**. During this phase, respirations slow, heart rate and blood pressure decrease, oxygen consumption by muscles decreases, and urine formation decreases. NREM accounts for about 75% to 85% of total sleep time.

TABLE 16.1	Stages of Sleep
Stage	**Description**
NREM stage 1	At the onset of sleep, the person is in a stage of drowsiness for about 1 to 7 minutes. During this time, the person can be easily awakened. This stage lasts for about 4% to 5% of total sleep time.
NREM stage 2	The person can still be easily awakened. The stage comprises the greatest amount of total sleep time, 45% to 55%.
NREM stage 3	The person may move into or out of a deeper sleep. Heart rate and blood pressure fall; gastrointestinal activity rises. This stage lasts for about 4% to 6% of total sleep time.
NREM stage 4	The deepest stage of sleep; this stage lasts a little longer than stage 1 or stage 3, about 12% to 15%. This is the stage during which nightmares occur in children. Sleepwalking is also a common behaviour during this stage. Heart rate and blood pressure remain low; gastrointestinal activity remains high.
REM	This stage is characterized by eye movement and a loss of muscle tone. Eye movement occurs in bursts of activity. Dreaming takes place in this stage. The mind is very active and resembles a normal waking state.

Rapid eye movement (REM) sleep is considered the active dreaming stage of sleep, although dreams may also occur in NREM sleep. As the name implies, the eyes move during this stage. Muscle tone diminishes and heart rate and breathing become irregular. Penile erections and clitoral enlargement may occur. Although adults spend about 25% of their sleep in REM sleep, newborns may spend as much as 80% of their sleep in this phase.

Sleep occurs in cycles, alternating between REM and NREM sleep about four to five times each night, with each sleep cycle lasting approximately 90 minutes. There is more time spent in NREM in early cycles, with REM sleep increasing in the later cycles. When the person moves from NREM to REM sleep, there is an increase of acetylcholine and further decreases in serotonin and norepinephrine. As REM sleep continues, the body progressively increases the levels of serotonin and norepinephrine until the amounts are adequate to stop REM sleep. For a brief time, the person may awaken until the next cycle begins.

Clients who are deprived of stage 4 NREM experience depression and a feeling of apathy and fatigue. Stage 4 NREM sleep appears to be linked to repair and restoration of the physical body, whereas REM sleep is associated with learning, memory, and the capacity to adjust to changes in the environment. The body requires the dream state associated with REM sleep to keep the psyche functioning normally. When deprived of REM sleep, people experience a sleep deficit and become frightened, irritable, paranoid, and even emotionally disturbed. Judgment is impaired, and reaction time is slowed. It is speculated that to make up for their lack of dreaming, these persons experience far more daydreaming and fantasizing throughout the day.

There is a wide variation in sleep patterns among adults. Some people do very well with less sleep, whereas others require above-average amounts to feel refreshed and mentally alert. Most people, even young adults, awaken at least once during the night;

the elderly awaken more frequently. The nurse can be a valuable ally to the client who is experiencing sleep disturbances by explaining these normal variations and by assisting the client to reach a desirable sleep pattern.

The acts of sleeping and waking are synchronized with many different bodily functions. Body temperature, blood pressure, hormone levels, and respiration all fluctuate on a cyclical basis throughout the 24-hour day, known as the **circadian rhythm**. Even without realizing it, people who are "day persons" or "night persons" structure their activities, even their occupations, around what they recognize as their best individual pattern of sleep and wakefulness. *Circadian dysrhythm* refers to the psychological and biological stress a person undergoes when travelling rapidly through several time zones, such as during a long airplane journey. "Jet lag" is a very real, and sometimes disabling, phenomenon, although not a permanent dysfunction. When this cycle becomes impaired, pharmacological or other interventions may be needed to readjust it. Circadian rhythms are based on many complex variables, including light–dark cycles and secretion of hormones such as melatonin.

Anxiety Management Through Pharmacological and Non-Pharmacological Strategies

16.4 Anxiety can be managed through pharmacological and non-pharmacological strategies.

Although stress itself may be incapacitating, it is often only a symptom of an underlying disorder. It is considered more productive to uncover and address the cause of the anxiety rather than to merely treat the symptoms with medications. Clients should be encouraged to explore and develop non-pharmacological coping strategies to deal with the underlying causes. Such strategies may include behavioural therapy, biofeedback techniques, meditation, and other complementary therapies. One model for stress management is shown in Figure 16.2.

When anxiety becomes severe enough to significantly interfere with daily activities of life, pharmacotherapy in addition to non-pharmacological strategies is indicated. In most types of stress, **anxiolytics**, which are drugs with the ability to relieve anxiety, are quite effective. Anxiolytics are usually meant to address generalized anxiety on a short-term basis. Longer-term pharmacotherapy for phobias and obsessive-compulsive and post-traumatic stress disorders may include mood disorder drugs (Chapter 17).

INSOMNIA

A sleep disorder is a disturbance in the normal pattern, quality, or quantity of sleep. More than 25% of Canadians suffer from sleep disorders, a percentage that increases with aging. Although about 70 specific types of sleep-related disorders have been identified, pharmacotherapy is beneficial in treating only a few of them.

Insomnia is the most common sleep disorder and the one that is the most frequent indication for pharmacotherapy. Insomnia

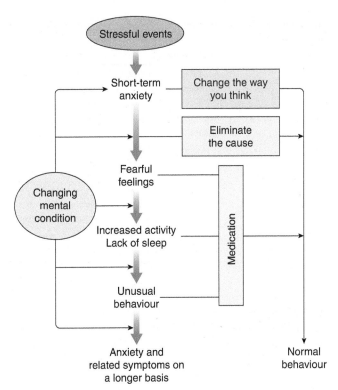

Figure 16.2 A model of anxiety in which stressful events or a changing mental condition can produce unfavourable symptoms, some of which may be controlled by medication.

can be simply defined as the lack of adequate sleep; however, the disorder can be better explained by the following terms:

- *Sleep-onset insomnia.* Inability to fall asleep within a reasonable time, usually more than 30 minutes
- *Sleep-maintenance insomnia.* Frequent awakenings during the night or the inability to fall back asleep
- *Sleep-offset insomnia.* Premature, early morning awakenings
- *Non-restorative sleep.* Persistent sleepiness during the day, despite adequate sleep duration.

The diagnosis of chronic insomnia is determined by its duration (at least 30 days or more) and the degree to which it affects activities of daily living. The most frequent symptom reported by clients is excessive daytime drowsiness.

Insomnia has multiple causes and often presents secondary to an underlying disorder. Examples of conditions that cause secondary insomnia are shown in Table 16.2.

The best approach to resolving secondary insomnia is to treat the underlying disorder. Insomnia not associated with another medical, psychiatric, or medication-related cause is considered to be *primary*.

A good medical history can sometimes distinguish between primary and secondary insomnia; however, for objective testing, clients are referred to sleep disorder specialists for polysomnography and actigraphy. Polysomnography is a series of tests that record physiological changes occurring during sleep, including eye movement, muscle tension, respiration, cardiac rhythm, and brain wave activity. Polysomnography can also determine the amount of REM and NREM sleep. Brain wave activity is

TABLE 16.2   Causes of Secondary Insomnia

Cause	Description
Drugs	Amphetamines, cocaine, caffeinated beverages, corticosteroids, sympathomimetics, antidepressants, alcohol use, nicotine or tobacco use
Medical disorder	Dementia, anxiety disorder, epilepsy, Parkinson's disease, Tourette's syndrome, psychosis, mania, migraines, asthma, sleep apnea, chronic or severe pain, chronic obstructive pulmonary disease, gastro-esophageal reflux, hyperthyroidism
Poor sleep hygiene	Noisy environment; too much light in the bedroom; large meals; working or exercising just prior to sleeping; partner who snores, talks, or moves frequently during sleep
Stressful situation	Major life event such as marriage, divorce, death of a loved one, chronic or terminal disease, stressful job

measured using an **electroencephalogram (EEG)**. Actigraphy is another frequently used diagnostic test that measures the motor activity of a client during waking and sleeping hours. The results of these comprehensive tests can be used to diagnose most sleep disorders.

Insomnia and the Role of Melatonin

16.5 Melatonin, a natural hormone produced in the pineal gland especially at night, is known to help induce restful sleep.

Melatonin is a natural hormone (N-acetyl-5-methoxytryptamine) produced in the pineal gland, especially at night. Its secretion is stimulated by darkness and inhibited by light. Tryptophan is converted to serotonin and finally to melatonin. As melatonin production rises, alertness decreases and body temperature starts to fall, both of which make sleep more inviting. Melatonin production is also related to age. Children manufacture more melatonin than elderly people; however, melatonin production begins to drop at puberty.

Supplemental melatonin, 0.5 to 3.0 mg at bedtime, is purported to decrease the time required to fall asleep and to produce a deep and restful sleep. Melatonin is sold over the counter (OTC) without a prescription in several countries, including Canada. There are several safety concerns about the use of melatonin. People with severe allergies, autoimmune diseases, and immune system cancers such as lymphoma and leukemia should not take melatonin because it could exacerbate such conditions by stimulating the immune system. Clients who are taking corticosteroids should not take melatonin because it may interfere with the efficacy of these hormones. Melatonin use in some children with seizure disorders may lead to increased seizure activity. Melatonin should not be given to healthy children, as they already produce it in abundance. The safety of melatonin use by pregnant or nursing women has not been established. Large doses of melatonin may inhibit ovulation. It is best used for people with "jet lag" or "shift workers," since it produces the naturally produced hormone. It is *not* a quick fix and does not cause sleepiness immediately. Furthermore, there is a large placebo effect with using melatonin.

The acts of sleeping and waking are synchronized to many different bodily functions. Body temperature, blood pressure, hormone levels, and respiration all fluctuate on a cyclical basis throughout the 24-hour day. When this cycle becomes impaired, pharmacological or other interventions may be needed to readjust it. Increased levels of the neurotransmitter serotonin help to initiate the various processes of sleep.

Insomnia, or sleeplessness, is a disorder sometimes associated with anxiety. There are several major types of insomnia. Short-term or behavioural insomnia may be attributed to stress caused by a hectic lifestyle or the inability to resolve day-to-day conflicts within the home environment or the workplace. Worries about work, marriage, children, and health are common reasons for short-term loss of sleep. When stress interrupts normal sleeping patterns, people cannot sleep because their minds are too active.

Foods or beverages that contain stimulants such as caffeine may interrupt sleep. People may also find that the use of tobacco products makes them restless and edgy. Alcohol, while often enabling a person to fall asleep, may produce vivid dreams and frequent awakening that prevent restful sleep. Ingestion of a large meal, especially one high in protein and fat, close to bedtime can interfere with sleep due to the increased metabolic rate needed to digest the food. Certain medications cause central nervous system (CNS) stimulation, and these should not be taken immediately before bedtime. Stressful conditions such as too much light, uncomfortable room temperature (especially one that is too warm), snoring, sleep apnea, and recurring nightmares also interfere with sleep. Long-term insomnia may be caused by depression, manic disorders, and chronic pain.

Non-pharmacological means should be attempted prior to initiating drug therapy for sleep disorders. Long-term use of sleep medications is likely to worsen insomnia and may cause physical or psychological dependence. Some clients experience a phenomenon referred to as **rebound insomnia**. This occurs when a sedative drug is discontinued abruptly or after it has been taken for a long time; sleeplessness and symptoms of anxiety then become markedly worse.

Older clients are more likely to experience medication-related sleep problems. Drugs may seem to help the insomnia of an elderly client for a night or two, only to produce generalized brain dysfunction as the medication accumulates in the system. The agitated client may then be mistakenly overdosed with further medication. Nurses, especially those who work in geriatric settings, are responsible for making accurate observations and reporting client responses to drugs so that the healthcare provider can determine the lowest effective maintenance dose. The need for PRN (as needed) medication for sleep requires individualized assessment by the nurse as well as follow-up evaluation and documentation of its effect on the client.

The stages of sleep are shown in Table 16.1.

CENTRAL NERVOUS SYSTEM DEPRESSANTS

CNS depressants are used to slow brain activity in clients who are experiencing anxiety or sleep disorders. These medications are grouped into three classes: benzodiazepines, barbiturates, and non-barbiturate/non-benzodiazepine CNS depressants.

Treating Anxiety and Insomnia with CNS Depressants

16.6 CNS depressants, including anxiolytics, sedatives, and hypnotics, are used to treat anxiety and insomnia.

CNS depressants are drugs that slow neuronal activity in the brain. CNS depression should be viewed as a continuum ranging from relaxation, to sedation, to the induction of sleep and anesthesia. Coma and death are the end stages of CNS depression. Some drug classes are capable of producing the full range of CNS depression from calming to anesthesia, whereas others are less efficacious. CNS depressants used for anxiety and sleep disorders are categorized into two major classes, the benzodiazepines and the barbiturates. A third class consists of miscellaneous drugs that are chemically unrelated to the benzodiazepines or barbiturates but have similar therapeutic uses. Other CNS depressants include the opioids (Chapter 23) and ethyl alcohol (Chapter 25).

Medications that depress the CNS are sometimes called **sedatives** because of their ability to sedate or relax a client. At higher doses, some of these drugs are called **hypnotics** because of their ability to induce sleep. Therefore, the term **sedative-hypnotic** is often used to describe a drug with the ability to produce a calming effect at lower doses and the ability to induce sleep at higher doses. *Tranquilizer* is an older term sometimes used to describe a drug that produces a calm or tranquil feeling.

Many CNS depressants can cause physical and psychological dependence, as discussed in Chapter 25. The withdrawal syndrome for some CNS depressants can cause life-threatening neurological reactions, including fever, psychosis, and seizures. Other withdrawal symptoms include increased heart rate and lowered blood pressure; loss of appetite; muscle cramps; impairment of memory, concentration, and orientation; abnormal sounds in the ears; blurred vision; and insomnia, agitation, anxiety, and panic. Obvious withdrawal symptoms typically last 2 to 4 weeks. Subtle ones can last for months.

BENZODIAZEPINES

The benzodiazepines are one of the most widely prescribed drug classes. The root word *benzo* refers to an aromatic compound, one having a carbon ring structure attached to different atoms or another carbon ring. Two nitrogen atoms incorporated into the ring structure are the reason for the *diazepine* (*di* = two; *azepine* = nitrogen) portion of the name.

Treating Anxiety and Insomnia with Benzodiazepines

16.7 Benzodiazepines are drugs of choice for generalized anxiety and insomnia.

The benzodiazepines, listed in Table 16.3, are drugs of choice for various anxiety disorders and for insomnia. Since the introduction of the first benzodiazepines—chlordiazepoxide and diazepam (Valium)—in the 1960s, the class has become one of the most widely prescribed in medicine. Although several benzodiazepines

TABLE 16.3 Benzodiazepines for Anxiety and Insomnia

Drug	Route and Adult Dose
Anxiety Therapy	
alprazolam (Xanax)	For anxiety: Orally (PO), 0.25–0.5 mg three times a day (tid) For panic attacks: 0.5 mg tid; dose may be increased every 3-4 days in increments <1 mg/day; mean effect dosage is 5-6 mg/day (some patients may require as much as 10 mg/day).
chlordiazepoxide (Librium)	Mild anxiety: PO, 5–10 mg tid or four times a day (qid) Preoperative anxiety: PO, 5–10 mg/day 3–4 times daily on the days preceding surgery Severe anxiety: PO, 20–25 mg tid or qid
clonazepam (Rivotril)	PO, 0.5–2 mg/day in divided doses (max 4 mg/day)
clorazepate	Anxiety: PO, 7.5–15 mg 2–4 times/day
diazepam (Valium)	Anxiety: PO, 2–10 mg 2–4 times a day if needed IM/IV: 2–10 mg, may repeat in 3–4 hours if needed
Pr lorazepam (Ativan)	PO, 0.5–6 mg/day in divided doses (max 10 mg/day)
midazolam (Versed)	2.5-5 mg SC 1-2 hours for severe agitation/anxiety
oxazepam (Serax)	PO, 10–30 mg tid or qid
Insomnia Therapy	
flurazepam (Dalmane)	PO, 15–30 mg hs
nitrazepam (Mogadon)	5-10 mg at bedtime
temazepam (Restoril)	PO, 7.5–30 mg hs
triazolam	PO, 0.125–0.25 mg hs (max 0.5 mg/day)

are available, all have the same actions and adverse effects and differ primarily in their onset and duration of action. The benzodiazepines are categorized as Controlled Drugs and Substances Act (CDSA) Schedule IV drugs, although they produce considerably less physical dependence and result in less tolerance than the barbiturates.

NCLEX Success Tips

Benzodiazepines should be avoided with mind-altering substances, alcohol, narcotics, and depressants because a side effect is drowsiness. Prolonged use will cause dependency.

Dose-related adverse reactions to benzodiazepines include drowsiness, confusion, ataxia, weakness, dizziness, nystagmus, vertigo, syncope, dysarthria, headache, tremor, and a glassy-eyed appearance. These dose-related reactions diminish as therapy continues.

Lorazepam (Ativan) is available in dosage ranges that allow more gradual tapering down of doses over 3 to 4 days.

The client should be instructed to avoid alcohol while taking chlordiazepoxide because alcohol potentiates the drug's CNS depressant effect. Taken at bedtime, it will induce sleep.

Antianxiety agents such as lorazepam and chlordiazepoxide are commonly used to ease symptoms during early alcohol withdrawal.

Mood swings are expected during the withdrawal period and aren't an indication for further medication administration. Piloerection isn't a symptom of alcohol withdrawal.

Temazepam (Restoril) is a sedative-hypnotic not used for alcohol withdrawal.

Benzodiazepines act by binding to the gamma-aminobutyric acid (GABA) receptor–chloride channel complex. These drugs intensify the effect of GABA, which is a natural inhibitory neurotransmitter found throughout the brain. Most are metabolized in the liver to active metabolites and are excreted primarily in urine. One major advantage of the benzodiazepines is that they do not produce life-threatening respiratory depression or coma if taken in excessive amounts. Death is unlikely unless the benzodiazepines are taken in large quantities in combination with other CNS depressants or the client suffers from sleep apnea.

Most benzodiazepines are given orally. Those that can be given parenterally, such as midazolam, diazepam, and lorazepam, should be used with caution due to their rapid onset of CNS effects and possible respiratory depression.

The benzodiazepines are drugs of choice for the short-term treatment of insomnia caused by anxiety, having replaced the barbiturates because of their greater margin of safety. Benzodiazepines shorten the length of time it takes to fall asleep and reduce the frequency of interrupted sleep. Although most benzodiazepines increase total sleep time, some reduce stage 4 sleep, and some affect REM sleep. In general, the benzodiazepines used to treat short-term insomnia are different from those used to treat generalized anxiety disorder.

Benzodiazepines have a number of other important indications. Diazepam is featured as a Prototype Drug in Chapter 21 for its use in treating seizure disorders. Other uses include treatment of alcohol withdrawal symptoms, central muscle relaxation, and induction of general anesthesia.

Nursing Considerations

The role of the nurse in benzodiazepine therapy involves careful monitoring of the client's condition and providing education as it relates to the prescribed drug regimen. Assess the client's need for antianxiety drugs, including intensity and duration of symptoms. The assessment should include identification of factors that precipitate anxiety or insomnia: physical symptoms, excessive CNS stimulation, excessive daytime sleep, or too little exercise or activity. Obtain a drug history, including hypersensitivity and the use of alcohol and other CNS depressants. Assess for the likelihood of drug abuse and dependence, and identify coping mechanisms used in managing previous episodes of stress, anxiety, and insomnia. These drugs should be used with caution in clients with suicidal tendency, as the risk for suicide may be increased. Assess for the existence of a primary sleep disorder, such as sleep apnea, as benzodiazepines depress respiratory drive.

Alterations in neurotransmitter activity produce changes in intraocular pressure; therefore, benzodiazepines are contraindicated in narrow-angle glaucoma. The presence of any organic brain disease is contraindicated, as these drugs alter the level of consciousness. Liver and kidney function should be monitored in long-term use, and these drugs should be used cautiously in those clients with impaired renal or liver function. Because benzodiazepines cross the placenta and are excreted in breast milk, they are not recommended in pregnant or nursing women (pregnancy category D).

The risk of respiratory depression should be taken into consideration when administering IV doses and when administering to clients with impaired respiratory function or those taking other CNS depressants. Assess for common side effects related to CNS depression such as drowsiness and dizziness, as these increase a client's risk for injury and may indicate a need for dose reduction. Should an overdose occur, flumazenil (Romazicon) is a specific benzodiazepine receptor antagonist that can be administered to reverse CNS depression.

Benzodiazepines are used illicitly for recreation, most often by adolescents, young adults, and individuals addicted to opioids or cocaine. Nurses should help clients to evaluate the social context of their environment and take any precautions necessary to safeguard the medication supply.

See Nursing Process Focus: Clients Receiving Benzodiazepine and Non-Benzodiazepine Antianxiety Therapy on page 172 for specific teaching points.

NCLEX Success Tips

Lorazepam, a Schedule IV drug, is a benzodiazepine that is used to treat anxiety. It is addictive and clients can develop a tolerance to it. It should not be used before other measures to reduce anxiety have been tried. If the client has severe anxiety, the client will be unable to learn new information that is needed to reduce anxiety. Temporary use of lorazepam can allow the client to learn. It is not possible to completely eliminate anxiety.

Lorazepam is a central nervous system depressant and has a pronounced sedative effect, especially in older adults. This puts the client at risk for injury and falls. When lorazepam is taken in combination with alcohol, the depressant effect increases, posing a further risk for falls and causing paradoxical excitement.

The nurse should instruct the client not to suddenly discontinue taking lorazepam. Lorazepam should be continued as prescribed and does adjusted by prescriber to ensure a safe, slow, tapering withdrawal from diazepam.

Ingesting 500 mg or more of caffeine can significantly alter the anxiolytic effects of lorazepam.

Lorazepam, when taken with a neuroleptic such as haloperidol (Haldol), potentiates the neuroleptic's sedating effect and is used to treat severely agitated clients.

Benzodiazepines are the drugs of choice for catatonia. Clinically significant improvement typically begins to occur about 24 hours after starting benzodiazepines. Clients who are unresponsive or insufficiently responsive to benzodiazepines may require electroconvulsive therapy (ECT).

PROTOTYPE DRUG | **Lorazepam (Ativan)**

Actions and Uses: Lorazepam is a benzodiazepine that acts by potentiating the effects of GABA, an inhibitory neurotransmitter, in the thalamic, hypothalamic, and limbic levels of the CNS. It is one of the most potent benzodiazepines. It has an extended half-life that allows for once- or twice-daily oral dosing. In addition to its use as an anxiolytic, lorazepam is used as a pre-anesthetic medication to provide sedation and for the management of status epilepticus.

Administration Alerts:

- When administering by the IV route, monitor respirations every 5 to 15 minutes. Have airway and resuscitative equipment accessible.
- Lorazepam is pregnancy category D.

Pharmacokinetics: Lorazepam is well absorbed after oral administration. It is widely distributed, crosses the blood-brain barrier and placenta, and enters breast milk. It is almost completely metabolized by the liver. Its half-life is 10 to 16 hours.

Adverse Effects and Interactions: The most common side effects of lorazepam are drowsiness and sedation, which may decrease with time. When given in higher doses or by the IV route, more severe effects, such as amnesia, weakness, disorientation, ataxia, sleep disturbance, blood pressure changes, blurred vision, double vision, nausea, and vomiting, may be observed.

Lorazepam interacts with multiple drugs. For example, concurrent use of CNS depressants, including alcohol, potentiates sedation effects and increases the risk for respiratory depression and death. Lorazepam may contribute to digoxin toxicity by increasing the serum digoxin level. Symptoms include visual changes, nausea, vomiting, dizziness, and confusion.

Use with caution with herbal supplements. For example, sedation-producing herbs such as kava, valerian, chamomile, or hops may have an additive effect with lorazepam. Stimulant herbs such as gotu kola and ma huang may reduce the drug's effectiveness.

BARBITURATES

Barbiturates are drugs derived from barbituric acid. They are powerful CNS depressants prescribed for their sedative, hypnotic, and antiseizure effects that have been used in pharmacotherapy since the early 1900s.

Use of Barbiturates as Sedatives

16.8 Because of their side effects and high potential for dependency, barbiturates are rarely used to treat insomnia.

Until the discovery of the benzodiazepines, barbiturates were the drugs of choice for treating anxiety and insomnia. While barbiturates are still indicated for several conditions, they are rarely if ever prescribed for treating anxiety or insomnia because of significant side effects and the availability of more effective medications. Table 16.4 provides a list of barbiturates. The risk of psychological and physical dependence is high—several barbiturates are Schedule II drugs. The withdrawal syndrome from barbiturates is extremely severe and can be fatal. Overdose results in profound respiratory depression, hypotension, and shock. Barbiturates have been used to commit suicide, and death due to overdose is not uncommon.

Barbiturates are capable of depressing CNS function at all levels. Like benzodiazepines, barbiturates act by binding to GABA receptor–chloride channel complexes, intensifying the effect of GABA throughout the brain. At low doses they reduce anxiety and cause drowsiness. At moderate doses they inhibit seizure activity (for example, status epilepticus; see Chapter 21) and promote sleep, presumably by inhibiting brain impulses travelling through the limbic system and the reticular activating system. At higher doses, some barbiturates can induce anesthesia (Chapter 24).

When taken for prolonged periods, barbiturates stimulate the microsomal enzymes in the liver that metabolize medications. Therefore, barbiturates can stimulate their own metabolism as well as that of hundreds of other drugs that use these enzymes for their breakdown. With repeated use, tolerance develops to the sedative effects of the drug; this includes cross-tolerance to other CNS depressants such as the opioids. Tolerance does not develop, however, to the respiratory depressant effects (see Nursing Process Focus: Clients Receiving Barbiturate Therapy for Seizures in Chapter 21, page 235).

Other CNS Depressants for Anxiety and Sleep Disorders

16.9 Some commonly prescribed CNS depressants used for anxiety and sleep disorders are not related to either benzodiazepines or barbiturates.

The final group of CNS depressants used for anxiety and sleep disorders consists of miscellaneous agents that are chemically unrelated to either benzodiazepines or barbiturates, as shown in Table 16.5. Some of the older drugs, such as paraldehyde and chloral hydrate, are now rarely prescribed. Several newer agents, such as buspirone (BuSpar) and zopiclone (Imovane), are commonly prescribed for their anxiolytic and hypnotic effects.

TABLE 16.4 Barbiturates for Sedation and Insomnia

Drug	Route and Adult Dose
Short Acting	
pentobarbital (Nembutal)	IM, 150–200 mg
secobarbital	Sedative: PO, 100–300 mg/day in three divided doses Hypnotic: PO, 100 mg at bedtime (limit to short-term use only; efficacy for sleep induction and maintenance is lost after 14 days)
Long Acting	
mephobarbital (Mebaral)	Sedative: PO, 32–100 mg tid or qid
phenobarbital (Phenobarb)	Sedative: PO/IV/IM, 30–120 mg/day in two to three divided doses; maximum 400 mg/day

(see page 163 for the Prototype Drug box)

TABLE 16.5 Non-Benzodiazepine/Non-Barbiturate Agents

Drug	Route and Adult Dose
buspirone (BuSpar)	PO, 7.5–15 mg in two divided doses; may increase by 5 mg/day every 2–3 days if needed (max 60 mg/day)
chloral hydrate	Sedative: PO, 250 mg tid after meals Hypnotic: PO, 500 mg–1 g 15–30 minutes before bedtime
paraldehyde	Sedative: PO, 5–10 mL PRN Rarely used; not a first-line therapy
Pr zopiclone (Imovane)	Hypnotic: PO, 5–7.5 mg hs

The mechanism of action for buspirone is unclear but appears to be related to dopamine D_2 receptors in the brain. The drug has agonist effects on presynaptic dopamine receptors and a high affinity for serotonin receptors. Buspirone is less likely than benzodiazepines to affect cognitive and motor performance and rarely interacts with other CNS depressants. Common side effects include dizziness, headache, and drowsiness. Dependence and withdrawal problems are less of a concern with buspirone. Therapy may take several weeks to achieve optimal results. Buspirone is pregnancy category B.

Zopiclone is a hypnotic agent with sedative, anxiolytic, anticonvulsant, and muscle relaxant properties. It exerts specific agonist action at central $GABA_A$ receptors. Zopiclone reduces time to onset of sleep and the frequency of nocturnal awakenings to increase duration of sleep. It decreases stage 1 and increases stage 2 NREM sleep while preserving or prolonging the deep stages (stages 3 and 4) and REM sleep. Zopiclone may be used to treat short-term and chronic insomnia in adults (including difficulty falling asleep and nocturnal awakening). Regardless, the treatment period should be as short as possible, and doses should be tapered if zopiclone is used for 3 weeks or longer. Side effects are usually mild and include bitter taste. Because of rapid absorption, zopiclone should be taken just prior to bedtime. Zopiclone is contraindicated in myasthenia gravis, respiratory failure, severe sleep apnea, and severe hepatic insufficiency.

As with other CNS depressants, these non-benzodiazepine/non-barbiturate agents should be used cautiously in clients with respiratory impairment, older adults, and those taking them concurrently with other CNS depressants. Lower dosage may be necessary.

Diphenhydramine (Benadryl) and hydroxyzine (Atarax) are antihistamines that produce drowsiness and may be beneficial in calming clients. They offer the advantage of not causing dependence, although their use is often limited by anticholinergic side effects. Diphenhydramine is a common component of OTC sleep aids.

PROTOTYPE DRUG   **Zopiclone (Imovane)**

Actions and Uses: Zopiclone is a hypnotic agent with sedative, anxiolytic, anticonvulsant, and muscle relaxant properties. It exerts specific agonist action at central $GABA_A$ receptors. It reduces time to onset of sleep and the frequency of nocturnal awakenings, while preserving or prolonging deep sleep. Zopiclone may be used to treat short-term and chronic insomnia in adults.

Pharmacokinetics: Zopiclone is absorbed rapidly and peaks within 2 hours. Absorption is not affected by food. The risk of drug interactions is low due to weak plasma protein binding. Its elimination half-life is 5 hours (may be longer in older adults). There is no accumulation of zopiclone or its metabolites, even in older adults. It is excreted from the kidneys and lungs.

Administration Alerts:
- Give drug immediately before bedtime.
- Do not take drug with alcohol.
- Taper off if used long term.
- Zopiclone is pregnancy category C.

Adverse Effects and Interactions: The most common side effects include dizziness, headache, residual somnolence, dyspepsia, dry mouth, bitter taste, nausea, and anterograde amnesia.

NURSING PROCESS FOCUS

Clients Receiving Benzodiazepine and Non-Benzodiazepine Antianxiety Therapy

Assessment	Potential Nursing Diagnoses/Identified Patterns
Prior to administration: • Obtain complete health history (both physical and mental), including allergies and drug history for possible drug interactions. • Identify factors that precipitate anxiety or insomnia. • Assess likelihood of drug abuse and dependence. • Establish baseline vital signs and level of consciousness.	• Risk for injury • Anxiety • Need for knowledge regarding drug therapy • Disturbed sleep • Coping pattern

Planning: Client Goals and Expected Outcomes

The client will:

- Experience an increase in psychological comfort
- Report absence of physical and behavioural manifestations of anxiety
- Demonstrate an understanding of the drug's action by accurately describing drug side effects and precautions

Implementation

Interventions (Rationales)	Client Education/Discharge Planning
• Monitor vital signs. Observe respiratory patterns, especially during sleep, for evidence of apnea or shallow breathing. (Benzodiazepines can reduce the respiratory drive in susceptible clients.) • Monitor neurological status, especially level of consciousness. (Confusion or lack of response may indicate overmedication.) • Ensure client safety. (Drug may cause excessive drowsiness.)	Instruct client: • To consult the healthcare provider before taking this drug if snoring is a problem. Snoring may indicate an obstruction in the upper respiratory tract resulting in hypoxia. • Regarding methods to monitor vital signs at home, especially respirations

- Monitor the client's intake of stimulants, including caffeine (in beverages such as coffee, tea, cola and other soft drinks, and in OTC analgesics such as Excedrin) and nicotine (from tobacco products and nicotine patches). (These products can reduce the drug's effectiveness.)
- Monitor affect and emotional status. (Drug may increase risk for mental depression, especially in clients with suicidal tendencies.)
- Avoid abrupt discontinuation of therapy. (Withdrawal symptoms, including rebound anxiety and sleeplessness, are possible with abrupt discontinuation after long-term use.)

- Instruct client to report extreme lethargy, slurred speech, disorientation, or ataxia.

Instruct client:
- To not drive or perform hazardous activities until effects of drug are known
- To request assistance when getting out of bed and ambulating until effect of medication is known

Instruct client to:
- Avoid taking OTC sleep-inducing antihistamines, such as diphenhydramine
- Consult the healthcare provider before self-medicating with any OTC preparation

Instruct client to:
- Report significant mood changes, especially depression
- Avoid consuming alcohol or taking other CNS depressants while on benzodiazepines because these increase depressant effect

Instruct client:
- To take drug exactly as prescribed
- To keep all follow-up appointments as directed by healthcare provider to monitor response to medication
- About non-pharmacological methods for re-establishing sleep regimen

Evaluation of Outcome Criteria

Evaluate effectiveness of drug therapy by confirming that client goals and expected outcomes have been met (see "Planning").

See Tables 16.3 (page 169) and 16.5 (page 171) for lists of drugs to which these nursing actions apply.

CHAPTER

16 Understanding the Chapter

Key Concepts Summary

The numbered key concepts provide a succinct summary of the important points from the corresponding numbered section within the chapter. If any of these points are not clear, refer to the numbered section within the chapter for review.

16.1 Generalized anxiety disorder is the most common type of anxiety; phobias, obsessive-compulsive disorder, panic attacks, and post-traumatic stress disorder are other important categories.

16.2 The limbic system and the reticular activating system are specific regions of the brain responsible for anxiety and wakefulness.

16.3 Sleep occurs in distinct stages.

16.4 Anxiety can be managed through pharmacological and non-pharmacological strategies.

16.5 Melatonin, a natural hormone produced in the pineal gland especially at night, is known to help induce restful sleep.

16.6 CNS depressants, including anxiolytics, sedatives, and hypnotics, are used to treat anxiety and insomnia.

16.7 Benzodiazepines are drugs of choice for generalized anxiety and insomnia.

16.8 Because of their side effects and high potential for dependency, barbiturates are rarely used to treat insomnia.

16.9 Some commonly prescribed CNS depressants used for anxiety and sleep disorders are not related to either benzodiazepines or barbiturates.

Chapter 16 Scenario

Seraphina Alvarez, age 55, is an elementary school teacher who has planned on retiring at the end of this academic year. She is the married mother of seven adult children, six of whom live within a 25-km radius and see her often. Her husband, Joe, has been retired for 3 years. He receives Old Age Security and a small pension from his former employment as a construction worker. Seraphina and Joe's oldest daughter's two children and two dogs came to live with them approximately 10 months ago because the daughter is unable to provide a home for them. The children—Joseph, age 15, and Mariah, age 12—are "good kids." They are good students who are active in school and church activities. They resent having to move from their long-time home and school and are acting out some. Seraphina also resents having to raise her grandchildren. It interferes with plans that she and her husband had made to travel after she retired. In fact, she may not be able to retire as planned because she and Joe need her income to meet the children's needs. She loves the children and tries very hard not to let her resentment show. She also has feelings of guilt that she did not do all she could or should have done to raise her daughter to be a responsible parent. As a result, she is unable to sleep well and reports having anxiety. Seraphina first turned to herbal remedies common in her culture and to prayer. Neither of these interventions has helped, but she is reluctant to discuss her problems with anyone else.

She sees her parish priest on a regular basis. He is very supportive of her and understanding of her feelings of resentment, but he does not realize that she is experiencing anxiety and insomnia.

Seraphina, whose health has always been good, has begun to have some health issues, including hypertension, diarrhea, and weight loss. She finds herself becoming more anxious, and her family has noticed that she is decreasing the time spent with family and friends and does not leave her home other than to go to work and to church. She has lost 16 kg (35 lb) in 2 months and appears to have lost her "zest" for living. Her diet consists of black coffee and fresh fruit. Joe frequently finds her sitting in a rocking chair on their front porch during the night, rather than being in bed.

Critical Thinking Questions

1. What current factors in Seraphina's life are interfering with her ability to get a good night's sleep?

2. What medications may Seraphina's healthcare provider order on a short-term or longer-term basis?

3. What part do herbal remedies play in anxiety control and sleep induction in the Latino culture? What specific herbs is Seraphina probably using?

See Answers to Critical Thinking Questions in Appendix B.

NCLEX Practice Questions

1 A nurse should advise a client who is receiving lorazepam (Ativan) about the adverse effects of this medication, which include

   a. Tachypnea

   b. Astigmatism

   c. Ataxia

   d. Euphoria

2 A client with insomnia is being treated with temazepam (Restoril). The nurse monitors for therapeutic effectiveness by noting which of the following? The client is

   a. Sleeping in 3-hour intervals, awakening for a short time, and then returning to sleep

   b. Feeling less anxiety during the activities of daily living

   c. Having fewer episodes of panic attacks when stressed

   d. Sleeping 7 hours without awakening

3 Which of these statements by a client would indicate that further instruction about alprazolam (Xanax) is needed?

   a. "I will stop smoking by undergoing hypnosis."

   b. "I will not drive immediately after I take this medication."

   c. "I will stop the medicine when I feel less anxious."

   d. "I will take my medication with food if my stomach feels upset."

4 The nurse should question the healthcare provider's order of phenobarbital for a client with which of the following conditions?

   a. Seizure disorder

   b. Panic disorder

   c. Prior to a bronchoscopy

   d. Prior to receiving a general anesthetic

5 A client who is receiving benzodiazepines is a two-pack per day cigarette smoker. The nurse expects to administer a/an _____ dose of this medication.

   a. Larger

   b. Smaller

   c. Extra

   d. Half

See Answers to NCLEX Practice Questions in Appendix A.

PROTOTYPE DRUGS

ANTIDEPRESSANTS
Tricyclic antidepressants
  Pr *amitriptyline* (Elavil)
Selective serotonin reuptake inhibitors

  Pr *fluoxetine* (Prozac)
Atypical antidepressants
MAO inhibitors
  Pr *phenelzine* (Nardil)

DRUGS FOR BIPOLAR DISORDER: MOOD STABILIZERS
  Pr *lithium* (Carbolith, Lithane)

Miscellaneous drugs

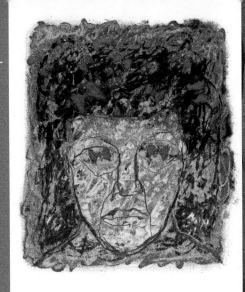

BSIP SA/Alamy Stock Photo

Ken Ross/VWPics/Alamy Stock Photo

CHAPTER 17
Pharmacotherapy of Emotional and Mood Disorders

LEARNING OUTCOMES

After reading this chapter, the student should be able to:

1. Compare and contrast the major categories of mood disorders and their symptoms.
2. Explain the pathophysiology of major depression and bipolar disorder.
3. Identify drug classes used for treating emotional and mood disorders.
4. Explain the therapeutic action of antidepressant drugs in relation to physiological aspects of neurotransmission.
5. For each of the drug classes listed in Prototype Drugs, identify a representative drug and explain its mechanism of action, primary actions, and important adverse effects.
6. Discuss the nurse's role in the pharmacological management of clients with depression or bipolar disorder.
7. Describe and explain, based on pharmacological principles, the rationale for nursing assessment, planning, and interventions for clients with mood disorders.
8. Use the nursing process to care for clients who are receiving drug therapy for emotional and mood disorders.

CHAPTER OUTLINE

▶ Depression
  ▶ Categories of Mood Disorders
  ▶ The Characteristics of Depression
  ▶ Assessment and Treatment of Depression
▶ Antidepressants
  ▶ Mechanism of Action of Antidepressants
  ▶ Treating Depression with Tricyclic Antidepressants
  ▶ Treating Depression with SSRIs
  ▶ Treating Depression with MAO Inhibitors
  ▶ Atypical Antidepressants
▶ Bipolar Disorder
  ▶ Lithium

KEY TERMS

atypical antidepressants, 188

bipolar disorder (manic depression), 189

depression, 176

electroconvulsive therapy (ECT), 178

hypomania, 189

major depressive disorder, 177

mania, 189

monoamine oxidase (MAO) inhibitors, 184

mood disorder, 176

mood stabilizer, 190

selective serotonin reuptake inhibitors (SSRIs), 182

serotonin syndrome (SES), 182

SSRI discontinuation syndrome, 183

tricyclic antidepressants (TCAs), 180

tyramine, 184

Mood disorders are common mental health disorders. A large percentage of all drug prescriptions filled in Canada are for mood disorders. Although mood changes are a normal part of life, when those changes become severe and result in impaired functioning within the family, work environment, or interpersonal relationships, an individual may be diagnosed as having a mood disorder. The two major categories of mood disorders are depression and bipolar disorder. A third emotional disorder, attention deficit/hyperactivity disorder, is discussed in Chapter 18.

DEPRESSION

Depression is a disorder characterized by a sad or despondent mood. Many symptoms are associated with depression, including lack of energy, sleep disturbances, abnormal eating patterns, and feelings of despair, guilt, and misery.

Categories of Mood Disorders

17.1 The two primary categories of mood disorders are depression and bipolar disorder.

Mood disorders form a cluster of mental health conditions that occur frequently in the population. They affect all cultures and people of all ages, from children to older adults. Mood disorders are a major cause of disability and can significantly strain social relationships. They are a leading cause of absenteeism and diminished productivity in the workplace.

The diagnosis of mood disorders is often challenging; the line between normal emotion and a mood disorder is sometimes unclear. Because healthcare providers see clients for such brief periods, they must rely on client self-reports or caregiver information, both of which are often unreliable. A **mood disorder** can be broadly defined as a persistent disturbance in mood that impairs a person's ability to effectively deal with normal activities of daily living (ADLs).

Mood disorders can present with a wide range of symptoms, which has resulted in classification of the disorder into the following categories.

- *Major depressive disorder.* When people use the word *depression*, they are most often referring to major depressive disorder. This is sometimes called clinical depression.

- *Dysthymic disorder.* This is mild, chronic depression that persists for at least 2 continuous years.

- *Bipolar disorder.* Formerly called manic depression, the client alternates between intense excitement (mania) and major depressive disorder.

- *Manic and hypomanic episodes.* Include mania symptoms that last for at least 1 week and significantly affect social functioning. Hypomania is less intense, lasting only 4 days, and has less impact on social or work functioning.

- *Cyclothymic disorder.* A mild form of bipolar disorder in which the client alternates between hypomania and mild depression. Largely undiagnosed, 33% of these clients will eventually develop bipolar disorder.

Mood disorders often coexist with other conditions. For example, about 50% of clients diagnosed with major depression also meet the criteria for an anxiety disorder. Among clients with mood disorder, 25% to 40% have a comorbid substance abuse condition. Those with chronic medical conditions such as hypertension or arthritis have a higher incidence of depression. The most serious of the comorbid conditions is completed or attempted suicide.

The Characteristics of Depression

17.2 Depression has many causes and methods of classification. The identification of depression and its etiology is essential for proper treatment. Major depressive disorder is characterized by a depressed mood, with accompanying symptoms, that lasts for at least 2 weeks.

Depression is one of the oldest known mental health conditions and one of the most frequently diagnosed. Despite this, the etiology of depression is not well understood. Several theories have been proposed to explain the causes of depression and why some people are predisposed to developing the disease. The etiology and pathogenesis are likely influenced by multiple, complex variables that may include biological, genetic, and environmental components.

Research attempting to identify the biological causes of depression has focused on the levels and function of neurotransmitters in the limbic system of the brain. The limbic system is the region that regulates emotions (see Chapter 15). Major depression has been associated with abnormally low levels of neurotransmitters such as norepinephrine, serotonin, and dopamine in this region. Although it is well known that some of the antidepressant medications act by increasing the levels of these neurotransmitters, scientists have yet to discover what role each specific neurotransmitter plays in the development of major depressive disorder. Does having depression deplete the brain of these neurotransmitters, or does a loss of neurotransmitters cause depression? The answers remain elusive.

Certain hormonal abnormalities are associated with depression, suggesting that the endocrine system also plays an important role in the pathogenesis of the disease. About half of persons who are depressed have abnormally high serum cortisol levels. Cortisol mobilizes the body for stress situations and is thought to reduce serotonin levels in the brain, bringing about symptoms of depression. Hypothyroidism is also associated with depression. In some clients, therapy with thyroid hormone (T_3) results in a marked improvement in mood.

It is well established that depression has a genetic component. Major depression is 1.5 to 3 times more common in persons who have a first-degree relative (parent or sibling) with depression when compared to the general population. In identical twins, when one twin is diagnosed with depression, the other twin has a 50% probability of acquiring the disorder. This relationship holds true whether the twins were raised together or separately. Even fraternal twins have a 19% chance of developing depression when the other twin is diagnosed, which is a percentage higher than that of the general population.

Environmental causes of depression include prolonged stress at work or at home, loss of a loved one, and other traumatic life events. Various childhood events have been associated with an increased risk of adult depression, including sexual or physical abuse and death of, separation from, or mental illness of a parent.

Major depressive disorder is the most common mood disorder in Canada, affecting about 6% of adults. According to the *Diagnostic and Statistical Manual of Mental Disorders,* 5th Edition (DSM-V), **major depressive disorder** is diagnosed when the client has a depressed mood that lasts for a minimum of 2 weeks and that is present for most of the day, every day, or almost every day. In addition, at least five of the symptoms shown in Table 17.1 must be present. Depressed moods caused by general medical conditions or by substances such as alcohol or other central nervous system (CNS) depressants do not warrant a diagnosis of major depressive disorder. For the purposes of this text, the terms *depression* and *major depressive disorder* are considered interchangeable unless otherwise specified.

The majority of depressed clients are not found in psychiatric hospitals but in mainstream everyday settings. Many go undiagnosed. The recognition of depression, in order for proper diagnosis and treatment to occur, is a collaborative effort among healthcare providers. Because depressed clients are present in multiple settings and in all areas of practice, every nurse should possess proficiency in the assessment and nursing care of clients afflicted with this disorder. Nurses may recognize depression in clients who are admitted for reasons other than depression or in their family members. A drug history of self-medication with remedies to enhance mood or sleep may alert the nurse to the possibility of depression.

People suffer from depression for a variety of reasons. Depression may be biological, or organic, in origin, associated with dysfunction of neurological processes leading to an imbalance of neurotransmitters. Family history of depression increases the risk for biological depression. In some cases, depression may be situational or reactive, meaning that it results from challenging circumstances, such as severe physical illness, loss of a job, death of a loved one, divorce, or financial difficulties, coupled with inadequate psychosocial support. Depression is the most common mental health disorder among older adults, encompassing a variety of physical, emotional, cognitive, and social considerations.

Some women experience intense mood shifts associated with hormonal changes during the menstrual cycle, pregnancy, childbirth, and menopause. For example, up to 80% of women experience depression 2 weeks to 6 months after the birth of a baby. Many women face additional stresses such as responsibilities at both work and home, single parenthood, and caring for children and aging parents. If mood is severely depressed and persists long enough, many women, including those with premenstrual distress disorder, postpartum depression, or menopausal distress, may benefit from medical treatment.

During the dark winter months, some clients experience a type of depression known as seasonal affective disorder (SAD). This type of depression is associated with a reduced release of the brain neurohormone melatonin. Exposing clients to specific wavelengths of light on a regular basis may relieve SAD depression and prevent future episodes. Some patients with SAD are effectively treated with antidepressants only during the winter months to help combat symptoms.

TABLE 17.1 Symptoms of Depression

CNS Symptoms	Behavioural Symptoms	General Symptoms
Feelings of despair, lack of self-worth, guilt, and misery	Staying in bed most of the day and night	Extremely tired; without energy
Obsessed with death; expresses desire to die or to commit suicide	Neglecting usual household chores	Vague physical symptoms (GI pain, joint or muscle pain, or headaches)
Delusions or hallucinations	Not going to work, or unable to function effectively at work Abnormal eating patterns (eating too much or not enough) Lack of interest in personal appearance or sex Avoiding psychosocial and interpersonal interactions	Physiological depression (constipation, sleep disorders, or decreased heart rate)

◀ **Cultural Influences on Depression and Its Management**

- Depression (and other mental illnesses) is often ignored in many Asian communities because of the tremendous amount of stigma attached to it. Emotions are largely suppressed. Asian clients tend to come to the attention of mental health workers late in the course of their illness and often come with a feeling of hopelessness.
- Close to one-quarter of elderly Chinese immigrants report symptoms of depression.
- The incidence of mental illness, including depression, and alcoholism is higher in many Aboriginal communities than in the general Canadian population. The rate of suicide among Aboriginal youth is five to six times higher than in the general population. Depression may be viewed as an imbalance within the individual and between the individual and the environment that arose from not living life in a good way. Traditional healers or elders may use rituals, charms, and other practices to help restore this balance.
- Some people of European origin deny that mental illness exists and therefore believe that depression will subside on its own.
- The ability to metabolize drugs used for emotional and mood disorders may vary significantly among ethnic groups due to differences in the genes for cytochrome P450 enzymes. Asian clients may require lower doses of antidepressants, lithium, and some other drugs.

Assessment and Treatment of Depression

17.3 Major depression may be treated with medications, psychotherapeutic techniques, or electroconvulsive therapy.

The first step in implementing appropriate treatment for depression is a complete health examination. Certain drugs, such as glucocorticoids and oral contraceptives, can cause the same symptoms as depression, and the healthcare provider should rule out this possibility. Depression may be mimicked by a variety of medical and neurological disorders, ranging from B vitamin deficiencies to thyroid gland problems to early Alzheimer's disease. If underlying causes for the depression are ruled out, a psychological evaluation is often performed by a psychiatrist or psychologist to confirm the diagnosis.

During health examinations, inquiries should be made about alcohol and drug use and whether the client has thoughts about death or suicide. Ask the client about a family history of depressive illness; if other family members have been treated, document the therapies received and whether they were effective. Assess for symptoms of depression. In general, severe depressive illness, particularly that which is recurrent, will require both medication and psychotherapy to achieve the best response. Counselling therapies help clients to gain insight and resolve their problems through verbal "give-and-take" with the therapist. Behavioural therapies help clients learn how to obtain more satisfaction and rewards through

their own actions and how to unlearn the behavioural patterns that contribute to or result from their depression.

Short-term psychotherapies that are helpful for some forms of depression are interpersonal and cognitive-behavioural therapies. Interpersonal therapy focuses on the client's disturbed personal relationships that both cause and exacerbate the depression. Cognitive-behavioural therapies help clients to change the negative styles of thought and behaviour that are often associated with their depression.

Psychodynamic therapies focus on resolving the client's internal conflicts. These therapies are often postponed until the depressive symptoms are significantly improved.

In clients with serious and life-threatening mood disorders that are unresponsive to pharmacotherapy, **electroconvulsive therapy (ECT)** has been the traditional treatment. Although ECT has been found to be safe, there are still deaths (1 in 10 000 clients) and other serious complications related to the seizure activity and anesthesia (Janicak, 2002). Recent studies suggest that repetitive transcranial magnetic stimulation (rTMS) is an effective somatic treatment for major depression. In contrast to ECT, it has minimal effects on memory, does not require general anesthesia, and produces its effects without a generalized seizure.

Even with the best professional care, the client with depression may take a long time to recover. Many clients with major depression have multiple bouts of the illness over the course of a lifetime. This can take its toll on the client's family, friends, and other caregivers who may sometimes feel burned out, frustrated, or even depressed themselves. They may experience episodes of anger toward the depressed loved one, only to subsequently suffer reactions of guilt over being angry. Although such feelings are common, they can be distressing, and the caregiver may not know where to turn for help, support, or advice. It is often the nurse who is best able to assist the family members of a person suffering from emotional and mood disorders. Family members may need counselling themselves.

ANTIDEPRESSANTS

Drugs for depression are called antidepressants. Antidepressants treat major depression by enhancing mood.

◀ **Depression across the Lifespan**

- Depression can occur at any age, but it is more prevalent in older adults.
- Drug dosages may require adjustment due to age-related changes in pharmacokinetics.
- Elderly clients are at increased risk for falls, confusion, and other side effects due to the sedating effects of some antidepressants and altered pharmacokinetics.
- Depressed teens and older adults have an increased risk for suicide.
- A healthy lifestyle should be promoted in all age groups to help reduce depressive symptoms and enhance antidepressant effectiveness.

Mechanism of Action of Antidepressants

17.4 The two basic mechanisms of action of antidepressants are blocking the enzymatic breakdown of norepinephrine and slowing the reuptake of serotonin.

Depression is associated with an imbalance of neurotransmitters in certain regions of the brain. Although medication does not completely restore these chemical imbalances, it does help to reduce depressive symptoms while the client develops effective means of coping. Antidepressants enhance the action of certain neurotransmitters in the brain, including norepinephrine and serotonin, which is also known by its chemical name, 5-hydroxytryptamine (5-HT). The two basic mechanisms of action are blocking the enzymatic breakdown of norepinephrine and slowing the reuptake of serotonin. The four primary classes of antidepressant drugs, also shown in Tables 17.2 and 17.3, are as follows:

1. Tricyclic antidepressants (TCAs)
2. Selective serotonin reuptake inhibitors (SSRIs)
3. Monoamine oxidase (MAO) inhibitors
4. Atypical antidepressants

TABLE 17.2 Antidepressants: An Overview

	Typical			Atypical		
	Monoamine Oxidase (MAO) Inhibitors	Tricyclic Antidepressants	Selective Serotonin Reuptake Inhibitors	Norepineph-rine (NE) Reuptake Inhibitors	NE and Dopamine Reuptake Inhibitors	Serotonin and NE Reuptake Inhibitors
Generic Drugs	phenelzine	imipramine	fluoxetine	reboxetine	bupropion	venlafaxine desvenlafaxine duloxetine
	tranylcypromine	clomipramine	sertraline	atomoxetine		
		amitriptyline	paroxetine			
		desipramine	fluvoxamine			
		doxepin	citalopram escitalopram			
		trimipramine				
Mechanism of Action	Inhibit MAO	Inhibit NE, serotonin, and dopamine reuptake	Inhibit serotonin reuptake	Inhibit NE reuptake	Inhibit NE and dopamine reuptake	Inhibit serotonin and NE reuptake
Therapeutic Effect	↑ NE ↑ serotonin ↑ dopamine ↑ NE	↑ NE ↑ serotonin ↑ dopamine ↑ NE	↑ serotonin	↑ NE	↑ NE ↑ dopamine	↑ NE ↑ serotonin
Key Side Effects	Orthostatic hypotension (hypertensive crisis with tyramine), headache, insomnia, diarrhea	Anticholinergic effects: sweating, sedation, orthostatic hypotension	Nervousness, insomnia, sexual dysfunction, weight gain	Dry mouth, hypotension, decreased libido, constipation, increased heart rate	Increased appetite	Nausea, headache, nervousness, hypertension
Serious Interactions	Tyramine, many over-the-counter and prescription drugs	MAO inhibitors	MAO inhibitors, warfarin	MAO inhibitors	MAO inhibitors	MAO inhibitors

TABLE 17.3 Antidepressants

Drug	Route and Adult Dose
Tricyclic Antidepressants (TCAs)	
amitriptyline (Elavil)	Adult: Orally (PO), begin with 25-50 mg single dose at bedtime or in divided doses; initial doses of 100 mg/day may be considered in hospitalized patients; may gradually increase up to 300 mg/day
amoxapine (Asendin)	Adult: PO, begin with 50 mg one to three times daily, may increase to 100 mg/day two to three times daily by the end of the first week based on response and tolerance (max 400 mg/day)
desipramine	Adult: PO, begin with 25-50 mg once daily or in divided doses; increase based on tolerance and response; maintenance 100-200 mg once daily or in divided doses (max 300 mg/day)
doxepin (Sinequan)	PO, begin with 25-50 mg as a single dose at bedtime or in divided doses; gradually increase based on response and tolerance; maintenance 100-300 mg/day
Pr imipramine (Impril)	PO, begin with 75 mg/day; may increase gradually to 150 mg/day; may be given in divided doses or as a single bedtime dose; maintenance 50-150 mg/day (max 200 mg/day)
trimipramine (Surmontil)	PO, begin with 25-50 mg/day at bedtime or in divided doses; gradually increase dose based on response and tolerance; may go up to 75-300 mg/day; always use lowest effective dose possible

(continued)

TABLE 17.3   Antidepressants (*continued*)

Selective Serotonin Reuptake Inhibitors (SSRIs)

citalopram (Celexa)	PO, start at 20 mg/day (max 40 mg/day)
Pr fluoxetine (Prozac)	PO, 20 mg/day in the a.m. (max 80 mg/day)
fluvoxamine (Luvox)	PO, start with 50 mg/day (max 300 mg/day)
paroxetine (Paxil)	PO, start at 20 mg/day (max 60 mg/day)
sertraline (Zoloft)	Adult: PO, start at 25-50 mg/day; gradually increase to effect (max 200 mg/day)

MAO Inhibitors

Pr phenelzine (Nardil)	PO, 15 mg three times a day (tid) (max 90 mg/day)
tranylcypromine (Parnate)	PO, begin with 20 mg/day in two doses; if symptoms don't improve after 2-3 weeks increase dosage by 10 mg/day; maintenance 10-20 mg/day (max 60 mg/day)

Atypical Antidepressants

bupropion (Wellbutrin)	Immediate release: 100 mg two to three times daily (max 450 mg/day) Extended release: 150 mg/day up to 300 mg/day (max 300 mg/day)
mirtazapine (Remeron)	PO, 15 mg/day in a single dose hs, may increase every 1–2 weeks (max 45 mg/day)
trazodone (Desyrel)	PO, 150 mg/day, may increase by 50 mg/day every 3–4 days up to 400–600 mg/day
venlafaxine (Effexor)	PO, 37.5-225 mg/day (max 375 mg/day)

Treating Depression with Tricyclic Antidepressants

17.5 TCAs are older medications used mainly for the treatment of major depression, obsessive-compulsive disorder, and panic attacks.

Tricyclic antidepressants (TCAs) are drugs named for their three-ring chemical structure. They were the mainstay of depression pharmacotherapy from the early 1960s until the 1980s and are still used today (they are also used to treat neuropathic pain).

Tricyclic antidepressants act by inhibiting the reuptake of norepinephrine and serotonin, and to a lesser extent dopamine, into presynaptic nerve terminals, as shown in Figure 17.1. TCAs are used mainly for major depression and occasionally for milder situational depression. Clomipramine (Anafranil) is approved for the treatment of obsessive-compulsive disorder, and other TCAs are sometimes used as unlabelled treatments for panic attacks. One use for TCAs, not related to psychopharmacology, is the treatment of childhood enuresis (bedwetting).

Shortly after their approval as antidepressants in the 1950s, it was found that the TCAs produced fewer side effects and were less dangerous than MAO inhibitors. However, TCAs have some unpleasant and serious side effects. The most common side effect is orthostatic hypotension, which occurs due to alpha₁ blockade on blood vessels. They also have many anticholinergic side effects, which often limit their use clinically. The most serious adverse effect occurs when TCAs accumulate in cardiac tissue. Although rare, cardiac dysrhythmias can occur.

Sedation is a frequently reported complaint at the initiation of therapy, though clients may become tolerant to this effect after several weeks of treatment. Most TCAs have a long half-life, which increases the risk for side effects for clients with delayed excretion. Anticholinergic effects, such as dry mouth, constipation, urinary retention, blurred vision, and tachycardia, are common and are often the reason for discontinuing therapy. These effects are less severe if the drug is gradually increased to the therapeutic dose over 2 to 3 weeks. Significant drug interactions can occur with CNS

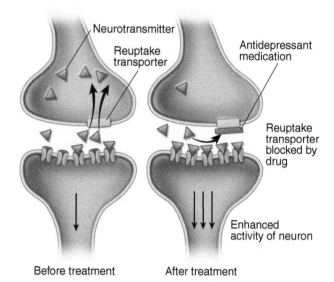

Figure 17.1 Mechanisms of action of antidepressants: (a) In adrenergic and serotonergic neurons the activity of the neurotransmitter is terminated by reuptake. (b) Tricyclic antidepressants and SSRIs produce their effects by inhibiting the reuptake of neurotransmitters. The neurotransmitter accumulates in the synaptic cleft and activates more receptors, thus causing an enhanced effect at the synapse.

depressants, sympathomimetics, anticholinergics, and MAO inhibitors. With the availability of newer antidepressants that have fewer side effects, TCAs are less likely to be used as first-line drugs in the treatment of depression.

NCLEX Success Tips

Tricyclic antidepressants (TCAs) put the client at risk for postural hypotension immediately after waking up in the morning.

Postural hypotension occurs due to the inhibitory effect of TCAs. TCAs have the ability to inhibit the body's natural vasoconstrictive reaction when the person stands. As such, the nurse must regularly monitor the client's vital signs—both lying and standing—and should teach the client to rise slowly and dangle his feet before standing.

The nurse should discourage the client from taking hot showers because heat causes vasodilatation, which could further exacerbate the dizziness, placing the client at risk for falls and subsequent injury.

The nurse should tell the client that electrocardiograms (ECGs) are done routinely for all clients taking TCAs because they may cause tachycardia, ECG changes, and cardiotoxicity.

Educating the client about these side effects will reassure the client and lessen his or her anxiety.

Drinking alcohol can increase the sedating effect of TCAs.

TCAs can potentially cause dry mouth and blurred vision because of their anticholinergic adverse effects. Weight gain—not loss—is also typical when taking TCAs.

Cardiovascular toxicity (cardiac arrhythmias) is a potential adverse effect with TCAs. The nurse should question the use of TCAs in a client with cardiac disease.

Nursing Considerations

The role of the nurse in TCA therapy involves careful monitoring of the client's condition and providing education as it relates to the prescribed drug regimen. Clients should be advised that the therapeutic effects of TCAs may take 2 to 6 weeks to occur. Although the neurotransmitter deficiencies are corrected quickly, subsequent changes in the receptors for the neurotransmitters occur more slowly over a period of weeks, resulting in a delay in the onset of therapeutic effects. Individual responses to drug therapy may vary and require assessment. Responses may be affected by variations in serum albumin levels (since TCAs are more than 90% bound to plasma proteins), genetic differences in metabolizing enzymes, and differences in receptor changes.

Suicide potential increases as blood levels of a TCA increase but have not yet reached their peak therapeutic level. While in the depths of depression, clients may lack the energy for suicide. As clients begin to recover from depression, their energy level rises and with it their ability to plan and enact suicide. The nurse needs to monitor the client closely for symptoms of suicidal ideation throughout treatment.

TCAs are contraindicated in clients in the acute recovery phase of a myocardial infarction (MI) and in clients with heart block or a history of dysrhythmias because of their effects on cardiac tissue. Because TCAs lower the seizure threshold, clients with epilepsy must be carefully monitored. Clients with urinary retention, narrow-angle glaucoma, or prostatic hypertrophy may not be good candidates for TCAs because of anticholinergic side effects. Annoying anticholinergic effects, coupled with the weight gain effect of TCAs, may lead to nonadherence. TCAs must be given with extreme caution to clients with asthma, cardiovascular disorders, gastrointestinal (GI) disorders, alcoholism, and other psychiatric disorders, including schizophrenia and bipolar disorder. Most TCAs are pregnancy category C or D, so they are used during pregnancy and lactation only when medically necessary. Should a client desire to become pregnant while taking a TCA, she should immediately discuss her depression medication with her healthcare provider. The TCAs should be withdrawn over several weeks and not be discontinued abruptly.

Significant drug interactions may occur with TCAs. Oral contraceptives may decrease the efficacy of TCAs. Cimetidine (Tagamet) interferes with their metabolism and excretion. TCAs

affect the efficacy of clonidine (Catapres). Concurrent use of alcohol and other CNS depressants may result in excessive sedation and should be avoided.

Client education as it relates to TCAs should include goals, reasons for obtaining baseline data such as vital signs and tests for cardiac and renal disorders, and possible side effects. Following are other important points to include when teaching clients about TCAs:

- Be aware that it may take several weeks or more to achieve the full therapeutic effect of the drug.
- Maintain follow-up appointments with the healthcare provider.
- Sweating, along with other anticholinergic side effects, may occur.
- Take medication exactly as prescribed, and report side effects if they occur.
- Do not take any prescription drugs, over-the-counter (OTC) drugs, or herbal products without first consulting with the healthcare provider.
- Change position slowly, especially when sitting or standing from a lying position.
- Do not drive or engage in hazardous activities until sedative effect is known; drowsiness may be considerable in the first weeks.
- Note that the TCA may be taken at bedtime if sedation occurs.
- Older adults may be more prone to the sedating effects and have an increased risk of falls.

NCLEX Success Tips

The nurse needs to inform a client taking imipramine (Impril) that it takes 2 to 4 weeks to reach a full clinical effect. The nurse should let the client know that he or she will gradually get better and the symptoms of depression will improve.

Sedation is a common adverse effect of imipramine, a tricyclic antidepressant, that usually decreases over time as tolerance develops.

Serious adverse effects include myocardial infarction, heart failure, and tachycardia.

Imipramine in combination with alcohol will produce additive central nervous system depression. If a client is experiencing excessive daytime sleepiness, he or she may be experiencing poor sleep or side effects of sedation.

The nurse should advise the client that while on imipramine the client should use sunscreen and protective clothing when exposed to the sun to avoid photosensitivity.

Dry eyes due to reduced lacrimation is a side effect. The nurse should encourage the client to use artificial tears to minimize this problem.

PROTOTYPE DRUG | **Imipramine (Tofranil)**

Actions and Uses: Imipramine blocks the reuptake of serotonin and norepinephrine into nerve terminals. It is mainly used for clinical depression; it is occasionally used for the treatment of nocturnal enuresis in children. The nurse may find imipramine prescribed for a number of unlabelled uses, including intractable pain, anxiety disorders, and withdrawal syndromes from alcohol and cocaine.

Administration Alerts:

• Paradoxical diaphoresis can be a side effect of TCAs; therefore, diaphoresis may not be a reliable indicator of other disease states such as hypoglycemia.

• Imipramine causes anticholinergic effects and may potentiate effects of anticholinergic drugs administered during surgery.

• Do not discontinue abruptly because rebound dysphoria, irritability, or sleeplessness may occur.

• Imipramine is pregnancy category C.

Pharmacokinetics: Imipramine is well absorbed after oral administration. It is widely distributed and crosses the placenta. It is 90% to 95% protein bound. It is highly metabolized by the liver, mostly on first pass. Its half-life is 8 to 16 hours.

Adverse Effects and Interactions: Side effects include sedation, drowsiness, blurred vision, dry mouth, and cardiovascular symptoms such as dysrhythmias, heart block, and extreme hypertension. Agents that mimic the action of norepinephrine or serotonin should be avoided because imipramine inhibits their metabolism and may produce toxicity. Some clients may experience photosensitivity. Concurrent use of other CNS depressants, including alcohol, may cause sedation. Cimetidine may inhibit the metabolism of imipramine, leading to increased serum levels and possible toxicity. Imipramine may decrease the antihypertensive effects of clonidine; clonidine may increase risk for CNS depression. Use of oral contraceptives may increase or decrease imipramine levels. Disulfiram may lead to delirium and tachycardia.

Use with caution with herbal supplements, such as evening primrose oil and ginkgo, which may lower the seizure threshold. St. John's wort used concurrently may cause serotonin syndrome.

Treating Depression with SSRIs

17.6 SSRIs act by selectively blocking the reuptake of serotonin in nerve terminals. Because of more tolerable side effects, SSRIs are drugs of choice in the pharmacotherapy of depression.

Selective serotonin reuptake inhibitors (SSRIs) are drugs that slow the reuptake of serotonin into presynaptic nerve terminals. They have become drugs of choice in the treatment of depression.

NCLEX Success Tip

Noncompliance with taking selective serotonin reuptake inhibitors (SSRIs) is a common problem due to the unwarranted sexual side effects associated with this group of medications. Side effects such as decreased libido, impotence, anorgasmia, and ejaculatory disturbances can occur frequently and are the main causes that lead to noncompliance with the regimen.

Sleep disturbances (insomnia) can occur with an SSRI. The nurse should encourage the client to take his or her medication every morning, which will not affect nighttime sleep and will prevent somnolence during the day.

Some individuals who start on SSRIs may develop hypomania or mania. The client will be very active and show no signs of fatigue, despite the limited number of hours of sleep. This situation requires immediate intervention, and the physician should be promptly informed.

Dry mouth is a possible side effect, but it is temporary. The nurse should instruct the client to take sips of water, suck on ice chips, or use sugarless gum or candy.

St. John's wort should not be taken with SSRIs because a severe reaction could occur.

Serotonin is a natural neurotransmitter in the CNS, found in high concentrations in certain neurons in the hypothalamus, limbic system, medulla, and spinal cord. It is important to several body activities, including the cycling between non–rapid eye movement (NREM) and rapid eye movement (REM) sleep, pain perception, and emotional states. Lack of adequate serotonin in the CNS can lead to depression. Serotonin is metabolized to a less active substance by the enzyme monoamine oxidase (MAO).

In the 1970s, it became increasingly clear that serotonin had a more substantial role in depression than once thought. Clinicians knew that the TCAs altered the sensitivity of serotonin to certain receptors in the brain, but they did not know how this was connected with depression. Ongoing efforts to find antidepressants with fewer side effects led to the development of another category of medications, the SSRIs.

While the tricyclic class inhibits the reuptake of both norepinephrine and serotonin into presynaptic nerve terminals, the SSRIs are selective for serotonin. Increased levels of serotonin in the synaptic gap induce complex neurotransmitter changes in presynaptic and postsynaptic neurons in the brain. Presynaptic receptors become less sensitive, whereas postsynaptic receptors become more sensitive. This concept is illustrated in Figure 17.2.

SSRIs have approximately the same efficacy at relieving depression as the MAO inhibitors and the TCAs. The major advantage of the SSRIs, and the one that makes them drugs of choice, is their greater safety. Sympathomimetic effects (increased heart rate and hypertension) and anticholinergic effects (dry mouth, blurred vision, urinary retention, and constipation) are less common with this drug class. Sedation is also experienced less frequently. Cardiac conduction (most commonly QT prolongation) changes are common with SSRIs. Babies born to women who are taking SSRIs are at greater risk for lung and heart defects. Drugs in the SSRI class have similar efficacy in inhibiting serotonin reuptake and improving depression. However, they differ in some effects due to differences in interactions with receptors other than serotonin. For example, sertraline (Zoloft) has dopamine reuptake inhibition properties that may improve attention and cognitive function as well as mood. Fluoxetine (Prozac) has norepinephrine reuptake inhibition action that may improve depression and also contribute to jitteriness, nervousness, and sleep problems that are common in early weeks of treatment. Fluoxetine may be associated with QT prolongation on the electrocardiogram (ECG). Clients who do not respond well to one SSRI may respond better to another.

The most common side effects of SSRIs relate to sexual dysfunction. Up to 70% of both men and women can experience decreased libido and lack of ability to reach orgasm. In men, delayed ejaculation and impotence may occur. For clients who are sexually active, these side effects may result in nonadherence with pharmacotherapy. Other common side effects of SSRIs include nausea, headache, anxiety, and insomnia.

Serotonin syndrome (SES) may occur when taking another medication that affects the metabolism, synthesis, or reuptake of

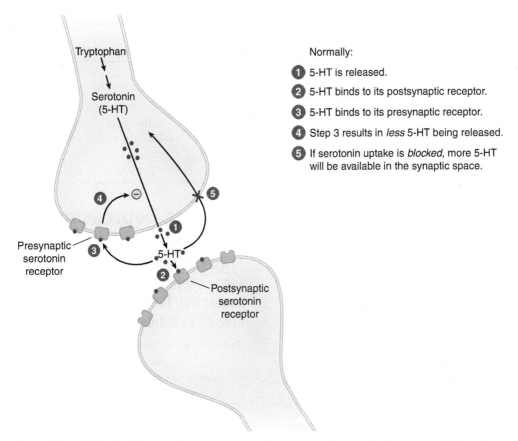

Normally:

1️⃣ 5-HT is released.

2️⃣ 5-HT binds to its postsynaptic receptor.

3️⃣ 5-HT binds to its presynaptic receptor.

4️⃣ Step 3 results in *less* 5-HT being released.

5️⃣ If serotonin uptake is *blocked*, more 5-HT will be available in the synaptic space.

Figure 17.2 SSRIs block the reuptake of serotonin into presynaptic nerve terminals: increased levels of serotonin induce complex changes in presynaptic and postsynaptic neurons of the brain; presynaptic receptors become less sensitive, whereas postsynaptic receptors become more sensitive.

serotonin, causing serotonin to accumulate in the body. Symptoms can begin as early as 2 hours after taking the first dose, or as late as several weeks after initiating pharmacotherapy. Symptoms of SES include mental status changes (confusion, anxiety, restlessness), hypertension, tremors, sweating, hyperpyrexia, and ataxia. Serotonin syndrome can be caused by the concurrent administration of an SSRI with an MAO inhibitor, a TCA, lithium, meperidine, or a number of other medications and herbals. Because deaths have been caused by administering meperidine and other drugs to clients who are receiving SSRIs, it is very important to always check for interactions. Early recognition of symptoms and early treatment can help to prevent deaths from SES. Conservative treatment is to discontinue the SSRI and provide supportive care. In severe cases, mechanical ventilation and muscle relaxants may be necessary.

Some clients may experience **SSRI discontinuation syndrome** when SSRI therapy is discontinued. Symptoms include lowered mood, dizziness, lethargy, paresthesia, nausea, vivid dreams, irritability, electric shock sensations, and confusion. Symptoms are more frequent with shorter half-life SSRIs, such as fluvoxamine (Luvox) or paroxetine. Symptoms may persist for up to 21 days despite slowly tapered SSRI withdrawal. Symptoms may be relieved within 24 hours by restarting the medication.

Nursing Considerations

The role of the nurse in SSRI therapy involves careful monitoring of the client's condition and providing education as it relates to the prescribed drug regimen. The nurse should assess the client's

need for antidepressant drugs, including intensity and duration of symptoms. The assessment should include identification of factors that led to the depression, such as life events or health changes. The nurse should obtain a careful drug history, including the use of CNS depressants, alcohol, and other antidepressants, especially MAO inhibitor therapy, as these may interact with SSRIs. The nurse should assess for hypersensitivity to SSRIs. The nurse should assess suicide ideation because the drugs may take several weeks before full therapeutic benefit is obtained. The medical history should include any disorders of sexual function since these drugs have a high incidence of side effects of this nature.

Although the SSRIs are safer than other antidepressants, serious adverse effects can still occur. Baseline liver function laboratory tests should be obtained because SSRIs are metabolized in the liver and hepatic disease can result in higher serum levels. A baseline body weight should be obtained, as SSRIs can cause weight gain.

Client education as it relates to SSRIs should include goals, reasons for obtaining baseline data such as vital signs and concurrent medications, and possible side effects. The nurse should inform the client that SSRIs take up to 5 weeks to reach their maximum therapeutic effectiveness. Following are other important points to include when teaching clients about SSRIs:

• Do not take any prescription or OTC drugs or herbal products without first consulting the healthcare provider.

• Maintain follow-up appointments with the healthcare provider.

- Report side effects to the healthcare provider as they occur.
- Do not drive or engage in hazardous activities until sedative effect is known; the SSRI may be taken at bedtime if sedation occurs.
- Do not discontinue drug abruptly after long-term use.
- Exercise and monitor caloric intake to avoid weight gain.

NCLEX Success Tips

Antidepressants can take 2 to 4 weeks before any improvement in symptoms occurs; effective blood concentrations are not reached until this time.

Anxiety and diarrhea are adverse effects of fluoxetine and they may be relieved by a decrease in dosage. It may be necessary to change to another selective serotonin reuptake inhibitors or to a different class of antidepressants.

Fluoxetine should be taken as early in the day as possible so as not to interfere with nighttime sleep; it may cause nervousness in some clients.

The presence of dizziness could indicate orthostatic hypotension, which may cause injury to the client from falling.

SSRIs such as fluoxetine are the medications of choice for panic disorder.

PROTOTYPE DRUG   **Fluoxetine (Prozac)**

Actions and Uses: Therapeutic actions of fluoxetine can be attributed to its ability to selectively inhibit serotonin reuptake into presynaptic nerve terminals. Its main use is clinical depression, although it may be prescribed for obsessive-compulsive disorder and eating disorders. Therapeutic actions include improved affect, mood enhancement, and increased appetite, with maximum effects observed after several days to weeks.

Administration Alerts:

- Fluoxetine is available in daily dose oral formulations.
- Fluoxetine is pregnancy category B.

Pharmacokinetics: Fluoxetine is well absorbed after oral administration. It is widely distributed and crosses the blood-brain barrier. It is 95% protein bound. Fluoxetine tends to be eliminated slowly and to accumulate in the body. Active metabolites may persist for weeks. This is of consequence when discontinuation of the drug is required and drugs that may interact with fluoxetine, or its metabolite norfluoxetine (also an antidepressant), are subsequently prescribed.

Adverse Effects and Interactions: Fluoxetine may cause headaches, nervousness, insomnia, nausea, and diarrhea. Foods high in the amino acid tryptophan should be avoided since tryptophan is the chemical precursor for serotonin synthesis. Concurrent use with selegiline (Eldepryl) may increase the risk of a hypertensive crisis. TCAs administered concurrently may produce serotonin syndrome. Symptoms of fluoxetine overdose include fever, confusion, shivering, sweating, and muscle spasms. Fluoxetine cannot be used if the client took an MAO inhibitor within the past 14 days. Concurrent use of benzodiazepines may cause increased adverse CNS effects. Concurrent use of beta blockers can cause

their decreased elimination, leading to hypotension or bradycardia. Concurrent use of phenytoin (Dilantin), clozapine (Clozaril), or theophylline (Theolair, Uniphyl) may lead to decreased elimination of these drugs and toxicity. Concurrent use of warfarin may lead to increased risk for bleeding due to competitive protein binding.

Concurrent use with meperidine (Demerol), fentanyl (Duragesic), or dextromethorphan may cause serotonin syndrome.

Use with caution with herbal supplements, such as St. John's wort and L-tryptophan, which may cause serotonin syndrome, and kava, which may increase the effects of fluoxetine.

Treating Depression with MAO Inhibitors

17.7 MAO inhibitors are usually prescribed in cases where other antidepressants have not been successful. They have more serious side effects than other antidepressants.

Monoamine oxidase (MAO) inhibitors inhibit monoamine oxidase, the enzyme that terminates the actions of neurotransmitters such as dopamine, norepinephrine, epinephrine, and serotonin. Because of their low safety margin, these drugs are reserved for clients who have not responded to TCAs or SSRIs.

As discussed in Chapter 12, the action of norepinephrine at adrenergic synapses is terminated through two means: reuptake into the presynaptic nerve and enzymatic destruction by the enzyme monoamine oxidase.

MAO inhibitors inhibit the breakdown of norepinephrine, dopamine, and serotonin in CNS neurons. The higher levels of these neurotransmitters in the brain intensify neurotransmission and alleviate the symptoms of depression. MAO is located within presynaptic nerve terminals, as shown in Figure 17.3.

The MAO inhibitors were the first drugs approved to treat depression, in the 1950s. They are as effective as TCAs and SSRIs in treating depression. However, because of drug-drug and food-drug interactions, hepatotoxicity, and the development of safer antidepressants, MAO inhibitors are now reserved for clients who are not responsive to other antidepressant classes.

Common side effects of the MAO inhibitors include orthostatic hypotension, headache, insomnia, and diarrhea. A primary concern is that these agents interact with a large number of foods and other medications, sometimes with serious effects. A hypertensive crisis can occur when an MAO inhibitor is used concurrently with other antidepressants or sympathomimetic drugs. Combining an MAO inhibitor with an SSRI can produce serotonin syndrome. If given with antihypertensives, the client can experience excessive hypotension. MAO inhibitors also potentiate the hypoglycemic effects of insulin and oral antidiabetic drugs. Hyperpyrexia is known to occur in clients who are taking MAO inhibitors with meperidine, dextromethorphan, and TCAs.

A hypertensive crisis can also result from an interaction between MAO inhibitors and foods containing **tyramine**, a form of the amino acid tyrosine. In many respects, tyramine resembles norepinephrine. Tyramine is usually degraded by MAO in the intestines. If a client is taking MAO inhibitors, however, tyramine enters the bloodstream in high amounts and displaces norepinephrine in

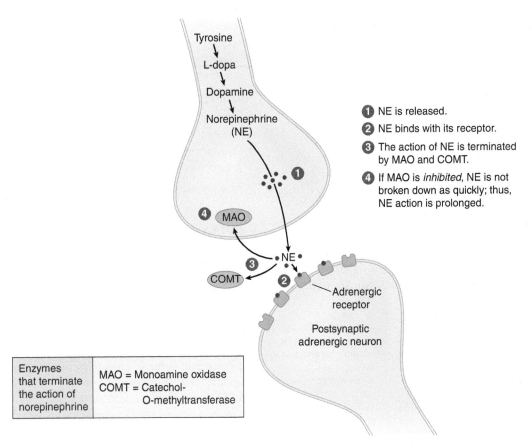

1. NE is released.
2. NE binds with its receptor.
3. The action of NE is terminated by MAO and COMT.
4. If MAO is *inhibited*, NE is not broken down as quickly; thus, NE action is prolonged.

Enzymes that terminate the action of norepinephrine	MAO = Monoamine oxidase COMT = Catechol-O-methyltransferase

Figure 17.3 Monoamine oxidase (MAO) inhibitors exert antidepressant effects by inhibiting the breakdown of norepinephrine by the enzyme monoamine oxidase.

TABLE 17.4	Foods Containing Tyramine
Fruits	Avocados, bananas, raisins, papaya products (including meat tenderizers), canned figs
Dairy products	Cheese (cottage cheese is okay), sour cream, yogurt
Alcohol	Beer, wine (especially red wine)
Meats	Beef or chicken liver, pâté, meat extracts, pickled or kippered herring, pepperoni, salami, sausage, bologna/hot dogs
Vegetables	Pods of broad beans (e.g., fava beans)
Sauces	Soy sauce
Yeast	All yeast and yeast extracts
Other foods to avoid	Chocolate

presynaptic nerve terminals. The result is a sudden increase in norepinephrine, causing acute hypertension. Symptoms usually occur within minutes of ingesting the food and include occipital headache, stiff neck, flushing, palpitations, diaphoresis, and nausea. Calcium channel blockers may be given as an antidote. Examples of foods containing tyramine are shown in Table 17.4.

Nursing Considerations

The role of the nurse in MAO inhibitor therapy involves careful monitoring of the client's condition and providing education as it relates to the prescribed drug regimen. Assess the client's need for antidepressant drugs, including intensity and duration of symptoms. The assessment should include identification of factors that led to

depression, such as life events or health changes. Assess suicide ideation because the drugs may take several weeks before full therapeutic benefit is obtained. Cardiovascular status should be assessed, as these agents may affect blood pressure. Phenelzine (Nardil) is contraindicated in cardiovascular disease, heart failure, cerebrovascular accident, hepatic or renal dysfunction, and paranoid schizophrenia. A complete blood count (CBC) should be obtained because MAO inhibitors can inhibit platelet function. Assess for the possibility of pregnancy; these agents are pregnancy category C and enter breast milk. A client taking an MAO inhibitor must refrain from foods that contain tyramine, which is found in many common foods (see Table 17.4). MAO inhibitors should be used with caution in epilepsy, as they may lower the seizure threshold.

The nurse should obtain a careful drug history; common drugs that may interact with an MAO inhibitor include other MAO inhibitors, insulin, caffeine-containing products, other antidepressants, meperidine, and possibly opioids and methyldopa. There must be at least a 14-day interval between the use of MAO inhibitors and these other drugs.

Some clients may not achieve the full therapeutic benefits of an MAO inhibitor for 4 to 8 weeks. Because depression continues during this time, clients may discontinue the drug if they do not feel it is helping them.

Because of the serious side effects possible with MAO inhibitors, client education is vital. The client's ability to comprehend restrictions and be compliant with them may be impaired in a severely depressed state. Client education should include goals, reasons for obtaining baseline data such as vital signs and laboratory studies, and a dietary consult for possible side effects. In addition, include the following points when educating clients and their caregivers about MAO inhibitors:

- Avoid foods containing tyramine (provide a list).
- Do not take any prescription or OTC drugs or herbal products without first consulting with the healthcare provider.
- Refrain from caffeine intake.
- Wear a MedicAlert bracelet identifying the MAO inhibitor medication.
- Be aware that it may take several weeks or more to obtain the full therapeutic effect of the drug.
- Maintain follow-up appointments with the healthcare provider.
- Do not drive or engage in hazardous activities until sedative effect is known; drug may be taken at bedtime if sedation occurs.
- Observe for and report signs of impending stroke or MI.

NCLEX Success Tip

The nurse should monitor the client's vital signs, paying particular attention to blood pressure. Administering the client's phenelzine before taking his or her vital signs could result in a dangerous situation if the client is experiencing a hypertensive crisis. Signs and symptoms of a hypertensive crisis include occipital headache, a stiff or sore neck, nausea, vomiting, sweating, dilated pupils and photophobia, nosebleed, tachycardia, bradycardia, and constricting chest pain.

PROTOTYPE DRUG   **Phenelzine (Nardil)**

Actions and Uses: Phenelzine produces its effects by irreversible inhibition of monoamine oxidase; therefore, it intensifies the effects of norepinephrine in adrenergic synapses. It is used to manage symptoms of depression not responsive to other types of pharmacotherapy and is occasionally used for panic disorder. Drug effects may persist for 2 to 3 weeks after therapy is discontinued.

Administration Alerts:
- Washout periods of 2 to 3 weeks are required before introducing other drugs.
- Abrupt discontinuation of this drug may cause rebound hypertension.
- Phenelzine is pregnancy category C.

Pharmacokinetics: Phenelzine is well absorbed from the GI tract. It is widely distributed, crosses the placenta, and enters breast milk. It is mostly metabolized by the liver. Its half-life is unknown.

Adverse Effects and Interactions: Common side effects are constipation, dry mouth, orthostatic hypotension, insomnia, nausea, and loss of appetite. It may increase heart rate and neural activity leading to delirium, mania, anxiety, and convulsions. Severe hypertension may occur when ingesting foods containing tyramine. Seizures, respiratory depression, circulatory collapse, and coma may occur in cases of severe overdose. Many other drugs affect the action of phenelzine. Concurrent use of TCAs and SSRIs should be avoided since the combination can cause temperature elevation and seizures. Opiates, including meperidine, should be avoided due to increased risk of respiratory failure or hypertensive crisis.

Use with caution with herbal supplements, such as ginseng, which could cause headache, tremors, mania, insomnia, irritability, and visual hallucinations. Concurrent use with ephedra, St. John's wort, or ma huang could lead to hypertensive crisis.

NURSING PROCESS FOCUS

Clients Receiving Antidepressant Therapy

Assessment	Potential Nursing Diagnoses/Identified Patterns
Prior to administration: • Obtain complete health history, including allergies, drug history, and possible drug interactions. • Obtain history of cardiac (including recent MI), renal, biliary, liver, and mental disorders, including ECG and blood studies (CBC, platelets, glucose, blood urea nitrogen [BUN], creatinine, electrolytes, liver function tests and enzymes) and urinalysis. • Assess neurological status, including seizure activity and identification of recent mood and behavioural patterns.	• Ineffective coping • Powerlessness • Disturbed thought processes related to side effects of drug • Adjustment difficulties • Need for knowledge related to drug therapy • Risk for self-directed violence • Urinary retention related to anticholinergic side effects of drug

Planning: Client Goals and Expected Outcomes

The client will:
- Report mood elevation and effectively engage in activities of daily living
- Report an absence of suicidal ideations and improvement in thought processes
- Demonstrate a decrease in anxiety (e.g., ritual behaviours)
- Demonstrate an understanding of the drug's action by accurately describing drug effects and precautions

Implementation

Interventions (Rationales)	Client Teaching/Discharge Planning
• Monitor vital signs, especially pulse and blood pressure. (Imipramine may cause orthostatic hypotension.) • Observe for serotonin syndrome in SSRI use. If suspected, discontinue drug and initiate supportive care. Respond according to intensive care unit/emergency department protocols. • Monitor for paradoxical diaphoresis, which must be considered a significant sign, especially serious when coupled with nausea/vomiting or chest pain. • Monitor cardiovascular status. Observe for hypertension and signs of impending stroke or MI and heart failure. • Monitor neurological status. Observe for somnolence and seizures. (TCAs may cause somnolence related to CNS depression and may reduce the seizure threshold.) • Monitor mental and emotional status. Observe for suicidal ideation. (Therapeutic benefits may be delayed. Outpatients should have no more than a 7-day medication supply, although once clients are stable they are usually dispensed a 30- or 90-day supply.) • Monitor for underlying or concomitant psychoses such as schizophrenia or bipolar disorders. (Antidepressants may trigger manic states.) • Monitor sleep-wake cycle. Observe for insomnia and/or daytime somnolence. • Monitor renal status and urinary output. (Antidepressants may cause urinary retention due to muscle relaxation in urinary tract. Imipramine is excreted through the kidneys. Fluoxetine is slowly metabolized and excreted, increasing the risk of organ damage. Urinary retention may exacerbate existing symptoms of prostatic hypertrophy.) • Use cautiously with older adults and the young. (Diminished kidney and liver function related to aging can result in higher serum drug levels and may require lower doses. Children, due to an immature CNS, respond paradoxically to CNS drugs.) • Monitor GI status. Observe for abdominal distention. (Muscarinic blockade reduces tone and motility of intestinal smooth muscle and may cause paralytic ileus.) • Monitor liver function. Observe for signs and symptoms of hepatotoxicity. • Monitor blood studies, including CBC, differential, platelets, prothrombin time (PT), partial thromboplastin time (PTT), and liver enzymes. • Monitor hematological status. Observe for signs of bleeding. (Imipramine may cause blood dyscrasias. Use with warfarin may increase bleeding time.) • Monitor immune/metabolic status. Use with caution in clients with diabetes mellitus or hyperthyroidism. (If given in hyperthyroidism agranulocytosis can occur. Imipramine may either increase or decrease serum glucose. Fluoxetine may cause initial anorexia and weight loss, but with prolonged therapy may result in weight gain of up to 10 kilograms/20 pounds.) • Observe for extrapyramidal and anticholinergic effects. In overdosage, 12 hours of anticholinergic activity is followed by CNS depression. • Do not treat overdosage with quinidine (Quinate), procainamide (Procan), atropine, or barbiturates. (Quinidine and procainamide can increase the possibility of dysrhythmia, atropine can lead to severe anticholinergic effects, and barbiturates can lead to excess sedation.)	Instruct client to: • Report any change in sensorium, particularly impending syncope. • Avoid abrupt changes in position. • Monitor vital signs (especially blood pressure), ensuring proper use of home equipment. • Consult the nurse regarding "reportable" blood pressure readings (e.g., lower than 80/50). • Inform client about the signs of serotonin syndrome, which can occur with overdosage and can be life threatening (see page 182 for description). • Instruct client to seek immediate medical attention for dizziness, headache, tremor, nausea/vomiting, anxiety, disorientation, hyperreflexia, diaphoresis, and fever. • Instruct client to immediately report severe headache, dizziness, paresthesias, bradycardia, chest pain, tachycardia, nausea/vomiting, or diaphoresis. Instruct client to: • Report significant changes in neurological status, such as seizures, extreme lethargy, slurred speech, disorientation, or ataxia and to discontinue the drug. • Take dose at bedtime to avoid daytime sedation. Instruct client: • To immediately report dysphoria or suicidal impulses • To commit to a "no self-harm" verbal contract • That it may take 10 to 14 days before improvement is noticed and about 1 month to achieve full therapeutic effect Instruct client to: • Take drug very early in the morning if insomnia occurs to promote normal timing of sleep onset. • Avoid driving or performing hazardous activities until effects of drug are known. • Take drug at bedtime if daytime drowsiness persists. Instruct client to: • Monitor fluid intake and output. • Notify the healthcare provider of edema, dysuria (hesitancy, pain, diminished stream), changes in urine quantity or quality (e.g., cloudy, with sediment). • Report fever or flank pain that may be indicative of a urinary tract infection related to urine retention. Instruct client that: • Older adults may be more prone to side effects such as hypertension and dysrhythmias. • Children on imipramine for nocturnal enuresis may experience mood alterations. Instruct client to: • Exercise, drink adequate amounts of fluid, and add dietary fibre to promote stool passage. • Consult the nurse regarding a bulk laxative or stool softener if constipation becomes a problem. Instruct client to: • Report nausea, vomiting, diarrhea, rash, jaundice, epigastric or abdominal pain or tenderness, or change in colour of stool.

- Monitor visual acuity. Use with caution in narrow-angle glaucoma. (Imipramine may cause an increase in intraocular pressure. Anticholinergic effects may produce blurred vision.)
- Ensure client safety. (Dizziness caused by postural hypotension increases the risk of fall injuries.)

- Adhere to laboratory testing regimen for blood tests and urinalysis as directed.
- Instruct client to report excessive bruising, fatigue, pallor, shortness of breath, frank bleeding, and/or tarry stools.
- Demonstrate guaiac testing on stool for occult blood.
- Instruct diabetics to monitor glucose level daily and consult the nurse regarding reportable serum glucose levels (e.g., less than 3.9 mmol/L and more than 7.8 mmol/L).
- Instruct client that anorexia and weight loss will diminish with continued therapy.

Instruct client to:
- Immediately report involuntary muscle movement of the face or upper body (e.g., tongue spasms), fever, anuria, lower abdominal pain, anxiety, hallucinations, psychomotor agitation, visual changes, dry mouth, and difficulty swallowing.
- Relieve dry mouth with (sugar-free) hard candies, chewing gum, and fluids.
- Avoid alcohol-containing mouthwashes, which can further dry oral mucous membranes.

Instruct client to:
- Report visual changes, headache, or eye pain.
- Inform eye care professional of imipramine therapy.

Instruct client to:
- Call for assistance before getting out of bed or attempting to ambulate alone.
- Avoid driving and performing hazardous activities until blood pressure is stabilized and effects of the drug are known.

Evaluation of Outcome Criteria

Evaluate effectiveness of drug therapy by confirming that client goals and expected outcomes have been met (see "Planning").

See Tables 17.2 (page 179) and 17.3 (page 179–180) for a list of drugs to which these nursing actions apply.

Atypical Antidepressants

17.8 Atypical antidepressants are newer drugs that may be used as first-choice drugs or when other drugs are not successful.

Several antidepressants have been classified as **atypical antidepressants** because of their unique or atypical structural or functional properties. Their efficacy in relieving depression is similar to the TCAs and SSRIs.

Bupropion (Wellbutrin), a norepinephrine and dopamine reuptake inhibitor (NDRI), is a unique agent that inhibits dopamine and norepinephrine reuptake without significant effects on the activity of monoamine oxidase, serotonin, or other neurotransmitters. One of the metabolites of bupropion that is concentrated in the brain may be an even more effective NDRI. Bupropion and its metabolites have no appreciable affinity for histamine, alpha-adrenergic, beta-adrenergic, dopamine, acetylcholine, or serotonin postsynaptic receptors. Therefore, side effects are generally more tolerable. Adverse effects include seizures, agitation, insomnia, tremor, headache, dry mouth, nausea, vomiting, and QT prolongation.

Serotonin and norepinephrine reuptake inhibitors (SNRIs), such as venlafaxine (Effexor), inhibit serotonin and norepinephrine reuptake. Venlafaxine has greater efficacy at higher doses. Depressive symptoms may improve earlier than with other antidepressants, often within 2 weeks of use. Common side effects include anxiety, headache, insomnia, abnormal dreams, dry mouth, drowsiness, dizziness, constipation, nervousness, sweating, chills, paresthesia, sexual dysfunction, loss of appetite, and nausea. Venlafaxine should be taken with meals to minimize nausea. Increased blood pressure occurs in some clients, so blood pressure should be monitored before and periodically during therapy.

Mirtazapine (Remeron) is a unique agent in that it does not inhibit the reuptake of norepinephrine, dopamine, or serotonin. Its most potent action is blocking histamine H_1 receptors. Through direct effects on specific serotonin and adrenergic subreceptors, norepinephrine and serotonin levels increase in the synapse. The antihistamine action of mirtazapine contributes to sedation, a common side effect. Increased appetite, weight gain, constipation, and dry mouth are other common side effects.

Norepinephrine reuptake inhibitors (NRIs), such as reboxetine, increase the action of norepinephrine by inhibiting the reuptake of norepinephrine into presynaptic neurons. These agents may improve symptoms in depressed clients who experience fatigue, apathy, impaired concentration, and slowness in information processing. Adverse effects include increased heart rate and other

◀ **St. John's Wort for Depression**

St. John's wort (*Hypericum perforatum*) is an herb found throughout Britain, Asia, Europe, and North America that is commonly used as an antidepressant. It gets its name from a legend that red spots once appeared on its leaves on the anniversary of St. John's beheading. The word *wort* is a British term for "plant." Researchers once claimed that it produced its effects in the same way MAO inhibitors do, by increasing the levels of serotonin, norepinephrine, and dopamine in the brain. More recent evidence suggests that it may inhibit serotonin reuptake. Some claim that it is just as effective as fluoxetine (Prozac), paroxetine (Paxil), and sertraline (Zoloft) for mild to moderate depression and with milder side effects. It may also be used as an anti-infective agent for conditions such as *Staphylococcus* and *Streptococcus* infections, for nerve pain such as neuralgia and sciatica, and for mental burnout. St. John's wort should not be taken concurrently with antidepressant medications.

An active ingredient in St. John's wort is a photoactive compound that, when exposed to light, produces substances that can damage myelin. Clients have reported feeling stinging pain on the hands after sun exposure while taking this herbal remedy. Advise clients who take this herb to apply sunscreen or to wear protective clothing when outdoors.

symptoms associated with excessive sympathetic nervous system stimulation. These agents are currently available only through Health Canada's Special Access Program.

Nurses should monitor clients for unusual responses when newer drugs are being used. Clients should be advised against using alcohol when taking atypical antidepressants to avoid harmful drug interactions. Caution clients not to drive if sedation effects persist.

BIPOLAR DISORDER

17.9 Bipolar disorder is a serious psychiatric disorder characterized by extreme mood swings from depression to euphoria.

Bipolar disorder (manic depression) is a relatively common and serious psychiatric disorder characterized by extreme mood swings from depression to euphoria. Suicide risk is high, and many clients stop taking their medication during the course of pharmacotherapy. The cause of the disorder is unknown, and symptoms may persist throughout the client's lifespan.

Mania is characterized by symptoms that are generally the opposite of depressive symptoms. The excessive CNS stimulation that is characteristic of mania can be recognized by the following symptoms:

- Inflated self-esteem or grandiosity; the belief that one's ideas are far superior to anyone else's
- Decreased need for sleep or food
- Distractibility; racing thoughts with attention too easily drawn to irrelevant external stimuli

- Increased psychomotor or goal-directed activity (either socially, at work or school, or sexually)
- Excessive pursuit of pleasurable activities without consideration of the negative consequences, such as shopping sprees, sexual indiscretions, or unsound business investments
- Increased talkativeness or pressure to keep talking
- With severe disease, delusions, paranoia, hallucinations, and bizarre behaviour

To be diagnosed with bipolar disorder, these symptoms must persist for at least 1 week and evidence of impaired functioning must be present. Suicide is a major risk in clients who have bipolar disorder; up to 50% of these clients attempt suicide, and 10% to 20% succeed in taking their lives. **Hypomania** is characterized by the same symptoms, but they are less severe and do not cause impaired functioning. In some cases, clients may experience a mixed episode in which depression and mania are experienced simultaneously.

Although the pathophysiology of bipolar disorder is incompletely understood, mania and hypomania likely result from abnormal functioning of neurotransmitters in the brain. Mania may involve an excess of excitatory neurotransmitters (such as glutamate or norepinephrine) or a deficiency of inhibitory neurotransmitters (such as gamma-aminobutyric acid). It is important to distinguish bipolar disorder from drug abuse, severe anxiety disorders, schizophrenia, dementia, or electrolyte disturbances, which can all produce symptoms similar to those of bipolar disorder.

Non-pharmacological interventions play important roles in the treatment of clients with bipolar disorder. Lack of sleep, excessive stress, and poor nutrition are triggers for manic episodes and should be addressed in the plan of care. Support groups and psychotherapy are helpful for many clients. ECT is very effective at treating acute manic and depressive episodes.

Pharmacotherapy of bipolar disorder is highly individualized and dependent on the severity of the condition and whether depression or mania is the predominant symptom. For clients with mild symptoms that cause only slight functional disruption, monotherapy with low doses of a mood stabilizer is indicated. More severely affected clients usually require combination therapy with a mood stabilizer plus an atypical antipsychotic. If the client is on antidepressant medications, these are usually tapered or discontinued because they can worsen mania or hypomania. Caution must be used in female clients of childbearing potential because some drugs used for bipolar disorder cause fetal malformations.

Like the treatment of major depression, nonadherence with drug therapy is a serious problem in clients with bipolar disorder. As many as 50% of clients discontinue their medication during the first year of therapy. Lack of awareness is the single most common reason for nonadherence; mania is simply not viewed as abnormal by the person experiencing it. In fact, people with mania are often able to work tirelessly on projects and accomplish many work- and home-related tasks. Surprisingly, the second most common reason for nonadherence is the presence of a comorbid substance abuse disorder, usually alcoholism. Psychotherapy and family support may be necessary to achieve proper adherence.

Lithium

17.10 Lithium is the conventional therapy for the treatment of bipolar disorder.

Drugs for bipolar disorder are called **mood stabilizers**, because they have the ability to moderate extreme shifts in emotion and relieve symptoms of mania and depression during acute episodes. The traditional treatment for bipolar disorder is lithium (Carbolith, Lithane) a mood stabilizer prescribed as monotherapy or in combination with other drugs. In recent years, valproic acid/divalproex (Depakene, Epival) has begun to replace lithium as the first-line therapy for bipolar disorder due to its improved safety profile.

NCLEX Success Tips

Lithium must be taken on a regular basis, preferably at the same time each day, to maintain therapeutic blood levels of the drug.

Lithium has a very narrow therapeutic index. That is, there is a fine line between the therapeutic dose and the toxic dose. If the client forgets to take a scheduled dose of lithium, he or she needs to wait until the next scheduled time to take it because taking twice the amount of lithium can cause lithium toxicity.

To be effective, lithium must gradually increase in the client's bloodstream to a therapeutic level. This process takes approximately 1 to 2 weeks. Once a therapeutic level is achieved, the symptoms of mania will disappear.

The reason for ongoing blood test is to periodically assess the client's lithium level to prevent toxicity.

Dosages for lithium, an antimania drug, are usually individualized to achieve a maintenance blood level of 0.6 to 1.2 mEq/L. Blood work for lithium levels should be done at least 12 hours after a client's last dose of lithium. Because lithium reaches peak blood levels in 1 to 3 hours, blood specimens for serum lithium concentration determinations are usually drawn before the first dose of lithium in the morning (which is usually 8 to 12 hours after the previous dose) or before breakfast. Stat lithium levels can be drawn at any time, usually when toxicity is suspected.

Clinical manifestations of lithium toxicity include muscle weakness, lack of coordination, vomiting, diarrhea, coarse hand tremors, twitching, lethargy, polyuria, and mental confusion.

The client needs to maintain a regular diet and regular salt intake. Lithium and sodium are eliminated from the body through the kidneys. An increase in salt intake leads to decreased plasma lithium levels because lithium is excreted more rapidly. A decrease in salt intake leads to increased plasma lithium levels.

The client needs to drink eight to ten 8-oz (240-mL) glasses of water daily in order to maintain fluid balance and decrease thirst. Decreased water intake can lead to an increase in the lithium level and, consequently, to a risk of toxicity.

PROTOTYPE DRUG | **Lithium (Carbolith, Lithane)**

Actions and Uses: Lithium is available for PO administration as tablets, syrup, and controlled-release and slow-release tablets. Onset of action may take 1 to 3 weeks. Dosing is highly individualized and is based on serum drug levels and clinical response. Lithium has a short half-life and must be taken in multiple doses each day.

Lithium is an effective drug for controlling acute manic episodes and for preventing the recurrence of mania or depression. In the client with mania, lithium decreases euphoria, hyperactivity, and other symptoms without causing sedation. Previously, lithium was used for all clients with mania; at the present time it is used primarily for those clients with classic euphoric mania. Lithium, rather than valproic acid, appears to be more effective in reducing suicide risk in persons diagnosed with bipolar disorder. Lithium may also be used for off-label indications, including alcoholism, bulimia, neutropenia, schizophrenia, prevention of vascular headaches, and hyperthyroidism. The precise mechanism of action of lithium is not known. It likely acts by changing neurotransmitter balance in specific brain regions. Lithium increases the synthesis of serotonin.

Pharmacokinetics: Lithium is given by the PO route and completely absorbed. It is distributed to all tissues and body fluids, crosses the blood-brain barrier and placenta, is secreted in breast milk, and is not bound to plasma protein. It is excreted by the kidneys, not metabolized. Peak level is between 4 and 12 hours.

Administration Alerts:

- Lithium has a narrow therapeutic index/toxic ratio; risk of toxicity is high.
- Acute overdosage may be treated by hemodialysis.
- Lithium is pregnancy category D.

Adverse Effects and Interactions: Many possible adverse effects are associated with the use of lithium. These are sometimes divided into those that occur at the initiation of therapy and those that occur with long-term therapy. Initial adverse effects are muscle weakness, lethargy, nausea, vomiting, polyuria, nocturia, headache, dizziness, drowsiness, tremors, and confusion. Many of the initial adverse effects are transient or may be easily managed. Long-term therapy can produce serious toxicity, including kidney impairment (proteinuria, albuminuria, or glycosuria), dysrhythmias, circulatory collapse, and leukocytosis. Lithium interferes with the synthesis of thyroid hormone and can cause hypothyroidism and goiter.

There are many potential drug interactions, some of which can be serious. Diuretics can increase the risk of lithium toxicity by promoting sodium loss; the body replaces lost sodium with lithium, which is also a salt. Nonsteroidal anti-inflammatory drugs and thiazide diuretics can increase lithium levels by increasing the renal reabsorption of lithium. Lithium may cause an increased hypothyroid effect of antithyroid drugs or drugs containing iodine. Concurrent administration with haloperidol may cause increased neurotoxicity. SES may result if lithium is administered with other drugs, such as SSRIs or dextromethorphan, or MAO inhibitors that potentiate the actions of serotonin.

Contraindications to the use of lithium include serious cardiovascular or renal impairment and severe dehydration or sodium depletion. Older adults and debilitated clients must be monitored carefully. Caution must be used when the drug is given to clients with cardiovascular disease, thyroid disease, history of a seizure disorder, diabetes, urinary retention, or a systemic infection. Lithium produces an increased incidence of congenital defects, especially those involving the heart, and is normally not used during pregnancy. Its use should be discouraged during lactation.

Nursing Considerations

Lithium is the only drug in this class. Lithium is classified as an antimanic agent as well as a mood stabilizer. See Table 17.5 for other commonly used mood stabilizers. Refer to the chapters on antiseizure drugs (Chapter 21), antipsychotics (Chapter 19), and anxiolytics (Chapter 16) for additional nursing considerations on adjunct medications.

TABLE 17.5 Drugs for Bipolar Disorder: Mood Stabilizers

Drug	Route and Adult Dose
Pr lithium (Carbolith, Lithane)	PO, initial: 300–600 mg tid; maintenance 900 to 1800 mg/day in three to four divided doses
Antiseizure Drugs	
carbamazepine (Tegretol)	PO, 200 mg twice a day (bid), gradually increased to 800–1200 mg/day in three to four divided doses; Bipolar: PO, start with 200 mg twice daily; may adjust by 200 mg/day increments (max 1600 mg/day)
lamotrigine (Lamictal)	PO, 50 mg/day for 2 weeks, then 50 mg bid for 2 weeks; may increase gradually up to 300–500 mg/day in two divided doses (max 700 mg/day)
valproic acid (Depakene, Epival)	PO, 250 mg tid (max 60 mg/kg/day)

(See page 175 for the Prototype Drug box.)

CHAPTER

17 Understanding the Chapter

Key Concepts Summary

The numbered key concepts provide a succinct summary of the important points from the corresponding numbered section within the chapter. If any of these points are not clear, refer to the numbered section within the chapter for review.

17.1 The two primary categories of mood disorders are depression and bipolar disorder.

17.2 Depression has many causes and methods of classification. The identification of depression and its etiology is essential for proper treatment. Major depressive disorder is characterized by a depressed mood, with accompanying symptoms, that lasts for at least 2 weeks.

17.3 Major depression may be treated with medications, psychotherapeutic techniques, or electroconvulsive therapy.

17.4 The two basic mechanisms of action of antidepressants are blocking the enzymatic breakdown of norepinephrine and slowing the reuptake of serotonin.

17.5 TCAs are older medications used mainly for the treatment of major depression, obsessive-compulsive disorder, and panic attacks.

17.6 SSRIs act by selectively blocking the reuptake of serotonin in nerve terminals. Because of more tolerable side effects, SSRIs are drugs of choice in the pharmacotherapy of depression.

17.7 MAO inhibitors are usually prescribed in cases where other antidepressants have not been successful. They have more serious side effects than other antidepressants.

17.8 Atypical antidepressants are newer drugs that may be used as first-choice drugs or when other drugs are not successful.

17.9 Bipolar disorder is a serious psychiatric disorder characterized by extreme mood swings from depression to euphoria.

17.10 Lithium is the conventional therapy for the treatment of bipolar disorder.

Chapter 17 Scenario

Jane is a 42-year-old woman married to Charlie and the mother of three young children. Before the children were born she was employed as a corporate attorney, but she and her husband decided prior to the birth of their first child that she would stay at home until the children completed high school. They are financially stable. Jane has been a soccer coach, Scouts leader, president of the ladies' group at her church, and involved in various other community organizations. Within the past month, she has not participated in any of her previous activities and she has not explained why. Jane is in good physical health and had her annual physical exam the previous month. She takes no routine medications or herbal products.

Critical Thinking Questions

1. What first step must Charlie take to aid his wife with her depression?

2. When Jane is evaluated by a mental health professional, they talk about how antidepressant drug therapy works. Provide a brief explanation of antidepressant therapy.

3. How can a nurse determine if a therapeutic effect from the antidepressant medication is being achieved with Jane?

See Answers to Critical Thinking Questions in Appendix B.

NCLEX Practice Questions

1 A healthcare provider has ordered imipramine (Impril) for each of the following clients. A nurse would question the order for

a. A client with seizure disorders

b. A client with depression

c. A client with enuresis

d. A client with neuropathic pain

2 A nurse determines that the client understands an important principle in self-administration of fluoxetine (Prozac) when the client makes which statement?

a. "I should not decrease my sodium or water intake."

b. "This drug can be taken concurrently with a monoamine oxidase inhibitor."

c. "It may take up to 1 month to reach full therapeutic effects."

d. "There are no problems associated with concurrent use of other central nervous system depressants."

3 A nurse is monitoring her client for early lithium (Carbolith, Lithane) toxicity. Which symptoms, if manifested by the client, would indicate that toxicity may be developing? Select all that apply.

a. Persistent gastrointestinal upset

b. Confusion

c. Polyuria

d. Convulsions

e. Ataxia

4 Which statement made by a client taking lithium (Carbolith, Lithane) would indicate to the nurse that further teaching is necessary?

a. "I will be sure to remain on a low-sodium diet."

b. "I will have blood levels drawn every 2 to 3 months, even when I have no symptoms."

c. "Lithium has a narrow margin of safety, so toxicity is a very real concern."

d. "I will not be able to breastfeed my baby."

5 A 17-year-old client is started on fluoxetine (Prozac) for treatment of depression. When teaching the client and his family about the medication, what information should the nurse include? Select all that apply.

a. Report any sedation to the provider, and exercise caution with activities requiring mental alertness.

b. Fluctuations in weight may be managed with a healthy diet and adequate amounts of exercise.

c. Report any thoughts of suicide to the provider immediately, especially during early initiation of the drug.

d. The drug may be safely stopped if unpleasant side effects occur and are reported to the provider at the next scheduled visit.

e. The drug may cause excessive thirst, but dramatic increase in fluid intake should be avoided.

See Answers to NCLEX Practice Questions in Appendix A.

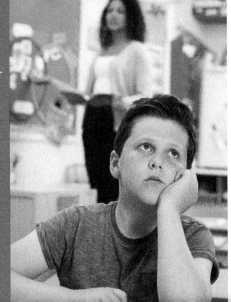

highwaystarz/Fotolia

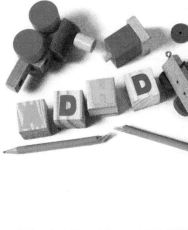

Andrzej Tokarski/Alamy Stock Photo

CHAPTER

18 Central Nervous System Stimulants and Pharmacotherapy of Attention Deficit and Hyperactive Disorders

LEARNING OUTCOMES

After reading the chapter, the student should be able to:

1. Describe the general actions and pharmacotherapeutic applications of central nervous system stimulants.

2. Identify the signs and symptoms of attention deficit/hyperactivity disorder.

3. Compare and contrast the central nervous system stimulants and non-stimulants in treating attention deficit/hyperactivity disorder.

4. Describe the nurse's role in the pharmacological management of attention deficit/hyperactivity disorder.

5. For each class of drugs listed in the Chapter Outline, identify the prototype and representative drugs and explain the mechanisms of drug action, primary indications, contraindications, significant drug interactions, pregnancy category, and important adverse effects.

6. Apply the nursing process to care for clients who are receiving pharmacotherapy with central nervous system stimulants.

CHAPTER OUTLINE

▸ Central Nervous System Stimulants

▸ Attention Deficit/ Hyperactivity Disorder

▸ Pharmacotherapy of Attention Deficit/ Hyperactivity Disorder

▸ Methylxanthines

The central nervous system (CNS) stimulants are a small group of drugs that have limited pharmacotherapeutic applications. Attention deficit/hyperactivity disorder (ADHD) is a condition that diminishes mental alertness and that may benefit from treatment with these medications. Some of the CNS stimulants such as cocaine and methamphetamine are widely abused. The purpose of this chapter is to examine the actions and pharmacotherapeutic applications of the CNS stimulants.

Central Nervous System Stimulants

18.1 Central nervous system stimulants increase alertness, enhance the ability to concentrate, and delay the symptoms of fatigue.

The **central nervous system (CNS) stimulants** are a diverse group of pharmacological agents. They are known to increase alertness, enhance the ability to concentrate, and delay the symptoms of fatigue. The stimulants range from widely accessible agents (caffeine) to Schedule I controlled substances (ecstasy). All CNS stimulants have the common action of raising the general alertness level of the brain. Wakefulness and the ability to focus or concentrate are increased. Mood is often elevated, and the person may temporarily become unaware of physical fatigue. For some of the controlled substances, mood elevation may progress to **euphoria**, an intense sense of happiness and well-being.

Because people generally view the sensations associated with CNS stimulation as desirable, many are driven to repeat the pleasurable experience. With continued use, physical and psychological dependence occur. Because of this, many CNS stimulants are highly regulated and are scheduled drugs (Table 18.1).

NCLEX Success Tips

Amphetamines are central nervous system (CNS) stimulants that cause sympathetic stimulation, including hypertension, tachycardia, vasoconstriction, and hyperthermia. They also stimulate norepinephrine release, which increases heart rate and blood flow. Pupils will be dilated. Diarrhea is a common adverse effect of amphetamines.

Amphetamines can potentially lead to abuse because they produce wakefulness and euphoria. Symptoms of amphetamine abuse include marked nervousness, restlessness, excitability, talkativeness, and excessive perspiration.

Amphetamine overdose can produce cardiac arrhythmias and respiratory collapse after monitoring is initiated; the haloperidol is indicated to antagonize the amphetamine affects.

Not all effects of these drugs on the CNS are pleasurable. Stimulants have the potential to cause adverse effects due to excessive excitation. Nervousness, dizziness, and irritability are common, and convulsions may occur at higher doses. Most of the stimulants also affect the cardiovascular system and can increase

TABLE 18.1 Central Nervous System Stimulants That Are Scheduled Drugs

Schedule	Central Nervous System Stimulants
I	3,4-methylenedioxymethamphetamine (MDMA, ecstasy), aminorex, cathinone, fenethylline, mephedrone, methcathinone, methaqualone (Quaalude), methylaminorex
II	Amphetamine (Adderall), dextroamphetamine (Dexedrine), cocaine, lisdexamfetamine (Vyvanse), methamphetamine (Desoxyn), methylphenidate (Concerta, Ritalin)
III	Chlorphentermine, clortermine, dronabinol (Marinol), phendimetrazine
IV	Cathine, diethylpropion, fencamfamin, fenproporex, modafinil (Alertec), phentermine
V	Pyrovalerone

Based on Lists of: *Scheduling Actions, Controlled Substances and Regulated Chemicals, Drug Enforcement Administration*, 2014. Retrieved from http://www.deadiversion.usdoj.gov/schedules/orangebook/orangebook.pdf. U.S. Department of Justice.

heart rate and cause dysrhythmias. Loss of appetite, or anorexia, occurs with some of the CNS stimulants.

Some medications produce CNS excitation as an adverse effect. For example, antihistamines are prescribed to treat allergy symptoms but may cause CNS stimulation and insomnia in some clients. Albuterol (Ventolin) inhalers are used for asthma but the drug may cause nervousness, tremors, and anxiety. Drugs that normally cause CNS depression, such as antidepressants, may cause paradoxical CNS excitement, especially in the very young or very old. Occasionally, drugs are purposefully taken in large amounts for their CNS stimulation adverse effects. For example, the primary over-the-counter (OTC) drug for treating cough, dextromethorphan, is abused by teenagers and can cause dizziness, restlessness, hallucinations, and seizures when taken in very high amounts.

The therapeutic applications of the CNS stimulants are limited. These include the following:

- ADHD
- Weight management
- Stimulation of respiration
- Migraine headaches

If CNS stimulants elevate mood, why are they not used to treat major depression? In fact, CNS stimulants have been used in the past to treat major depression. CNS stimulants, however, are nonselective in their CNS actions; the excitement produced by these drugs affects all parts of the brain. They produce many potentially serious adverse effects, including physical and psychological dependence. The tricyclic antidepressants (TCAs) and the selective serotonin reuptake inhibitors (SSRIs) have been demonstrated to be more effective and safer than stimulants in the treatment of depression. These drugs are able to elevate mood without causing CNS excitation.

Attention Deficit/Hyperactivity Disorder

18.2 Attention deficit/hyperactivity disorder is characterized by inattention, hyperactivity, and impulsive behaviour.

Attention deficit/hyperactivity disorder (ADHD) is a neuropsychiatric condition that presents in children before age 7 and can extend into adulthood. It is characterized by symptoms of impulsive behaviour, lack of attention, and hyperactivity. The client diagnosed with ADHD must exhibit symptoms of inattention and hyperactivity, as shown in Table 18.2 (American Psychiatric Association, 2013).

ADHD affects 5% of girls and 12% of boys under 18 years of age in Canada. Statistically, boys are about twice as likely as girls to develop signs and symptoms of ADHD, although the incidence is rising rapidly in girls. ADHD is diagnosed based on criteria set out in the *Diagnostic and Statistical Manual of Mental Disorders*, 5th edition (DSM-V), and includes subtypes related to inattention, impulsivity, and hyperactivity.

TABLE 18.2 Symptoms That May Lead to a Diagnosis of Attention Deficit/Hyperactivity Disorder

Inattention

1. Often does not give close attention to details or makes careless mistakes in schoolwork, work, or other activities.
2. Often has trouble keeping attention on tasks or play activities.
3. Often does not seem to listen when spoken to directly.
4. Often does not follow instructions and fails to finish schoolwork, chores, or duties in the workplace (not due to oppositional behaviour or failure to understand instructions).
5. Often has trouble organizing activities.
6. Often avoids, dislikes, or does not want to do things that take a lot of mental effort for a long period of time (such as schoolwork or homework).
7. Often loses things needed for tasks and activities (e.g., toys, school assignments, pencils, books, or tools).
8. Is often easily distracted.
9. Is often forgetful in daily activities.

Hyperactivity/Impulsivity

1. Often fidgets with hands or feet or squirms in seat.
2. Often gets up from seat when remaining in seat is expected.
3. Often runs about or climbs when and where it is not appropriate (adolescents or adults may feel very restless).
4. Often has trouble playing or enjoying leisure activities quietly.
5. Is often "on the go" or often acts as if "driven by a motor."
6. Often talks excessively.
7. Often blurts out answers before questions have been finished.
8. Often has trouble waiting one's turn.
9. Often interrupts or intrudes on others (e.g., butts into conversations or games).

Symptoms of ADHD such as impulsive behaviour, distractibility, lack of attention, and hyperactivity during the school-aged years can lead to poor performance and lack of interest in school activities. The symptoms of inattention and hyperactivity also contribute to difficulty with peer and family relationships. Hyperactive children usually have increased motor activity with impulsivity and a tendency to interrupt at inappropriate times. This behaviour can result in disciplinary action by teachers and parents. Some additional symptoms noted include difficulty remembering details and the placement of personal items, changing tasks without completing prior tasks, and disturbances in sleep.

Symptoms continue into adulthood in 35% to 55% of persons diagnosed with childhood ADHD. Symptoms in adults include workaholic tendencies, being overwhelmed, talking excessively, low tolerance for frustration, chronic boredom, short temper, quitting jobs abruptly, personal relationship problems, and multiple driving violations. Adults with ADHD are more likely to have an "addictive" personality, which may be exhibited in behaviour that includes smoking and using illegal substances. Adult ADHD is treated with the same therapies used for childhood ADHD.

Considerable attention has focused on the causes of ADHD, and it is clear that the disorder's etiology is complex and involves multiple variables. Studies on twins have indicated that genetics is an important contributor to the development of ADHD. An identical twin has a 92% probability of presenting with ADHD if his or her twin has been diagnosed with the disorder, and about 25% of families that have a member who has been diagnosed with ADHD will have other relatives also diagnosed. This percentage is significantly higher than that in the general population, which is approximately 5%.

Brain injury has been studied as a contributing factor in the development of ADHD because some children who experience head trauma will exhibit symptoms of the disorder. The percentage of brain injuries that lead to a diagnosis of ADHD is small but remains relevant in assessing for the condition as the client ages.

Environmental agents such as lead can contribute to the development of ADHD in children. Children who live in buildings built before 1972 have a higher risk for developing lead poisoning. Other environmental agents that contribute to the development of ADHD include alcohol consumption and cigarette smoking by the mother during pregnancy. Food additives and sugar intake by the child have been implicated as causes of ADHD, but research studies have failed to find a strong link.

There are differences in the anatomy and physiology of children with ADHD and control subjects. Children with a known diagnosis of ADHD possess a smaller brain volume in the frontal lobes, temporal grey matter, caudate nucleus, and cerebellum. Children who are affected by ADHD have a deficiency in the catecholamines dopamine and norepinephrine. The brain of a child with ADHD also has decreased development in the area of self-regulation. This factor yields the development of symptoms such as irritability, aggression, learning disability, and motor disorders when the child is stimulated.

Pharmacotherapy of Attention Deficit/Hyperactivity Disorder

18.3 Psychostimulants are central nervous system stimulants indicated for the treatment of attention deficit/hyperactivity disorder.

The nurse is often involved in the screening and mental health assessment of children with suspected ADHD. When a child is referred for testing, both the child and the family members are assessed. Data are collected on the child's physical, psychological, and developmental health situation to create an individualized plan of care.

Once ADHD is diagnosed, the nurse is instrumental in educating the parents and child, based on his or her developmental level, about the disorder and the importance of medication management and adherence. Parents should be educated about the importance of appropriate expectations and behavioural consequences and coping mechanisms that may be used to manage the demands of a child who is hyperactive. Self-esteem must be fostered in the child so that ego strengths can develop.

Drugs for Attention Deficit/Hyperactivity Disorder

Traditionally, the drugs used to treat ADHD in children have been CNS stimulants. These drugs stimulate specific areas of the CNS that heighten alertness and increase focus. A non–CNS stimulant has also been approved to treat ADHD. Agents used to treat ADHD are shown in Table 18.3.

TABLE 18.3 Drugs for Attention Deficit/ Hyperactivity Disorder

Drug	Route and Adult Dose
CNS Stimulants	
dextroamphetamine (Dexedrine)	3–5 years old: orally (PO), start with 2.5 mg daily (qd); may increase in increments by 2.5 mg at weekly intervals until optimal response is obtained (max 40 mg/day) >6 years old: PO, 5 mg qd to bid; increase by 5 mg at weekly intervals (max 40 mg/day)
Pr methylphenidate (Ritalin, Concerta, Biphentin)	Ritalin: PO, 5–10 mg before breakfast and lunch, with gradual increase of 5–10 mg/ week as needed (max 60 mg/day) Concerta: 18-36 mg/day in the morning (max 72 mg/day); sustained-release formulation available (Concerta XR) Biphentin: 10-20 mg/day; may be adjusted in 10 mg increments at weekly intervals (max 80 mg/day)
Non-stimulants for ADHD	
atomoxetine (Strattera)	PO; start with 40 mg in a.m. for 7-14 days; if tolerated, may increase dose at 7-14 day intervals to 60 mg/day, then to 80 mg/day. If optimal response is not obtained after 2-4 weeks, may increase to a maximum of 100 mg/day
guanfacine XR (Intuniv XR)	PO; Start with 1 mg qd, maintain dose for minimum of 7 days before adjusting by no more than 1 mg/week; age 6–12, maximum dose is 4 mg/day; age 13–17, maximum dose is 7 mg/day; sustained-release formulations available

◀ Zero Drug Tolerance in Schools

Methylphenidate (Ritalin, Concerta, Biphentin) is an effective drug used to treat ADHD and is often promoted by teachers and school counsellors as an adjunct to improving academic performance and social adjustment. However, schools may have a "zero drug tolerance" policy that creates a hostile environment for students who must take this drug. Zero tolerance policies generally prohibit the possession of *any* drug and define the school's right to search and seizure and the right to demand that students submit to random drug testing or screening as a condition of participating in sports and extracurricular activities. In some districts, students found in violation of such policies may be expelled or arrested.

Methylphenidate is a Schedule III controlled substance considered to have a high abuse potential. Students who take this drug should be made aware of the academic and social consequences of unauthorized possession of this medication. Most schools have strict guidelines regarding medication administration and require original prescriptions and containers of drugs to be supplied to the school health office. Students should carry an official notice from the healthcare provider regarding methylphenidate therapy that can be produced in the event of random drug testing.

NCLEX Success Tip

Atomoxetine (Strattera) is a selective norepinephrine reuptake inhibitor antidepressant. It may take more than 2 to 3 weeks to see the full effects of this medication. Nausea and dizziness are transient side effects. Monoamine oxidase inhibitors (MAOIs) are contraindicated with atomoxetine.

CNS stimulants are the main course of treatment for ADHD. Stimulants reverse many of the symptoms, helping clients to focus on tasks. The most widely prescribed drug for ADHD is methylphenidate. Another CNS stimulant that is rarely prescribed due to its abuse potential is dextroamphetamine (Dexedrine). These are Schedule III controlled substances and pregnancy category C.

Clients who are taking CNS stimulants must be carefully monitored. CNS stimulants used to treat ADHD may create paradoxical hyperactivity. Adverse reactions include insomnia, nervousness, anorexia, and weight loss. Occasionally, a client may suffer from dizziness, depression, irritability, nausea, or abdominal pain.

Non–CNS stimulants have been tried for ADHD; however, they exhibit less efficacy. Clonidine (Catapres) is sometimes prescribed when clients are extremely aggressive and active or have difficulty falling asleep. Atypical antidepressants, such as bupropion (Wellbutrin), and TCAs, such as desipramine (Norpramin) and imipramine (Impril), are considered second-choice drugs when CNS stimulants fail to work or are contraindicated.

A recent addition to the treatment of ADHD in children and adults is atomoxetine. Although its exact mechanism is not known, it is classified as a norepinephrine reuptake inhibitor. Clients on atomoxetine showed improved ability to focus on tasks and reduced hyperactivity. Efficacy appears to be equivalent to methylphenidate, although the drug is too new for long-term comparisons. Common side effects include headache, insomnia, upper abdominal pain, decreased appetite, and cough. Unlike methylphenidate, it is not a scheduled drug; therefore, parents who are hesitant to place their child on stimulants now have a reasonable alternative.

Guanfacine (Intuniv XR) has emerged as another medication option for children diagnosed with ADHD, and it is similar in mechanism of action to clonidine. Guanfacine was originally developed as an antihypertension medication but is currently also indicated for ADHD. It is an alpha$_2$ agonist and can be used alone or in combination with CNS stimulants. Because guanfacine reduces sympathetic tone, blood pressure and heart rate should be monitored carefully. This medication should be discontinued slowly, as rebound hypertension can occur. Guanfacine is available in a sustained-release formulation so that it may be taken only once per day. It is essential that the pills are swallowed whole, as breaking or crushing them will alter the timing of release of guanfacine and affect the duration of the medication. Guanfacine interacts with other antihypertensive medications and with CNS depressants, leading to enhanced sedative and hypnotic effects.

Nursing Considerations

Methylphenidate, dextroamphetamine, and lisdexamfetamine (Vyvnase) are the only drugs in this class. See Nursing Process Focus: Clients Receiving Methylphenidate (Ritalin, Concerta, Biphentin) and the Prototype Drug box for more information.

NCLEX Success Tips

Weight loss is a common side effect of methylphenidate. Because the client's symptoms are often controlled with the stimulant, the first action should be to increase the client's oral intake before the medication's side effects begin.

The weight loss is directly due to the medication's side effects, so the client will continue to lose weight unless an intervention is made. A change of medication should be the last resort since methylphenidate is the most effective medication for ADHD.

The single-dose form of methylphenidate should be taken 10 to 14 hours before bedtime to prevent problems with insomnia, which can occur when the daily or last dose of the medication is taken within 6 hours (for multiple dosing) or 10 to 14 hours (for single dosing) before bedtime. It is recommended that a missed dose be taken as soon as possible; the dose should be skipped if it is not remembered until the next dose is due.

Methylphenidate hydrochloride must never be stopped abruptly; it requires tapering off of the dosage as directed by a physician. Improvement does not mean the client may stop taking the mediation.

ADHD is typically managed by psychostimulant medications, such as methylphenidate, along with behaviour modification.

Antianxiety medications, such as buspirone (BuSpar), are not appropriate for treating ADHD.

Loss of appetite is one of the more common adverse effects associated with methylphenidate. Parents can try to cook foods that they know their child will eat and try to give them meal replacement milk shakes at other times.

PROTOTYPE DRUG	Methylphenidate (Ritalin, Concerta, Biphentin)

Actions and Uses: Methylphenidate activates the reticular activating system, causing heightened alertness in various regions of the brain, particularly those centres associated with focus and attention. Activation is partially achieved by the release of

neurotransmitters such as norepinephrine, dopamine, and serotonin. Impulsiveness, hyperactivity, and disruptive behaviour are usually reduced within a few weeks. These changes promote improved psychosocial interactions and academic performance.

Pharmacokinetics: Methylphenidate is slowly and incompletely absorbed from the gastrointestinal (GI) tract. Distribution is unknown. It is mostly metabolized by the liver. Its half-life is 2 to 4 hours.

Administration Alerts:
- Sustained-release tablets must be swallowed whole. Breaking or crushing these tablets causes immediate release of the entire dose.
- Methylphenidate is pregnancy category C.

Adverse Effects and Interactions: In a non-ADHD client, methylphenidate causes nervousness and insomnia. All clients are at risk for irregular heartbeat, high blood pressure, and liver toxicity. Methylphenidate is a Schedule III drug, indicating its potential to cause dependence when used for extended periods. Periodic drug-free "holidays" are recommended to reduce drug dependence and to assess the client's condition (for example, summer school break for children).

Methylphenidate interacts with many drugs. For example, it may decrease the effectiveness of antiseizure medications and anticoagulants. Concurrent therapy with clonidine may increase adverse effects. Antihypertensives or other CNS stimulants could potentiate the vasoconstrictive action of methylphenidate. MAOIs may produce hypertensive crisis.

Methylxanthines

18.4 Methylxanthines are central nervous system stimulants used for their ability to increase alertness or their effects on the respiratory system.

Methylxanthines are substances similar to xanthine, a chemical produced during the breakdown of deoxyribonucleic acid (DNA). Unlike the other CNS stimulants discussed in this chapter, the methylxanthines are not used for their effects on the brain. Instead, the methylxanthines are associated with treating clients with chronic obstructive pulmonary disease (COPD), asthma, and other restrictive lung diseases due to their ability to relax bronchial smooth muscle. The methylxanthines include caffeine, theophylline (Theolair, Uniphyl), and theobromine. Caffeine is the prototype drug for the methylxanthines.

Theophylline and theobromine are formed by the metabolic breakdown of caffeine in the liver. Theophylline is not used to treat ADHD, but it is administered to produce bronchodilation in clients with acute bronchospasm. It decreases wheezing and obstructed airways in asthma and bronchitis. It is important to note that the medication is a CNS stimulant that can produce restlessness, insomnia, and irritability. Close monitoring is required to prevent drug toxicity. Once widely prescribed, theophylline use has declined due to the development of safer drugs for clients with asthma. Theobromine is a natural substance found in chocolate that once was used as a drug to treat hypertension and other vascular disorders. Although similar to caffeine, it has very little CNS stimulant activity.

NURSING PROCESS FOCUS

Clients Receiving Methylphenidate (Ritalin)

Assessment	Potential Nursing Diagnoses/Identified Patterns
Prior to administration: • Obtain complete health history, including allergies, drug history, and possible drug interactions. • Obtain history of neurological, cardiac, renal, biliary, and mental disorders, including blood studies: complete blood count (CBC), platelets, liver enzymes. • Assess neurological status, including identification of recent behavioural patterns. • Assess growth and development.	• Risk for growth retardation related to methylphenidate • Risk for unsuccessful interpersonal relationships • Inadequate nutrition • Need for knowledge regarding drug therapy • Disturbed sleep pattern

Planning: Client Goals and Expected Outcomes

The client will:

• Experience subjective improvement in attention/concentration and reduction in impulsivity and/or psychomotor symptoms ("hyperactivity")
• Demonstrate understanding of the drug's action by accurately describing drug effects and precautions

Implementation

Interventions (Rationales)	Client Education/Discharge Planning
• Monitor mental status and observe for changes in level of consciousness and adverse effects such as persistent drowsiness, psychomotor agitation or anxiety, dizziness, trembling, or seizures. • Use with caution in epilepsy. (Drug may lower the seizure threshold.) • Monitor vital signs. (Stimulation of the CNS induces the release of catecholamines, with a subsequent increase in heart rate and blood pressure.) • Monitor GI and nutritional status. (CNS stimulation causes anorexia and elevates basal metabolic rate [BMR], producing weight loss.) Other GI side effects include nausea/vomiting and abdominal pain. • Monitor laboratory tests such as CBC, differential, and platelet count. (Drug is metabolized in the liver and excreted by the kidneys; impaired organ function can increase serum drug levels. Drug may cause leukopenia and/or anemia.) • Monitor effectiveness of drug therapy. • Monitor growth and development. (Growth rate may stall in response to nutritional deficiency caused by anorexia.) • Monitor sleep-wake cycle. (CNS stimulation may disrupt normal sleep patterns.)	• Instruct client to report any significant increase in motor behaviour, changes in sensorium, or feelings of dysphoria • Instruct client to discontinue drug immediately if seizures occur and to notify healthcare provider Instruct client to: • Immediately report rapid heartbeat, palpitations, or dizziness • Monitor blood pressure and pulse, ensuring proper use of home equipment Instruct client to: • Report any distressing GI side effects • Take drug with meals to reduce GI upset and counteract anorexia; eat frequent small nutrient- and calorie-dense snacks • Weigh self weekly and report significant losses more than 0.5 kg Instruct client to: • Report shortness of breath, profound fatigue, pallor, bleeding or excessive bruising (these are signs of blood disorder) • Report nausea; vomiting; diarrhea; rash; jaundice; abdominal pain, tenderness, or distention; or change in colour of stool (these are signs of liver disease) • Adhere to laboratory testing regimen for blood tests and urinalysis as directed Instruct client to: • Schedule regular drug holidays • Not discontinue drug abruptly, as rebound hyperactivity or withdrawal symptoms may occur; taper the dose prior to starting a drug holiday • Keep a behaviour diary to chronicle symptoms and response to drug • Safeguard medication supply due to abuse potential • Instruct client that reductions in growth rate are associated with drug usage. Drug holidays may decrease this effect. Instruct client that: • Insomnia may be adverse reaction • Sleeplessness can sometimes be counteracted by taking the last dose no later than 4 p.m. • Drug is not intended to treat fatigue; warn the client that fatigue may accompany washout period

Evaluation of Outcome Criteria

Evaluate effectiveness of drug therapy by confirming that client goals and expected outcomes have been met (see "Planning").

NCLEX Success Tip

Regular coffee contains caffeine, which acts as a psychomotor stimulant and leads to feelings of anxiety and agitation; hence, clients with alcohol withdrawal should avoid coffee.

PROTOTYPE DRUG | **Caffeine**

Actions and Uses: Caffeine is a methylxanthine naturally found in more than 60 plant species. Caffeine has potent psychoactive properties. When taken orally, it quickly restores mental alertness and aids in wakefulness. In addition to its consumption in beverages and food, caffeine is also available in OTC products designed to increase alertness and delay fatigue.

Caffeine also has a number of off-label indications. In clients with asthma, orally administered caffeine will produce bronchodilation and smooth muscle relaxation. Caffeine produces a mild diuresis due to increased blood flow to the glomerulus and has been used as an OTC diuretic product. Caffeine can be administered intravenously to relieve headache associated with lumbar puncture.

Caffeine itself has no analgesic properties. However, it enhances pain relief when administered with a narcotic analgesic. Caffeine is also combined with ergotamine (Cafergor) in the treatment of migraine headaches. It may be administered parenterally in emergency situations to treat circulatory collapse.

Pharmacokinetics: Caffeine can be given by the PO, IM, or IV route and is rapidly absorbed and widely distributed. It crosses the blood-brain barrier and the placenta and is secreted in breast milk. It is 36% protein bound. Half-life is 3 to 5 hours. Caffeine is metabolized in the liver to theobromine and theophylline, both of which are active metabolites that enhance the CNS and respiratory stimulant effects of caffeine and are excreted by the kidneys. When higher doses are administered, the medulla, respiratory centre, and vagus nerve are stimulated and produce a relaxation of smooth muscle, which is particularly evident in the bronchi and coronary and systemic blood vessels.

Administration Alerts:

- Caffeine should not be administered during acute myocardial infarction or to clients with cardiac dysrhythmias because the drug increases the workload of the heart.

- Caffeine increases the secretion of gastric acid; therefore, clients who have peptic ulcer disease should limit their caffeine intake.

- Clients with anxiety disorders, insomnia, or panic attacks should not be administered caffeine because it may worsen these conditions.

- Caffeine should be used cautiously in clients with diabetes mellitus, hiatal hernia, hypertension, and heart disease. Clients with hepatic or renal impairment should receive lower doses because the drug may accumulate to toxic levels.

Adverse Effects and Interactions: Caffeine may cause adverse effects at therapeutic doses, many of which are extensions of its pharmacological actions. Excessive CNS stimulation may cause nervousness, insomnia, tremors, and restlessness. The cardiovascular effects of caffeine include tingling of the face, palpitations, tachycardia, bradycardia, and ventricular ectopic beats. GI effects noted with the administration of caffeine are related to the stimulation of the vagus nerve and include nausea, vomiting, epigastric pain, hematemesis, and kernicterus in neonates. Clonic seizures can occur in rare instances. Caffeine withdrawal can produce symptoms of irritability, headache, lethargy, or anxiety.

Caffeine administered with cimetidine (Tagamet) will increase the effect of cimetidine. Beta-adrenergic agonists administered with caffeine will result in increased cardiovascular stimulation. Additive effects are likely if the drug is taken concurrently with other CNS stimulants. Clients who are taking drugs for insomnia or anxiety should limit their intake of caffeine. Caffeine is a substrate of hepatic cytochrome CYP1A2. Drugs that enhance or inhibit this enzyme may interact with caffeine. Food and fluids that contain caffeine will increase the insomnia or restlessness that is normally noted with methylxanthines.

CHAPTER

18 Understanding the Chapter

Key Concepts Summary

The numbered key concepts provide a succinct summary of the important points from the corresponding numbered section within the chapter. If any of these points are not clear, refer to the numbered section within the chapter for review.

18.1 Central nervous system stimulants increase alertness, enhance the ability to concentrate, and delay the symptoms of fatigue.

18.2 Attention deficit/hyperactivity disorder is characterized by inattention, hyperactivity, and impulsive behaviour.

18.3 Psychostimulants are central nervous system stimulants indicated for the treatment of attention deficit/hyperactivity disorder.

18.4 Methylxanthines are central nervous system stimulants used for their ability to increase alertness or their effects on the respiratory system.

Chapter 18 Scenario

Jonathon Hogan has had trouble at school beginning in kindergarten and for the past year. His teachers have consistently reported that he is easily distracted and wanders around the classroom even during a lesson. Getting him to do his homework after school has been a struggle. Jonathon loves art and does well at video games. Because he is a happy-go-lucky child, his parents have assumed that Jonathon's right-brain dominance has created trouble with left-brain logical work. With more homework now in grade 2, Jonathon is struggling to keep up in school. The school nurse suspects that he may have ADHD. She has recommended an appointment with Jonathon's healthcare provider and has told his parents that Adderall may help Jonathan to focus on his schoolwork.

Critical Thinking Questions

1. What is ADHD and why would Jonathon be experiencing more difficulty as he becomes older?
2. How might dextroamphetamine and amphetamine (Adderall) help Jonathon with his ADHD?
3. What caregiver education would be appropriate regarding dextroamphetamine and amphetamine (Adderall)?

See Answers to Critical Thinking Questions in Appendix B.

NCLEX Practice Questions

1 An elementary school nurse is providing education to the faculty on the use of central nervous system stimulants used to treat attention deficit/hyperactivity disorder. Of the following instructions, which is most important for the nurse to convey to the faculty?

   a. Have the child bring the drug dose in a lunch bag and come to the office to take it in order to avoid being teased.

   b. Request that the parents leave an extra copy of the prescription at the school in case the dose runs out.

   c. Suggest that parents have two prescriptions filled, one for home and one to keep at school.

   d. Keep the drugs in a locked drawer clearly labelled with the student's name, and keep only the number of doses allowed by school policy.

2 Which therapeutic outcome would the nurse consider most significant in evaluating a client who started atomoxetine (Strattera) 6 months ago?

   a. Decrease in attention

   b. Decrease in hyperactivity

   c. Development of mydriasis

   d. Elevated liver enzymes

3 A client who has overdosed on amphetamine in combination with dextroamphetamine (Adderall XR) is admitted to the emergency department. The nurse would anticipate which medications to be administered in counteracting the effects of the overdosage?

   a. Chlorpromazine

   b. Phenytoin (Dilantin)

   c. Propofol (Diprivan)

   d. Dexamethasone (Decadron)

4 A high school student taking atomoxetine (Strattera) for attention deficit/hyperactivity disorder visits the school nurse's office and confides, "I am so depressed. The world would be better off without me." Which action should the nurse take for this client?

   a. Tell the client to stop taking atomoxetine immediately and not to resume until he or she has checked with the provider.

   b. Assure the client that these are normal symptoms, because the drug may take 3 or 4 weeks to work.

   c. Alert the family or caregiver that immediate attention and treatment are needed for these symptoms.

   d. Have the client increase intake of caffeine by consuming cola products, coffee, or tea to counteract the depressive effect.

5 A client who is taking methylphenidate (Concerta, Ritalin, Biphentin) for attention deficit/hyperactivity disorder reports having insomnia. Which intervention will assist in the promotion of sleep?

   a. Having a glass of wine with dinner

   b. Eating a chocolate bar at bedtime

   c. Taking the drug before 4 p.m.

   d. Switching to decaffeinated coffee

See Answers to NCLEX Practice Questions in Appendix A.

PROTOTYPE DRUGS

CONVENTIONAL (TYPICAL) ANTIPSYCHOTICS

Phenothiazines
Pr *chlorpromazine*

Non-phenothiazines
Pr *haloperidol (Haldol)*

ATYPICAL ANTIPSYCHOTICS

Pr *clozapine (Clozaril)*
risperidone (Risperdal)
Pr *aripiprazole (Abilify)*

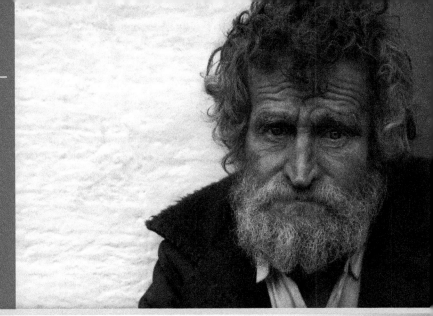

Kuzma/Shutterstock

CHAPTER

19

Pharmacotherapy of Psychoses

LEARNING OUTCOMES

After reading this chapter, the student should be able to:

1. Identify drug classes used for treating psychoses.
2. Explain the therapeutic action of antipsychotic drugs in relation to physiological aspects of neurotransmission.
3. For each of the drug classes listed in Prototype Drugs, identify a representative drug and explain its mechanism of action, primary actions, and important adverse effects.
4. Discuss the rationale for selecting a specific antipsychotic drug for the treatment of schizophrenia.
5. Explain the importance of client drug adherence in the pharmacotherapy of schizophrenia.
6. Describe the nurse's role in the pharmacological management of schizophrenia.
7. Explain the symptoms associated with extrapyramidal side effects of antipsychotic drugs and the nurse's role in preventing and managing these side effects.
8. Describe and explain, based on pharmacological principles, the rationale for nursing assessment, planning, and interventions for clients with psychoses.
9. Use the nursing process to care for clients who are receiving drug therapy for psychoses.

CHAPTER OUTLINE

▸ The Nature of Psychoses

▸ Signs and Symptoms of Schizophrenia

▸ Pharmacological Management of Psychoses

▸ Conventional (Typical) Antipsychotic Agents

  ▸ Treating Psychoses with Phenothiazines

  ▸ Treating Psychoses with Non-Phenothiazines

▸ Atypical Antipsychotic Agents

  ▸ Treating Psychoses with Atypical Antipsychotics

  ▸ Treating Psychoses with Dopamine System Stabilizers

akathisia, 206

atypical antipsychotics, 210

conventional (typical)
   antipsychotics, 205

delusions, 202

dopamine D$_2$ receptor, 203

dopamine system stabilizers
   (DSS), 213

dystonias, 206

extrapyramidal signs
   (EPS), 206

hallucinations, 202

negative symptoms, 203

neuroleptic malignant syndrome
   (NMS), 206

neuroleptics, 205

paranoia, 203

positive symptoms, 203

pseudo-parkinsonism, 206

psychosis, 202

schizoaffective disorder, 203

schizophrenia, 202

tardive dyskinesia, 206

Severe mental illness can be incapacitating for the client and intensely frustrating for caregivers and the healthcare providers treating the client. Prior to the 1950s, clients with severe mental illness were institutionalized as soon as symptoms appeared, and often remained that way for their entire lives, with little or no hope of ever improving to the point of being able to function in society. The introduction of chlorpromazine in the 1950s, and the subsequent development of newer drugs, revolutionized the treatment of mental illness. Many people with schizophrenia and other mental illnesses can now lead normal or near-normal lives as functioning members of society, as long as their healthcare provider is able to successfully manage their condition. This chapter examines the nature and pharmacotherapy of psychotic illness.

The Nature of Psychoses

19.1 Psychoses are severe mental and behavioural disorders characterized by disorganized mental capacity and an inability to recognize reality.

Psychosis is a general term used in medicine to describe a loss of contact with reality. A psychosis is a symptom of a mental illness and is not considered a disease in itself. Characteristics of psychosis are relatively easy to recognize and include the following:

- *Delusions:* **Delusions** are firm ideas and beliefs that are false and not founded in reality. Delusions sometimes are religious in nature, with the individual believing that he or she is a higher power, or a messenger of a higher power. Delusions may be grandiose, with the person believing that he or she is a king, queen, or great leader. Some clients with psychosis exhibit paranoid delusions, an extreme suspicion that they are being followed and that others are trying to harm them.

- *Hallucinations:* **Hallucinations** involve seeing, hearing, or feeling something that is not really there. Hallucinations most often are auditory; clients may hear voices telling them to harm themselves or others, that they are worthless or ugly, or that their behaviour is unacceptable. Some clients may have visual hallucinations, seeing persons or objects that are not present.

- *Lack of insight and judgment:* Clients are often unaware of their bizarre behaviour and truly believe that the voices they hear and the delusions they experience are real.

- *Mood and affect:* During psychotic episodes, the client's mood and affect may vary widely and be socially inappropriate. The client may laugh at sad events or show no emotion at all. The client may rapidly shift between happy and sad moods for no apparent reason.

Psychotic behaviour ranges from total inactivity to extreme agitation and combativeness. Because clients are unable to distinguish what is real from what is illusion, they are often labelled as insane.

Psychoses are classified as acute or chronic. Acute psychotic episodes occur over hours or days, whereas chronic psychoses develop over months or years. Sometimes a specific cause, such as brain tumors, overdoses of certain medications, extreme depression, electrolyte disorders, chronic alcoholism, or psychoactive drugs, may be attributed to the psychosis. Treating the underlying disorder may cause the psychosis to disappear.

Unfortunately, the vast majority of psychoses have no identifiable cause. These include psychoses associated with schizophrenia, bipolar disorder, and severe clinical depression.

To function in society, clients with chronic psychoses require long-term pharmacotherapy. Clients must see their healthcare provider at regular intervals, and medication must be taken for life. Family members and social support groups are important sources of help for clients who cannot function normally in society without continuous drug therapy. One major difficulty is that family relationships may be fractured secondary to the symptoms of psychosis, the length of time symptoms have been evident, and the tendency for the clients to become nonadherent to drug therapy. If these clients stop taking the antipsychotic medications, then symptoms of psychosis will most assuredly promptly reappear.

Signs and Symptoms of Schizophrenia

19.2 Schizophrenia is a type of psychosis characterized by abnormal thoughts and thought processes, disordered communication, withdrawal from other people and the outside environment, and a high risk for suicide.

Schizophrenia is a type of psychosis characterized by abnormal thoughts and thought processes, disordered communication, withdrawal from other people and the outside environment, and a

Lifespan Considerations

◀ **Schizophrenia Across the Lifespan**

- Schizophrenia can occur in childhood, but it usually begins in early adulthood.
- Incidence is slightly higher in males.
- Symptoms may compromise the ability of adults to fulfill role expectations and maintain employment.
- Rates of suicide are 15% to 25% higher than the national average among teens and adults with schizophrenia.
- Drug dosages may require adjustment due to age-related changes in pharmacokinetics.
- Side effects may decrease drug adherence in all age groups.
- Older adults may experience more severe adverse effects.

When observing clients with schizophrenia, nurses should look for both positive and negative symptoms. **Positive symptoms** are those that add on to normal behaviour. These include hallucinations, delusions, and a disorganized thought or speech pattern. **Negative symptoms** are those that subtract from normal behaviour. These symptoms include a lack of interest, motivation, responsiveness, or pleasure in daily activities. Negative symptoms are characteristic of the indifferent personality exhibited by many schizophrenics. Proper diagnosis of positive and negative symptoms is important for selection of the appropriate antipsychotic drug. See Table 19.1 for categories of symptoms of schizophrenia.

The cause of schizophrenia has not been determined, although several theories have been proposed. There appears to be a genetic component to schizophrenia since many clients suffering from schizophrenia have family members who have been afflicted with the same disorder. Another theory suggests that the disorder is caused by imbalances in neurotransmitters in specific areas of the brain. This theory suggests the possibility of overactive dopaminergic pathways in the basal nuclei, an area of the brain that controls motor activity. The basal ganglia (nuclei) are responsible for starting and stopping synchronized motor activity, such as leg and arm motions during walking.

Symptoms of schizophrenia seem to be associated with the **dopamine D_2 receptor**. The basal nuclei are particularly rich in D_2 receptors, whereas the cerebrum contains very few. All antipsychotic drugs act by entering dopaminergic synapses and competing with dopamine for D_2 receptors. By blocking about 65% of the D_2 receptors, antipsychotic drugs reduce the symptoms of schizophrenia. If 80% of receptors are blocked, motor abnormalities begin to occur. Figure 19.1 illustrates antipsychotic drug action at the dopaminergic receptor.

Schizoaffective disorder is a condition in which the client exhibits symptoms of both schizophrenia and mood disorder. For example, an acute schizoaffective reaction may include distorted perceptions, hallucinations, and delusions followed by extreme depression. Over time, both positive and negative psychotic symptoms will appear. It is challenging to differentiate schizoaffective disorder from bipolar disorder or major depression with psychotic features, as clients with affective disorders may also experience psychotic episodes.

Many conditions can cause bizarre behaviour, and these should be distinguished from schizophrenia. Chronic use of amphetamines or cocaine can create a paranoid syndrome. Certain complex partial

high risk for suicide. Several subtypes of schizophrenic disorders are based on clinical presentation.

Schizophrenia is the most common psychotic disorder, affecting 0.5% to 1% of the population. Symptoms generally begin to appear in early adulthood, with a peak incidence in men 15 to 24 years of age and in women 25 to 34 years of age. Symptoms may be mild with no lasting impairment, but the majority experience repeated episodes with worsening symptoms and outcomes. Clients experience many different symptoms that may change over time. The following symptoms may appear quickly or take several months or years to develop:

- Hallucinations, delusions, or **paranoia**
- Strange behaviour, such as communicating in rambling statements or made-up words
- Alternating rapidly between extreme hyperactivity and stupor
- Attitude of indifference or detachment toward life activities
- Acting strangely or irrationally
- Deterioration of personal hygiene and job or academic performance
- Marked withdrawal from social interactions and interpersonal relationships

TABLE 19.1 Categories of Symptoms of Schizophrenia

Positive Symptoms	Negative Symptoms	Cognitive Symptoms
Hallucinations	Apathy	Deficits in long-term memory
Delusions	Withdrawal from other persons and the social environment	Inability to focus attention
Illusions	Lack of ability to perform activities of daily living	Diminished "working memory": an inability to remember recently learned information and use it right away
Paranoia	Diminished or missing affect	Difficulty following instructions
Agitation, anxiety	Poor judgment	Difficulty following the thread of a conversation
Disorganized thoughts and speech	Lack of awareness or insight	Difficulty in identifying the steps needed to complete a task and placing them in the proper sequence
Aggressiveness, combativeness	Little or no functional speech	

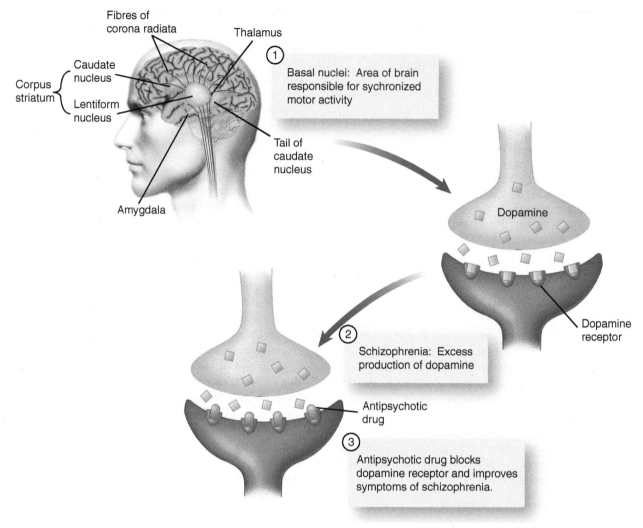

Figure 19.1   Mechanism of action of antipsychotics: antipsychotic drug molecules occupy D$_2$ receptors on the postsynaptic neuron, preventing dopamine from stimulating the receptors.

◀ **Cultural Views and Treatment of Mental Illness**

Some cultures have very different perspectives on the cause and treatment of mental illness. The foundation of many of these mental health treatments involves herbs and spiritual healing methods. First Nations people may be treated by the community traditional "medicine man," who may treat mental symptoms with a sweat lodge and herbs. Some African Canadians may be treated by a traditional voodoo priest or other traditional healer, and herbs are frequently used to treat mental symptoms. Amulets, or charms, that are worn on a string or chain may be used by members of some cultures to protect the wearer from evil spirits that are believed to cause mental illness.

seizures (Chapter 21) can cause unusual symptoms that are sometimes mistaken for psychoses. Brain neoplasms, infections, and hemorrhage can also cause bizarre, psychotic-like symptoms.

Pharmacological Management of Psychoses

19.3 Pharmacological management of psychoses is difficult because the adverse effects of the drugs may be severe, and clients often do not understand the need for medication.

Management of severe mental illness is difficult. Many clients do not see their behaviour as abnormal and have difficulty understanding the need for medication. When that medication produces undesirable side effects, such as severe twitching or loss of sexual function, adherence diminishes and clients exhibit symptoms of their pre-treatment illness. Agitation, distrust, and extreme frustration are common, as clients cannot comprehend why others are unable to think and see the same as them.

From a pharmacological perspective, therapy has both a positive and a negative side. While many symptoms of psychosis can be controlled with current drugs, adverse effects are common and often severe. The antipsychotic agents do not cure mental illness, and symptoms remain in remission for only as long as the client chooses to take the drug. In addition, many of the antipsychotics are being targeted by the government for appropriate use, since these medications are often prescribed for symptoms in which they either don't respond or there is a better alternative therapy available. In terms of efficacy, there is little difference among the various antipsychotic drugs; there is no single drug of choice for schizophrenia. Selection of a specific drug is based on the needs of the client, the occurrence of side effects, and clinician experience. For example, clients with Parkinson's disease need an antipsychotic with minimal extrapyramidal side effects. Those who operate machinery need a drug that does not cause sedation. Men who are sexually active may want a drug without negative effects on ejaculation. The experience and skills of the physician and mental health nurse are particularly valuable in achieving successful psychiatric pharmacotherapy.

CONVENTIONAL (TYPICAL) ANTIPSYCHOTIC AGENTS

The two basic categories of drug for psychoses are conventional antipsychotics and atypical antipsychotics. The **conventional antipsychotics**, sometimes called first-generation or **typical antipsychotics**, include the phenothiazines and phenothiazine-like drugs. They are listed in Table 19.2. Within each category, agents are named by their chemical structure. Conventional antipsychotics are most effective at treating the positive signs of schizophrenia, such as hallucinations and delusions, and have been the treatment of choice for psychoses for 50 years. However, they are not used as a first choice in many cases because of their many side effects. Antipsychotic drugs are sometimes referred to as **neuroleptics**.

NCLEX Success Tips

An adverse reaction to phenothiazines, tardive dyskinesia refers to choreiform tongue movements that are commonly irreversible and may interfere with speech.

TABLE 19.2 Conventional Antipsychotic Drugs: Phenothiazines

Drug	Route and Adult Dose
Pr chlorpromazine	Orally (PO), 30–800 mg/day in two to four divided doses; initiate at lower doses and titrate as needed; usual dose is 200–800 mg/day, but some patients may require 1–2 g (however, therapeutic gain is limited at doses > 1 g daily) Intramuscularly (IM), begin with 25 mg; may repeat (25–50 mg) in 1 to 4 hours; gradually increase to a maximum of 400 mg/day every 4 to 6 hours until patient is controlled (usual dose is 200–800 mg/day)
fluphenazine (Modecate)	Subcutaneous (SC): start with 12.5–25 mg every 2 to 4 weeks; increase in 12.5 mg increments (max 100 mg)
perphenazine	PO, start with 4–8 mg three times a day; reduce dose as soon as possible to minimum effective dose (max 24 mg/day); higher doses can be used in the hospital setting
thioridazine	PO, 50–100 mg tid (max 800 mg/day)
trifluoperazine	PO, start with 2–5 mg twice daily (bid); titrate dose gradually based on response and tolerance; usual dose is 15 or 20 mg/day in divided doses

Shortly after phenothiazine administration, a quieting and calming effect occurs, but the client is easily aroused, alert, and responsive and has good motor coordination.

Although most phenothiazines produce some effects within minutes to hours, their antipsychotic effects may not appear until several weeks after the start of therapy.

Treating Psychoses with Phenothiazines

19.4 The phenothiazines have been effectively used for the treatment of psychoses for more than 50 years; however, they have a high incidence of side effects. Extrapyramidal signs (EPS) and neuroleptic malignant syndrome (NMS) are two particularly serious conditions.

The first effective drug used to treat schizophrenia was chlorpromazine, a low-potency phenothiazine agent. Several phenothiazines are now available to treat mental illness. All are efficacious at blocking the excitement associated with the positive symptoms of schizophrenia, although they differ in their potency and side effect profiles. False perceptions, such as hallucinations and delusions, often begin to diminish within days. Other symptoms, however, may require as long as 7 to 8 weeks of pharmacotherapy to improve. Because of the high rate of recurrence of psychotic episodes, pharmacotherapy should be considered long term, often for the life of the client. Phenothiazines are thought to act by preventing dopamine and serotonin from occupying their receptor sites in certain regions of the brain. This mechanism is illustrated in Figure 19.1.

NCLEX Success Tips

Fluphenazine decanoate (Modecate), if dropped on the skin, can cause skin irritation.

Droperidol increases the risk of extrapyramidal effects when given in conjunction with phenothiazines such as fluphenazine.

Antipsychotic effects of fluphenazine may take several weeks to appear. Tardive dyskinesia is a possible adverse reaction, but it is not transient and should be reported immediately. Clients taking fluphenazine should increase their fluid intake.

Although they revolutionized the treatment of severe mental illness, the phenothiazines exhibit numerous adverse effects that can limit pharmacotherapy. These are listed in Table 19.3. Anticholinergic effects such as dry mouth, postural hypotension, and urinary retention are common. Ejaculation disorders occur in a high percentage of clients taking phenothiazines; delay in achieving orgasm (in both men and women) is a common cause for nonadherence. Menstrual disorders are common. Each phenothiazine has a slightly different side effect spectrum. For example, perphenazine has a lower incidence of anticholinergic effects. Thioridazine frequently causes sedation, whereas this side effect is less common with trifluoperazine.

Unlike many other drugs whose primary action is on the central nervous system (CNS) (e.g., amphetamines, barbiturates, anxiolytics, alcohol), antipsychotic drugs do not cause dependence.

TABLE 19.3 Adverse Effects of Conventional Antipsychotic Agents

Effect	Description
Acute dystonia	Severe spasms, particularly the back muscles, tongue, and facial muscles; twitching movements
Akathisia	Constant pacing with repetitive, compulsive movements
Pseudo-parkinsonism	Tremor, muscle rigidity, stooped posture, shuffling gait
Tardive dyskinesia	Bizarre tongue and face movements such as lip smacking and wormlike motions of the tongue; puffing of cheeks; uncontrolled chewing movements
Anticholinergic effects	Dry mouth, tachycardia, blurred vision
Sedation	Usually diminishes with continued therapy
Hypotension	Particularly severe when quickly moving from a recumbent to an upright position
Sexual dysfunction	Impotence and diminished libido
Neuroleptic malignant syndrome	High fever, confusion, muscle rigidity, and high serum creatine kinase; can be fatal

They also have a wide safety margin between a therapeutic and a lethal dose; deaths due to overdoses of antipsychotic drugs are uncommon.

One particularly serious set of adverse reactions to antipsychotic drugs is called extrapyramidal signs (this is more common with first-generation antipsychotics, such as phenothiazines). **Extrapyramidal signs (EPS)** include acute dystonia, akathisia, pseudo-parkinsonism, and tardive dyskinesia. Acute **dystonias** occur early in the course of pharmacotherapy and involve severe muscle spasms, particularly of the back, neck, tongue, and face. **Akathisia**, the most common EPS, is an inability to rest or relax. The client paces, has trouble sitting or remaining still, and has difficulty sleeping. Symptoms of antipsychotic-induced **pseudo-parkinsonism** include tremor, muscle rigidity, stooped posture, and a shuffling gait. Long-term use of phenothiazines may lead to **tardive dyskinesia**, which is characterized by unusual tongue and face movements such as lip smacking and wormlike motions of the tongue. If extrapyramidal effects are reported early and the drug is withdrawn or the dosage is reduced, the side effects can be reversible. With higher doses given for prolonged periods, the extrapyramidal symptoms may become permanent. The nurse must be vigilant in observing and reporting EPS, as prevention is the best treatment.

NCLEX Success Tip

Tardive dyskinesia usually occurs later in treatment, typically months to years later. Extrapyramidal adverse effects (dystonia, akathisia) and drug-induced parkinsonism, although common, are not life threatening.

With the conventional antipsychotics, it is not always possible to control the disabling symptoms of schizophrenia without producing some degree of extrapyramidal effects. In these clients, drug therapy may be warranted to treat EPS. Concurrent pharmacotherapy with an anticholinergic drug may prevent some of the extrapyramidal signs (see Chapter 13). For acute dystonia, benztropine may be given parenterally. Levodopa-carbidopa (Sinemet) is usually avoided since its ability to increase dopamine function antagonizes the action of the phenothiazines. Beta-adrenergic blockers and benzodiazepines are sometimes given to reduce signs of akathisia. Amantadine, an antiviral, may be given to reduce signs of tardive dyskinesia.

Nursing Considerations

The role of the nurse in phenothiazine therapy involves careful monitoring of the client's condition and providing education as it relates to the prescribed drug regimen. Assessment information that must be gathered on clients who are beginning antipsychotic pharmacotherapy includes a complete health history, including any long-term physical problems (e.g., seizure disorders, cardiovascular disease), medication use, allergies, and lifestyle information (e.g., use of alcohol, illegal drugs, caffeine, tobacco, herbal preparations). This allows the physician to individualize treatment and minimize the possibility of adverse reactions.

Assessment also includes a complete physical examination, including liver and kidney function tests, vision screening, and mental status, to provide a baseline of the client's health status. If the client is a child, the nurse should assess for hyperexcitability, dehydration, and gastroenteritis as well as for chickenpox or measles because such conditions increase the chance of EPS. If possible, phenothiazines should not be given to children under 12 years of age. If the client is elderly, the nurse should also determine whether a lower dose may be indicated due to the slower metabolism in older adults.

Contraindications to the use of phenothiazine and phenothiazine-like drugs include CNS depression, bone marrow suppression, coma, alcohol withdrawal syndrome, lactation, age (children under age 6 months), presence of Reye's syndrome, blood dyscrasia, and hepatic disease. This class of drug must be used with caution in asthma, emphysema, respiratory infections, and pregnancy (only when benefits outweigh risks) and in older adults and children.

The nurse should monitor the client for extrapyramidal symptoms. Symptoms include lip smacking; spasms of the face, tongue, or back muscles; facial grimacing; involuntary upward eye movements; jerking motions; extreme restlessness; stooped posture; shuffling gait; and tremors at rest. Observations of EPS by the nurse should be reported to the physician immediately. These symptoms may be reason to discontinue the drug.

A possible life-threatening side effect of antipsychotic drugs is **neuroleptic malignant syndrome (NMS)**. In this condition, the client suffers a toxic reaction to therapeutic doses of an antipsychotic drug. The client exhibits elevated temperature, unstable blood pressure, profuse sweating, dyspnea, muscle rigidity, and incontinence. The nurse should observe for these symptoms and report them immediately to the healthcare provider.

In addition, the nurse should assess the client for drowsiness and sedation, which are both common side effects of this type of medication due to CNS depression. The nurse should evaluate the client's safety and ability to function.

Client and family education is an especially important aspect of care for clients with mental illness. Client education as it relates to phenothiazines should include goals, reasons for obtaining baseline data, and possible side effects. The nurse should educate the family regarding symptoms indicative of

EPS and NMS and instruct them to report such symptoms to the physician immediately. If adherence is a problem, the nurse can supply clients and families with dose calendars and reminder signs. Because these drugs are prescribed for long-term use, the nurse should teach the client the importance of taking the drug as directed and to contact the healthcare provider immediately if side effects occur or if symptoms begin to return. See Nursing Process Focus: Clients Receiving Conventional Phenothiazine and Non-Phenothiazine Therapy on page 209 for additional specific points that the nurse should include when teaching clients and caregivers about these drugs.

PROTOTYPE DRUG | Chlorpromazine

Actions and Uses: Chlorpromazine provides symptomatic relief of positive symptoms of schizophrenia and controls manic symptoms in clients with schizoaffective disorder. Many clients must take chlorpromazine for 7 or 8 weeks before they experience improvement. Extreme agitation may be treated with IM injections, which begin to act within minutes. Chlorpromazine can also control severe nausea and vomiting.

Administration Alerts:

- Sustained-release forms should not be crushed or opened.
- When the drug is administered IM, give deep IM, only in the upper outer quadrant of the buttocks; client should remain supine for 30 to 60 minutes after injection, and then rise slowly.
- The drug must be gradually withdrawn over 2 to 3 weeks, and nausea/vomiting, dizziness, tremors, or dyskinesia may occur.
- IV forms should be used only during surgery or for severe hiccups.
- Chlorpromazine is pregnancy category C (contraindicated during lactation).

Pharmacokinetics: Chlorpromazine PO is variably absorbed. Chlorpromazine IM is well absorbed. It is widely distributed, crosses the blood-brain barrier and placenta, and enters breast milk. It is about 90% protein bound. It is highly metabolized by the liver and gastrointestinal (GI) mucosa. Its half-life is 30 hours.

Adverse Effects and Interactions: Strong blockade of alpha-adrenergic receptors and weak blockade of cholinergic receptors explain some of chlorpromazine's adverse effects. Common side effects are dizziness, drowsiness, and orthostatic hypotension.

EPS occur mostly in older adults, women, and pediatric clients who are dehydrated. NMS may also occur. Clients who are taking chlorpromazine and exposed to warmer temperatures should be monitored more closely for symptoms of NMS.

Chlorpromazine interacts with several drugs. For example, concurrent use with sedative medications such as phenobarbital (Phenobarb) can cause excessive sedation and should be avoided. Taking chlorpromazine with tricyclic antidepressants can elevate blood pressure. Concurrent use of chlorpromazine with antiseizure medication can lower the seizure threshold.

Herbal supplements should be used only on the advice of the healthcare provider. Some products, such as kava and St. John's wort, increase the risk and severity of dystonia.

Treating Psychoses with Non-Phenothiazines

19.5 The non-phenothiazine conventional antipsychotics have the same therapeutic applications and side effects as the phenothiazines.

The conventional non-phenothiazine antipsychotic class consists of drugs whose chemical structures are dissimilar to the phenothiazines. They are listed in Table 19.4. Introduced shortly after the phenothiazines, initial expectations were that non-phenothiazines would produce fewer side effects. Unfortunately, this appears to not be the case. The spectrum of side effects for the non-phenothiazines is identical to that for the phenothiazines, although the degree to which a particular effect occurs depends on the specific drug. In general, the non-phenothiazine agents cause less sedation and fewer anticholinergic side effects than chlorpromazine, but they exhibit an equal or even greater incidence of extrapyramidal signs. Concurrent therapy with other CNS depressants must be carefully monitored due to the potential additive effects.

Drugs in the non-phenothiazine class have the same therapeutic effects and efficacy as the phenothiazines. They are also believed to act by the same mechanism as the phenothiazines, that is, by blocking postsynaptic D_2 receptors. As a class, they offer no significant advantages over the phenothiazines in the treatment of schizophrenia.

Nursing Considerations

The role of the nurse in conventional non-phenothiazine therapy involves careful monitoring of the client's condition and providing education as it relates to the prescribed drug regimen. Assessment of clients who are taking a conventional non-phenothiazine antipsychotic includes a complete drug history, including current and past medications to establish any previous allergic reactions or adverse effects from these medications. Elderly clients must be

TABLE 19.4 Conventional Antipsychotic Drugs: Non-Phenothiazines

Drug	Route and Adult Dose
Pr haloperidol (Haldol)	PO, 0.2–5 mg bid or tid
loxapine (Xylac)	PO, start with 10 mg twice daily; increase dose until psychotic symptoms are controlled; usual maintenance dose is 60–100 mg/day in divided doses 2–4 times daily (max. 250 mg/day); therapy should be maintained at lowest effective dose
	IM, 12.5–50 mg every 4–6 hours or longer; individualize dose early in therapy; some patients respond satisfactorily to twice daily dosing
pimozide (Orap)	PO, start with 1–2 mg/day in divided doses; increase dosage as needed every other day (max. 10 mg/day)
thiothixene (Navane)	PO, 2 mg tid; may increase up to 15 mg/day (max 60 mg/day)

assessed more carefully than younger clients due to the possibility of unusual adverse reactions such as confusion, depression, and hallucinations that are drug induced.

A complete baseline assessment, including physical assessment, mental status (orientation, affect, cognition), vital signs, laboratory studies (complete blood count [CBC], liver and renal function tests), pre-existing medical conditions (especially cardiac, kidney, and liver function), and vision screening should be performed. The nurse should also assess the available support system because many psychiatric clients are unable to self-manage their drug regimen. Contraindications for this class of drug include Parkinson's disease, CNS depression, alcoholism, seizure disorders, and age less than 3 years.

When monitoring and teaching about side effects, the nurse should inform the client and caregivers that sedation is a less severe side effect than with phenothiazines, but that there is a greater EPS incidence with non-phenothiazine antipsychotics. A possible life-threatening adverse effect of antipsychotic drugs is NMS. Refer to information in Nursing Considerations in section 19.4 for information regarding EPS and NMS.

Because of the anticholinergic side effects of these drugs, the nurse should monitor for dry mouth, urinary retention, constipation, and hypotension with resultant tachycardia. Adherence with this classification of drug is equally as important as with the phenothiazines. The nurse should assess for alcohol and illegal drug use, which cause an increased depressant effect when used with antipsychotic drugs. The nurse should also caution the client that any form of caffeine used with these drugs would likely increase anxiety.

When assessing older clients, the nurse should check for unusual reactions to haloperidol (Haldol). Older adults need smaller doses and more frequent monitoring with a gradual dose increase. There is a great occurrence of tardive dyskinesia in elderly women. This category of drug is not safe for use in children under 2 years of age.

Client education as it relates to conventional non-phenothiazines should include goals, reasons for obtaining baseline data, and possible side effects. The nurse should instruct the family regarding symptoms indicative of EPS and NMS, telling them to report such symptoms to the healthcare provider immediately. See Nursing Process Focus: Clients Receiving Conventional Phenothiazine and Non-Phenothiazine Therapy for additional teaching points.

NCLEX Success Tips

An antipsychotic agent such as haloperidol can cause muscle spasms in the neck, face, tongue, back, and legs, as well as torticollis (twisted neck position). The nurse should be aware of these adverse reactions and promptly assess for related reactions. Posturing, which may occur in clients with schizophrenia, isn't the same as neck and jaw spasms.

Haloperidol, an antipsychotic drug, is used to decrease agitation in acute psychosis, dyskinesia in clients with Tourette's syndrome, and dementia in elderly clients.

Tardive dyskinesia may occur after prolonged haloperidol use.

Elderly clients with dementia have increased risk for falls due to balance problems, medication use, and decreased eyesight. Haloperidol may cause extrapyramidal side effects, which increase the risk for falls.

When given intramuscularly, haloperidol is considered most restrictive because it is intrusive, and a client usually does not receive the drug voluntarily. Oral haloperidol is considered less restrictive because the client usually accepts the pill voluntarily.

Haloperidol, a traditional antipsychotic drug, is associated with a high rate of extrapyramidal adverse effects.

PROTOTYPE DRUG **Haloperidol (Haldol)**

Actions and Uses: Haloperidol is classified chemically as a butyrophenone. Its primary use is for the management of acute and chronic psychotic disorders. It may be used to treat clients with Tourette's syndrome and children with severe behaviour problems such as unprovoked aggressiveness and explosive hyperexcitability. It is approximately 50 times more potent than chlorpromazine, but it has equal efficacy in relieving symptoms of schizophrenia. Haldol LA is a long-acting preparation that lasts for approximately 3 weeks following IM or subcutaneous (SC) administration. This is particularly beneficial for clients who are uncooperative or unable to take oral medications.

Administration Alerts:

- The drug must not be abruptly discontinued or severe adverse reactions may occur.
- The client must take medication as ordered for therapeutic results to occur.
- If the client does not comply with oral therapy, injectable extended-release haloperidol should be considered.
- Haloperidol is pregnancy category C.

Pharmacokinetics: Haloperidol is well absorbed after oral or IM administration. It is widely distributed, crosses the placenta, and enters breast milk. It is about 90% protein bound. It is mostly metabolized by the liver. Its half-life is 21 to 24 hours.

Adverse Effects and Interactions: Haloperidol produces less sedation and hypotension than chlorpromazine, but the incidence of EPS is high. Elderly clients are more likely to experience side effects and often are prescribed half of the adult dose until the side effects of therapy can be determined. Although the incidence of NMS is rare, it can occur.

Haloperidol interacts with many drugs. For example, the following drugs decrease the effects and absorption of haloperidol: aluminum- and magnesium-containing antacids, levodopa (also increases chance of levodopa toxicity), lithium (Carbolith, Lithane; increases chance of severe neurological toxicity), phenobarbital, phenytoin (Dilantin; also increases chance of phenytoin toxicity), rifampin (Rifadin, Rofact), and beta blockers (may increase blood levels of haloperidol thus leading to possible toxicity). Haloperidol inhibits the action of centrally acting antihypertensives.

Herbal supplements, such as kava, may increase the effect of haloperidol. Herbal supplements should be used only on the advice of the healthcare provider.

NURSING PROCESS FOCUS

Clients Receiving Conventional Phenothiazine and Non-Phenothiazine Therapy (Typical Antipsychotics)

Assessment	Potential Nursing Diagnoses/Identified Patterns
Prior to administration: • Obtain complete health history (medical and psychological), including allergies, drug history, and possible drug interactions. • Obtain baseline lab studies (electrolytes, CBC, blood urea nitrogen [BUN], creatinine, white blood cell [WBC] count, liver enzymes, drug screens). • Assess for hallucinations, level of consciousness, and mental status. • Assess client support systems.	• Ineffective therapeutic regimen management related to nonadherence with medication regimen, presence of side effects, and need for long-term medication use • Anxiety related to symptoms of psychosis • Risk for injury related to side effects of medication • Nonadherence related to length of time before medication reaches therapeutic levels, desire to use alcohol or illegal drugs • Deficient knowledge related to no previous contact with psychosis or its treatment

Planning: Client Goals and Expected Outcomes

The client will:
• Report a reduction of psychotic symptoms, including delusions, paranoia, irrational behaviour, hallucinations
• Demonstrate an understanding of the drug's action by accurately describing side effects, precautions, and measures to take to decrease any side effects
• Immediately report side effects or adverse reactions
• Adhere to recommended treatment regimen

Implementation

Interventions (Rationales)	Client Education/Discharge Planning
• Monitor for decrease of psychotic symptoms. (If client continues to exhibit symptoms of psychosis, he or she may not be taking drug as ordered, may be taking an inadequate dose, or may not be affected by the drug; it may need to be discontinued and another antipsychotic begun.) • Monitor for side effects such as drowsiness, dizziness, lethargy, headaches, blurred vision, skin rash, diaphoresis, nausea/vomiting, anorexia, diarrhea, menstrual irregularities, depression, hypotension, and hypertension. • Monitor for anticholinergic side effects such as orthostatic hypotension, constipation, anorexia, genitourinary problems, respiratory changes, and visual disturbances. • Monitor for EPS and NMS. (Presence of EPS may be sufficient reason for client to discontinue antipsychotic. NMS is life threatening and must be reported and treated immediately.) • Monitor for alcohol/illegal drug use. (Client may decide to use alcohol or illegal drugs as a means of coping with symptoms of psychosis, so may stop taking the antipsychotic. Used concurrently, these will cause increased CNS depressant effect.) • Monitor caffeine use. (Use of caffeine-containing substances will negate effects of antipsychotics.) • Monitor for cardiovascular (CV) changes, including hypotension, tachycardia, and electrocardiogram (ECG) changes. (Haloperidol has fewer cardiotoxic effects than other antipsychotics and may be preferred for client with existing CV problems.) • Monitor for smoking. (Heavy smoking may decrease metabolism of haloperidol, leading to decreased efficacy.) • Monitor elderly clients closely. (Older adults may need lower doses and a more gradual dosage increase. Elderly women are at greater risk for developing tardive dyskinesia.)	Instruct client and caregiver to: • Notice increases or decreases in symptoms of psychosis, including hallucinations, abnormal sleep patterns, social withdrawal, delusions, and paranoia • Contact physician if no decrease of symptoms occurs over a 6-week period • Instruct client and caregiver to report side effects • Inform client and caregiver that impotence, gynecomastia, amenorrhea, and enuresis may occur Instruct client to: • Avoid abrupt changes in position • Not drive or perform hazardous activities until effects of the drug are known • Report vision changes • Comply with required laboratory tests • Increase dietary fibre, fluids, and exercise to prevent constipation • Relieve symptoms of dry mouth with sugarless hard candy or gum and frequent drinks of water • Notify physician immediately if urinary retention occurs Instruct client and caregiver to: • Recognize tardive dyskinesia, dystonia, akathisia, pseudo-parkinsonism • Immediately seek treatment for elevated temperature, unstable blood pressure, profuse sweating, dyspnea, muscle rigidity, incontinence • Instruct client to refrain from alcohol and illegal drug use; refer client to community support groups for persons with addictions, as appropriate, and to mental health support groups for general support

- Monitor lab results, including red blood cell (RBC) and WBC counts, and drug levels.
- Monitor for use of medication. (All antipsychotics must be taken as ordered for therapeutic results to occur.)
- Monitor for seizures. (Drug may lower seizure threshold.)
- Monitor client's environment. (Drug may cause client to perceive a brownish discoloration of objects or photophobia. Drug may also interfere with the ability to regulate body temperature.)

Instruct client or caregiver of:
- Common caffeine-containing products
- Acceptable substitutes, such as decaffeinated coffee and tea, caffeine-free colas
- Instruct client and caregiver that dizziness and falls, especially upon sudden position changes, may indicate CV changes. Teach safety measures.
- Instruct client to stop or decrease smoking. Refer to smoking cessation programs, if indicated.
- Instruct caregiver to observe for unusual reactions such as confusion, depression, and hallucinations and for symptoms of tardive dyskinesia and to report immediately.
- Instruct elderly client or caregiver on ways to counteract anticholinergic effects of medication, while taking into account any other existing medical problems.
- Advise client and caregiver of necessity of having regular lab studies done.
- Instruct client and caregiver that medication must be continued as ordered, even if no therapeutic benefits are felt, because it may take several months to achieve full therapeutic benefits.
- Instruct client and caregiver that seizures may occur and review appropriate safety precautions.

Instruct client and caregiver to:
- Wear dark glasses to avoid discomfort from photophobia
- Avoid temperature extremes
- Be aware that perception of brownish discoloration of objects may appear, but it is not harmful

---

Evaluation of Outcome Criteria

Evaluate effectiveness of drug therapy by confirming that client goals and expected outcomes have been met (see "Planning").

See Table 19.2 (page 205) and 19.3 (page 206) for lists of drugs to which these nursing actions apply.

TABLE 19.5 Atypical Antipsychotic Drugs	
Drug	**Route and Adult Dose**
aripiprazole (Abilify)	PO, start with 2-5 mg/day (max is 30 mg/day; typical range is 2-15 mg/day) IM, 400 mg once monthly
Pr clozapine (Clozaril)	PO, start with 12.5 mg once or twice daily; increase as tolerated (max. 900 mg/day)
lurasidone (Latuda)	PO, initial 20-40 mg/day; increase dose based on response and tolerance (max 160 mg/day)
olanzapine (Zyprexa)	Adult: PO, start with 5–10 mg/day, may increase by 2.5–5 mg every week (range 10–15 mg/day, max 20 mg/day)
paliperidone (Invega)	PO, 3-6 mg/day (max 12 mg/day) IM, start with: 150 mg on day 1 followed by 100 mg 1 week later; maintenance dose is 50-150 mg monthly
quetiapine (Seroquel)	PO, start with 25 mg bid; may increase to a target dose of 300–400 mg/day in divided doses; there is also an extended release formulation available
risperidone (Risperdal)	PO, start with 1–6 mg/day (or in divided doses); increase based on response; recommended dosage range is 2–8 mg/day IM, start with 25 mg every 2 weeks (max 50 mg every 2 weeks)
ziprasidone (Zeldox)	PO, 20-40 mg bid; may increase to 60-80 mg bid (max 100 mg bid)

ATYPICAL ANTIPSYCHOTIC AGENTS

Atypical antipsychotics treat both positive and negative symptoms of schizophrenia. They have become drugs of choice for treating psychoses. These agents are listed in Table 19.5.

Treating Psychoses with Atypical Antipsychotics

19.6 Atypical antipsychotics are often preferred because they address both positive and negative symptoms of schizophrenia and produce less dramatic side effects.

The approval of clozapine, the first atypical antipsychotic, marked the first major advance in the pharmacotherapy of psychoses since the discovery of chlorpromazine decades earlier. Clozapine and the other drugs in this class are called atypical, or second-generation, antipsychotics because they have a broader spectrum of action than the conventional antipsychotics, controlling both the positive and the negative symptoms of schizophrenia. Furthermore, at therapeutic doses they exhibit their antipsychotic actions without producing the EPS of the conventional agents. Some drugs, such as clozapine, are especially useful for clients in whom other drugs have proven unsuccessful.

The mechanism of action of the atypical agents is largely unknown, but they are thought to act by blocking several different receptor types in the brain. Like the phenothiazines, the atypical agents block dopamine D_2 receptors. However, the atypical agents also block serotonin (5-HT) and alpha-adrenergic receptors, which is thought to account for some of their properties. Because they are only loosely bound to D_2 receptors, fewer extrapyramidal side effects occur than with the conventional antipsychotics.

Although there are fewer side effects with atypical antipsychotics, adverse effects are still significant and clients must be carefully monitored. Although most antipsychotics cause weight gain, the atypical agents are associated with obesity and its risk factors. Risperidone (Risperdal) and some of the other antipsychotic drugs increase prolactin levels, which can lead to menstrual disorders, decreased libido, and osteoporosis in women. In men, high prolactin levels can cause lack of libido and impotence. There is also concern that some atypical agents alter glucose metabolism, which could lead to type 2 diabetes.

Nursing Considerations

The role of the nurse in atypical antipsychotic therapy involves careful monitoring of the client's condition and providing education as it relates to the prescribed drug regimen. Assessment of the client who is taking atypical antipsychotics includes a complete health history, including seizure activity, cardiovascular status, psychological disorders, and neurological and blood diseases. Baseline lab tests, including CBC, WBC with differential, electrolytes, BUN, creatinine, and liver enzymes, should be obtained. With clozapine, a WBC with differential should be continued every week for the first 6 months, then every 2 weeks for the next 6 months, then every 4 weeks until the drug is discontinued. The nurse should assess for hallucinations, mental status, dementia, and bipolar disorder, initially and throughout therapy. The nurse should obtain the client's drug history to determine possible drug interactions and allergies.

Atypical antipsychotics, except for clozapine, are contraindicated during pregnancy and lactation, as they can cause harm to the developing fetus and the infant. The nurse should instruct female clients to have a negative pregnancy test within 6 weeks of beginning therapy and to use reliable birth control during treatment. Female clients should also be instructed to notify their physician if they plan to become pregnant. In addition, clozapine is contraindicated in coma or severe CNS depression, uncontrolled epilepsy, history of clozapine-induced agranulocytosis, and leukopenia (WBC count less than 5000/mm³).

Precautions must be taken when atypical antipsychotics are given to clients with cardiovascular disorders and conditions that predispose the client to hypotension. Additional precautions include the concurrent use of other CNS depressants (including alcohol), renal or hepatic disorders, exposure to extreme heat, older and younger age (older adults and children), prostatic hypertrophy, glaucoma, and a history of paralytic ileus.

Client education as it relates to atypical antipsychotic drugs should include goals, reasons for obtaining baseline data, and possible side effects. The nurse should include the following points when educating clients and their families about atypical antipsychotic medications:

- Avoid abrupt changes in position to decrease dizziness and postural hypotension.
- Take drug strictly as prescribed; do not make any dosage changes or stop taking the medication without the approval of the healthcare provider. Medication may take a minimum of 6 weeks before any therapeutic effects are noted.
- Have routine lab studies performed as ordered.
- Call the physician if no improvement in behaviour is noted after 6 weeks of therapy.
- Avoid use of alcohol, illegal drugs, caffeine, and tobacco.
- If significant side effects occur, continue taking the medication but contact the physician immediately.
- Increase intake of fruits, vegetables, and fluids if constipation occurs.

NCLEX Success Tips

The client's white blood cell count should be monitored at least weekly during clozapine treatment because this drug can cause agranulocytosis. This is a condition caused by a deficiency of granulocytes (a type of white blood cell), and it increases the individual's susceptibility to infection. Agranulocytosis may be manifested as sore throat, fever, and the sudden onset of other flulike symptoms. These manifestations must be brought to the attention of psychiatrists immediately. Mandatory weekly white blood cell counts are used to detect developing agranulocytosis, which can be fatal and occurs in 1% to 2% of clients taking clozapine. This medication is associated with a risk of seizures; the risk is dose dependent.

Orthostatic hypotension may occur with initial use of clozapine. Dizziness upon standing with or without fainting can also occur during clozapine treatment.

Sedation and drowsiness are common adverse effects of clozapine. Usually, taking the majority of the dose at bedtime is helpful.

Excessive salivation, or sialorrhea, is commonly associated with clozapine therapy. The client can use a washcloth to wipe the saliva instead of spitting.

Clozapine can cause tachycardia. If the pulse rate is greater than 140 bpm, the nurse should withhold medication and notify the physician.

Clozapine is the one atypical antipsychotic associated with severe anticholinergic adverse effects such as constipation.

PROTOTYPE DRUG | Clozapine (Clozaril)

Actions and Uses: Therapeutic effects of clozapine include remission of a range of psychotic symptoms, including delusions, paranoia, and irrational behaviour. Of severely ill clients, 25% show improvement within 6 weeks of starting clozapine; 60% show improvement within 6 months. Clozapine acts by interfering with the binding of dopamine to its receptors in the limbic system. Clozapine also binds to alpha-adrenergic, serotonergic, and cholinergic sites throughout the brain.

Administration Alerts:

- The client should be given only a 1-week supply of clozapine at a time to ensure return for weekly lab studies.
- Dose must be increased gradually.
- Clozapine is pregnancy category B.

Pharmacokinetics: Clozapine is well absorbed after oral administration. It is widely distributed and crosses the placenta and blood-brain barrier. It is about 95% protein bound. It is mostly metabolized on first pass by the liver. Its half-life is 8 to 12 hours.

Adverse Effects and Interactions: Because seizures and agranulocytosis are associated with clozapine use, a course of therapy with conventional antipsychotics is recommended before starting clozapine therapy. Common side effects are dizziness, drowsiness, headache, constipation, transient fever, salivation, flu-like symptoms, and tachycardia. As with the conventional agents, elderly clients exhibit a higher incidence of orthostatic hypotension and anticholinergic side effects. Clozapine may also cause bone marrow suppression, which has proven fatal in some cases.

Clozapine interacts with many drugs. For example, it should not be taken with alcohol, other CNS depressants, or drugs that suppress bone marrow function, such as anticancer drugs.

Concurrent use with antihypertensives may lead to hypotension. Benzodiazepines taken with clozapine may lead to severe hypotension and a risk for respiratory arrest. Concurrent use of digoxin (Lanoxin, Toloxin) or warfarin (Coumadin) may cause increased levels of those drugs, which could lead to increased cardiac problems or hemorrhage, respectively. If phenytoin is taken concurrently with clozapine, seizure threshold will be decreased.

Use with caution with herbal supplements, such as kava, which may increase CNS depression.

NURSING PROCESS FOCUS

Clients Receiving Atypical Antipsychotic Therapy

Assessment	Potential Nursing Diagnoses/Identified Patterns
Prior to administration: • Obtain complete health history (medical and psychological), including allergies, drug history, and possible drug interactions. • Obtain baseline lab studies, especially RBC and WBC counts. • Assess for hallucinations, mental status, and level of consciousness. • Assess client support systems.	• Anxiety related to symptoms of psychosis, side effects of medication • Risk for injury related to side effects of medication, psychosis • Nonadherence related to lack of understanding or knowledge, desire to use alcohol and caffeine-containing products • Risk for violence, self-directed or directed at others

Planning: Client Goals and Expected Outcomes

The client will:
• Adhere to recommended treatment regimen
• Report a reduction of psychotic symptoms, including delusions, paranoia, irrational behaviour, hallucinations
• Demonstrate an understanding of the drug's actions by accurately describing side effects, precautions, and measures to take to decrease any side effects

Implementation

Interventions (Rationales)	Client Education/Discharge Planning (Rationales)
• Monitor RBC and WBC counts. (If WBC levels drop below 3500/mm³, the client may be developing life-threatening agranulocytosis; drug will need to be stopped immediately.) • Monitor for hematological side effects. (Neutropenia, leukopenia, agranulocytosis, and thrombocytopenia may occur secondary to possible bone marrow suppression caused by drug.) • Observe for side effects such as drowsiness, dizziness, depression, anxiety, tachycardia, hypotension, nausea/vomiting, excessive salivation, urinary frequency or urgency, incontinence, weight gain, muscle pain or weakness, rash, fever. • Monitor for anticholinergic side effects, such as mouth dryness, constipation, and urinary retention. (Severe urinary retention may be corrected only by use of an indwelling catheter.) • Monitor for decrease of psychotic symptoms. (If client continues to exhibit symptoms of psychosis, he or she may not be taking medication as ordered, may be taking an inadequate dose, or may not be affected by the drug; it may need to be discontinued and another antipsychotic begun.) • Monitor for alcohol or illegal drug use. (Used concurrently, these will cause increased CNS depression. Client may decide to use alcohol or illegal drugs as a means of coping with symptoms of psychosis, so may stop taking the drug.)	• When using clozapine, advise client and caregiver of importance of having weekly lab studies performed. All other atypicals do not require this level of monitoring. • Instruct client to report immediately any sore throat, signs of infection, fatigue without apparent cause, bruising. • Instruct client and caregiver to report side effects. Instruct client and caregiver to: • Increase dietary fibre, fluids, and exercise to prevent constipation • Relieve symptoms of dry mouth with sugarless hard candy or chewing gum and frequent drinks of water • Notify physician immediately if urinary retention occurs Instruct client and caregiver to: • Notice increases or decreases in symptoms of psychosis, including hallucinations, abnormal sleep patterns, social withdrawal, delusions, and paranoia • Contact physician if no decrease of symptoms occurs over a 6-week period • Instruct client to refrain from alcohol or illegal drug use. Refer client to Alcoholics Anonymous (AA), Narcotics Anonymous (NA), or other support group as appropriate.

- Monitor caffeine use. (Use of caffeine-containing substances will inhibit effects of antipsychotics.)
- Monitor for smoking. (Heavy smoking may decrease blood levels of drug.)
- Monitor elderly closely. (Older clients may be more sensitive to anticholinergic side effects.)
- Monitor for EPS and NMS. (Presence of EPS may be sufficient reason for client to discontinue medication. NMS is life threatening and must be reported and treated immediately.)

Instruct client and caregiver of:
- Common caffeine-containing products
- Acceptable substitutes, including decaffeinated coffee and tea, caffeine-free soda
- Instruct client to stop or decrease smoking. Refer to smoking cessation programs if indicated
- Instruct elderly clients on ways to counteract anticholinergic effects of medication, while taking into account any other existing medical problems

Instruct client and caregiver to:
- Recognize tardive dyskinesia, dystonia, akathisia, pseudo-parkinsonism
- Seek immediate treatment for elevated temperature, unstable blood pressure, profuse sweating, dyspnea, muscle rigidity, incontinence

Evaluation of Outcome Criteria

Evaluate effectiveness of drug therapy by confirming that client goals and expected outcomes have been met (see "Planning").

See Table 19.5 (page 210) for a list of drugs to which these nursing actions apply.

Treating Psychoses with Dopamine System Stabilizers

19.7 Dopamine system stabilizers are the newest antipsychotic class. It is hoped that this new class will have equal efficacy to other antipsychotic classes, with fewer serious side effects.

Dopamine system stabilizers (DSS) are so named because they exhibit both antagonist and partial agonist activities on dopamine receptors. The balance between these two activities appears to account for the decrease in observed adverse effects, relative to other antipsychotics. Aripiprazole (Abilify) is the only approved drug in this class at the current time. It is hoped that this new class will have the same efficacy as other antipsychotic classes, with fewer serious adverse effects.

NCLEX Success Tip
Headaches, transient anxiety, and insomnia are the most common adverse effects of aripiprazole.

PROTOTYPE DRUG | Aripiprazole (Abilify)

Actions and Uses: Aripiprazole controls both positive and negative symptoms of schizophrenia and improves cognition with only minimal risk of EPS. Aripiprazole is classified as a second-generation atypical antipsychotic because of its ability to control both negative and positive symptoms. Sustenna is available as a long-acting injection.

Aripiprazole appears to have the same level of effectiveness as other atypical antipsychotics but with a lower incidence of adverse effects. An advantage over other atypical drugs is that there is little or no weight gain, hypotension, dysrhythmias, anticholinergic effects, or prolactin release with aripiprazole. This drug does not appear to lower the seizure threshold.

Pharmacokinetics: Aripiprazole is thought to act through a combination of partial agonist activity at dopamine type 2 (D_2 and D_3) and serotonin type 2 ($5\text{-}HT_{1A}$) receptors and antagonist activity at $5\text{-}HT_{2A}$ receptors. Route of administration is PO and IM. It is widely distributed, and it is not known if it crosses the blood-brain barrier or is secreted into breast milk. It is metabolized by the liver and excreted in feces and sometimes in urine. Peak effect occurs within 3 to 5 hours, and half-life is 75 to 146 hours.

Administration Alerts:
- Lactation, seizure disorders, and hypersensitivity are contraindications to the use of aripiprazole.
- Precautions must be taken when administering aripiprazole to persons with cardiovascular or cerebrovascular disease or any condition that predisposes them to hypotension.

Adverse Effects and Interactions: Frequently reported adverse effects include drowsiness, insomnia, agitation, hypertension or hypotension, lightheadedness, anxiety, headache, restlessness, EPS, akathisia, nausea, vomiting, and constipation. Life-threatening adverse effects include seizures, NMS, and tachycardia.

Aripiprazole is a substrate for several hepatic cytochrome P450 (CYP) enzymes and induces others; therefore, it may interact with drugs that undergo hepatic metabolism. For example, many of the selective serotonin reuptake inhibitors (SSRIs) inhibit CYP2D6, which can cause reduced metabolism of aripiprazole, raised serum levels, and possible toxicity. Concurrent use of other antipsychotics or lithium may increase the incidence of EPS. Alcohol and other CNS depressants will cause increased CNS depression. Decreased excretion of aripiprazole may occur with the use of drugs such as fluoxetine (Prozac) or paroxetine (Paxil). Grapefruit juice may increase the serum levels of aripiprazole and cause toxicity.

19   Understanding the Chapter

Key Concepts Summary

The numbered key concepts provide a succinct summary of the important points from the corresponding numbered section within the chapter. If any of these points are not clear, refer to the numbered section within the chapter for review.

19.1   Psychoses are severe mental and behavioural disorders characterized by disorganized mental capacity and an inability to recognize reality.

19.2   Schizophrenia is a type of psychosis characterized by abnormal thoughts and thought processes, disordered communication, withdrawal from other people and the outside environment, and a high risk for suicide.

19.3   Pharmacological management of psychoses is difficult because the adverse effects of the drugs may be severe, and clients often do not understand the need for medication.

19.4   The phenothiazines have been effectively used for the treatment of psychoses for more than 50 years; however, they have a high incidence of side effects. Extrapyramidal signs (EPS) and neuroleptic malignant syndrome (NMS) are two particularly serious conditions.

19.5   The non-phenothiazine conventional antipsychotics have the same therapeutic applications and side effects as the phenothiazines.

19.6   Atypical antipsychotics are often preferred because they address both positive and negative symptoms of schizophrenia and produce less dramatic side effects.

19.7   Dopamine system stabilizers are the newest antipsychotic class. It is hoped that this new class will have equal efficacy to other antipsychotic classes, with fewer serious side effects.

Chapter 19 Scenario

George Watkins is a 47-year-old African-Canadian male who was admitted to the psychiatric unit this morning. He was diagnosed with schizophrenia at age 20. He is dishevelled looking, with long, dirty, stringy hair. His clothes are mismatched and dirty. Although it is summer, he is wearing an overcoat and a winter hat pulled down over his ears.

Sheri Watkins, George's wife, states that George quit his job as an assembly line supervisor about 2 weeks ago. Sheri and George have been married since they were both 18. Their marriage is basically strong but has had its difficult times, especially when George's schizophrenia is active. About 3 to 4 weeks before each hospitalization for psychosis, he stopped taking his antipsychotic medication. He has taken different antipsychotic medications over the course of his schizophrenia, but none has proved to be successful over a long period.

Mr. and Mrs. Watkins, George's parents, tell you that their son had a "normal" childhood. He was active in sports, starred on the high school

football team, was an honour student, was a Scout, and had many friends. They have always enjoyed many social occasions with their large extended family. George is always welcome at family gatherings, but relatives tend to avoid him when his behaviour becomes bizarre. They all know that he has schizophrenia but do not fully understand the implications of the diagnosis.

Critical Thinking Questions

1. What are the most likely reasons George gives for discontinuing his medication?

2. What clues do his family and friends have that would indicate that his schizophrenia may be getting out of control?

3. What can be done to prevent George's schizophrenia from getting out of control in the future?

See Answers to Critical Thinking Questions in Appendix B.

NCLEX Practice Questions

1 The client states that he has not taken his antipsychotic drug for the past 2 weeks because it was causing sexual dysfunction. The nurse is aware that the name *antipsychotic* indicates that it is important to continue the medication as prescribed because

  a. Hypertensive crisis may occur with abrupt withdrawal.

  b. Muscle twitching may occur with abrupt withdrawal.

  c. Parkinson-like symptoms will occur with withdrawal.

  d. Symptoms of psychosis are likely to return if the medication is withdrawn.

2 Prior to discharge, the nurse provides the client and caregivers with teaching related to the adverse effects of phenothiazines. Which of the following points should be included?

  a. The client may experience social withdrawal and slowed activity.

  b. Severe muscle spasms may occur early in therapy.

  c. Tardive dyskinesia is likely early in therapy.

  d. Medications should be taken as prescribed to prevent adverse effects.

3 A nurse expects that a client experiencing extrapyramidal symptoms during therapy with phenothiazines will be prescribed

  a. Benztropine (Cogentin)

  b. Diazepam (Valium)

  c. Haloperidol (Haldol)

  d. Lorazepam (Ativan)

4 Which of the following are nursing implications of the administration of haloperidol (Haldol) to a client exhibiting psychotic behaviour? Select all that apply.

  a. Take medication 1 hour before or 2 hours after antacids.

  b. The incidence of extrapyramidal symptoms is high.

  c. Treatment is therapeutic if ordered on an as-needed basis.

  d. Haldol is contraindicated in Parkinson's disease, seizure disorders, alcoholism, and severe mental depression.

  e. Crush the sustained release form for easier swallowing.

5 Which statement made by a client who taking risperidone (Risperdal) indicates that further teaching is necessary?

  a. "I'll monitor my weight every month."

  b. "I can increase my intake of fluids and fibre if I have any gastrointestinal problems."

  c. "I'll have my blood pressure monitored regularly."

  d. "There is no problem if I want to drink alcohol on the weekends."

See Answers to NCLEX Practice Questions in Appendix A.

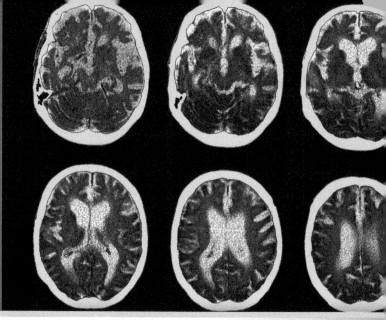

ZEPHYR/Science Photo Library/Getty Images

CHAPTER 20

Pharmacotherapy of Degenerative Diseases of the Nervous System

LEARNING OUTCOMES

After reading this chapter, the student should be able to:

1. Identify drug classes used for treating Parkinson's disease.

2. Explain the therapeutic action of antiparkinson drugs, focusing on the roles of dopamine and acetylcholine in the brain.

3. For each of the drug classes listed in Prototype Drugs, identify a representative drug and explain its mechanism of action, primary actions, and important adverse effects.

4. Explain the therapeutic action of drugs used for treating Alzheimer's disease and the efficacy of existing medications.

5. Discuss the nurse's role in the pharmacological management of clients with Parkinson's disease and Alzheimer's disease.

6. Describe and explain, based on pharmacological principles, the rationale for nursing assessment, planning, and interventions for clients receiving drug therapy for degenerative diseases of the central nervous system (CNS).

7. Use the nursing process to care for clients who are receiving drug therapy for degenerative diseases of the CNS.

CHAPTER OUTLINE

▶ Degenerative Diseases of the Central Nervous System

▶ Parkinson's Disease

  ▶ Characteristics of Parkinson's Disease

▶ Drugs for Parkinsonism

  ▶ Treating Parkinsonism with Dopaminergic Drugs

  ▶ Treating Parkinsonism with Anticholinergics

▶ Alzheimer's Disease

  ▶ Characteristics of Alzheimer's Disease

▶ Drugs for Alzheimer's Disease

  ▶ Treating Alzheimer's Disease with Acetylcholinesterase Inhibitors

▶ Multiple Sclerosis

Alzheimer's disease (AD), 223

amyloid plaques, 223

bradykinesia, 218

corpus striatum, 218

dementia, 223

hippocampus, 223

immunomodulator, 227

neurofibrillary tangles, 223

parkinsonism, 218

substantia nigra, 218

Degenerative diseases of the central nervous system (CNS) are often difficult to deal with pharmacologically. Medications are unable to stop or reverse the progressive nature of these diseases; they can only offer symptomatic relief. Parkinson's disease and Alzheimer's disease, the two most common debilitating and progressive conditions, are the focus of this chapter.

Degenerative Diseases of the Central Nervous System

20.1 Degenerative diseases of the nervous system, such as Parkinson's disease and Alzheimer's disease, cause a progressive loss of neuron function.

Degenerative diseases of the CNS include a diverse set of disorders that differ in their causes and outcomes. Some, such as Huntington's disease, are quite rare, affect younger clients, and are caused by chromosomal defects. Others, such as Alzheimer's disease, affect millions of people, mostly elderly clients, and have a devastating economic and social impact. Table 20.1 lists the major degenerative disorders of the CNS.

TABLE 20.1 Degenerative Diseases of the Central Nervous

Disease	Description
Alzheimer's disease	A chronic, progressive disease that profoundly diminishes memory, reasoning ability, and thinking skills and leaves the patient totally dependent on others for all aspects of care; usually affects persons over age 60.
Amyotrophic lateral sclerosis (Lou Gehrig's disease)	A degenerative disease of the motor neurons characterized by weakness and atrophy of the muscles of the hands, forearms, and legs, spreading to involve most of the body and face; symptoms usually begin during the middle years, with death occurring within 2–5 years.
Huntington's disease (formerly called Huntington's chorea)	A rare hereditary condition characterized by progressive chorea and mental deterioration resulting in dementia; symptoms usually begin in the 30s–50s with death occurring within 15 years.
Multiple sclerosis	A chronic debilitating autoimmune disease characterized by fatigue, muscle weakness, difficulty with balance and walking, and vision, hearing, and speech abnormalities; symptomatic periods alternate with remissions; symptoms vary depending upon which portion of the nervous system is experiencing inflammation.
Parkinson's disease	A debilitating disease characterized by resting tremor, muscle rigidity, hypokinesia, masklike faces, and a slow, shuffling gait. Symptoms usually appear in the 60s.

CONNECTIONS Special Considerations

◀ Degenerative Diseases of the Central Nervous System

- There is no cure for degenerative diseases of the nervous system.
- Drugs alleviate the symptoms but do not halt the progression.
- As symptoms advance, more medication is needed. While treatment enables people to function better, it can cause unpleasant side effects.
- Clients often require assistance to ensure that they receive their medications.
- Safety is an important consideration, as physical and cognitive changes increase the risk for falls and other injuries.

The etiology of most neurological degenerative diseases is unknown. Most progress from very subtle signs and symptoms early in the course of the disease to profound neurological and cognitive deficits. In their early stages, these disorders may be quite difficult to diagnose. With the exception of Parkinson's disease, pharmacotherapy provides only minimal benefit. Currently, medication is unable to cure any of the degenerative diseases of the CNS.

PARKINSON'S DISEASE

Parkinson's disease is a degenerative disorder of the CNS caused by death of neurons that produce the brain neurotransmitter dopamine. It is the second most common degenerative disease of the nervous system, affecting nearly 100 000 Canadians. Pharmacotherapy is often successful at reducing some of the distressing symptoms of this disease.

CONNECTIONS Lifespan Considerations

◀ Age-Related Incidence

- The incidence of Parkinson's disease increases with age. Most clients with Parkinson's disease are over the age of 50; 20% may be diagnosed under the age of 50 and 5% to 10% may be diagnosed under the age of 40.
- According to the Alzheimer's Society of Canada, nearly 750 000 Canadians were living with Alzheimer's disease and other dementias in 2011. That represents 14.9% of Canadians who are 65 years and older.

Characteristics of Parkinson's Disease

20.2 Parkinson's disease is characterized by symptoms of tremors, muscle rigidity, and postural instability and ambulation caused by the destruction of dopamine-producing neurons within the corpus striatum. The underlying biochemical problem is lack of dopamine activity and a related hyperactivity of acetylcholine.

Parkinson's disease affects primarily clients older than 50 years of age; however, even teenagers can develop the disorder. Men are affected slightly more than women. The disease is progressive, with the expression of full symptoms often taking many years. The symptoms of Parkinson's disease, or parkinsonism, are summarized as follows:

- *Tremors:* The hands and head develop a palsy-like motion or shakiness when at rest; pill-rolling is a common behaviour in progressive states, in which clients rub the thumb and forefinger together in a circular motion.

- *Muscle rigidity:* Stiffness may resemble symptoms of arthritis; clients often have difficulty bending over or moving their limbs. Some clients develop a rigid poker face. These symptoms may be less noticeable at first but progress to become obvious in later years.

- *Bradykinesia:* **Bradykinesia** is the most noticeable of all symptoms; clients may have difficulty chewing, swallowing, or speaking. Clients with Parkinson's disease have difficulty initiating movement and controlling fine muscle movements. Walking often becomes difficult. Clients shuffle their feet without taking normal strides.

- *Postural instability:* Clients may be humped over slightly and easily lose their balance. Stumbling results in frequent falls with associated injuries.

Although Parkinson's disease is a progressive, neurological disorder that primarily affects muscle movement, other health problems often develop in these clients, including anxiety, depression, sleep disturbances, dementia, and disturbances of the autonomic nervous system such as difficulty urinating and performing sexually. Several theories have been proposed to explain the development of **parkinsonism**. Because some clients with Parkinson's symptoms have a family history of this disorder, a genetic link is highly probable. Numerous environmental toxins also have been suggested as a cause, but results have been inconclusive. Potentially harmful agents include carbon monoxide, cyanide, manganese, chlorine, and pesticides. Viral infections, head trauma, and stroke have also been proposed as causes of parkinsonism.

Symptoms of parkinsonism develop due to the degeneration and destruction of dopamine-producing neurons within an area of the brain known as the substantia nigra. Under normal circumstances, neurons in the **substantia nigra** supply dopamine to the **corpus striatum**, a region of the brain that controls unconscious muscle movement.

Balance, posture, muscle tone, and involuntary muscle movement depend on the proper balance of the neurotransmitters dopamine (inhibitory) and acetylcholine (stimulatory) in the corpus striatum. If dopamine is absent, acetylcholine has a more dramatic stimulatory effect in this area. For this reason, drug therapy for parkinsonism focuses not only on restoring dopamine function, but also on blocking the effect of acetylcholine within the corpus striatum. Therefore, when the brain experiences a loss of dopamine within the substantia nigra or an overactive cholinergic influence in the corpus striatum, parkinsonism results.

Extrapyramidal signs (EPS) develop for the same neurochemical reasons as Parkinson's disease. Recall from Chapter 19 that antipsychotic drugs act through a blockade of dopamine receptors. Therefore, treatment with certain antipsychotic drugs may induce parkinsonism-like symptoms, or EPS, by interfering with the same neural pathway and functions affected by the lack of dopamine.

EPS may occur suddenly and become a medical emergency. With acute EPS, the client's muscles may spasm or become locked up. Fever and confusion are other signs and symptoms of this reaction. For acute EPS in a healthcare facility, short-term medical treatment can be provided by administering diphenhydramine (Benadryl). If recognized outside the healthcare setting, the client should be taken to the emergency room immediately, as untreated acute episodes of EPS can be fatal.

DRUGS FOR PARKINSONISM

Antiparkinson agents are given to alleviate symptoms but do not cure the disease. These drugs restore the balance of dopamine and acetylcholine in specific regions of the brain. These drugs include dopaminergic agents and anticholinergics (cholinergic blockers).

Treating Parkinsonism with Dopaminergic Drugs

20.3 The most commonly used medications for parkinsonism attempt to restore levels of dopamine in the corpus striatum of the brain. Levodopa, enhanced by combination with carbidopa, is the drug of choice for Parkinson's disease.

The goal of pharmacotherapy for Parkinson's disease is to increase the ability of the client to perform normal daily activities such as eating, walking, dressing, and bathing. Although pharmacotherapy does not cure this disorder, symptoms may be dramatically reduced in some clients.

Drug therapy attempts to restore the functional balance of dopamine and acetylcholine in the corpus striatum of the brain. Dopaminergic drugs are used to increase dopamine levels in this region. These agents are listed in Table 20.2. The drug of choice for parkinsonism is levodopa in combination with carbidopa (Sinemet). Levodopa, a dopaminergic drug, has been used more extensively than any other medication for this disorder. As shown in Figure 20.1, levodopa is a precursor for dopamine synthesis. Supplying it directly leads to increased biosynthesis of dopamine within the nerve terminals. Whereas levodopa can cross the

TABLE 20.2 Dopaminergic Drugs Used for Parkinsonism

Drug	Route and Adult Dose
amantadine	Orally (PO), 100 mg daily (qd) or twice a day (bid) (max 400 mg/day in divided doses)
bromocriptine	PO, 1.25 mg bid (max 100 mg/day)
Pr carbidopa-levodopa (Sinemet)	PO, tablets are available in 1:4 ratio as well as a 1:10 ratio; frequency ranges from 3–8 times/day (max 2000 mg of levodopa and 200 mg of carbidopa)
entacapone (Comtan)	PO, 200 mg with each dose of levodopa-carbidopa (max 8 times daily; max dose 1600 mg/day)
pramipexole (Mirapex)	PO (immediate release), 0.125 mg tid; usual maintenance dose is 0.5–1.5 mg tid; PO (extended release), 0.375 mg qd; gradually increase to 0.75 mg/day if needed (max 4.5 mg/day)
ropinirole (Requip)	PO, start with 0.25 mg tid; based on individual patient response the dosage should be titrated weekly (max 24 mg/day)
selegiline	PO, 5 mg/dose bid; doses greater than 10 mg/day are potentially toxic

blood-brain barrier, dopamine cannot; therefore, dopamine itself is not used for therapy. The effectiveness of levodopa can be "boosted" by combining it with carbidopa. Carbidopa does not cross the blood-brain barrier but acts outside the CNS to decrease the metabolism of levodopa to dopamine. Therefore, the combination of levodopa and carbidopa makes more levodopa available to enter the CNS.

NCLEX Success Tips

Amantadine is an anticholinergic drug used to relieve drug-induced extrapyramidal adverse effects, such as muscle weakness, involuntary muscle movement, pseudo-parkinsonism, and tardive dyskinesia. Amantadine is also used as an influenza A treatment/prophylaxis. It is one of the agents that may be given on a mass scale during influenza outbreaks.

Other anticholinergic agents used to control extrapyramidal reactions include benztropine (Cogentin), trihexyphenidyl, and diphenhydramine.

Both fluphenazine (Modecate) and amantadine can have orthostatic hypotensive effects. Clients, especially the elderly, should be educated about this side effect. Telling the client to change positions slowly will help ease the dizziness. If the dizziness is prolonged, the client should report those results to his or her practitioner.

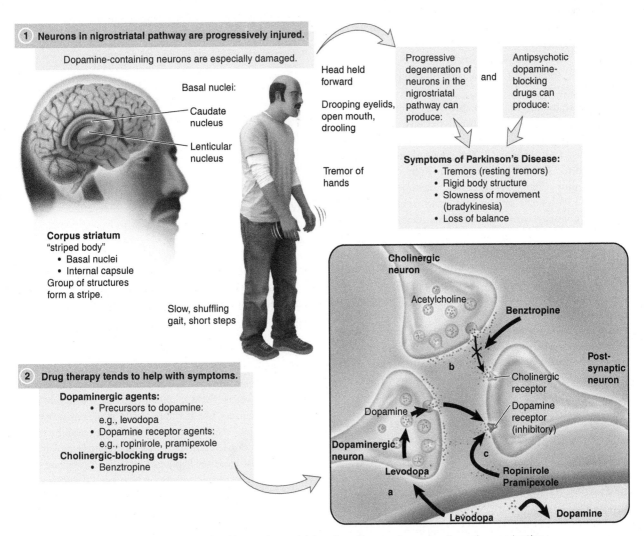

Figure 20.1 Mechanism of action of antiparkinson drugs: (a) levodopa therapy increases dopamine production; (b) anticholinergic (cholinergic blocker) decreases the amount of acetylcholine reaching the receptor; (c) ropinirole and pramipexole (dopamine agonists) activate the dopamine receptor.

Several additional approaches to enhancing dopamine are used in treating parkinsonism. Entacapone (Comtan) and selegiline inhibit enzymes that normally destroy levodopa and/or dopamine. Bromocriptine, pramipexole (Mirapex), and ropinirole (Requip) directly activate the dopamine receptor and are called dopamine agonists. Amantadine, an antiviral agent, causes the release of dopamine from its nerve terminals. All of these drugs are considered adjuncts to the pharmacotherapy of Parkinson's disease because they are not as effective as levodopa.

Nursing Considerations

The role of the nurse in dopaminergic therapy involves careful monitoring of the client's condition and providing education as it relates to the prescribed drug regimen. Prior to the initiation of drug therapy, the client's health history should be taken. Those with narrow-angle glaucoma, undiagnosed skin lesions, or history of hypersensitivity should not take dopaminergic agents. Dopaminergics should be used cautiously in clients with severe cardiac, renal, liver, or endocrine diseases; mood disorders; or a history of seizures or ulcers and in those who are pregnant or lactating. Initial lab testing should include a complete blood count and liver and renal function studies. These tests should be obtained throughout the treatment regimen. Baseline information should include vital signs (especially blood pressure), mental status, and symptoms of Parkinson's disease. Lastly, all other medications taken by the client should be fully evaluated for compatibility with dopaminergic agonists.

During initial treatment, blood pressure, pulse, and respirations should be closely monitored because these drugs may cause hypotension and tachycardia. Additional lab testing for diabetes and acromegaly should be done if the client is expected to take the drug long term. The nurse should especially monitor clients for excessive daytime sleepiness, eye twitching, involuntary movements, hand tremors, fatigue, anxiety, mood changes, confusion, agitation, nausea, vomiting, anorexia, dry mouth, and constipation. Muscle twitching and mood changes may indicate toxicity and should be reported at once. The nurse may need to assist clients with drug administration and activities of daily living, including ambulation, at least initially. It is normal for the client's urine and perspiration to darken in colour.

Client education as it relates to dopaminergic drugs should include goals, reasons for obtaining baseline data, and possible side effects. The following are additional points to include when instructing the client and caregivers regarding dopaminergics:

- Increase fibre and fluid consumption to prevent constipation.
- Avoid foods high in pyridoxine (vitamin B_6), such as beef, liver, ham, pork, egg yolks, sweet potatoes, and oatmeal, because they will decrease the effects of these medications.
- Report significant reactions or side effects immediately.
- It may be several months before the full therapeutic effect of pharmacotherapy is achieved.
- Do not abruptly discontinue taking the drug because parkinsonian crisis may occur.
- Change positions slowly to prevent dizziness and fainting.

NCLEX Success Tips

The nurse should contact the physician before administering carbidopa-levodopa because this medication can cause symptoms of depression in clients with a diagnosis of depression.

The nurse should also determine if the client is on an monoamine oxidase (MAO) inhibitor because concurrent use with carbidopa-levodopa can cause a hypertensive crisis.

PROTOTYPE DRUG | **Carbidopa-Levodopa (Sinemet)**

Actions and Uses: Levodopa restores the neurotransmitter dopamine in extrapyramidal areas of the brain, thus relieving some Parkinson's symptoms. To increase its effect, levodopa is combined with carbidopa, which prevents its enzymatic breakdown in the periphery. As many as 6 months may be needed to achieve maximum therapeutic effects.

Administration Alerts:
- The client may be unable to self-administer medication and may need assistance.
- Administer exactly as ordered.
- Abrupt withdrawal of the drug can result in parkinsonian crisis or neuroleptic malignant syndrome (NMS).
- Carbidopa-levodopa is pregnancy category C.

Pharmacokinetics: Levodopa is well absorbed after oral administration, but absorption may be decreased with high-fat, high-calorie, or high-protein meals. It is widely distributed, crosses the blood-brain barrier and placenta, and enters breast milk. Carbidopa does not cross the blood-brain barrier but it enters breast milk. Levodopa (half-life 1 hour) and carbidopa (half-life 1 to 2 hours) are mostly metabolized by the liver.

Adverse Effects and Interactions: Side effects of levodopa include uncontrolled and purposeless movements such as extending the fingers and shrugging the shoulders, involuntary movements, loss of appetite, nausea, and vomiting. Muscle twitching and spasmodic winking are early signs of toxicity. Orthostatic hypotension is common in some clients. The drug should be discontinued gradually since abrupt withdrawal can produce acute parkinsonism.

Levodopa interacts with many drugs. For example, tricyclic antidepressants decrease the effects of levodopa, increase postural hypotension, and may increase sympathetic activity, with resulting hypertension and sinus tachycardia. Levodopa cannot be used if a monoamine oxidase (MAO) inhibitor was taken within 14 to 28 days because concurrent use may precipitate hypertensive crisis. Haloperidol (Haldol) taken concurrently may antagonize the therapeutic effects of levodopa. Methyldopa may increase toxicity. Antihypertensives may cause increased hypotensive effects. Antiseizure drugs may decrease the therapeutic effects of levodopa. Antacids containing magnesium, calcium, or sodium bicarbonate may increase levodopa absorption, which could lead to toxicity. Pyridoxine (vitamin B_6) reverses the antiparkinson effects of levodopa.

Use with caution with herbal supplements, such as kava, which may worsen symptoms of Parkinson's disease.

NURSING PROCESS FOCUS

Clients Receiving Carbidopa-Levodopa (Sinemet)

Assessment	Potential Nursing Diagnoses/Identified Patterns
Prior to administration: • Obtain complete health history, including allergies, drug history, and possible drug interactions. • Obtain baseline evaluation of severity of Parkinson's disease to determine medication effectiveness. • Obtain baseline vital signs, especially blood pressure and pulse.	• Risk for falls • Need for knowledge related to drug therapy • Impaired physical mobility • Self-care deficit: feeding, toileting • Constipation

Planning: Client Goals and Expected Outcomes

The client will:

• Report increased ease of movement and decreased symptoms of Parkinson's disease
• Demonstrate an understanding of the drug's action by accurately describing drug side effects, precautions, and measures to take to decrease any side effects
• Immediately report side effects and adverse reactions
• Adhere to the medication regimen

Implementation

Interventions (Rationales)	Client Education/Discharge Planning
• Monitor vital signs closely when dose is being adjusted. (Hypotension could occur as a result of dose adjustment. Dysrhythmias can occur in clients predisposed to cardiac problems.) • Provide for client safety. (Orthostatic hypotension may occur.) • Monitor for behaviour changes. (Drug increases risk for depression and suicidal thoughts and may cause other mood disturbances such as aggressiveness and confusion.) • Monitor for symptoms of overdose. (Muscle twitching and blepharospasm are early symptoms.) • Monitor for improved functional status followed by a loss of therapeutic effects (on-off phenomenon) due to changes in dopamine levels that may last only minutes, or days. (Usually this occurs in clients on long-term levodopa therapy.) • Evaluate diet. (Absorption of levodopa decreases with high-protein meals and high consumption of pyridoxine-containing foods.) • Monitor glucose levels in clients with diabetes mellitus. (Loss of glycemic control may occur in the diabetic client.) • Monitor for decreased kidney or liver function. (Decrease in these functions may slow metabolism and excretion of drug, possibly leading to overdose or toxicity.) • Monitor for side effects in older adults. (Elderly clients may experience more rapid and severe side effects, especially those affecting the cardiovascular system.) • Monitor for other drug-related changes. (Drug may cause urine and perspiration to darken in colour, but it is not a sign of overdose or toxicity.)	Instruct client and caregiver to: • Report signs of hypotension: dizziness, lightheadedness, feeling that heart is racing or skipping beats, and dyspnea • Have electrocardiograms (ECGs) and vital signs taken periodically Instruct client: • To change position slowly and to resume normal activities slowly • How to prevent and protect self from falls Instruct client and caregiver to: • Watch for and report immediately any signs of changes in behaviour or mood • Seek counselling or a support group to help deal with these feelings; assist client to find such resources if needed • Instruct client and caregiver to be aware of newly occurring muscle twitching, including muscles of eyelids, and to report it immediately • Instruct client and caregiver to report rapid, unpredictable changes in motor symptoms to healthcare provider immediately, and that this can be corrected with changes in levodopa dosage schedule Instruct client to: • Take drug on empty stomach, but food may be eaten 15 minutes after, to decrease gastrointestinal (GI) upset • Avoid taking levodopa with high-fat, high-calorie, or high-protein meals • Avoid high consumption of foods containing vitamin B_6 (pyridoxine), such as bananas, wheat germ, green vegetables, liver, legumes • Watch for vitamin B_6 in multivitamins, fortified cereals, and antinauseants, and avoid such products Instruct diabetic client to: • Consistently monitor blood glucose both by self and with periodic lab studies • Report symptoms of hypoglycemia or hyperglycemia • Instruct client to keep all appointments for liver and kidney function tests during therapy • Instruct elderly clients to report any symptoms involving cardiovascular system: changes in heart rate, dizziness, faintness, edema, palpitations • Inform client that urine may darken and sweat may be dark coloured, but not to be alarmed

Evaluation of Outcome Criteria

Evaluate effectiveness of drug therapy by confirming that client goals and expected outcomes have been met (see "Planning").

Treating Parkinsonism with Anticholinergics

20.4 Centrally acting anticholinergic drugs are sometimes used to relieve symptoms of parkinsonism, although they are less effective than levodopa.

A second approach to changing the balance between dopamine and acetylcholine in the brain is to give anticholinergics, or cholinergic blockers. By blocking the effect of acetylcholine, anticholinergics inhibit the hyperactivity of this neurotransmitter in the corpus striatum of the brain. These agents are shown in Table 20.3.

NCLEX Success Tips

Benztropine is an anticholinergic medication administered to reduce the extrapyramidal adverse effects of chlorpromazine and other antipsychotic medications.

Benztropine blocks cholinergic activity in the CNS. Overactivity of acetylcholine and lower levels of dopamine are the causes of extrapyramidal effects. Constipation caused by medication is best managed by diet, fluids, and exercise.

Dystonic adverse effects of haloperidol, especially oculogyric crises, are painful and frightening. Intramuscular (IM) benztropine is the fastest and most effective drug for managing dystonia. IM benztropine should be administered to prevent asphyxia or aspiration in a client who is experiencing muscle rigidity caused by haloperidol.

To minimize the risk of adverse drug reactions, the client should take benztropine as a single dose at bedtime.

An antiparkinson agent such as amantadine may be used to control pseudo-parkinsonism; diphenhydramine or benztropine may be used to control other extrapyramidal effects.

Anticholinergics such as atropine were the first agents used to treat parkinsonism. The numerous peripheral side effects have limited the uses of this drug class. The anticholinergics now used for parkinsonism are centrally acting and produce fewer side effects. Although they act on the CNS, autonomic effects such as dry mouth, blurred vision, tachycardia, urinary retention, and constipation are still troublesome. The centrally acting anticholinergics are not as effective as levodopa at relieving severe symptoms of parkinsonism. They are used early in the course of the disease when symptoms are less severe, in clients who cannot tolerate levodopa, and in combination therapy with other antiparkinson drugs.

Nursing Considerations

The following content provides nursing considerations that apply to anticholinergics when given to treat parkinsonism. For the complete nursing process applied to anticholinergic therapy, see Nursing Process Focus: Clients Receiving Anticholinergic Therapy in Chapter 14 on page 148.

The role of the nurse in anticholinergic therapy for parkinsonism involves careful monitoring of the client's condition and providing education as it relates to the prescribed drug regimen. As with clients taking dopaminergic drugs, the nurse needs to carefully evaluate and monitor clients who are taking anticholinergic drugs. Before a client begins treatment, a thorough health history should be obtained. Clients under the age of 3 years and those with known hypersensitivity, narrow-angle glaucoma, myasthenia gravis, or obstruction of the urinary or gastrointestinal (GI) tract should not take cholinergic blockers. These drugs should be used carefully in older adults (due to slowed metabolism), in clients who have dysrhythmias or benign prostatic hypertrophy (BPH), and in pregnant or lactating women. Before treatment begins, the nurse should obtain a medication history and a complete physical that includes complete blood count, liver and renal function studies, vital signs, mental status, and progression of Parkinson's disease to establish baseline data. These tests should be repeated throughout the treatment to help determine effectiveness of the drug.

Client education as it relates to anticholinergics should include goals, reasons for obtaining baseline data, and possible side effects. The following are important points to include when teaching clients and caregivers about anticholinergics:

- To help relieve dry mouth, take frequent drinks of cool liquids, suck on sugarless hard candy or ice chips, and chew sugarless gum.
- Take with food or milk to prevent GI upset.
- Be evaluated by an eye specialist periodically, as anticholinergics may promote glaucoma development.
- Avoid driving and other hazardous activities because drowsiness may occur. Do not abruptly discontinue taking the drug, as withdrawal symptoms such as tremors, insomnia, and restlessness may occur.
- Avoid use of alcohol.
- Notify the healthcare provider if the following side effects or adverse reactions occur: disorientation, depression, hallucinations, confusion, memory impairment, nervousness, psychoses, vision changes, nausea/vomiting, urinary retention, dysuria.
- Wear dark glasses and avoid bright sunlight as necessary.

NCLEX Success Tip

The nurse should teach the client and family the importance of not discontinuing benztropine abruptly. Rather, the drug should be tapered slowly over a 1-week period. Benztropine should not be used with over-the-counter cough and cold preparations because of the risk of an additive anticholinergic effect. Antacids delay the absorption of benztropine, and alcohol in combination with benztropine causes an increase in central nervous system depression; concomitant use should be avoided.

TABLE 20.3 Anticholinergic Drugs Used for Parkinsonism	
Drug	**Route and Adult Dose**
Pr benztropine (Cogentin)	PO, 0.5–1 mg/day; gradually increase as needed (max 6 mg/day)
diphenhydramine (Benadryl) (see Chapter 42, page 504, for the Prototype Drug box)	PO, 25–50 mg tid or qid (max 300 mg/day)
procyclidine	PO, 2.5 mg tid after meals; gradually increase dose if needed (max 30 mg/day in 3 or 4 divided doses)
trihexyphenidyl	PO, start with 1 mg/day; increase by 2 mg increments at intervals of 3–5 days; usual dose is 6-10 mg/day in 3 to 4 divided doses; doses of 12–15 mg/day may be required

---

PROTOTYPE DRUG Benztropine (Cogentin)

Actions and Uses: Benztropine acts by blocking excess cholinergic stimulation of neurons in the corpus striatum. It is used for relief of parkinsonism symptoms and for the treatment of EPS brought on by antipsychotic pharmacotherapy. This medication suppresses tremors but does not affect tardive dyskinesia.

Administration Alerts:

- The client may be unable to self-administer medication and may need assistance.
- Benztropine may be taken in divided doses, two to four times a day, or the entire day's dose may be taken at bedtime.
- If muscle weakness occurs, dose should be reduced.
- Benztropine is pregnancy category C.

Pharmacokinetics: Benztropine is well absorbed after oral or IM administration. Distribution, metabolism, excretion, and half-life are unknown.

Adverse Effects and Interactions: As expected from its autonomic action, benztropine can cause typical anticholinergic side effects such as sedation, dry mouth, constipation, and tachycardia.

Benztropine interacts with many drugs. For example, benztropine should not be taken with tricyclic antidepressants, MAO inhibitors, phenothiazines, procainamide (Procan), or quinidine (Quinate) because of combined sedative effects. Over-the-counter (OTC) cold medicines and alcohol should be avoided. Other drugs that enhance dopamine release or activation of the dopamine receptor may produce additive effects. Haloperidol will cause decreased effectiveness.

Antihistamines, phenothiazines, tricyclics, disopyramide, and quinidine may increase anticholinergic effects, and antidiarrheals may decrease absorption.

ALZHEIMER'S DISEASE

Alzheimer's disease is a devastating, progressive, degenerative disease that generally begins after age 60. By age 85, as much as 25% of the population may be affected. Pharmacotherapy has limited success in improving the cognitive function of clients with Alzheimer's disease.

Characteristics of Alzheimer's Disease

20.5 Alzheimer's disease is a progressive, degenerative disease of older adults. Primary symptoms include disorientation, confusion, and memory loss.

An estimated 750 000 Canadians over the age of 65 have Alzheimer's disease and other dementias. **Alzheimer's disease (AD)** is responsible for about 65% of all dementia. **Dementia** is a degenerative disorder characterized by progressive memory loss, confusion, and an inability to think or communicate effectively. Consciousness and perception are usually unaffected. Known causes of dementia include multiple cerebral infarcts, severe infections, and toxins. Although the cause of most dementia is unknown, it is usually associated with cerebral atrophy or other structural changes within the brain. The client generally lives 5 to 10 years following diagnosis; AD is the fourth leading cause of death.

Despite extensive, ongoing research, the cause of Alzheimer's disease remains unknown. The early-onset familial form of this disorder, which accounts for about 10% of cases, is associated with gene defects on chromosome 1, 14, or 21. Chronic inflammation and excess free radicals may cause neuron damage. Environmental, immunological, and nutritional factors, as well as viruses, are considered possible sources of brain damage.

Although the cause may be unknown, structural damage in the brain of clients with AD has been well documented. **Amyloid plaques** and **neurofibrillary tangles** found within the brain at autopsy are present in nearly all clients with AD. It is suspected that these structural changes are caused by chronic inflammatory or oxidative cellular damage to the surrounding neurons. There is a loss in both the number and the function of neurons.

Clients with AD experience a dramatic loss of ability to perform tasks that require acetylcholine as the neurotransmitter. Because acetylcholine is a major neurotransmitter within the **hippocampus**, an area of the brain responsible for learning and memory, and other parts of the cerebral cortex, neuronal function within these brain areas is especially affected. Therefore, an inability to remember and to recall information is among the early symptoms of AD. Symptoms of this disease are as follows:

- Impaired memory and judgment
- Confusion or disorientation
- Inability to recognize family or friends
- Aggressive behaviour
- Depression
- Psychoses, including paranoia and delusions
- Anxiety

DRUGS FOR ALZHEIMER'S DISEASE

Drugs for AD are used to slow memory loss and other progressive symptoms of dementia. Some drugs are given to treat associated symptoms such as depression, anxiety, or psychoses. The acetylcholinesterase inhibitors are the most widely used class of drug for treating AD. These agents are shown in Table 20.4. Memantine (Ebixa), the first of a new class of drug called glutamergic inhibitors, was approved in 2003.

NCLEX Success Tips

Memantine and donepezil (Aricept) are commonly given together. Neither medicine will improve dementia, but they may slow the progression. Neither medicine is more effective than the other; they act differently in the brain. Both medicines have a half-life of 60 or more hours.

Abrupt cessation of donepezil may result in rapid deterioration of client functioning, which often is not reversible, even when the agent is added back to therapy.

When compared with other similar medications, donepezil has fewer adverse effects. The drug helps to slow the progression of the disease if started in the early stages.

TABLE 20.4   Agents Used for Alzheimer's Disease

Drug	Route and Adult Dose
Pr donepezil (Aricept)	PO, 5–10 mg/day
galantamine (Reminyl)	PO, ER tablet: start with 8 mg/day and if tolerated increase to 16 mg/day after 4 weeks; if tolerated can further increase to 24 mg/day (normal range is 16–24 mg/day)
memantine (Ebixa)	PO, 5 mg/day; increase dose by 5 mg/day to a target dose of 20 mg/day; doses > 5 mg/day should be given in 2 divided doses
rivastigmine (Exelon)	PO, start with 1.5 mg bid with food; may increase by 1.5 mg bid every 2 weeks (q2wk) if tolerated; target dose of 3–6 mg bid (max 12 mg bid)

Treating Alzheimer's Disease with Acetylcholinesterase Inhibitors

20.6 Acetylcholinesterase inhibitors are used to slow the progression of Alzheimer's disease symptoms. These agents have minimal efficacy and do not cure the dementia.

Health Canada has approved only a few drugs for AD. The most effective of these medications act by intensifying the effect of acetylcholine at the cholinergic receptor, as shown in Figure 20.2. Acetylcholine is naturally degraded in the synapse by the enzyme acetylcholinesterase (AchE). When AchE is inhibited, acetylcholine levels become elevated and produce a more profound effect on the receptor. As described in Chapter 13, the acetylcholinesterase inhibitors are indirect-acting cholinergics.

When treating AD, the goal of pharmacotherapy is to improve function in three domains: activities of daily living, behaviour, and cognition. Although the acetylcholinesterase inhibitors improve all three domains, their efficacy is modest at best. These agents do not cure AD; they only slow its progression. Therapy is begun as soon as the diagnosis of AD is established. These agents are ineffective in treating the severe stages of this disorder, probably because so many neurons have died; increasing the levels of acetylcholine is only effective if there are functioning neurons present. Often, as the disease progresses, the acetylcholinesterase inhibitors are discontinued; their therapeutic benefit is not enough to outweigh their expense or the risk for side effects.

All acetylcholinesterase inhibitors used to treat AD have equal efficacy. Side effects are those expected of drugs that enhance the parasympathetic nervous system (Chapter 12). The GI system is most affected, with nausea, vomiting, and diarrhea being reported. Of the agents available for AD, rivastigmine (Exelon) is associated with weight loss, a potentially serious side effect in some elderly clients. When discontinuing therapy, doses of the acetylcholinesterase inhibitors should be lowered gradually.

Although acetylcholinesterase inhibitors are the mainstay of treatment for AD dementia, several other agents are being investigated for their possible benefit in delaying the progression of AD. Because at least some of the neuronal changes in AD are caused by oxidative cellular damage, antioxidants such as vitamin E are being examined for their effects in clients with AD. Other agents currently being examined are anti-inflammatory agents (such as the COX-2 inhibitors), estrogen, and *Ginkgo biloba*.

Agitation occurs in the majority of clients with AD. This may be accompanied by delusions, paranoia, hallucinations, or other psychotic symptoms. Atypical antipsychotic agents such as risperidone and olanzapine may be used to control these episodes. Conventional antipsychotics such as haloperidol are occasionally prescribed, though extrapyramidal side effects often limit their use. The pharmacotherapy of psychosis is discussed in Chapter 19.

Although not as common as agitation, anxiety and depression may occur in clients with AD. Anxiolytics such as buspirone (BuSpar) or some of the benzodiazepines are used to control excessive anxiousness (Chapter 16). Mood stabilizers, such as sertraline (Zoloft), citalopram (Celexa), or fluoxetine (Prozac), are given when major depression interferes with daily activities (Chapter 17).

Nursing Considerations

The following content provides nursing considerations that apply to acetylcholinesterase inhibitors when given to treat Alzheimer's disease. For the complete nursing process applied to acetylcholinesterase inhibitor therapy, see Nursing Process Focus: Clients Receiving Cholinergic Therapy in Chapter 13 on page 140.

The role of the nurse in acetylcholinesterase inhibitor therapy involves carefully monitoring the client's condition and providing education as it relates to the prescribed drug regimen. Prior to the initiation of drug therapy, the client's health history should be taken. Young children and those with hypersensitivity should not take acetylcholinesterase inhibitors. Clients with narrow-angle glaucoma or undiagnosed skin lesions should not take rivastigmine. All acetylcholinesterase inhibitors should be used cautiously in clients with severe cardiac, renal, liver, or respiratory diseases (such as asthma or chronic obstructive pulmonary disease), a history of seizures, GI bleeding or peptic ulcers, and those who are pregnant or lactating. Lab testing, including a complete blood count and liver and renal function tests, should be done initially and throughout the treatment regimen. Baseline vital signs should be taken. During initial treatment, vital signs should be closely monitored, as these medications may cause hypotension. A full assessment of mental status and other signs of Alzheimer's disease should be done to provide a baseline and determine effectiveness of medication. All other medications taken by the client should be fully evaluated for interactions with acetylcholinesterase inhibitors.

The nurse should monitor clients for side effects or reactions such as changes in mental status, mood changes, dizziness, confusion, insomnia, nausea, vomiting, and anorexia. Client education as it relates to acetylcholinesterase inhibitors should include goals, reasons for obtaining baseline data, and possible side effects.

Nurses may care for clients with AD in acute or long-term care facilities or may provide support and education for caregivers in the home. Families and clients who are able to understand must be made aware that currently available medications may

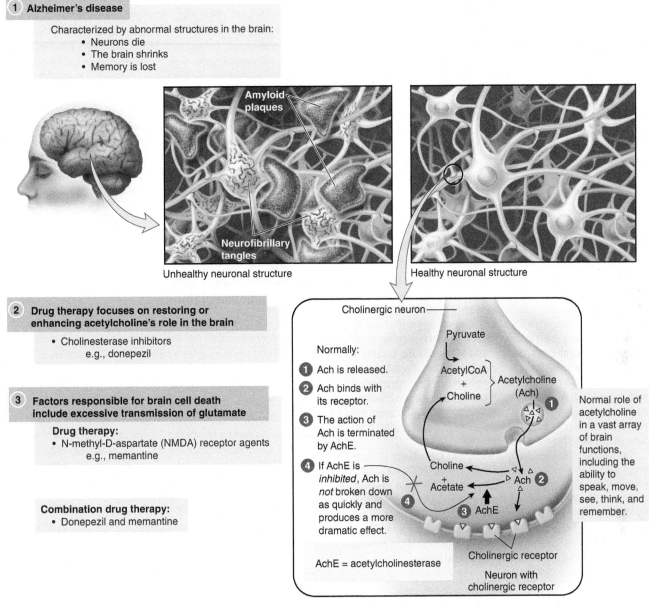

1 Alzheimer's disease

Characterized by abnormal structures in the brain:
- Neurons die
- The brain shrinks
- Memory is lost

Amyloid plaques

Neurofibrillary tangles

Unhealthy neuronal structure

Healthy neuronal structure

2 Drug therapy focuses on restoring or enhancing acetylcholine's role in the brain
- Cholinesterase inhibitors
  e.g., donepezil

3 Factors responsible for brain cell death include excessive transmission of glutamate

Drug therapy:
- N-methyl-D-aspartate (NMDA) receptor agents
  e.g., memantine

Combination drug therapy:
- Donepezil and memantine

Cholinergic neuron

Pyruvate

Normally:

1 Ach is released.

2 Ach binds with its receptor.

3 The action of Ach is terminated by AchE.

4 If AchE is *inhibited*, Ach is *not* broken down as quickly and produces a more dramatic effect.

AchE = acetylcholinesterase

AcetylCoA + Choline

Acetylcholine (Ach)

Choline + Acetate

AchE

Cholinergic receptor

Neuron with cholinergic receptor

Normal role of acetylcholine in a vast array of brain functions, including the ability to speak, move, see, think, and remember.

Figure 20.2 Alzheimer's disease drugs work by intensifying the effect of acetylcholine at the receptor.

slow the progression of the disease but not effect a cure. In addition, the nurse should include the following points when educating clients and caregivers about acetylcholinesterase inhibitors:

- Take with food or milk to decrease GI upset.
- Take the drug strictly as prescribed or serious side effects may result.
- Report any changes in mental status or mood.
- Report the following side effects to the healthcare provider: dizziness, confusion, insomnia, constipation, nausea, urinary frequency, GI bleeding, vomiting, seizures, and anorexia.
- Make appointments with the healthcare provider on a regular basis.
- To help relieve dry mouth, take frequent drinks of cool liquids, suck on sugarless hard candy, or chew sugarless gum.
- Increase fibre and fluid consumption to prevent constipation.

- Recognize symptoms of overdose: severe nausea/vomiting, sweating, salivation, hypotension, bradycardia, convulsions, and increased muscle weakness, including respiratory muscles; if noted, contact the healthcare provider immediately.

PROTOTYPE DRUG | **Donepezil (Aricept)**

Actions and Uses: Donepezil is an acetylcholinesterase inhibitor that improves memory in cases of mild to moderate Alzheimer's dementia by enhancing the effects of acetylcholine in neurons in the cerebral cortex that have not yet been damaged. Clients should receive pharmacotherapy for at least 6 months prior to assessing maximum benefits of drug therapy. Improvement in memory may be observed as early as 1 to 4 weeks following initiation of the medication. The therapeutic effects of donepezil are often

◀ *Ginkgo biloba* **for Treatment of Dementia**

Ginkgo biloba has been used for many years to improve memory. In Europe, an extract of this herb is already approved for the treatment of dementia. In one study, 120 mg of ginkgo taken daily was shown to improve mental functioning and stabilize Alzheimer's disease. In other studies, clinical results were seen between 4 weeks and 6 months of treatment and were found to be relevant. Clients need to speak with their healthcare provider before taking this herb. Although most clients can take ginkgo without problems, those on anticoagulants may have an increased risk for bleeding.

◀ **Living with Alzheimer's or Parkinson's Disease**

Both Alzheimer's and Parkinson's disease are progressive, degenerative, neurological disorders. While Alzheimer's disease leads to impairments in memory, thinking, and reasoning, Parkinson's disease can lead to the inability to hold small items due to tremors and rigidity. It is because of these progressive symptoms that clients need all the help and support that caregivers can provide. While non-pharmacological management such as providing a safe environment can help, medications are available to slow the progression and minimize symptoms. Caregivers will need to provide assistance with activities of daily living, including making sure that these clients receive their medications.

For clients with Alzheimer's disease, the side effects of some drugs used to control dementia can disrupt sleep. Additionally, people with dementia often suffer sleep apnea. In addition to providing a routine and structured environment, new research suggests that as little as a few hours of bright light, especially in the evening, may help people living with Alzheimer's disease to maintain a normal sleeping pattern. Clients who received light therapy in the evening also experienced an improvement in their sleep cycle.

short lived, and the degree of improvement is modest at best. It is important to note that once donepezil is discontinued, any benefit that was gained may be lost. Even if it is then added back, the client might not be able to gain back the benefit the medication once had. An advantage of donepezil over other drugs in its class is that its long half-life permits it to be given once daily.

Administration Alerts:

- Give medication prior to bedtime.
- Medication is most effective when given on a regular schedule.
- Donepezil is pregnancy category C.

Pharmacokinetics: Donepezil is well absorbed after oral administration. Distribution is unknown. It is about 96% protein bound. It is mostly metabolized by the liver, with less than 20% excreted unchanged by the kidneys. Its half-life is 70 hours.

Adverse Effects and Interactions: Common side effects of donepezil are vomiting, diarrhea, and darkened urine. CNS side effects include insomnia, syncope, depression, headache, and irritability. Musculoskeletal side effects include muscle cramps, arthritis, and bone fractures. Generalized side effects include headache, fatigue, chest pain, increased libido, hot flashes, urinary incontinence, dehydration, and blurred vision. Hepatotoxicity has not been observed. Clients with bradycardia, hypotension, asthma, hyperthyroidism, or active peptic ulcer disease should be monitored carefully. Anticholinergics will be less effective. Donepezil interacts with several other drugs. For example, bethanechol (Duvoid) causes a synergistic effect. Phenobarbital (Phenobarb), phenytoin (Dilantin), dexamethasone (Dexasone), and rifampin (Rifadin, Rofact) may speed elimination of donepezil. Quinidine or ketoconazole (Nizoral) may inhibit metabolism of donepezil. Because donepezil acts by increasing cholinergic activity, other drugs with cholinergic effects should not be administered concurrently.

MULTIPLE SCLEROSIS

20.7 Multiple sclerosis is a chronic neurodegenerative disease that is treated with immunomodulator drugs.

Multiple sclerosis (MS) is a neurodegenerative disease characterized by demyelination, the destruction or removal of the myelin sheath from a nerve or nerve fibre. The destruction is secondary to an inflammatory response that leads to random areas of demyelination, known as plaques, in the white matter of the CNS. The exact cause of MS is unknown. It is believed that a pathogen, such as a latent virus, may trigger an abnormal autoimmune response in clients who are genetically susceptible. MS is a leading cause of neurological disability in the 20- to 40-year-old age group, although it may affect persons of any age (Figure 20.3).

(a) Normal neuron

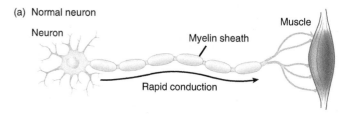

(b) Early stage of multiple sclerosis

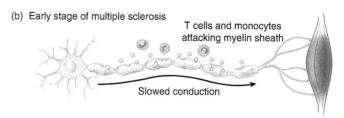

(c) Late stage of multiple sclerosis

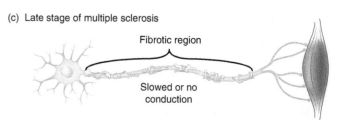

Figure 20.3 Multiple sclerosis.

MS has a typical pattern of progression that is characterized by periods of symptom exacerbation alternating with periods of remission during which symptoms completely disappear. Remissions may last several months or even years. Less commonly, progression may be continuous without any clear remission periods.

Diagnosis of MS is often difficult because its symptoms mimic those of other neurological disorders. The early symptoms are frequently vague and nonspecific and include weakness, visual disturbances, paresthesias, mild affective disturbances, and difficulty with bladder control. Cognitive impairment is common. It should be determined if the symptoms are worsening or are intermittent. Also of note is whether the activity level of the client has decreased, along with worsening fatigue, things that aggravate the symptoms (e.g., hot showers or baths, overexertion, stress), and any changes in personality or behaviour. A diagnosis is made after other neurological disorders have been ruled out. Imaging studies such as magnetic resonance imaging are useful in identifying the areas of demyelination in the brain.

Like other neurodegenerative disorders, there are no drugs available that can cure MS or reverse the progressive demyelination of nerves. Existing drugs for MS are only partially effective, and some have serious adverse effects. In general, pharmacotherapy for MS has the following three goals:

- Modify the progression of the disease
- Treat acute exacerbations
- Manage symptoms

Drugs for Modifying the Progression of Multiple Sclerosis

Although the exact cause of MS remains unknown, it is considered an autoimmune disease. The body has mounted an immune attack against its own tissues—in this case, the myelin surrounding nerves. Strategies for slowing the progression of MS have therefore focused on modifying the abnormal immune response of these clients through the application of immunomodulators. **Immunomodulator** is a general term that refers to drugs that affect body defences. There are two basic types of immunomodulators: those that stimulate or boost the immune response and those that suppress some aspect of immune function. Both types are used in MS pharmacotherapy. For detailed information on the immunomodulators, the student should refer to Chapter 40.

The immunomodulators are used to prevent exacerbations in clients with MS. They can decrease the number of new plaques being formed within the CNS, delay future disability, and help clients to maintain their present quality of life. Immunomodulators are initiated soon after the diagnosis of MS is confirmed. The earlier treatment is begun, the better chance the client has of avoiding or delaying permanent neurological deficits. Treatment should continue indefinitely and be stopped only if toxicity develops or there is no apparent benefit. The immunomodulators have equal efficacy in treating MS. Selection is frequently based on the clinical experiences of the healthcare provider and client tolerance.

CHAPTER 20 Understanding the Chapter

Key Concepts Summary

The numbered key concepts provide a succinct summary of the important points from the corresponding numbered section within the chapter. If any of these points are not clear, refer to the numbered section within the chapter for review.

20.1 Degenerative diseases of the nervous system, such as Parkinson's disease and Alzheimer's disease, cause a progressive loss of neuron function.

20.2 Parkinson's disease is characterized by symptoms of tremors, muscle rigidity, and postural instability and ambulation caused by the destruction of dopamine-producing neurons within the corpus striatum. The underlying biochemical problem is lack of dopamine activity and a related hyperactivity of acetylcholine.

20.3 The most commonly used medications for parkinsonism attempt to restore levels of dopamine in the corpus striatum of the brain. Levodopa, enhanced by combination with carbidopa, is the drug of choice for Parkinson's disease.

20.4 Centrally acting anticholinergic drugs are sometimes used to relieve symptoms of parkinsonism, although they are less effective than levodopa.

20.5 Alzheimer's disease is a progressive, degenerative disease of older adults. Primary symptoms include disorientation, confusion, and memory loss.

20.6 Acetylcholinesterase inhibitors are used to slow the progression of Alzheimer's disease symptoms. These agents have minimal efficacy and do not cure the dementia.

20.7 Multiple sclerosis is a chronic neurodegenerative disease that is treated with immunomodulator drugs.

Chapter 20 Scenario

Mary Lee is a 73-year-old retired high school principal with a PhD in educational administration. She has been married to Robert for almost 50 years, and they have three grown children. Mary's physical health has been good. She has mild hypertension and had colon cancer successfully removed 20 years ago. She has an annual physical and cancer screenings as recommended for her age. Robert makes an appointment with Mary's healthcare provider because he has noticed signs of decreasing mental acuity in Mary over the past year. Mary's physical exam is negative, but the healthcare provider suspects that she is experiencing the early stage of AD. Mary is started on donepezil (Aricept), 5 mg at bedtime.

Critical Thinking Questions

1. What information should be included in the initial assessment in order to determine a diagnosis for Mary?
2. What recommendations will the healthcare provider most likely make to Mary and her husband?
3. What should Robert be alert for with regard to the donepezil?

See Answers to Critical Thinking Questions in Appendix B.

NCLEX Practice Questions

1 A client is receiving levodopa-carbidopa (Sinemet) for parkinsonism. Which drug would the nurse expect to be added to the client's drug regimen to help control tremors?

a. Amantadine

b. Benztropine (Cogentin)

c. Haloperidol (Haldol)

d. Donepezil (Aricept)

2 Which statement made by the client would alert the nurse that the antiparkinson medication is effective?

a. "I'm sleeping a lot more, especially during the day."

b. "My appetite has improved."

c. "I'm able to shower by myself."

d. "My skin doesn't itch anymore."

3 A nurse is counselling the caregivers of a client with Alzheimer's disease. Which statement by a caregiver would indicate that the session had been effective?

a. "I should give this medication as symptoms of AD become noticeable."

b. "If constipation occurs, I will notify the healthcare provider immediately."

c. "The medication may improve symptoms, but it will not cure the disease."

d. "I will take the client's vital signs before every dose of the medication."

4 Which of the following would a nurse know to be a major disadvantage of the use of donepezil (Aricept) to treat the symptoms of early Alzheimer's disease? Select all that apply.

a. It must be administered four times per day.

b. It causes constipation.

c. It may cause vision difficulties.

d. It may cause potentially life-threatening cardiac dysrhythmias.

e. It can be purchased over the counter.

5 Dopamine precursors and anticholinergics are all used in the management of Parkinson's disease because they

a. Increase dopamine activity in the basal ganglia

b. Induce regeneration of neurons in the basal ganglia

c. Prevent progression of the disease

d. Produce excitation of basal ganglia structures

See Answers to NCLEX Practice Questions in Appendix A.

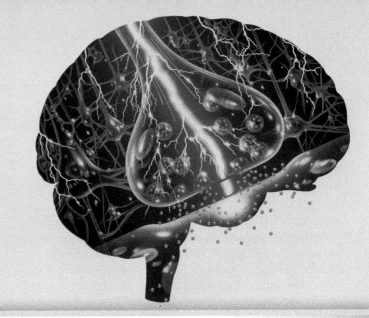

John Bavosi/SPL/Science Source

CHAPTER

21

Pharmacotherapy of Seizures

LEARNING OUTCOMES

After reading this chapter, the student should be able to:

1. Understand the causes of epilepsy.
2. Differentiate among the following terms: *epilepsy*, *seizures*, and *convulsions*.
3. Identify drug classes used for treating epilepsy and seizures.
4. For each of the drug classes listed in Prototype Drugs, identify a representative drug and explain its mechanism of action, primary actions, and important adverse effects.
5. Describe the nurse's role in the pharmacological management of clients with epilepsy.
6. Describe and explain, based on pharmacological principles, the rationale for nursing assessment, planning, and interventions for clients with epilepsy.
7. Explain the importance of client adherence in the pharmacotherapy of epilepsy.
8. Use the nursing process to care for clients who are receiving drug therapy for epilepsy.

CHAPTER OUTLINE

▸ Seizures

  ▸ Causes of Seizures

  ▸ Types of Seizures

  ▸ General Concepts of Epilepsy Pharmacotherapy

  ▸ Treating Seizures with Barbiturates and Miscellaneous GABA Agents

  ▸ Treating Seizures with Benzodiazepines

▸ Drugs That Suppress Sodium Influx

  ▸ Treating Seizures with Hydantoins and Phenytoin-Like Drugs

▸ Drugs That Suppress Calcium Influx

  ▸ Treating Seizures with Succinimides

Epilepsy is a common neurological disease. **Epilepsy** may be defined as any disorder characterized by recurrent seizures. The symptoms of epilepsy depend on the type of seizure and may include blackout, fainting spells, sensory disturbances, jerking body movements, and temporary loss of memory. Epilepsy affects approximately 0.6% of Canadians. This chapter examines the pharmacotherapy used to treat the different types of seizures.

SEIZURES

A **seizure** is a disturbance of electrical activity in the brain that may affect consciousness, motor activity, and sensation. The symptoms of seizure are caused by abnormal or uncontrollable neuronal discharges within the brain. These abnormal discharges can be measured using an electroencephalogram (EEG), a valuable tool in diagnosing seizure disorders. Figure 21.1 compares normal and abnormal EEG recordings.

The terms *convulsion* and *seizure* are not synonymous. **Convulsions** specifically refer to involuntary, violent spasms of the large skeletal muscles of the face, neck, arms, and legs. Although some types of seizures do indeed involve convulsions, other seizures do not. Therefore, it may be stated that all convulsions are seizures but not all seizures are convulsions. Because of this difference, agents used to treat epilepsy should correctly be called antiseizure medications, rather than anticonvulsants.

Causes of Seizures

21.1 Seizures are associated with many causes, including head trauma, brain infection, fluid and electrolyte imbalance, hypoxia, stroke, brain tumours, and high fever in children.

A seizure is considered a symptom of an underlying disorder rather than a disease in itself. There are many different causes of seizure activity. Seizures can result from acute situations or occur on a chronic basis, as with epilepsy. In some cases, the exact etiology may not be identified. The following are known causes of seizures:

- *Infectious diseases:* Acute infections such as meningitis and encephalitis can cause inflammation in the brain.

- *Trauma:* Physical trauma such as direct blows to the skull may increase intracranial pressure; chemical trauma such as the presence of toxic substances or the ingestion of poisons may cause brain injury.

- *Metabolic disorders:* Changes in fluid and electrolytes such as hypoglycemia, hyponatremia, and water intoxication may cause seizures by altering electrical impulse transmission at the cellular level.

- *Vascular diseases:* Changes in oxygenation, such as that caused by respiratory hypoxia and carbon monoxide poisoning, and changes in perfusion, such as that caused by hypotension,

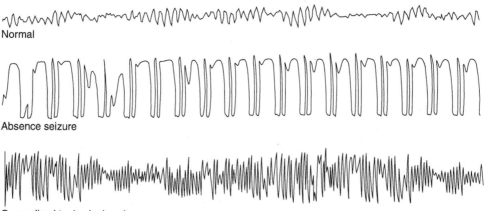

Normal

Absence seizure

Generalized tonic-clonic seizure

Figure 21.1 EEG recordings showing the differences between normal, absence seizure, and generalized tonic-clonic seizure tracings.

cerebral vascular accidents, shock, and cardiac dysrhythmias, may be causes.

- *Pediatric disorders:* Rapid increase in body temperature may result in a febrile seizure.
- *Neoplastic disease:* Tumours, especially rapidly growing ones, may occupy space, increase intracranial pressure, and damage brain tissue by disrupting blood flow.

Certain medications for mood disorders, psychoses, and local anesthesia, when given in high doses, may cause seizures because of increased levels of stimulatory neurotransmitters. Seizures may also occur from drug abuse, as with cocaine, or during withdrawal syndromes from alcohol or sedative-hypnotic drugs.

Pregnancy is a major concern for clients with epilepsy. Additional barrier methods of birth control should be practised to avoid unintended pregnancy, as some antiseizure medications decrease the effectiveness of oral contraceptives. Most antiseizure drugs are pregnancy category D. Clients should consult with their healthcare provider prior to pregnancy to determine the most appropriate plan of action for seizure control, given their seizure history. Because some antiseizure drugs may cause folate deficiency, a condition correlated with increased risk for neural tube defects, vitamin supplements may be necessary. Pregnant women may experience seizures with eclampsia, a pregnancy-induced hypertensive disorder.

In some cases, the cause of the seizures cannot be found. Clients may have a lower tolerance to environmental triggers, and seizures may occur when the client is sleep deprived, is exposed to strobe or flickering lights, or experiences small fluid and electrolyte imbalances. Seizures represent the most common serious neurological problem affecting children, with an overall incidence approaching 2% for febrile seizures and 1% for idiopathic epilepsy. Seizures that result from acute situations generally do not reoccur after the situation has been resolved. If a brain abnormality exists after the acute situation resolves, continuing seizures are likely.

Seizures can have a significant impact on quality of life. They may cause serious injury if they occur while a person is driving a vehicle or performing a dangerous activity. Without

pharmacotherapy, epilepsy can severely limit participation in school, employment, and social activities and can affect self-esteem. Chronic depression may accompany poorly controlled seizures. However, proper treatment can eliminate seizures completely in many clients. Important considerations in nursing care include identifying clients at risk for seizures, documenting the pattern and type of seizure activity, and implementing safety precautions. In collaboration with the client, healthcare provider, and pharmacist, the nurse is instrumental in achieving positive therapeutic outcomes. Through a combination of pharmacotherapy, client-family support, and education, effective seizure control can be achieved by the majority of clients.

Types of Seizures

21.2 The three broad categories of seizure are partial seizures, generalized seizures, and special epileptic syndromes. Each seizure type has a characteristic set of signs, and different drugs are used for different types.

The differing presentation of seizures relates to the areas of the brain affected by the abnormal electrical activity. Symptoms of a seizure can range from sudden, violent shaking and total loss of consciousness (LOC) to muscle twitching or slight tremor of a limb. Staring into space, altered vision, and difficulty speaking are other symptoms a person may exhibit during a seizure. Determining the cause of recurrent seizures is important in order to plan appropriate treatment options.

Methods of classifying epilepsy have evolved over time. The terms *grand mal* and *petit mal* epilepsy have, for the most part, been replaced by more descriptive and detailed categorization. Epilepsies are typically identified using the International Classification of Epileptic Seizures nomenclature as partial (focal), generalized, or special epileptic syndromes. Types of partial or generalized seizures may be recognized based on symptoms observed during a seizure episode. Some symptoms are subtle and reflect the simple nature of neuronal misfiring in specific areas of the brain; others are more complex.

Partial Seizures

Partial (focal) seizures involve a limited portion of the brain. They may start on one side and travel only a short distance before they stop. The area where the abnormal electrical activity starts is known as an abnormal focus (plural = *foci*).

Simple partial seizures have an onset that may begin as a small, limited focus and subsequently progress to a generalized seizure. Clients with simple partial seizures may feel for a brief moment that their precise location is vague, and they may hear and see things that are not there. Some clients smell and taste things that are not present or have an upset stomach. Others may become emotional and experience a sense of joy, sorrow, or grief. The arms, legs, or face may twitch.

Complex partial seizures (formerly known as psychomotor or temporal lobe seizures) show sensory, motor, or autonomic symptoms with some degree of altered or impaired consciousness. Total loss of consciousness may not occur during a complex partial seizure, but a brief period of somnolence or confusion may follow the seizure. Such seizures are often preceded by an aura that is often described as an unpleasant odour or taste. Seizures may start with a blank stare, and clients may begin to chew or swallow repetitively. Some clients fumble with clothing; others may try to take off their clothes. Most clients will not pay attention to verbal commands and act as if they are having a psychotic episode. After the seizure, clients do not remember the seizure incident.

Generalized Seizures

As the name suggests, **generalized seizures** are not localized to one area but travel throughout the entire brain on both sides. The seizure is thought to originate bilaterally and symmetrically within the brain.

Absence seizures (formerly known as petit mal seizures) most often occur in children and last for only a few seconds. Absence seizures involve a loss or reduction of normal activity. Staring and transient loss of responsiveness are the most common signs, but there may be slight motor activity with eyelid fluttering or myoclonic jerks. Because these episodes are subtle and last for only a few seconds, absence epilepsy may go unrecognized for a long time or be mistaken for daydreaming or attention deficit disorder.

Atonic seizures are sometimes called drop attacks because clients often stumble and fall for no apparent reason. Episodes are very short, lasting only a matter of seconds.

Tonic-clonic seizures are the most common type of seizure in all age groups. Seizures may be preceded by an aura, a warning that some clients describe as a spiritual feeling, a flash of light, or a special noise. Intense muscle contractions indicate the tonic phase. A hoarse cry may occur at the onset of the seizure due to air being forced out of the lungs, and clients may temporarily lose bladder or bowel control. Breathing may become shallow and even stop momentarily. The clonic phase is characterized by alternating contraction and relaxation of muscles. The seizure usually lasts 1 to 2 minutes, after which the client becomes drowsy, disoriented, and sleeps deeply (known as the postictal state).

Special Epileptic Syndromes

Special epileptic seizures include the febrile seizures of infancy, reflex epilepsies, and other forms of myoclonic epilepsies. Myoclonic epilepsies often go along with other neurological abnormalities or progressive symptoms.

Febrile seizures typically cause tonic-clonic motor activity lasting for 1 or 2 minutes with rapid return of consciousness. They occur in conjunction with a rapid rise in body temperature and usually occur only once during any given illness. Febrile seizures are most likely to occur in the 3-month to 5-year age group, and as many as 5% of all children experience febrile seizures. Preventing the onset of high fever is the best way to control these seizures.

Myoclonic seizures are characterized by large, jerking body movements. Major muscle groups contract quickly, and clients appear unsteady and clumsy. They may fall from a sitting position or drop whatever they are holding. Infantile spasms exemplify a type of generalized, myoclonic seizure distinguished by short-lived

muscle spasms involving the trunk and extremities. Such spasms are often not identified as seizures by parents or healthcare providers because the movements are much like the normal infantile Moro (startle) reflex.

Status epilepticus is a medical emergency that occurs when a seizure is repeated continuously. It could occur with any type of seizure, but usually generalized tonic-clonic seizures are exhibited. When generalized tonic-clonic seizures are prolonged or continuous, the time in which breathing is affected by muscle contraction is lengthened and hypoxia may develop. The continuous muscle contraction also can lead to hypoglycemia, acidosis, and hypothermia due to increased metabolic needs, lactic acid production, and heat loss during contraction. Carbon dioxide retention also leads to acidosis. If not treated, status epilepticus could lead to brain damage and death. Medical treatment involves the intravenous (IV) administration of antiseizure medications. Steps must also be taken to ensure that the airway remains open.

General Concepts of Epilepsy Pharmacotherapy

21.3 Antiseizure drugs act by distinct mechanisms: potentiation of GABA and delaying the influx of sodium or calcium ions into neurons. Pharmacotherapy may continue for many years, and withdrawal from these agents must be done gradually to avoid seizure recurrence.

The choice of drug for epilepsy pharmacotherapy depends on the type of seizure the client is experiencing, the client's previous medical history, diagnostic studies, and the pathological processes causing the seizures. Once a medication is selected, the client is placed on a low initial dose. The amount is gradually increased until seizure control is achieved or the side effects of the drug prevent additional increases in dose. Serum drug levels may be obtained to assist the healthcare provider in determining the most effective drug concentration. If seizure activity continues, a

---

CONNECTIONS | **Lifespan Considerations**

◀ **Epilepsy across the Lifespan**

- Epilepsy affects 0.6% of the Canadian population.
- Epilepsy can occur at any age.
- About 30% of new cases begin in childhood, particularly in early childhood and around the time of adolescence.
- Another period of relatively high onset occurs after the age of 65 years.
- Drug dosages may require adjustment due to age-related changes in pharmacokinetics.
- Side effects may decrease drug adherence in all age groups.
- Older adults may experience more severe adverse effects.

Based on Epilepsy Canada, http://www.epilepsy.ca/eng/content/epidemio.html.

different medication is added in small dose increments while the dose of the first drug is slowly reduced. Because seizures are likely to occur with abrupt withdrawal, antiseizure medication is withdrawn over a period of 6 to 12 weeks.

In most cases, effective seizure management can be obtained using a single drug. In some clients, two antiseizure medications may be necessary to control seizure activity, although additional side effects may become evident. Some antiseizure drug combinations may actually increase the incidence of seizures. The nurse should consult current drug guides regarding compatibility before administering a second antiseizure agent.

Once seizures have been controlled, clients are continued indefinitely on the antiseizure drug. After several years of being seizure-free, clients may question the need for their medication. In general, withdrawal of antiseizure drugs should be attempted only after at least 3 years of being seizure-free and only under the close direction of the healthcare provider. Doses of medications are reduced slowly, one at a time, over a period of several months. If seizures recur during the withdrawal process, pharmacotherapy is resumed, usually with the same drug. The nurse must strongly urge clients to maintain adherence with pharmacotherapy and not attempt to discontinue antiseizure drug use without professional guidance. Table 21.1 shows antiseizure drugs, based on the type of seizure.

With a valid diagnosis of epilepsy, there is no substitute for effective antiseizure pharmacotherapy. There are situations, however, when the medicines cannot be tolerated. Sometimes another medical therapy, such as the ketogenic diet, is used, along with natural remedies.

Antiseizure pharmacotherapy is directed at controlling the movement of electrolytes across neuronal membranes or affecting neurotransmitter balance. In a resting state, neurons are normally surrounded by a higher concentration of sodium, calcium, and chloride ions. Potassium levels are higher inside the cell. An influx of sodium or calcium into the neuron *enhances* neuronal activity, whereas an influx of chloride *suppresses* neuronal activity.

The goal of antiseizure pharmacotherapy is to suppress neuronal activity just enough to prevent abnormal or repetitive firing. To this end, there are three general mechanisms by which antiseizure drugs act:

1. Stimulating an influx of chloride ions, an effect that potentiates the inhibitory neurotransmitter, gamma-aminobutyric acid (GABA)
2. Delaying an influx of sodium ions
3. Delaying an influx of calcium ions

Drugs That Potentiate GABA

Several important antiseizure drugs act by changing the action of **gamma-aminobutyric acid (GABA)**, the primary inhibitory neurotransmitter in the brain. These agents mimic the effects of GABA by stimulating an influx of chloride ions that interact with the GABA receptor–chloride channel complex. A model of this receptor is shown in Figure 21.2. When the receptor is stimulated, chloride ions move into the cell, thus suppressing the ability of neurons to fire.

Barbiturates, benzodiazepines, and several miscellaneous drugs reduce seizure activity by intensifying GABA action. The major effect of enhancing GABA activity is CNS depression. These agents are shown in Table 21.2. The antiseizure properties of phenobarbital (Phenobarb) were discovered in 1912, and the drug is still one of the most commonly prescribed for epilepsy.

Treating Seizures with Barbiturates and Miscellaneous GABA Agents

21.4 Barbiturates act by potentiating the effects of GABA. Phenobarbital is used for tonic-clonic and febrile seizures.

As a class, barbiturates have a low margin of safety, cause profound CNS depression, and have a high potential for dependence. Phenobarbital, however, is able to suppress abnormal neuronal discharges. It is inexpensive, long acting, and produces many side effects. When given orally, several weeks may be necessary to achieve optimum antiseizure activity.

TABLE 21.1 Drugs for the Management of Specific Types of Seizure

	Partial Seizures		Generalized Seizures	
	Simple, Complex	Absence	Atonic, Myoclonic	Tonic-Clonic, Status Epilepticus
Benzodiazepines				
diazepam (Valium)				✓
lorazepam (Ativan)				✓
Phenytoin-Like Agents				
phenytoin (Dilantin)	✓			✓
carbamazepine (Tegretol)	✓			✓
valproic acid (Depakene, Epival)	✓	✓	✓	✓
Succinimides				
ethosuximide (Zarontin)		✓	✓	

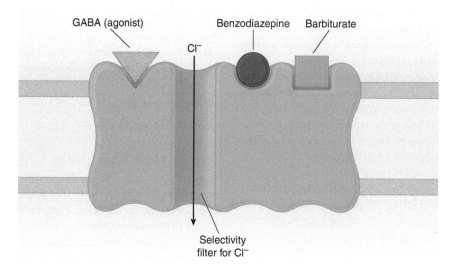

Figure 21.2 Model of the GABA receptor–chloride channel complex.

TABLE 21.2 Antiseizure Drugs That Potentiate GABA Action	
Drug	**Route and Adult Dose**
Barbiturates	
pentobarbital (Nembutal) **Pr** phenobarbital (Phenobarb)	Intramuscularly (IM), 150–200 mg in two divided doses; IV, 100 mg, may increase to 500 mg if necessary For seizures: Orally (PO), 60–200 mg/day or 50–100 mg 2 to 3 times daily For status epilepticus: IV, 20 mg/kg (infused at 50–100 mg/min); if necessary may repeat once after 10 minutes with an additional 5–10 mg/kg
Benzodiazepines (when used for seizures)	
clonazepam (Rivotril) clorazepate **Pr** diazepam (Valium) lorazepam (Ativan) (see Chapter 16, page 170, for the Prototype Drug box)	PO, 1.5 mg/day in three divided doses, increased by 0.5–1.0 mg every 3 days until seizures are controlled PO, 7.5 mg three times a day (tid) For status epilepticus: IM/IV, 5–10 mg (repeat as needed at 10- to 15-min intervals up to 30 mg max; if necessary, may repeat in 2–4 hours); IV push, administer emulsion at 5 mg/min For seizures: PO, 2–10 mg 2 to 4 times daily For status epilepticus: IV, 4 mg injected slowly at 2 mg/min; if inadequate response after 10 min, may repeat once
Miscellaneous Agents (for seizure control)	
gabapentin (Neurontin) primidone topiramate (Topamax)	PO, 300 mg tid; increase dosage based on response and tolerance; usual dose is 900–1800 mg/day administered in three divided doses PO, 250 mg/day; increased by 250 mg/week up to max of 2 g in two to four divided doses PO, start with 25 mg/day; increase to 25 mg bid in a few weeks; may increase further in weekly increments of 50 mg/day up to maximum amount of 200 mg bid

Other barbiturates are occasionally used for epilepsy. Amobarbital is an intermediate-acting barbiturate that is given by the IM or IV route to terminate status epilepticus. Unlike phenobarbital, which is a Schedule IV drug, amobarbital is a Schedule II drug and has a higher risk for dependence; it is not given orally as an antiseizure drug.

Several non-benzodiazepine/non-barbiturate agents act by the GABA mechanism. An example of these newer drugs, first approved in the 1990s, is gabapentin (Neurontin).

Nursing Considerations

The role of the nurse in barbiturate therapy for seizures involves careful monitoring of the client's condition and providing education as it relates to the prescribed drug regimen. Of those drugs that mimic or enhance GABA production, barbiturates produce the most pronounced adverse effects, including sedation and respiratory depression.

Barbiturates are metabolized in the liver and excreted primarily in urine. These drugs should be used with caution in clients with impaired hepatic or renal capacity; liver and kidney function must be monitored regularly with long-term usage. Barbiturates cross the placenta and are excreted in breast milk; therefore, they are not recommended for pregnant or nursing women. Assess female clients of childbearing age for pregnancy or intent to become pregnant. There is an increased risk of congenital malformations when the drug is taken during the first trimester (pregnancy category D). These drugs may also produce folic acid deficiency, which is associated with an increased risk of neural tube birth defects, including spina bifida and hydrocephalus. Barbiturates may also decrease the effectiveness of oral contraceptives.

Barbiturates produce biochemical changes at the cellular level that result in accelerated metabolism and subsequent depletion of nutrients such as vitamins D and K. Alterations in vitamin synthesis can result in reduced bone density (vitamin D deficiency) and impaired blood coagulability (vitamin K deficiency). Bleeding caused by vitamin K deficiency may present as simple bruising or petechiae or may manifest as a more serious adverse reaction, such as epistaxis, gastrointestinal (GI) bleeding, menorrhagia, or hematuria. Older adults can be particularly at risk for significant vitamin deficiency caused by barbiturates due to nutritional imbalances that may already exist because of aging. Diminished renal, hepatic, and respiratory function associated with aging also places older adults at risk of CNS depression. GABA-enhancing drugs may produce an idiosyncratic response in children, resulting in restlessness and psychomotor agitation.

The risk for respiratory depression must be considered when administering IV doses of barbiturates and when administering to clients with impaired respiratory function and those taking other CNS depressants. Monitor for common side effects such as drowsiness, dizziness, and postural hypotension, which increase a client's risk for injury. CNS depressants should not be stopped abruptly; abrupt cessation can result in potentially life-threatening rebound seizure activity. Clients should avoid consuming alcohol while taking barbiturates. The use of the herb *Ginkgo biloba* may decrease the antiseizure effect of these drugs. Concurrent use of other antiseizure drugs may also decrease their antiseizure effect.

Clients taking gabapentin should be monitored for dizziness and drowsiness. Drugs with GABA-intensifying action are not recommended for pregnant or nursing women (pregnancy category C).

See Nursing Process Focus: Clients Receiving Barbiturate Therapy for Seizures for specific teaching points.

PROTOTYPE DRUG Phenobarbital (Phenobarb)

Actions and Uses: Phenobarbital is a long-acting barbiturate used for the management of a variety of seizures. It is also used for insomnia. Phenobarbital should not be used for pain relief, as it may increase a client's sensitivity to pain.

Phenobarbital acts biochemically in the brain by enhancing the action of the neurotransmitter GABA, which is responsible for suppressing abnormal neuronal discharges that can cause epilepsy.

Pharmacokinetics: Phenobarbital PO is slowly absorbed. Distribution is unknown. It is mostly metabolized by the liver. About 25% is excreted unchanged in urine. The half-life is 2 to 6 days in adults and 1.5 to 3 days in children.

Administration Alerts:

- Parenteral phenobarbital is a soft tissue irritant. IM injections may produce local inflammatory reaction. IV administration is rarely used because extravasation may produce tissue necrosis.
- Phenobarbital is pregnancy category D.

Adverse Effects and Interactions: Phenobarbital is a Schedule IV drug that may cause dependence. Common side effects include drowsiness, vitamin deficiencies (vitamin D, folate, and vitamin B_{12}), and laryngospasm. With overdose, phenobarbital may cause severe respiratory depression, CNS depression, coma, and death.

Phenobarbital interacts with many other drugs. For example, it should not be taken with alcohol or other CNS depressants. These substances potentiate the action of barbiturates, increasing the risk for life-threatening respiratory depression or cardiac arrest. Phenobarbital increases the metabolism of many other drugs, reducing their effectiveness.

NURSING PROCESS FOCUS

Clients Receiving Barbiturate Therapy for Seizures

Assessment	Potential Nursing Diagnoses/Identified Patterns
Prior to administration: • Obtain complete health history, including allergies and drug history, to determine possible drug interactions. • Assess neurological status, including identification of recent seizure activity.	• Disturbed sensory perception • Risk for injury related to drug side effects • Risk for imbalanced nutrition: less than body requirements • Deficient knowledge related to drug therapy • Disturbed sleep pattern

Planning: Client Goals and Expected Outcomes

The client will:

- Experience the absence of seizures or a reduction in the number or severity of seizures
- Avoid physical injury related to seizure activity or medication-induced somnolence
- Demonstrate an understanding of the drug's action by accurately describing drug effects and precautions

Implementation	
Interventions (Rationales)	**Client Education/Discharge Planning**
• Monitor vital signs, especially blood pressure and depth and rate of respirations. (These drugs can cause severe respiratory depression.) • Monitor neurological status. Monitor changes in level of consciousness. (Excessive somnolence may occur.) Observe for persistent seizures. • Monitor for signs of hepatic or renal toxicity. (Barbiturates are metabolized by the liver and excreted by the kidneys.) • Ensure client safety. (Barbiturates can cause drowsiness and dizziness.) • Monitor effectiveness of drug therapy. • Monitor children for paradoxical response to drug, which may cause hyperactivity. • Monitor for signs of vitamin deficiency (vitamin D, vitamin K, folate, and other B vitamins). • Obtain consultation with dietitian per healthcare provider's order as needed.	• Instruct client to withhold medication for any difficulty in breathing or respirations below 12 breaths per minute Instruct client to: • Report any significant change in sensorium such as lethargy, stupor, auras, visual changes, and other effects that may indicate an impending seizure • Report dizziness, which may indicate hypotension • Be aware that the drug will cause initial drowsiness, which may diminish with continued therapy • Keep a seizure diary to chronicle symptoms Instruct client to: • Observe for signs of toxicity such as nausea; vomiting; diarrhea; rash; jaundice; abdominal pain, tenderness, or distention; change in colour of stool; flank pain; hematuria • Adhere to a regular schedule of laboratory testing for liver and kidney function as ordered by the healthcare provider Instruct client to: • Request assistance when getting out of bed and ambulating until effect of drug is known • Avoid driving and hazardous activities until effect of drug is known Instruct client to: • Be aware that full therapeutic effect of oral barbiturate may take 2 to 3 weeks • Not discontinue drug abruptly or reduce dosage, as increased seizure activity and/or withdrawal symptoms may occur Instruct client: • Regarding the role of vitamins and nutrition in maintaining health • To immediately report signs of vitamin deficiency: vitamin K—easy bleeding, tarry stools, bruising, pallor; vitamin D—joint pain, bone deformities; vitamin B_6—skin changes, dandruff, peripheral neuropathy, fatigue
Evaluation of Outcome Criteria	
Evaluate effectiveness of drug therapy by confirming that client goals and expected outcomes have been met (see "Planning").	

See Table 21.2, "Barbiturates" (page 234), for a list of drugs to which these nursing actions apply.

Treating Seizures with Benzodiazepines

21.5 Benzodiazepines reduce seizure activity by intensifying GABA action. Their use is limited to short-term adjuncts to other more effective agents.

Like barbiturates, benzodiazepines intensify the effect of GABA in the brain. The benzodiazepines bind to the GABA receptor directly, suppressing abnormal neuronal foci. These agents are listed in Table 21.2.

Benzodiazepines used in treating epilepsy include clonazepam (Rivotril), clorazepate, lorazepam (Ativan), and diazepam (Valium). Indications include absence seizures and myoclonic seizures.

Parenteral diazepam is used to terminate status epilepticus. Because tolerance may begin to develop after only a few months of therapy with benzodiazepines, seizures may recur unless the dose is periodically adjusted. These agents are generally not used alone in seizure pharmacotherapy, but instead serve as adjuncts to other antiseizure drugs for short-term seizure control.

The benzodiazepines are one of the most widely prescribed classes of drugs, used not only to control seizures but also for anxiety, skeletal muscle spasms, and alcohol withdrawal symptoms.

Nursing Considerations

The following content provides nursing considerations that apply to benzodiazepines when given to treat seizure disorders. For the complete nursing process applied to benzodiazepine therapy, see Nursing Process Focus: Clients Receiving Benzodiazepine and Non-Benzodiazepine Antianxiety Therapy in Chapter 16, page 172.

The role of the nurse in benzodiazepine therapy for seizures involves careful monitoring of the client's condition and providing education as it relates to the prescribed drug regimen. Assess the client's need for seizure medication. The assessment should include identification of factors associated with the seizures, such as frequency, symptoms, and previous therapies. A drug history should be obtained, including the use of CNS depressants and over-the-counter (OTC) drugs. Assess for the likelihood of drug abuse and dependence, as benzodiazepines are Schedule IV drugs. Assess women of childbearing age for pregnancy, intent to become pregnant, and lactation status, as these drugs are pregnancy category D and are secreted into breast milk. Benzodiazepines may also decrease the effectiveness of oral contraceptives.

Alterations in neurotransmitter activity produce changes in intraocular pressure; therefore, benzodiazepines are contraindicated in narrow-angle glaucoma. Liver and kidney function should be monitored in long-term use and these drugs should be used cautiously in those with impaired renal or liver function.

The risk for respiratory depression should be taken into consideration, especially when administering IV doses and when administering to clients with impaired respiratory function and those taking other CNS depressants. Assess for common side effects related to CNS depression, such as drowsiness and dizziness. Should an overdose occur, flumazenil (Romazicon) is a specific benzodiazepine receptor antagonist that can be administered to reverse CNS depression.

Intravenous benzodiazepines such as diazepam and lorazepam are used in the treatment of status epilepticus or continuous seizures. When administering these drugs by the IV route, it is important to have supplemental oxygen and resuscitation equipment available. Monitor respiratory effort and oxygen saturation. Because the desired action is to terminate seizure activity, severe respiratory depression would be treated with intubation and ventilation rather than by reversing the benzodiazepine effects with flumazenil. Because IV administration may cause hypotension, tachycardia, and muscular weakness, monitoring of heart rhythm, heart rate, and blood pressure is necessary. These drugs have a tendency to precipitate from solution and are irritating to veins. They should not be mixed with other drugs or IV fluid additives and should be given in a large vein if possible.

Client education as it relates to benzodiazepines should include goals, reasons for obtaining baseline data, and possible side effects. Following are points to include when teaching regarding benzodiazepines:

- Avoid alcohol and other CNS depressants, including herbal and OTC drugs, unless advised by the healthcare provider.
- Tobacco use (and nicotine patches) can decrease benzodiazepine effectiveness.
- Benzodiazepines can potentiate the action of digoxin (Lanoxin, Toloxin), thus raising blood levels.
- Do not drive or perform hazardous activities until effects of the drug are known.
- Do not discontinue the drug abruptly, as this may result in rebound seizure activity.
- Take with food if GI upset occurs.
- Benzodiazepines are used illegally for recreation; clients should evaluate the social context of their environment and take any precautions necessary to safeguard their medication supply.

PROTOTYPE DRUG | **Diazepam (Valium)**

Actions and Uses: Diazepam binds to the GABA receptor–chloride channels throughout the CNS. It produces its effects by suppressing neuronal activity in the limbic system and subsequent impulses that might be transmitted to the reticular activating system. Effects of this drug are suppression of abnormal neuronal foci that may cause seizures, calming without strong sedation, and skeletal muscle relaxation. When used orally, maximum therapeutic effects may take 1 to 2 weeks. Tolerance may develop after about 4 weeks. When given by the IV route, effects occur in minutes and its anticonvulsant effects last about 20 minutes.

Pharmacokinetics: Diazepam PO is rapidly absorbed. It is widely distributed, crosses the blood-brain barrier and placenta, and enters breast milk. It is highly metabolized by the liver. Its half-life is 20 to 50 hours in adults.

Administration Alerts:

- When administering IV, monitor respirations every 5 to 15 minutes. Have airway and resuscitative equipment accessible.
- Diazepam is pregnancy category D.

Adverse Effects and Interactions: Diazepam should not be taken with alcohol or other CNS depressants because of combined sedation effects. Other drug interactions include cimetidine (Tagamet), oral contraceptives, valproic acid (Depakene, Epival), and metoprolol (Lopressor), which potentiate diazepam's action, and levodopa-carbidopa (Sinemet) and barbiturates, which decrease diazepam's action. Diazepam increases the levels of phenytoin (Dilantin) in the bloodstream and may cause phenytoin toxicity. When given IV, hypotension, muscular weakness, tachycardia, and respiratory depression are common. Because of tolerance and dependency, use of diazepam is reserved for short-term seizure control or for status epilepticus.

Use with caution with herbal supplements, such as kava and chamomile, which may cause an increased effect.

DRUGS THAT SUPPRESS SODIUM INFLUX

This class of drug dampens CNS activity by delaying an influx of sodium ions across neuronal membranes. Hydantoins and several other related antiseizure drugs act by this mechanism.

Sodium channels guide the movement of sodium across neuronal membranes into the intracellular space. Sodium movement is the major factor that determines whether a neuron will undergo an action potential. If these channels are temporarily inactivated, neuronal activity will be suppressed. With hydantoin and phenytoin-like drugs, sodium channels are not blocked; they are just desensitized. If channels are blocked, neuronal activity completely stops, as occurs with local anesthetic drugs. These agents are shown in Table 21.3.

TABLE 21.3 Hydantoins and Phenytoin-Like Drugs

Drug	Route and Adult Dose
Hydantoins	
fosphenytoin (Cerebyx)	IV, initial dose 15–20 mg phenytoin equivalents (PE)/kg at 100–150 mg PE/min
Pr phenytoin (Dilantin)	For status epilepticus: IV loading dose, 10–15 mg/kg at a maximum rate of 50 mg/min; initial maintenance dose IV or PO of 100 mg every 6-8 hours For convulsions: PO (immediate release), 100 mg tid with dosage adjustments at no less than 7- to 10-day intervals; maintenance dose is 300–400 mg/day; (extended release), loading dose of 1 g divided into 3 doses (begin maintenance dosage 24 hours after loading dose); initial dose 100 mg tid; adjust dosage at no less than 7- to 10-day intervals; maintenance dose is 100 mg 3 to 4 times daily; doses up to 200 mg tid may be necessary
Phenytoin-Like Agents	
carbamazepine (Tegretol)	For epilepsy: PO, start with 400 mg/day in two divided doses (tablets or extended release tablets) or four divided doses (oral suspension); increase by up to 200 mg/day at weekly intervals (max 1600 mg/day)
lamotrigine (Lamictal)	PO, 50 mg/day for 2 weeks, then 50 mg bid for 2 weeks; may increase gradually up to 300–500 mg/day in two divided doses (max 700 mg/day); usually used in combination with other agents to control seizures
Pr valproic acid (Depakene, Epival)*	PO/IV, 10–15 mg/kg/day in divided doses when total daily dose is greater than 250 mg; increase 5–10 mg every week until seizures are controlled (max 60 mg/kg/day)

*Other formulations of valproic acid include its salts, valproate, and divalproex sodium.

Treating Seizures with Hydantoins and Phenytoin-Like Drugs

21.6 Hydantoin and phenytoin-like drugs act by delaying sodium influx into neurons. Phenytoin is a broad-spectrum drug used for all types of epilepsy except absence seizures.

The oldest and most commonly prescribed hydantoin is phenytoin. Approved in the 1930s, phenytoin is a broad-spectrum drug that is useful in treating all types of epilepsy except absence seizures. It is able to provide effective seizure suppression without the abuse potential or CNS depression associated with barbiturates. Clients vary significantly in their ability to metabolize phenytoin; therefore, dosages are highly individualized. Because of the very narrow range between a therapeutic dose and a toxic dose, clients must be carefully monitored. The other hydantoins are used much less frequently than phenytoin.

Several widely used drugs share a mechanism of action similar to the hydantoins, including carbamazepine (Tegretol) and valproic acid, which is also available as valproate and divalproex sodium. Carbamazepine is a drug of choice for tonic-clonic and partial seizures because it produces fewer adverse effects than phenytoin or phenobarbital. Valproic acid is a drug of choice for absence seizures. Both carbamazepine and valproic acid are also used for bipolar disorder (Chapter 17). Newer antiseizure drugs, such as lamotrigine, have more limited uses.

Nursing Considerations

The role of the nurse in hydantoin and phenytoin-like drug therapy involves careful monitoring of the client's condition and providing education as it relates to the prescribed drug regimen. Some of these drugs are monitored via serum drug levels, so regular laboratory testing is required. When serum drug levels stray outside the normal range, dosage adjustments are made.

Common signs of hydantoin toxicity include dizziness, ataxia, diplopia, and lethargy. These drugs affect vitamin K metabolism; therefore, blood dyscrasias and bleeding may ensue. Because hydantoins may increase serum glucose levels, a complete blood count (CBC) and urinalysis should be obtained. Urinalysis is also important to identify the presence of hematuria; phenytoin may change urine colour to pink, red, or brown. These drugs should be used cautiously in clients with hepatic or renal disease.

There have been several cases of fatal hepatotoxicity in clients taking valproic acid. The risk is higher for clients taking multiple antiseizure drugs, those with existing liver disease, those with organic brain disease, and those under 2 years of age. Extreme caution must be taken when administering valproic acid to these clients.

Pregnancy tests must be conducted on all women of childbearing age before beginning therapy since drugs in this class are pregnancy class D (phenytoin, carbamazepine, and valproic acid) or class C (felbamate and lamotrigine). Hydantoins may also decrease the effectiveness of oral contraceptives. Additional contraindications include heart block and seizures due to hypoglycemia.

Client education as it relates to hydantoin and phenytoin-like drugs should include goals, reasons for obtaining baseline data, and possible side effects. See Nursing Process Focus: Clients Receiving Antiseizure Drug Therapy for specific teaching points.

Phenytoin is metabolized in the liver. A client taking phenytoin to control seizures must undergo routine blood testing to monitor for therapeutic serum phenytoin levels. Typically, the client takes the medication for 1 year after the original seizure, then is re-evaluated for continued therapy. During phenytoin therapy, the client may drive and operate machinery. This drug may cause a decreased heart rate and hypotension.

Antiseizure medications are often the cause of toxic epidermal necrolysis.

Phenytoin can lead to excessive gum tissue growth, known as gingival hyperplasia. However, brushing the teeth two or three times daily helps retard such growth. Some clients may require excision of excessive gum tissue every 6 to 12 months.

Phenytoin therapy may contribute to a folic acid deficiency.

Phenytoin is a known teratogenic agent, causing numerous fetal problems. Therefore, a pregnant client should be advised to talk to the physician to see if changing the medication is possible. Additionally, anticonvulsant requirements usually increase during pregnancy.

A therapeutic phenytoin level is 10 to 20 mg/dL. Symptoms of toxicity include confusion and ataxia.

Administer an intravenous bolus by slow (50 mg/minute) intravenous push method; too rapid an injection may cause hypotension and circulatory collapse. Continuous monitoring of electrocardiogram (ECG), blood pressure, and respiratory status is essential when administering phenytoin intravenously. Early toxicity may cause drowsiness, nausea, vomiting, nystagmus, ataxia, dysarthria, tremor, and slurred speech. Later effects may include hypotension, arrhythmias, respiratory depression, and coma. Death may result from respiratory and circulatory depression. Phenytoin would not be administered by intravenous push in veins on the back of the hand; larger veins are needed to prevent discolouration associated with purple glove syndrome. Mix intravenous doses in normal saline solution and use the solution within 30 minutes; doses mixed in dextrose 5% in water will precipitate. Use of an inline filter is recommended.

PROTOTYPE DRUG | **Phenytoin (Dilantin)**

Actions and Uses: Phenytoin acts by desensitizing sodium channels in the CNS that are responsible for neuronal responsivity. Desensitization prevents the spread of disruptive electrical charges in the brain that produce seizures. It is effective against most types of seizure except absence seizures. Phenytoin has antidysrhythmic activity similar to lidocaine (Xylocaine; class IB). An unlabelled use is for digitalis-induced dysrhythmias.

Administration Alerts:

- When administering by the IV route, mix with saline only and infuse at the maximum rate of 50 mg/minute. Mixing it with other medications or dextrose solutions produces precipitate.
- Always prime or flush IV lines with saline before hanging phenytoin as a piggyback since traces of dextrose solution in an existing main IV or piggyback line can cause microscopic precipitate formation, which becomes emboli if infused. Use an IV line with filter when infusing this drug.
- Injectable phenytoin is a soft tissue irritant that causes local tissue damage following extravasation.
- To reduce the risk of soft tissue damage, do not give by the IM route; inject into a large vein or via central venous catheter.
- Avoid using hand veins to prevent serious local vasoconstrictive response (purple glove syndrome).
- Phenytoin is pregnancy category D.

Pharmacokinetics: Phenytoin is slowly absorbed from the GI tract. It is widely distributed, crosses the placenta, and enters breast milk and cerebrospinal fluid (CSF). It is mostly metabolized by the liver. Its half-life is about 22 hours.

Adverse Effects and Interactions: Phenytoin may cause dysrhythmias, such as bradycardia or ventricular fibrillation, severe hypotension, and hyperglycemia. Severe CNS reactions include headache, nystagmus, ataxia, confusion and slurred speech, paradoxical nervousness, twitching, and insomnia. Peripheral neuropathy may occur with long-term use. Phenytoin can cause multiple blood dyscrasias, including agranulocytosis and aplastic anemia. It may cause severe skin reactions, such as rashes, including exfoliative dermatitis, and Stevens-Johnson syndrome. Connective tissue reactions include lupus erythematosa, hypertrichosis, hirsutism, and gingival hypertrophy.

Phenytoin interacts with many other drugs, including oral anticoagulants, glucocorticoids, H_2-receptor antagonists, antituberculin agents, and food supplements such as folic acid, calcium, and vitamin D. It impairs the efficacy of drugs such as digoxin (Lanoxin, Toloxin), doxycycline (Vibramycin), furosemide (Lasix), estrogens and oral contraceptives, and theophylline (Theolair, Uniphyl). Phenytoin can trigger seizures when combined with tricyclic antidepressants.

Use with caution with herbal supplements, such as herbal laxatives (buckthorn, cascara sagrada, and senna), which may increase potassium loss.

NCLEX Success Tips

Valproic acid, an anticonvulsant agent, is used as a mood stabilizer for clients with bipolar disorder. It is also commonly used to treat manic symptoms. Therefore, a decrease in the valproic acid level could explain the increase in manic symptoms. Common side effects include drowsiness and gastrointestinal upset. The client needs to be cautioned not to drive or perform tasks requiring alertness and to take the medication with food or milk or eat frequent, small meals. Alcohol as well as over-the-counter drugs and sleep-inducing agents must be avoided to prevent oversedation. Increased appetite is common with this drug.

Valproic acid and propranolol (Inderal) are often prescribed to help manage explosive anger.

Chewing the pill or capsule form of valproic acid can cause mouth and throat irritation and is contraindicated. It is important to take the pills at the same time each day to maintain therapeutic effectiveness of the drug. Taking the pills with food is appropriate if the client is experiencing gastrointestinal upset. Valproic acid may cause clotting problems; therefore, bruising should be reported.

Periodic determinations of the valproic acid level are necessary to determine the effectiveness of the drug. Blood tests are required to evaluate the serum level and to check for possible hematological effects.

Valproic acid can cause changes in liver function and blood dyscrasias. Aspartate transaminase is routinely monitored to evaluate for hepatic toxicity, which may manifest with jaundice and abdominal pain. Extended-release tablets should not be split or crushed; doing so changes their absorption.

The therapeutic level of valproic acid is 50 to 100 mg/mL (347 to 693 mmol/L).

Because valproic acid is associated with thrombocytopenia and hypofibrinogenemia, routine follow-up blood work would consist of monitoring platelet and fibrinogen levels for decreases.

PROTOTYPE DRUG	**Valproic Acid (Depakene, Epival)**

Actions and Uses: The mechanism of action of valproic acid is the same as phenytoin, although effects on GABA and calcium channels may cause some additional actions. It is useful for a wide range of seizure types, including absence seizures and mixed types of seizure. Other uses include prevention of migraine headaches and treatment of bipolar disorder.

Administration Alerts:

- Valproic acid is a GI irritant. Extended-release tablets must not be chewed, as mouth soreness will occur.
- Valproic acid syrup must not be mixed with carbonated beverages because they will trigger immediate release of the drug, which causes severe mouth and throat irritation.
- Capsules may be opened and sprinkled on soft foods.
- Valproic acid is contraindicated in clients with liver disease.
- Valproic acid is pregnancy category D.

Pharmacokinetics: Valproic acid is well absorbed from the GI tract. It is widely distributed, crosses the blood-brain barrier and placenta, and enters breast milk. It is mostly metabolized by the liver. Its half-life is 8 to 17 hours in adults.

Adverse Effects and Interactions: Side effects include sedation, drowsiness, GI upset, and prolonged bleeding time. Other effects include visual disturbances, muscle weakness, tremor, psychomotor agitation, bone marrow suppression, weight gain, abdominal cramps, rash, alopecia, pruritus, photosensitivity, erythema multiforme, and fatal hepatotoxicity.

Valproic acid interacts with many drugs. For example, acetylsalicylic acid (ASA), cimetidine, chlorpromazine, erythromycin (ERYC), and felbamate (Felbatol) may increase valproic acid toxicity. Concomitant warfarin (Coumadin), ASA, or alcohol use can cause severe bleeding. Alcohol, benzodiazepines, and other CNS depressants potentiate CNS depressant action. Lamotrigine, phenytoin, and rifampin (Rifadin, Rofact) lower valproic acid levels. Valproic acid increases serum phenobarbital and phenytoin levels. Use of clonazepam concurrently with valproic acid may induce absence seizures.

NURSING PROCESS FOCUS

Clients Receiving Antiseizure Drug Therapy

Assessment	Potential Nursing Diagnoses/Identified Patterns
Prior to administration: • Obtain complete health history, including allergies and drug history, to determine possible drug interactions. • Assess neurological status, including identification of recent seizure activity. • Assess growth and development.	• Risk for injury related to drug side effects • Deficient knowledge related to drug therapy • Nonadherence

Planning: Client Goals and Outcomes

The client will:

- Experience the absence of seizures or a reduction in the number or severity of seizures
- Avoid physical injury related to seizure activity or medication-induced sensory changes
- Demonstrate an understanding of the drug's action by accurately describing drug effects and precautions

Implementation

Interventions (Rationales)	Client Education/Discharge Planning
• Monitor neurological status, especially changes in level of consciousness and/or mental status. (Sedation may indicate impending toxicity.) • Protect the client from injury during seizure events until therapeutic effects of drugs are achieved. • Monitor effectiveness of drug therapy. Observe for developmental changes, which may indicate a need for dose adjustment. • Monitor for adverse effects. Observe for hypersensitivity, nephrotoxicity, and hepatotoxicity. • Monitor oral health. Observe for signs of gingival hypertrophy, bleeding, or inflammation (phenytoin specific). • Monitor gastrointestinal status. (Valproic acid is a GI irritant and anticoagulant.)	Instruct the client to: • Report any significant change in sensorium, such as slurred speech, confusion, hallucinations, or lethargy • Report any changes in seizure quality or unexpected involuntary muscle movement, such as twitching, tremor, or unusual eye movement • Instruct client to avoid driving and other hazardous activities until effects of the drug are known Instruct client to: • Keep a seizure diary to record symptoms during dosage adjustment phases and whenever seizures occur • Take the medication exactly as ordered, including the same manufacturer's drug each time the prescription is refilled (switching brands may result in alterations in seizure control)

- Conduct guaiac stool testing (FOBT) for occult blood. (Phenytoin's CNS depressant effects decrease GI motility, producing constipation.)
- Monitor nutritional status. (Phenytoin's action on electrolytes may cause decreased absorption of folic acid, vitamin D, magnesium, and calcium. Deficiencies in these vitamins and minerals lead to anemia and osteoporosis. Valproic acid may cause an increase in appetite and weight.)

- Take a missed dose as soon as remembered, but not to take double doses (doubling doses could result in toxic serum level)
- Instruct client to report side effects specific to drug regimen

Instruct client to:
- Use a soft toothbrush and oral rinses as prescribed by the dentist
- Avoid mouthwashes containing alcohol
- Report changes in oral health such as excessive bleeding or inflammation of the gums
- Maintain a regular schedule of dental visits

Instruct client to:
- Take drug with food to reduce GI upset
- Immediately report any severe or persistent heartburn, upper GI pain, nausea, or vomiting
- Increase exercise, fluid and fibre intake to facilitate stool passage
- Instruct client in dietary or drug administration techniques specific to prescribed medications.
- Instruct client to report significant changes in appetite or weight gain.

Evaluation of Outcome Criteria

Evaluate effectiveness of drug therapy by confirming that client goals and expected outcomes have been met (see "Planning").

See Tables 21.3 (page 238) and 21.4 (page 241) for lists of drugs to which these nursing actions apply.

DRUGS THAT SUPPRESS CALCIUM INFLUX

Succinimides are medications that suppress seizures by delaying calcium ion influx into neurons. They are generally only effective against absence seizures.

Treating Seizures with Succinimides

21.7 Succinimides act by delaying calcium influx into neurons. Ethosuximide is a drug of choice for absence seizures.

Neurotransmitters, hormones, and some medications bind to neuronal membranes, stimulating the entry of calcium ions. Without calcium influx, neuronal transmission would not be possible. Succinimides delay entry of calcium into neurons by blocking calcium channels, increasing the electrical threshold, and reducing the likelihood that an action potential will be generated. By raising the seizure threshold, succinimides keep neurons from firing too quickly, thus suppressing abnormal foci. The succinimides are shown in Table 21.4.

Ethosuximide (Zarontin) is the most commonly prescribed drug in this class. It remains a drug of choice for absence seizures, although valproic acid is also effective for these types of seizures. Some of the newer antiseizure agents, such as lamotrigine, are being investigated for their roles in treating absence seizures.

Nursing Considerations

The role of the nurse in succinimide therapy involves careful monitoring of the client's seizure activity and providing education as it relates to the prescribed drug regimen. Obtain a medical history confirming the baseline seizure activity. Baseline renal and hepatic function tests should be obtained because these drugs are metabolized by the liver and excreted by the kidneys. Succinimides should be used cautiously in clients with liver or renal insufficiency. Succinimides are pregnancy category C.

Review the client's current drug history to determine if any medications interact with succinimides. Succinimides may alter the effectiveness of other antiseizure drugs. Many drugs that alter CNS activity, such as phenothiazines and antidepressants, lower the seizure threshold and can decrease the effectiveness of succinimides.

The nurse should observe for common adverse reactions during therapy, including drowsiness, headache, fatigue, dizziness, depression or euphoria, nausea and vomiting, diarrhea, weight loss, and abdominal pain. Life-threatening adverse reactions include severe mental depression with overt suicidal intent, Stevens-Johnson syndrome, and blood dyscrasias such as agranulocytosis, pancytopenia, and leukopenia.

Seizure activity should be monitored during therapy to confirm the drug's efficacy. Symptoms of overdose include CNS depression, stupor, ataxia, and coma. These symptoms may occur when ethosuximide is given alone or in combination with other

TABLE 21.4 Succinimides

Drug	Route and Adult Dose
Pr ethosuximide (Zarontin)	500 mg/day (individualize dose based on client response by increasing in small increments); doses >1500 mg/day should be given in divided doses
methsuximide (Celontin)	PO, 300 mg/day; may increase every 4–7 days (max 1.2 g/day in 2–4 divided doses)

CONNECTIONS Natural Therapies

◀ The Ketogenic Diet

The ketogenic diet is used when seizures cannot be controlled through pharmacotherapy or there are unacceptable side effects of the medications. Before antiepileptic drugs were developed, this diet was a primary treatment for epilepsy. The ketogenic diet may be used for babies, children, or adults. With adults, however, it is harder to produce the ketones that are necessary for the therapeutic effect.

The ketogenic diet is a stringently calculated diet that is high in fat and low in carbohydrates and protein. It limits water intake to avoid ketone dilution and carefully controls caloric intake. Each meal has the same ketogenic ratio of 4 g of fat to 1 g of protein and carbohydrate. Extra fat is usually given in the form of cream. Research suggests that the diet produces success rates similar to the use of medication, with one-third of the children using it becoming seizure-free, one-third having their seizures reduced, and one-third not responding.

The diet appears to be equally effective for every seizure type, though drop attacks (atonic seizures) may be the most rapid responders. It also helps children with Lennox-Gastaut syndrome and shows promise in babies with infantile spasms. Side effects include hyperlipidemia, constipation, vitamin deficiencies, kidney stones, acidosis, and possibly slower growth rates. Those interested in trying the diet must consult with their healthcare provider; this is not a do-it-yourself diet and may be harmful if not carefully monitored by skilled professionals.

anticonvulsants. Combined usage must be monitored carefully, with regular testing for serum levels of each drug.

Client education as it relates to succinimides should include goals, reasons for obtaining baseline data, and possible side effects. Following are the points the nurse should include when teaching clients about succinimides:

- Immediately report changes in mood, mental depression, and suicidal urges.
- Do not drive or perform hazardous activities until effect of the drug is known.

- Do not discontinue the drug abruptly, as this may result in rebound seizure activity.
- Take with food if GI upset occurs.
- Immediately report symptoms suggestive of infection (e.g., fever, sore throat, malaise).
- Report weight loss and anorexia.

PROTOTYPE DRUG | Ethosuximide (Zarontin)

Actions and Uses: Ethosuximide is a drug of choice for absence (petit mal) seizures. It depresses the activity of neurons in the motor cortex by elevating the neuronal threshold. It is usually ineffective against psychomotor or tonic-clonic seizures; however, it may be given in combination with other medications, which better treat these conditions. It is available in tablet and flavoured syrup formulations.

Administration Alerts:

- Abrupt withdrawal of this medication may induce grand mal seizures.
- Ethosuximide is pregnancy category C.

Pharmacokinetics: Ethosuximide is rapidly absorbed. It is mostly metabolized by the liver. Its half-life is 60 hours in adults and 30 hours in children.

Adverse Effects and Interactions: Ethosuximide may impair mental and physical abilities. Psychosis or extreme mood swings, including depression with overt suicidal intent, can occur. Behavioural changes are more prominent in clients with a history of psychiatric illness. CNS effects include dizziness, headache, lethargy, fatigue, ataxia, sleep pattern disturbances, attention difficulty, and hiccups. Bone marrow suppression and blood dyscrasias are possible, as is systemic lupus erythematosa.

Other reactions include gingival hypertrophy and tongue swelling. Common side effects are abdominal distress and weight loss.

Drug interactions include phenytoin, since ethosuximide increases phenytoin serum levels. Valproic acid causes ethosuximide serum levels to fluctuate (increase or decrease).

CHAPTER
21 Understanding the Chapter

Key Concepts Summary

The numbered key concepts provide a succinct summary of the important points from the corresponding numbered section within the chapter. If any of these points are not clear, refer to the numbered section within the chapter for review.

21.1 Seizures are associated with many causes, including head trauma, brain infection, fluid and electrolyte imbalance, hypoxia, stroke, brain tumours, and high fever in children.

21.2 The three broad categories of seizure are partial seizures, generalized seizures, and special epileptic syndromes. Each seizure type has a characteristic set of signs, and different drugs are used for different types.

21.3 Antiseizure drugs act by distinct mechanisms: potentiation of GABA and delaying the influx of sodium or calcium ions into neurons. Pharmacotherapy may continue

for many years, and withdrawal from these agents must be done gradually to avoid seizure recurrence.

21.4 Barbiturates act by potentiating the effects of GABA. Phenobarbital is used for tonic-clonic and febrile seizures.

21.5 Benzodiazepines reduce seizure activity by intensifying GABA action. Their use is limited to short-term adjuncts to other more effective agents.

21.6 Hydantoin and phenytoin-like drugs act by delaying sodium influx into neurons. Phenytoin is a broad-spectrum drug used for all types of epilepsy except absence seizures.

21.7 Succinimides act by delaying calcium influx into neurons. Ethosuximide is a drug of choice for absence seizures.

Chapter 21 Scenario

Jorge Alvarez is a 3-year-old boy who has been hospitalized following a seizure. Since being admitted 2 days ago he has experienced three subsequent tonic-clonic seizures that lasted 2 to 2.5 minutes each. Before having a seizure Jorge notices a flash of light. He then loses consciousness, emits a hoarse cry, and has intense muscle contractions. During the clonic phase he is incontinent of bowel and bladder. His postictal phase is characterized by drowsiness, disorientation, and deep sleep.

On admission, Jorge was scheduled for a sleep-and-awake EEG. His EEG revealed a high-voltage spike discharge, which is diagnostic of a tonic-clonic seizure. The laboratory studies performed on Jorge included a serum lead level to rule out lead intoxication and a serum glucose

level to rule out hypoglycemia. Both the lead level and the blood glucose level were in the normal range.

Jorge has been started on the following medications to assist in controlling his tonic-clonic seizures: carbamazepine (Tegretol) 300 mg PO tid and phenytoin (Dilantin) 120 mg PO tid.

Critical Thinking Questions

1. Jorge's mother expresses concern about what to do if Jorge has a seizure. Create a list of home safety tips that could be given to her.

2. How will you instruct Jorge's mother with regard to his medication administration?

See Answers to Critical Thinking Questions in Appendix B.

NCLEX Practice Questions

1 A 10-year-old child has been evaluated for a learning disability and has been diagnosed with absence seizures. Ethosuximide (Zarontin) has been ordered and the nurse is teaching the client and family about the drug. Because of the client's age, it is important to include instructions to

a. Curtail after-school sports activities because the drug's metabolism may be increased with physical activity.

b. Increase intake of calcium-rich foods and vitamin D to prevent bone loss.

c. Monitor height and weight weekly to be sure GI side effects are not hindering nutrition and normal growth.

d. Increase fluid intake to avoid dehydration caused by the drug.

2 The nurse is caring for a 42-year-old client who was recently diagnosed with partial seizures and has been prescribed oxcarbazepine (Trileptal). Which laboratory study would the nurse expect to be ordered?

a. CBC with differential

b. Serum albumin and glucose levels

c. Sedimentation rate and platelet count

d. Serum sodium and renal function studies

3 An 80-year-old client is prescribed carbamazepine (Tegretol) for a newly diagnosed seizure disorder. The nurse will implement safety measures because this client is at an increased risk for which adverse effects?

a. Dementia and confusion

b. Insomnia and forgetfulness related to sleep deprivation

c. Stroke and decreased motor function

d. Sedation and falls

4 A 23-year-old client has been taking gabapentin (Neurontin) for control of partial seizures. He is admitted to the emergency department with slurred speech, dyspnea, reports of double vision, and sedation. The admitting nurse suspects the client has

a. Not taken his drug for several days

b. Taken an overdose of the drug, either accidentally or deliberately

c. Taken the drug with grapefruit or grapefruit juice

d. Continued to smoke despite prior client education that smoking interacts with the drug

5 A nurse who is monitoring a client taking phenytoin (Dilantin) notes symptoms of nystagmus, confusion, and ataxia. Considering these findings, the nurse would suspect that the dose of the drug should be

a. Reduced

b. Increased

c. Maintained

d. Discontinued

See Answers to NCLEX Practice Questions in Appendix A.

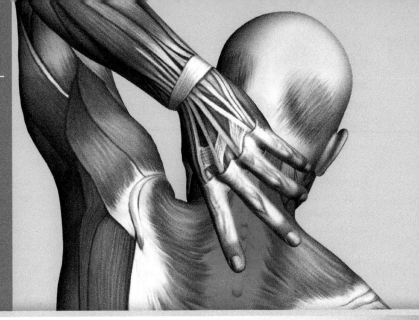

ForeverLee/Fotolia

PROTOTYPE DRUGS

CENTRALLY ACTING MUSCLE RELAXANTS	DIRECT-ACTING ANTISPASMOTICS
Pr *cyclobenzaprine* (Flexeril)	Pr *dantrolene* (Dantrium)

CHAPTER

22 Pharmacotherapy of Muscle Spasms and Spasticity

LEARNING OUTCOMES

After reading this chapter, the student should be able to:

1. Discuss non-pharmacological therapies used to treat muscle spasms and spasticity.
2. Explain the therapeutic actions of centrally acting skeletal muscle relaxants and direct-acting antispasmodics in relation to the pathophysiology of muscle spasms and spasticity.
3. Discuss the nurse's role in the pharmacological and non-pharmacological treatment of clients with muscle spasms and spasticity.
4. For each of the drug classes listed in Prototype Drugs, identify a representative drug and explain its mechanism of action, therapeutic effects, and important adverse effects.
5. Describe and explain, based on pharmacological principles, the rationale for nursing assessment, planning, and interventions for clients with muscle spasms and spasticity.
6. Use the nursing process to care for clients who are receiving therapy for muscle spasms.

CHAPTER OUTLINE

▶ Muscle Spasms

  ▶ Causes of Muscle Injury and Spasms

  ▶ Pharmacological and Non-Pharmacological Treatment of Muscle Spasms

▶ Centrally Acting Skeletal Muscle Relaxants

  ▶ Treating Muscle Spasms at the Level of the Central Nervous System

▶ Spasticity

  ▶ Causes and Treatment of Spasticity

  ▶ Treating Muscle Spasms Directly at the Muscle Tissue

KEY TERMS

clonic spasm, 246

dystonia, 248

muscle spasms, 246

spasticity, 248

tonic spasm, 246

Disorders associated with movement are some of the most difficult conditions to treat because their underlying mechanisms may be related to disorders of the nervous, muscular, endocrine, and skeletal systems. Proper body movement depends not only on intact neural pathways, but also on proper functioning of muscles, which in turn depends on the levels of minerals such as sodium, potassium, and calcium in the bloodstream. This chapter focuses on the pharmacotherapy of muscular disorders associated with muscle spasms and spasticity. Many of the drugs used to treat muscle spasms are distinct from those used for spasticity.

Skeletal muscle contraction is regulated by the activity of upper motor neurons that originate in the brain and project to the spinal cord. Upper motor neurons synapse with alpha motor neurons (or lower motor neurons) in the ventral horn of the spinal cord. Alpha motor neurons in turn project to motor end plates on skeletal muscle cells where they release acetylcholine, which leads to muscle contraction. Alpha motor neurons have an excitatory effect on skeletal muscle cells and, when stimulated, typically cause contraction of skeletal muscle cells as part of an alpha motor unit.

Neurons that originate in the brain regulate the activity of alpha motor neurons through excitatory and inhibitory mechanisms. The role of these neurons is to ensure that alpha motor neuron and skeletal muscle function are controlled such that skeletal muscles can contract and relax in an orderly and coordinated manner. In conditions in which upper motor neurons are damaged, this regulation becomes less effective through reduced inhibition of alpha motor neurons. As a result, alpha motor neurons become more active, leading to muscle spasticity, hypertonia, and hyperreflexia.

In conditions in which alpha motor neurons become damaged, skeletal muscle cells cannot be stimulated to contract, leading to hypotonia and hyporeflexia.

MUSCLE SPASMS

Muscle spasms are involuntary contractions of a muscle or group of muscles. The muscles become tightened, develop a fixed pattern of resistance, and exhibit a diminished level of functioning.

Causes of Muscle Injury and Spasms

22.1 Muscle spasms, involuntary contractions of a muscle or group of muscles, most commonly occur because of localized trauma to skeletal muscle.

Muscle spasms are a common condition usually associated with excessive use of and local injury to the skeletal muscle. Other causes of muscle spasms include epilepsy, hypocalcemia, pain, debilitating neurological disorders, genetic susceptibilities, and drug toxicities. Drug-induced muscle injury may lead to symptoms of muscle weakness or spasms that emerge over time. Causative agents may include lipid-lowering agents (such as statins), penicillamine (used for rheumatoid arthritis), antimalarials, colchicine, corticosteroids, antipsychotic drugs, alcohol, and cocaine.

Clients with muscle spasms may experience inflammation, edema, pain at the affected muscle, loss of coordination, and reduced mobility. Muscle spasms can be **tonic**, when a muscle remains contracted for a single, usually prolonged time, or **clonic**, when a muscle rapidly contracts and relaxes. Treatment of muscle spasms involves both non-pharmacological and pharmacological therapies.

Pharmacological and Non-Pharmacological Treatment of Muscle Spasms

22.2 Muscle spasms can be treated with non-pharmacological and pharmacological therapies.

Treating a client with complaints of muscle spasms requires a thorough history and physical exam to determine the cause of the spasms. After a determination has been made, non-pharmacological therapies are normally used in conjunction with medications. Non-pharmacological measures may include immobilization of the affected muscle, application of heat or cold, hydrotherapy, ultrasound, supervised exercises, massage, acupuncture manipulation, and review of diet.

Pharmacotherapy for muscle spasms may include combinations of analgesics, anti-inflammatory agents, and centrally acting skeletal muscle relaxants. Most skeletal muscle relaxants relieve symptoms of muscular stiffness and rigidity resulting from muscular injury. They help to improve mobility in cases where clients have restricted movement. The therapeutic goals are to minimize pain and discomfort, increase range of motion, and improve the client's ability to function independently.

CENTRALLY ACTING SKELETAL MUSCLE RELAXANTS

The origin of action of many drugs used to treat muscle spasms is within the central nervous system (CNS). These drugs inhibit motor neurons in the brain and spinal cord, reducing the activity of alpha motor neurons and allowing skeletal muscles to relax.

Treating Muscle Spasms at the Level of the Central Nervous System

22.3 Many muscle relaxants treat muscle spasms at the level of the CNS, generating their effect within the brain and/or spinal cord, usually by inhibiting upper motor neuron activity, causing sedation, or altering simple reflexes.

Skeletal muscle relaxants act at various levels within the CNS. Although their exact mechanisms are not fully known, it is believed that they generate their effects within the brain and/or spinal cord by inhibiting upper motor neuron activity, causing CNS depression, or altering simple reflexes.

Antispasmodic drugs are used to treat local spasms resulting from muscular injury and may be prescribed alone or in combination with other medications to reduce pain and increase range of motion. Commonly used centrally acting medications include baclofen (Lioresal), cyclobenzaprine (Flexeril), tizanidine (Zanaflex), and benzodiazepines such as diazepam (Valium), clonazepam (Rivotril), and lorazepam (Ativan), as summarized in Table 22.1. All of the centrally acting agents have the potential to cause sedation.

NCLEX Success Tips

Baclofen is a centrally acting skeletal muscle relaxant that helps relieve the muscle spasms common in multiple sclerosis (MS). MS is a progressive disease characterized by demyelination of the brain and spinal cord. This disease causes a number of manifestations, including muscle spasticity. Drowsiness is an adverse effect of baclofen, and driving should be avoided if the medication produces a sedative effect.

To prevent a baclofen withdrawal, pump refills are scheduled several days before anticipated low-volume alarms. The nurse should make it a high priority to have the pump refilled as soon as possible. Discontinuing baclofen suddenly can result in a high fever, muscle rigidity, change in level of consciousness, and even death.

Baclofen's principal clinical indication is for the paraplegic or quadriplegic client with spinal cord lesions, most commonly caused by multiple sclerosis or trauma. For these clients, baclofen significantly reduces the number and severity of painful flexor spasms.

The nurse should ask the client with multiple sclerosis about areas of muscle weakness because baclofen may increase the weakness. The nurse should ask the client about a history of muscle spasms. Baclofen is effective against involuntary spasms resistant to passive movement for clients with multiple sclerosis and paralysis. Baclofen is not effective against the spasticity of cerebral origin, such as with cerebral palsy, Parkinson's disease, and stroke. The nurse should ask about the client's liver and renal function because baclofen is metabolized and excreted by these organs. The nurse should check the laboratory values reflecting the function of the kidneys and liver, which includes serum creatinine and blood urea nitrogen levels because baclofen is metabolized and excreted by these organs. The nurse should also check blood glucose levels because baclofen can increase blood glucose. Clients with diabetes taking antidiabetic medication may need to adjust the dosage.

Baclofen, structurally similar to the inhibitory neurotransmitter gamma-aminobutyric acid (GABA), produces its effect by a mechanism that is not fully known. It can inhibit neuronal activity within the brain and the spinal cord, although there is some question as to whether the spinal effects of baclofen are associated with GABA. It has been postulated to reduce spasticity by inhibiting the release of excitatory neurotransmitters at the level of the spinal cord through a presynaptic inhibition mechanism. It may be used to reduce muscle spasms in clients with multiple sclerosis, cerebral palsy, or spinal cord injury. Common side effects of baclofen are drowsiness, dizziness, weakness, and fatigue. Baclofen is often a drug of first choice due to its wide safety margin. Baclofen can be delivered through a number of routes, including oral and intrathecal. Intrathecal may be the route of choice, as it requires a lower dose and can more directly access spinal neurons compared to an oral route.

Tizanidine is a centrally acting alpha$_2$-adrenergic agonist that inhibits motor neurons mainly at the spinal cord level. Clients who are receiving high doses report drowsiness; therefore, it also affects some neural activity in the brain. Although uncommon, one adverse effect of tizanidine is hallucinations. The most frequent side effects are dry mouth, fatigue, dizziness, and sleepiness. Tizanidine is as effective as baclofen and is considered by some to be a drug of first choice. As with baclofen, tizanidine can also be delivered via the oral route. It is indicated for patients with multiple sclerosis, cerebral palsy, and spinal diplegia and has been used off label to manage migraine headaches and as an anticonvulsant.

As discussed in Chapter 16, benzodiazepines inhibit both sensory and motor neuron activity by enhancing the effects of GABA. Common adverse side effects include drowsiness and ataxia (loss of coordination). Benzodiazepines are usually prescribed for muscle relaxation when baclofen and tizanidine fail to produce adequate relief.

TABLE 22.1 Centrally Acting Skeletal Muscle Relaxants

Drug	Route and Adult Dose
baclofen (Lioresal)	Orally (PO), 5 mg three times a day (tid) (max 80 mg/day)
cyclobenzaprine (Flexeril)	PO, 5 mg tid; may increase up to 10 mg tid if needed (do not use for longer than 2–3 weeks)
chlorzoxazone (Paraflex, Parafon Forte)	PO, 250–500 mg tid–qid (max 3 g/day)
clonazepam (Rivotril)	PO, 0.25 mg bid; increase in increments of 0.125–0.25 mg bid (max 4.5–6 mg/day)
diazepam (Valium) (see Chapter 21, page 237, for the Prototype Drug Box)	PO, 2–10 mg 3 to 4 times daily if needed; Intramuscularly/intravenously (IM/IV), 5–10 mg initially, then 5–10 mg in 3 to 4 hours if necessary
lorazepam (Ativan) (see Chapter 16, page 170, for the Prototype Drug Box)	PO, 1–2 mg bid–tid (max 10 mg/day)
methocarbamol (Robaxin)	PO, 1.5 g 4 times a day for 2–3 days (up to 8 g/day may be given in severe conditions), then decrease to 4–4.5 g/day in 3–6 divided doses
orphenadrine (Norflex)	PO, 100 mg bid
tizanidine (Zanaflex)	PO, start with 2 mg up to tid (at 6–8 hour intervals) as needed; may titrate to optimal effect in 2–4 mg increments per dose (with a minimum of 1–4 days between dose increases); max 36 mg/day

CONNECTIONS | Natural Therapies

◀ Cayenne for Muscular Tension

Several herbals are claimed to have muscle relaxant properties. These include celery seed, chamomile, goldenrod, rosemary, saw palmetto, wild yam, yarrow, and cayenne.

Cayenne (*Capsicum annum*), also known as chili pepper, paprika, or red pepper, has been used as a remedy for muscle tension. Applied in a cream base, it is commonly used to relieve muscle spasms in the shoulder and arm. Capsaicin, the active ingredient in cayenne, diminishes the chemical messengers that travel through the sensory nerves, therefore decreasing the sensation of pain. Because its effects accumulate over time, creams that contain capsaicin (0.025% to 0.075%) need to be applied regularly, up to four times daily, to be effective. Although no known medical condition exists that would prevent the use of cayenne, it should never be applied over broken skin. Topical use of full-strength cayenne should be limited to no more than 2 days because it may cause skin inflammation, blisters, and ulcers. It also needs to be kept away from eyes and mucous membranes to avoid burns. Hands must be washed thoroughly after use. Cayenne is also available in capsules (30 to 120 mg), taken three times daily, or as a tea.

During certain surgical procedures it is necessary to produce total skeletal muscle relaxation in the patient. Skeletal muscle relaxants such as succinylcholine (Quelicin) and tubocurarine are administered in combination with general anesthetics to induce skeletal muscle relaxation, which aids in intubation and other invasive procedures. These drugs are also administered to facilitate endoscopy, to enhance the management of mechanical ventilation, and to control the severity of muscle contractions resulting from electroshock therapy.

The skeletal muscle relaxants used as surgical adjuncts have the ability to produce complete muscle paralysis; therefore, mechanical ventilation may be necessary. Continuous monitoring is required. Most of these drugs have very rapid onsets of action and brief half-lives; drug effects rapidly diminish following the surgical procedure.

PROTOTYPE DRUG | Cyclobenzaprine (Flexeril)

Actions and Uses: Cyclobenzaprine relieves muscle spasms of local origin without interfering with general muscle function. This drug acts by depressing motor activity primarily in the brainstem but with limited effects occurring also in the spinal cord. It increases circulating levels of norepinephrine by blocking presynaptic uptake. Its mechanism of action is similar to the tricyclic antidepressants (see Chapter 17). It causes muscle relaxation in cases of acute muscle spasticity, but it is not effective in cases of cerebral palsy or diseases of the brain and spinal cord in which upper motor neurons have been damage. This medication is meant to provide therapy for only 2 to 3 weeks.

Pharmacokinetics: Cyclobenzaprine is well absorbed from the gastrointestinal (GI) tract. It has an onset of action of 1 hour and peaks in 3 to 8 hours. It is 93% protein bound and is metabolized by the liver. The half-life is 1 to 3 days.

Administration Alerts:
- The drug is not recommended for pediatric use.
- Maximum effects may take 1 to 2 weeks.
- Cyclobenzaprine is pregnancy category B.

Adverse Effects and Interactions: Adverse reactions to cyclobenzaprine include drowsiness, blurred vision, dizziness, dry mouth, rash, and tachycardia. One reaction, although rare, is swelling of the tongue. Alcohol, phenothiazines, and other CNS depressants may cause additive sedation. Cyclobenzaprine should not be used within 2 weeks of an monoamine oxidase (MAO) inhibitor since hyperpyretic crisis and convulsions may occur. It should be used with caution in clients with myocardial infarction (MI), dysrhythmias, or severe cardiovascular disease.

Treatment of Overdose: The IV administration of 1 to 3 mg of physostigmine salicylate is reported to reverse symptoms of poisoning by drugs with anticholinergic activity. Physostigmine may be helpful in the treatment of cyclobenzaprine overdose.

SPASTICITY

Spasticity is a condition in which certain muscle groups remain in a continuous state of contraction, usually as a result of damage to the CNS. The contracted muscles become stiff with increased muscle tone. Other signs and symptoms may include mild to severe pain, exaggerated deep tendon reflexes, muscle spasms, scissoring (involuntary crossing of the legs), and fixed joints.

Causes and Treatment of Spasticity

22.4 Spasticity, a condition in which selected muscles are continuously contracted, results from damage to the CNS. Effective treatment for spasticity includes both physical therapy and medications.

Spasticity usually results from damage to the motor area of the cerebral cortex that controls muscle movement. Etiologies most commonly associated with this condition include neurological disorders such as cerebral palsy, severe head injury, spinal cord injury or lesions, and stroke. **Dystonia**, a chronic neurological disorder, is characterized by involuntary muscle contraction that forces body parts into abnormal, occasionally painful movements or postures. It affects the muscle tone of the arms, legs, trunk, neck, eyelids, face, and vocal cords. Spasticity can be very distressing and can have a negative impact on a client's quality of life, whether the condition is short or long term. In addition to causing pain, impaired physical mobility reduces the ability to perform activities of daily living (ADLs) and diminishes the client's sense of independence.

Effective treatment for spasticity includes both physical therapy and medications. Medications alone are not adequate in reducing the complications of spasticity. Regular and consistent physical therapy exercises have been shown to decrease the severity of symptoms. Types of treatment include muscle stretching to help prevent contractures, muscle group strengthening exercises, and repetitive motion exercises for improving accuracy. In extreme cases, surgery for tendon release or to sever the nerve-muscle pathway is occasionally used. Drugs effective in the treatment of spasticity include several classifications of antispasmodics that act in the CNS, at neuromuscular junctions, or in muscle tissue.

Treating Muscle Spasms Directly at the Muscle Tissue

22.5 Some antispasmodic drugs used for spasticity act directly on muscle tissue, relieving spasticity by interfering with the release of calcium ions.

Drugs that are effective in the treatment of spasticity include two centrally acting drugs, baclofen and diazepam, and a direct-acting drug, dantrolene (Dantrium). The direct-acting drugs produce an antispasmodic effect at the level of the neuromuscular junction, as shown in Figure 22.1.

Dantrolene relieves spasticity by interfering with the release of calcium ions from the sarcoplasmic reticulum in skeletal muscle. Other direct-acting drugs include botulinum toxin type A and type B (Botox), used to offer significant relief of symptoms in people with dystonia, and quinine, used to treat leg cramps. Direct-acting drugs are summarized in Table 22.2.

Botulinum toxin is an unusual drug because, in higher quantities, it acts as a poison. *Clostridium botulinum* is the bacterium responsible for producing the toxin that causes the food poisoning known as botulism. At lower doses, however, botulinum toxin is safe and effective as a muscle relaxant for clients with dystonia. For example, it is used to reduce spasticity, such as a clenched fist or bent elbow that can occur after a stroke or due to cerebral palsy, and for blepharospasm (excessive blinking), strabismus (crossed eyes), and eyelid tics. It produces its effect by blocking the release of acetylcholine from cholinergic nerve terminals (Chapters 12 and 13).

In 2001, Health Canada approved botulinum toxin type A (Botox Cosmetic) injections for temporary improvement in the appearance of moderate to severe frown lines (vertical lines between the brows) in adult clients. It works to relax frown muscles by blocking nerve impulses that trigger wrinkle-causing muscle contractions, creating a smooth appearance between the brows. Administered in a few tiny injections of purified protein, this minimally invasive treatment is

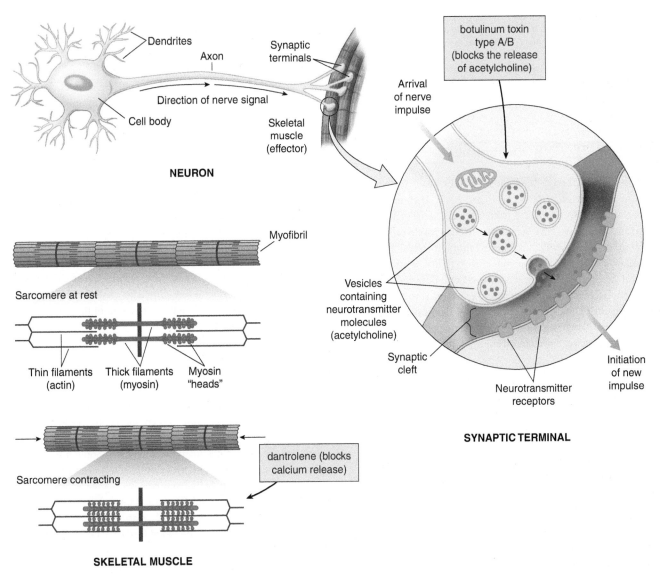

Figure 22.1 Mechanism of action of direct-acting antispasmodics.

TABLE 22.2 Direct-Acting Antispasmodic Drugs

Drug	Route and Adult Dose
botulinum toxin type A (Botox Cosmetic, Botox PWS)	Dosing depends on the subtype being used; subtypes include abobotulinumtoxinA, incobotulinumtoxinA, and onabotulinumtoxinA
botulinum toxin type B	2500–5000 U/dose injected directly into target muscle; doses should be divided among muscle groups
Pr dantrolene (Dantrium)	PO, 25 mg daily (qd); increase to 25 mg bid–qid; may increase every 4–7 days up to max of 400 mg bid–tid
quinine	PO, 260–300 mg at bedtime (hs)

simple and quick and delivers dramatic results with minimal discomfort. Results can be seen in as soon as 24 to 48 hours, and the effect lasts up to 4 months. Injections should not be repeated more than once every 3 months. Side effects include headache, nausea, flu-like symptoms, temporary eyelid drooping, mild pain, erythema at the injection site, and muscle weakness.

NCLEX Success Tips

The most common adverse reaction to dantrolene is muscle weakness. The drug may also depress liver function or cause idiosyncratic hepatitis. Muscle weakness is rarely severe enough to cause slurring of speech, drooling, or enuresis. Although excessive tearing and urine retention are adverse reactions associated with dantrolene use, they aren't as common as muscle weakness.

Dantolene can be used intravenously in the treatment of malignant hyperthermia. In malignant hyperthermia, unless the body is cooled and the influx of calcium into the muscle cells is reversed, lethal cardiac arrhythmia and hypermetabolism occur. The client's body temperature can rise as high as 109°F (42.8°C) as body muscles contract.

PROTOTYPE DRUG | **Dantrolene (Dantrium)**

Actions and Uses: Dantrolene is often used for spasticity, especially for spasms of the head and neck. It directly relaxes muscle spasms by interfering with the release of calcium ions from the sarcoplasmic reticulum of skeletal muscle cells via type 1 ryanodine receptor. Dantrolene is especially useful for muscle spasms when they occur after spinal cord injury or stroke and in cases of cerebral palsy, multiple sclerosis, and occasionally for the treatment of muscle pain after heavy exercise. It is also used for the treatment of malignant hyperthermia. Dantrolene appears to have promise in managing some arrhythmias related to actions on type 2 ryanodine receptors in cardiomyocytes.

Pharmacokinetics: Taken orally, dantrolene is 35% absorbed, has an onset of action of 1 hour, peaks in 5 to 12 hours, and has a variable duration of action. It is metabolized by the liver. Its half-life is 9 hours.

Administration Alerts:

- Use the oral suspension within several days, as it does not contain a preservative.

- IV solution has a high pH and therefore is extremely irritating to tissue.

- Dantrolene is pregnancy category C.

Adverse Effects and Interactions: Adverse effects include muscle weakness, drowsiness, dry mouth, dizziness, nausea, diarrhea,

tachycardia, erratic blood pressure, photosensitivity, and urinary retention.

Dantrolene interacts with many other drugs. For example, it should not be taken with over-the-counter (OTC) cough preparations and antihistamines, alcohol, or other CNS depressants. Verapamil (Isoptin) and other calcium channel blockers taken with dantrolene increase the risk of ventricular fibrillation and cardiovascular collapse. Clients with impaired cardiac or pulmonary function or hepatic disease should not take this drug.

Because of the extreme weakness associated with botulinum, therapies may be needed to improve muscle strength. To circumvent major problems with mobility or posture, botulinum toxin is often applied to small muscle groups. Sometimes this drug is administered with centrally acting oral medications to increase functional use of a range of muscle groups.

Drawbacks to botulinum therapy are its delayed and limited effects. The treatment is mostly effective within 6 weeks and lasts for only 3 to 6 months. Another drawback is pain; botulinum is injected directly into the muscle. Pain associated with injections is usually blocked by a local anesthetic.

Nursing Considerations

The role of the nurse in antispasmodic therapy involves careful monitoring of the client's condition and providing education as it relates to the prescribed drug regimen. Assess adherence with drug use, side effects, and expected outcomes. Centrally acting drugs such as cyclobenzaprine and chlorzoxazone (Paraflex, Parafon Forte) should be avoided in clients with liver disease. All centrally acting drugs cause CNS depression as evidenced by drowsiness and dizziness; therefore, clients should be advised to avoid hazardous activities such as driving until the effects of the drug are known. Clients should also be advised to avoid alcohol, benzodiazepines, opioids, and antihistamines, as they can intensify the CNS depressant effects of the drugs. Clients should be warned against abrupt discontinuation of treatment because this may result in seizures.

Although dantrolene is a direct-acting muscle relaxant, it has similar effects and precautions as centrally acting drugs and is contraindicated in clients with liver disease, compromised pulmonary function, or cardiac dysfunction. The nurse should also be aware that a client with spasticity may not be able to self-medicate and caregiver assistance may be required.

Client education as it relates to centrally acting and direct-acting antispasmodics should include goals, reasons for obtaining baseline data such as health history and blood work, and possible side effects and interactions. See Nursing Process Focus: Clients Receiving Drugs for Muscle Spasms or Spasticity for specific points the nurse should include when teaching clients regarding this class of drug.

NURSING PROCESS FOCUS

Clients Receiving Drugs for Muscle Spasms or Spasticity

Assessment	Potential Nursing Identified Patterns
Prior to administration: • Obtain complete health history, including allergies, drug history, and possible drug interactions. • Obtain complete physical examination. • Establish baseline level of consciousness (LOC), vital signs, muscle tone, range of motion, and degree of muscle spasm.	• Pain (acute/chronic) related to muscle spasms • Mobility impairment related to acute/chronic pain and spasms • Risk for injury and discomfort related to drug side effects • Need for knowledge regarding to drug therapy and supportive therapies

Planning: Client Goals and Expected Outcomes

The client will:

• Report a decrease in pain, increase in range of motion, and reduction of muscle spasm
• Exhibit no adverse effects from the therapeutic regimen
• Demonstrate an understanding of the therapeutic regime
• Demonstrate an understanding of the drug by accurately describing the drug's purpose, action, side effects, and precautions

Implementation

Interventions (Rationales)	Client Education/Discharge Planning
• Monitor LOC and vital signs. (Some skeletal muscle relaxants alter the client's LOC. Others within this class may alter blood pressure and heart rate.) • Monitor pain. • Determine location, duration, and precipitating factors of the client's pain. (Drugs should diminish client's pain.) • Monitor for withdrawal reactions. (Abrupt withdrawal of baclofen may cause visual hallucinations, paranoid ideation, and seizures.) • Monitor muscle tone, range of motion, and degree of muscle spasm. (This will determine effectiveness of drug therapy.) • Provide additional pain relief measures such as positional support, gentle massage, and moist heat or ice packs. (Drugs alone may not be sufficient in providing pain relief.) • Monitor for side effects such as drowsiness, dry mouth, dizziness, nausea, vomiting, faintness, headache, nervousness, diplopia, and urinary retention (cyclobenzaprine). • Monitor for side effects such as muscle weakness, dry mouth, dizziness, nausea, diarrhea, tachycardia, erratic blood pressure, photosensitivity, and urinary retention. (These adverse effects occur with certain drugs in this class.)	Instruct client to: • Avoid driving and other activities requiring mental alertness until effects of the medication are known • Report any significant change in sensorium, such as slurred speech, confusion, hallucinations, or extreme lethargy • Report palpitations, chest pain, dyspnea, unusual fatigue, weakness, and visual disturbances • Avoid using other CNS depressants such as alcohol that will intensify sedation Instruct client to: • Report the development of new sites of muscle pain • Use relaxation techniques, deep breathing, and meditation methods to facilitate relaxation and reduce pain • Advise client to avoid abrupt discontinuation of treatment. • Instruct client to perform gentle range of motion exercises, only to the point of mild physical discomfort, throughout the day. • Instruct client to use complementary pain interventions such as positioning, gentle massage, and the application of heat or cold to the painful area. Instruct client to: • Report side effects • Take medication with food to decrease GI upset • Report signs of urinary retention such as a feeling of urinary bladder fullness, distended abdomen, and discomfort Instruct client: • To use mouth rinses, sips of water, or sugarless candy or gum to help with dry mouth • That medication may cause a decrease in muscle strength and dosage may need to be reduced • To use sunscreen and protective clothing when outdoors

---

Evaluation of Outcome Criteria

Evaluate the effectiveness of drug therapy by confirming that client goals and expected outcomes have been met (see "Planning").

See Tables 22.1 (page 247) and 22.2 (page 250) for lists of drugs to which these nursing actions apply.

CHAPTER

22 Understanding the Chapter

Key Concepts Summary

The numbered key concepts provide a succinct summary of the important points from the corresponding numbered section within the chapter. If any of these points are not clear, refer to the numbered section within the chapter for review.

22.1 Muscle spasms, involuntary contractions of a muscle or group of muscles, most commonly occur because of localized trauma to skeletal muscle.

22.2 Muscle spasms can be treated with non-pharmacological and pharmacological therapies.

22.3 Many muscle relaxants treat muscle spasms at the level of the CNS, generating their effect within the brain and/

or spinal cord, usually by inhibiting upper motor neuron activity, causing sedation, or altering simple reflexes.

22.4 Spasticity, a condition in which selected muscles are continuously contracted, results from damage to the CNS. Effective treatment for spasticity includes both physical therapy and medications.

22.5 Some antispasmodic drugs used for spasticity act directly on muscle tissue, relieving spasticity by interfering with the release of calcium ions.

Chapter 22 Scenario

Andrew is a 27-year-old landscaper who was building a landscaping wall yesterday. His job requires lifting, bending, and twisting. He states that, on arising today, his back hurt and he could not move from side to side. The nurse has performed a physical assessment on Andrew, which revealed tightened muscles in the lumbosacral region and limited mobility. The patient describes his pain as a level 7 on a scale of 1 to 10.

Critical Thinking Questions

1. What are the etiology and pathophysiology of Andrew's muscle spasms? What are other possible causes of muscle spasms?

2. Andrew has been prescribed cyclobenzaprine (Flexeril) to relieve his back spasms. What is the action of this medication and why has it been prescribed?

3. How should Andrew be instructed regarding the administration of this medication?

See Answers to Critical Thinking Questions in Appendix B.

NCLEX Practice Questions

1 A 67-year-old patient experienced a severe back strain while lifting groceries from his car. He is given a prescription for cyclobenzaprine (Flexeril). The nurse will include which precautions in the teaching plan for this patient? Select all that apply.

a. Report any palpitations or rapid pulse rate immediately.

b. Take frequent walks throughout the day to relieve soreness.

c. Rinse the mouth frequently with an alcohol-based mouthwash to relieve excess secretions.

d. Be cautious with driving and other activities requiring alertness.

e. Immediately report any facial or tongue swelling.

2 A patient with spastic cerebral palsy is being treated with oral baclofen (Lioresal). Which patient statement indicates the need for more teaching?

a. "I will be cautious about activities because I may feel weak."

b. "It may take several months before I experience the full effects of the drug."

c. "If I experience unpleasant side effects, I can stop taking the drug."

d. "I will be sure to get enough fluid and fibre in my diet."

3 A patient has been taught to apply capsaicin to increase mobility and relieve pain. Which instruction is most important for the nurse to give to this patient?

a. Apply the medication liberally above and below the site of pain.

b. Apply with a gloved hand to only the site of pain.

c. Apply to areas of redness and inflammation.

d. Apply liberally with a bare hand.

4 A patient has been treated for cervical dystonia with an injection of botulinum toxin type A (Botox). Which of the following symptoms will the nurse teach the patient to immediately report?

a. Fever, aches, or chills

b. Difficulty swallowing, blurred vision, or ptosis

c. Moderate levels of muscle weakness on the affected side

d. Continuous spasms and pain on the affected side

5 A female patient, age 45, is receiving dantrolene (Dantrium) for treatment of painful muscle spasms associated with multiple sclerosis. What will the nurse teach the patient? Select all that apply.

a. Increase fluid and fibre intake to prevent constipation.

b. Inform the healthcare provider if you are taking estrogen products.

c. Sip water or ice, or suck on hard candy to relieve xerostomia.

d. Be sure to obtain 20 minutes of sun exposure per day to boost vitamin D levels.

e. Return periodically to the provider to monitor liver function.

See Answers to NCLEX Practice Questions in Appendix A.

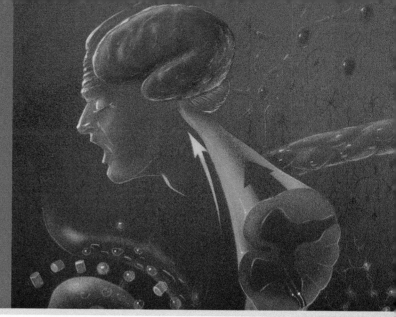

Patrick McDonnell/Science Source

CHAPTER 23

Pharmacotherapy of Pain and Migraine

LEARNING OUTCOMES

After reading this chapter, the student should be able to:

1. Identify key principles of pain management.
2. Describe the assessment and classification of pain.
3. Explain the phases of pain physiology: transduction, transmission, perception, and modulation
4. Identify drug classes used for treating pain.
5. Explain the therapeutic action of analgesics in relation to physiological mechanisms of pain.
6. For each of the drug classes listed in Prototype Drugs, identify a representative drug and explain its mechanism of action, primary actions, and important adverse effects.
7. Relate the importance of pain assessment to effective pharmacotherapy.
8. Discuss the nurse's role in using pharmacological and non-pharmacological therapies for clients who are experiencing pain.
9. Compare and contrast the types of opioid receptors and their importance to pharmacology.
10. Explain the role of opioid antagonists in the diagnosis and treatment of acute opioid toxicity.
11. Describe the long-term treatment of opioid dependence.
12. Compare the pharmacotherapeutic approaches of preventing migraines to those of aborting migraines.
13. Describe and explain, based on pharmacological principles, the rationale for nursing assessment, planning, and interventions for clients who are experiencing pain.
14. Use the nursing process to care for clients who are receiving analgesics and antimigraine drugs.

CHAPTER OUTLINE

Pain is a physiological and emotional experience characterized by unpleasant feelings, usually associated with trauma or disease. On a simple level, pain may be viewed as a defence mechanism that helps people to avoid potentially damaging situations and encourages them to seek medical help. Although the neural and chemical mechanisms for pain are straightforward, many psychological and emotional processes can modify this sensation. Anxiety, fatigue, and depression can increase the perception of pain. Positive attitudes and support from caregivers may reduce the perception of pain. Clients are more likely to tolerate their pain if they know the source of the sensation and the medical course of treatment designed to manage the pain. For example, if clients know that the pain is temporary, such as during labour or after surgery, they are more likely to be accepting of the pain.

General Principles of Pain Management

23.1 The primary goal of pain management is to reduce pain to a level that allows the client to continue normal daily activities.

Pain management is one of the most important tasks for healthcare providers. It is also one of the most difficult because the experience of pain by clients and its assessment by the healthcare provider are subjective. The perception of pain can clearly be influenced by comorbid conditions such as anxiety, fatigue, and depression. For example, knowing that healthcare providers and caregivers are attentive and actively engaged in pain management may lower clients' anxiety, thus reducing pain perception and increasing pain tolerance. Listening carefully, showing respect, and helping clients to understand their treatment options are important steps in attaining optimum pain relief.

The immediate goal of pain management is to reduce pain to a level that allows the client to perform reasonable activities of daily living (ADLs) such as sleeping, eating, and normal physical activities. For some disorders, the client should understand that the total elimination of pain may not be a realistic goal or that the pain may require a long period of treatment. Several key principles underlie the nursing management of pain:

- The client should be considered the expert on his or her own pain; the nurse should always believe the client's self-assessment of pain.

- Pain management is a client right and should be based on the client's goals. The client should be screened for pain during an initial assessment and periodically thereafter. If pain cannot be managed effectively, a pain management specialist should be consulted.

- Non-pharmacological interventions such as massage or the application of heat or cold should be encouraged in pain management. A combination of therapies is optimum because different modalities work by different mechanisms, thus improving the effectiveness of pain management.

- Dosing should be individualized and adjusted to produce the established pain management goal in each client.

- Adverse effects from pain medications should be anticipated and prevented whenever possible. Should they appear, adverse effects should be addressed immediately.

- Around-the-clock dosing for moderate to severe pain should be implemented because it is much easier to *maintain* a pain-free level than to *eliminate* existing or escalating pain.

Pharmacological Therapies

Dozens of over-the-counter (OTC) and prescription pain medications are available, and the selection of a specific medication depends on many factors. Foremost is the severity of the pain. The drug selected must be capable of providing adequate pain relief. Second, the choice of analgesic depends on potential adverse events and drug interactions and contraindications. A key point is that every analgesic, even an OTC pain reliever, has the potential to cause serious adverse effects in susceptible clients. This reinforces the need to use non-pharmacological therapies for pain relief whenever possible.

The two broad categories of analgesics are the opioids and non-opioids. A third category of drugs for the management of pain is the adjuvant analgesics. The adjuvant analgesics have no pain relief activity when used alone, but they are able to enhance the analgesic action of opioids and non-opioids.

The drug class of choice for severe pain is the opioids. Minor to moderate pain is treated with non-opioids such as nonsteroidal anti-inflammatory drugs (NSAIDs), centrally acting agents, or acetaminophen (Tylenol). There are dozens of opioids and NSAIDs to choose from, and it is difficult for beginning students, and even experienced healthcare providers, to learn the subtle differences of drugs within each class. Although the large number of analgesics appears overwhelming, many of them are quite similar, and prescribers most often use only a few drugs in each class.

The pharmacological management of acute and chronic pain is based on the analgesic ladder proposed by the World Health Organization. Pain ratings of less than 4 are treated with non-opioid analgesics, complementary and alternative therapies (CATs), or a combination of the two. When pain ratings become moderate (4 to 6), oral opioids are added to the baseline treatment. When pain is severe (7 to 10), parenteral opioids are used. If chronic pain has neuropathic qualities, adjuvant analgesics are added.

Management of Cancer Pain

Clients with intractable cancer pain require more invasive techniques because rapidly growing tumours often press on vital tissues and nerves. Furthermore, chemotherapy and surgical treatments for cancer can cause severe pain. Radiation therapy may provide pain relief by shrinking solid tumours that may be pressing on nerves. Surgery may be used to reduce pain by removing part of or the entire tumour. Injection of alcohol or another neurotoxic substance into neurons is occasionally performed to cause nerve blocks. Nerve blocks irreversibly stop impulse transmission along the treated nerves and have the potential to provide total pain relief. Injection of local anesthetics or steroid hormones as nerve blocks can provide relief for months and is used for pain resulting from pressure on spinal nerves.

Patient-Controlled Analgesia

Patient-controlled analgesia (PCA) is a method of drug delivery that uses an infusion pump to deliver a prescribed amount of opioid by client self-administration. By pressing a button, the client can self-administer the opioid, thus relieving the anxiety of waiting for an as-needed drug administration. The client does not have unlimited access to the drug; the infusion pump is programmed by the nurse to deliver a prescribed amount of drug over a designated time period. If the client attempts to self-administer the drug too often, the client is locked out until the next dose interval. The program is adjusted depending on the client's response to the drug. Morphine is the opioid usually used for PCA; however, hydromorphone (Dilaudid), meperidine (Demerol), or fentanyl (Duragesic) may be used.

PCA allows clients to participate in their own care. Frequent, small doses of analgesics give a more consistent serum drug level than would be obtained by administering larger doses three to four times per day. PCA requires that the client be conscious and capable of understanding the operation of the pump. Clients should be taught not to be overly concerned about activating the pump because the program is set to prevent the possibility of overdose. Nurses, family members, and visitors should not use the device to give the client more medication, but should consult with the healthcare provider if they feel that the client's pain is not relieved.

Assessment and Classification of Pain

23.2 The ways to assess and classify pain include acute or chronic and nociceptor or neuropathic.

The psychological reaction to pain is a subjective experience. The same degree and type of pain may be described as excruciating and unbearable by one client but not be mentioned during physical assessment by

another. Several numerical scales and survey instruments are available to help healthcare providers standardize the assessment of pain and measure the progress of subsequent drug therapy. Successful pain management depends on accurate assessment of both the degree of pain experienced by the client and the potential underlying disorders that may be causing the pain. Selection of the correct therapy is dependent on the nature and character of the pain.

Pain can be classified as either acute or chronic. Acute pain is an intense pain that occurs over a defined time, usually from injury to recovery. Chronic pain persists for longer than 6 months, can interfere with daily activities, and is associated with feelings of helplessness or hopelessness.

Pain can also be classified according to its source. Injury to *tissues* produces **nociceptor pain**. This type of pain may be further subdivided into somatic pain, which produces sharp, localized sensations, or visceral pain, which is described as a generalized dull, throbbing, or aching pain. In contrast, **neuropathic pain** is caused by injury to *nerves* and typically is described as burning, shooting, or numb pain. Whereas nociceptor pain responds quite well to conventional pain relief medications, neuropathic pain has less therapeutic success.

Pain transmission processes allow multiple targets for pharmacological intervention.

Pain physiology may be divided into four phases: transduction, transmission, perception, and modulation. These phases are illustrated in Figure 23.1.

Pain Transduction

Pain transduction begins when nociceptor nerve endings in the peripheral nervous system are stimulated. This occurs when local tissue injury causes the release of chemical mediators of inflammation, including prostaglandins, leukotrienes, histamine, bradykinin, and substance P. These substances sensitize peripheral nociceptors, making them easier to activate.

Pain Transmission

The nerve impulse signalling the pain travels from the nociceptor to the spinal cord along two types of sensory neurons called A and C fibres. A fibres are wrapped in myelin, a lipid substance that speeds nerve transmission, and carry signals for intense, well-defined pain. On the other hand, **C fibres** are unmyelinated and thus carry information more slowly and conduct poorly localized pain, which is often perceived as burning or a dull ache.

A fibres have three subtypes: alpha, beta, and delta. A alpha fibres have the fastest transmission and respond to touch and pressure on muscle; A beta fibres are slower and respond to touch and pressure on skin. Finally, **A delta fibres** are the slowest of the A fibres and respond to tissue injury, producing the sensation of sharp pain.

The sensory nerve fibres enter the dorsal horn of the spinal cord and have adjacent synapses in an area called the substantia gelatinosa. The **gate control theory** proposes a gating mechanism for the transmission of pain in the spinal cord. Signals from faster A alpha or A beta fibres reach the spinal cord and close the gate before those of C fibres reach the region (or gate), in effect blocking the transmission of these types of pain impulses. The gate control theory, proposed in 1965, has withstood the test of time and has been found to be more complex than originally proposed. The "gates" can also be closed when flooded with

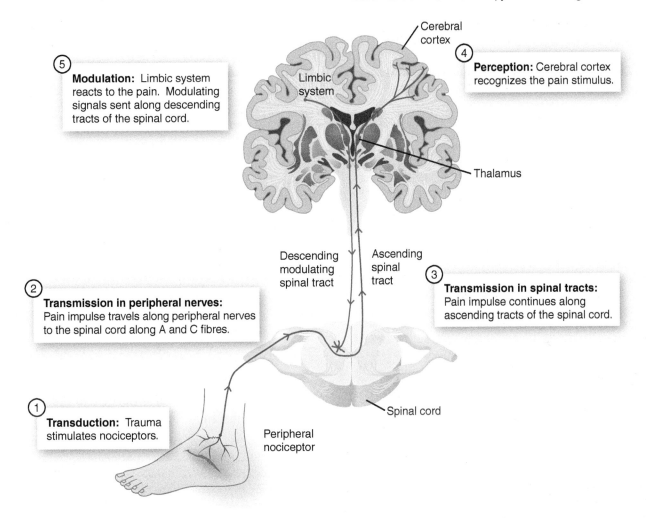

Figure 23.1 Phases of pain physiology.

⑤ **Modulation:** Limbic system reacts to the pain. Modulating signals sent along descending tracts of the spinal cord.

④ **Perception:** Cerebral cortex recognizes the pain stimulus.

Cerebral cortex

Limbic system

Thalamus

Descending modulating spinal tract

Ascending spinal tract

② **Transmission in peripheral nerves:** Pain impulse travels along peripheral nerves to the spinal cord along A and C fibres.

③ **Transmission in spinal tracts:** Pain impulse continues along ascending tracts of the spinal cord.

Spinal cord

① **Transduction:** Trauma stimulates nociceptors.

Peripheral nociceptor

non-nociceptor impulses. Gate control explains the effectiveness of massage, transcutaneous electrical nerve stimulation, and possibly acupuncture in reducing pain.

Once a pain impulse reaches the spinal cord, neurotransmitters are responsible for passing the message along to the next neuron. At the spinal cord level, glutamate is the neurotransmitter for A fibres, whereas both glutamate and substance P are neurotransmitters for C fibres. Impulse transmission from the spinal cord to the brain is moderated by both excitatory and inhibitory neurotransmitters. The activity of substance P may be affected by other neurotransmitters released from neurons in the central nervous system (CNS). One group of neurotransmitters functions as endogenous opioids, or natural pain modifiers; these include **endorphins** and enkephalins.

Pain Perception

Perception, the conscious experience of pain, occurs in the brain. Numerous cortical structures and pathways are involved in perception, including the reticular activating system, the somatosensory system, and the limbic system. When the pain impulse reaches the brain, it may respond to the sensation with a wide variety of possible actions, ranging from signalling the skeletal muscles to jerk away from a sharp object to mental depression in those experiencing chronic pain.

Pain Modulation

Modulation involves descending nervous impulses travelling down the spinal cord that inhibit afferent pain transmission via a feedback mechanism. Neurotransmitters such as serotonin, norepinephrine, and endogenous opioids (endorphins and enkephalins) inhibit pain transmission.

The four phases of pain physiology allow for multiple targets for pharmacological intervention. The two primary classes of analgesics

CONNECTIONS **Lifespan Considerations**

◀ Pain in Infants and Older Adults

- Infants and older adults are the most likely Canadians to be undermedicated for pain.
- Infants older than 1 month can clear opioids as well as adults do.
- Premature infants can experience severe pain; they receive normal pain signals but have underdeveloped mechanisms to moderate pain signals.
- Due to age-related changes in pharmacokinetics, older adults may experience more frequent and serious side effects from analgesics.

◀ Cultural Influences on Pain Expression and Perception

How a person responds to pain and the type of pain management chosen may be culturally determined. Establishment of a therapeutic relationship is of the utmost importance in helping a client to attain pain relief. Respect the client's attitudes and beliefs about pain as well as their preferred treatment. An assessment of the client's needs, beliefs, and customs by listening, showing respect, and allowing the client to help develop and choose treatment options to attain pain relief is the most culturally sensitive approach.

When assessing pain, the nurse must remember that some clients may openly express their feelings and need for pain relief while others believe that the expression of pain symptoms, such as crying, is a sign of weakness. Pain management also varies according to cultural and religious beliefs. Traditional pain medications may or may not be the preferred method for pain control. For example, some Aboriginal peoples and some Asian Canadians may prefer to use alternative therapies such as herbs, thermal therapies, acupuncture, massage, and meditation. Prayer plays an important role within some Canadian cultural groups, including some African Canadians.

act at different locations: the NSAIDs act at the peripheral level, whereas the opioids act on the CNS. Drugs that affect or mimic the inhibitory neurotransmitters are used as adjuvant analgesics.

Non-Pharmacological Techniques for Pain Management

23.3 Non-pharmacological techniques such as massage, biofeedback therapy, and meditation are often important adjuncts to effective pain management.

Although drugs are quite effective at relieving pain in most clients, they can have significant side effects. For example, at high doses, acetylsalicylic acid (ASA, Aspirin) causes gastrointestinal (GI) bleeding, and the opioids cause significant drowsiness and have the potential for dependence. Non-pharmacological techniques may be used in place of drugs or as an adjunct to pharmacotherapy to assist clients in obtaining adequate pain relief. When used concurrently with medication, non-pharmacological techniques may allow for lower doses and possibly fewer drug-related adverse effects. Some techniques used for reducing pain are as follows:

- Acupuncture
- Biofeedback therapy
- Massage
- Heat or cold
- Meditation
- Relaxation therapy
- Art or music therapy
- Imagery
- Chiropractic manipulation
- Hypnosis
- Therapeutic touch
- Transcutaneous electrical nerve stimulation (TENS)
- Energy therapies such as reiki and qigong

Clients with intractable cancer pain sometimes require more invasive techniques, as rapidly growing tumours press on vital tissues and nerves. Furthermore, chemotherapy and surgical treatments for cancer can cause severe pain. Radiation therapy may provide pain relief by shrinking solid tumours that may be pressing on nerves. Surgery may be used to reduce pain by removing part or all of the tumour. Injection of alcohol or another neurotoxic substance into neurons is occasionally performed to cause nerve blocks. Nerve blocks irreversibly stop impulse transmission along the treated nerves and have the potential to provide total pain relief.

The Neural Mechanisms of Pain

23.4 Neural mechanisms include the pain transmission via A delta or C fibres and the release of substance P.

The process of pain transmission begins when pain receptors are stimulated. These receptors, called **nociceptors**, are free nerve endings strategically located throughout the body. As discussed, the nerve impulse signalling the pain is sent to the spinal cord along two types of sensory neurons, called A delta and C fibres. Once pain impulses reach the spinal cord, a neurotransmitter called **substance P** is thought to be responsible for continuing the pain message, although other neurotransmitter candidates have been proposed. Spinal substance P is critical because it controls whether pain signals will continue to the brain. The activity of substance P may be affected by other neurotransmitters released from neurons in the CNS. One group of neurotransmitters called **endogenous opioids** includes endorphins, dynorphins, and enkephalins. Figure 23.2 shows one point of contact where endogenous opioids modify sensory information at the level of the spinal cord. If the pain impulse reaches the brain, it may respond to the sensation with many possible actions, ranging from signalling the skeletal muscles to jerk away from a sharp object, to mental depression caused by thoughts of death or disability in those suffering from chronic pain.

The fact that the pain signal begins at nociceptors located within peripheral tissues and proceeds through the CNS provides several targets for the pharmacological intervention of pain transmission.

OPIOID (NARCOTIC) ANALGESICS

Analgesics are medications used to relieve pain. The two basic categories of analgesics are the opioids and the non-opioids. An opioid analgesic is a natural or synthetic morphine-like substance capable of reducing severe pain. Opioids are **narcotic** substances, meaning that they produce numbness and stupor-like symptoms.

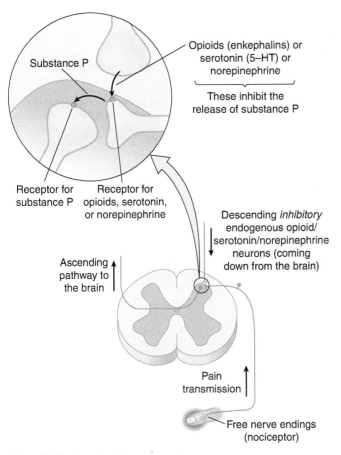

Figure 23.2 Neural pathways for pain.

TABLE 23.1 Responses Produced by Activation of Specific Opioid Receptors		
Response	**Mu Receptor**	**Kappa Receptor**
Analgesia	X	X
Decreased GI motility	X	X
Euphoria	X	
Miosis		X
Physical dependence	X	
Respiratory depression	X	
Sedation	X	X

specifically refer to opioid substances. Because narcotics have addictive and high abuse potential, drug products that contain narcotics are designated Controlled Drugs and Substances Act (CDSA) Schedule I, and their administration is documented on the narcotic control record.

Opioids exert their actions by interacting with at least six types of receptors: mu (types 1 and 2), kappa, sigma, delta, and epsilon. From the perspective of pain management, the **mu** and **kappa receptors** are the most important. Drugs that stimulate a particular receptor are called opioid agonists; those that block a receptor are called opioid antagonists. The types of actions produced by activating mu and kappa receptors are shown in Table 23.1.

Some opioid agonists, such as morphine, activate both mu and kappa receptors. Other opioids, such as pentazocine (Talwin), exert mixed opioid agonist-antagonist effects by activating the kappa receptor but blocking the mu receptor. Opioid blockers such as naloxone (Narcan) inhibit both mu and kappa receptors. This is the body's natural way of providing the mechanism for a diverse set of body responses from one substance. Figure 23.3 illustrates opioid actions on the mu and kappa receptors.

Classification of Opioids

23.5 Opioids are natural or synthetic substances extracted from the poppy plant that exert their effects through interaction with mu and kappa receptors.

Terminology associated with the narcotic analgesic medications is often confusing. Several of these drugs are obtained from opium, a milky extract from the unripe seeds of the poppy plant that contains more than 20 different chemicals with pharmacological activity. These natural substances are called **opiates**. Opium consists of 9% to 14% morphine and 0.8% to 2.5% codeine. In a search for safer analgesics, chemists have created several dozen synthetic drugs with activity similar to that of the opiates. **Opioid** is a general term referring to any of these substances, natural or synthetic, and is often used interchangeably with the term *opiate*.

Narcotic is a general term used to describe morphine-like drugs that produce analgesia and CNS depression. Narcotics may be natural, such as morphine, or synthetic, such as meperidine (Demerol). In common usage, a narcotic analgesic is the same as an opioid, and the terms are often used interchangeably. In the context of drug enforcement, however, the term *narcotic* is often used to describe a much broader range of illegal drugs of addiction such as hallucinogens, heroin, amphetamines, and marijuana. In medical environments, restrict the use of the term *narcotic* to

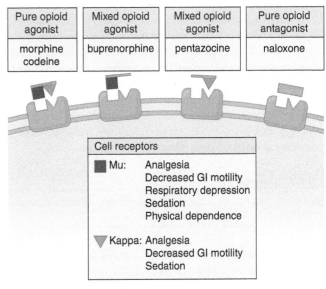

Figure 23.3 Opioid receptors.

Pharmacotherapy with Opioids

23.6 Opioids are the drugs of choice for severe pain. They also have other important therapeutic effects, including dampening of the cough reflex and slowing of the motility of the GI tract.

Opioids are drugs of choice for moderate to severe pain that cannot be controlled with other classes of analgesics. More than 20 different opioids are available as medications, and they may be classified by similarities in their chemical structure, by their mechanism of action, or by their efficacy, as shown in Table 23.2. The most clinically useful method is classifying by efficacy, which places opiates into categories of strong or moderate narcotic activity. Morphine is the prototype drug for severe pain and the drug to which all other opiates are compared.

NCLEX Success Tip

Hydromorphone (Dilaudid) is about five times more potent than morphine, from which it is prepared. Therefore, it is administered only in small doses. Hydromorphone can cause dependency in any dose; however, fear of dependency developing in the postoperative period is unwarranted. The dose is determined by the client's need for pain relief. As with opioid analgesics, excretion depends on normal liver function.

Opiates produce many important effects other than analgesia. They are effective at suppressing the cough reflex and at slowing the motility of the GI tract for cases of severe diarrhea. As powerful CNS depressants, opioids can cause sedation, which may be either a therapeutic effect or a side effect depending on the client's disease state. Some clients experience euphoria and intense relaxation, which are reasons why opiates are sometimes abused. There are many adverse effects, including respiratory depression, sedation, nausea, and vomiting.

All of the narcotic analgesics have the potential to cause physical and psychological dependence, as discussed in Chapter 25. Dependence is more likely to occur when taking high doses for extended periods. Many healthcare providers and nurses are hesitant to administer the proper amount of opioid analgesics for fear of causing client dependence or of producing serious adverse effects such as sedation or respiratory depression. Because of this undermedication, clients may not receive complete pain relief. When used according to accepted medical practice, clients can, and indeed should, receive the pain relief they need without fear of addiction or adverse effects. Clients who are addicted to narcotics will often need higher doses of the drugs for adequate pain relief. Because tolerance to the respiratory depression effects occurs rapidly when narcotics are taken regularly, higher than average doses can safely be given. Pain relief is a priority.

NCLEX Success Tip

Assessment findings in a client abusing opiates include agitation, slurred speech, euphoria, and constricted pupils.

It is common practice to combine opioids and non-narcotic analgesics into a single tablet or capsule. The two classes of analgesics work synergistically to relieve pain, and the dose of narcotic

TABLE 23.2 Opioids for Pain Management	
Drug	**Route and Adult Dose**
Opioid Agonists with Moderate Efficacy	
codeine	Orally (PO), immediate release, 15–60 mg q4h prn (max 360 mg/day); sustained release, 50 mg every 12 hours (titrate at intervals of > 48 hours until adequate analgesia has been achieved); doses > 600 mg/day should not be used
oxycodone (OxyNeo [sustained release], OxyIR [immediate release])	PO, immediate release, 5–15 mg every 4–6 hours as needed; extended release, start with 10 mg every 12 hours; dose is titrated to effect
oxycodone + acetaminophen (Percocet)	PO, 5–10 mg qid prn, usually every 4–12 hours (supplied as 5 mg oxycodone + 325 mg acetaminophen) (max 4 g acetaminophen/day)
Opioid Agonists with High Efficacy	
hydromorphone (Dilaudid)	PO, 1–8 mg q4–6h prn
meperidine (Demerol)	PO/IM/SC, 50–150 mg every 3 to 4 hours (q3–4h) prn
methadone (Metadol)	PO, start with 2.5mg every 8–12 hours; IV, start with 2.5-10 mg every 8–12 hours
Pr morphine (Kadian, M-Eslon, MS Contin, MS-IR, Statex)	PO, 10–30 mg q4h prn (also sustained release [SR], per rectum [PR], subcutaneous/intramuscular/intravenous [SC/IM/IV])
Opioids with Mixed Agonist-Antagonist Effects	
butorphanol	Nasal spray, 1–2 mg q3–4h prn
nalbuphine (Nubain)	SC/IM/IV, 10 mg every 3 to 6 hours (q3–6h) prn (max 160 mg/day)
pentazocine (Talwin)	SC/IM/IV, 30 mg q3–4h (max 360 mg/day)
Opioid Antagonists	
Pr naloxone (Narcan)	IV/IM/SC, 0.4–2 mg; may be repeated every 2–3 min up to 10 mg if necessary
naltrexone (ReVia)	For alcohol dependence: PO, 50 mg/day; for opioid dependence: PO, 25 mg/day; for both indications can give IM 380 mg once every 4 weeks

can be kept small to avoid dependence and opioid-related side effects. Combination products containing narcotics are designated CDSA Schedule I. Caffeine is often added to enhance absorption and distribution of the analgesic. Caffeine may also help to relieve headache by constricting cerebral blood vessels. Some common combination analgesics are as follows:

- Percocet or oxycocet (oxycodone [HCl], 5 mg; acetaminophen, 325 mg)

- Percodan (oxycodone, 4.8 mg; acetylsalicylic acid, 325 mg)

- A.C. & C. tablets (acetylsalicylic acid, 325 mg; caffeine, 15 mg; codeine, 8 mg)

- Atasol 30 (acetaminophen, 325 mg; caffeine, 30 mg; codeine, 30 mg)

- Tylenol with Codeine No. 2 (acetaminophen, 300 mg; caffeine, 15 mg; codeine, 15 mg)

Some opioids are used primarily for conditions other than pain. For example, alfentanil (Alfenta), fentanyl, remifentanil (Ultiva), and sufentanil (Sufenta) are used for general anesthesia; these are discussed in Chapter 24. Codeine is most often prescribed as a cough suppressant and is covered in Chapter 38. Opiates used in treating diarrhea are presented in Chapter 35.

Nursing Considerations

The role of the nurse involves careful monitoring of the client's condition and providing education as it relates to the prescribed drug regimen. When providing care for clients who are taking opioids, perform an initial assessment to determine the presence or history of severe respiratory disorders, increased intracranial pressure (ICP), seizures, and liver or renal disease. Obtain an allergy history before administering these drugs. A complete blood count (CBC) and liver and renal studies, including aspartate aminotransferase (AST), alanine aminotransferase (ALT), amylase, and bilirubin, should be obtained to rule out the presence of disease. The character, duration, location, and intensity of pain should be determined before the administration of these agents. Obtain a history of current medication usage, especially alcohol and other CNS depressants because these drugs will increase respiratory depression and sedation. Contraindications include hypersensitivity and conditions precluding IV opioid administration, such as acute asthma or upper airway obstruction.

Through activation of primarily mu receptors, opioids may cause profound respiratory depression. Vital signs, especially respirations, should be obtained prior to and throughout the treatment regimen. Opioids should not be administered if respirations are below 12 breaths per minute. Narcotic antagonists such as naloxone should be readily available if respirations fall below 10 breaths per minute. Watch for decreasing level of consciousness (LOC) and ensure safety by keeping the bed in a low position with side rails raised. Assistance may be needed with ambulation and ADLs.

CONNECTIONS ⟩ Lifespan Considerations

◀ The Influence of Age on Pain Expression and Perception

Pain control in both children and older adults can be challenging. Knowledge of developmental theories, the aging process, behavioural cues, subtle signs of discomfort, and verbal and nonverbal responses to pain are a must when it comes to effective pain management. Older clients may have a decreased perception of pain or simply ignore pain as a "natural" consequence of aging. Because these clients are frequently undermedicated, a thorough assessment is a necessity. As with adults, it is important that the nurse believe children's self-reports when assessing for pain. Developmentally appropriate pain rating tools are available and should be used on a continuous basis. Comfort measures should also be used.

When administering opioids for pain relief, always closely monitor older adults and children. Smaller doses are usually indicated, and side effects may be heightened. Closely monitor decreased respirations, LOC, and dizziness. Body weight should be taken prior to the start of opioid administration and doses calculated accordingly. Bed or crib rails should be kept raised, and the bed should be in the low position at all times to prevent injury from falls. Some opioids, such as meperidine, should be used cautiously in children. Many older adults take multiple drugs (polypharmacy); therefore, it is important to obtain a complete list of all medications taken and check for interactions.

Another severe adverse reaction, increased ICP, occurs as an indirect result of the respiratory depression effect. When respiration is suppressed, the carbon dioxide (CO_2) content of blood is increased, which dilates the cerebral blood vessels and causes ICP to rise. Similarly, orthostatic hypotension may also occur due to the blunting of the baroreceptor reflex and dilation of the peripheral arterioles and veins.

The nurse should continually monitor urinary output for urinary retention. This may occur due to the effect of increasing tone in the bladder sphincter and through suppression of the bladder stimuli.

Side effects such as constipation, nausea, and vomiting occur due to a combination of actions on the GI tract. By suppressing intestinal contractions, increasing the tone of the anal sphincter, and inhibiting secretion of fluids into the intestine, constipation may occur. Nausea or vomiting may occur due to the direct stimulation of the chemoreceptor trigger zone of the medulla. If this occurs, an antiemetic may be indicated. Opioids may be contraindicated for clients who are suffering from diarrhea caused by infections, especially following antibiotic therapy (pseudomembranous colitis). Pathogens in the GI tract produce toxins that are shed during diarrhea; constipation causes toxins to build up in the body.

Client education as it relates to opioids should include goals, reasons for obtaining baseline data such as vital signs and laboratory tests and procedures, and possible side effects. See Nursing Process Focus: Clients Receiving Opioid Therapy on page 263 for important points to include when teaching clients regarding this class of drug.

NCLEX Success Tips

When given to treat acute myocardial infarction (MI), morphine eliminates pain, reduces venous return to the heart, reduces vascular resistance, reduces cardiac workload, and reduces the oxygen demand of the heart.

The preferred opioid analgesic to treat cholecystitis is meperidine. Elderly clients should not be given meperidine because of the risk of acute confusion and seizures in this population. A nurse should question the prescription for morphine because it is believed to cause biliary spasm in case of cholecystitis or pancreatitis.

PROTOTYPE DRUG | Morphine (Kadian, M-Eslon, MS Contin, MS-IR, Statex)

Actions and Uses: Morphine binds with both mu and kappa receptor sites to produce profound analgesia. It causes euphoria, constriction of the pupils, and stimulation of cardiac muscle. It is used for symptomatic relief of serious acute and chronic pain after non-narcotic analgesics have failed, as a pre-anesthetic medication, to relieve shortness of breath associated with heart failure and pulmonary edema, and for acute chest pain connected with myocardial infarction (MI).

Administration Alerts:

- Oral solution may be given sublingually.
- Oral solution comes in multiple strengths; carefully observe drug orders and labels before administering.
- Morphine causes peripheral vasodilation, which results in orthostatic hypotension and flushing of the face and neck.
- Morphine is pregnancy category D in long-term use or with high doses.

Pharmacokinetics: Morphine is variably absorbed following PO administration. It is well absorbed by other routes. It is widely distributed, crosses the placenta, and enters breast milk. It is up to 35% protein bound. It is mostly metabolized by the liver. The half-life of morphine is 2 to 4 hours in adults. Half-life is 10 to 20 hours in premature neonates, 7.6 hours in neonates, 6.2 hours in infants 1 to 3 months, 3 hours in children 6 months to 2.5 years, and 1 to 2 hours in children 3 to 6 years.

Adverse Effects and Interactions: Morphine may cause dysphoria (restlessness, depression, and anxiety), hallucinations, nausea, constipation, dizziness, and an itching sensation. Overdose may result in severe respiratory depression or cardiac arrest. Tolerance develops to the analgesic, sedative, and euphoric effects of the drug. Cross-tolerance also develops between morphine and other opioids such as heroin, methadone (Metadol), and meperidine. Physical and psychological dependence develop when high doses are taken for prolonged periods of time. Morphine may intensify or mask the pain of gallbladder disease, due to biliary tract spasms.

Morphine interacts with several drugs. For example, concurrent use of CNS depressants such as alcohol, other opioids, general anesthetics, sedatives, and antidepressants such as monoamine oxidase (MAO) inhibitors and tricyclic antidepressants (TCAs) potentiates the action of opiates, increasing the risk for severe respiratory depression and death.

Use with caution with herbal supplements, such as yohimbe, which may potentiate the effect of morphine.

NCLEX Success Tips

A client can provide informed consent only when competent to do so. A client who has been given morphine may not be considered competent to give consent.

Morphine can cause respiratory depression, leading to respiratory arrest. The nurse should assess the client's respiratory rate before administration and throughout the course of analgesic treatment.

For greatest analgesic effectiveness, the nurse should administer an opioid agonist, such as morphine, before the client's pain becomes severe. If the nurse waits until the pain becomes severe, the medication will be less effective, taking longer to provide relief. Giving morphine as seldom as possible to avoid dependency would cause needless client suffering.

The Joint Commission of the United States and the Institute for Safe Medication Practices Canada recommend not to use the abbreviation *MSO₄* because it can apply to morphine as well as to magnesium sulfate.

Morphine is a narcotic. Clients need to understand that when pain is present and morphine is used therapeutically, there is less likelihood of addiction. If morphine is taken in the absence of pain, addiction can result.

Constipation, nausea, vomiting, and pruritus are all treatable adverse effects of morphine.

Contraindications to the use of opioid analgesics include known drug allergy and severe asthma.

Many clients will claim to be allergic to morphine because it causes itching. Itching is a pharmacological effect due to histamine release and not an allergic reaction. Diphenhydramine (Benadryl) can be administered for pruritus.

Morphine sulfate may also increase intracranial pressure if the client is not ventilating properly, which could result in an accumulation of CO_2, a potent vasodilator.

Morphine sulfate acts as an analgesic and sedative. It also reduces myocardial oxygen consumption, blood pressure, and heart rate. Morphine also reduces anxiety and fear due to its sedative effects and by slowing the heart rate.

Pharmacotherapy with Opioid Antagonists

23.7 Opioid antagonists may be used to reverse the symptoms of opioid toxicity or overdose, such as sedation and respiratory depression.

Opioid overdose can occur as a result of overly aggressive pain therapy or as a result of substance abuse. Any opioid may be abused for its psychoactive effects; however, morphine, meperidine, and heroin are preferred due to their potency. Although heroin is currently available as a legal analgesic in many countries, it is deemed too dangerous for therapeutic use by Health Canada and is a major drug of addiction. Once injected or inhaled, heroin rapidly crosses the blood-brain barrier to the brain, where it is metabolized to morphine. Therefore, the effects and symptoms of heroin administration are actually caused by the activation of mu and kappa receptors by morphine. The initial effect is an intense euphoria, called a rush, followed by several hours of deep relaxation.

Acute opioid intoxication is a medical emergency, with respiratory depression being the most serious problem. Infusion with the opioid antagonist naloxone may be used to reverse respiratory depression and other acute symptoms. In cases where the client is unconscious and the healthcare provider is unclear what drug has been taken, opioid antagonists may be given to diagnose the overdose. If the opioid antagonist fails to quickly reverse the acute symptoms, the overdose was likely due to a non-opioid substance.

Nursing Considerations

The role of the nurse in opioid antagonist therapy involves careful monitoring of the client's condition and providing education as it relates to the prescribed drug regimen. The primary indication for use of an opioid antagonist is established or suspected opioid-induced respiratory depression. An opioid antagonist may also be used to reverse opioid-induced pruritus. However, in clinical practice it is not often used for pruritus as its use would completely reverse the full pain relief achieved with the opioid. The primary nursing response is to assess the client's respiratory status and administer the opioid antagonist if respirations are below 10 breaths per minute. Resuscitative equipment should be immediately accessible. Obtaining key medical information is a priority; the presence or history of cardiovascular disease should be included. Opioids increase cardiac workload, so they must be used with caution in clients with cardiovascular disease. Assess the social context of the client's environment for the potential for opioid dependency. Opioid antagonists should be used cautiously in clients who are physically dependent on opioids because drug-induced withdrawal may be more severe than spontaneous opioid withdrawal. Caution is also advised in pregnant or lactating women and in children.

The nurse should assess the client's pain level before administration of these drugs and during therapy. During and immediately after the administration of opioid antagonists, check vital signs every 3 to 5 minutes (especially respiratory function and blood pressure). Obtain an arterial blood gas and electrocardiogram (ECG) when ordered. Monitor for the following side effects: drowsiness, tremors, hyperventilation, ventricular tachycardia, and loss of analgesia. If giving these drugs to drug-dependent clients, monitor for signs of opioid withdrawal such as cramping, vomiting, hypertension, and anxiety.

Opioid antagonists such as naltrexone (ReVia) are also used for the treatment of opioid addiction. The nurse must monitor for side effects during treatment, many of which reflect the opioid withdrawal syndromes. Symptoms include increased thirst, chills, fever, joint/muscle pain, CNS stimulation, drowsiness, dizziness, confusion, seizures, headache, nausea, vomiting, diarrhea, rash, rapid pulse and respirations, pulmonary edema, and wheezing. Vital signs should be taken every 3 to 5 minutes. Respiratory function should be continually assessed, and cardiac status should be monitored for tachycardia and hypertension. As with naloxone, resuscitative equipment should always be available.

Client education regarding opioid antagonists should include goals, reasons for obtaining baseline data such as vital signs and tests and procedures, and possible drug side effects. See Nursing Process Focus: Clients Receiving Opioid Therapy for specific teaching points.

NCLEX Success Tip

Naloxone is the antidote for morphine. The signs of overdose on morphine are a respiration rate of 2 to 4 breaths per minute, bradycardia, and hypotension. The client may need repeated doses of naloxone to prevent or treat a recurrence of the respiratory depression. Naloxone is usually effective in a few minutes; however, its effects last only 1 to 2 hours and ongoing monitoring of the client's respiratory rate will be necessary.

PROTOTYPE DRUG | Naloxone (Narcan)

Actions and Uses: Naloxone is a pure opioid antagonist, blocking both mu and kappa receptors. It is used for complete or partial reversal of opioid effects in emergency situations when acute opioid overdose is suspected. Given by the IV route, it will immediately cause opioid withdrawal symptoms in clients who are physically dependent on opioids. It is also used to treat postoperative opioid depression and opioid pruritus. It is occasionally given as adjunctive therapy to reverse hypotension caused by septic shock.

Administration Alerts:
- Administer for respiratory rate of fewer than 10 breaths per minute. Keep resuscitative equipment accessible.
- Naloxone is pregnancy category B.

Pharmacokinetics: Naloxone is well absorbed following IM or SC administration. Given by the IV route, it begins to reverse opioid-initiated CNS and respiratory depression within minutes. It is widely distributed and crosses the blood-brain barrier and placenta. It is metabolized by the liver. Half-life is 60 to 90 minutes in adults and up to 3 hours in neonates.

Adverse Effects and Interactions: Naloxone itself has minimal toxicity. However, in reversing the effects of opioids, the client may experience rapid loss of analgesia, increased blood pressure, tremors, hyperventilation, nausea/vomiting, and drowsiness. It should not be used for respiratory depression caused by non-opioid medications.

Drug interactions include a reversal of the analgesic effects of opioid agonists and agonist-antagonists.

NURSING PROCESS FOCUS

Clients Receiving Opioid Therapy

Assessment	Potential Nursing Diagnoses/Identified Patterns
Prior to administration: • Obtain complete health history, including allergies, drug history, and possible drug interactions. • Assess pain (quality, intensity, location, duration). • Assess respiratory function. • Assess LOC before and after administration. • Obtain vital signs.	• Need for knowledge related to drug therapy • Acute pain related to injury, disease, or surgical procedure • Ineffective breathing pattern related to action of medication • Constipation • Disturbed sleep pattern related to surgical pain

Planning: Client Goals and Expected Outcomes

The client will:

- Report pain relief or a reduction in pain intensity
- Demonstrate an understanding of the drug's action by accurately describing drug side effects and precautions
- Immediately report effects such as untoward or rebound pain, restlessness, anxiety, depression, hallucination, nausea, dizziness, and itching

Implementation	
Interventions (Rationales)	**Client Education/Discharge Planning**
• Opioids may be administered PO, SC, IM, IV, or PR.	Instruct client:
• Opioids are CDSA Schedule I controlled substances. (Opioids produce both physical and psychological dependence.)	• To take necessary steps to safeguard drug supply; avoid sharing medications with others
• Monitor liver function via laboratory tests. (Opioids are metabolized in the liver. Hepatic disease can increase blood levels of opioids to toxic levels.)	• That oral *capsules* may be opened and mixed with cool foods; extended-release *tablets*, however, may not be chewed, crushed, or broken
• Monitor vital signs, especially depth and rate of respirations and pulse oximetry.	• That oral solution given sublingually may be in a higher concentration than solution for swallowing
• Withhold the drug if the client's respiratory rate is below 12, and notify the healthcare provider.	Instruct client to:
• Keep resuscitative equipment and a narcotic-antagonist such as naloxone accessible. (Opioid antagonists may be used to reverse respiratory depression, decreased LOC, and other symptoms of narcotic overdose.)	• Report nausea; vomiting; diarrhea; rash; jaundice; abdominal pain, tenderness, or distention; or change in colour of stool
• Monitor neurological status; perform neurochecks regularly.	• Adhere to laboratory testing regimen for liver function as ordered by the healthcare provider
• Monitor changes in LOC. (Decreased LOC and sluggish pupillary response may occur with high doses.)	Instruct client or caregiver to:
• Observe for seizures. (Drug may increase ICP.)	• Monitor vital signs regularly, particularly respirations
• If ordered prn, administer medication upon client request or when nursing observations indicate client expressions of pain.	• Withhold medication for any difficulty in breathing or respirations below 12 breaths per minute; report symptoms to the healthcare provider
• Monitor renal status and urinary output. (These drugs may cause urinary retention, which may exacerbate existing symptoms of prostatic hypertrophy.)	Instruct client to:
• Monitor for other side effects such as restlessness, dizziness, anxiety, depression, hallucinations, nausea, and vomiting. (Hives or itching may indicate an allergic reaction due to the production of histamine.)	• Report headache or any significant change in sensorium, such as an aura or other visual effects that may indicate an impending seizure
• Monitor for constipation. (Drug slows peristalsis.)	• Recognize seizures and methods to ensure personal safety during a seizure
• Ensure client safety.	• Report any seizure activity immediately
• Monitor ambulation until response to drug is known. (Drug can cause sedation and dizziness.)	Instruct client to:
• Monitor frequency of requests and stated effectiveness of narcotic administered. (Opioids cause tolerance and dependence.)	• Alert the nurse immediately upon the return or increase of pain
	• Notify the nurse regarding the drug's effectiveness
	Instruct client or caregiver to:
	• Measure and monitor fluid intake and output
	• Report symptoms of dysuria (hesitancy, pain, diminished stream), changes in urine quality, or scanty urine output
	• Report fever or flank pain, which may be indicative of a urinary tract infection
	Instruct client or caregiver to:
	• Recognize side effects and symptoms of an allergic or anaphylactic reaction
	• Immediately report any shortness of breath, tight feeling in the throat, itching, hives or other rash, feelings of dysphoria, nausea, or vomiting
	• Avoid the use of sleep-inducing OTC antihistamines without first consulting the healthcare provider
	Instruct client to:
	• Maintain an adequate fluid and fibre intake to facilitate stool passage
	• Use a stool softener or laxative as recommended by the healthcare provider
	Instruct client to:
	• Request assistance when getting out of bed
	• Avoid driving and performing hazardous activities until effects of the drug are known
	Instruct client and caregiver:
	• Regarding cross-tolerance issues
	• To monitor medication supply to observe for hoarding, which may signal an impending suicide attempt
	• When educating clients suffering from terminal illnesses, address the issue of drug dependence from the perspective of reduced life expectancy.

Evaluate effectiveness of drug therapy by confirming that client goals and expected outcomes have been met (see "Planning").

See Table 23.2 (page 260) for a list of drugs to which these nursing actions apply.

Treatment for Opioid Dependence

23.8 Opioid withdrawal can result in severe symptoms, and dependence is often treated with methadone maintenance.

Although effective at relieving pain, the opioids have a greater risk for dependence than almost any other class of medication. Tolerance develops relatively quickly to the euphoric effects of opioids, causing users to escalate their doses and take the drug more frequently. The higher and more frequent doses can rapidly cause physical dependence.

When physically dependent clients attempt to discontinue drug use, they experience extremely uncomfortable symptoms that convince many to continue their drug-taking behaviour in order to avoid the suffering. As long as the drug is continued, they feel "normal," and many can continue work and social activities. In cases where the drug is abruptly discontinued, about 7 days of withdrawal symptoms are experienced before the client overcomes the physical dependence.

The intense craving characteristic of psychological dependence may occur for many months, and even years, following discontinuation of opioids. This often results in a return to drug-seeking behaviour unless significant support systems are established.

One common method of treating opioid dependence is to switch the client from IV, PO, and inhalation forms of illegal drugs to methadone. Although an opioid, oral methadone does not cause the euphoria that is common with the other opioids. Methadone does not cure the dependence, and the client must continue taking the drug to avoid withdrawal symptoms. This therapy, called **methadone maintenance**, may continue for many months or years until the client decides to enter a total withdrawal treatment program. Methadone maintenance allows clients to return to productive work and social relationships without the physical, emotional, and criminal risks associated with illegal drug use.

A newer treatment approach that is used in some countries is to administer buprenorphine (Butrans), an opioid agonist-antagonist, by the sublingual route. Buprenorphine is used early in opioid addiction therapy to prevent opioid withdrawal symptoms. A combination agent, Suboxone, contains both buprenorphine and naloxone and is used later in the maintenance of opioid addiction.

NON-OPIOID ANALGESICS

The non-opioid analgesics include acetaminophen, NSAIDs, and a few centrally acting agents.

Pharmacotherapy with NSAIDs

23.9 Non-opioid analgesics, such as ASA, acetaminophen, and NSAIDs are effective in treating mild to moderate pain, inflammation, and fever.

The NSAIDs inhibit **cyclooxygenase**, which is an enzyme responsible for the formation of prostaglandins. When cyclooxygenase is inhibited, inflammation and pain are reduced.

NSAIDs are the drugs of choice for mild to moderate pain, especially for pain associated with inflammation. These drugs have many advantages over the opioids. Acetylsalicylic acid (ASA), ibuprofen (Advil, Motrin), naproxen (Aleve), and diclofenac (Voltaren gel) are available OTC and are inexpensive. They are available in many different formulations, including those designed for children. They are safe and produce adverse effects only at high doses. The NSAIDs have antipyretic and anti-inflammatory activity, as well as analgesic properties. Some of the NSAIDs, such as the selective COX-2 inhibitors, are used primarily for their anti-inflammatory properties. The role of the NSAIDs in the treatment of inflammation and fever is discussed in Chapter 42. Table 23.3 highlights the common non-opioid analgesics.

The NSAIDs act by inhibiting pain mediators at the nociceptor level. When tissue is damaged, chemical mediators, including histamine, potassium ion, hydrogen ion, bradykinin, and prostaglandins, are released locally. Bradykinin is associated with the sensory impulse of pain. Prostaglandins can induce pain through the formation of free radicals.

NCLEX Success Tips

Gastric upset is an adverse effect of NSAIDs. Taking these drugs with food and fluids minimizes this effect.

Antacids may interfere with the absorption of NSAIDs.

NSAIDs can decrease the antihypertensive effect of angiotensin-converting enzyme (ACE) inhibitors and predispose clients to the development of acute renal failure. Common lab tests used to evaluate how well the kidneys are working are blood urea nitrogen (BUN), creatinine, and creatinine clearance.

Ibuprofen prolongs bleeding time and is contraindicated in clients with leukemia.

Prostaglandins are formed with the help of two enzymes called cyclooxygenase type 1 (COX-1) and cyclooxygenase type 2 (COX-2). ASA inhibits both COX-1 and COX-2. Because the COX-2 enzyme is more specific for the synthesis of those prostaglandins that cause pain and inflammation,

TABLE 23.3 Non-Opioid Analgesics

Drug	Route and Adult Dose
acetaminophen (Tylenol) (see Chapter 42, page 492, for the Prototype Drug box)	PO, 325–650 mg q4–6h (max 4 g/day)
NSAIDs	
Selective COX-2 Inhibitors	
celecoxib (Celebrex)	PO, 100–200 mg once (qd) or twice daily (bid)
Ibuprofen and Ibuprofen-Like: Non-Salicylates	
diclofenac (Voltaren)	PO, 50 mg bid to qid (max 200 mg/day)
diflunisal	PO, start with 1 g followed by 500 mg every 12 hours; maintenance doses of 500 mg every 8 hours may be necessary (max 1.5g/day)
etodolac	PO, 200–400 mg every 6-8 hours as needed
flurbiprofen	PO, 50–100 mg tid to qid (max 300 mg/day)
ibuprofen (Advil, Motrin)	PO, 400-600 mg every 6-8 hours (max 1800 mg/day)
indomethacin (Indocin)	PO, 25–50 mg bid or tid (max 200 mg/day)
ketoprofen	PO, 12.5–50 mg tid to qid (max 300 mg/day)
ketorolac (Toradol)	PO, 10 mg every 4-6 hours as needed (max 40 mg/day), not to exceed 5 days; IM, start with 10-30 mg as a single dose; can repeat every 4-6 hours as needed (max 120 mg/day); not to exceed 2 days
meloxicam (Mobicox)	PO, 7.5–15 mg daily (qd) (max 15 mg/day)
naproxen (Aleve, Naprosyn)	PO, 500 mg followed by 200–250 mg tid to qid (max 1000 mg/day)
piroxicam	PO, 10–20 mg qd to bid (max 20 mg/day)
sulindac	PO, 150–200 mg bid (max 400 mg/day)
Salicylates	
Pr acetylsalicylic acid (Aspirin)	PO, 325–625 mg q4h (max 4 g/day)
Centrally Acting Agents	
tramadol (Ultram, Tridural, Ralivia)	PO, 50-100 mg every 4-6 hours (max 400 mg/day)

the selective COX-2 inhibitors provide more specific pain relief and produce fewer side effects than ASA. Figure 23.4 illustrates the mechanisms involved in pain at the nociceptor level.

Several important non-opioid analgesics are not classified as NSAIDs. Acetaminophen is a non-opioid analgesic that has equal efficacy to ASA and ibuprofen in relieving pain. Acetaminophen is one of the most widely used analgesics, yet its mechanism of action remains unclear. Possible mechanisms of action, including potential interaction with opioid, serotonergic, adrenergic, cholinergic, and COX systems, are currently being investigated. Acetaminophen is featured as an antipyretic Prototype Drug in Chapter 42. Clonidine (Catapres) and tramadol (Ultram, Tridural, Ralivia) are centrally acting analgesics. Tramadol has weak opioid activity, though it is not thought to relieve pain by this mechanism.

Nursing Considerations

The role of the nurse in NSAID therapy involves careful monitoring of the client's condition and providing education as it relates to the prescribed drug regimen. Because NSAIDs are readily available, inexpensive, and taken orally, clients sometimes forget that these medications can have serious side effects. The inhibition of COX-1 by ASA makes it more likely to cause gastric ulcers and bleeding and acute renal failure. Ibuprofen exerts less of an effect on COX-1 inhibition, so it produces less gastric bleeding than ASA.

When caring for clients who are taking high doses of these drugs, a thorough assessment for pregnancy and the presence or history of hypersensitivity, bleeding disorders, gastric ulcers, and severe renal or hepatic disease should be done. NSAIDs are not recommended for clients with these conditions. Hemoglobin and renal and liver function studies (BUN, creatinine, AST, ALT) should be performed before and during pharmacotherapy. An assessment of the location, character, and intensity of pain should be done initially for baseline data and throughout treatment to determine drug effectiveness. ASA has many drug interactions, so a complete client drug list should be obtained (see Nursing Process Focus: Clients Receiving NSAID Therapy on page 268). Contraindications include hypersensitivity to ASA or other NSAIDs and bleeding disorders such as hemophilia, von Willebrand's disease, telangiectasia, and favism (due to a genetic glucose-6-phosphate dehydrogenase [G6PD] enzyme deficiency). When taking high doses of these medications, it is important that clients are monitored for nephrotoxicity (dysuria, hematuria, oliguria), blood dyscrasias, hepatitis, and allergic responses (rash and urticaria). Monitor clients for the following side effects: nausea, abdominal pain, anorexia, dizziness, and drowsiness. To decrease GI upset, the medication may be taken with food and plenty of fluids. Tablets with enteric coating should not be crushed.

Nurses should exercise extreme caution in administering ASA to children and teenagers. ASA has been implicated in the development of Reye's syndrome in conjunction with flu-like illnesses. Febrile, dehydrated children can rapidly develop ASA toxicity. Use ASA with caution in clients who are pregnant or lactating. Pregnancy category C (D in third trimester) denotes potential harm to the fetus.

Client education for non-opioid analgesics should include goals; reasons for obtaining baseline data such as vital signs, diagnostic procedures, and laboratory tests; and possible side effects. See Nursing Process Focus: Clients Receiving NSAID Therapy on page 268 for specific points to include when teaching clients regarding this class of drug.

PROTOTYPE DRUG | **Acetylsalicylic Acid (Aspirin)**

Actions and Uses: Acetylsalicylic acid (ASA) inhibits prostaglandin synthesis involved in the processes of pain and inflammation and produces mild to moderate relief of fever. It has limited effects on peripheral blood vessels, causing vasodilation and sweating. ASA has significant anticoagulant activity, and this property is responsible for its ability to reduce the risk of mortality following MI and to reduce the incidence of stroke. ASA has also been found to reduce

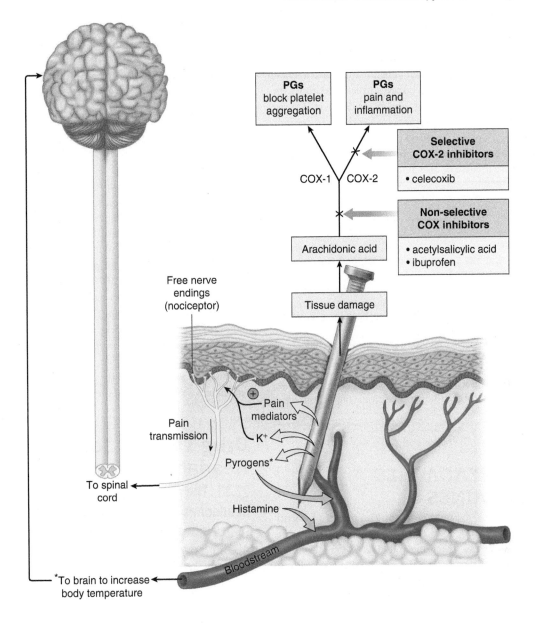

Figure 23.4 Mechanisms of pain at the nociceptor level.

the risk of colorectal cancer, although the mechanism by which it affords this protective effect is unknown.

Administration Alerts:

- Platelet aggregation inhibition caused by ASA is irreversible. ASA should be discontinued 1 week prior to elective surgery.
- ASA is excreted in the urine and affects urine testing for glucose and other metabolites, such as vanillylmandelic acid (VMA).
- ASA is pregnancy C/D (depending on the trimester).

Pharmacokinetics: ASA is well absorbed after oral administration. It is widely distributed, crosses the placenta, and enters breast

milk. It is mostly metabolized by the liver. The amount excreted unchanged in urine varies according to urine pH (increases as urinary pH increases). Its half-life is 2 to 3 hours for low doses but can be up to 30 hours at high doses if liver metabolism is saturated.

Adverse Effects and Interactions: At high doses, such as those used to treat severe inflammatory disorders, ASA may cause gastric discomfort and bleeding because of its antiplatelet effects. Enteric-coated tablets and buffered preparations are available for clients who experience GI side effects.

Because ASA increases bleeding time, it should not be given to clients who are receiving anticoagulant therapy such as warfarin (Coumadin) and heparin. ASA may potentiate the action of oral hypoglycemic agents. The effects of NSAIDs, uricosuric agents (such as probenecid [Benuryl]), beta blockers, spironolactone (Aldactone), and sulfa drugs may be decreased when combined with ASA.

Concurrent use of phenobarbital (Phenobarb), antacids, and glucocorticoids may decrease ASA effects. Insulin, methotrexate, phenytoin (Dilantin), sulfonamides, and penicillin may increase effects. When taken with alcohol, pyrazolone derivatives, steroids, or other NSAIDs, there is an increased risk for gastric ulcers.

Use with caution with herbal supplements, such as feverfew, which may increase the risk of bleeding.

NCLEX Success Tips

A symptom of acetylsalicylic acid toxicity is tinnitus, and it must be reported to the nurse.

Acetylsalicylic acid has an antiplatelet effect, and bleeding time can consequently be prolonged.

Acetylsalicylic acid is thought to exert its anti-inflammatory effect by inhibiting prostaglandin and other substances that sensitize pain receptors. In low doses, it interferes with clotting by keeping a platelet-aggregating substance from forming.

Acetylsalicylic acid is given following a transient ischemic attack (TIA) in order to reduce platelet aggregation. It will decrease the chances of a TIA or stroke occurring by about 22%. Acetylsalicylic acid should be taken with a full glass of water. Side effects of aspirin include bleeding and gastric irritation. Acetylsalicylic acid is never administered to children.

TENSION HEADACHES AND MIGRAINES

Headaches are some of the most common complaints of clients. Living with headaches can interfere with activities of daily life, thus causing great distress. The pain and the inability to focus and concentrate result in work-related absences and the inability to take care of home and family. When the headaches are persistent, or occur as migraines, drug therapy is warranted.

Classification of Headaches

23.10 Headaches are classified as tension headaches or migraines. Migraines may be preceded by auras, and symptoms include nausea and vomiting.

Of the several varieties of headache, the most common is the **tension headache**. This occurs when muscles of the head and neck become very tight due to stress, causing a steady and lingering pain. Although quite painful, tension headaches are self-limiting and generally considered an annoyance rather than a medical emergency. Tension headaches can usually be effectively treated with OTC analgesics such as ASA, acetaminophen, or NSAIDs.

The most painful type of headache is the **migraine**, which is characterized by throbbing or pulsating pain, sometimes preceded by an aura. **Auras** are sensory cues that let the client know that a migraine attack is coming. Examples of sensory cues are jagged lines, flashing lights, and special smells, tastes, or sounds. Most migraines are accompanied by nausea and vomiting. Triggers for migraines include nitrates, monosodium glutamate (MSG) found in many Asian foods, red wine, perfumes, food additives, caffeine, chocolate, and aspartame. By avoiding foods that contain these substances, some clients can prevent the onset of a migraine attack.

Drug Therapy for Migraine Headaches

23.11 The goals of pharmacotherapy for migraine headaches are to stop migraines in progress and to prevent them from occurring. Triptans, ergot alkaloids, and a number of drugs from other classes are used for migraines.

There are two primary goals for the pharmacological therapy of migraines. The first is to stop migraines in progress, and the

NURSING PROCESS FOCUS

Clients Receiving NSAID Therapy

Assessment	Potential Nursing Diagnoses/Identified Patterns
Prior to administration: • Obtain complete health history, including allergies, drug history, and possible drug interactions. • Determine pain history and preferred analgesic and non-analgesic pain management strategies. • Determine current pain and analgesic usage patterns. • Identify infectious agents or other factors responsible for inflammation or pain.	• Acute pain related to injury or surgical procedure • Chronic pain related to back injury • Need for knowledge related to drug therapy • Ineffective health maintenance related to chronic pain

Planning: Client Goals and Expected Outcomes

The client will:
- Report pain relief or a reduction in pain intensity
- Demonstrate an understanding of the drug's action by accurately describing drug side effects and precautions
- Report ability to manage activities of daily living
- Immediately report effects such as unresolved, untoward, or rebound pain; persistent fever; blurred vision; tinnitus; bleeding; changes in colour of stool or urine

Implementation

Interventions (Rationales)	Client Education/Discharge Planning
• NSAIDs may be administered PO or PR. When using suppositories, monitor integrity of rectum; observe for rectal bleeding. • Monitor vital signs, especially temperature. (Increased pulse and blood pressure may indicate discomfort; increased pulse and decreased blood pressure accompanied by pallor and/or dizziness may indicate bleeding.) • Monitor for signs of GI bleeding or hepatic toxicity. (NSAIDs can be a local irritant to the GI tract and are metabolized in the liver.) • Monitor GI elimination; conduct guaiac stool testing for occult blood. • Monitor CBC for signs of anemia related to blood loss. • Assess for character, duration, location, and intensity of pain and the presence of inflammation. • Monitor for hypersensitivity reaction. • Monitor urinary output and edema in feet/ankles. (Medication is excreted through the kidneys. Long-term use may lead to renal dysfunction.) • Monitor for sensory changes indicative of drug toxicity: tinnitus, blurred vision. • Evaluate blood salicylate levels.	Inform client of the following: • Enteric-coated tablets must not be cut or crushed. Regular tablets may be broken or pulverized and mixed with food. • Administer liquid ASA immediately after mixing because it breaks down rapidly. • Different drugs and formulations, such as multiple NSAIDs, should not be taken concurrently. Consult the healthcare provider regarding appropriate OTC analgesics for specific types of pain. • ASA is an anticoagulant. The body needs time to manufacture new platelets to make clots that promote wound healing. Consult the nurse regarding ASA therapy following surgery. • Advise laboratory personnel of ASA therapy when providing urine samples. Instruct client to: • Report rapid heartbeat, palpitations, dizziness, or pallor • Monitor blood pressure and temperature ensuring proper use of home equipment Instruct client to: • Report any bleeding, abdominal pain, anorexia, heartburn, nausea, vomiting, jaundice, or a change in the colour or character of stools • Know the proper method of obtaining stool samples and home testing for occult blood • Adhere to a regimen of laboratory testing as ordered by the healthcare provider • Take NSAIDs with food to reduce stomach upset • Instruct client to notify nurse if pain and/or inflammation remains unresolved. • Advise client to take only the prescribed amount to decrease the potential for adverse effects. Advise client to: • Immediately report shortness of breath, wheezing, throat tightness, itching, or hives. If these occur, stop taking ASA immediately and inform the healthcare provider. • Immediately report changes in urination, flank pain, or pitting edema • Return to healthcare provider for prescribed follow-up appointments • Immediately report any sensory changes in sight or hearing, especially blurred vision or ringing in the ears

Evaluation of Outcome Criteria

Evaluate effectiveness of drug therapy by confirming that client goals and expected outcomes have been met (see "Planning").

See Table 23.3 (page 266) under "NSAIDs" for a list of drugs to which these nursing actions apply.

second is to prevent migraines from occurring. For the most part, the drugs used to abort migraines are different from those used for prophylaxis. Drug therapy is most effective if it is started before a migraine has reached a severe level. Drugs for migraines are listed in Table 23.4.

The two major drug classes used as antimigraine agents, the triptans and the ergot alkaloids, are both serotonin (5-HT) agonists. Serotonergic receptors are found throughout the CNS and in the cardiovascular and GI systems. At least five receptor subtypes have been identified. In addition to the triptans, other drugs acting at serotonergic receptors include the popular antianxiety agents fluoxetine (Prozac) and buspirone (BuSpar).

Pharmacotherapy of migraine termination generally begins with acetaminophen or NSAIDs. If OTC analgesics are unable to abort the migraine, the drugs of choice are often the triptans. The first of the triptans, sumatriptan (Imitrex), was marketed in the 1990s. Triptans are selective for the 5-HT$_1$ receptor subtype, and they are thought to act by constricting certain intracranial vessels. They are effective in aborting migraines with or without aura. Although oral forms of the triptans are most convenient, clients who experience nausea and vomiting during the migraine may require an alternate dosage form. Intranasal formulations and pre-filled syringes of triptans are available for clients who are able to self-administer the medication.

TABLE 23.4 Antimigraine Drugs

Drug	Route and Adult Dose
Drugs for Terminating Migraines	
Ergotamine Alkaloids	
dihydroergotamine (Migranal)	IM/SC, 1 mg; may be repeated at 1-hour intervals to a total of 3 mg (max 6 mg/week)
ergotamine	Sublingual, 2 mg (1 tablet) under tongue at first sign of migraine, then 2 mg every 30 minutes if needed; (max 6 mg per 24 hours or 10 mg/week)
ergotamine with caffeine (Cafergor)	
Triptans	
almotriptan (Axert)	PO, 6.25–12.5 mg; may repeat in 2 hours if necessary (max 2 tabs/day)
eletriptan (Relpax)	PO, 20–40 mg; may repeat in 2 hours if necessary (max 40 mg/day)
naratriptan (Amerge)	PO, 1–2.5 mg; may repeat in 4 hours if necessary (max 5 mg/day)
rizatriptan (Maxalt)	PO/ODT, 5–10 mg; may repeat in 2 hours if necessary (max 30 mg/day); 5 mg with concurrent propranolol (max 15 mg/day)
Pr sumatriptan (Imitrex)	PO/SC/intranasal, 25 mg for 1 dose; may repeat in 2 hours if necessary (max 100 mg)
zolmitriptan (Zomig)	PO/ODT/nasal inhalation, 2.5–5 mg; may repeat in 2 hours if necessary (max 10 mg/day)
Beta-Adrenergic Blockers	
atenolol (Tenormin) (see Chapter 50, page 618, for the Prototype Drug box)	PO, 25–50 mg qd (max 100 mg/day)
metoprolol (Lopresor) (see Chapter 50, page 619, for the Prototype Drug box)	PO, 50–100 mg qd–bid (max 450 mg/day)
propranolol (Inderal) (see Chapter 55, page 704, for the Prototype Drug box)	PO, 80–240 mg qd in divided doses; may need 160–240 mg/day
timolol	For migraine prophylaxis: PO, start with 10 mg bid; increase to max 30 mg/day
Calcium Channel Blockers	
nifedipine (Adalat) (see Chapter 51, page 640, for the Prototype Drug box)	PO, 10–20 mg tid (max 180 mg/day)
nimodipine (Nimotop)	PO, 60 mg q4h for 21 days, start therapy within 96 hours of subarachnoid hemorrhage
verapamil (Isoptin) (see Chapter 55, page 705, for the Prototype Drug box)	PO, 40–80 mg tid (max 360 mg/day)
Tricyclic Antidepressants	
amitriptyline (Elavil)	PO, 10–25 mg at bedtime; increase at weekly increments of 10–25 mg based on response and tolerance (max 150 mg/day)
imipramine (Impril) (see Chapter 17, page 181, for the Prototype Drug box)	PO, 75–100 mg/day (max 300 mg/day)
Miscellaneous Agents	
valproic acid (Depakene, Epival) (see Chapter 21, page 239, for the Prototype Drug box)	PO, 250 mg bid (max 1000 mg/day)
riboflavin (vitamin B$_2$)	As a supplement: PO, 5–10 mg/day
onabotulinumtoxinA (Botox), a drug often used to erase facial wrinkles, was approved by Health Canada in 2011 to prevent and treat chronic headache and migraines (see Chapter 22).	Dose depends on condition and toxin used

For clients who are unresponsive to triptans, the ergot alkaloids may be used to abort migraines. The first purified alkaloid, ergotamine, was isolated from the ergot fungus in 1920, although the actions of the ergot alkaloids had been known for thousands of years. Ergotamine is an inexpensive drug that is available in oral, sublingual, and suppository forms. Modification of the original molecule has produced a number of other pharmacologically useful drugs, such as dihydroergotamine (Migranal). Dihydroergotamine is given parenterally and as a nasal spray. Because the ergot alkaloids interact with adrenergic and dopaminergic receptors, as well as serotonergic receptors, they produce multiple actions and side effects. Many ergot alkaloids are pregnancy category X drugs.

Drugs for migraine prophylaxis include various classes of drug that are discussed in other chapters of this text. These include beta-adrenergic blockers, calcium channel blockers, antidepressants, and antiseizure drugs. Because all of these drugs have the potential to produce side effects, prophylaxis is only initiated if the incidence of migraines is high and the client is unresponsive to the drugs used to abort migraines. Of the various drugs, propranolol (Inderal) is one of the most commonly prescribed. Amitriptyline (Elavil) is preferred for clients who may have a mood disorder or suffer from insomnia in addition to their migraines.

Nursing Considerations

The role of the nurse in antimigraine therapy involves careful monitoring of the client's condition and providing education as it relates to the prescribed drug regimen. Before starting clients on antimigraine medications, gather information about the frequency and intensity of the migraine headaches and the presence or history of MI, angina, and hypertension. Also determine pregnancy status and gather information about the presence or history of renal and liver disease and diabetes. Laboratory tests to determine renal and liver disease should be obtained.

The baseline frequency of migraine headaches along with apical pulse, respirations, and blood pressure should be obtained. Because migraines may be stress related, the client's stress level and coping mechanisms should be investigated. Always assess for hypersensitivity and the use of other medications. With triptans, clients should not take MAO inhibitors or selective serotonin reuptake inhibitors (SSRIs), which cause an increase in effect.

The nurse should assess the client's neurological status, including LOC, blurred vision, nausea and vomiting, and tingling in the extremities. These signs or symptoms may indicate that a migraine is beginning. A quiet, calm environment with decreased noise and subdued lighting should be provided, and care should be organized to limit disruptions and decrease neural stimulation. Cold packs can be applied to help lessen the uncomfortable effects of the migraine. Monitor for possible side effects, including dizziness, drowsiness, vasoconstriction, warming sensations, tingling, lightheadedness, weakness, and neck stiffness. Use with caution during pregnancy or lactation. Sumatriptan is excreted in breast milk. Advise the client that the drug could be harmful to the fetus or infant. Because of the vasoconstriction action of the drugs, they are contraindicated in the following conditions: hypertension; myocardial ischemia and coronary artery disease (CAD); history of MI, dysrhythmias, or heart failure; high-risk CAD profile; and diabetes.

The ergot alkaloids promote vasoconstriction, which terminates ongoing migraines. Side effects may include nausea,

CONNECTIONS | Natural Therapies

◀ Feverfew for Migraines

Feverfew (*Tanacetum parthenium*) is an herb that originated in southeastern Europe and is now found all over Europe, Australia, and North America. The common name feverfew is derived from its antipyretic properties. The leaves contain the active ingredients, the most prevalent of which is a lactone known as parthenolide. Standardization of this herb is based on the percent of parthenolide in the product.

Feverfew has an overall spectrum of action resembling that of ASA. The herb has been shown to exert anti-inflammatory and antispasmodic effects, as well as to inhibit platelet aggregation. Feverfew extract has also been shown to contain a novel type of mast cell inhibitor that inhibits anti-immunoglobulin E–induced histamine release. In clinical trials, feverfew was associated with a reduction in the number and severity of migraine attacks, as well as a reduction in vomiting. The most common adverse effect is mouth ulceration, which occurs in about 10% of feverfew users.

vomiting, weakness in the legs, myalgia, numbness and tingling in fingers and toes, angina-like pain, and tachycardia. Toxicity may be evidenced by constriction of peripheral arteries: cold, pale, numb extremities and muscle pain. Sumatriptan is metabolized in the liver and excreted by the kidneys; impaired organ function can increase serum drug levels. The client should be advised against and monitored for constant usage because these medications can cause physical dependence.

Client education regarding drug therapy for migraines should include goals; reasons for obtaining baseline data such as vital signs, laboratory tests, and procedures (such as computed tomography or magnetic resonance imaging of the brain, or lumbar puncture for samples of cerebrospinal fluid); and possible side effects. The following are teaching points to include when educating clients regarding the ergot alkaloids:

- Take dose immediately after the onset of symptoms.
- Control, avoid, or eliminate factors that trigger a headache or migraine, such as fatigue, anxiety, and alcohol.
- Report the signs of ergot toxicity, which may include muscle pain, numbness, and cold extremities.
- Do not overuse any of these drugs, as physical dependence may result.

See Nursing Process Focus: Clients Receiving Triptan Therapy for specific teaching points about this subclass of drugs.

NCLEX Success Tips

Sumatriptan is contraindicated in clients with ischemic heart disease—such as angina, myocardial infarction, or coronary artery disease—because it is a vasoconstrictor, just like all triptan therapies.

Sumatriptan is used for the abortive treatment of migraines, not prophylactic treatment, and it is effective in treating acute migraines with or without aura.

Sumatriptan relieves migraine headaches by constricting cerebral arterial vessels.

NURSING PROCESS FOCUS

Clients Receiving Triptan Therapy

Assessment	Potential Nursing Diagnoses/Identified Patterns
Prior to administration: • Obtain complete health history, including allergies, drug history, and possible drug interactions. • Determine pain and analgesic usage patterns. • Identify infectious agents or other factors responsible for inflammation or pain. • Assess LOC before and after administration.	• Acute pain related to severe headache • Need for knowledge related to drug therapy • Ineffective coping related to chronic pain • Ineffective health maintenance related to inability to manage ADLs

Planning: Client Goals and Expected Outcomes

The client will:

• Report pain relief or a reduction in pain intensity
• Demonstrate an understanding of the drug's action by accurately describing drug side effects and precautions
• Immediately report effects such as shortness of breath, chest tightness or pressure, jaw pain, untoward or worsened rebound headache, seizures or other neurological changes

Implementation

Interventions (Rationales)	Client Education/Discharge Planning
• Administer the first dose of the medication under supervision. • Monitor vital signs, especially blood pressure and pulse. (Triptans have vasoconstrictor action.) • Observe for changes in severity, character, or duration of headache. (Sudden severe headaches of "thunderclap" quality can signal subarachnoid hemorrhage. Headaches that differ in quality and are accompanied by such signs as fever, rash, or stiff neck may herald meningitis.) • Monitor neurological status; perform neurochecks regularly • Monitor for possible side effects: dizziness, drowsiness, warming sensation, tingling, lightheadedness, weakness, or neck stiffness due to vasoconstriction. (Such symptoms can result from decreased blood flow to the brain related to reduced carotid arterial blood supply.) • Monitor dietary intake of foods that contain tyramine. (These foods may trigger an acute migraine.) • Monitor kidney and liver function via laboratory tests.	• Instruct client that the first dose may need to be given under medical supervision because of potential cardiac side effects. Reassure the client that this is merely a precautionary measure. • Instruct client to monitor vital signs, especially blood pressure and pulse, ensuring proper use of home equipment. • Instruct client that changes in the character of migraines could signal other potentially more serious disorders. • Provide the client with written materials on warning signs of stroke; discuss other conditions such as meningitis, which may cause headache. Instruct client: • That feeling dizzy or lightheaded can be the result of the drug's action on the CNS or coronary ischemia • To immediately report episodes of severe dizziness or impending syncope • To review emergency response and safety measures in the event of a seizure Advise client: • To immediately report side effects to the healthcare provider • Regarding emergent symptoms suggestive of stroke or MI that may require immediate emergency intervention and transport to a hospital • Instruct client to avoid or limit foods containing tyramine such as pickled foods, beer, wine, and aged cheeses. Provide client with a list of tyramine-containing foods. Instruct client to: • Report nausea; vomiting; diarrhea; rash; jaundice; abdominal pain, tenderness, distention; or change in colour of stool • Adhere to laboratory testing regimen for liver function as ordered by healthcare provider

Evaluation of Outcome Criteria

Evaluate effectiveness of drug therapy by confirming that client goals and expected outcomes have been met (see "Planning").

See Table 23.4 (page 270) under "Triptans" for a list of drugs to which these nursing actions apply.

PROTOTYPE DRUG | **Sumatriptan (Imitrex)**

Actions and Uses: Sumatriptan belongs to a relatively new group of antimigraine drugs known as the triptans. The triptans act by causing vasoconstriction of cranial arteries; this vasoconstriction is moderately selective and does not usually affect overall blood pressure. This medication is available in oral, intranasal, and SC forms. SC administration terminates migraine attacks in 10 to 20 minutes; the dose may be repeated 60 minutes after the first injection, to a maximum of two doses per day. If taken orally, sumatriptan should be administered as soon as possible after the migraine is suspected or has begun.

Pharmacokinetics: Sumatriptan is well absorbed after SC and intranasal administration. Absorption is variable after oral administration due to first-pass metabolism. Distribution is unknown. It is mostly metabolized by the liver. Its half-life is 2 hours.

Administration Alerts:
• Sumatriptan may produce cardiac ischemia in susceptible persons with no previous cardiac events. Healthcare providers may opt to administer the initial dose of sumatriptan in the healthcare setting.

• The drug's systemic vasoconstrictor activity may cause hypertension and result in dysrhythmias or MI. Keep resuscitative equipment accessible.

• Sumatriptan selectively reduces carotid arterial blood flow. Monitor changes in LOC and observe for seizures.

• Sumatriptan is pregnancy category C.

Adverse Effects and Interactions: Some dizziness, drowsiness, or a warming sensation may be experienced after taking sumatriptan; however, these effects are not normally severe enough to warrant discontinuation of therapy. Because of its vasoconstricting action, the drug should be used cautiously, if at all, in clients with recent MI or a history of angina pectoris, hypertension, or diabetes.

Sumatriptan interacts with several drugs. For example, an increased effect may occur when taken with MAO inhibitors or SSRIs. Further vasoconstriction can occur when taken with ergot alkaloids and other triptans.

CHAPTER
23 Understanding the Chapter

Key Concepts Summary

The numbered key concepts provide a succinct summary of the important points from the corresponding numbered section within the chapter. If any of these points are not clear, refer to the numbered section within the chapter for review.

23.1 The primary goal of pain management is to reduce pain to a level that allows the client to continue normal daily activities.

23.2 The ways to assess and classify pain include acute or chronic and nociceptor or neuropathic.

23.3 Non-pharmacological techniques such as massage, biofeedback therapy, and meditation are often important adjuncts to effective pain management.

23.4 Neural mechanisms include the pain transmission via A delta or C fibres and the release of substance P.

23.5 Opioids are natural or synthetic substances extracted from the poppy plant that exert their effects through interaction with mu and kappa receptors.

23.6 Opioids are the drugs of choice for severe pain. They also have other important therapeutic effects, including dampening of the cough reflex and slowing of the motility of the GI tract.

23.7 Opioid antagonists may be used to reverse the symptoms of opioid toxicity or overdose, such as sedation and respiratory depression.

23.8 Opioid withdrawal can result in severe symptoms, and dependence is often treated with methadone maintenance.

23.9 Non-opioid analgesics, such as ASA, acetaminophen, and NSAIDs are effective in treating mild to moderate pain, inflammation, and fever.

23.10 Headaches are classified as tension headaches or migraines. Migraines may be preceded by auras, and symptoms include nausea and vomiting.

23.11 The goals of pharmacotherapy for migraine headaches are to stop migraines in progress and to prevent them from occurring. Triptans, ergot alkaloids, and a number of drugs from other classes are used for migraines.

Chapter 23 Scenario

Larry Smith is being seen for an outpatient pre-surgery workup the evening before scheduled urological surgery. The nurse conducts a thorough history and examination related to Mr. Smith's back pain and current pain management. His anticipated hospital stay is 2 days postsurgery.

Mr. Smith is a 64-year-old male. Vital signs are blood pressure, 108/64 mm Hg; pulse, 88 beats/minute; and respirations, 16 breaths/minute. He has a well-healed midline scar on his back from lumbar vertebrae surgery, with a shorter scar over his right iliac crest. He moves a bit slowly with some limited lumbar range of motion. He also uses a cane for ambulating any distance. He describes his pain as a constant dull ache in the lower back that increases with prolonged standing or walking. Mr. Smith also reports a feeling of "cold electricity" down both legs, with the left greater than the right, which increases with standing and walking, as well as numbness of the middle toes on his left foot. He has been using mixed opioid and non-opioid analgesics for the past 8 years and previously had used SSRI antidepressants as

adjuvant for his pain. His current healthcare provider weaned him off morphine about a year ago. He now takes methadone 20 mg twice a day. When the pain is not relieved he uses Percocet (oxycodone and acetaminophen) for breakthrough pain. His use of Percocet is 1 to 2 per day. Constipation is an ongoing problem, requiring stool softeners and occasional laxatives.

Critical Thinking Questions

1. How should Mr. Smith's postoperative pain be managed? Is there a referral the nurse can make to facilitate effective pain management?

2. How could the nurse best communicate Mr. Smith's needs to the postoperative nursing staff?

3. What should be included in the care plan for postoperative management of analgesic adverse effects?

See Answers to Critical Thinking Questions in Appendix B.

NCLEX Practice Questions

1 A nurse is monitoring a client for adverse effects associated with morphine. Which adverse effects would be expected? Select all that apply.

  a. Respiratory depression

  b. Hypertension

  c. Urinary retention

  d. Constipation

  e. Nausea

2 Several days postoperative bowel surgery, the client is eating soft food, ambulating regularly, and using oxycodone + acetaminophen (Percocet) for pain. What should the nursing care plan include?

  a. Monitoring vital signs for respiratory depression

  b. Inserting a urinary catheter for urinary retention

  c. Weaning pain medication to prevent addiction

  d. Increasing dietary fibre and fluids and administering a stool softener if needed

3 A client who has migraines self-administered sumatriptan (Imitrex) for the first time yesterday. Today, the client informs the nurse that after taking the medication, he began to experience chest pain. The client further states that the drug was effective in relieving the headache. The nurse should

  a. Encourage the client to continue using the drug because it is effective.

  b. Advise the client to tell the healthcare provider about the chest pain at the next visit.

  c. Instruct the client to contact the healthcare provider to report the chest pain today and to refrain from using the sumatriptan until he has talked to the healthcare provider.

  d. Encourage the client to lie down in a quiet room and use cold packs during the next migraine.

4 A client with diabetes reports increasing pain and numbness in his legs. "It feels like pins and needles all the time, especially at night." Which drug would the nurse expect to be prescribed for this client?

  a. Ibuprofen (Motrin)

  b. Gabapentin (Neurontin)

  c. Naloxone (Narcan)

  d. Methadone (Metadol)

5 A nurse is caring for several clients who are receiving opioids for pain relief. Which client is at the highest risk of developing hypotension, respiratory depression, and mental confusion?

  a. A 23-year-old female, postoperative ruptured appendix

  b. A 16-year-old male, post–motorcycle injury with lacerations

  c. A 54-year-old female, post–myocardial infarction

  d. An 86-year-old male, postoperative femur fracture

See Answers to NCLEX Practice Questions in Appendix A.

PROTOTYPE DRUGS

LOCAL ANESTHETICS
Amides
  Pr *lidocaine*
    (Xylocaine)
Esters

GENERAL ANESTHETICS
Inhalation agents
Gases
  Pr *nitrous oxide*
Volatile liquids
  Pr *halothane*
    (Fluothane)
Intravenous agents

Barbiturate and
  barbiturate-like agents
  Pr *propofol (Diprivan)*
Opioids
Benzodiazepines

**ADJUNCTS TO
ANESTHESIA**
Barbiturate and
  barbiturate-like agents
Opioids
Neuromuscular blocking
  agents
  Pr *succinylcholine
    (Quelicin)*
Miscellaneous agents

CHAPTER

24 Pharmacology of Local and General Anesthesia

LEARNING OUTCOMES

After reading this chapter, the student should be able to:

1. Identify drug classes used for local and general anesthesia.
2. Compare and contrast the five major clinical techniques for administering local anesthetics.
3. Describe differences in therapeutic action between the two major chemical classes of local anesthetics.
4. Explain why epinephrine and sodium hydroxide are sometimes included in local anesthetic cartridges.
5. Explain the therapeutic action of drugs used for general anesthesia with reference to effects on the central nervous system (CNS).
6. Compare and contrast the two primary ways that general anesthesia may be induced.
7. For each of the drug classes listed in Prototype Drugs, identify a representative drug and explain its mechanism of action, primary actions, and important adverse effects.
8. Discuss the nurse's role in the pharmacological management of clients who are receiving anesthetics.
9. Describe and explain, based on pharmacological principles, the rationale for nursing assessment, planning, and interventions for clients who are receiving anesthetics.
10. Use the nursing process to care for clients who are receiving anesthetics.

CHAPTER OUTLINE

▶ Regional Loss of Sensation Using Local Anesthetics

▶ Local Anesthetics

  ▶ Mechanism of Action of Local Anesthetics

  ▶ Classification of Local Anesthetics

  ▶ Characteristics of General Anesthesia

▶ General Anesthetics

  ▶ Pharmacotherapy with Inhaled General Anesthetics

▶ Intravenous Anesthetics

  ▶ Pharmacotherapy with IV Anesthetics

▶ Non-Anesthetic Drugs as Adjuncts to Surgery

amides, 278

balanced anesthesia, 280

esters, 278

general anesthesia, 276

local anesthesia, 276

monitored anesthesia care (MAC), 276

neuromuscular blockers, 284

regional anesthesia, 276

surgical anesthesia, 280

Certain medical procedures produce a significant degree of pain and would not be possible without anesthesia. There are four types of anesthesia. The type of anesthesia selected depends on the degree of sedation and analgesia needed to conduct the procedure.

General anesthesia is the loss of sensation throughout the entire body, accompanied by loss of consciousness. General anesthesia is necessary for major surgical procedures.

The application of **local anesthesia** results in loss of sensation to a limited body region without loss of consciousness. It affects only the immediate area that surrounds where the anesthetic is administered. **Regional anesthesia** is similar, except that it encompasses a larger body area, such as an entire limb. Local and regional anesthesias produce fewer adverse effects than general anesthesia and are thus the methods of choice where applicable.

A fourth type of anesthesia is **monitored anesthesia care (MAC)**, which uses sedatives, analgesics, and other low-dose drugs that allow clients to remain responsive and breathe without assistance during the medical procedure. This type of anesthesia is used during diagnostic procedures and minor surgeries to supplement local and regional anesthesias. Subtypes of MAC are based on the degree of sedation produced:

- *Minimal sedation (anxiolysis).* Clients respond to verbal commands. Airway, ventilation, and cardiovascular functions are normal.

- *Moderate (conscious) sedation.* Clients respond to verbal or light tactile prompting. Airway, ventilation, and cardiovascular functions are usually adequate.

- *Deep sedation/analgesia.* Clients are aroused by repeated or painful stimulation. Airway and ventilation intervention may be required. Cardiovascular functions are usually adequate.

This chapter examines drugs used for both local and general anesthesia.

Regional Loss of Sensation Using Local Anesthetics

24.1 Regional loss of sensation is achieved by administering local anesthetics topically or through the infiltration, nerve block, spinal, or epidural methods.

Local anesthesia is loss of sensation to a relatively small part of the body without loss of consciousness. This technique may be necessary when a relatively brief dental or medical procedure is performed.

Although local anesthesia often results in a loss of sensation to a small, limited area, it sometimes affects relatively large portions of the body, such as an entire limb. Because of this, some local anesthetic treatments are more accurately called surface anesthesia or regional anesthesia, depending on how the drugs are administered and their resulting effects.

The five major routes for applying local anesthetics are shown in Figure 24.1. The method employed is dependent on the location and extent of the desired anesthesia. For example, some local anesthetics are applied topically before a needlestick or minor skin surgery. Others are used to block sensations to large areas such as a limb or the lower abdomen. The different methods of local and regional anesthesia are summarized in Table 24.1.

LOCAL ANESTHETICS

Local anesthetics are drugs that produce a rapid loss of sensation to a limited part of the body. They produce their therapeutic effect by blocking the entry of sodium ions (Na^+) into neurons.

Mechanism of Action of Local Anesthetics

24.2 Local anesthetics act by blocking sodium channels in neurons. Epinephrine is sometimes added to prolong the duration of anesthetic action.

The mechanism of action of local anesthetics is well known. Recall that the concentration of sodium ions is normally higher on the outside of neurons than on the inside. A rapid influx of sodium ions into cells is necessary for neurons to fire and conduct an action impulse.

Local anesthetics act by blocking sodium channels, as illustrated in Figure 24.2. Because the blocking of sodium channels is a nonselective process, both sensory and motor impulses are affected. Therefore, both sensation and muscle activity will temporarily diminish in the area treated with the local anesthetic. Because of their mechanism of action, local anesthetics are sometimes called sodium channel blockers.

During a medical or surgical procedure, it is essential that the duration of action of the anesthetic is long enough to complete the procedure. Small amounts of epinephrine (Adrenalin) are sometimes added to the anesthetic solution to constrict blood vessels in the immediate area where the local anesthetic is applied. In addition to reducing bleeding in the area, this keeps the anesthetic in the area longer, thus extending the duration of action of the drug. The addition of epinephrine to lidocaine (Xylocaine), for example, increases the duration of the local anesthetic effect from 20 minutes to as long as 60 minutes. This is important for dental or surgical procedures that take longer than 20 minutes; otherwise, a second injection of the anesthetic would be necessary.

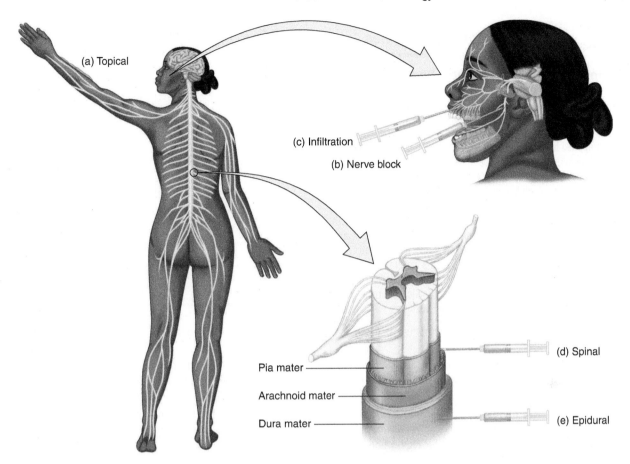

Figure 24.1 Techniques for applying local anesthesia: (a) topical; (b) nerve block; (c) infiltration; (d) spinal; (e) epidural.

TABLE 24.1 Methods of Local Anesthetic Administration

Route	Formulation/Method	Description
Topical (surface)	Creams, sprays, suppositories, drops, and lozenges	Applied to mucous membranes including the eyes, lips, gums, nasal membranes, and throat; very safe unless absorbed
Infiltration (field block)	Direct injection into tissue immediate to the surgical site	Drug diffuses into tissue to block a specific group of nerves in a small area close to the surgical site
Nerve block	Direct injection into tissue that may be distant from the operation site	Drug affects nerve bundles serving the surgical area; used to block sensation in a limb or large area of the face
Spinal	Injection into the cerebrospinal fluid (CSF)	Drug affects large, regional area such as the lower abdomen and legs
Epidural	Injection into epidural space of spinal cord	Most commonly used in obstetrics during labour and delivery

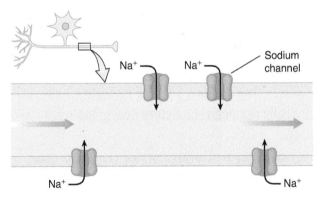

(a) Normal nerve conduction

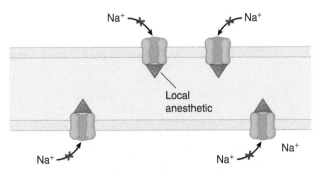

(b) Local anesthetic blocking sodium channels

Figure 24.2 Mechanism of action of local anesthetics: (a) Na^+ enters neuron for normal nerve conduction; (b) local anesthetic blocks sodium channels and prevents nerve conduction.

CONNECTIONS | Natural Therapies

◀ Clove and Anise as Natural Dental Remedies

One natural remedy for tooth pain is oil of clove. Extracted from the plant *Eugenia*, eugenol is the chemical in clove that is thought to produce its numbing effect. It works especially well for cavities. The herb is applied by soaking a piece of cotton and packing it around the gums close to the painful area. Dentists sometimes recommend it for temporary relief of a toothache. Clove oil has an antiseptic effect that has been reported to kill bacteria, fungi, and helminths.

Another natural remedy is oil of anise, from *Pimpinella anisum*, that is used for jaw pain caused by nerve pressure or gritting of teeth. Anise oil is an antispasmodic agent, which means that it relaxes intense muscular pressure around the jaw angle, cheeks, and throat area. It has extra benefits in that it is also a natural expectorant, cough suppressant, and breath freshener. The pharmacological effects of anise are thought to be due to the chemical anethole, which is similar in structure to natural catecholamines.

TABLE 24.2 Select Local Anesthetics

Chemical Classification	Drug
Esters	benzocaine (Zilactin, Anbesol)
	chloroprocaine (Nesacaine)
	cocaine
	tetracaine (Pontocaine)
Amides	articaine (Septanest)
	bupivacaine (Marcaine)
	dibucaine (Nupercaine, Nupercainal)
	Pr lidocaine (Xylocaine)
	mepivacaine (Carbocaine)
	prilocaine (Citanest)
	ropivacaine (Naropin)
Miscellaneous agents	cetylpyridinium and benzocaine (Cepacol)
	pramoxine (Tronothane)

Sodium hydroxide is sometimes added to anesthetic solutions to increase the effectiveness of the anesthetic in regions that have extensive local infection or abscesses. Bacteria tend to acidify an infected site, and local anesthetics are less effective in an acidic environment. Adding alkaline substances such as sodium hydroxide or sodium bicarbonate neutralizes the region and creates a more favourable environment for the anesthetic.

Classification of Local Anesthetics

24.3 Local anesthetics are classified as amides or esters. The amides, such as lidocaine, have generally replaced the esters due to their greater safety.

Local anesthetics are classified by their chemical structure; the two major classes are **esters** and **amides**. The terms *ester* and *amide* refer to types of chemical linkages found within the anesthetic molecules, as illustrated in Figure 24.3. Although esters and amides have equal efficacy, important differences exist. A small number of miscellaneous agents are neither esters nor amides. Local anesthetic agents are listed in Table 24.2.

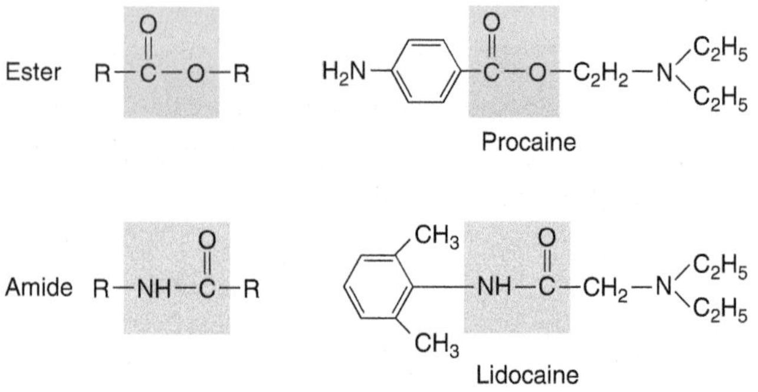

Cocaine was the first local anesthetic widely used for medical procedures. Cocaine is a natural ester found in the leaves of the *Erythroxylum coca* plant native to the Andes Mountains of Peru. As late as the 1880s, cocaine was routinely used for eye surgery, nerve blocks, and spinal anesthesia. Although still available for local anesthesia, cocaine is a Controlled Drugs and Substances Act (CDSA) Schedule I drug and is rarely used therapeutically in Canada. The abuse potential of cocaine is discussed in Chapter 25.

Another ester, procaine (Novocain), was the drug of choice for dental procedures from the mid-1900s to the 1960s, until the development of the amide anesthetics led to a significant decline in its use, which is now often non-existent. One ester, benzocaine (Zilactin, Anbesol) is used as a topical, over-the-counter (OTC) agent for treating a large number of painful conditions, including sunburn, insect bites, hemorrhoids, sore throat, and minor wounds.

Amides have largely replaced the esters because they produce fewer side effects and generally have a longer duration of action. Lidocaine is the most widely used amide for short surgical procedures requiring local anesthesia.

Adverse effects of local anesthetics are uncommon. Allergy is rare. When it does occur, it is often due to sulfites, which are added as preservatives to prolong the shelf life of the anesthetic, or to methylparaben, which may be added to retard bacterial growth in anesthetic solutions. Early signs of adverse effects of local anesthetics include symptoms of CNS stimulation such as restlessness or anxiety. Later effects, such as drowsiness and unresponsiveness, are due to CNS depression. Cardiovascular effects, including hypotension and dysrhythmias, are possible. Clients with a history of cardiovascular disease are often given forms of local anesthetics that contain no epinephrine in order to reduce the potential effects of this sympathomimetic on the heart and blood pressure. CNS and cardiovascular side effects are not expected unless the local anesthetic is absorbed rapidly or is accidentally injected directly into a blood vessel.

Figure 24.3 Chemical structure of ester and amide local anesthetics.

Stomatitis occurs 7 to 10 days after chemotherapy. To decrease the pain of stomatitis, the nurse can provide a solution of hydrogen viscous lidocaine for the client to use as a mouth rinse. (Commercially prepared mouthwashes contain alcohol and may cause dryness and irritation of the oral mucosa.)

Nursing Considerations

The role of the nurse in local anesthetic administration involves careful monitoring of the client's condition and providing education as it relates to the prescribed drug regimen. Although these medications are usually administered by the physician to anesthetize an area for medical procedures, the nurse often assists. The nurse's role may include preparing the area to be anesthetized and monitoring the effectiveness of the medication by assessing pain and comfort levels. Document the presence of broken skin, infection, burns, and wounds at the site of anesthetic administration.

Contraindications for these drugs include hypersensitivity to local anesthetics; sepsis and blood dyscrasias; untreated sinus bradycardia; and severe degrees of atrioventricular, sinoatrial, and intraventricular heart block in the absence of a pacemaker. Local anesthetics should be used with caution over large body areas, in clients with extensive surface trauma, and in severe skin disorders because the medication may be absorbed and result in systemic effects. Unless specifically formulated for optic use, local anesthetics should not be used on the eyes.

CONNECTIONS Lifespan Considerations

◀ Effects of Anesthesia on Children and Older Adults

Children are usually more sensitive to anesthesia than adults because their body systems are not fully developed. Therefore, medication dosages must be calculated carefully. Some drugs used for anesthesia, such as neuromuscular blockers, are not recommended for use by children under the age of 2 years.

Children who are undergoing surgery have fears and concerns about surgery and anesthesia. A child's age and developmental level play a role in his or her thoughts about receiving anesthesia. Children younger than 1 year are usually not concerned about what will be happening and will easily separate from family members. Fear of needles, the unknown, and being separated from primary caregivers begins to happen during the toddler stage and continues throughout childhood. Children are often perceptive to the anxieties of their parents; therefore, it is imperative that caregivers remain calm. Holding the child during induction of anesthesia may help to alleviate fears. Local anesthetic creams can be applied to the skin to decrease the pain of needlesticks.

Older adults are also more affected by anesthesia than younger adults. Because of the changes in drug metabolism that occur with advancing age, these clients are particularly sensitive to the effects of barbiturate and general anesthetics. This increases the chance of side effects; therefore, elderly clients should be monitored closely. Older adults are also especially sensitive to the effects of local anesthetics. Sedative-hypnotic drugs used preoperatively may cause increased confusion or excitement in older adults.

PROTOTYPE DRUG | Lidocaine (Xylocaine)

Actions and Uses: Lidocaine, the most frequently used injectable local anesthetic, acts by blocking neuronal pain impulses. It is injected as a nerve block for spinal and epidural anesthesia. Its actions are achieved by blocking sodium channels located within the membranes of neurons.

Lidocaine may be given by the intravenous (IV), intramuscular (IM), or subcutaneous (SC) route to treat dysrhythmias, as discussed in Chapter 55. A topical form is also available.

Pharmacokinetics: Lidocaine is well absorbed. It is widely distributed, crosses the blood-brain barrier and placenta, and concentrates in adipose tissue. Lidocaine is mostly metabolized by the liver. Its half-life is biphasic, with an initial phase from 7 to 30 minutes and a final phase from 1.5 to 2 hours.

Administration Alerts:
- Solutions of lidocaine that contain preservatives or epinephrine are intended for local anesthesia only and must never be given parenterally for dysrhythmias.
- Topical lidocaine should not be applied to large skin areas or to broken or abraded areas, as significant absorption may occur. It should not be allowed to come in contact with the eyes.
- For spinal or epidural block, use only preparations specifically labelled for IV use.
- Lidocaine is pregnancy category B.

Adverse Effects and Interactions: When used for anesthesia, side effects are uncommon. An early symptom of toxicity is CNS excitement, leading to irritability and confusion. Serious adverse effects include convulsions, respiratory depression, and cardiac arrest. Until the effect of the anesthetic diminishes, clients may injure themselves by biting or chewing areas of the mouth that have no sensation following a dental procedure.

Side effects of lidocaine include lightheadedness, euphoria, shaking, low blood pressure, drowsiness, confusion, weakness, blurred or double vision, and dizziness. Serious reactions such as seizures, bradycardia, and heart block are possible if lidocaine reaches toxic levels. The nurse should recognize these potential adverse effects, and the lidocaine infusion should be decreased while lidocaine blood levels are checked to determine if the client's complaint is due to lidocaine toxicity.

Characteristics of General Anesthesia

24.4 General anesthesia produces a complete loss of sensation accompanied by loss of consciousness. This is usually achieved through the use of multiple medications.

General anesthesia is a loss of sensation that occurs throughout the entire body, accompanied by a loss of consciousness. General anesthetics are applied when it is necessary for clients to remain still and without pain for a longer period of time than could be achieved with local anesthetics.

NURSING PROCESS FOCUS

Clients Receiving Local Anesthesia

Assessment	Potential Nursing Diagnoses/Identified Patterns
Prior to administration: • Assess for allergies to amide-type local anesthetics. • Check for the presence of broken skin, infection, burns, and wounds where medication is to be applied. • Assess for character, duration, location, and intensity of pain where medication is to be applied.	• Risk for aspiration • Risk for injury • Need for knowledge related to drug use

Planning: Client Goals and Expected Outcomes

The client will:

• Experience no pain during surgical procedure
• Experience no side effects or adverse reactions to anesthesia

Implementation

Interventions (Rationales)	Client Education/Discharge Planning
• Monitor for cardiovascular side effects. (These may occur if anesthetic is absorbed.) • Monitor skin or mucous membranes for infection or inflammation. (Condition could be worsened by drug.) • Monitor for length of effectiveness. (Local anesthetics are effective for 1 to 3 hours.) • Obtain information about and monitor use of other medications. • Provide for client safety. (There is potential for injury related to lack of sensation in the area being treated.) • Monitor for gag reflex. (Xylocaine viscous may interfere with swallowing reflex.)	• Instruct client to report any unusual heart palpitations. If using medication on a regular basis, instruct client to see a healthcare provider regularly. • Instruct client to report irritation or increase in discomfort in areas where medication is used. • Instruct client to report any discomfort during procedure. • Instruct client to report use of any medication to healthcare provider. • Inform client about having no feeling in anesthetized area and taking extra caution to avoid injury, including heat-related injury. Instruct client to: • Not eat within 1 hour of administration • Not chew gum while any portion of mouth or throat is anesthetized to prevent biting injuries

Evaluation of Outcome Criteria

Evaluate the effectiveness of drug therapy by confirming that client goals and expected outcomes have been met (see "Planning").

See Table 24.2 (p. 278) for a list of drugs to which these nursing actions apply.

The goal of general anesthesia is to provide a rapid and complete loss of sensation. Signs of general anesthesia include total analgesia and loss of consciousness, memory, and body movement. Although these signs are similar to those of sleeping, general anesthesia and sleep are not exactly the same. General anesthetics depress all nervous activity in the brain, whereas sleeping depresses only very specific areas. In fact, some brain activity actually increases during sleep, as described in Chapter 16.

General anesthesia is rarely achieved with a single drug. Instead, multiple medications are used to rapidly induce unconsciousness, cause muscle relaxation, and maintain deep anesthesia. This approach, called **balanced anesthesia**, allows the dose of inhalation anesthetic to be lower, thus making the procedure safer for the client.

General anesthesia is a progressive process that occurs in distinct phases. The most efficacious medications can quickly induce all four stages, whereas others are only able to induce stage 1. Stage 3 is where most major surgery occurs; therefore, it is called **surgical anesthesia**. When seeking surgical anesthesia, it is

desirable to progress through stage 2 as rapidly as possible since this stage produces distressing symptoms. These stages are shown in Table 24.3.

TABLE 24.3   Stages of General Anesthesia

Stage	Characteristics
1	Loss of pain: The client loses general sensation but may be awake. This stage proceeds until the client loses consciousness.
2	Excitement and hyperactivity: The client may be delirious and try to resist treatment. Heart rate and breathing may become irregular and blood pressure can increase. IV agents are administered here to calm the client.
3	Surgical anesthesia: Skeletal muscles become relaxed and delirium stabilizes. Cardiovascular and breathing activities stabilize. Eye movements slow and the client becomes still. Surgery is performed during this stage.
4	Paralysis of the medulla region in the brain (responsible for controlling respiratory and cardiovascular activity): If breathing or the heart stops, death could result. This stage is usually avoided during general anesthesia.

GENERAL ANESTHETICS

General anesthetics are drugs that rapidly produce unconsciousness and total analgesia. These drugs are usually administered by the IV or inhalation route. To supplement the effects of a general anesthetic, adjunct drugs are given before, during, and after surgery.

Pharmacotherapy with Inhaled General Anesthetics

24.5 Inhaled general anesthetics are used to maintain surgical anesthesia. Some, such as nitrous oxide, have low efficacy, whereas others, such as halothane, can induce deep anesthesia.

There are two primary methods of inducing general anesthesia. Intravenous agents are usually administered first because they act within a few seconds. After the client loses consciousness, inhaled agents are used to maintain the anesthesia. During short surgical procedures or those requiring lower stages of anesthesia, the IV agents may be used alone.

Inhaled general anesthetics, shown in Table 24.4, may be gases or volatile liquids. These agents produce their effects by preventing the flow of sodium into neurons in the CNS, thus delaying nerve impulses and producing a dramatic reduction in neural activity. The exact mechanism for how this occurs is not exactly known, although it is likely that gamma-aminobutyric acid (GABA) receptors in the brain are activated. It is not the same mechanism known for local anesthetics. There is some evidence suggesting that the mechanism may be related to how some antiseizure drugs work; however, this is still not conclusive. There is not a specific receptor that binds to general anesthetics, and they do not seem to affect neurotransmitter release.

NCLEX Success Tip

Desflurane (Suprane) and sevoflurane (Sevorane) are volatile liquid anesthesia agents that are used for outpatient surgeries primarily because they are rapidly eliminated. They have the added benefits of being better tolerated and nonirritating to the respiratory tract, and they have predictable cardiovascular effects.

Gaseous General Anesthetics

The only gas used routinely for anesthesia is nitrous oxide, commonly called laughing gas. Nitrous oxide is used for dental procedures and for brief obstetrical and surgical procedures. It may also be used in conjunction with other general anesthetics, making it possible to decrease their dosages with greater effectiveness.

TABLE 24.4 Inhaled General Anesthetics

Type	Drug
Volatile liquid	desflurane (Suprane)
	Pr halothane (Fluothane)
	isoflurane (Forane)
	sevoflurane (Sevorane)
Gas	**Pr** nitrous oxide

Nitrous oxide should be used cautiously in myasthenia gravis, as it may cause respiratory depression and prolonged hypnotic effects. Clients with cardiovascular disease, especially those with increased intracranial pressure, should be monitored carefully because the hypnotic effects of the drug may be prolonged or potentiated.

Nursing Considerations

Nitrous oxide has a rapid onset and recovery with minimal side effects (e.g., nausea and vomiting). The nurse's responsibilities are to determine the knowledge level of the client and to reassure the client to alleviate anxiety. Postoperatively, monitor the client's level of consciousness (LOC), vital signs, and pain level and give medication to prevent nausea and vomiting. See Nursing Process Focus: Clients Receiving General Anesthesia on page 283 for more information, including specific teaching points.

PROTOTYPE DRUG | **Nitrous Oxide**

Actions and Uses: The main action of nitrous oxide is analgesia caused by suppression of pain mechanisms in the CNS. It causes cerebral vasodilation and increased cerebral blood flow. This agent has a low potency and does not produce complete loss of consciousness or profound relaxation of skeletal muscle. Because nitrous oxide does not induce surgical anesthesia (stage 3), it is commonly combined with other surgical anesthetic agents. Nitrous oxide is ideal for dental procedures because the client remains conscious and can follow instructions while experiencing full analgesia.

Pharmacokinetics: Nitrous oxide is rapidly absorbed. It is widely distributed and crosses the blood-brain barrier and placenta. (It can cause CNS depression in the fetus.) Elimination is primarily by the lungs and kidneys. Half-life is variable.

Administration Alert: Establish an IV if one is not already in place in case emergency medications are needed.

Adverse Effects: When used in low to moderate doses, nitrous oxide produces few adverse effects. At higher doses, clients exhibit some adverse signs of stage 2 anesthesia such as anxiety, excitement, and combativeness. Lowering the inhaled dose will quickly reverse these adverse effects. As nitrous oxide is exhaled, the client may temporarily have some difficulty breathing at the end of a procedure. Nausea and vomiting following the procedure are more common with nitrous oxide than with other inhalation anesthetics. Nitrous oxide has the potential to be abused (sometimes by medical personnel) because of the relaxed, sedated state that it produces.

Volatile Liquid General Anesthetics

The volatile anesthetics are liquid at room temperature but are converted into a vapour and inhaled to produce their anesthetic effects. Commonly administered volatile agents are halothane (Fluothane), and isoflurane (Forane). The most potent of these is halothane. Some general anesthetics enhance the sensitivity of the heart to drugs such as epinephrine, norepinephrine, dopamine, and serotonin. Most volatile liquids depress cardiovascular and respiratory function. Because it has less effect on the heart and does not damage the liver, isoflurane has become the most widely used inhalation anesthetic. The volatile anesthetics are excreted almost entirely by the lungs, through exhalation.

Nursing Considerations

General anesthesia is primarily used for lengthy surgical procedures, and it involves significant risks. The client should be informed that anesthesia will be administered by highly trained personnel, either an anesthesiologist or a nurse anesthetist, and that the nurse will have a major role in monitoring the client and ensuring client safety. A comprehensive assessment must be done in each phase of surgical experience. General preoperative information such as vital signs, lab tests, health history, level of knowledge concerning the procedure, and the presence of anxiety should be obtained. Preoperatively, the client should be assessed for the use of alcohol or other CNS depressants within the previous 24 hours, as these substances will enhance anesthetic effects. Information concerning the use of other medications should also be obtained.

Use of halothane is contraindicated in clients who have had this drug within the previous 14 to 21 days, as it can cause halothane hepatitis if used frequently. Halothane is also contraindicated in pregnancy (category D) and in clients with diminished hepatic functioning, as it can be hepatotoxic. Caution should be used in clients with cardiac conditions, especially bradycardia and dysrhythmias, as the medication decreases blood pressure and sensitizes the myocardium to catecholamines, which can lead to serious dysrhythmias.

In the immediate postoperative period, monitor the client for side effects of the general anesthesia such as nausea and vomiting, CNS depression, respiratory difficulty, and vital sign changes. Also monitor for complications related to the procedure, such as bleeding or impeding shock.

See Nursing Process Focus: Clients Receiving General Anesthesia on page 283 for more details, including specific teaching points.

PROTOTYPE DRUG	Halothane (Fluothane)

Actions and Uses: Halothane produces a potent level of surgical anesthesia that is rapid in onset. Although potent, halothane does not produce as much muscle relaxation or analgesia as other volatile anesthetics. Therefore, halothane is primarily used with other anesthetic agents, including muscle relaxants and analgesics. Nitrous oxide is sometimes combined with halothane. Clients recover from anesthesia rapidly after halothane is discontinued.

Pharmacokinetics: Halothane is rapidly absorbed. It is widely distributed and crosses the blood-brain barrier. Elimination is primarily by the lungs and kidneys. Half-life is variable.

Adverse Effects and Interactions: Halothane moderately sensitizes the heart muscle to epinephrine; therefore, dysrhythmias are a concern. This agent lowers blood pressure and respiration rate. It also increases the risk of aspirating stomach contents into the lungs. Because of potential hepatotoxicity, use of halothane has declined.

Malignant hyperthermia is rare but can be a fatal adverse effect triggered by all inhalation anesthetics. It causes muscle rigidity and severe temperature elevation (up to 43°C). This risk is greatest when halothane is used with succinylcholine (Quelicin).

Levodopa-carbidopa (Sinemet) taken concurrently increases the level of dopamine in the CNS and should be discontinued 6 to 8 hours before halothane administration.

Skeletal muscle weakness, respiratory depression, or apnea may occur if halothane is administered concurrently with polymyxins, lincomycin, or aminoglycosides.

INTRAVENOUS ANESTHETICS

Several miscellaneous drugs are used as parenteral anesthetics. Propofol (Diprivan) and ketamine (Ketalar) are two of the widely used IV anesthetics. The two drugs are not related chemically, but both have short durations and can induce anesthesia rapidly.

NCLEX Success Tips

Propofol, a non-barbiturate anesthetic, causes less nausea and vomiting than other induction agents because of a direct antiemetic action. If propofol is used in clients with extensive burns who are particularly susceptible to zinc deficiency, the nurse should arrange for zinc supplementation. Propofol causes urinary zinc losses.

Pharmacotherapy with IV Anesthetics

24.6 IV anesthetics are used either alone, for short procedures, or to supplement inhalation anesthetics.

Intravenous anesthetics, shown in Table 24.5, are important supplements to general anesthesia. Although occasionally used alone, they are often administered with inhaled general anesthetics. Concurrent administration of IV and inhaled anesthetics allows the dose of the inhaled agent to be reduced, thus lowering the potential for serious side effects. Furthermore, when combined, IV anesthetics provide more analgesia and muscle relaxation than could be provided by the inhaled anesthetic alone. When IV anesthetics are administered without other anesthetics, they are generally reserved for medical procedures that take less than 15 minutes.

NCLEX Success Tips

Diazepam (Valium) is used for short-term management of muscle spasms because it's potentially addictive. To prevent adverse reactions, which are common, IV diazepam should be administered no faster than

TABLE 24.5   Intravenous Anesthetics

Chemical Classification	Drug
Barbiturate and barbiturate-like agents	**Pr** propofol (Diprivan)
	diazepam (Valium)
Benzodiazepines	lorazepam (Ativan)
	midazolam (Versed)
Opioids	alfentanil (Alfenta)
	fentanyl (Duragesic)
	remifentanil (Ultiva)
	sufentanil (Sufenta)
Others	ketamine (Ketalar)

5 mg/minute in an adult and should be given over at least 3 minutes in children. Diazepam shouldn't be mixed with other drugs in an infusion because of the high risk of incompatibility. To help prevent extravasation, the nurse should avoid administering diazepam in a small vein. IV diazepam may cause cardiorespiratory depression; to detect this adverse reaction, the nurse should monitor the client's vital signs carefully during administration. IV lorazepam is the benzodiazepine of choice for treating prolonged seizure activity. IV benzodiazepines act to potentiate the action of the GABA neurotransmitter, stopping seizure activity. If an IV is not available, rectal diazepam is the benzodiazepine of choice. Most adverse reactions to diazepam and other benzodiazepines involve the central nervous system. The client is more likely to experience sedation than bradycardia, skin rash, or hypotension. Diazepam is a benzodiazepine that causes symptoms of withdrawal when stopped abruptly. The nurse should assess the client for tremors, agitation, irritability, insomnia, vomiting, sweating, tachycardia, headache, anxiety, and confusion. Drugs employed as IV anesthetics include barbiturates, opioids, and benzodiazepines. Opioids offer the advantage of superior analgesia. Combining the opioid fentanyl with the antipsychotic agent droperidol produces a state known as neurolept analgesia. In this state, clients are conscious but insensitive to pain and unconnected with surroundings. A similar conscious, dissociated state is produced with ketamine. For this reason, ketamine has been misused as a date rape drug and is now reclassified from a Schedule F to a CDSA Schedule I drug in Canada. Clients who receive these drugs therapeutically or illicitly may express awareness of events that occurred while under the drug's influence, yet at the same time have a sense of uncertainty and unreality about them.

Nursing Considerations

The role of the nurse in drug therapy with IV anesthetics involves careful monitoring of the client's condition and providing education as it relates to the anesthetic in use. IV sedation is used to decrease anxiety and fear secondary to confinement of the mask used for inhalation anesthesia. A thorough assessment must be completed prior to selecting an anesthetic or combination of anesthetics. Clients may be given medications other than anesthesia, including antianxiety agents, sedatives, analgesics, opioids, and anticholinergics, during preoperative, perioperative, or postoperative periods. Obtain a complete medical history from the client. IV anesthetics are contraindicated in clients with drug sensitivity since allergic reactions ranging from hives to respiratory arrest can result. Because they are administered intravenously, suitability of an IV access site should be assessed.

Clients with cardiovascular disease should be monitored carefully, as IV anesthetics can cause depression of the myocardium, leading to dysrhythmias. Clients with respiratory disorders should also be monitored carefully because respiratory depression may result in high levels of anesthetic in the blood.

The use of general anesthetics results in CNS depression. During the postoperative period, monitor the client for vital sign changes, hallucinations, confusion, and excitability. Other side effects or reactions that should be assessed include respiratory difficulties, shivering and trembling, nausea or vomiting, headache, and somnolence. Preoperative teaching is vital to understanding the anesthetic and the entire surgical experience. It also helps to allay fears and anxiety of the client and caregivers.

See Nursing Process Focus: Clients Receiving General Anesthesia for specific teaching points.

PROTOTYPE DRUG | **Propofol (Diprivan)**

Actions and Uses: The exact mechanism by which propofol produces anesthesia is not clear. It is believed to act by activating GABA receptors, which causes a general inhibition of CNS activity. Propofol has become the most widely used IV anesthetic due to its effectiveness and relative safety profile. It is indicated for the induction and maintenance of general anesthesia. In the intensive care unit (ICU), the drug may be administered to intubated, mechanically ventilated adult clients to provide continuous sedation and control of stress responses.

Pharmacokinetics: Propofol is administered by the IV route and is widely distributed to body tissues. It has almost immediate onset of action and a duration of action of 10 to 115 minutes. It is highly protein bound, metabolized at the liver, and excreted by the kidneys. Emergence from anesthesia is rapid, and few adverse effects occur during recovery. Unlike other anesthetics that cause nausea and vomiting, propofol has an antiemetic effect that can prevent nausea and vomiting in clients who are receiving chemotherapy.

Administration Alerts:

- Propofol is contraindicated in clients who have a known hypersensitivity reaction to the medication or its emulsion, which contains soybean and egg products. The emulsion supports rapid microorganism growth; unused portions must be discarded.

NURSING PROCESS FOCUS

Clients Receiving General Anesthesia

Assessment	Potential Nursing Diagnoses/Identified Patterns
Prior to administration: - Obtain complete health history, including allergies, drug history, and possible drug interactions. - Assess for presence or history of severe respiratory, cardiac, renal, or liver disorders. - Obtain baseline vital signs. - Assess for any musculoskeletal disorders or injuries that may impair movement and require special positioning during anesthesia. - Obtain blood work: complete blood count and chemistry panel. - Assess client's knowledge of procedure and level of anxiety.	- Anxiety related to surgical procedure - Impaired gas exchange - Need for knowledge related to drug use - Nausea related to drug side effect - Disturbed sensory perception - Ineffective breathing pattern - Decreased cardiac output

---

Planning: Client Goals and Expected Outcomes

The client will:

- Experience adequate anesthesia during surgical procedure
- Experience no side effects or adverse reaction to anesthesia
- Demonstrate an understanding of perioperative procedures

Implementation

Interventions (Rationales)	Client Education/Discharge Planning
• Preoperatively, assess knowledge level of preoperative and postoperative procedures. Ensure that the client has accurate information and questions are answered. (Teaching will reduce client anxiety.) • Preoperatively, assess emotional state. (Clients who are fearful or extremely anxious may be more difficult to induce and maintain under anesthesia.) • Monitor preoperative status. • Postoperatively, monitor for respiratory difficulty and adequate oxygen–carbon dioxide (O_2-CO_2) exchange. (Anesthetics cause respiratory depression.) • Monitor recovery from anesthesia. Evaluate LOC, nausea, vomiting, and pain. • Monitor vital signs. (Respiratory status may be impaired leading to prolonged apnea, respiratory depression, and cyanosis. Blood pressure may drop to shock levels.)	• Give preoperative and postoperative instructions • Explain what the client will see, hear, and feel prior to surgery • Explain the recovery room process • Explain what the client and family will see and hear postoperatively • Take client on tour of operative facilities, if possible • Instruct client about using stress reduction techniques such as deep breathing, imagery, and distraction Instruct client to: • Remain nothing by mouth (NPO) as ordered prior to surgery to prevent risk of aspiration, nausea, and vomiting • Stop taking medications 24 hours prior to surgery as ordered by the healthcare provider • Refrain from alcohol 24 hours prior to surgery • Inform client to report shortness of breath, difficulty breathing, or dizziness • Instruct client about possible side effects and to report any discomfort immediately • Advise client to report heart palpitations, dizziness, difficulty breathing, or faintness

---

Evaluation of Outcome Criteria

Evaluate the effectiveness of drug therapy by confirming that client goals and expected outcomes have been met (see "Planning").

See Tables 24.4 (p. 281) and 24.5 (p. 282) for lists of drugs to which these nursing actions apply.

- Obstetrical clients and those with increased intracranial pressure should not be administered propofol.
- The drug should be used with caution in clients with cardiac or respiratory impairment.
- Propofol is not recommended for induction of anesthesia in children younger than 3 years.
- Although not a controlled substance, incidences of propofol abuse have occurred, including the high-profile case of Michael Jackson, who used this medication (among others) to induce sleep.

Adverse Effects and Interactions: Injection site pain, apnea, respiratory depression, and hypotension are common adverse effects. Propofol has been associated with a collection of metabolic abnormalities and organ system failures, referred to as propofol infusion syndrome (PRIS). The syndrome is characterized by severe metabolic acidosis, hyperkalemia, lipemia, rhabdomyolysis, hepatomegaly, and cardiac and renal failure. PRIS is usually associated with prolonged, high-dose infusions of the drug. Deaths have resulted from this syndrome.

The dose of propofol should be reduced in clients who are receiving preanesthetic medications such as opioids or benzodiazepines. Use with other CNS depressants can cause additive CNS and respiratory depression.

NON-ANESTHETIC DRUGS AS ADJUNCTS TO SURGERY

24.7 Numerous non-anesthetic medications, including opioids, antianxiety agents, barbiturates, and neuromuscular blockers, are administered as adjuncts to surgery.

A number of drugs are used either to complement the effects of general anesthetics or to treat anticipated side effects of the anesthesia. These agents, shown in Table 24.6, are called adjuncts to anesthesia. They may be given prior to, during, or after surgery.

The preoperative drugs given to relieve anxiety and provide mild sedation include barbiturates and benzodiazepines. Opioids such as morphine (Kadian, M-Eslon, MS Contin, MS-IR, Statex) may be given to counteract pain that the client will experience after surgery. Anticholinergics such as atropine may be administered to dry secretions and to suppress the bradycardia caused by some anesthetics.

During surgery, the primary adjuncts are the **neuromuscular blockers**. So that surgical procedures can be carried out safely, it is necessary to administer drugs that cause skeletal muscles to totally relax. Administration of these drugs also allows the amount of anesthetic to be reduced. Neuromuscular blocking agents are classified as depolarizing blockers

TABLE 24.6 Select Adjuncts to Anesthesia

Chemical Classification	Drug
Barbiturate and barbiturate-like agents	butabarbital (Butisol)
	pentobarbital (Nembutal)
	secobarbital
Opioids	alfentanil (Alfenta)
	fentanyl (Duragesic)
	fentanyl/droperidol (Innovar)
	remifentanil (Ultiva)
	sufentanil (Sufenta)
Miscellaneous agents	bethanechol (Duvoid): anticholinergic
	droperidol (Inapsine): dopamine blocker
	promethazine (Phenergan): dopamine blocker
	Pr succinylcholine (Quelicin): neuromuscular blocker
	tubocurarine: neuromuscular blocker

or non-depolarizing blockers. The only depolarizing blocker is succinylcholine, which works by binding to acetylcholine receptors at neuromuscular junctions to cause total skeletal muscle relaxation. Succinylcholine is used in surgery for ease of tracheal intubation. Mivacurium (Mivacron) is the shortest acting of the non-depolarizing blockers, whereas tubocurarine is a longer acting neuromuscular blocking agent. The non-depolarizing blockers cause muscle paralysis by competing with acetylcholine for cholinergic receptors at neuromuscular junctions. Once on the receptor, the non-polarizing blockers prevent muscle contraction. When drugs that decrease sensation and cause skeletal muscles to relax are administered, the client is unable to resist being positioned in a way that would otherwise cause discomfort and perhaps injury. It is important that the nurse assess for and document any musculoskeletal disorders or injuries and limitations to joint movement that may require special positioning during anesthesia.

Succinylcholine, a depolarizing blocking agent, is the drug of choice when short-term muscle relaxation is desired—for example, during electroconvulsive therapy (ECT) or intubation. Vecuronium (Norcuron), pancuronium, and atracurium are non-depolarizing blocking agents used for intermediate- or long-term muscle relaxation. Succinylcholine is an ultra short-acting depolarizing agent used for rapid sequence intubation. Bradycardia can occur, especially in children. Atropine is the drug of choice in treating or preventing succinylcholine-induced bradycardia. Lidocaine is used in adults only. Epinephrine (Adrenalin) bolus and isoproterenol are not used in rapid sequence intubation because of their profound cardiac effects.

Postoperative drugs include analgesics for pain and antiemetics such as promethazine (Phenergan) or ondansetron (Zofran) for the nausea and vomiting that sometimes occur during recovery from the anesthetic. Occasionally a cholinergic such as bethanechol (Duvoid) is administered to stimulate the smooth muscle of the bladder wall to contract to expel urine and the smooth muscle of the bowel to begin peristalsis following surgery.

Nursing Considerations

The role of the nurse in neuromuscular blocker therapy involves careful monitoring of the client's condition and providing education as it relates to the drug therapy. Neuromuscular blocking agents are used so that the client experiences complete skeletal muscle relaxation during the surgical procedure. Continuous use is not recommended because of potential side effects. Clients should be aware that these drugs are used only in a controlled acute care setting, usually surgery, by a skilled professional.

In preparation for use of succinylcholine, assess for the presence or history of hepatic or renal dysfunction, neuromuscular disease, fractures, myasthenia gravis, malignant hyperthermia, glaucoma, and penetrating eye injuries. Use of this drug is contraindicated in these conditions. Use in children under 2 years of age is contraindicated because the drug can cause dysrhythmias and malignant hyperthermia.

Mivacurium is used for intubation and is contraindicated for persons with renal or hepatic disease, fluid and electrolyte imbalances, neuromuscular disorders, respiratory disease, and obesity. It should be used cautiously in older adults and children. It should not be used during pregnancy or lactation. An anesthesiologist may administer it during cesarean section.

Prior to use of any neuromuscular blocker, assess physical status to rule out potential expected problems, including vital signs, reflexes, muscle tone and response, pupil size and reactivity, electrocardiogram (ECG), lung sounds, bowel sounds, affect, and LOC. Monitor for a decrease in blood pressure, tachycardia, prolonged apnea, bronchospasm, respiratory depression, paralysis, and hypersensitivity.

PROTOTYPE DRUG | Succinylcholine (Quelicin)

Actions and Uses: Like the natural neurotransmitter acetylcholine, succinylcholine acts on cholinergic receptor sites at neuromuscular junctions. At first, depolarization occurs and skeletal muscles contract. After repeated contractions, however, the membrane is unable to repolarize as long as the drug stays on the receptor. Effects are first noted as muscle weakness and muscle spasms. Eventually paralysis occurs. Succinylcholine is rapidly broken down by the enzyme pseudocholinesterase; when the IV infusion is stopped, the duration of action is only a few minutes. Use of succinylcholine reduces the amount of general anesthetic needed for procedures.

Administration Alert:
• Succinylcholine is pregnancy category C.

Pharmacokinetics: Succinylcholine is widely distributed. It is metabolized mostly by the liver. A small amount is excreted unchanged in the urine. Its half-life is unknown.

Adverse Effects and Interactions: Succinylcholine can cause complete paralysis of the diaphragm and intercostal muscles; therefore, mechanical ventilation is necessary during surgery. Bradycardia and respiratory depression are expected adverse effects. If doses are high, the ganglia are affected, causing tachycardia, hypotension, and urinary retention. Clients with certain genetic mutations may experience rapid onset of extremely high fever with muscle rigidity—a serious condition known as malignant hyperthermia.

Additive skeletal muscle blockade will occur if succinylcholine is given concurrently with clindamycin (Dalacin), aminoglycosides, furosemide (Lasix), lithium (Carbolith, Lithane), quinidine (Quinate), or lidocaine.

Increased effect of succinylcholine may occur if given concurrently with phenothiazines, oxytocin (Pitocin), or thiazide diuretics. Decreased effect of succinylcholine occurs if given with diazepam (Valium).

If this drug is given concurrently with halothane or nitrous oxide, an increased risk of bradycardia, dysrhythmias, sinus arrest, apnea, and malignant hyperthermia exists. If succinylcholine is given concurrently with cardiac glycosides, there is increased risk of cardiac dysrhythmias. If narcotics are given concurrently with succinylcholine, there is increased risk of bradycardia and sinus arrest.

CHAPTER 24

Understanding the Chapter

Key Concepts Summary

The numbered key concepts provide a succinct summary of the important points from the corresponding numbered section within the chapter. If any of these points are not clear, refer to the numbered section within the chapter for review.

24.1 Regional loss of sensation is achieved by administering local anesthetics topically or through the infiltration, nerve block, spinal, or epidural methods.

24.2 Local anesthetics act by blocking sodium channels in neurons. Epinephrine is sometimes added to prolong the duration of anesthetic action.

24.3 Local anesthetics are classified as amides or esters. The amides, such as lidocaine, have generally replaced the esters due to their greater safety.

24.4 General anesthesia produces a complete loss of sensation accompanied by loss of consciousness. This is usually achieved through the use of multiple medications.

24.5 Inhaled general anesthetics are used to maintain surgical anesthesia. Some, such as nitrous oxide, have low efficacy, whereas others, such as halothane, can induce deep anesthesia.

24.6 IV anesthetics are used either alone, for short procedures, or to supplement inhalation anesthetics.

24.7 Numerous non-anesthetic medications, including opioids, antianxiety agents, barbiturates, and neuromuscular blockers, are administered as adjuncts to surgery.

Chapter 24 Scenario

Elena is a 37-year-old woman who is scheduled for a vaginal hysterectomy after a positive Pap smear returned with results suggestive of cancer. While in the holding area of the operating room suite, Elena states that she is fearful of general anesthesia. The preoperative nurse caring for Elena notices that she is very anxious. Upon further assessment and conversation, Elena states that her mother died of breast cancer when she was young.

The client's vital signs are as follows: blood pressure 138/88 mm Hg, temperature 36.3°C, pulse 94 beats/minute, and respiration 20 breaths/minute. She denies pain and states that she is concerned she will wake up during the surgery. She is to receive balanced anesthesia.

Critical Thinking Questions

1. In your own words, how would you describe balanced anesthesia to Elena?

2. How does nitrous oxide differ from IV anesthetic agents?

3. How should the nurse educate a client regarding the use of IV propofol?

See Answers to Critical Thinking Questions in Appendix B.

NCLEX Practice Questions

1 A surgical nurse is alerted that the client receiving general anesthesia has become excitable and hyperactive, with irregular heart and respiratory rates. The nurse knows that the client has entered which stage of general anesthesia?

  a. Stage 1

  b. Stage 2

  c. Stage 3

  d. Stage 4

2 A nurse should question the administration of propofol (Diprivan) for

  a. A client with an allergy to eggs or soy products

  b. A client with an allergy to iodine

  c. A client with kidney disease

  d. A client with Addison's disease

3 During the administration of nitrous oxide, a client develops anxiety, excitement, and combativeness. The nurse would anticipate which change in the client's anesthesia is needed?

  a. The nitrous oxide dose will be increased.

  b. Propofol (Diprivan) will be given along with the nitrous oxide.

  c. Succinylcholine (Quelicin) will be given to the client.

  d. The nitrous oxide dose will be decreased.

4 A nurse is providing preoperative instructions to a client who will be receiving ketamine (Ketalar). Which statement by the client would indicate that teaching is successful?

  a. "The medication will decrease anxiety during surgery."

  b. "I will experience increased energy due to this drug."

  c. "I may experience a feeling of being separated from the environment."

  d. "The drug will cause me to have dry mouth after the operation."

5 A client who is having a scalp laceration sutured will be receiving local anesthesia with lidocaine (Xylocaine) that contains epinephrine. The nurse knows that the purpose of this drug combination is to

  a. Increase the duration of the anesthetic action

  b. Increase vasodilation at the site of the laceration

  c. Decrease blood pressure in individuals who are hypertensive

  d. Ensure that infection at the wound site will not occur

See Answers to NCLEX Practice Questions in Appendix A.

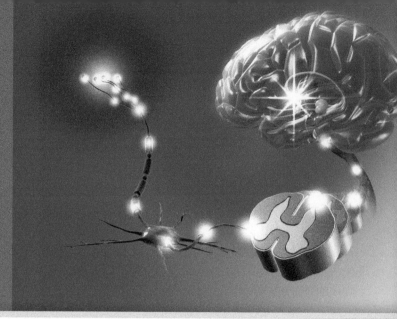

Marc Phares/Science Source

CHAPTER 25

Pharmacotherapy in Substances of Abuse and Addiction

LEARNING OUTCOMES

After reading this chapter, the student should be able to:

1. Describe underlying causes of addiction.
2. Differentiate psychological and physical dependence.
3. Compare withdrawal syndromes for the various addictive substance classes.
4. Describe signs of drug tolerance, drug dependence, and withdrawal.
5. Describe the major characteristics of addiction, dependence, and tolerance resulting from the following substances: alcohol, nicotine, marijuana, hallucinogens, central nervous system (CNS) stimulants, sedatives, and opioids.
6. Describe the role of the nurse in delivering care to individuals with drug addictions.

CHAPTER OUTLINE

Throughout history, individuals have self-administered both natural substances and prescription drugs to increase performance, assist with relaxation, alter psychological state, or simply fit in with the crowd. **Substance abuse** is the self-administration of a drug in a manner that does not conform to the norms within one's given culture or society. Many of these substances are addictive. Substance addiction has a tremendous economic, social, and public health impact on society. With the 2013 publication of the *Diagnostic and Statistical Manual of Mental Disorders,* 5th Edition (DSM-5), a newer term was introduced to describe this condition to avoid the word *abuse* entirely: *substance use disorder* (American Psychological Association, 2013). Because most nurses are still familiar with the term *substance abuse,* that term will continue to be used in this chapter for clarity.

Although the terms *drugs of addiction* and *substances of addiction* are sometimes used interchangeably, *substances of addiction* is more accurate because some abused agents are not considered drugs. For example, glue is not classified as a drug. The term *substance of addiction* may be preferable to *abused substance* since it shifts the focus to labelling the substance rather than the behaviour of the individual who is suffering from the stigma and despair of living with an addiction.

This chapter introduces the types of drugs commonly abused by clients and the pharmacological management of withdrawal syndromes.

Overview of Substances of Addiction

25.1 A wide variety of addictive substances may be used by individuals, all of which share the common characteristic of altering brain physiology and/or perception.

Characteristics of substance abuse vary widely from drug to drug and person to person. Diagnosis of the disorder is often difficult, even for experienced healthcare professionals. Recognition of abuse is relatively easy for substances such as heroin, cocaine, or hallucinogens. However, what about for legal substances such as alcohol, tobacco, or marijuana? It is apparent that, with the exception of certain illegal substances, there is often not a clear distinction among proper use, misuse, and substance abuse.

There are certain characteristics, however, that assist in the proper diagnosis of substance abuse. Nurses should be aware of these characteristics because they may be the first to recognize the following when obtaining a client's history:

1. Craving for a specific substance despite an understanding that the substance is lowering the client's quality of life (physical dependence)

2. Failure to maintain normal work or home relationships because a substance is being used repeatedly

3. Recognition that, over time, increased amounts of the substance are needed to produce the desired effect (tolerance)

4. Repeated, unsuccessful attempts have been made to discontinue using the substance

5. Recognition that behavioural changes such as agitation, drowsiness, anxiety, and pain (withdrawal syndrome) occur when the substance is discontinued

6. Increased amount of time is devoted to obtaining or using the substance, which reduces time available for work, home, or leisure activities.

Addictive substances belong to a number of diverse chemical classes. They have few structural similarities but have the common ability to affect the nervous system, particularly the brain. Some substances, such as opium, marijuana, cocaine, nicotine, caffeine, and alcohol, are obtained from natural sources. Others are synthetic or **designer drugs** created in illicit laboratories for the express purpose of making fortunes in illicit drug trafficking.

Although the public often associates substance addiction with illicit drugs, this is not necessarily the case; alcohol and nicotine are the two most common substances of addiction. Prescription medications such as methylphenidate (Ritalin, Concerta, Biphentin) and meperidine (Demerol) are sometimes addictive. Substances used illicitly that are frequent sources of addiction include marijuana, volatile inhalants such as aerosols and paint thinners, cocaine, sedatives sold on the street, and hallucinogens such as lysergic acid diethylamide (LSD) and phencyclidine hydrochloride (PCP).

Several drugs once used therapeutically are now illicit due to their high potential for addiction. Cocaine was once widely used as a local anesthetic, but today nearly all cocaine acquired by users is obtained illicitly. LSD is now illicit, although in the 1940s and 1950s it was used in psychotherapy. Phencyclidine was popular in the early 1960s as an anesthetic but was withdrawn from the market in 1965 because clients reported hallucinations, delusions, and anxiety after recovering from anesthesia. Many amphetamines once used for bronchodilation were discontinued in the 1980s after psychotic episodes were reported.

Neurobiological and Psychosocial Components of Substance Addiction

25.2 Addiction is an overwhelming compulsion to continue repeated drug use that has both neurobiological and psychosocial components.

Behaviours such as eating, drinking, and engaging in sexual activity that are necessary for survival of the species are reinforced through stimulation of "reward pathways" in the brain that provide pleasure. In this way, the brain naturally encourages behaviours that lead to pleasure. The addictive process is hypothesized to involve stimulation of these reward pathways by an addictive substance that mimics and even surpasses that of its naturally occurring chemical counterpart. With repeated self-administration of the addictive substance, tolerance develops, and with it develops the perceived need to continue to use the substance in order to experience pleasure. **Addiction** is an overwhelming compulsion that drives someone to repetitive drug-taking behaviour despite serious health and social consequences. It is impossible to accurately predict whether a person will become addicted to a substance. Attempts to predict a person's addictive tendency using psychological profiles or genetic markers have largely been unsuccessful. Substance addiction depends on multiple complex, interacting variables. These variables focus on the following categories:

- Agent or drug factors: cost, availability, dose, mode of administration (e.g., oral, intravenous [IV], inhalation), speed of onset and termination, length of drug use
- User factors: genetic factors (e.g., metabolic enzymes, innate tolerance), propensity for risk-taking behaviour, prior experiences with drugs, disease that may require a scheduled drug
- Environmental factors: social and community norms, role models, peer influences, educational opportunities

NCLEX Success Tips

Addiction indicates that an individual cannot control his or her use of psychoactive substances. It is a complex condition in which the drug is used for psychological effect and not analgesia. Addiction is not a concern when giving narcotics to manage cancer pain. This term, *addiction*, has been replaced by the term *dependence*. Drug dependence occurs when the client must take a usual or increasing amount of the drug to prevent the onset of abstinence symptoms, cannot keep drug intake under control, and continues to use even though physical, social, and emotional processes are compromised.

Abuse refers to the excessive use of a substance that differs from societal norms.

In the case of prescription drugs, addiction may begin with a legitimate need for pharmacotherapy. For example, narcotic analgesics may be indicated for pain relief, or sedatives may be indicated for a sleep disorder. These drugs may result in a favourable experience, such as pain relief or sleep, and clients will want to repeat these positive experiences.

It is a common misunderstanding, even among some health professionals, that the therapeutic use of scheduled drugs creates large numbers of addicted clients. In fact, prescription drugs rarely cause addiction when used according to accepted medical protocols. The risk for addiction associated with prescription drugs is primarily a function of the dose and the length of therapy. Because of this, medications that have the potential for addiction are usually prescribed at the lowest effective dose and for the shortest time necessary to treat the medical problem. Nurses should administer these medications as prescribed for the relief of client symptoms without undue fear of producing dependency. As mentioned in Chapters 1 and 2, numerous laws have been passed in an attempt to limit drug addiction.

Physical and Psychological Dependence

25.3 Certain substances can cause both physical and psychological dependence, which result in continued drug-seeking behaviour despite negative health and social consequences.

Whether a substance is addictive is related to how easily an individual can stop taking the substance on a repetitive basis. When a person has an overwhelming desire to take a drug and cannot stop, this is referred to as substance dependence. Substance dependence is classified by two categories: physical dependence and psychological dependence.

Physical dependence refers to an altered physical condition caused by the nervous system adapting to repeated substance use. Over time, the body's cells start to respond as though it is normal for the substance to be continually present. With physical dependence, uncomfortable symptoms known as withdrawal result when the agent is discontinued. Opioids, such as morphine (Kadian, M-Eslon, MS Contin, MS-IR, Statex) and heroin, may produce physical dependence rather quickly with repeated doses, particularly when taken intravenously. Alcohol, sedatives, some stimulants, and nicotine are other examples of substances that may produce physical dependence easily with extended use.

NCLEX Success Tip

Addiction is characterized by a drive to take a medication for the psychic effect rather than the therapeutic effect. Physical dependence is a response to ongoing exposure to a medication and is manifested by withdrawal symptoms when the drug is discontinued abruptly.

In contrast, **psychological dependence** produces no signs of physical discomfort after the agent is discontinued. The user, however, has an overwhelming desire to continue using the substance despite obvious negative economic, physical, or social consequences. This intense craving may be associated with the client's home environment or social contacts. Strong psychological craving for a substance may continue for months or even years and is often responsible for relapses during substance addiction therapy and a return to drug-seeking behaviour. Psychological dependence usually requires relatively high doses for a prolonged time, such as with marijuana and antianxiety drugs; however, psychological dependence may develop quickly, perhaps after only one use with crack—a potent, inexpensive form of cocaine.

To summarize, physical dependence refers to the state in which an individual must take the substance to feel physically normal; not taking the drug results in withdrawal symptoms. Psychological dependence refers to an individual's need to derive an alteration in mood from a substance.

Withdrawal Syndrome

25.4 The withdrawal syndrome is a set of uncomfortable symptoms that occur when a substance to which an individual is addicted is no longer available. The severity of the withdrawal syndrome varies among the different drug classes.

Once a client becomes physically dependent and the substance is discontinued, a **withdrawal syndrome** will occur. Symptoms of withdrawal syndrome may be particularly severe for clients who are physically dependent on alcohol and sedatives. Because of the severity of the symptoms, the process of withdrawal from these agents is best accomplished in a substance addiction treatment facility. Examples of the types of withdrawal syndromes experienced with different addictive substances are shown in Table 25.1.

NCLEX Success Tips

Symptoms of opioid withdrawal include yawning, rhinorrhea, sweating, chills, piloerection (goose bumps), tremors, restlessness, irritability, leg spasms, bone pain, diarrhea, and vomiting. Symptoms of withdrawal occur within 36 to 72 hours of usage and subside within a week. Withdrawal from heroin is seldom fatal and usually does not necessitate medical intervention.

Synesthesia (a blending of senses) is associated with lysergic acid diethylamide use, and formication (feeling of bugs crawling beneath the skin) is associated with cocaine use.

Prescription drugs may be used to reduce the severity of withdrawal symptoms. For example, alcohol withdrawal can be treated with a short-acting benzodiazepine such as oxazepam (Serax), and opioid withdrawal can be treated with methadone (Metadol). Symptoms of nicotine withdrawal may be relieved by nicotine replacement therapy in the form of patches or chewing gum. No specific pharmacological intervention is indicated for withdrawal from CNS stimulants, hallucinogens, marijuana, or inhalants.

With chronic use of addictive substances, clients will often associate their conditions and surroundings, including social contacts with other users, with the taking of the drug. Users tend to revert back to drug-seeking behaviour when they return to the company of other users of addictive substances. Counsellors often encourage users to refrain from associating with past social contacts or engaging in relationships with other people with addictions to lessen the possibility of relapse. The formation of new social contacts as a result of association with self-help groups such as Alcoholics Anonymous helps some clients to transition to a drug-free lifestyle.

Tolerance

25.5 Tolerance is a biological condition that occurs with repeated use of certain substances and results in higher doses being needed to achieve the same initial response. Cross-tolerance occurs between closely related drugs.

Tolerance is a biological condition that occurs when the body adapts to a substance after repeated administration. Over time, higher doses of the agent are required to produce the same initial effect. For example, at the start of pharmacotherapy, a client may

TABLE 25.1 Withdrawal Symptoms of Select Substances of Abuse

Drug Class	Symptoms	Treatment
Alcohol	Tremors, fatigue, anxiety, abdominal cramping, hallucinations, confusion, seizures, delirium	Benzodiazepines, antiseizure drugs; disulfiram (Antabuse) and naltrexone (ReVia) after withdrawal is over
Anabolic steroids	Mood swings, fatigue, restlessness, anorexia, insomnia, reduced sex drive, depression, and psychological craving for steroids	Behavioural therapy, symptomatic treatment such as antidepressants
Barbiturates and other sedative–hypnotics	Insomnia, anxiety, weakness, abdominal cramps, tremor, anorexia, seizures, hallucinations, and delirium	Same as alcohol
Benzodiazepines	Insomnia, irritability, abdominal pain, nausea, sensitivity to light and sound, headache, fatigue, and tremors	Gradual tapering of dosage over several weeks or months; for acute benzodiazepine intoxication, flumazenil (Romazicon) is administered by rapid IV infusion (15–20 seconds)
Cocaine and amphetamines	Mental depression, anxiety, agitation, irritability, extreme fatigue, hunger, disturbed sleep, psychological craving	Behavioural therapy; no specific pharmacological treatment available
Hallucinogens	Dependent on the specific drug; may include anxiety, mental depression, insomnia, paranoid delusions, panic attacks, lethargy	Treatment usually is not necessary; symptoms resolve in about 12 hours; PCP excretion is very pH dependent and acidification of the urine increases the clearance rate of PCP by about 100-fold.
Marijuana	Irritability, restlessness, insomnia, tremor, chills, weight loss	No treatment
Nicotine	Irritability, anxiety, restlessness, headaches, increased appetite, insomnia, inability to concentrate, decrease in heart rate and blood pressure	Nicotine replacement therapy, varenicline (Champix) or bupropion (Zyban)
Opioids	Excessive sweating, restlessness, dilated pupils, agitation, goose bumps, tremor, violent yawning, increased heart rate and blood pressure, nausea, vomiting, abdominal cramps and pain, muscle spasms with kicking movements, weight loss	Methadone maintenance; buprenorphine (Butrans) therapy; clonidine (Catapres) reduces anxiety, agitation, cramping, and sweating; oxazepam reduces muscle spasms and insomnia; antiemetics for nausea and vomiting; detoxification can be completed in 2–3 days; withdrawal may be done more rapidly using naltrexone in combination with propofol (Diprivan) anesthetic, the antiemetic ondansetron (Zofran), the antidiarrheal octreotide (Sandostatin), and clonidine and benzodiazepines for other symptoms

◀ Pediatric Use of Volatile Inhalants

Many parents are concerned about their children smoking tobacco or marijuana or becoming addicted to crack or amphetamines. Yet few parents consider that the most common sources of addictive substances lie in their own homes. Inhaling volatile chemicals, known as huffing, is most prevalent in the 10- to 12-year-old age group and then declines with age; one in five children has tried huffing by grade 8. Virtually any organic compound can be huffed, including nail polish remover, spray paint, household glue, correction fluid, propane, gasoline, and even whipped cream propellants. These agents are readily available, inexpensive, and can be used anytime and anywhere. Children can die after a single exposure or suffer brain damage, which may be manifested as slurred or slow speech, tremor, memory loss, or personality changes. Nurses who work with pediatric clients should be aware of the widespread nature of this type of addiction and should advise parents to keep close watch on volatile substances.

find that 2 mg of a sedative is effective at inducing sleep. After taking the medication for several months, the client notices that it takes 4 mg or perhaps 6 mg to fall asleep. Development of drug tolerance is common for substances that affect the nervous system. Tolerance should be thought of as a natural consequence of continued drug use and not be considered evidence of addiction.

NCLEX Success Tip

Tolerance occurs when the body requires higher doses of substances—such as alcohol, opioids, or benzodiazepines—to achieve desired effects.

Tolerance does not develop at the same rate for all actions of a drug. For example, clients usually develop tolerance to the nausea and vomiting produced by narcotic analgesics after only a few doses. Tolerance to the mood-altering effects of these drugs and to their ability to reduce pain develops more slowly but eventually may be complete. Tolerance to the drug's ability to constrict the pupils never develops. Clients will often endure annoying side effects of drugs, such as the sedation caused by antihistamines, if they know that tolerance will develop quickly to these effects.

Once tolerance to a substance develops, it often extends to closely related drugs. This phenomenon is known as **cross-tolerance**. For example, a heroin addict will be tolerant to the analgesic effects of other opioids such as morphine and meperidine. Clients who have developed tolerance to alcohol will show tolerance to other CNS depressants such as barbiturates, benzodiazepines, and some general anesthetics. This has important clinical implications for the nurse, as doses of these related medications will have to be adjusted accordingly to obtain maximum therapeutic benefit.

NCLEX Success Tip

Cross-tolerance occurs when a drug with a similar action causes a decreased response to another drug. A drug that can prevent withdrawal symptoms from another drug describes cross-dependence.

The terms *immunity* and *resistance* are often confused with tolerance. These terms more correctly refer to the immune system and infections and should not be used interchangeably with tolerance. For example, microorganisms become resistant to the effects of an antibiotic—they do not become tolerant. Clients become tolerant to the effects of pain relievers—they do not become resistant.

CNS Depressants

25.6 CNS depressants, which include sedatives, opioids, and ethyl alcohol, decrease the activity of the central nervous system.

CNS depressants form a group of drugs that cause clients to feel sedated or relaxed. Drugs in this group include barbiturates, non-barbiturate sedative-hypnotics, benzodiazepines, alcohol, and opioids. Although the majority of these are available by prescription, they are controlled under the Controlled Drugs and Substances Act (CDSA) due to their addictive potential.

Sedatives

Sedatives, also known as tranquilizers, are primarily prescribed for sleep disorders and certain forms of epilepsy. The two primary classes of sedatives are the barbiturates and the non-barbiturate sedative-hypnotics. Their actions, indications, safety profiles, and addictive potential are roughly equivalent. Physical dependence, psychological dependence, and tolerance develop when these agents are taken for extended periods at high doses. Individuals sometimes obtain these drugs by faking prescriptions or by sharing medication with friends. They are commonly combined with other substances of addiction, such as CNS stimulants or alcohol. Addicted individuals often alternate between amphetamines, which keep them awake for several days, and barbiturates, which are needed to help them relax and fall sleep.

Many sedatives have a long duration of action: effects may last an entire day, depending on the specific drug. Clients may appear dull or apathetic. Higher doses resemble alcohol intoxication, with slurred speech and motor incoordination. Barbiturates commonly used in addiction include pentobarbital (Nembutal) and secobarbital. The medical use of barbiturates and non-barbiturate sedative-hypnotics has declined markedly over the past 20 years. The use of barbiturates in treating sleep disorders is discussed in Chapter 16, and their use in epilepsy is presented in Chapter 21.

Overdoses of barbiturates and non-barbiturate sedative-hypnotics are extremely dangerous. The drugs suppress the respiratory centres in the brain, and the user may stop breathing or lapse into a coma. Death may result from barbiturate overdose. There is no specific antidote for barbiturates. Withdrawal symptoms from these drugs resemble those of alcohol withdrawal and may be life-threatening.

Benzodiazepines are another group of CNS depressants that have the potential for addiction. They are one of the most widely prescribed classes of drug and have largely replaced the barbiturates for certain disorders. Their primary indication is anxiety (Chapter 16), although they are also used to prevent seizures (Chapter 21) and treat muscle spasms (Chapter 22). Common benzodiazepines include alprazolam (Xanax), diazepam (Valium), temazepam (Restoril), triazolam (Halcion), midazolam (Versed), lorazepam (Ativan), and clonazepam (Rivotril).

NCLEX Success Tip

Diazepam, like any benzodiazepine, cannot be stopped abruptly. The client must be slowly tapered off of the medication to decrease withdrawal symptoms, which would be similar to those of withdrawal from alcohol. Alcohol in combination with a benzodiazepine produces an increased central nervous system depressant effect, and therefore, it should be avoided. Diazepam can cause drowsiness, so the client should be warned about driving until tolerance develops. Diazepam has muscle relaxant properties and will help tight, tense muscles feel better.

Although benzodiazepines are the most frequently prescribed drug class, benzodiazepine abuse is not common. Individuals who abuse benzodiazepines may appear carefree, detached, sleepy, or disoriented. Death due to overdose is rare, even with high doses. The antidote for benzodiazepines is flumazenil (Romazicon). Users may combine these agents with alcohol, cocaine, or heroin to augment their drug experience. If combined with these other agents, overdose may be lethal. The benzodiazepine withdrawal syndrome is less severe than that of barbiturates and alcohol.

Opioids

Opioids, also known as narcotic analgesics, are prescribed for severe pain, persistent cough, and diarrhea. The opioid class includes natural substances obtained from the unripe seeds of the poppy plant, such as opium, morphine, and codeine, and synthetic drugs such as meperidine, oxycodone (OxyNeo, OxyIR), fentanyl (Duragesic), methadone, and heroin. The therapeutic effects of the opioids are discussed in detail in Chapter 23.

The effects of *oral* opioids begin within 30 minutes and may last for more than a day. *Parenteral* forms produce immediate effects, including the brief, intense rush of euphoria sought by heroin addicts. Individuals experience a range of CNS effects, from extreme pleasure to slowed body activities and profound sedation. Signs include constricted pupils, an increase in the pain threshold, and respiratory depression.

NCLEX Success Tip

Scheduled use of long-acting opioids and an around-the-clock dosing are necessary to achieve a steady level of analgesia. Whatever the route or frequency, a prescription should be available for "breakthrough" pain medication to be administered in addition to the regularly scheduled medication. Oral drug administration is the route of choice for economy, safety, and ease of use. Even severe pain requiring high doses of opioids can be managed orally as long as the client can swallow medication and has a functioning gastrointestinal system.

Addiction to opioids can occur rapidly, and withdrawal can produce intense symptoms. While extremely unpleasant, withdrawal from opioids is not life-threatening, compared to barbiturate withdrawal. Methadone is a narcotic sometimes used to treat opioid addiction. Although methadone has addictive properties of its own, it does not produce the same degree of euphoria as other opioids and its effects are longer lasting. Heroin addicts are switched to methadone to prevent unpleasant withdrawal symptoms. Since methadone is taken orally, clients are no longer exposed to serious risks associated with IV drug use, such as hepatitis and AIDS. Clients sometimes remain on methadone maintenance for a lifetime. Withdrawal from methadone is more prolonged than with heroin or morphine, but the symptoms are less intense.

NCLEX Success Tips

Tolerance to a regular opioid dose can develop with frequent use. The client experiences increased discomfort, asks for medication more frequently, and exhibits anxious and restless behaviour. These actions are often misinterpreted as indicative of developing dependence or addiction.

Pseudo-addiction is a term used to describe the iatrogenic syndrome of drug-seeking behaviour that develops as a direct consequence of inadequate pain management.

Ethyl Alcohol

Ethyl alcohol, commonly known as alcohol, is one of the most commonly abused drugs. Alcohol is readily available to adults as beer, wine, and liquor. The economic, social, and health consequences of alcohol abuse are staggering. Despite the enormous negative consequences associated with long-term use, small quantities of alcohol consumed on a daily basis have been found to reduce the risk for stroke and heart attack.

Alcohol is classified as a CNS depressant because it slows the region of the brain responsible for alertness and wakefulness. Alcohol easily crosses the blood-brain barrier, so its effects are observed within 5 to 30 minutes of consumption. Effects of alcohol are directly proportional to the amount consumed and include relaxation, sedation, memory impairment, loss of motor coordination, reduced judgment, and decreased inhibition. Alcohol also imparts a characteristic odour to the breath and increases blood flow in certain areas of the skin, causing a flushed face, pink cheeks, or red nose. Although flushing and lack of coordination are easily recognized, the nurse must be aware that other substances and disorders may cause similar symptoms. For example, many antianxiety agents, sedatives, and antidepressants can cause drowsiness, memory difficulties, and loss of motor coordination. Certain mouthwashes contain alcohol and cause the breath to smell alcoholic. During assessment, the skilled nurse must consider these factors before suspicion of alcohol use can be confirmed.

The presence of food in the stomach will slow the absorption of alcohol, thus delaying the onset of drug action. Metabolism, or detoxification, of alcohol by the liver occurs at a slow, constant rate, which is not affected by the presence of food. The average rate is about 15 mL per hour—the practical equivalent of one alcoholic beverage per hour. If consumed at a higher rate, alcohol will accumulate in the blood and produce greater effects on the brain. Acute overdoses of alcohol produce vomiting, severe hypotension, respiratory failure, and coma. Death due to alcohol poisoning is not uncommon. The nurse should teach clients to never combine alcohol with the use of other CNS depressants, as their effects are cumulative and profound sedation or coma may result.

Chronic alcohol consumption produces both psychological and physiological dependence and results in a large number of adverse health effects. The organ most affected by chronic alcohol use is the liver. Alcoholism is a common cause of cirrhosis, a debilitating and often fatal failure of the liver to perform its vital functions. Liver failure results in abnormalities in blood clotting and nutritional deficiencies, and sensitizes the client to the effects of all medications metabolized by the liver. For alcoholic clients, the nurse should begin therapy with lower than normal doses until the adverse effects of the medication can be assessed.

The alcohol withdrawal syndrome is severe and may be life-threatening. The use of anticonvulsants in the treatment of alcohol withdrawal is discussed in Chapter 15. Long-term treatment for alcohol addiction includes behavioural counselling and self-help groups such as Alcoholics Anonymous. Disulfiram (Antabuse) may be given to discourage relapses. Disulfiram inhibits acetaldehyde dehydrogenase, the enzyme that metabolizes alcohol. If alcohol is consumed while taking disulfiram, the client becomes violently ill within 5 to 10 minutes, with headache, shortness of breath, nausea/vomiting, and other unpleasant symptoms. Disulfiram is effective only in highly motivated clients, since the success of pharmacotherapy is entirely dependent on client adherence. Alcohol sensitivity continues for up to 2 weeks after disulfiram has been discontinued. As a pregnancy category X drug, disulfiram should never be taken during pregnancy. See Figure 25.1 for the metabolism of alcohol.

Cannabinoids

25.7 Cannabinoids, which include marijuana, are the most frequently used class of addictive substances. They cause less physical dependence and tolerance than the CNS depressants.

Cannabinoids are agents obtained from the hemp plant *Cannabis sativa*, which thrives in tropical climates. Cannabinoid agents are usually smoked and include marijuana, hashish, and hash oil. Although more than 61 cannabinoid chemicals have been identified, the ingredient responsible for most of the psychoactive properties is delta-9-**tetrahydrocannabinol (THC)**.

Marijuana

Marijuana, also known as grass, pot, weed, reefer, or dope, is a natural product obtained from *C. sativa*. It is the most commonly

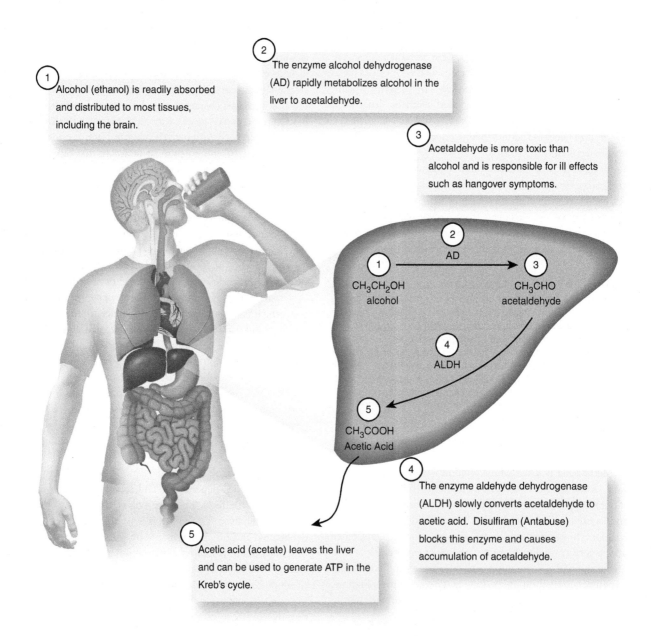

Figure 25.1   The metabolism of alcohol.

used illicit drug in Canada. Use of marijuana slows motor activity, decreases coordination, and causes disconnected thoughts, feelings of paranoia, and euphoria. It increases thirst and craving for food, particularly chocolate and other candies. One hallmark symptom of marijuana use is red or bloodshot eyes, caused by dilation of blood vessels. THC accumulates in the gonads.

When inhaled, marijuana produces effects that occur within minutes and last up to 24 hours. Because marijuana smoke is inhaled more deeply and held within the lungs for a longer time than cigarette smoke, marijuana smoke introduces four times more particulates (tar) into the lungs than tobacco smoke. Smoking marijuana on a daily basis may increase the risk for lung cancer and other respiratory disorders. Chronic use is associated with a lack of motivation in achieving or pursuing life goals.

Unlike many addictive substances, marijuana produces little physical dependence and/or tolerance. Withdrawal symptoms are mild, if they are experienced at all. Metabolites of THC, however, remain in the body for months to years, allowing laboratory specialists to easily determine whether someone has used marijuana. For several days after use, THC can also be detected in the urine. Despite numerous attempts to demonstrate therapeutic applications for marijuana, results have been controversial and the medical value of the drug remains to be proven.

Medical marijuana is a controversial topic; most healthcare providers and politicians are reluctant to endorse a drug that impairs judgment and may harm users, although those who support legalizing marijuana seem to be attracting supporters among politicians. THC appears to reduce the pressure in the eyeball, a condition called glaucoma. Clients who receive antineoplastic drugs have reported that THC reduces the severe nausea and vomiting associated with these drugs. The ability of THC to reduce muscle spasticity may lead to applications for clients with multiple sclerosis and other spasticity disorders. In most cases, current drugs for these conditions have been demonstrated to be more effective and safer. Although the medical value of marijuana remains to be conclusively proven, several countries, including Canada, have approved the medical use of marijuana despite its being a Schedule I drug.

Hallucinogens

25.8 Hallucinogens, including LSD, cause an altered state of thought and perception similar to that found in dreams. Their effects are extremely variable and unpredictable.

Hallucinogens consist of a diverse class of chemicals that have in common the ability to produce an altered, dreamlike state of consciousness. Sometimes called **psychedelics**, the prototype substance for this class is LSD. All hallucinogens are Schedule I drugs; they have no medical use.

LSD

For nearly all drugs of addiction, predictable symptoms occur in every user. Effects from hallucinogens, however, are highly variable and dependent on the mood and expectations of the user and the surrounding environment in which the substance is used. Two clients taking the same agent will report completely different symptoms, and the same client may report different symptoms with each use. Users who take LSD or psilocybin, also known as magic mushrooms or shrooms, may experience symptoms such as laughter, visions, religious revelations, and deep personal insights. The structures of these hallucinogens are shown in Figure 25.2. Common occurrences are hallucinations and afterimages being projected onto people as they move. Users also report unusually bright lights and vivid colours. Some users hear voices; others report smells. Many experience a profound sense of truth and deep-directed thoughts. Unpleasant experiences can be terrifying and may include anxiety, panic attacks, confusion, severe depression, and paranoia.

LSD, also called acid, the beast, blotter acid, and California sunshine, is derived from a fungus that grows on rye and other grains. LSD is nearly always administered orally and can be manufactured in capsule, tablet, or liquid form. A common and inexpensive method of distributing LSD is to place drops of the drug on paper, often containing the images of cartoon characters or graphics related to the drug culture. After drying, the paper that contains the LSD is ingested to produce the drug's effects.

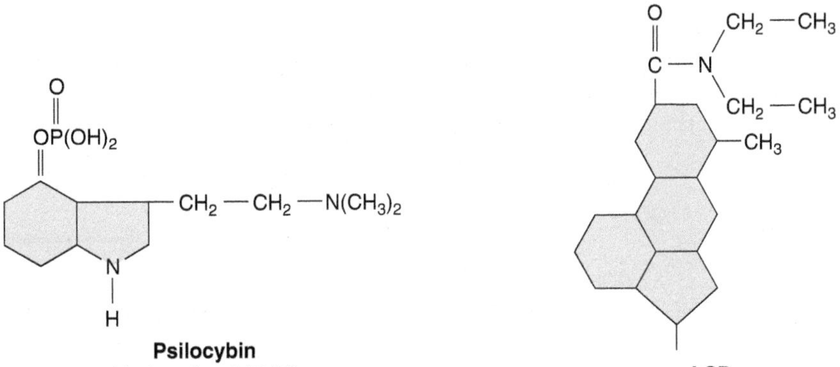

Figure 25.2 Comparison of the chemical structures of psilocybin (derived from a mushroom) and LSD (derived from a fungus).

Source: Pearson Education/PH College.

LSD is distributed throughout the body immediately after use. Effects are experienced within an hour and may last from 6 to 12 hours. LSD affects the central and autonomic nervous systems, increasing blood pressure, elevating body temperature, dilating pupils, and increasing heart rate. Repeated use may cause impaired memory and inability to reason. In extreme cases, clients may develop psychoses. One unusual adverse effect is flashbacks, in which the user experiences the effects of the drug again, sometimes weeks, months, or years after the drug was initially taken. While tolerance is observed, little or no dependence occurs with the hallucinogens.

Other Hallucinogens

In addition to LSD, other hallucinogens that are abused include the following:

- Mescaline: found in the peyote cactus of Mexico and Central America (Figure 25.3)
- MDMA (3,4-methylenedioxymethamphetamine; XTC or Ecstasy): an amphetamine originally synthesized for research purposes that has since become extremely popular among teens and young adults
- DOM (2,5-dimethoxy-4-methylamphetamine; STP): a recreational drug often linked with rave parties
- MDA (3,4-methylenedioxyamphetamine): called the love drug due to a belief that it enhances sexual desire
- PCP (phenylcyclohexylpiperidine; angel dust or phencyclidine): produces a trance-like state that may last for days and results in severe brain damage
- Ketamine (date rape drug or special K): produces unconsciousness and amnesia; primary approved use is as an anesthetic

CNS Stimulants

25.9 CNS stimulants, including amphetamines, methylphenidate, caffeine, and cocaine, increase the activity of the CNS and produce increased wakefulness.

Stimulants include a diverse family of drugs known for their ability to increase the activity of the CNS. Some are available by prescription for the treatment of narcolepsy, obesity, and attention deficit disorder. As drugs of addiction, CNS stimulants are taken to produce a sense of exhilaration, improve mental and physical performance, reduce appetite, prolong wakefulness, or simply "get high." Stimulants include the amphetamines, methylphenidate, cocaine, and caffeine.

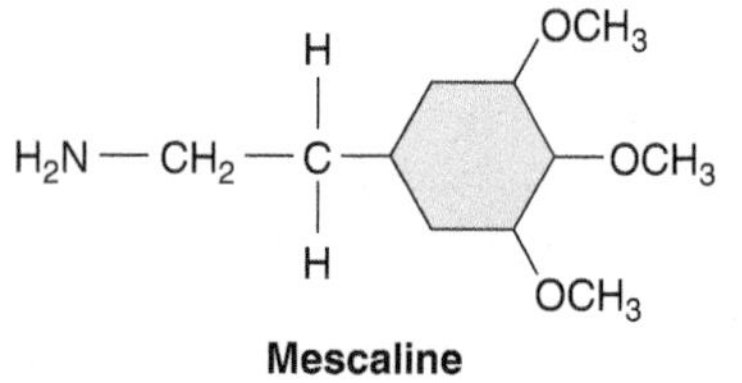

Mescaline

Figure 25.3 The chemical structure of mescaline (derived from the peyote cactus).

Source: Pearson Education/PH College.

Amphetamines and Methylphenidate

CNS stimulants have effects similar to the neurotransmitter norepinephrine (see Chapter 12). Norepinephrine affects awareness and wakefulness by activating neurons in a part of the brain called the **reticular formation**. High doses of amphetamines give the user a feeling of self-confidence, euphoria, alertness, and empowerment; however, just as short-term use induces favourable feelings, long-term use often results in feelings of restlessness, anxiety, and fits of rage, especially when the user is coming down from a high induced by the drug.

Most CNS stimulants affect cardiovascular and respiratory activity, resulting in increased blood pressure and increased respiration rate. Other symptoms include dilated pupils, sweating, and tremors. Overdoses of some stimulants lead to seizures and cardiac arrest.

NCLEX Success Tips

Amphetamines are a nervous system stimulant that are subject to abuse because of their ability to produce wakefulness and euphoria. An overdose increases tension and irritability. Amphetamines stimulate norepinephrine, which increases the heart rate and blood flow. Diarrhea is a common adverse effect.

Amphetamines use can lead to hypertension, tachycardia, vasoconstriction, and hyperthermia. Pupils will be dilated.

Amphetamines and dextroamphetamines were once widely prescribed for depression, obesity, drowsiness, and congestion. In the 1960s it became recognized that the medical uses of amphetamines did not outweigh their risk of dependence. Due to the development of safer medications, the current therapeutic uses of these drugs are extremely limited. Illicit laboratories can easily produce amphetamines and sell them for tremendous profit.

Dextroamphetamine (Dexedrine) may be used for short-term weight loss, when all other attempts to reduce weight have been exhausted, and to treat narcolepsy. Methamphetamine, commonly called ice, is often used as a recreational drug for users who like the rush that it gives them. It usually is administered in powder or crystal form, but it may also be smoked. Most users obtain it from illicit methamphetamine laboratories. A structural analogue of methamphetamine, methcathinone (street name: Cat) is made illicitly and is snorted, taken orally, or injected IV.

Methylphenidate is a CNS stimulant widely prescribed for children who are diagnosed with **attention deficit disorder (ADD)**. Methylphenidate has a calming effect in children who are inattentive or hyperactive. It stimulates the alertness centre in the brain, and the child is able to focus on tasks for longer periods of time. This explains the paradoxical calming effects that this stimulant has on children, which is usually opposite to its effects on adults.

NCLEX Success Tip

ADD is typically managed by psychostimulant medications, such as methylphenidate, along with behaviour modification.

Methylphenidate is a CDSA Schedule III drug that has many of the same effects as cocaine and amphetamines. It is sometimes abused by adolescents and adults seeking euphoria. Tablets are crushed and used intranasally or dissolved in liquid and injected IV. Methylphenidate is sometimes mixed with heroin, a combination called a speedball.

Cocaine

Cocaine is a natural substance obtained from leaves of the coca plant, which grows in the Andes Mountain region of South America. Documentation suggests that the plant has been used by Andean cultures since 2500 BCE. Natives in this region chew the coca leaves or make tea from the dried leaves. Because it is taken orally and is absorbed slowly, and because the leaves contain only 1% cocaine, users do not suffer the ill effects caused by chemically pure extracts from the plant. In the Andean culture, use of coca leaves is not considered substance abuse because it is part of the social norms of that society.

Cocaine is a CDSA Schedule I drug that produces actions similar to the amphetamines, although its effects are usually more rapid and intense. It is the second most commonly used illicit drug in Canada. Routes of administration include snorting, smoking, and injecting. In small doses, cocaine produces feelings of intense euphoria, a decrease in hunger, analgesia, illusions of physical strength, and increased sensory perception. Larger doses will magnify these effects and also cause rapid heartbeat, sweating, dilation of the pupils, and an elevated body temperature. After the feelings of euphoria diminish, the user is left with a sense of irritability, insomnia, depression, and extreme distrust. Some users report the sensation that insects are crawling under their skin. Users who snort cocaine develop a chronic runny nose, a crusty redness around the nostrils, and deterioration of the nasal cartilage. Overdose can result in dysrhythmias, convulsions, stroke, or death due to respiratory arrest. The withdrawal syndrome for amphetamines and cocaine is much less intense than that for alcohol and barbiturates.

Caffeine

Caffeine is a natural substance found in the seeds, leaves, or fruits of more than 63 plant species throughout the world. Significant amounts of caffeine are consumed in chocolate, coffee, tea, soft drinks, and ice cream. Caffeine is sometimes added to over-the-counter (OTC) pain relievers because it has been shown to increase the effectiveness of these medications. Caffeine travels to almost all parts of the body after ingestion, and several hours are needed for the body to metabolize and eliminate the drug. Caffeine has a pronounced diuretic effect.

Caffeine is considered a CNS stimulant because it produces increased mental alertness, restlessness, nervousness, irritability, and insomnia. The physical effects of caffeine include bronchodilation, increased blood pressure, increased production of stomach acid, and changes in blood glucose levels. Repeated use of caffeine may result in physical dependence and tolerance. Withdrawal symptoms include headaches, fatigue, depression, and impaired performance of daily activities.

Nicotine

25.10 Nicotine is a powerful and highly addictive cardiovascular and CNS stimulant that has serious adverse effects with chronic use.

Nicotine is sometimes considered a CNS stimulant, and although it does increase alertness, its actions and long-term consequences place it into a class by itself. Nicotine is unique among addictive substances in that it is not illicit but is strongly addictive and highly carcinogenic. Furthermore, use of tobacco can cause harmful effects to those in the immediate area due to secondhand smoke.

Tobacco Use and Nicotine

The most common method by which nicotine enters the body is through the inhalation of cigarette, pipe, or cigar smoke. Tobacco smoke contains more than 1000 chemicals, a significant number of which are carcinogens. The primary addictive substance present in cigarette smoke is nicotine. Effects of inhaled nicotine may last from 30 minutes to several hours.

Nicotine affects many body systems, including the nervous, cardiovascular, and endocrine systems. Nicotine stimulates the CNS directly, causing increased alertness and ability to focus, feelings of relaxation, and lightheadedness. Stimulation of dopamine release in the pleasure area of the brain may contribute to its addictive potential. The cardiovascular effects of nicotine include an accelerated heart rate and increased blood pressure caused by activation of nicotinic receptors located throughout the autonomic nervous system (see Chapter 12). These cardiovascular effects can be particularly serious in clients who are taking oral contraceptives: the risk for a fatal heart attack is five times greater in smokers than in non-smokers. Muscular tremors may occur with moderate doses of nicotine, and convulsions may result from very high doses. Nicotine affects the endocrine system by increasing the basal metabolic rate, leading to weight loss. Nicotine also reduces appetite. Chronic use leads to bronchitis, emphysema, and lung cancer.

Both psychological and physical dependence occur relatively quickly with nicotine. Once started on tobacco, clients tend to continue their drug use for many years despite overwhelming medical evidence that their quality of life will be adversely affected and their lifespan shortened. Discontinuation of tobacco results in a withdrawal syndrome that includes agitation,

---

CONNECTIONS Natural Therapies

◀ Herbal Stimulants and Ephedra

Recovering from addiction may be a difficult experience. Individuals claim that discretionary use of some herbal stimulants may ease the symptoms associated with recovery. Examples are kola, damiana, Asiatic and Siberian ginseng, and gotu kola. These agents are thought to stimulate the CNS, providing just enough of an effect to reduce the tension and stresses associated with drug craving.

Ephedra is an herbal stimulant. In addition to its stimulant effects of increasing wakefulness and alertness, the herb affects the cardiovascular system to potentially cause increases in blood pressure and heart rate. Ephedra is an ingredient in a variety of products marketed as dietary supplements for weight loss, energy enhancement, and body-building purposes. It has been implicated in several deaths and serious adverse effects, such as heart attack and stroke, and may be removed from the market due to safety concerns. Nurses should advise their clients to never take this herbal stimulant until they have consulted with their physician.

◀ Ethnic Groups and Smoking

Although smoking rates continue to decline in Canada, 22% of men and 17% of women are smokers. In the past 5 years, smoking rates for youth have declined from 28% to 18%. The incidence of tobacco use varies among racial and ethnic groups. Smoking prevalence is lower among foreign-born (16%) than native-born (25%) Canadians. The highest smoking rates are among Canadian Aboriginal peoples (59%). The lowest rates are among Asian Canadians (11%). Each year, 42% of Canadian smokers attempt to quit. Smoking and tobacco use contribute to the leading causes of death: heart disease, cancer, and stroke. Clients who smoke should be informed about their increased risk for disease and the strategies and resources available to support smoking cessation.

impaired concentration, weight gain, anxiety, headache, and an extreme craving for the drug. The syndrome peaks at 24 to 48 hours after the last dose and may continue over several weeks. Symptoms vary in intensity among clients and are not related to dose or duration of use; those who are light smokers or who have smoked for a shorter length of time do not necessarily have less intense withdrawal symptoms. Approximately 90% of individuals who successfully stop smoking do so without any treatment.

Nicotine replacement therapy (NRT) is based on the assumption that the blood level of nicotine is what drives people to continue smoking. When blood nicotine levels fall, the person begins to experience early symptoms of withdrawal, which are quickly eliminated by smoking another cigarette. Indeed, blood nicotine levels have clearly been shown to influence smoking behaviour. For example, if a smoker is switched to low-nicotine cigarettes, he or she will take longer and more frequent puffs. NRT delivery systems include transdermal patches (Figure 25.4), nasal sprays, and chewing gum that raise serum nicotine levels and help clients to deal with the unpleasant withdrawal symptoms. Tobacco

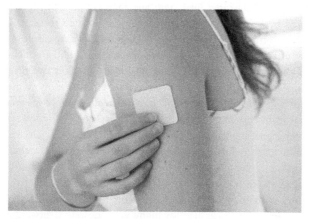

Figure 25.4 Nicotine replacment therapy: transdermal patch. Courtesy Ruth Jenkinson/Dorling Kindersley.

use, however, has a strong psychological component and simply replacing nicotine with patches or gum is ineffective for a large number of clients. Only 25% of clients who attempt to stop smoking remain tobacco-free a year later.

Recently, prescription medications have been used to promote smoking cessation. Bupropion (Zyban), a drug classified as an antidepressant, reduces cravings for nicotine and has been found to double the likelihood of becoming tobacco-free if it is taken for 3 to 6 months. Therapy generally begins 1 to 2 weeks before smoking cessation to lessen the severity of withdrawal symptoms. Bupropion is sometimes given concurrently with NRT. When used for depression, bupropion is marketed by the trade name of Wellbutrin. Varenicline (Champix) is a newer drug approved by Health Canada to manage nicotine withdrawal in clients seeking smoking cessation. Both bupropion and varenicline carry a black box warning that advises clients of serious neuropsychiatric events that can occur during therapy or shortly following discontinuation of the drug.

Inhalants

25.11 Inhalant abuse occurs when clients breathe the fumes of vaporized substances.

Inhalants are a diverse group of substances that have in common the ability to vaporize or form a gas at room temperature. Some are already in gaseous form, whereas others are liquids that have the property of volatility (rapid evaporation when exposed to air). Sometimes the liquids are heated to increase the speed or extent of vaporization. Most drugs in this class are placed in a paper or plastic bag or soaked on a cloth and deeply inhaled. Inhaling the fumes is known as huffing.

Inhalants differ greatly in their chemical structures and include nearly any chemical that can be vaporized. Products abused as inhalants include adhesives and glues, aerosols, cleaning agents, solvents, and fuels. These products are readily available and can be purchased at hardware or office supply stores. The highest use of inhalants is among teens and preteens, probably because these agents can be found in nearly every household. Legal anesthetics such as nitrous oxide that are sometimes abused by medical personnel are also classified as inhalants and are discussed in Chapter 24.

The inhalation route affords almost instantaneous drug action and, because most inhalants are lipid soluble, the substances quickly enter the brain. The specific psychoactive effects depend on the inhalant used but generally include lightheadedness, drowsiness, exhilaration, and euphoria. Hallucinations are common. Symptoms of inhalant abuse often resemble alcohol intoxication. Because most psychoactive effects of inhalants are transient and disappear within minutes, the user may repeat the drug use multiple times over a period of several hours. Coma and death are possible with repeated exposure or high doses.

Because most inhalant abuse is sporadic, physical dependence is not observed, and it is unknown whether tolerance develops. Some of the inhalants cause hangover-like symptoms after the psychoactive effects wear off. When chronic abuse does occur, it is generally in adult males. Chronic effects can be serious and permanent, with the most obvious effects on the nervous system.

Cognitive impairment, tremors, loss of coordination, hallucinations, psychosis, and dementia may be observed. Nephrotoxicity is common with certain inhalants. The breathing reflex may be diminished, and clients may suffocate from placing a plastic bag over their heads.

Treatment for inhalant abuse is symptomatic. Long-term behavioural therapy may be needed to reinforce to the client that permanent damage will result from chronic, continued abuse.

Anabolic Steroids

25.12 Anabolic steroids are abused for their ability to increase muscle strength.

All of the drugs presented thus far in this chapter have in common the ability to affect the CNS and produce psychoactive effects. Many produce euphoria, some induce relaxation, and others enhance alertness. In most cases, the user views the drug experience as pleasurable and the drug effects are experienced soon after it is taken, sometimes within seconds. Anabolic steroids, however, are not taken for their CNS actions, and their desirable effects may be delayed for weeks or months. In this respect they are different from other abused substances.

Anabolic steroids are very similar to testosterone, the primary male sex hormone or androgen. The term *anabolic* means growth or building up. Because these substances can add to skeletal muscle mass and increased strength, they are usually abused in an attempt to enhance athletic performance. Do these drugs actually boost performance? The answer is a qualified yes. The most important aspects of athletic performance are skill, training, and confidence. If these factors are equal among performers, anabolic steroids may indeed provide an extra boost in performance, which is all important in a competitive sport such as track, downhill skiing, or swimming where a few hundredths of a second can mean the difference between first and sixth place. On the other hand, no amount of steroid is able to overcome lack of athletic skill or inadequate training. Most sports organizations have banned the use of these drugs, and athletes may be eliminated from competition if they test positive for anabolic steroids. Some abusers take anabolic steroids to enhance their appearance and self-confidence rather than for athletic competition.

Anabolic steroids have legitimate medical uses as replacement therapy for men who secrete deficient quantities of testosterone, and they are occasionally used to treat certain cancers. Doses used by abusers, however, are 10 to 100 times higher than those required for therapeutic use.

Anabolic steroids may be taken as tablets or intramuscular (IM) injections, or applied as ointments or a transdermal patch. Abusers may take two or more different types of steroids concurrently, sometimes by different routes, a practice called "stacking." The drugs may be taken in a cyclical pattern called "pyramiding" in which the dose is progressively increased over 6 to 12 weeks, then slowly decreased to zero. Abusers believe that this is a safer and more effective way to obtain benefits from the drugs.

One of the ironies of steroid abuse is that the very drug that is being taken to enhance appearance and performance eventually produces serious consequences that have the opposite effect. Men may believe that anabolic steroids make them appear more masculine, but the drugs can cause infertility, impotence, testicular atrophy, and breast enlargement (gynecomastia). Women who take anabolic steroids will develop masculine characteristics, excessive growth of body hair (hirsutism), shrinking of breast size, menstrual irregularities, and deepening of the voice. The most serious adverse effects, in both men and women, include hepatic cysts, elevated cholesterol, myocardial infarction, and stroke. Personality changes include aggression, violent behaviour, depression, insomnia, anorexia, and decreased libido.

The Nurse's Role in Substance Addiction

25.13 The nurse serves an important role in educating clients about the consequences of substance addiction and in recommending appropriate treatment.

The nurse serves a key role in the prevention, diagnosis, and treatment of substance addiction. A thorough medical history must include questions about the use of addictive substances. In the case of IV drug users, the nurse must consider the possibility of HIV infection, hepatitis, and associated diagnoses. Clients are often reluctant to report their drug use for fear of embarrassment or being arrested. The nurse must be knowledgeable about the signs of substance dependence and withdrawal symptoms and must develop a keen sense of perception during the assessment stage. A trusting nurse-client relationship is essential to helping clients deal with their dependence.

It is often difficult for a healthcare provider not to condemn or stigmatize a client for his or her substance addiction. Nurses are all too familiar with the devastating medical, economic, and social consequences of heroin and cocaine. Yet compassion and encouragement may help to motivate the client who uses illicit and addictive substances to receive treatment. A list of social agencies that deal with dependency should be readily available to provide to clients. When possible, the nurse should attempt to involve family members and other close social contacts in the treatment. Educating the client and family members about the long-term consequences of the use of substances of addiction is essential.

25

Understanding the Chapter

Key Concepts Summary

The numbered key concepts provide a succinct summary of the important points from the corresponding numbered section within the chapter. If any of these points are not clear, refer to the numbered section within the chapter for review.

25.1 A wide variety of addictive substances may be used by individuals, all of which share the common characteristic of altering brain physiology and/or perception.

25.2 Addiction is an overwhelming compulsion to continue repeated drug use that has both neurobiological and psychosocial components.

25.3 Certain substances can cause both physical and psychological dependence, which result in continued drug-seeking behaviour despite negative health and social consequences.

25.4 The withdrawal syndrome is a set of uncomfortable symptoms that occur when a substance to which an individual is addicted is no longer available. The severity of the withdrawal syndrome varies among the different drug classes.

25.5 Tolerance is a biological condition that occurs with repeated use of certain substances and results in higher doses being needed to achieve the same initial response. Cross-tolerance occurs between closely related drugs.

25.6 CNS depressants, which include sedatives, opioids, and ethyl alcohol, decrease the activity of the central nervous system.

25.7 Cannabinoids, which include marijuana, are the most frequently used class of addictive substances. They cause less physical dependence and tolerance than the CNS depressants.

25.8 Hallucinogens, including LSD, cause an altered state of thought and perception similar to that found in dreams. Their effects are extremely variable and unpredictable.

25.9 CNS stimulants, including amphetamines, methylphenidate, caffeine, and cocaine, increase the activity of the CNS and produce increased wakefulness.

25.10 Nicotine is a powerful and highly addictive cardiovascular and CNS stimulant that has serious adverse effects with chronic use.

25.11 Inhalant abuse occurs when clients breathe the fumes of vaporized substances.

25.12 Anabolic steroids are abused for their ability to increase muscle strength.

25.13 The nurse serves an important role in educating clients about the consequences of substance addiction and in recommending appropriate treatment.

Chapter 25 Scenario

J.C. Wilkins has come to the counselling clinic to get information and advice about her pregnancy and drug use. She is a 19-year-old woman who has been living with her boyfriend for the past 18 months. Since she moved in with her boyfriend, she has been a daily user of heroin.

J.C. has a long history of substance abuse. When she was 14 years old, her stepfather sexually abused her on a regular basis. To cope with the guilt and shame, she began using alcohol and marijuana. On her sixteenth birthday, J.C. ran away from home and never returned. Since then she has done anything and everything possible to survive, including selling herself for sex.

To support herself and her heroin addiction, J.C. has become a prostitute. She states that she usually drinks at least four to five beers before she walks the streets at night. If she cannot score enough heroin, she will smoke crack or take Valium just to "mellow out." J.C. says that her drug abuse is only to calm her nerves and get her through the night. In periods when she was not able to obtain drugs, she states that she felt sick, with trembling and perfuse sweating. However, she is convinced that she can stop taking drugs any time she wishes.

J.C. reports that she has not had a menstrual period in 2 months and her breasts are swollen and tender. She is certain that she is pregnant, although she has not been tested and is confused about what to do. She is hopeful that her unemployed boyfriend is the father but is not totally sure. She believes that if she stops working, he will abandon her and there will be no means to support herself or a baby.

Critical Thinking Questions

1. How would you classify J.C.'s substance abuse? Physical dependence or psychological dependence, or both? Explain.
2. Create a list of abused substances reported by J.C. What symptoms of withdrawal would you expect with each?
3. What effect will J.C.'s substance abuse have on her unborn baby? Should J.C. stop using drugs while pregnant? Why or why not?
4. As the nurse, describe your approach in dealing with this client.
5. Addiction depends on multiple variables such as drug factors, user factors, and environmental factors. Considering the case study, describe how each variable attributes to J.C.'s substance abuse.

See Answers to Critical Thinking Questions in Appendix B.

NCLEX Practice Questions

1 A client returned from major surgery 3 hours ago and is requesting medication for pain. In considering the best action for this client, the nurse knows that

   a. Prescription drugs rarely cause addiction when used according to accepted medical protocol
   b. All drugs should be withheld until the client's past substance abuse history is evaluated
   c. It is best to wait until the client can no longer tolerate the pain to avoid addiction problems
   d. Clients often request analgesia when it is not really needed

2 Which of the following statements made by a client recovering from a substance use disorder would indicate high potential for relapse?

   a. "I need the help of a support system to stop using."
   b. "After I stop using, I will no longer have a desire to use drugs."
   c. "The people I hang out with don't make any difference to whether or not I use drugs."
   d. "Talking with other recovering addicts will help me cope."

3 A nurse is teaching a client who will begin varenicline (Champix) for smoking cessation. Which of the following instructions will the nurse give the client? Select all that apply.

   a. Doses will be increased over a week's period and the drug used for up to 6 months.

   b. Smoking may continue because the drug blocks the harmful effects of nicotine.
   c. The drug is not known to cause any adverse effects and has an excellent safety profile.
   d. Any unusual rashes, skin reactions, or facial edema should be reported immediately.
   e. Any unusual changes in behaviour, including depression, hostility, or thoughts of suicide, should be reported immediately.

4 Which parameter is most critical when a nurse is assessing a client with an overdose of sedatives?

   a. Cardiac stimulation
   b. Respiratory suppression
   c. Hepatic dysfunction
   d. Depression of consciousness

5 A 22-year-old heroin addict is exhibiting withdrawal symptoms. Which symptoms of withdrawal would the nurse expect to see?

   a. Somnolence, lethargy, and fatigue
   b. Dry skin, rash, and itching
   c. Paranoia, hallucinations, and delusions
   d. Chills, runny nose, and muscle spasms

See Answers to NCLEX Practice Questions in Appendix A.

UNIT

6

Pharmacology of Alterations in the Endocrine System

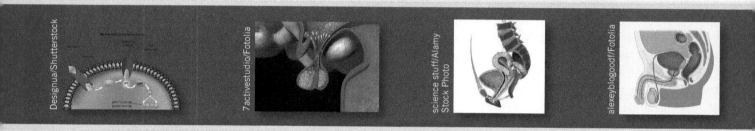

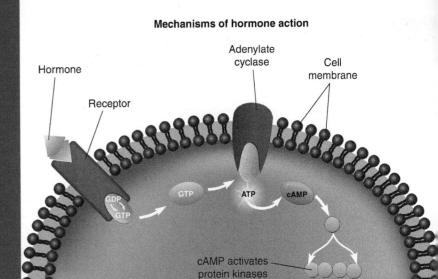

Mechanisms of hormone action

Hormone

Receptor

Adenylate cyclase

Cell membrane

GDP
GTP

GTP

ATP

cAMP

cAMP activates protein kinases

Designua/Shutterstock

Brief Review of the Endocrine System

LEARNING OUTCOMES

After reading this chapter, the student should be able to:

1. Describe the general structure and functions of the endocrine system.

2. Compare and contrast the nervous and endocrine systems in the control of homeostasis.

3. Explain circumstances in which hormone receptors may be upregulated or downregulated.

4. Through the use of a specific example, explain the concept of negative feedback mechanism in the endocrine system.

5. Explain the three primary types of stimuli that regulate hormone secretion.

6. Identify indications for hormone pharmacotherapy.

CHAPTER OUTLINE

▶ Overview of the Endocrine System

▶ Hormone Receptors

▶ Negative Feedback Mechanism

▶ Hormone Pharmacotherapy

KEY TERMS

downregulation, 304

endocrine system, 304

hormones, 304

negative feedback, 304

replacement therapy, 306

target cells, 304

upregulation, 304

Like the nervous system, the endocrine system is a major controller of homeostasis. Whereas a nerve exerts instantaneous control over a single muscle fibre or gland, a hormone from the endocrine system may affect all body cells and take as long as several days to produce an optimum response. Hormonal balance is kept within a narrow range: too little or too much of a hormone may produce profound physiological changes. This chapter reviews endocrine anatomy and physiology and its relevance to pharmacotherapy.

Overview of the Endocrine System

26.1 The endocrine system controls homeostasis through the secretion of hormones.

The **endocrine system** consists of various glands that secrete **hormones**, chemical messengers that the body releases in response to a change in the body's internal environment. The role of hormones is to maintain homeostasis in the body. For example, when the level of glucose in the blood rises above normal, the pancreas secretes insulin to return glucose levels to normal. The various endocrine glands and their hormones are illustrated in Figure 26.1.

After secretion from an endocrine gland, hormones enter the blood and are transported throughout the body. Compared to the nervous system, which reacts to body changes within milliseconds, the endocrine system responds relatively slowly. A few hormones, such as epinephrine, act within seconds, whereas others, such as testosterone, may take several days or even months to produce noticeable changes. Although slower in onset, the effects of hormones have a longer duration than those of the nervous system.

Hormone Receptors

26.2 Hormones must bind to specific receptors to cause physiological changes.

The cells affected by a hormone are called its target cells. **Target cells** have specific protein receptors on their plasma membrane that bind to the hormone. For some hormones, the receptors are in the cytoplasm or nucleus of the target cell. Once binding occurs, a change is produced in the cell, resulting in an action that is characteristic for the hormone. For example, when epinephrine binds to receptors on smooth muscle cells, they contract. When prolactin binds to secretory cells in the breast, milk production occurs.

Although a hormone travels throughout the body via blood circulation, it only affects cells that have receptors for that specific hormone. Epinephrine does not affect breast secretory cells because these cells have no epinephrine receptors. Prolactin does not cause muscular contraction because smooth muscle cells do not have prolactin receptors.

In some cases, the target cells for a hormone are limited and specific. For example, the only receptors for thyroid-stimulating hormone are in the thyroid gland. However, some hormones, such as insulin and cortisol, have receptors on nearly every cell in the body; therefore, these hormones have widespread effects.

The number of protein receptors for a hormone is dynamic and changes with the needs of the body. Cells can create more receptors on their plasma membrane to capture hormone molecules as they pass by, a process called **upregulation**. This may occur if the cell is receiving signals that a hormone action is needed, such as the need for production of more breast milk or additional secretion of thyroid hormone. Once the hormone is upregulated (secreted in large quantities), the cell no longer needs to capture every hormone molecule so it makes fewer receptors on its surface, a process called **downregulation**. Receptors are very efficient at capturing hormone molecules; although most hormones are secreted only in small amounts, they produce profound changes.

Downregulation has important implications for pharmacotherapy. When a hormone is administered as pharmacotherapy for long periods, the body recognizes an abundance of the hormone, and cells will downregulate the number of receptors for that hormone. This causes a desensitization of the target cells; that is, they are less responsive to the effects of the hormone. When therapy is discontinued, the cells will need time, usually several days, to synthesize more protein receptors and adjust to the new hormone level.

It is important to understand that the amount of hormone secreted by an endocrine gland is only partially responsible for the therapeutic response. Other critical components include the number of receptors and their sensitivity. During pharmacotherapy, increasing the dose of a hormone will produce little additional pharmacological effect if all of the receptors are already occupied or if they are no longer sensitive to the hormone.

Negative Feedback Mechanism

26.3 Most hormone action is regulated through negative feedback.

Because hormones can produce profound effects on the body, their secretion and release is carefully regulated by several levels of control. The most important mechanism is **negative feedback**, which is illustrated in Figure 26.2.

A hormone causes an output or action in its target cell or tissue. As the levels of hormone rise, so does its action. The increased output or action is monitored by sensors. Once homeostasis is restored, the sensor signals the endocrine tissue to stop secreting the hormone; that is, the target tissue provides negative feedback.

Depending on the specific hormone, the negative feedback mechanism may be based on three primary types of stimuli: neuronal, humoral, and hormonal. In some cases, regulation involves multiple stimuli.

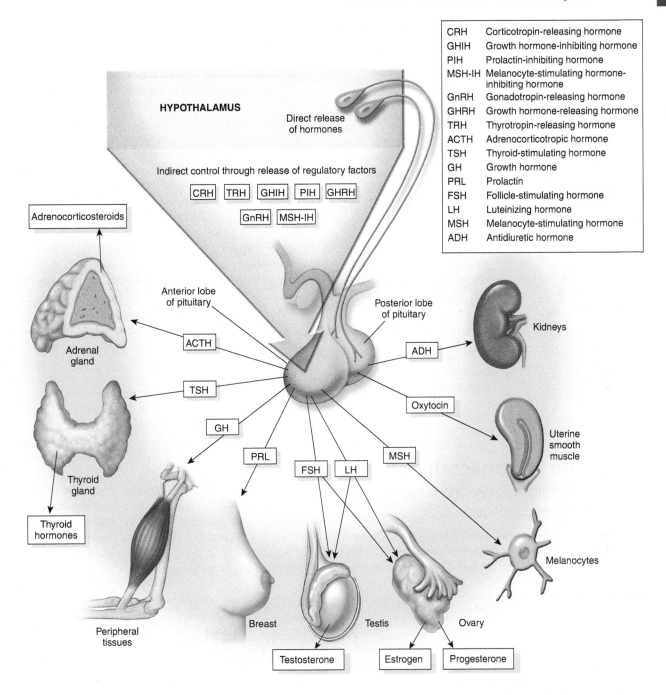

CRH	Corticotropin-releasing hormone
GHIH	Growth hormone-inhibiting hormone
PIH	Prolactin-inhibiting hormone
MSH-IH	Melanocyte-stimulating hormone-inhibiting hormone
GnRH	Gonadotropin-releasing hormone
GHRH	Growth hormone-releasing hormone
TRH	Thyrotropin-releasing hormone
ACTH	Adrenocorticotropic hormone
TSH	Thyroid-stimulating hormone
GH	Growth hormone
PRL	Prolactin
FSH	Follicle-stimulating hormone
LH	Luteinizing hormone
MSH	Melanocyte-stimulating hormone
ADH	Antidiuretic hormone

Figure 26.1 Hormones and the endocrine system.

Neuronal Stimuli

A few hormones are regulated by nerve impulses. The best example is epinephrine, which is released when a neuronal impulse from the sympathetic nervous system reaches the adrenal medulla. Another example is the release of oxytocin from the pituitary gland.

Humoral Stimuli

Some endocrine glands sense the levels of specific substances in the blood and release the hormone when the substance rises above or falls below the normal range. For example, pancreatic islet cells can sense the level of glucose in the blood. If glucose levels become too high, insulin is secreted. Another example is the release of parathyroid hormone when blood calcium levels fall.

Hormonal Stimuli

In the endocrine system, it is common for one hormone to control the secretion of another hormone. In some cases, the sequence involves three hormones. For example, thyrotropin-releasing hormone (TRH, from the hypothalamus) stimulates thyroid-stimulating hormone (TSH, from the pituitary), which causes the release of thyroid hormone (TH, from the thyroid gland). In a loop typical of the endocrine system, the last hormone in the pathway (TH) provides negative feedback to shut off secretion of the initial hormone (TRH).

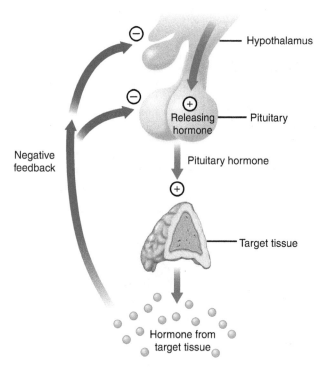

Figure 26.2 Negative feedback mechanism.

Hormone Pharmacotherapy

26.4 Hormone pharmacotherapy is indicated for a diverse variety of conditions.

The goals of hormone pharmacotherapy vary widely. In many cases, a hormone is administered as **replacement therapy** for clients who are unable to secrete sufficient quantities of their own endogenous

hormones. Examples of replacement therapy include the administration of thyroid hormone after the thyroid gland has been surgically removed, supplying insulin to clients whose pancreas is not functioning, or administering growth hormone to children with short-stature disorder. The pharmacological goal of replacement therapy is to supply the same physiological, low-level amounts of the hormone that would normally be present in the body. Select endocrine disorders and their drug therapy are summarized in Table 26.1.

Some hormones are used in cancer chemotherapy to shrink the size of hormone-sensitive tumours. For example, certain breast cancers are strongly dependent on estrogen for their growth. Giving the "opposite" hormone, testosterone, will shrink the tumour. In a similar manner, estrogen is used to shrink the size of testicular cancer, which is dependent on testosterone for its growth. Exactly how these hormones produce their antineoplastic action is largely unknown. When hormones are used as antineoplastics, their doses far exceed physiological levels normally present in the body. Hormones are nearly always used in combination with other antineoplastic medications.

Another goal of hormonal pharmacotherapy may be to produce an exaggerated response that is part of the normal action of the hormone. Administering hydrocortisone (Cortef) to suppress inflammation takes advantage of the normal action of the corticosteroids but at higher amounts than would normally be present in the body. Hydrocortisone is indicated for acute inflammatory disorders such as lupus or rheumatoid arthritis. As another example, supplying estrogen or progesterone at specific times during the uterine cycle can prevent ovulation and pregnancy. In this example, the client is given natural hormones; however, they are taken at a time when levels in the body are normally low.

Endocrine pharmacotherapy also involves the use of "antihormones." These hormone antagonists block the actions of endogenous hormones. For example, propylthiouracil (PTU) is given to block the effects of an overactive thyroid gland. Tamoxifen (Nolvadex) is given to block the actions of estrogen in estrogen receptor–dependent breast cancers.

TABLE 26.1   Select Endocrine Disorders and Their Pharmacotherapy

Gland	Hormone(s)	Disorder	Drug Therapy Examples
Adrenal cortex	Corticosteroids	Hypersecretion: Cushing's syndrome	ketoconazole (Nizoral) and mitotane (Lysodren)
		Hyposecretion: Addison's disease	hydrocortisone, prednisone
Gonads	Ovaries: estrogen	Hyposecretion: menstrual and metabolic dysfunction	conjugated estrogens and estradiol
	Ovaries: progesterone	Hyposecretion: dysfunctional uterine bleeding	medroxyprogesterone (Provera), progesterone (Prometrium), and norethindrone (Micronor)
	Testes: testosterone	Hyposecretion: hypogonadism	testosterone
Pancreatic islets	Insulin	Hyposecretion: diabetes mellitus	insulin and oral antidiabetic agents
Parathyroid	Parathyroid hormone	Hypersecretion: hyperparathyroidism	surgery (no drug therapy)
		Hyposecretion: hypoparathyroidism	vitamin D and calcium supplements
Pituitary	Antidiuretic hormone	Hyposecretion: diabetes insipidus	desmopressin (DDAVP, Nocdurna) and vasopressin (Pressyn)
		Hypersecretion: syndrome of inappropriate antidiuretic hormone (SIADH)	conivaptan (Vaprisol) and tolvaptan (Samsca)
	Growth hormone	Hyposecretion: small stature	somatropin (Genotropin, Humatrope, Omnitrope, Saizen, Serostim)
		Hypersecretion: acromegaly (adults)	octreotide (Sandostatin)
	Oxytocin	Hyposecretion: delayed delivery or lack of milk ejection	oxytocin (Pitocin)
Thyroid	Thyroid hormone (T_3 and T_4)	Hypersecretion: Graves' disease	propylthiouracil (PTU) and I-131
		Hyposecretion: myxedema (adults), cretinism (children)	thyroid hormone and levothyroxine (Synthroid, Eltroxin)

26 Understanding the Chapter

Key Concepts Summary

The numbered key concepts provide a succinct summary of the important points from the corresponding numbered section within the chapter. If any of these points are not clear, refer to the numbered section within the chapter for review.

26.1 The endocrine system controls homeostasis through the secretion of hormones.

26.2 Hormones must bind to specific receptors to cause physiological changes.

26.3 Most hormone action is regulated through negative feedback.

26.4 Hormone pharmacotherapy is indicated for a diverse variety of conditions.

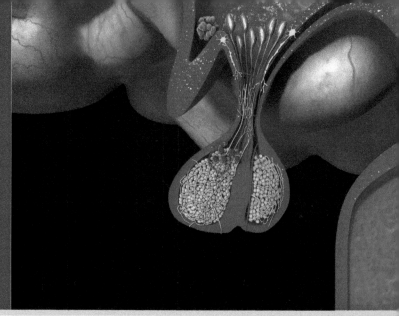

7activestudio/Fotolia

CHAPTER

27 Pharmacotherapy of Hypothalamic and Pituitary Disorders

LEARNING OUTCOMES

After reading this chapter, the student should be able to:

1. Explain the principal actions of the hormones secreted by the hypothalamus and pituitary gland.
2. Identify indications for hypothalamic hormone therapy.
3. Explain the pharmacotherapy of growth hormone disorders in children and adults.
4. Explain the pharmacotherapy of antidiuretic hormone disorders.
5. For each of the classes shown in the Prototype Drugs list, identify the prototype and representative drugs and explain the mechanism of drug action, primary actions, and important adverse effects.
6. Apply the nursing process to the care of clients who are receiving pharmacotherapy for disorders of the hypothalamus and pituitary gland.

CHAPTER OUTLINE

▸ Functions of the Hypothalamus

▸ Functions of the Pituitary Gland

▸ Pharmacotherapy of Growth Hormone Disorders

▸ Disorders of the Hypothalamus and Pituitary Gland

  ▸ Pharmacotherapy with Pituitary and Hypothalamic Hormones

  ▸ Antidiuretic Hormone

In the specialty of endocrinology, understanding the complex relationship between the hypothalamus and pituitary gland is important because these organs regulate so many homeostatic functions. The two collaborate to secrete hormones that control functions of the gonads, adrenal glands, thyroid gland, kidneys, and milk-producing tissues of the breast. The functioning of these two glands serves as the control centre that provides integration between the nervous and endocrine systems. This chapter examines drugs that directly affect the functions of the pituitary and hypothalamus.

Functions of the Hypothalamus

27.1 The hypothalamus controls many diverse body processes and secretes hormones that influence pituitary function.

Roughly the size of an almond, the hypothalamus lies in the centre of the diencephalon of the brain, just superior to the brainstem. The general purpose of the hypothalamus is to maintain homeostasis. To achieve this, the hypothalamus receives input from numerous vital regions of the nervous system, recognizes imbalances, and makes adjustments to bring the body back to homeostasis. Examples of the multiple and diverse functions of this organ include control of body temperature, thirst, appetite, fatigue, circadian rhythms, anger, and the rate of overall body metabolism. The hypothalamus also controls vital functions of the autonomic nervous system such as heart rate, vasoconstriction, digestion, and sweating. For the purposes of this chapter, only the endocrine functions of the hypothalamus are presented. Figure 27.1 describes the hormones associated with the hypothalamus and pituitary gland.

Every hormone has target cells that possess receptors for that specific hormone. For the hormones secreted by the hypothalamus, there is only one target organ: the pituitary gland. All hypothalamic hormones travel by the blood a short distance to the pituitary, which lies immediately below the hypothalamus. Upon reaching their receptors, the hypothalamic hormones simply increase or decrease the release of hormones by the pituitary gland. Because of this, hormones from the hypothalamus are called releasing hormones or inhibiting hormones. The major hypothalamic hormones and their actions on the pituitary gland are given in Table 27.1.

There are very few indications for the administration of hypothalamic hormones: rather than give hypothalamic hormones, it is more effective (and less expensive) to administer pituitary hormones or the secretions of a target endocrine organ such as thyroid hormone, estrogen, testosterone, or corticosteroids.

The hypothalamic hormones that do have clinical applications are analogues or antagonists of gonadotropin-releasing hormone (GnRH). Initially the effect of the GnRH analogues is to increase the production of interstitial cell-stimulating hormone (in males) or follicle-stimulating hormone (in females), which increases the secretion of sex hormones. With continued therapy, however, the pituitary becomes insensitive to the effects of GnRH, and the production of sex hormones falls to near castration levels. Indications for these drugs include the following:

- Endometriosis, a common cause of female infertility
- Central precocious puberty, the premature onset of puberty in children

TABLE 27.1 Hormones Secreted by the Hypothalamus and Pituitary Glands

Hypothalamic Hormone	Pituitary Hormone	Target Organ	Principal Actions
Corticotropin-releasing hormone (CRH)	Adrenocorticotropic hormone (ACTH)	Adrenal cortex	Stimulates release of corticosteroids
Gonadotropin-releasing hormone (GnRH)	Follicle-stimulating hormone (FSH)	Ovaries, testes	Stimulates release of estrogen and ovarian follicle development in females, and sperm production in males
	Luteinizing hormone (LH)	Ovaries, testes	Triggers ovulation and secretion of estrogen and progesterone in females, increases testosterone secretion in males
Growth hormone-inhibiting hormone (GHIH) Growth hormone-releasing hormone (GHRH)	Growth hormone (GH)	Most body cells	Regulates growth and development of bones, muscles, cartilage, organs; general body metabolism
None	Melanocyte-stimulating hormone (MSH)	Skin	Stimulates pigmentation
Prolactin-inhibiting hormone (PIH) Prolactin-releasing hormone (PRH)	Prolactin	Mammary glands	Regulates lactation
Thyrotropin-releasing hormone (TRH)	Thyroid-stimulating hormone (TSH)	Thyroid gland	Stimulates release of thyroid hormone

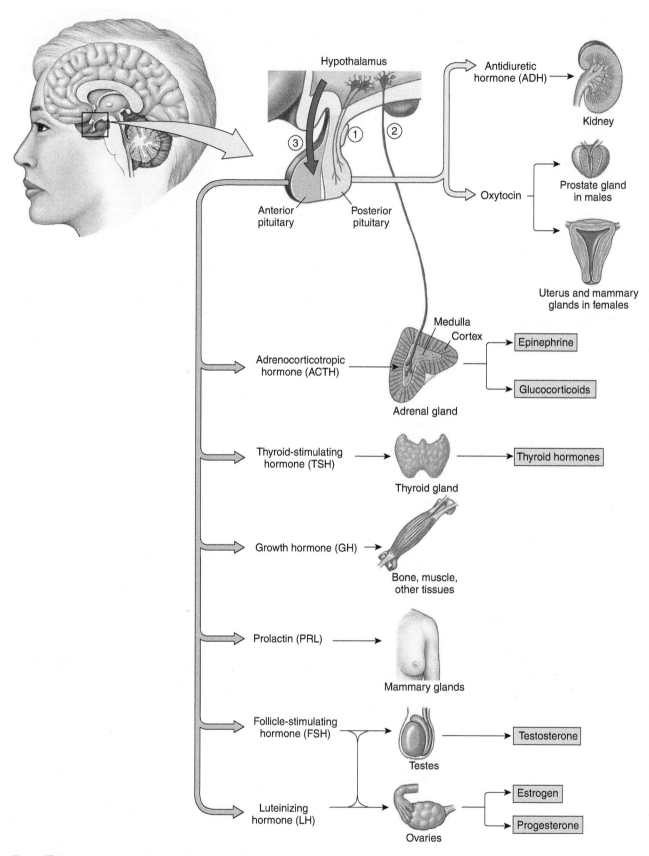

Figure 27.1 Hormones associated with the hypothalamus and pituitary gland.
Source: Pearson Education

- Palliative treatment of advanced prostate cancer
- Uterine leiomyomata, a benign tissue of smooth muscle sometimes called fibroids

Functions of the Pituitary Gland

27.2 The pituitary gland secretes hormones that control many diverse body functions.

Although the pituitary gland is often referred to as the "master gland," its function is largely controlled by releasing or inhibiting hormones from the hypothalamus. The pituitary gland is divided into anterior and posterior lobes, which have very different structures and functions.

The **anterior pituitary gland** (adenohypophysis) comprises glandular tissue that manufactures and secretes hormones that control major body functions and systems. Four of these are called **tropic hormones**, a term that refers to the ability of these hormones to regulate the secretory actions of other endocrine glands. The anterior pituitary hormones are synthesized and stored in the pituitary until they receive a message from the hypothalamus. The message from the hypothalamus is usually to *enhance* the release of the hormones, as is the case for growth hormone–releasing hormone (GHRH), thyrotropin-releasing hormone (TRH), prolactin-releasing hormone (PRH), corticotropin-releasing hormone (CRH), and gonadotropin-releasing hormone (GnRH). Two of the hypothalamic secretions, growth hormone–inhibiting hormone (GHIH) and prolactin-inhibiting hormone (PIH), *prevent* the release of pituitary hormones.

The **posterior pituitary gland** (neurohypophysis), by contrast, consists of nervous tissue and is basically an extension of the hypothalamus. It secretes two hormones: antidiuretic hormone (ADH) and oxytocin. These hormones are manufactured in the hypothalamus and travel down neurons to the posterior pituitary where they are stored until factors stimulate their release. The primary stimulus causing ADH secretion is an increased serum osmolality, or a high concentration of solutes in the blood. Oxytocin release is stimulated by touch receptors in the nipples of lactating women. Pharmacotherapy with oxytocin is presented in Chapter 31.

Regulation of hormone levels is an essential function because too little or too much of any of these endocrine secretions can cause profound symptoms. Many are controlled by negative feedback loops. As circulating levels of a hormone rise above normal, a message is sent to the hypothalamus, pituitary, or other endocrine gland to shut down the manufacture and secretion of the hormone. This prevents excess hormone levels. When hormones are administered as drug therapy, they can influence this normal negative feedback mechanism. One of the most important examples of this phenomenon is the negative feedback suppression of the adrenal glands caused by administration of corticosteroid medications.

Because of the widespread effects of the hormones secreted and controlled by the hypothalamus and pituitary glands, disorders of these glands are quite complex. In general, the pathologies of endocrine glands can be categorized as causing hypofunction or hyperfunction of the particular gland. Pituitary disorders can be the result of tumours, surgery, radiation therapy, infection, injury, infarction (loss of blood supply), or bleeding (hemorrhage) in the area. Congenital defects may also result in absent or impaired function of a hormone or in the lack of an enzyme necessary for hormone production.

Pharmacotherapy of Growth Hormone Disorders

27.3 Growth hormone deficiency in adults and children can be treated by administering recombinant growth hormone.

Growth hormone (GH), also called somatotropin or somatropin, is produced and secreted by the anterior pituitary gland. This hormone was once believed to be of importance only during periods of active growth, but it is now recognized that adults produce nearly as much GH as children. Although its major targets are bone and skeletal muscle, GH stimulates many types of body cells to increase in size and replicate. It is considered an anabolic (tissue-building) hormone. The primary effects of GH are as follows:

- Increases length and width of bone
- Stimulates cartilage growth
- Stimulates the growth and development of most visceral and endocrine organs, skeletal and cardiac muscle, and skin and connective tissue
- Enhances cellular uptake of amino acids and increased protein synthesis
- Breaks down adipose tissue to release fatty acids for use as fuel
- Decreases use of glucose; impairs glucose tolerance and induces insulin resistance in peripheral tissues

Many of the effects of GH are dependent on **insulin-like growth factor (IGF)**, a family of peptides that promote cartilage and bone growth. IGFs are produced in the liver and released when hepatic cells become activated by GH. Secretion of GH fluctuates during the day, peaking 1 to 4 hours after the onset of sleep. These nighttime bursts in GH are greater in children than in adults.

The overall regulation of serum GH levels resides in the hypothalamus, with the secretion of GHRH and GHIH. A large number of secondary factors, such as exercise and sleep, influence the release of GH.

In children, GH deficiency results in dwarfism. **Dwarfism** is associated with normal birth length followed by a slowing of the growth rate. These children have normal intelligence, short stature, immature facial features, obesity, and delayed skeletal maturation. In this context, **short stature** is defined as well below the fifth percentile for age and gender, or more than two standard deviations below the mean (average) height for age and gender. Acquired GH deficiency develops later in childhood and can be caused by a hypothalamic-pituitary tumour or an infection. Children who have been severely neglected or emotionally deprived can develop a psychosocial dwarfism, with poor growth, a pot belly, and poor nutritional habits. GH levels often return to normal once the child is removed from the dysfunctional environment.

Adult GH deficiency is associated with reduced muscle mass, increased cardiovascular mortality, central adiposity and increased visceral fat, insulin resistance, and dyslipidemia. This hormonal deficiency may develop during adulthood, or it may be a continuation of childhood deficiency. Several forms of recombinant human GH formulations (Humatrope and Genotropin) have been approved for use in adults with body wasting–type disorders. Treatment can result in increased lean body mass, decreased fat mass, increased bone mineral density, and decreased lipid levels.

Human GH has been abused for its anabolic effects. Athletes have used the drug to build muscle, increase strength, and maintain less body fat. It has also been called an antiaging drug because it promotes younger looking skin, improved memory, and reduced wrinkles. The administration of GH for these purposes is illegal, and prolonged use may lead to long-term adverse effects in clients. Despite potential adverse health effects, products advertised as "human growth hormone supplements" are readily marketed without a prescription. These do not contain any GH (which must be administered parenterally) but instead contain a mixture of oral (PO) supplements that are claimed to stimulate the pituitary gland. The safety and effectiveness of these products have not been evaluated adequately.

Octreotide is a synthetic growth hormone antagonist structurally related to **somatostatin** (growth hormone–inhibiting hormone). In addition to inhibiting growth hormone, octreotide promotes fluid and electrolyte reabsorption from the gastrointestinal (GI) tract and prolongs intestinal transit time. It has limited applications in treating growth hormone excess in adults (**acromegaly**) and in treating the severe diarrhea sometimes associated with metastatic carcinoid tumours. Acromegaly may also be treated with pegvisomant (Somavert), which is a growth hormone receptor antagonist.

NCLEX Success Tip

Consider the multiple therapeutic effects of octreotide and the common adverse effects related to the GI tract. The drug is to be used cautiously in clients with pre-existing gallbladder disease. Used concurrently with PO antidiabetic drugs or insulin, it can cause hypoglycemia. Additive bradycardia may occur when octreotide is given with beta blockers and calcium channel blockers. Use caution in treating clients with renal and liver impairment.

DISORDERS OF THE HYPOTHALAMUS AND PITUITARY GLAND

Because of its critical role in controlling other endocrine tissues, lack of adequate pituitary secretion can have multiple, profound effects on body function. Pharmacotherapy involves administration of the missing hormone, perhaps for the life of the client. See Table 27.2 for hypothalamic and pituitary agents.

Pharmacotherapy with Pituitary and Hypothalamic Hormones

27.4 Only a few pituitary and hypothalamic hormones, including growth hormone and corticotropin (ACTH), have clinical applications as drugs.

Of the 15 different hormones secreted by the pituitary and hypothalamus, only a few are used in pharmacotherapy. There are several reasons why hormones are not widely used. Some of these

TABLE 27.2   Hypothalamic and Pituitary Agents

Drug	Route and Adult Dose
Hypothalamic Agents	
gonadorelin (Lutrepulse)	Subcutaneous/intravenous (SC/IV), start with 5 µg every 90 minutes via suitable pulsatile pump; dosage adjustments may be made every 21 days if necessary; increased dose may be necessary if no response after three treatment intervals; treatment should be continued for 2 weeks after ovulation to maintain the corpus luteum
nafarelin (Synarel)	Inhalation, one spray (200 µg) into one nostril each morning and one spray into the other nostril each evening between days 2 and 4 of the menstrual cycle (max 400 µg/day)
octreotide (Sandostatin)	SC, 100–600 µg/day in two to four divided doses; may switch to intramuscular (IM) depot injection after 2 weeks at 20 mg every 4 weeks for 2 months
protirelin	IV, 500 µg bolus over a period of 15–30 seconds
Anterior Pituitary Agents	
corticotropin (ACTH)	Gel/injection, 40-80 units every 24-72 hours
cosyntropin (Cortrosyn)	IM Depot, initial for acute treatment, 1 mg/day for 3 days; maintenance dose is 0.5-1 mg every 2-3 days or twice weekly, or 2 mg once weekly or less frequently (titrate to lowest effective dose at the longest effective dosing interval)
menotropin (Menopur, Repronex)	IM/SC, start with 150 units once daily for the first 5 days of treatment; subsequent dose adjustments should not be made more frequently than once every 2 days and should not exceed 75-150 units per adjustment (max daily dose 450 units; treatment for more than 12 days is not recommended)
Pr somatropin (Genotropin, Humatrope, Omnitrope, Saizen, Serostim)	Dose depends on which brand is used and the weight of the individual
thyrotropin (Thyrogen)	IM, 0.9 mg followed 24 hours later by a second 0.9 mg
Posterior Pituitary Agents	
desmopressin (DDAVP, Nocdurna)	IV/SC/IM, 1-4 µg (0.25-1 mL) once daily; intranasal (100 µg/mL nasal solution), usual dose range is 10-40 µg daily (0.1 to 0.4 mL) as a single dose or divided into 2 or 3 doses; PO, start with 0.1 mg tid (max 1.2 mg/day in three divided doses)
oxytocin (Pitocin) (see Chapter 31, page 376, for the Prototype Drug box)	IV, 1 mU/minute, may increase by 1 mU/minute every 15 minutes (max 20 mU/minute)
Pr vasopressin (Pressyn)	IM/SC, 5–10 U aqueous solution 2–4 times per day (5–60 U/day) or 1.25-2.5 U in oil every 2–3 days

hormones can be obtained only from natural sources and can be quite expensive when used in therapeutic quantities. Furthermore, it is usually more effective to give drugs that directly affect secretion at the target organs. Two pituitary hormones, prolactin and oxytocin, affect the female reproductive system. Of those remaining, growth hormone and antidiuretic hormone have the most clinical utility.

PROTOTYPE DRUG | Somatropin (Genotropin, Humatrope, Omnitrope, Saizen, Serostim)

Actions and Uses: Somatropin is prepared through recombinant DNA technology and is identical to endogenous human GH. It is available in several different formulations that vary by dose and regimen. The preferred route of administration is subcutaneous, although some forms may be given via the intramuscular (IM) route. GH produces growth of long bones in children prior to epiphyseal closure. The gain in growth is very rapid at the initiation of therapy but slows over time. Treatment may continue until the desired height is achieved, epiphyseal closure occurs, or the client fails to respond to treatment. If treatment does not result in growth, it is stopped, and the diagnosis is re-evaluated. The metabolic effects of the drug include increased protein synthesis, reduced carbohydrate use, and increased use of fatty acids for energy.

GH is used in the management of a number of growth-related disorders, including the following:

- Growth failure in children due to GH deficiency or Prader-Willi syndrome (Genotropin)
- Short stature associated with Turner syndrome (Genotropin, Humatrope, Norditropin)
- Adult GH deficiency (Genotropin, Humatrope, Norditropin, Saizen)
- Acquired immunodeficiency syndrome (AIDS) wasting, cachexia, and severe thermal injuries (Serostim)
- Short bowel syndrome in clients who are receiving specialized nutrition support (Zorbtive)

Although the various brand name products of GH have the same effectiveness, they differ in potency and are not interchangeable. Some are available in prefilled syringes, whereas others are longer acting. The nurse should check the package insert for specific dosing instructions.

Pharmacokinetics: Somatropin has the same amino acid sequence as endogenous human GH and produces the same effects as the naturally occurring form of the hormone. The effects of GH are mediated by IGF. Somatropin is administered by the SC or IV route, and it is well absorbed following injection and well distributed in the body bound to proteins. The primary site for metabolism is the liver, although the kidneys play a role in this. Peak action after administration is variable and could be days or weeks, with a half-life of 3.8 to 5 hours. The drug is excreted by the kidneys.

Administration Alerts:

- Somatropin is contraindicated for use in clients with closed epiphyses. It is also contraindicated in clients with severe

obesity, respiratory impairment, or sleep apnea due to potentially fatal respiratory impairment.

- Somatropin is contraindicated in clients with intracranial tumour due to the risk for increased growth or recurrence of the tumour.
- The drug is contraindicated in clients who are sensitive to glycerin. Somatropin should be used with caution in clients with severe renal or hepatic disease due to reduced clearance and in clients with diabetes mellitus due to hyperglycemia and insulin resistance.
- Somatropin should be used with caution in pregnant or lactating clients because safety has not been established. Somatropin is pregnancy category B or C, depending on the specific formulation.

Adverse Effects and Interactions: Adverse effects of somatropin include hyperglycemia and insulin resistance, which is made worse in clients with pre-existing diabetes mellitus. It can also cause hypothyroidism. Edema of the hands and feet, headache, and hypertension often occur initially but may resolve with continued therapy. Joint pain, muscle aches, and pain at the injection site are common. Carpal tunnel syndrome may occur with use of Serostim. Development of antibodies to GH may rarely occur. Hypercalciuria, possibly asymptomatic, may occur in the first few months of therapy.

Corticosteroids interfere with the bone growth–promoting action of GH; therefore, the two drugs should not be given concurrently. Concurrent use with anabolic steroids, androgens, estrogens, or thyroid hormone may increase the rate of epiphyseal closure. Clients who are receiving insulin should be monitored carefully because somatropin decreases the actions of insulin.

Antidiuretic Hormone

27.5 Pharmacotherapy is used to treat deficient or excess secretion of antidiuretic hormone.

As its name implies, **antidiuretic hormone (ADH)** conserves water in the body. ADH is secreted from the posterior pituitary gland when the hypothalamus senses that plasma volume has decreased or that the osmolality of the blood has become too high. This is an example of a negative feedback mechanism. ADH acts on the collecting ducts in the kidney to increase water reabsorption. The increased amount of water in the body reduces the serum osmolality to normal levels, and the ADH secretion stops. **Diabetes insipidus (DI)** is a rare disease caused by a deficiency of ADH. Clients with this disorder have an intense thirst and produce very dilute urine due to the large volume of water lost by the kidneys. Nephrogenic DI is caused by the inability of the kidneys to respond to ADH, and replacement therapy is not effective. Neurogenic DI is the result of inadequate production or secretion of ADH in the brain. ADH is also called vasopressin (Pressyn) because it has the capability to raise blood pressure when secreted in large amounts. Vasopressin is available as a drug for the treatment of DI.

Desmopressin (DDAVP) is the most common form of ADH in use for neurogenic DI. It has a duration of action of 8 to 20 hours, whereas vasopressin has a duration of only 2 to 8 hours. Desmopressin is available as a nasal spray and is easily self-administered;

vasopressin must be administered by the IM or SC route. The client may also more easily increase or decrease the dosage of desmopressin depending on urine output. Desmopressin is also available in SC, IV, and PO forms. Desmopressin and lypressin do not have the intense vasoconstricting effects of vasopressin. Desmopressin also produces an increase in plasma factor VIII and von Willebrand factor and therefore is indicated for the management of bleeding in clients with hemophilia A and von Willebrand's disease (type 1).

Nursing Considerations

The role of the nurse in ADH therapy involves careful monitoring of the client's condition and providing education as it relates to the prescribed drug treatment. The therapeutic goal for clients who are receiving ADH therapy is focused on maintaining fluid and electrolyte status. For clients who are taking antidiuretic hormones, assess for fluid and electrolyte imbalances and assess urine specific gravity prior to administration. A low specific gravity indicates lack of urine concentration and suggests ADH deficiency. Periodically assess urine specific gravity during pharmacotherapy to determine whether the therapeutic effect is being achieved. Closely monitor the client's vital signs, especially pulse and blood pressure, as ADH can affect plasma volume and is a potent vasoconstrictor.

Body weight, intake, and output must be monitored because these drugs may cause excess water retention. Also monitor the neurological status of the client. Symptoms of water intoxication may first present as headache accompanied by confusion and drowsiness. The use of vasopressin is contraindicated in clients with pre-existing heart disease. Furthermore, it should be used cautiously in elderly clients because of the possibility of undiagnosed heart disease.

Client education as it relates to ADH should include goals, reasons for obtaining baseline data such as vital signs and tests for cardiac and renal function, and possible side effects. The client should be instructed to check weight at least two times per week and report significant changes to the healthcare provider. See Nursing Process Focus: Clients Receiving Antidiuretic Hormone Therapy for additional points to include when teaching about this class of drug.

PROTOTYPE DRUG　**Vasopressin (Pressyn)**

Actions and Uses: Two ADH preparations are available for the treatment of diabetes insipidus: vasopressin and desmopressin (DDAVP, Nocdurna). Vasopressin is a synthetic hormone that has a structure identical to that of human ADH. It acts on the renal collecting tubules to increase their permeability to water, thus enhancing water reabsorption. Although it acts within minutes, vasopressin has a short half-life that requires it to be administered three to four times per day. Vasopressin is formulated in peanut oil to increase its duration of action. Vasopressin is usually given IM or IV, although an intranasal form is available for mild DI. Desmopressin has a longer duration of action than vasopressin and results in fewer serious adverse effects. Desmopressin is occasionally used by the intranasal route for enuresis (bedwetting).

Pharmacokinetics: Vasopressin is widely distributed in extracellular fluid. It is rapidly metabolized by the liver and kidneys. Its half-life is 10 to 20 minutes.

Administration Alerts:

- Vasopressin should never be administered IV because it is an oil.
- Vasopressin aqueous injection may be given by continuous IV infusion after it is diluted in normal saline or D5W.
- Vasopressin is pregnancy category X.

Adverse Effects and Interactions: Vasopressin has a strong vasoconstrictor action that is unrelated to its antidiuretic properties, thus hypertension is possible. The drug can precipitate angina episodes and myocardial infarction in clients with coronary artery disease. Excessive fluid retention can cause water intoxication, including symptoms of headache, restlessness, drowsiness, and coma. Water intoxication can usually be avoided by teaching the client to decrease water intake during vasopressin therapy.

Vasopressin injection interacts with several other drugs. For example, alcohol, epinephrine (Adrenalin), heparin, lithium (Carbolith, Lithane), and phenytoin (Dilantin) may decrease the antidiuretic effects of vasopressin. Neostigmine (Prostigmin) may increase vasopressor actions. Carbamazepine (Tegretol) and thiazide diuretics may increase antidiuretic activity.

NCLEX Success Tip

Consider the effects on fluid balance and related manifestations (physical and diagnostic) when administering exogenous ADH. Apply the nursing process for potential complications and the client assessment when administering ADH. Consider the cardiac effects of vasopressin.

NURSING PROCESS FOCUS

Clients Receiving Antidiuretic Hormone Therapy

Assessment	Potential Nursing Diagnoses/Identified Patterns
Prior to administration: • Obtain complete health history, including allergies, drug history, and possible drug interactions. • Obtain complete physical examination. • Assess for the presence or history of neurosurgery, pituitary tumours, head injury, and nocturia. • Obtain laboratory studies, including urine specific gravity, urine/serum osmolarity, and serum electrolytes.	• Safety from injury related to side effects of drug therapy • Risk for fluid imbalance • Risk for sleep disturbances related to effects of drug therapy and frequent nocturia • Need for knowledge regarding drug therapy and adverse effects

---

Planning: Client Goals and Expected Outcomes

The client will:

- Exhibit normal fluid and electrolyte balance
- Report uninterrupted sleep patterns
- Identify and report side effects to the healthcare provider
- Demonstrate an understanding of the drug's action

Implementation

Interventions (Rationales)	Client Education/Discharge Planning
• Monitor vital signs. (Changes may indicate alterations in body fluid status such as hypervolemia or hypovolemia.) • Monitor cardiovascular status such as peripheral pulses, heart sounds, skin temperature and colour, and electrocardiogram (ECG). (ADH has potent vasoconstriction properties and may cause hypertension and dysrhythmias.) • Administer fluid replacement as directed. (IV infusions should be regulated to maintain body fluid balance.) • Encourage oral fluid intake to satisfy thirst only. (Excessive fluid intake may trigger a diabetes insipidus episode.) • Monitor intake/output ratio and weigh client daily. (ADH may result in fluid retention that can lead to water intoxication. Daily weight is an indicator of fluid retention.) • Monitor for presence of nocturia or nocturnal enuresis. Determine the client's ability to satisfy physiological sleep needs. (Less frequent nighttime urination is an indication of the effectiveness of ADH therapy.) • Monitor for symptoms of fluid volume overload such as headache, restlessness, shortness of breath, tachycardia, hypertension, and low urinary output. (These are signs of water intoxication.) • Monitor status of nasal mucous membranes if nasal preparations are prescribed. (Intranasal use can cause changes in the nasal mucosa, resulting in unpredictable drug absorption.) • Monitor laboratory studies, including urine and serum osmolarity, urine specific gravity, and serum electrolytes. (These assess fluid volume status.)	• Instruct the client to report irregular heartbeat, shortness of breath, dizziness, or headache • Instruct the client in the importance of follow-up care and to take medication exactly as prescribed Instruct client to: • Monitor fluid balance and report vomiting, diarrhea, profuse sweating, and frequent urination • Consume fluid to satisfy thirst and to report excessive unquenchable thirst Instruct client: • To weigh self daily and report excessive gains or losses • In titration techniques based on urinary output Instruct client to: • Keep a sleep log, recording the number of times per night he or she is awakened to urinate • Avoid potentially hazardous activities due to possible drowsiness until therapeutic effect of drug is achieved and drowsiness is no longer a risk • Have frequent rest periods or daytime naps if sleep deprivation is present until therapeutic effect is achieved • Instruct client to report headaches, shortness of breath, palpitations, and low urine output. Instruct client: • To report worsening of condition since route of administration may need to be changed • To report drainage or irritation of the nasal mucosa if taking nasal preparation • In subcutaneous injection methods, as appropriate Instruct client: • To measure urine specific gravity • In the importance of keeping all laboratory appointments

---

Evaluation of Outcome Criteria

Evaluate effectiveness of drug therapy by confirming that client goals and expected outcomes have been met (see "Planning").

See Table 27.2 under "Posterior Pituitary Agents" for a list of drugs to which these nursing actions apply.

27 Understanding the Chapter

Key Concepts Summary

The numbered key concepts provide a succinct summary of the important points from the corresponding numbered section within the chapter. If any of these points are not clear, refer to the numbered section within the chapter for review.

27.1 The hypothalamus controls many diverse body processes and secretes hormones that influence pituitary function.

27.2 The pituitary gland secretes hormones that control many diverse body functions.

27.3 Growth hormone deficiency in adults and children can be treated by administering recombinant growth hormone.

27.4 Only a few pituitary and hypothalamic hormones, including growth hormone and corticotropin (ACTH), have clinical applications as drugs.

27.5 Pharmacotherapy is used to treat deficient or excess secretion of antidiuretic hormone.

Chapter 27 Scenario

Raj, an 8-year-old boy, was referred to the pediatric endocrinology clinic for evaluation of his short stature. He had been healthy and developmentally normal until 3 years ago. Since that time, his growth has been extremely slow and almost imperceptible. On his initial exam, Raj's weight and height were 17 kg and 108 cm, respectively. His height standard deviation score was –4.0 with a body mass index of 14.6. The remainder of his physical examination was normal.

When the pediatrician reviewed the results of hormonal assay tests with Raj's parents, everyone was relieved to find out that although there is a problem, it is not due to a tumour or other life-threatening disorder. Raj has a congenital deficiency in growth hormone (GH), and the pediatrician begins to discuss replacement therapy with the parents. They agree that Raj should have this therapy and want to start it as soon as possible. Somatropin (Humatrope) has been ordered. As the nurse working with Raj and his family, address each of the following questions.

Critical Thinking Questions

1. What teaching will you need to provide to Raj's parents regarding drug therapy for his disorder?

2. Raj's father states, "I hope my health insurance will cover this medication." What would you say in response to this comment?

3. The parents ask about the adverse effects that might occur with this therapy. How would you respond?

See Answers to Critical Thinking Questions in Appendix B.

NCLEX Practice Questions

1 A teaching plan for a parent whose child is receiving somatropin (Genotropin) should include which important information?

a. The client must adhere to therapy to prevent mental retardation.

b. The medication cannot be given orally; it can only be given parenterally.

c. If growth hormone is used in adolescence, it can add up to 15 cm (6 in.) in height.

d. Growth hormone therapy requires frequent blood work.

2 Which of the following findings would a nurse consider to be effects of somatropin? Select all that apply.

a. Increase in the length and width of long bones

b. Organ, muscle, and connective tissue growth

c. Increased synthesis of proteins

d. Lowering of serum glucose levels

e. Increase in fat deposits around the abdomen

3 A client with neurogenic diabetes insipidus is being started on an oral dose of desmopressin (DDAVP, Nocdurna). Which instruction should the nurse include in the teaching plan?

  a. Use the drug only if urine output is excessive.

  b. Use twice the prescribed dose if you miss a dose.

  c. Obtain and record your weight each morning.

  d. Use an NSAID such as ibuprofen (Advil, Motrin) if leg cramping occurs during walking.

4 A client with metastatic colon cancer is experiencing bowel-related complications of the cancer and treatment. Octreotide (Sandostatin) has been ordered. The nurse will anticipate which therapeutic effect from this drug?

  a. Decrease in the number of diarrheal stools per day

  b. Slowing of the metastatic spread of the cancer

  c. Increase in lean body mass and fat deposits

  d. Episodes of hypo- or hyperglycemia

5 Prior to starting a client on vasopressin for control of esophageal varices, the nurse will obtain the client's past health history. If present, which condition might indicate the need to verify the order with the prescriber?

  a. Glaucoma

  b. Alcoholism

  c. Chronic obstructive pulmonary disease (COPD)

  d. Angina

See Answers to NCLEX Practice Questions in Appendix A.

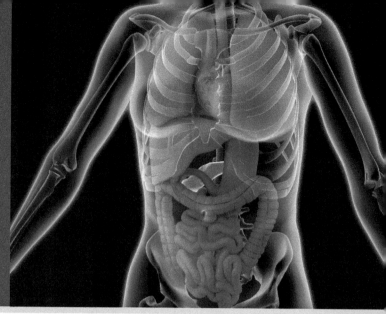

PROTOTYPE DRUGS

INSULINS	ORAL ANTIHYPER-GLYCEMICS
Pr *regular insulin* (Humulin R, Novolin ge Toronto)	Pr *metformin* (Glucophage) Pr *glyburide (DiaBeta)*

Roger Harris/Science Photo Library/Getty Images

CHAPTER

28 Pharmacotherapy of Diabetes Mellitus

LEARNING OUTCOMES

After reading this chapter, the student should be able to:

1. Describe the endocrine and exocrine functions of the pancreas.

2. Compare and contrast type 1 and type 2 diabetes mellitus in relation to their pathophysiology and treatment.

3. Compare and contrast types of insulin, including onset, peak, and duration of action.

4. Describe the signs and symptoms of insulin overdose and underdose.

5. Compare and contrast the pharmacology of the different types of diabetes.

6. Describe the nurse's role in the pharmacological management of diabetes mellitus.

7. For each of the drug classes listed in Prototype Drugs, identify a representative drug and explain its mechanism of action, therapeutic effects, and important adverse effects.

8. Use the nursing process to care for clients who are receiving drug therapy for diabetes mellitus.

CHAPTER OUTLINE

▶ Normal Functions of the Pancreas

▶ Etiology and Characteristics of Type 1 and Type 2 Diabetes Mellitus

▶ Pharmacotherapy with Insulin

▶ Pharmacotherapy with Oral Antihyperglycemics

KEY TERMS

The pancreas serves unique and vital functions by supplying essential digestive enzymes while also secreting the hormones responsible for glucose homeostasis. From a pharmacological perspective, the most important disorder associated with the pancreas is diabetes mellitus (DM). According to the Canadian Diabetes Association (CDA), in 2015 more than 3.4 million Canadians, or 9.3% of the population, had diabetes. This is expected to increase to 5 million, or 12.1%, by 2025 (Canadian Diabetes Association as of January 27, 2016). See Table 28.1 for recent Canadian statistics on diabetes. Diabetes is a disease caused by genetic and environmental factors that impairs the cellular use of glucose. Because glucose is essential to every cell in the body, the effects of diabetes are widespread. Diabetes merits special consideration in pharmacology because the nurse will encounter many clients with this disorder.

Normal Functions of the Pancreas

28.1 The pancreas is both an endocrine and an exocrine gland. Insulin is released when blood glucose increases, and glucagon is released when blood glucose decreases.

Located behind the stomach and between the duodenum and spleen, the pancreas is an essential organ to both the digestive and the endocrine systems. It is responsible for the secretion of several enzymes into the duodenum that assist in the chemical digestion of nutrients. This is its **exocrine** function.

Clusters of cells in the pancreas, called **islets of Langerhans**, are responsible for its endocrine function: the secretion of glucagon and insulin. Alpha cells secrete **glucagon**, and beta cells secrete **insulin**, as illustrated in Figure 28.1. As do other endocrine organs, the pancreas secretes these hormones directly into blood capillaries, where they are available for transport to body tissues. Insulin and glucagon play key roles in keeping glucose levels within a normal range in the blood.

Insulin secretion is regulated by a number of chemical, hormonal, and neural factors. One important regulator is the level of glucose in the blood. After a meal, when blood glucose levels rise, the islets of Langerhans are stimulated to secrete insulin, which causes glucose to leave the blood and enter cells. High insulin levels and falling blood glucose levels provide negative feedback to the pancreas to stop secreting insulin.

Insulin affects carbohydrate, lipid, and protein metabolism in most cells of the body. One of its most important actions is to assist in glucose transport: without insulin, glucose cannot enter cells. Activation of insulin receptors leads to internal cellular mechanisms that directly affect glucose uptake by regulating the number and operation of protein molecules in the cell membrane that transport glucose into the cell. A cell may be literally swimming in glucose, but glucose cannot enter and be used as an energy source by the cell without insulin present. Insulin is said to have a **hypoglycemic effect** because its presence causes glucose to *leave* the blood and serum glucose to *fall*. The brain is an important exception because it does not require insulin for glucose transport. As a result, the brain relies almost exclusively on glucose for its energy needs because it is unable to synthesize glucose and will exhaust its supply after just a few minutes of activity.

TABLE 28.1 Diabetes: Recent Canadian Statistics

Key Canadian Statistic	2015	2025
Estimated diabetes prevalence (n/%)	3.4 million/9.3%	5 million/12.1%
Estimated prediabetes prevalence in Canada (n/%) (age 20+)	5.7 million/22.1%	6.4 million/23.2%
Estimated cost of diabetes in Canada ($)	$14 billion	$17.4 billion
Estimated diabetes prevalence increase (%)	44% from 2015 to 2025	
Estimated diabetes cost increase (%)	25% from 2015 to 2025	

Data from Canadian Diabetes Association as of April 15, 2016.

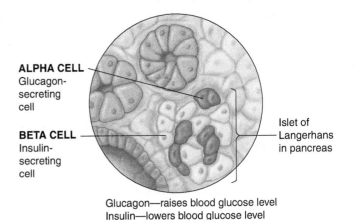

Glucagon—raises blood glucose level
Insulin—lowers blood glucose level

Figure 28.1 Glucagon- and insulin-secreting cells in the islets of Langerhans.

Pearson Education.

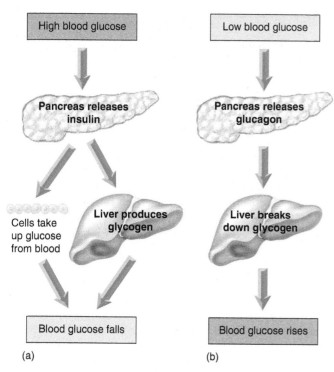

Figure 28.2   Relationship among insulin, glucagon, and blood glucose.

Islet cells in the pancreas also secrete glucagon. Glucagon is an antagonist to insulin. When levels of glucose are low, glucagon is secreted, and its primary function is to maintain adequate blood glucose levels between meals. Glucagon has a **hyperglycemic effect** because its presence causes blood glucose to rise. Figure 28.2 illustrates the relationship among blood glucose, insulin, and glucagon.

Blood glucose levels are usually kept within a normal range by insulin and glucagon; however, other hormones and drugs can affect glucose metabolism. Hyperglycemic hormones include epinephrine, thyroid hormones, growth hormone, and corticosteroids. Common drugs that can raise blood glucose levels include phenytoin, nonsteroidal anti-inflammatory drugs (NSAIDs), and diuretics. Drugs with a hypoglycemic effect include alcohol, lithium (Carbolith, Lithane), angiotensin-converting enzyme (ACE) inhibitors, and beta-adrenergic blockers. Blood glucose levels should be monitored periodically in clients who are receiving medications that have hypoglycemic effects.

Because diabetes is essentially a disorder of carbohydrate metabolism, it is important to understand the way in which the body obtains, metabolizes, and stores glucose. Of all the different molecules available, the body prefers to use glucose as its primary energy source. Most other tissues can use fatty acids and proteins for energy production, if necessary, but they too prefer to use glucose. One of the most important roles of the liver and pancreas is to regulate the body's fuel supply so that all tissues of the body have sufficient energy to perform their functions.

Although the normal range for serum glucose during fasting is considered to be 4–7 mmol/L, it is usually tightly regulated by the body to remain between 5–8 mmol/L even after meals. Two pancreatic hormones contribute to maintaining a stable serum glucose level: insulin, which acts to decrease blood glucose levels, and glucagon, which acts to increase blood glucose levels.

Following a meal, glucose is rapidly absorbed from the gastrointestinal (GI) tract, and serum levels rise. Some of the glucose is taken up by cells and used for immediate energy needs, but about two-thirds is stored in liver and muscle cells as glycogen, the storage form of glucose. When glucose levels fall between meals, glycogen is broken down in a process called **glycogenolysis**, and glucose is released into the bloodstream. Maintaining a stable serum glucose level is simply a matter of storing glucose during times of excess and returning it to the bloodstream in times of deficiency. The importance of maintaining this delicate balance, however, cannot be overstated. Too much glucose or too little glucose can have lethal consequences.

Following a meal, the pancreas recognizes the rising serum glucose levels and releases insulin. Without insulin, glucose is not able to enter cells of the body. The cells may be surrounded by high amounts of glucose, but they are unable to use it until insulin arrives. It may be helpful to visualize insulin as a transporter or "gatekeeper." When present, insulin swings open the gate, transporting glucose inside cells; if there is no insulin, there is no entry. The physiological actions of insulin are summarized as follows:

- Promotes the entry of glucose into cells
- Provides for the storage of glucose, as glycogen
- Inhibits the breakdown of fat and glycogen
- Increases protein synthesis and inhibits **gluconeogenesis**, which is the production of new glucose from noncarbohydrate molecules.

Insulin is produced in beta cells of the pancreas known as islets of Langerhans, whereas alpha cells in the pancreas secrete glucagon. Glucagon maintains stable blood glucose levels between meals and during periods of fasting and has actions that are opposite to those of insulin. It removes glucose from its storage in the liver and sends it to the blood (glycogenolysis), raising serum glucose within minutes.

The level of glucose in the blood regulates the release of both insulin and glucagon. A hypoglycemic state (low serum glucose) stimulates the release of glucagon and inhibits the release of insulin, whereas a hyperglycemic state (high serum glucose) has the opposite effect: it stimulates the release of insulin and inhibits the release of glucagon.

Additional factors that decrease blood glucose levels are fasting, exercise, and alcohol. Factors that increase blood glucose levels include stress from infection, injury, or surgery, which triggers release of epinephrine and norepinephrine; large meals or overconsumption of carbohydrates; growth hormone; and corticosteroids.

Diabetes mellitus is a group of metabolic diseases in which there is deficient insulin secretion or decreased sensitivity of insulin receptors on target cells, resulting in hyperglycemia. DM includes type 1, type 2, gestational diabetes, and other specific types such as those found in Cushing's syndrome or those that are chemically induced. Discussion in this chapter is limited to type 1 and type 2 DM and gestational diabetes.

Etiology and Characteristics of Type 1 and Type 2 Diabetes Mellitus

28.2 Type 1 diabetes mellitus is caused by a lack of insulin secretion and is characterized by serious, chronic conditions affecting the cardiovascular and nervous systems. Type 2 DM is caused by a lack of sensitivity of insulin receptors at the target cells and a deficiency in insulin secretion. If untreated, the same chronic conditions result as in type 1 DM.

Type 1 diabetes mellitus was previously called *juvenile-onset diabetes* because it is often diagnosed between the ages of 11 and 13 years. Because the symptoms of type 1 DM can occur for the first time in adulthood, this was not the most accurate name for this disorder. This type of diabetes is also referred to as insulin-dependent DM. Type 1 DM accounts for only 5% to 10% of all cases of diabetes and is one of the most common diseases of childhood. Type 1 DM results from autoimmune destruction of pancreatic beta cells, causing an absolute lack of insulin secretion. The disease is thought to be caused by an interaction of genetic, immunological, and environmental factors. Children and siblings of those with DM have a higher risk of developing the disorder. The signs and symptoms of type 1 DM are consistent from client to client, with the most diagnostic sign being sustained hyperglycemia. The typical signs and symptoms are as follows:

- Hyperglycemia
- Polyuria: excessive urination
- Polyphagia: increased hunger
- Polydipsia: increased thirst
- Glucosuria: high levels of glucose in the urine
- Weight loss
- Fatigue
- Bedwetting in children who previously didn't wet the bed during the night
- Irritability and other mood changes
- Blurred vision

Untreated DM produces long-term damage to arteries, which leads to heart disease, stroke, kidney disease, and blindness. Lack of adequate circulation to the feet may cause gangrene of the toes, which may require amputation. Nerve degeneration is common and produces symptoms ranging from tingling in the fingers or toes to complete loss of sensation of a limb. Because glucose is unable to enter cells, lipids are used as an energy source and **keto acids** are produced as waste products. These keto acids can give the client's breath an acetone-like, fruity odour. More important, high levels of keto acids lower the pH of the blood, causing **diabetic ketoacidosis (DKA)**, which may progress to coma and possible death if untreated.

There are a number of differences between type 1 and type 2 DM. Because **type 2 diabetes mellitus (DM)** usually begins in middle age, it has been referred to as maturity-onset

◀ Pediatric Type 2 Diabetes

The rapid rise in the incidence of type 2 diabetes mellitus (DM) in children is a growing concern for healthcare providers. The disease is reaching epidemic proportions, especially in certain ethnic groups such as Aboriginals and those of African, Hispanic, and Asian descent. Children who develop type 2 diabetes are most often overweight and sedentary. Although insulin and metformin are the two drugs commonly used to treat pediatric type 2 DM, other drugs are sometimes prescribed. Insulin is the most effective agent, although children often respond negatively to daily injections. Metformin (Glucophage) has been shown to be safe and effective in children, although drugs from other classes may need to be added to the regimen over time. The guidelines for pharmacotherapy of pediatric type 2 DM will likely change as research determines the best therapies for this age group.

diabetes. This is an inaccurate description of this disorder, however, because increasing numbers of children are being diagnosed with type 2 DM (see Lifespan Considerations: Pediatric Type 2 Diabetes). Approximately 90% to 95% of all diabetics are type 2. Adults and children who develop type 2 DM are most often overweight and sedentary. Aboriginal children are in a high-risk group for type 2 DM, perhaps because their diets are high in carbohydrates and fats and they may experience higher stress levels.

Unlike in type 1 DM, the pancreas in type 2 DM is capable of secreting insulin, although the amount may be deficient in some clients (see Table 28.2 for a comparison of type 1 and type 2 diabetes). There is a relative deficiency of endogenous insulin. The fundamental problem in type 2 DM is that insulin receptors in the target tissues have become insensitive to the hormone. This phenomenon is referred to as **insulin resistance**. The pancreas may

TABLE 28.2 Comparison of Type 1 and Type 2 Diabetes Mellitus

Diabetes Mellitus	Type 1	Type 2
Cause	Destruction of beta cells with lack of insulin	Insulin resistance; insulin deficiency may develop
Incidence	5–10%	90–95%
Age at onset	Children, young adults, usually younger than 35 years	Usually older than 35 years
Symptom onset	Rapid	Gradual
Body weight	Usually underweight	Usually overweight or obese
Symptoms	Polyuria, polydipsia, polyphagia, weight loss	Same as type 1, plus blurred vision, fatigue, recurrent infections
Ketosis	Often present with poor control	Infrequent
Pharmacological treatment	Insulin replacement	Oral antidiabetes drugs with or without insulin

CONNECTIONS Lifespan Considerations

◀ Pregestational Diabetes

All women with pre-existing type 1 or type 2 diabetes should receive preconception care to optimize glycemic control, assess complications, review medications, and begin folate supplementation. Care by an interdisciplinary diabetes healthcare team composed of diabetes nurse educators, dietitians, obstetricians, and diabetologists, both prior to conception and during pregnancy, has been shown to minimize maternal and fetal risks in women with pre-existing type 1 or type 2 diabetes.

be producing significant amounts of insulin, but the target cells do not recognize it, the insulin binds less effectively to the receptors, and less effect is achieved.

Another important difference is that proper diet and exercise can sometimes increase the sensitivity of insulin receptors to the point that drug therapy is unnecessary for type 2 DM. Eighty percent of people with type 2 DM are obese, and the degree of obesity directly affects the degree of insulin resistance. People with central or visceral obesity are at increased risk for developing insulin resistance and type 2 DM. They will need a medically supervised plan to reduce weight gradually and to exercise safely. This is an important lifestyle change for such clients, and they will need to maintain these changes for a lifetime. Clients with poorly managed type 2 DM often suffer from the same chronic complications as clients with type 1 DM (e.g., retinopathy, neuropathy, and nephropathy).

Insulin

Insulin was discovered in 1921–1922 by Canadian researchers Frederick Banting and Charles Best. Prior to that time, type 1 diabetics were unable to adequately maintain normal blood

CONNECTIONS Lifespan Considerations

◀ Gestational Diabetes Mellitus

The diagnostic criteria for gestational diabetes mellitus (GDM) remain controversial. The preferred approach is to begin with a 50-g glucose challenge test and, if appropriate, proceed with a 75-g oral glucose tolerance test; a diagnosis of GDM can be made if ≥1 value is abnormal (fasting blood glucose ≥5.3 mmol/L, 1-hour postprandial plasma glucose ≥10.6 mmol/L, 2-hour postprandial plasma glucose ≥9.0 mmol/L). The alternative is a one-step approach of a 75-g oral glucose tolerance test; a diagnosis of GDM can be made if ≥1 value is abnormal (fasting blood glucose ≥5.1 mmol/L, 1 hour ≥10.0 mmol/L, 2 hours ≥8.5 mmol/L).

Untreated GDM leads to increased maternal and perinatal morbidity, whereas treatment for GDM is associated with outcomes similar to control populations.

Source: Canadian Diabetes Association Clinical Practice Guidelines Expert Committee. Canadian Diabetes Association 2013 Clinical Practice Guidelines for the Prevention and Management of Diabetes in Canada. *Can J Diabetes* 2013; 37(suppl 1):S1-S212. Page 183. Elsevier.

glucose, experienced many complications, and usually died at a young age. Increased insulin availability and improvements in insulin products, personal blood glucose monitoring devices, and the insulin pump have made it possible for clients to maintain better control of their blood glucose levels. The level of glycosylated hemoglobin (A1C) in the blood may be assessed periodically to estimate overall glucose control across a 3-month period. A1C levels indicate the percentage of hemoglobin to which glucose has become bound, a process referred to as glycosylation. Higher levels of A1C are found in people with persistently elevated blood glucose. As exposure to glucose in the blood increases, the percentage of A1C increases. A target A1C level of less than 7% is desirable to prevent complications.

NCLEX Success Tip

Be aware of the personal impact of managing a complex disease, the impact of finances, and the client's ability to manage his or her disease safely, including which additional supports might be required to maintain safety.

CONNECTIONS Special Considerations

◀ What Does the Diabetes Charter Mean for Canada?

The Diabetes Charter for Canada (the Charter) clearly outlines the support that Canadians with diabetes require to live to their full potential. Commitments within the Charter address the unique needs of people living with diabetes in Canada. For example:

- Canada is home to immigrants from populations at higher risk of type 2 diabetes. The three largest visible minority groups in 2011—South Asians, Chinese, and Blacks—account for 61.3% of the total visible minority population.
- Aboriginal people represent 4.3% of the Canadian population.
  - First Nations people, who make up more than 60% of Aboriginal people in Canada, have prevalence rates three to five times that of non–First Nations populations.
  - The prevalence of diabetes in the Métis population was 7.3%, compared to 5% in the non-Aboriginal population in 2008–2009.
- More than 60% of Canadian adults are overweight or obese.
- Close to one-third (31.5%) of children and adolescents are overweight or obese.
- There are significant variances in the rates of diabetes and prediabetes across Canada, with the highest rates in the Atlantic provinces. The Atlantic provinces also have higher rural populations compared to other provinces in Canada, and accessing care for people with diabetes is more challenging in rural areas than in urban areas.

The Charter outlines the rights of people with diabetes to information, education, and care that take into account a person's culture and language.

Data from Canadian Diabetes Association as of April 15, 2016.

Lifespan Considerations

◀ Gestational Diabetes

Gestational diabetes mellitus (GDM) is a temporary condition that is diagnosed during pregnancy and usually is not present after the post-partum period, approximately 6 weeks after delivery. It affects approximately 2% to 4% of all pregnancies (in the non-Aboriginal population) and involves an increased risk for developing diabetes in both mother and child. Placental lactogen and destruction of maternal insulin by the placenta contribute to GDM by increasing insulin resistance in the mother. The incidence of GDM has been on the rise in the past decade, and many healthcare providers recommend performing glucose tests at about 24 to 28 weeks' gestation to rule out GDM. Following diagnosis of GDM, changes in dietary and exercise habits are implemented. If these changes are ineffective in controlling blood glucose level, the client will be prescribed a regimen of insulin injections. Educate clients about the potential problems to the fetus and to themselves during the pregnancy, labour, birth, and postpartum periods if the treatment prescribed by the healthcare provider is not followed. A child born to a mother diagnosed with GDM has a 40% chance of being obese and developing type 2 DM in later life. The mother has the increased risk of both developing GDM in future pregnancies and developing diabetes herself. Oral antihyperglycemic agents are contraindicated during pregnancy because of their potential teratogenic effects on the fetus.

Data from Canadian Diabetes Association as of April 15, 2016.

Lifespan Considerations

◀ Diabetes in the Geriatric Population

The geriatric population also has specific problems with regard to maintaining a normal blood glucose level. If geriatric clients have been diabetic for most of their lives, they may choose to ignore their recommended therapy because they feel it will make little difference at this time in their lives. Also, elderly clients frequently display cognitive impairment that distorts their judgment and their desire to maintain their prescribed diet. Monitor these clients closely, because diet is a major factor in the control of blood glucose levels. In the frail elderly client, while avoiding symptomatic hyperglycemia, glycemic targets should be A1C ≤8.5% and fasting plasma glucose or preprandial plasma glucose of 5.0 to 12.0 mmol/L, depending on the level of frailty. Prevention of hypoglycemia should take priority over attainment of glycemic targets because the risks of hypoglycemia are magnified in this client population.

Pharmacotherapy with Insulin

28.3 Type 1 DM is treated by dietary restrictions, exercise, and insulin injections. The many types of insulin preparations vary as to their onset of action, time to peak effect, and duration.

Because clients with type 1 DM have a total lack of endogenous insulin secretion, replacement therapy with insulin is required for survival. Insulin requirements vary in response to fluctuations in

blood glucose that occur with daily activities such as exercise, eating, and sleep. The goal of insulin therapy is to prevent long-term complications of diabetes by keeping blood glucose levels within the target ranges, shown in Table 28.3. Therefore, insulin administration is planned in conjunction with current blood glucose level, nutrient intake, and exercise. The fundamental principle of insulin pharmacotherapy is that the right amount of insulin must be available to cells when glucose is present in the blood. Without insulin present, glucose from a meal can build up to high levels in the blood, a condition called hyperglycemia. This situation may occur when a client forgets to administer insulin in conjunction with a meal. Administering insulin when glucose is not available can lead to hypoglycemia and coma. For this reason, insulin is normally withheld when clients are fasting for laboratory tests. Clients are counselled that they must consume food once they have received their insulin. Regular, moderate exercise increases the cellular responsiveness to insulin, lowering the amount of insulin needed to maintain normal blood glucose levels. During heavy, prolonged exercise, such as in competitive sports, individuals may become hypoglycemic and need to consume food or drink to raise their blood glucose to normal levels. Those who regularly engage in

TABLE 28.3 Recommended Glycemic Targets for Clients with Diabetes

Test	Child and Adolescent Type 1 Diabetes		Adult
A1C (%)	<6 years 6–12 years 13–18 years	<8.0 <7.5 <7.0	<7.0
FBG/preprandial PG (mmol/L)	<6 years 6–12 years 13–18 years	6.0–10.0 4.0–10.0 4.0–7.0	4.0–7.0
Two-hour postprandial PG (mmol/L)	<6 years* 6–12 years* 13–18 years	– – 5.0–10.0	5.0–10.0
Considerations	Caution is required to minimize hypoglycemia because of the potential association between severe hypoglycemia and later cognitive impairment. Consider A1C target of <8.5% if excessive hypoglycemia occurs. 　Targets should be graduated to the child's age. Consider A1C target of <8.0% if excessive hypoglycemia occurs. 　Appropriate for most adolescents.†		If an A1C target ≤7.0% cannot be achieved with a postprandial PG target of 5.0–10.0 mmol/L, further postprandial PG lowering to 5.0–8.0 mmol/L should be achieved.

A1C, Glycosylated hemoglobin; *FBG*, fasting blood glucose; *PG*, plasma glucose.

Adolescent = 13–18 years

*Postprandial monitoring is rarely done in young children except for those on pump therapy for whom targets are not available.

†In adolescents in whom it can be safely achieved, consider aiming toward normal PG range (i.e., A1C ≤6%, FBG/preprandial PG 4.0–6.0 mmol/L, and 2-hour postprandial PG 5.0–8.0 mmol/L).

Data from Canadian Diabetes Association as of April 18, 2016.

strenuous activities should eat food or consume a sports drink just prior to commencing the activity, as a preventive measure. Nurses play an important role in educating clients about managing and adhering to their insulin therapy.

Several types of insulin are available, differing in their source, onset, and duration of action. Until the 1980s, the source of all insulin was beef or pork pancreas. However, almost all insulin today is human insulin obtained through recombinant DNA technology. Human insulin can be modified to alter its pharmacokinetics, such as a more rapid onset of action (lispro) or a more prolonged duration of action (glargine). Human insulin is more effective, causes fewer allergies, and has a lower incidence of resistance than animal-source insulin. However, a small number of clients may still use pork insulin (or beef insulin, through a special access program) because they experience hypoglycemia without clearly recognizable symptoms and wide and sudden swings in blood glucose levels when using human insulin. Health Canada monitors adverse effects associated with taking insulin.

Doses and routes of insulin are highly individualized for each client. Some clients may need two or more doses daily. Because the GI tract destroys insulin, insulin must be given by injection. The most common route of administration for insulin is subcutaneous (SC) injection. Some clients have an insulin pump that is programmed to deliver small doses of insulin at predetermined intervals, with larger boluses programmed manually at mealtimes. The pump delivers insulin through a small pliable catheter that is anchored in the subcutaneous tissue of the abdomen. Dry powder insulin for inhalation is now available. Bolus doses are delivered through a special inhalation device. Inhaled insulin may be used as an adjunct to SC or oral antihyperglycemic therapy. The inhalation route is contraindicated in clients with lung disorders. Common insulin preparations are listed in Table 28.4.

The fundamental principle to remember about insulin therapy is that the right amount of insulin must be available to cells when glucose is present in the blood. The primary adverse effect of insulin therapy is hypoglycemia. Symptoms of hypoglycemia occur when a client with type 1 DM has more insulin in the blood than is needed for the amount of circulating blood glucose. This may occur when the insulin level peaks, during exercise, when the client receives too much insulin because of a medication error, or when the client skips a meal. Some of the symptoms of hypoglycemia are the same as those of DKA. Those symptoms that differ and help in determining whether a client is hypoglycemic include pale, cool, and moist skin with blood glucose less than 4 mmol/L and a sudden onset of symptoms. Left untreated, severe hypoglycemia may result in death.

Other adverse effects of insulin include localized allergic reactions at the injection site, generalized urticaria, and swollen lymph glands. Some clients will experience the **Somogyi phenomenon**. This is a rapid decrease in blood glucose, usually during the night, that stimulates the release of hormones that elevate blood glucose (epinephrine, cortisol, and glucagon), resulting in an elevated morning blood glucose level. Additional insulin above the client's normal dose may produce a rapid rebound hypoglycemia.

TABLE 28.4 Insulin Preparations

Type	Onset (How quickly it starts working)	Peak (When it is most effective)	Duration (How long it works)	Timing of Injection (When it should be given)
Bolus insulins				
Rapid-acting analogues aspart (Novorapid), glulisine (Apidra), lispro (Humalog)	10–15 minutes	1–2 hours	3–5 hours	Given with one or more meals per day. To be given 0–15 minutes before or after meals.
Short-acting Humulin R/Novolin ge Toronto	30 minutes	2–3 hours	6.5 hours	Given with one or more meals per day. Should be injected 30–45 minutes before the start of the meal.
Basal insulins				
Intermediate-acting Humulin N/NPH	1–3 hours	5–8 hours	Up to 18 hours	Often started once daily at bedtime. May be given once or twice daily. Not given at any time specific to meals.
Long-acting analogues Glargine (Lantus) Detemir (Levemir)	90 minutes	Not applicable	Lantus: Up to 24 hours Levemir: 16–24 hours	Often started once daily at bedtime. Levemir may be given once or twice daily. Not given at any time specific to meals.
Premixed insulins				
Premixed regular insulin Humulin 30/70 and Novolin ge 30/70, 40/60, 50/50	Varies according to types of insulin	Contains a fixed ratio of insulin (% of rapid-acting or short-acting insulin to % of intermediate-acting insulin). See above for information on peak actions based on insulin contained.		Given with one or more meals per day. Should be injected 30–45 minutes before the start of the meal.
Premixed insulin analogues NovoMix 30 and Humalog Mix 25, Mix 50	Varies according to types of insulin			Given with one or more meals per day. Should be injected 0–15 minutes before or after meals.

Canadian Diabetes Association as of April 18, 2016 http://www.diabetes.ca/diabetes-and-you/healthy-living-resources/blood-glucose-insulin/getting-started-with-insulin. Used by permission.

The hormone glucagon may be administered as an emergency replacement therapy for diabetic clients when they are in a hypoglycemic state and have impaired glucagon secretion. Glucagon (1 mg) may be given by intravenous (IV), intramuscular (IM), or SC route to reverse hypoglycemic symptoms in 20 minutes or less, depending on the route. Prefilled 50-mL syringes of dextrose 50% in water (D50W) for IV infusion are commonly available to treat hypoglycemia in hospitalized clients. Agency guidelines for D50W infusion must be followed.

Nursing Considerations

The role of the nurse in insulin therapy involves careful monitoring of the client's condition and providing education as it relates to the prescribed drug treatment. Be familiar with the onset, peak, and duration of action of the prescribed insulin (see Table 28.4) as well as any other important aspects of the specific insulin, and convey this information to the client.

Assess the client for signs and symptoms of hypoglycemia as well as the adequacy of glucose monitoring. Hypoglycemia is most likely to occur when insulin reaches its peak effect or during exercise or acute illness. Obtain food for the client and determine that the client is ready to eat before administering insulin. Insulin is normally withheld when clients are fasting for tests or procedures. Assess the client's level of understanding of the symptoms of insulin reaction, hypoglycemia, and DKA. Teach the client to recognize key symptoms and what action to take in response to them. Contraindications to insulin include sensitivity to an ingredient in the formulation and hypoglycemia that would be worsened by administration of insulin. Use insulin with caution in pregnant clients and in those with severe stress or infection. Clients with these conditions usually have increased insulin requirements and must be monitored more carefully.

Two of the most frequently prescribed types of insulin are NPH and regular insulin. Intermediate or NPH insulin is used to provide a longer-acting source of insulin compared with regular insulin and other types of short-acting insulin. NPH insulin is normally administered 30 minutes before the first meal of the day, but in some instances a second, smaller dose is taken before the evening meal or at bedtime. Some clients are prescribed insulin that is premixed, such as 70% NPH with 30% regular or rapid-acting insulin. If the client is prescribed a premixed insulin solution, it is important that proper instruction be given, especially if the client will be using additional regular or rapid-acting insulin on a sliding scale.

In some circumstances, regular insulin may be given by the IV route, but other types of insulin, including NPH, are to be given only as SC injections. Intermediate insulin cannot be given by the IV route. Rapid-acting insulin lispro (Humalog) is being used more frequently. Its onset of action is 10 to 15 minutes, which is much faster than the onset of 30 to 60 minutes associated with regular insulin. The peak effect of rapid-acting insulin lispro occurs in 30 to 60 minutes, and its duration of action is 5 hours or less. It is often used with insulin infusion pumps.

Insulin glargine (Lantus) is a recombinant human insulin analogue. It must not be mixed in the syringe with any other insulin and must be administered via SC injection. Insulin glargine exhibits a constant, long-duration hypoglycemic effect with no defined peak. It is prescribed once daily, at bedtime.

Long-acting insulin is prescribed for some clients. Protamine zinc insulin (PZI) has an onset of 4 to 8 hours, a peak of 14 to 24 hours, and a duration of 36 hours. Extended insulin zinc suspension has an onset of 4 to 6 hours, a peak of 10 to 30 hours, and a duration of 36 hours. A premixed insulin, Novolin Mix (70/30), has an onset of 4 to 8 hours, a peak of 16 to 18 hours, and a duration greater than 36 hours. Insulins that are available in Canada are listed with their onset of action, peak effects, and duration of action in Table 28.4.

When administering insulin, ensure that the units on the syringe match the units on the insulin vial. For example, when U-100 insulin is ordered, the vial must be U-100 and the syringe must also be calibrated for U-100. Although U-100 is the most frequently used strength of insulin, U-500 is available for clients who have developed insulin resistance and need a much higher dose to manage their blood glucose. When U-500 insulin is given, a syringe calibrated for U-500 is necessary. It is also imperative to understand that not all types of insulin are compatible and may not be mixed together in a single syringe. Clear insulin must be drawn into the syringe first to reduce the possible contamination of the clear insulin by an insulin containing a suspension.

Client education at it relates to insulin therapy should include goals, reasons for obtaining baseline data such as vital signs, the existence of underlying hypoglycemic disorders, and possible drug side effects. Include the following points when teaching clients about insulin therapy:

- Closely monitor blood glucose before each meal and before insulin administration, as directed by the healthcare provider.
- Always carry a source of simple sugar in case of hypoglycemic reactions. If blood glucose is less than 4 mmol/L, take a fast-acting carbohydrate (15-g glucose tablets, 3 tsp sugar, or 1/2 cup orange juice). Repeat in 15 minutes if blood glucose level is still less than 4 mmol/L. If there is more than 1 hour until the next meal, eat a snack of a starch and protein (cheese and 6 crackers, or half of a peanut butter sandwich).
- Immediately report nervousness, confusion, excessive sweating, rapid pulse, or tremors because these are signs of overdosage (hypoglycemia).
- Immediately report increased thirst or urine output, decreased appetite, or excessive fatigue because these are signs of underdosage (hyperglycemia).
- When in doubt about whether symptoms indicate hypoglycemia or hyperglycemia, treat for hypoglycemia. Hypoglycemia progresses rapidly, whereas hyperglycemia progresses slowly.
- Rotate insulin sites to prevent lipodystrophy.
- Do not inject insulin into areas that are raised, swollen, dimpled, or itching.
- Keep insulin vials that are currently in use at room temperature because insulin at that temperature is less irritating to skin and helps to prevent lipodystrophy.
- When not needed, refrigerate insulin to keep it stable.
- Strictly follow the prescribed diet (e.g., calorie restrictions, food exchanges, carbohydrate counting) unless otherwise instructed.
- Wear a MedicAlert bracelet to alert emergency personnel of DM. Notify caregivers, co-workers, and others who may be able to render assistance.

- Use only an insulin syringe calibrated to the same strength as the insulin.
- Use only the type of insulin prescribed by the healthcare provider.

NCLEX Success Tip

Teaching and learning are important components. Be aware of all the content that clients with diabetes must clearly understand in order to demonstrate safety in managing their disease. These types of questions often require the writer to identify the gap in knowledge of the person being taught.

PROTOTYPE DRUG	Regular Insulin (Humulin R, Novolin ge Toronto)

Actions and Uses: Regular insulin is prepared from pork pancreas or as human insulin through recombinant DNA technology. It is classified as short-acting insulin, with an onset of 30 to 60 minutes, a peak effect in 2 to 3 hours, and a duration of 5 to 7 hours. Its primary action is to promote the entry of glucose into cells. For the emergency treatment of acute ketoacidosis, it may be given by the SC or IV route. Regular insulin is also available as Humulin 70/30 (a mixture of 30% regular insulin and 70% insulin NPH) or as Humulin 50/50 (a mixture of 50% of both regular and insulin NPH).

Administration Alerts:

- Hypoglycemic reactions may occur quickly if regular insulin is not supported by sufficient food or is given when the client is hypoglycemic.
- Regular insulin is the only type of insulin that may be used for IV injection.
- Injection sites must be rotated. When the client is hospitalized, use sites not normally used while the client is at home.
- Insulin is administered approximately 30 minutes before meals so it will be absorbed and available when the client begins to eat.
- Regular insulin is pregnancy category B.

Pharmacokinetics: Regular insulin is rapidly absorbed from SC tissue. It is widely distributed. It is metabolized in the liver, spleen, kidney, and muscle. The half-life of insulin in diabetes is 1.5 hours.

Adverse Effects and Interactions: The most serious adverse effect of insulin therapy is hypoglycemia. Hypoglycemia may result from taking too much insulin, not timing the insulin injection properly with food intake, or skipping a meal. Dietary carbohydrates must have reached the blood when insulin is injected; otherwise, the drug will remove too much glucose and signs of hypoglycemia—tachycardia, confusion, sweating, and drowsiness—will ensue. If severe hypoglycemia is not treated quickly with glucose, convulsions, coma, and death may follow.

Regular insulin interacts with many drugs. For example, the following substances may potentiate hypoglycemic effects: alcohol, salicylates, monoamine oxidase (MAO) inhibitors, and anabolic steroids. The following substances may antagonize hypoglycemic effects: corticosteroids, thyroid hormones, and epinephrine.

Serum glucose levels may be increased with furosemide (Lasix) or thiazide diuretics. Symptoms of hypoglycemic reaction may be masked with beta-adrenergic blockers.

Use with caution with herbal supplements, such as garlic and ginseng, which may potentiate the hypoglycemic effects of insulin.

NCLEX Success Tip

Consider the implications of the peak, duration, and action of the variety of insulins and the appropriate nursing interventions. Understand the effects of other medications on blood glucose levels and the potential for signs and symptoms of hypoglycemia and hyperglycemia.

CONNECTIONS ◖ Lifespan Considerations

◂ Psychosocial Impacts on the Young Diabetic

For the child or adolescent who has diabetes, there are psychosocial and cultural considerations of adherence to medication and dietary regimens. Even if diagnosed early in life (with learned behaviours regarding the disease parameters), the elementary school years can be difficult for some children with diabetes. Social events such as birthday parties, field trips, and after-school snack time, where sweet treats are the norm, serve as a physical and psychological temptation. During adolescence, when the teenager wants to fit in with a peer group, the diabetic treatment can become more difficult. It is during this time that failure to take insulin or to follow dietary guidelines becomes an issue that may negatively affect present and future health. Some teens may have insulin pumps and can more easily take extra insulin to cover foods not usually on their diet. The ability to do this helps teens to feel less different from their peers, but when carried to excess this practice can also lead to problems. The nurse plays a vital role in educating the client and family and in making referrals to community agencies that may assist in helping the young person to keep blood sugar in control while preserving self-esteem.

CONNECTIONS ◖ Special Considerations

◂ Carbohydrate Counting: Flexible Carbohydrate Plan

Carbohydrate counting provides meal flexibility while improving A1C levels. In carbohydrate counting, the insulin dose is adjusted based on carbohydrate content: the more carbohydrates, the more rapid the absorption rate and the more insulin that will be required. The client is prescribed an insulin-to-carbohydrate ratio. At every meal, the client counts carbohydrates and adjusts the insulin dose. For example, if the client is having two slices of bread, and one slice of bread is 15 g of carbohydrate requiring 1 unit of insulin, 2 units of rapid-acting insulin are required.

The client is also prescribed a *correction factor*. Clients with diabetes do not always achieve their before-meal target glucose level of 6 mmol/L. If blood glucose is 12 mmol/L before a meal, for example, the correction factor is applied. If the prescribed correction factor is to increase the insulin dose by 1 unit for every 3 mmol/L above the target glucose level, the client would inject an additional 2 units of insulin at that mealtime.

NURSING PROCESS FOCUS

Clients Receiving Insulin Therapy

Assessment	Potential Nursing Diagnoses and Identified Patterns
Prior to administration: • Obtain complete health history, including allergies, drug history, and possible drug interactions. • Assess vital signs. If the client has a fever or elevated pulse, assess further to determine the cause because infection can alter the amount of insulin required. • Assess blood glucose level. • Assess appetite and presence of symptoms that indicate the client may not be able to consume or retain the next meal. • Assess subcutaneous areas for potential insulin injection sites. • Assess knowledge of insulin and ability to self-administer insulin.	• Impaired sensory perception (neuropathy) related to complications of diabetes • Risk for impaired skin integrity • Need for knowledge regarding drug therapy • Risk for fluid imbalance • Risk for infection related to blood glucose elevations and impaired circulation • Risk for injury (hypoglycemia) related to adverse effects of drug therapy • Need for knowledge and skills for self-injection • Need for knowledge related to dietary modifications (e.g., carbohydrate counting)

Planning: Client Goals and Expected Outcomes

The client will:

• Immediately report irritability, dizziness, diaphoresis, hunger, behaviour changes, and changes in level of consciousness (LOC)
• Demonstrate ability to self-administer insulin
• Demonstrate an understanding of lifestyle and dietary modifications necessary for successful maintenance of drug therapy
• Describe management of emergencies (hypoglycemia and hyperglycemia)

Implementation

Interventions (Rationales)	Client Education and Discharge Planning
• Increase frequency of blood glucose monitoring if the client is experiencing fever, nausea, vomiting, or diarrhea. (Illness usually requires adjustments in insulin doses.) • Check urine for ketones if blood glucose is more than 14 mmol/L. (Ketones will spill into the urine at this glucose level and provide an early sign of diabetic ketoacidosis.) • Monitor weight on a routine basis. (Changes in weight will alter insulin needs.) • Monitor vital signs. (Increased pulse and blood pressure are early signs of hypoglycemia. Clients with diabetes may have circulatory problems and/or impaired kidney function that can increase blood pressure.) • Monitor potassium level. (Insulin causes potassium to move into the cell and may cause hypokalemia.) • Check blood glucose and feed client some form of simple sugar at the first sign of hypoglycemia. (Using a simple sugar will raise blood sugar immediately.)	• Instruct client to increase blood glucose monitoring when experiencing fever, nausea, vomiting, or diarrhea Teach client: • When and how to check urine for glucose and ketones • That ketoacidosis normally develops slowly but is a serious problem that needs to be corrected • Instruct client to weigh self on a routine basis at the same time each day and to report significant changes • Teach client how to take blood pressure and pulse and to report significant changes, such as the first sign of heart irregularity • Instruct client to report the first sign of heart irregularity Advise client: • To check blood glucose and eat a simple sugar at the first sign of hypoglycemia; if symptoms do not improve, call 911 • Not to skip meals and to follow a diet specified by the healthcare provider • That exercise may increase insulin needs • To check blood glucose before and after exercise and to keep a simple sugar nearby while exercising • Before strenuous exercise, to eat some form of simple sugar or complex carbohydrate as a prophylaxis against hypoglycemia

Evaluation of Outcome Criteria

The client will:

• Have no report or symptoms of irritability, dizziness, diaphoresis, hunger, behaviour changes, and changes in LOC
• Demonstrate ability to self-administer insulin
• Demonstrate ability and understanding of lifestyle and dietary modifications necessary for successful maintenance of drug therapy
• Correctly describe management of emergencies (hypoglycemia and hyperglycemia)

See Table 28.6 for a list of drugs to which these nursing actions apply.

Pharmacotherapy with Oral Antihyperglycemics

28.4 Type 2 DM is controlled through lifestyle changes and oral antihyperglycemic drugs.

Type 2 DM is often controlled with oral antihyperglycemic agents, which are prescribed after diet and exercise have failed to reduce blood glucose to normal levels. Insulin also may be necessary for type 2 diabetics who are unable to take or are unresponsive to oral agents. Insulin is commonly required temporarily by type 2 diabetics at times of increased stress such as surgery, illness, or loss.

All oral antihyperglycemics have the common action of lowering blood glucose levels when taken on a regular basis. Antihyperglycemics are sometimes referred to as oral hypoglycemics, although this term is less accurate because the goal of therapy is to lower glucose to normal levels, never to induce hypoglycemia. Many antihyperglycemics have the potential to cause hypoglycemia; therefore, periodic laboratory tests are conducted to monitor blood glucose levels. Oral antihyperglycemics are not effective for type 1 DM. The different classes of oral antihyperglycemics are listed in Table 28.5, and Table 28.6 details the different oral antihyperglycemic drugs and their routes of administration, doses, and adverse effects.

Classification of oral antihyperglycemic drugs is based on their chemical structure and mechanism of action. The six classes of oral antihyperglycemic medications used for type 2 DM are sulfonylureas, biguanides, thiazolidinediones, alpha-glucosidase inhibitors, meglitinides, and incretin enhancers. Therapy is usually initiated with a single agent. If therapeutic goals are not achieved with monotherapy, two agents are administered concurrently. Failure to achieve normal blood glucose levels with two oral antihyperglycemics usually indicates a need for insulin.

Type 2 diabetics may be advised to maintain a preprandial blood glucose level at or just below 6.0 mmol/L. In healthy persons, the beta cells secrete insulin in response to small increases in blood glucose, which is referred to as an *acute insulin response.* This response is diminished at 6.4 mmol/L, and the higher the glucose level the less likely it is that the beta cells will respond by

secreting insulin. Because clients with type 2 DM need to secrete some insulin, keeping the blood glucose level below 6.0 mmol/L before meals optimizes the secretion of insulin. Management of blood glucose levels is individualized and takes into account the client's response to treatment.

Clients with type 2 DM need to recognize the symptoms of **hyperosmolar nonketotic coma (HNKC)**, which is a life-threatening emergency. As with the onset of DKA in those with type 1 DM, HNKC develops slowly and is caused by insufficient circulating insulin. It is seen most often in older adults. The skin appears flushed, dry, and warm, as in DKA. Unlike DKA, HNKC does not affect breathing. Blood glucose levels may rise above 50 mmol/L and reach 100 mmol/L. HNKC has a higher mortality rate than DKA.

NCLEX Success Tip

As you work through the oral antihyperglycemic medications, be aware of the action of the medication—where does it do its work? This will help you to recall potential adverse effects. For example, any medication that triggers the pancreas to secrete more insulin will place the client at risk for hypoglycemia.

Note: Not all agents cause the pancreas to secrete more insulin; therefore hypoglycemia with some agents is very rare (whereas with others it is more common).

Sulfonylureas

The sulfonylureas were the first oral antihyperglycemics available, and they are divided into first- and second-generation categories. Although drugs from both generations are equally effective at lowering blood glucose, the second-generation drugs exhibit fewer drug-drug interactions. The sulfonylureas act by stimulating the release of insulin from pancreatic islet cells and by increasing the sensitivity of insulin receptors on target cells. The most common adverse effect of sulfonylureas is hypoglycemia, which is usually caused by taking too much medication or not eating enough food. Persistent hypoglycemia from these agents may be prolonged and may require administration of dextrose to

---

TABLE 28.5   Summary of Antidiabetic Drug Classes

Drug	Action(s)	Nursing Considerations
Alpha-glucosidase inhibitors	Interferes with carbohydrate breakdown and absorption; acts locally in GI tract with little systemic absorption	Common GI effects; hypoglycemia can occur if combined with another oral drug; if this occurs, treat with glucose, not sucrose; take with meals
Biguanides	Decreases production and release of glucose from the liver; increases cellular uptake of glucose; lowers lipid levels; promotes weight loss	Common GI adverse effects; risk for lactic acidosis (rare); avoid alcohol; low risk for hypoglycemia
Incretin enhancers	Slows the breakdown of insulin, keeping it circulating in the blood longer; slows the rate of digestion, which increases satiety	Well tolerated; minor nausea, vomiting, and diarrhea; some weight loss is likely; low risk for hypoglycemia
Meglitinides	Stimulates insulin release	Can cause hypoglycemia, GI effects; well tolerated; administer shortly before meals
Sulfonylureas	Stimulates insulin release; decreases insulin resistance	Can cause hypoglycemia, GI disturbances, rash; cross sensitivity with sulfa drugs and thiazide diuretics; possible disulfiram response with alcohol
Thiazolidinediones	Decreases production and release of glucose from the liver; increases insulin sensitivity in fat and muscle tissue	Can cause fluid retention and worsening of heart failure; therapeutic effects take several weeks to develop

TABLE 28.6 Antidiabetic Drugs for Type 2 Diabetes

Drug	Route and Adult Dose (Maximum Dose Where Indicated)	Adverse Effects
Alpha-Glucosidase Inhibitors		
acarbose (Glucobay)	Orally (PO), start with 50 mg once daily with the first bite of a main meal; increase dosage to 50 mg bid after a few weeks to usual dosage of 50 mg tid (max 300 mg/day)	*Flatulence, diarrhea, abdominal distention* Hypoglycemia (tremors, palpitations, sweating)
Biguanides		
metformin immediate release (Glucophage) extended release (Glucophage XR, Glumetza)	PO, 500 mg 2 times/day or 850 mg once daily; increase to 1000–2550 mg in two to three divided doses/day (max 2.55 g/day) Glumetza: 500 mg/day; dosage may be increased by 500 mg weekly (max 2 g/day) Glucophage XR: 500 mg once daily (max 2 g/day)	*Flatulence, diarrhea, nausea, anorexia, abdominal pain, bitter or metallic taste, decreased vitamin B_{12} levels* Lactic acidosis
Incretin Enhancers (GLP-1 Agonists)		
albiglutide (Tanzeum)	Subcutaneous (SC), 30–50 mg once weekly	*Nausea, vomiting, diarrhea, headache, nervousness* Hypoglycemia (tremors, palpitations, sweating), antibody formation, pancreatitis (exenatide), renal impairment (exenatide), thyroid tumours (liraglutide, albiglutide)
exenatide (Byetta)	SC, 5–10 mcg 2 times/day 60 minutes prior to morning and evening meals	
dulaglutide (Trulicity)	SC, 0.75–1.5 mg once weekly	
liraglutide (Victoza)	SC, 0.6–1.8 mg once daily, any time of day	
Incretin Enhancers (DPP-4 Inhibitors)		
alogliptin (Nesina)	PO, 25 mg once daily	*Headache, upper respiratory and urinary tract infections* Hypoglycemia (tremors, palpitations, sweating), anaphylaxis, peripheral edema, exfoliative dermatitis, Stevens–Johnson syndrome
linagliptin (Tradjenta)	PO, 5 mg once daily	
saxagliptin (Onglyza)	PO, 2.5–5 mg once daily	
sitagliptin (Januvia)	PO, 100 mg once daily	
Meglitinides		
nateglinide (Starlix)	PO, 60–120 mg tid, 1–30 minutes prior to meals	*Flulike symptoms, upper respiratory infection, back pain* Hypoglycemia (tremors, palpitations, sweating), anaphylaxis, pancreatitis
repaglinide (GlucoNorm)	PO, 0.5–4 mg twice to four times daily (bid–qid), 1–30 minutes prior to meals (max 16 mg/day)	
Sulfonylureas, First Generation		
chlorpropamide (Diabinese)	PO, 100–500 mg/day (max 750 mg/day)	*Nausea, heartburn, dizziness, headache, drowsiness* Hypoglycemia (tremors, palpitations, sweating), cholestatic jaundice, blood dyscrasias
tolbutamide (Orinase)	PO, 250–1500 mg 1–2 times/day (max 3 g/day)	
Sulfonylureas, Second Generation		
glimepiride (Amaryl)	PO, 1–4 mg/day (max 8 mg/day)	*Nausea, heartburn, dizziness, headache, drowsiness* Hypoglycemia (tremors, palpitations, sweating), cholestatic jaundice, blood dyscrasias
gliclazide (Diamicron)	IR (immediate release), start with 80 mg bid; usual dosage range is 80-320 mg/day; doses > 160 mg should be divided into two doses (max 320 mg/day) MR (modified release), start with 30 mg qd (max 120 mg/day)	
glyburide (DiaBeta)	PO, 1.25–10 mg 1–2 times/day (max 20 mg/day)	
Thiazolidinediones		
pioglitazone (Actos)	PO: 15–30 mg/day (max: 45 mg/day)	*Upper respiratory infection, myalgia, headache, edema, weight gain* Hypoglycemia (tremors, palpitations, sweating), hepatotoxicity, bone fractures, heart failure, myocardial infarction
rosiglitazone (Avandia)	PO: 4–8 mg 1–2 times/day (max: 8 mg/day)	
Miscellaneous Drugs		
canagliflozin (Invokana)	PO, 100 mg once daily (max 300 mg/day) taken before first meal	*Female genital mycotic infections, urinary tract infection, and nasopharyngitis* Hypotension, renal impairment, hyperkalemia, hypoglycemia
dapagliflozin (Farxiga)	PO, 5–10 mg once daily in the morning, with or without food	
empagliflozin (Jardiance)	PO, 10–25 mg once daily in the morning, with or without food	

Note: Italics indicates common adverse effects. Underline indicates serious adverse effects.

return glucose to normal levels. Other side effects include weight gain, hypersensitivity reactions, GI distress, and hepatotoxicity. When alcohol is taken with these agents, some clients experience a serious disulfiram (Antabuse)-like reaction, including flushing, angina, palpitations, vertigo, and nausea. Serious reactions, such as seizures and possibly death, also may occur. Clients with diabetes who take any first- or second-generation sulfonylurea should be advised to avoid alcohol intake.

Sulfonylureas should be used with caution in elderly people with type 2 DM because the risk of hypoglycemia increases exponentially with age. In general, initial doses of sulfonylureas used for elderly clients should be half of those used for younger people, and doses should be increased more slowly (Canadian Diabetes Association, 2016).

NCLEX Success Tip

A client with diabetes who takes any first- or second-generation sulfonylurea should be advised to avoid alcohol intake. Sulfonylureas in combination with alcohol can cause serious disulfiram-like reactions, including flushing, angina, palpitations, and vertigo. Serious reactions, such as seizures and possibly death, may also occur.

Biguanides

Metformin, the only drug in this class, acts by decreasing the hepatic production of glucose (gluconeogenesis) and reducing insulin resistance. It does not promote insulin release from the pancreas. Most side effects are minor and GI related, such as anorexia, nausea, and diarrhea. Unlike the sulfonylureas, metformin does not cause hypoglycemia or weight gain. Rarely, metformin has been reported to cause lactic acidosis in clients with impaired liver function because of accumulation of the medication in the liver.

NCLEX Success Tips

The nurse should verify that the physician has requested to withhold the metformin prior to any procedure requiring dye, such as a cardiac catheterization, due to the increased risk of lactic acidosis. Metformin will usually be withheld for up to 48 hours following a procedure involving dye while it clears the client's system. The physician may prescribe sliding scale insulin during this time, if needed.

Metformin is currently approved by the FDA and Health Canada to treat type 2 diabetes in children. Other oral medications used to treat diabetes augments insulin production or decreases carbohydrate absorption, but those medications are primarily used in adults.

When taken in combination with ACE inhibitors, metformin commonly causes hypoglycemia.

Lactic acidosis is a rare but serious adverse effect of metformin when combined with alcohol use. Ideally, one should stop metformin for 2 days before and 2 days after drinking alcohol. Signs and symptoms of lactic acidosis are weakness, fatigue, unusual muscle pain, dyspnea, unusual stomach discomfort, dizziness or lightheadedness, and bradycardia or cardiac arrhythmias.

Metformin works by decreasing the production of glucose in the liver and improving insulin sensitivity. These two mechanisms reduce insulin and blood glucose level. Reducing insulin levels reduces androgens and helps to restore menstruation.

Before metformin begins, and at least annually thereafter, assess the client's renal function; if renal impairment is detected, a different antidiabetic agent may be indicated.

A black box warning for metformin is to instruct the client to stop the drug and immediately notify the prescriber about unexplained hyperventilation, muscle pain, malaise, dizziness, lightheadedness, unusual sleepiness, unexplained stomach pain, feelings of coldness, slow or irregular heart rate, or other nonspecific symptoms of early lactic acidosis.

Alpha-Glucosidase Inhibitors

The alpha-glucosidase inhibitors, such as acarbose (Glucobay), act by blocking enzymes in the small intestine responsible for breaking down complex carbohydrates into monosaccharides. Because carbohydrates must be in the monosaccharide form to be absorbed, digestion of glucose is delayed. These agents are usually well tolerated and have minimal side effects. The most common side effects are GI related, such as abdominal cramping, diarrhea, and flatulence. Liver function should be monitored, as a small incidence of liver impairment has been reported. Although alpha-glucosidase inhibitors do not produce hypoglycemia when used alone, hypoglycemia may occur when these agents are combined with insulin or a sulfonylurea. Concurrent use of garlic and ginseng may increase the hypoglycemic action of alpha-glucosidase inhibitors.

NCLEX Success Tip

The client indicates a need for additional teaching if the client has hypoglycemia and states that he or she will eat sugar. Acarbose delays glucose absorption. So, when treating hypoglycemia, the client should take an oral form of dextrose rather than a product containing table sugar. The alpha-glucosidase inhibitors work by delaying carbohydrate digestion and glucose absorption, not by stimulating the pancreas to release more insulin. It's safe for the client to be on a regimen that includes insulin and an alpha-glucosidase inhibitor. The client should take the drug at the start of a meal.

Thiazolidinediones

The thiazolidinediones, or glitazones, reduce blood glucose by decreasing insulin resistance and inhibiting hepatic gluconeogenesis. Optimal lowering of blood glucose may take 3 to 4 months of therapy. The most common adverse effects are fluid retention, headache, and weight gain. Hypoglycemia does not occur with drugs in this class. Liver function should be monitored because thiazolidinediones may be hepatotoxic. One such drug, troglitazone (Rezulin), was withdrawn from the market because of drug-related deaths due to hepatic failure. Because of their tendency to promote fluid retention, thiazolidinediones are contraindicated in clients with serious heart failure or pulmonary edema. Rosiglitazone (Avandia) has been associated with a significant increase in heart attack and cardiovascular death.

Meglitinides

The meglitinides are a newer class of oral antihyperglycemic that act by stimulating the release of insulin from pancreatic islet cells in a manner similar to that of the sulfonylureas. Both agents in this class have a short a duration of action of 2 to 4 hours. Their efficacy is equal to that of the sulfonylureas, and they are well tolerated. Hypoglycemia is the most common adverse effect.

Incretin Enhancers

The incretins are hormones secreted by the intestine in response to a meal, when blood glucose is elevated. Incretins signal the pancreas to increase insulin secretion and the liver to stop producing glucagon. Both of these actions lower blood glucose levels. Diabetic clients are unable to secrete incretins in adequate amounts, thus disrupting an important glucose control mechanism. Drugs may be used to modify the incretin system in diabetics in two ways: by mimicking the actions of incretins or by reducing their destruction.

Glucagon-like peptide-1 (GLP-1) agonists are an example of a drug that influences incretin release. Their actions include increasing the amount of insulin secreted by the pancreas, decreasing the amount of glucagon secreted by the pancreas, delaying gastric emptying, and increasing satiety.

Dipeptidyl peptidase-4 (DDP-4) inhibitors reduce the destruction of incretins by inhibiting the DDP-4 enzyme, whose normal function is to break down incretins. Levels of incretin hormones increase, thus decreasing blood glucose levels in clients with type 2 diabetes.

Sodium-glucose cotransporter-2 (SGLT2) inhibitors are a newer class of antihyperglycemics that were approved by Health Canada in 2014. They allow more glucose to leave the blood and be excreted in urine. These drugs have the advantage of promoting weight loss. They are contraindicated in clients with severe renal impairment. The added glucose in the urine serves as a substrate for bacterial and fungal growth.

Pramlintide (Symlin) is a new injectable drug for type 1 and type 2 DM that resembles human amylin, a hormone produced by the pancreas after meals that helps the body to regulate blood glucose. Pramlintide slows the absorption of glucose and inhibits the action of glucagon. Pramlintide lowers blood glucose levels and promotes weight loss.

Because various oral antihyperglycemics work by different mechanisms to lower blood sugar and have different pharmacokinetic properties, combinations of antidiabetic agents have been developed to maximize therapeutic effects and minimize adverse effects. One such combination drug is sitagliptin and metformin (Janumet). The nurse can monitor the Drug Product Database and MedEffect Canada on Health Canada's website to identify drugs in these classes that have been approved, received warnings, or been withdrawn from the market. In addition, periodically reviewing the Canadian Diabetes Association website will inform the nurse of new therapies and recommendations.

NCLEX Success Tip

Understand the unique action and adverse effects of each of the classes of antihyperglycemics as they relate to the client across the drug lifespan and the related lab values.

Nursing Considerations

The role of the nurse in oral antihyperglycemic therapy involves carefully assessing and monitoring the client's condition and providing education as it relates to the prescribed drug treatment. Assessment of the client with type 2 diabetes includes a physical examination, health history, psychosocial history, and lifestyle history. A thorough assessment is needed because diabetes can affect multiple body systems. Psychosocial factors and lifestyle, as well as the knowledge base regarding diabetes, can affect the client's ability to keep his or her blood glucose within the normal range.

Lifestyle factors and health history help to determine the type of drug to be prescribed.

Provide clients with information about the importance of keeping blood glucose levels within the target range. Target blood levels are shown in Table 28.3. Blood glucose should be monitored daily. Urinary ketones should be monitored during periods of acute illness and when blood glucose is higher than 14.0 mmol/L. Urine ketone test strips remain the most commonly used method for ketone testing; however, this method may provide false-positive or false-negative results. Monitor intake and output and review laboratory studies for liver function abnormalities. Monitor the client for signs and symptoms of illness or infection, as illness can affect the client's medication needs. These drugs should be used cautiously in those with impaired renal and hepatic function and in those who are malnourished, because these conditions interfere with absorption and metabolism of the oral antihyperglycemics. Caution should be exercised in clients with pituitary or adrenal disorders because hormones from these sources affect blood glucose levels. Oral antihyperglycemics are contraindicated in clients with hypersensitivity, ketoacidosis, and diabetic coma. They are also contraindicated in clients who are pregnant or lactating, as their safety has not been established and these drugs may be secreted in breast milk.

Oral antihyperglycemics should be taken as directed by the prescriber. Some oral antidiabetic drugs are given 30 minutes before breakfast so that the drug will have reached the plasma when the client begins to eat.

Client education as it relates to oral antihyperglycemic drugs should include goals, importance of diet and exercise, reasons for obtaining baseline data such as vital signs and cardiac and renal function tests, and recognition of symptoms of hypoglycemia. Include the following points when teaching clients about oral antihyperglycemics:

- Always carry a source of simple sugar in case of hypoglycemic reactions. If blood glucose is less than 4 mmol/L, take a fast-acting carbohydrate (15-g glucose tablets, 1/2 cup orange juice). Repeat in 15 minutes if blood glucose levels are still less than 4 mmol/L. If there is more than 1 hour until the next meal, eat a snack of a starch and protein (cheese and 6 crackers, half of a peanut butter sandwich).

- Wear a MedicAlert bracelet to alert emergency personnel to the diabetes. Notify caregivers, co-workers, and others who may be able to render assistance.

- Avoid the use of alcohol to avoid a disulfiram-like reaction.

- Maintain a specified diet and exercise plan while on antidiabetic drugs.

- Swallow tablets whole and do not crush sustained-release tablets.

- Take medication 30 minutes before breakfast, or as directed by the healthcare provider.

- Immediately report nervousness, confusion, excessive sweating, rapid pulse, or tremors because these are signs of overdosage (hypoglycemia).

- Immediately report increased thirst or urine output, decreased appetite, or excessive fatigue because these are signs of underdosage (hyperglycemia).

CONNECTIONS Natural Therapies

◀ Stevia for Hyperglycemia

Stevia (*Stevia rebaudiana*) is an herb indigenous to Paraguay that may be helpful to diabetics. The powdered extract is readily available as a food supplement and can be used in place of sugar. Its sweetening power is 300 times that of sugar, but it does not appear to have a negative effect on blood glucose or insulin secretion. In animal experiments, stevia significantly elevated the glucose clearance, an effect that may be beneficial to diabetics. Encourage all diabetic clients to discuss this supplement and other herbal products with a healthcare provider before taking them.

NCLEX Success Tip

Like other oral antidiabetic agents ordered in a single daily dose, glyburide should be taken with breakfast. If the client takes glyburide later, such as in mid-morning, after dinner, or at bedtime, the drug won't provide adequate coverage for all meals consumed during the day.

PROTOTYPE DRUG Glyburide (DiaBeta)

Actions and Uses: Glyburide is a second-generation sulfonylurea offering the advantages of higher potency, once-a-day dosing, fewer side effects, and fewer drug-drug interactions than some of the first-generation drugs in this class. Glyburide stimulates the pancreas to secrete more insulin and also increases the sensitivity of insulin receptors at target tissues. Some degree of pancreatic function is required for glyburide to lower blood glucose. Maximum effects are achieved if the drug is taken 30 minutes prior to the first meal of the day.

Administration Alerts:

- Sustained-release tablets must be swallowed whole and not crushed or chewed.
- Sulfonylureas, including glyburide, should not be given after the last meal of the day.
- Administer medication as directed by the healthcare provider.
- Glyburide is pregnancy category C.

Pharmacokinetics: Glyburide is well absorbed after oral administration. It is widely distributed and crosses the placenta. It is 99% plasma protein bound. It is metabolized by the liver. Its half-life is about 10 hours.

Adverse Effects and Interactions: Hypoglycemia is less frequent with glyburide than with first-generation sulfonylureas. Elderly clients are prone to hypoglycemia because many have decreased renal and hepatic function, which can cause an increase in the amount of medication circulating in the blood. For this reason, elderly clients are often prescribed a reduced dosage.

Clients should stay out of direct sunlight since rashes and photosensitivity are possible. Some clients experience mild GI-related effects such as nausea, vomiting, or loss of appetite. Glyburide and other sulfonylureas have the potential to interact with a number of drugs; therefore, the client should always consult with a healthcare provider before adding a new medication or herbal supplement. Ingestion of alcohol will result in distressing symptoms that include headache, flushing, nausea, and abdominal cramping.

Glyburide interacts with several drugs. For example, there is a cross-sensitivity with sulfonamides and thiazide diuretics. Oral anticoagulants, chloramphenicol (Chloromycetin), and MAO inhibitors may potentiate the hypoglycemic actions of glyburide.

Use with caution with herbal supplements, such as ginseng and garlic, which may increase hypoglycemic effects.

NURSING PROCESS FOCUS

Clients Receiving Oral Antihyperglycemic Therapy

Assessment Data	Potential Nursing Diagnoses and Identified Patterns
Prior to administration: - Obtain complete health history, including allergies, drug history, and possible drug interactions. - Assess for pain location and level. - Assess knowledge of drug. - Assess ability to conduct blood glucose testing.	- Risk for impaired skin integrity and infection related to blood glucose elevations and impaired circulation - Need for knowledge regarding drug therapy - Need for knowledge regarding glucose testing - Risk for hypoglycemia related to adverse effects of drug therapy - Need for knowledge related to lifestyle and dietary modifications

Planning: Client Goals and Expected Outcomes

The client will:

- Demonstrate an understanding of the drug's action by accurately describing drug side effects and precautions
- Describe signs and symptoms that should be reported immediately, including nausea, diarrhea, jaundice, rash, headache, anorexia, abdominal pain, tachycardia, seizures, and confusion
- Demonstrate an ability to accurately self-monitor blood glucose and maintain blood glucose within a normal range

Implementation

Interventions (Rationales)	Client Education and Discharge Planning
• Monitor blood glucose at least daily, and monitor urinary ketones if blood glucose is higher than 14 mmol/L. (Ketones will spill into the urine at high blood glucose levels and provide an early sign of diabetic ketoacidosis.) • Monitor for signs of lactic acidosis if client is receiving a biguanide. (Mitochondrial oxidation of lactic acid is inhibited, and lactic acidosis may result.) • Review laboratory tests for any abnormalities in liver function. (These drugs are metabolized in the liver and may cause elevations in aspartate aminotransferase and lactate dehydrogenase. Metformin decreases absorption of vitamin B_{12} and folic acid, which may result in deficiencies of these substances.) • Obtain accurate history of alcohol use, especially if client is receiving a sulfonylurea or biguanide. (These drugs may cause a disulfiram-like reaction.) • Monitor for signs and symptoms of increased stress, illness, or infection. (These symptoms may increase blood glucose levels.) • Monitor blood glucose frequently, especially at the beginning of therapy and in elderly clients. • Monitor clients who also take a beta blocker carefully because early signs of hypoglycemia may not be apparent. • Monitor weight, weighing at the same time of day each time. (Changes in weight will affect the amount of drug needed to control blood glucose.) • Monitor vital signs. (Increased pulse and blood pressure are early signs of hypoglycemia.) • Monitor skin for rashes and itching. (These are signs of an allergic reaction to the drug.) • Monitor activity level. (Dose may require adjustment with change in physical activity.)	• Teach client how to monitor blood glucose and test urine for ketones, especially when ill. • Instruct client to report signs of lactic acidosis such as hyperventilation, muscle pain, fatigue, and increased sleeping. • Instruct client to report the first sign of yellow skin, pale stools, or dark urine. • Advise client to abstain from alcohol and to avoid liquid over-the-counter medications, which may contain alcohol. • Instruct client to report the first signs of fatigue, muscle weakness, and nausea. • Discuss importance of adequate rest and healthy routines. Teach client: • Signs and symptoms of hypoglycemia, such as hunger, irritability, and sweating • At first sign of hypoglycemia, to check blood glucose and eat a simple sugar; if symptoms do not improve, call 911 • To monitor blood glucose before breakfast and supper • Not to skip meals and to follow a diet specified by the healthcare provider • To weigh self each week, at the same time of day, and report any significant loss or gain • How to take accurate blood pressure, temperature, and pulse • The importance of immediately reporting skin rashes and itching that is unaccounted for by dry skin • To increase activity level, which will help to lower blood glucose • To closely monitor blood glucose when involved in vigorous physical activity

Evaluation of Outcome Criteria

The client:

- Demonstrates an understanding of the drug's action by accurately describing drug side effects and precautions
- Describes signs and symptoms that should be reported immediately, including nausea, diarrhea, jaundice, rash, headache, anorexia, abdominal pain, tachycardia, seizures, and confusion
- Demonstrates an ability to accurately self-monitor blood glucose and maintain blood glucose within a normal range

See Table 28.5 for a list of drugs to which these nursing actions apply.

CHAPTER 28

Understanding the Chapter

Key Concepts Summary

The numbered key concepts provide a succinct summary of the important points from the corresponding numbered section within the chapter. If any of these points are not clear, refer to the numbered section within the chapter for review.

28.1 The pancreas is both an endocrine and an exocrine gland. Insulin is released when blood glucose increases, and glucagon is released when blood glucose decreases.

28.2 Type 1 diabetes mellitus is caused by a lack of insulin secretion and is characterized by serious, chronic conditions affecting the cardiovascular and nervous systems.

Type 2 DM is caused by a lack of sensitivity of insulin receptors at the target cells and a deficiency in insulin secretion. If untreated, the same chronic conditions result as in type 1 DM.

28.3 Type 1 DM is treated by dietary restrictions, exercise, and insulin injections. The many types of insulin preparations vary as to their onset of action, time to peak effect, and duration.

28.4 Type 2 DM is controlled through lifestyle changes and oral antihyperglycemic drugs.

Chapter 28 Scenario

Ellen is a 44-year-old woman who works full time as an art teacher in a local high school. She also teaches art courses on the weekends at the local seniors centre. She visited her healthcare provider last week for her annual physical exam and to update her tuberculosis screening (PPD skin test) for the coming school year. The office called her this morning with her laboratory reports and requested that she make an appointment to discuss the results tomorrow. Her serum glucose level is elevated at 14 mmol/L and she will need further testing to rule out type 2 diabetes.

Ellen has follow-up testing, with the results of a fasting serum glucose level returning at 8 mmol/L and a 2-hour 75-g oral glucose test returning at 13 mmol/L. A diagnosis of new-onset type 2 diabetes is confirmed. Ellen expresses disbelief and tells you, the nurse, "I can't believe it! I watch what I eat; I don't eat a lot of sugar, cookies, or candy. I drink only diet soda. I don't have any of the symptoms you hear about. And no one in my family has ever had diabetes." A health history and the results of Ellen's recent physical examination confirm overall good health. Her height is 167.6 cm (66 in.) and her weight is 79.5 kg (175 lb) with a body mass index (BMI) of 28.2 kg/m^2, placing her in the "overweight" category. Vital signs, physical exam, and all other laboratory workup are within acceptable limits. Ellen admits that she has been thirstier lately, "But it's summertime and I always drink more when it's hot." She has also been urinating more frequently but attributes that to her increased fluid intake.

Ellen's healthcare provider will start her on glyburide (DiaBeta) and metformin (Glucophage) and will recheck her serum glucose in 1 month. In the meantime, she is to begin capillary blood glucose testing before meals and at bedtime and to bring her blood glucose log to the next visit. She is given dietary instructions, and you will be providing instruction on her medications.

Critical Thinking Questions

1. Why are two oral antidiabetic drugs prescribed for Ellen?
2. What essential teaching does Ellen need about her glyburide (DiaBeta) and metformin (Glucophage)?
3. Ellen asks why she is not being started on insulin. Why is insulin not being used at this time?
4. Ellen tells you that she occasionally enjoys a glass of wine with her dinner and wants to know if this is allowed. How will you answer?

See Answers to Critical Thinking Questions in Appendix B.

NCLEX Practice Questions

1 A client with type 1 diabetes will use a combination insulin that includes NPH and regular insulins. The nurse explains the importance of knowing the peak times for both insulins. Why is this important information for the client to know?

a. The client will be able to estimate the time for the next injection of insulin based on these peaks.

b. The risk of a hypoglycemic reaction is greatest around the peak of insulin activity.

c. It is best to plan activities or exercise around peak insulin times for the best use of glucose.

d. Additional insulin may be required at the peak periods to prevent hyperglycemia.

2 Before administering a morning lispro insulin (Humalog) injection, which activity should the nurse perform? Select all that apply.

a. Obtain a morning urine sample for glucose and ketones.

b. Check the client's finger-stick glucose level.

c. Ensure that breakfast trays are present on the unit and the client may eat.

d. Obtain the client's pulse and blood pressure.

e. Assess for symptoms of hypoglycemia.

3 The nurse would consider which of the following assessment findings adverse effects to metformin therapy?

a. Hypoglycemia

b. Gastrointestinal distress

c. Lactic acidosis

d. Weight loss

4 A client was started on rosiglitazone (Avandia) for type 2 diabetes. He tells the nurse that he has been taking it for 5 days, but his glucose levels are unchanged. What would the nurse's best response be?

a. "You should double the dose. That should help."

b. "You need to give the drug more time. It can take several weeks before it becomes fully effective."

c. "You will need to add a second drug since this one has not been effective."

d. "You most likely require insulin now."

5 A young woman calls the clinic and reports that her mother had an insulin overdose and was found unconscious. The young woman gave her a glucagon injection 20 minutes ago, and her mother woke up but is still groggy and "does not make sense." What should the nurse tell the daughter?

a. "Let her wake up on her own, then give her something to eat."

b. "Place some hard candies in her mouth."

c. "Just let her sleep. People are sleepy after hypoglycemic episodes."

d. "Give her another injection and call the paramedics."

See Answers to NCLEX Practice Questions in Appendix A.

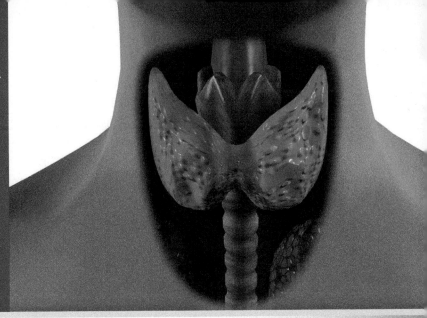

Hank Grebe/Purestock/Alamy Stock Photo

PROTOTYPE DRUGS

levothyroxine (Eltroxin, Synthroid)

propylthiouracil (PTU)

CHAPTER

29

Pharmacotherapy of Thyroid and Parathyroid Disorders

LEARNING OUTCOMES

After reading this chapter, the student should be able to:

1. Explain the functions of thyroid hormone.
2. Explain the negative feedback control of thyroid function.
3. Explain how thyroid disorders are diagnosed.
4. Describe the pathophysiology of thyroid disorders.
5. Describe the pharmacotherapy of thyroid disorders.
6. For each of the classes shown in the Prototype Drugs list, identify the prototype and representative drugs and explain the mechanism(s) of drug action, primary actions, and important adverse effects.
7. Apply the nursing process to the care of clients who are receiving pharmacotherapy for thyroid disorders.

CHAPTER OUTLINE

▶ Normal Function of the Thyroid Gland

▶ Diagnosis of Thyroid Disorders

▶ Hypothyroid Disorders

▶ Pharmacotherapy of Hypothyroid Disorders

▶ Hyperthyroid Disorders

▶ Pharmacotherapy of Hyperthyroid Disorders

basal metabolic rate, 336

cretinism, 338

exophthalmos, 341

follicular cells, 336

goiter, 337

Graves' disease, 341

Hashimoto's thyroiditis, 338

myxedema, 338

myxedema coma, 338

parafollicular cells, 336

thyroid crisis, 342

thyroid-stimulating hormone (TSH), 336

thyroid-stimulating immunoglobulins (TSIs), 341

thyroid storm, 342

thyrotoxicosis, 342

thyrotropin-releasing hormone (TRH), 336

thyroxine (T$_4$), 336

thyroxine-binding globulin (TBG), 336

triiodothyronine (T$_3$), 336

The thyroid gland affects the function of virtually every organ of the body. It synthesizes and secretes hormones that increase overall body metabolism and protein synthesis. Adequate secretion of these hormones is also necessary for normal growth and development in infants and children, including mental development and attainment of sexual maturity. The thyroid strongly affects functions of the cardiovascular, respiratory, gastrointestinal (GI), and neuromuscular systems. Thyroid disorders are common, affecting women 5 to 10 times more often than men. This chapter presents the pharmacotherapy of thyroid imbalances.

Normal Function of the Thyroid Gland

29.1 Thyroid hormones contain iodine and stimulate the basal metabolic rate of nearly all tissues.

The thyroid gland secretes hormones that affect nearly every cell in the body. By stimulating the enzymes involved with glucose oxidation, thyroid gland hormones regulate **basal metabolic rate**, the baseline speed by which cells perform their functions. By increasing oxidation of energy sources (glucose, fats, and proteins), thyroid hormone increases oxygen consumption and body temperature. The gland also helps to maintain blood pressure and regulate growth and development.

The thyroid gland has two basic cell types that secrete different hormones. **Parafollicular cells** secrete calcitonin, a hormone that is involved with calcium homeostasis. **Follicular cells** in the gland secrete thyroid hormone, which is actually a combination of two different hormones: thyroxine (T$_4$) and **triiodothyronine (T$_3$)**. Iodine is essential for the synthesis of these hormones and is provided through the dietary intake of common iodized salt. The names of these hormones refer to the number of bound iodine atoms in each molecule, either three (T$_3$) or four (T$_4$). Once secreted into the bloodstream, 99% of T$_3$ and T$_4$ is protein bound to **thyroxine-binding globulin (TBG)**, a protein manufactured in the liver.

Thyroxine (T$_4$) is the major hormone secreted by the thyroid gland. At the target tissues, however, thyroxine is converted to T$_3$ through the enzymatic cleavage of one iodine atom. T$_3$ is thought to enter the target cells, where it binds to intracellular receptors within the nucleus.

Thyroid function is regulated through multiple levels of hormonal control. Falling thyroxine levels in the blood signal the hypothalamus to secrete **thyrotropin-releasing hormone (TRH)**. TRH stimulates the pituitary gland to secrete **thyroid-stimulating hormone (TSH)**, which then stimulates the thyroid gland to release thyroid hormone. Rising levels of thyroid hormone in the blood trigger a negative feedback response to shut off secretion of TRH and TSH. The negative feedback mechanism for the thyroid gland is shown in Figure 29.1.

Most circulating thyroid hormone is in the form of T$_4$. To enter target cells, however, T$_4$ is converted in peripheral tissues to T$_3$, which is three to five times more biologically active. This offers an additional level of control (tissue level) of thyroid hormone function.

The two thyroid hormones are metabolized by the liver and excreted by the kidneys, with small amounts excreted in the stool. Iodine is conserved in the process and returned to the thyroid gland for the production of more hormone molecules. Therefore, only a small daily intake of iodine is needed to meet the demands of the thyroid gland. High amounts of iodine are found in shellfish, but the main dietary source is iodized salt. Thyroid hormones are the only known use for iodine in the body.

Thyroid hormone stimulates the basal metabolic rate of all tissues except the brain, anterior pituitary, spleen, lymph nodes, testes, and lungs. In the presence of large amounts of thyroid hormone, the basal metabolic rate of cells can increase by 60% to 100%. This increases the oxidation of energy sources (glucose, fats, and proteins), which in turn increases oxygen consumption and generates large amounts of heat. The rapid metabolic rate increases the body's demands for vitamins. Thyroid hormone affects GI function and motility, appetite, and body weight. Thyroid hormone increases the number of beta$_1$- and beta$_2$-adrenergic receptors and enhances their affinity to catecholamines (norepinephrine, epinephrine, and dopamine). The increase in sympathetic activity leads to increased heart rate and force of contraction, cardiac output, and cardiac demands for oxygen. Thyroid hormones also stimulate the secretion of growth hormone and are therefore essential for the normal growth and development of the skeletal and nervous systems. Thyroid hormone affects reflexes, thought processes, and overall level of consciousness (LOC). Signs and symptoms of thyroid hormone deficiency and excess are presented in Table 29.1.

Disorders of the thyroid result from hypofunction or hyperfunction of the thyroid gland. Hormonal imbalances may occur due to disease within the thyroid gland itself or be caused by abnormalities of the pituitary or hypothalamus. Table 29.2 lists the commonly used thyroid and antithyroid drugs.

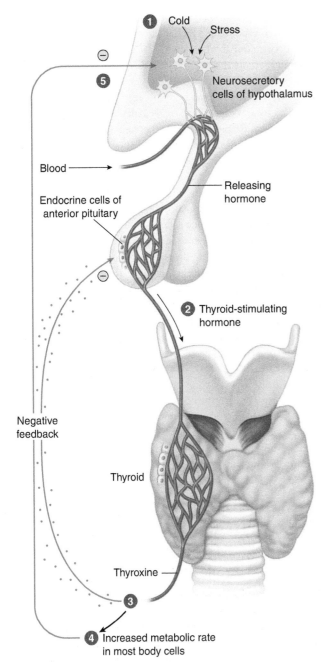

Figure 29.1 Feedback mechanisms of the thyroid gland: (1) stimulus; (2) release of TSH; (3) release of thyroid hormone; (4) increased basal metabolic rate; (5) negative feedback.

TABLE 29.1 Signs and Symptoms of Thyroid Emergencies

Thyroid Storm	Myxedema Coma
Tachycardia	Bradycardia
Hyperthermia	Hypothermia
Tachypnea	Hypoventilation
Hypercalcemia	Hyponatremia
Hyperglycemia	Hypoglycemia
Metabolic acidosis	Respiratory and metabolic acidosis
Cardiovascular collapse: cardiogenic shock, hypovolemia, arrhythmias	Cardiovascular collapse: decreased vascular tone
Depressed LOC	Depressed LOC
Emotional lability	Seizures, coma
Psychosis	Hyporeflexia
Tremors, restlessness	

TABLE 29.2 Thyroid and Antithyroid Drugs

Drug	Route and Adult Dose
Hypothyroid Agents	
levothyroxine (Eltroxin, Synthroid)	Orally (PO), 50-200 µg daily (qd) (in healthy adults, approximately 1.7 µg/kg/day)
liothyronine (Cytomel)	PO, 25–75 µg qd
desiccated thyroid (Armour Thyroid, Thyroid)	start with 15-30 mg /day; maintenance dose is usually 60-120 mg/day
Antithyroid Agents	
potassium iodide and iodine (Lugol's solution, Thyro-Block)	PO, 50–250 mg three times a day (tid) 10–14 days before surgery
propylthiouracil (PTU)	PO, start with 50-100 mg every 8 hours; may increase up to 500 mg/day
radioactive iodide (Iodotope)	PO, 0.8–150 millicurie (curies are units of radioactivity)

Diagnosis of Thyroid Disorders

29.2 An accurate diagnosis of thyroid hormone dysfunction is based on the client's symptoms and the results of diagnostic tests.

Because the thyroid gland is located close to the skin surface, palpation of the thyroid gland is conducted for routine screening of enlargements and nodules. Serum laboratory tests for T_3, T_4, and TSH are commonly used for diagnosis. TSH is the preferred laboratory value for diagnosing and monitoring the progression of thyroid disease. Primary hypothyroidism is characterized by a low serum T_4 level and an elevated TSH level.

Abnormal laboratory values must be carefully evaluated because a number of conditions, including stress in critically ill adults, can affect TSH and T_4 levels. In addition, these laboratory values are influenced by abnormalities in serum protein levels because both T_3 and T_4 are heavily protein bound. Any condition that affects protein levels requires careful analysis of these test results. Another laboratory test useful in the diagnosis of thyroid pathology is antithyroid antibody titer. Clients with Hashimoto's

Thyroid disorders can be caused by a congenital defect, or they may develop later in life. They may have an insidious or sudden onset. An increase in the size of the thyroid gland is referred to as a **goiter**. This can occur with normal, high, or low levels of thyroid hormone. Goiters may be diffuse, involving the entire gland, or nodular. When they become considerably enlarged, goiters can compress the trachea and esophagus, causing difficulty swallowing, a choking sensation, and possibly inspiratory stridor (abnormal high-pitched sounds when breathing). They may also compress the superior vena cava, causing distention of the neck veins and facial edema.

thyroiditis, an autoimmune type of thyroid disease, will show abnormal levels of antithyroid antibody titer.

The diagnostic tool of choice for detecting malignancy of a thyroid nodule is the fine-needle biopsy. Ultrasonography can be used to assess masses, cysts, and enlargement of the thyroid gland. The radioactive iodine uptake test measures the rate of iodine uptake by the thyroid gland after administration of ioflupane (^{123}I) tracer. This test can detect areas of increased and decreased function. Computed tomography (CT) and magnetic resonance imaging (MRI) scans can be used to determine tracheal compression or pressure on neighbouring structures caused by thyroid gland enlargement.

An accurate diagnosis of thyroid hormone dysfunction is essential. Proper treatment of the disorder will depend on whether the abnormality lies within the thyroid gland itself or is the result of a defect in the negative feedback control by the hypothalamus or pituitary.

Hypothyroid Disorders

29.3 Hypothyroidism, or thyroid deficiency, can occur as a congenital or acquired disorder.

Hypothyroidism may occur as a congenital disorder, or it may be acquired in adulthood. Congenital hypothyroidism is a common, preventable cause of mental retardation. The infant appears normal at birth due to hormones supplied by the mother while in utero. If untreated, congenital hypothyroidism results in a condition known as **cretinism**, marked by profound mental retardation and impaired growth. Almost half of normal brain development occurs during the first 6 months of life, and thyroid hormone is essential for this to occur. Studies show that if thyroid replacement therapy is begun in the first 6 weeks of life, normal growth and development take place and cretinism can be prevented. In the United States and Canada, screening for hypothyroidism is conducted on all neonates.

Hypothyroidism in older children and adults results in a general slowing of metabolic processes and **myxedema**, a mucous type of edema caused by an accumulation of hydrophilic substances in connective tissues. Primary hypothyroidism, the most common type in children and adults, results from dysfunction of the thyroid gland. Secondary hypothyroidism is due to pathology of the pituitary gland. Tertiary hypothyroidism is a result of a disorder of the hypothalamus. Causes of hypothyroidism include thyroidectomy or ablation of the thyroid gland with radiation, the use of lithium (in the treatment of bipolar disorder), or treatment with antithyroid drugs. Large amounts of iodine or substances that contain iodine, such as kelp tablets, certain cough syrups, the cardiac drug amiodarone (Cordarone), or iodine-containing radiographic contrast media, can block thyroid hormone production and cause goiter and hypothyroidism. Iodine deficiency is rarely a cause of hypothyroidism in Canada due to the widespread use of iodized salt.

The most common cause of hypothyroidism is an autoimmune disorder known as **Hashimoto's thyroiditis**. This is predominantly a disease of women, striking women 5 to 10 times more often than men. Because hypothyroidism during the first trimester of pregnancy has been shown to cause mental and developmental problems in the fetus, it is recommended that all women receive screening for hypothyroidism early in a pregnancy. By the second trimester, when the

fetus is able to synthesize thyroid hormone, this threat disappears. Women also experience a high incidence of postpartum thyroiditis, which occurs after approximately 10% of pregnancies.

Hypothyroidism affects nearly all major organ systems, with manifestations arising from two factors: a hypometabolic state and myxedematous changes in body tissues. The hypometabolic state is marked by a gradual onset of weakness and fatigue, a tendency to gain weight despite a decreased appetite, and cold intolerance. Hypotension, bradycardia, hypoventilation, and subnormal temperature may occur. In time, the skin becomes rough and dry and may have a yellowish cast; the hair becomes coarse and brittle; and GI motility slows, causing chronic constipation, flatulence, and abdominal distention. Mental dullness, lethargy, slowed reflexes, and memory problems may occur.

As fluid accumulates in tissues, the face takes on a puffy look, especially around the eyes; the tongue enlarges; and the voice may be husky. Fluid can accumulate in the pericardial or pleural spaces, causing effusions, cardiac dilation, and bradycardia. **Myxedema coma** or crisis is a life-threatening end-stage condition of hypothyroidism, characterized by coma, hypothermia, cardiovascular collapse, hypoventilation, hyponatremia, hypoglycemia, and lactic acidosis. This condition occurs most often in elderly women. Even with early detection and treatment, the mortality rate is 30% for those who develop myxedema coma. Treatment consists of supportive measures, correction of electrolyte and acid-base imbalances, treatment of hypotension, and immediate thyroid replacement therapy. If hypothermia is present, active rewarming is contraindicated because this may precipitate vasodilation and lead to cardiovascular collapse.

Pharmacotherapy of Hypothyroid Disorders

29.4 Hypothyroidism is treated by replacement therapy with thyroid hormone.

Hypothyroidism is treated by replacement therapy with T_3 or T_4. The standard replacement regimen consists of levothyroxine (T_4; Eltroxin, Synthroid), although combined therapy with levothyroxine plus liothyronine (T_3; Cytomel) is an option. Although T_4 is less biologically active than T_3, it is readily converted to T_3 in peripheral tissues. In most cases, thyroid replacement therapy is lifelong.

In children with cretinism, therapy should continue for 3 years, after which it should be stopped for 1 month. During this time, thyroid hormone levels are monitored to assess the status of the deficiency and to determine if further treatment is needed.

In adults, serum TSH levels are used to evaluate the progress of therapy. When initiating therapy in older adults, the precaution is to "go low and go slow" because there is a risk for inducing acute coronary syndromes in susceptible individuals.

NCLEX Success Tips

Levothyroxine is the agent of choice for thyroid hormone replacement therapy because its standard hormone content provides predictable results. Thyroid USP desiccated and liothyronine are no longer used for thyroid hormone replacement therapy because they may cause fluctuating plasma drug levels, increasing the risk of adverse effects.

Serum cholesterol levels are also elevated in clients with hypothyroidism.

As the metabolic rate increases with the thyroid replacement therapy, there is more demand on the heart, and angina and palpitations may occur. There is also an increase in temperature, a loss in weight, and increased energy levels.

The nurse should instruct the client to take levothyroxine on an empty stomach to promote regular absorption in the morning and to help prevent insomnia and to mimic normal hormone release. Levothyroxine must be given at the same time each day on an empty stomach, preferably 30 minutes to 1 hour before breakfast.

Sweating, insomnia, rapid pulse, dyspnea, irritability, fever, and weight loss are all signs indicating levothyroxine overdose.

Diminished or absent appetite (anorexia), constipation, and fatigue and sleepiness would suggest thyroid insufficiency.

Radioactive iodine is usually used for hyperthyroidism but is contraindicated in pregnancy.

A saturated solution of potassium iodide (SSKI; Lugol's solution, Thyro-Block) should be diluted well in milk, water, juice, or a carbonated beverage before administration to help disguise the strong, bitter taste. Also, this drug is irritating to mucosa if taken undiluted. The client should sip the diluted preparation through a drinking straw to help prevent staining of the teeth.

SSKI is frequently administered before a thyroidectomy because it helps decrease the vascularity of the thyroid gland. A highly vascular thyroid gland is friable, a condition that presents a hazard during surgery. Preparation of the client for surgery includes depleting the gland of thyroid hormone and decreasing vascularity.

Potassium iodide reaches its maximum effect in 1 to 2 weeks.

Propylthiouracil (PTU) blocks the conversion of thyroxine to triiodothyronine, the more biologically active thyroid hormone. PTU effects are also seen in 1 to 2 weeks.

To relieve symptoms of hyperthyroidism in the interim, clients are usually given a beta-adrenergic blocker such as propranolol.

CONNECTIONS Natural Therapies

◀ Treatments for Thyroid Disease

Thyroid disease is a serious condition that usually requires medical attention. As a preventive measure, one can consume substances that contain precursors to thyroid hormone. Since T_3 and T_4 both require iodine, dietary intake of this mineral must be sufficient. Iodized salt usually contains enough iodine for proper thyroid function; however, kelp and seafood, particularly shellfish, are additional, natural sources of iodine. T_3 and T_4 also contain the amino acid tyrosine, which is usually obtained from protein sources such as meat or eggs. Other rich sources of tyrosine include avocados, bananas, lima beans, and various seeds. Supplementation with L-tyrosine is usually not necessary.

A number of natural therapies have been used to treat overactive thyroid glands. Lemon balm (*Melissa officinalis*) is a beautiful perennial plant that has a slight lemon odour when the leaves are crushed. Although native to the Mediterranean region, it is widely cultivated in Europe, Asia, and North America. The leaves have traditional medicinal use as a sedative and antispasmodic, which has been reported for hundreds of years. It has been shown to block the antibodies responsible for destroying the thyroid gland in Graves' disease, although this effect has yet to be confirmed in clinical studies. Lemon balm is usually taken as a tea, several times daily, although capsules, extracts, and tinctures are available.

CONNECTIONS Special Considerations

◀ Shift Workers, Hypothyroidism, and Drug Adherence

Many body processes such as temperature, blood pressure, certain hormone levels, biochemical processes, and alertness fluctuate on a 24-hour schedule known as the circadian rhythm. Circadian processes are thought to be triggered by daylight. Normal circadian cycles may be interrupted in those people who work varied shifts. Likewise, medications that must be given at a specified time to enhance their potential effect can be a concern for shift workers.

Thyroid medication is best given at the same time each day; however, this can be a challenge for shift workers, especially if they rotate shifts. These drugs are best given after awakening in the morning, as they can disturb sleep patterns. For a shift worker, the time of awakening may vary depending on the shift worked. It is essential that the client be aware of this challenge and work with the healthcare provider to reach a medication schedule that allows optimization of the drug effects.

Nursing Considerations

The role of the nurse in thyroid hormone therapy involves careful monitoring of the client's condition and providing education as it relates to the prescribed drug treatment. Assess the client for signs and symptoms of thyroid disease. Also assess and monitor the client's vital signs, as cardiovascular complications may occur as a result of drug therapy.

Levothyroxine is a commonly used thyroid hormone replacement. Thoroughly assess cardiovascular function because this drug may cause cardiovascular collapse in clients with undiagnosed heart disease due to an increase in basal metabolic rate. This action may precipitate dysrhythmias in clients with undiagnosed heart disease, especially in elderly clients ("start low and go slow"). The drug should also be used with caution in clients with impaired renal function because the increased metabolic rate increases the workload of the kidney. Clients with diabetes mellitus, diabetes insipidus, or Addison's disease experience a worsening of symptoms because of the initial increase in basal metabolism. The drug is contraindicated in clients with adrenal insufficiency, as it may result in severe adrenal crisis.

Desiccated thyroid (Armour Thyroid, Thyroid) is made of dried beef and pork thyroid glands. It is used less frequently than levothyroxine because it does not produce reliable results. Desiccated thyroid will cause the same cardiac complications as levothyroxine. *Liothyronine sodium* is a short-acting synthetic form of the natural thyroid hormone that can be administered intravenously (IV) to individuals with myxedema coma. The short duration of action allows for rapid dosage adjustments in critically ill clients.

Thyroid hormones have their optimum effect when taken on an empty stomach. Clients should be taught the signs and symptoms of hyperthyroidism such as nervousness, weight loss, diarrhea, and intolerance to heat. The client should notify the healthcare provider at the first sign of any of these symptoms.

Client education as it relates to thyroid hormones should include goals, reasons for obtaining baseline data such as vital signs and tests for cardiac and renal function, and possible side effects. See Nursing Process Focus: Clients Receiving Thyroid Hormone Replacement for specific teaching points.

NCLEX Success Tip

Consider the interactions and potential resulting complications of thyroid hormone therapy with other commonly administered medications, such as warfarin (Coumadin), digoxin (Lanoxin, Toloxin), calcium, and iron. There are dietary implications with large amounts of various fruits and vegetables.

NURSING PROCESS FOCUS

Clients Receiving Thyroid Hormone Replacement

Assessment	Potential Nursing Diagnoses/Identified Patterns
Prior to administration: • Obtain complete health history, including allergies, drug history, and possible drug interactions. • Obtain complete physical examination. • Assess for the presence or history of symptoms of hypothyroidism. • Obtain electrocardiogram (ECG) and laboratory studies, including T_4, T_3, and serum TSH levels and liver function tests.	• Activity intolerance related to disease process • Fatigue related to impaired metabolic status • Need for knowledge regarding drug therapy and adverse effects • Risk for altered body image related to side effects of drug therapy

Planning: Client Goals and Expected Outcomes

The client will:

• Demonstrate an understanding of the drug's action by accurately describing drug side effects and precautions
• Exhibit normal thyroid hormone levels
• Report a decrease in hypothyroid symptoms
• Experience no significant adverse effects from drug therapy
• Demonstrate an understanding of hypothyroidism and the need for lifelong therapy

Implementation

Interventions (Rationales)	Client Education/Discharge Planning
• Monitor vital signs. (Changes in metabolic rate will be manifested as changes in blood pressure, pulse, and body temperature.) • Monitor for decreasing symptoms related to hypothyroidism, such as fatigue, constipation, cold intolerance, lethargy, depression, and menstrual irregularities. (Decreasing symptoms will determine that the drug is achieving a therapeutic effect.) • Monitor for symptoms related to hyperthyroidism, such as nervousness, insomnia, tachycardia, dysrhythmias, heat intolerance, chest pain, and diarrhea. (Symptoms of hyperthyroidism indicate the drug is at a toxic level.) • Monitor T_3, T_4, and TSH levels. (This helps to determine the effectiveness of pharmacotherapy.) • Monitor blood glucose levels, especially in individuals with diabetes mellitus. (Thyroid hormone increases metabolic rate, and glucose use may be altered.) • Provide supportive nursing care to cope with symptoms of hypothyroidism, such as constipation, cold intolerance, and fatigue, until the drug has achieved therapeutic effect. • Monitor weight at least weekly. (Weight loss is expected due to increased metabolic rate. Weight changes help to determine the effectiveness of drug therapy.) • Monitor client for signs of decreased adherence with therapeutic treatment.	• Instruct client to report dizziness, palpitations, and intolerance to temperature changes • Instruct client about the signs of hypothyroidism and to report symptoms • Instruct client about the signs of hyperthyroidism and to report symptoms • Instruct client about the importance of ongoing monitoring of thyroid hormone levels and to keep all laboratory appointments • Instruct the diabetic client to monitor blood glucose levels and adjust insulin doses as directed by the healthcare provider Instruct client to: • Increase activity and fluid and fibre intake to reduce constipation • Wear additional clothing and maintain a comfortable room environment for cold intolerance • Plan activities and include rest periods to avoid fatigue • Instruct client to weigh self weekly and to report significant changes • Instruct client about the disease and the importance of lifelong therapy and follow-up care

---

Evaluation of Outcome Criteria

Evaluate effectiveness of drug therapy by confirming that client goals and expected outcomes have been met (see "Planning").

See Table 29.2, under "Hypothyroid Agents," for a list of drugs to which these nursing actions apply.

PROTOTYPE DRUG | **Levothyroxine (Eltroxin, Synthroid)**

Actions and Uses: Levothyroxine is a synthetic form of T_4, with actions identical to endogenous thyroid hormone. It is used for primary or secondary hypothyroidism; congenital hypothyroidism; hypothyroid state resulting from the surgical removal of the thyroid gland, radiation, or antithyroid drugs; management of thyroid cancer; or treatment of myxedema coma. The drug is given by the PO route for routine replacement therapy and intravenously (IV) for myxedema coma.

The actions of levothyroxine are identical to endogenous thyroid hormone. The drug increases the metabolic rate, thereby increasing oxygen consumption, respiration, and heart rate; increases the rate of fat, protein, and carbohydrate metabolism; and promotes growth and maturation. Because levothyroxine is converted to T_3, it is not necessary to also give T_3.

Pharmacokinetics: Levothyroxine is given by the PO or IV route and has variable absorption (50% to 80%) from the GI tract. During distribution, the drug is gradually released to peripheral tissues. It crosses the placenta in pregnancy, is secreted in breast milk, and is more than 99% protein bound. The primary metabolic organ for levothyroxine is the liver. The kidney is primarily responsible for excretion, although some might be excreted in the bile or feces. If administered PO, onset of action is slow. Duration of action is 1 to 3 weeks and it has a half-life of 6 to 7 days.

Administration Alerts:

- The use of levothyroxine is contraindicated if the client is hypersensitive to the drug, is experiencing thyrotoxicosis, or has severe cardiovascular conditions or acute myocardial infarction (MI).

- If thyroid hormone is given to clients with adrenal insufficiency, it may cause a serious adrenal crisis; therefore, the insufficiency should be corrected prior to administration of levothyroxine.

- Levothyroxine should be used with caution in clients with cardiac disease, angina pectoris, cardiac dysrhythmias, hypertension, and impaired kidney function, and in older adults. Symptoms of diabetes mellitus may worsen with administration of thyroid hormone, and doses of antidiabetic drugs may require adjustment.

Adverse Effects and Interactions: At therapeutic doses, adverse effects of levothyroxine therapy are rare. At high doses, treatment may cause central nervous system (CNS) excitability such as tremors, headache, nervousness, or insomnia. Cardiovascular adverse effects include palpitations, tachycardia, angina, and cardiac arrest. Other possible adverse events include allergic skin reactions, diarrhea, nausea, and vomiting. Synthroid 100-μg and 300-μg tablets contain tartrazine, which may cause an allergic reaction in some clients, especially those who are sensitive to acetylsalicylic acid (Aspirin).

A large number of medications can interact with thyroid hormone and result in either increased or decreased effects. Drugs that decrease the absorption of levothyroxine include cholestyramine (Questran, Olestyr), colestipol (Colestid), calcium- or aluminum-containing antacids, sucralfate, and iron supplements. Several drugs are known to accelerate the metabolism of levothyroxine, including phenytoin (Dilantin), carbamazepine (Tegretol), rifampin (Rifadin, Rofact), phenobarbital (Phenobarb), and sertraline (Zoloft). Levothyroxine increases the effects of warfarin, resulting in an increased risk for bleeding. Digoxin decreases the effectiveness of levothyroxine. Thyroid hormone sensitizes cardiac responsive to catecholamines; therefore, administration of epinephrine (Adrenalin) or norepinephrine must be carefully monitored in these clients to prevent dysrhythmias.

Hyperthyroid Disorders

29.5 Hyperthyroidism, or Graves' disease, is an autoimmune disorder accompanied by ophthalmopathy and goiter.

Symptoms of hyperthyroidism have been recorded in medical documents dating back to the 12th century. The most common cause of hyperthyroidism is **Graves' disease**, named after the Irish doctor, Robert Graves, who described the disorder in 1835. The condition is characterized by the excessive secretion of thyroid hormone.

The two most visible signs of Graves' disease are goiter and **exophthalmos**, an outward bulging of the eyes. Up to one-third of those with Graves' disease develop ophthalmopathy, leading to severe eye problems. These problems include paralysis of the ocular muscles, damage to the optic nerve with some vision loss, and corneal ulceration due to the inability of the eyelids to close. These eye problems are aggravated by smoking, which should be strongly discouraged in persons with Graves' disease. The ophthalmopathy usually stabilizes with treatment, but not all eye changes are reversible with therapy. A rare skin disorder, pretibial myxedema, may also occur, with thickening of the skin, plaques, and nodules over the shins and dorsal surface of the feet. Like the ophthalmic changes, these skin changes may persist despite effective treatment of the disease.

Causes of Graves' disease include adenoma and excessive intake of thyroid hormone. The onset is usually between the ages of 20 and 40 years, and it occurs five times more often in women than in men. Graves' disease is an autoimmune disorder in which the thyroid gland is stimulated by **thyroid-stimulating immunoglobulins (TSIs)**. It may occur concurrently with other autoimmune disorders, and there is a familial tendency to the condition.

The manifestations of hyperthyroidism are caused by the hypermetabolic state and the increase in sympathetic nervous system activity. The symptoms include nervousness, irritability and fatigability, insomnia, weight loss despite a large appetite, tachycardia, palpitations, hypertension, shortness of breath, increased sweating, muscle cramps, hyperthermia, and heat intolerance. A fine muscle tremor may occur. Approximately 15% of older adults with new-onset atrial fibrillation, a common cardiac dysrhythmia, have thyrotoxicosis.

Very high levels of circulating thyroid hormone may cause **thyrotoxicosis. Thyroid crisis**, or **thyroid storm**, is a rare, life-threatening form of thyrotoxicosis. If untreated, it is associated with mortality rates of 80% to 90%. Even with treatment, mortality from thyroid storm exceeds 20%. It occurs most often in teenage and young adult women with undiagnosed or untreated cases of hyperthyroidism and can be precipitated by the stress of an acute infection, diabetic ketoacidosis, trauma, or manipulation of the thyroid gland during surgery. Manifestations include high fever, cardiovascular effects (tachycardia, heart failure, angina, and MI), and CNS effects (agitation, restlessness, delirium, progressing to coma). It is treated with supportive measures, efforts to reduce body temperature without causing shivering, fluid, glucose and electrolyte replacement, and beta-adrenergic blockers. Aspirin should not be used to lower the body temperature of a person in thyroid storm because it displaces thyroid hormone from its protein-binding sites in the serum, increasing the level of free, or active, thyroid hormone, which worsens the condition. Antithyroid drugs may be used to decrease thyroid hormone production.

Pharmacotherapy of Hyperthyroid Disorders

29.6 Hyperthyroidism is treated with surgery or drugs that reduce the production of thyroid hormone.

Hypersecretion of thyroid hormone results in symptoms that are the opposite of hypothyroidism: increased body metabolism,

tachycardia, weight loss, elevated body temperature, and anxiety. As mentioned, the most common type of hyperthyroidism is Graves' disease. Other causes of hyperthyroidism are adenomas of the thyroid, pituitary tumours, and pregnancy. If the cause of the hypersecretion is found to be a tumour, or if the disease cannot be controlled through pharmacotherapy, removal of the thyroid gland is indicated.

The two most common drugs for hyperthyroidism, propylthiouracil (PTU) and methimazole (Tapazole), are called thioamides. These agents prevent the incorporation of iodine into the thyroid hormone molecule and block the conversion of T_4 to T_3 in peripheral tissues. Methimazole has a much longer half-life that offers the advantage of less frequent dosing, but side effects can be more severe. Although both thioamides are pregnancy category D agents, methimazole crosses the placenta more readily than PTU and is contraindicated in clients who are pregnant.

A third antithyroid drug, sodium iodide I-131, is a radioisotope used to destroy overactive thyroid glands by emitting ionizing radiation. Shortly after oral administration, I-131 accumulates in the thyroid gland, where it destroys follicular cells. The goal of pharmacotherapy with I-131 is to destroy just enough of the thyroid gland so that thyroid function returns to normal levels. Full benefits may take several months. Although most clients require only a single dose, others may need additional treatments. Small diagnostic doses of I-131 are used in nuclear medicine to determine the degree of iodide uptake in the various parts of the thyroid gland.

Non-radioactive sodium iodide is used to treat other thyroid conditions. Lugol's solution is a mixture of 5% elemental iodine and 10% potassium iodide that is used to suppress thyroid function 10 to 15 days prior to thyroidectomy. Sodium iodide is administered IV (along with PTU) to manage an acute, life-threatening form of hyperthyroidism known as thyrotoxic crisis, or thyroid storm. Potassium iodide is administered to protect the thyroid from radiation damage after a nuclear exposure. Doses of the antithyroid drugs are listed in Table 29.3.

NCLEX Success Tips

Clients receiving antithyroid drug should be able to sleep and rest well at night since the level of thyroid hormones is reduced in the blood. Excess energy throughout the day, loss of weight, and perspiring through the day are symptoms of hyperthyroidism, indicating the drug has not produced its outcome.

TABLE 29.3 Antithyroid Drugs

Drug Name	Dose for Adults (Maximum Dose Where Indicated)	Adverse Effects
methimazole (Tapazole)	PO, 5–15 mg tid (max 60 mg/day)	*Nausea, rash, pruritus, urticaria, fever, numbness in fingers, peripheral neuropathy, leukopenia, hypothyroidism* Agranulocytosis, bradycardia, hepatotoxicity
potassium iodide and iodine (Lugol's solution, Thyro-Block)	PO, 125 mg daily	*Diarrhea, nausea, vomiting, stomach pain, fever, weakness, irregular heartbeat, hypothyroidism* Angioneurotic edema, iodine poisoning
propylthiouracil (PTU)	PO, start with 50-100 mg every 8 hours; may increase up to 500 mg/day	*Nausea, rash, pruritus, headache, fever, numbness in fingers, diarrhea, myelosuppression, hypothyroidism* Agranulocytosis
radioactive iodide (^{131}I)	PO, 0.8–150 millicurie (a curie is a unit of radioactivity)	*Adverse effects are uncommon* Thyroiditis, hypothyroidism, hypersensitivity

Note: *Italics* indicate common adverse effects. Underline indicates severe adverse effects.

The most serious adverse effects of PTU are leukopenia and agranulocytosis, which usually occur within the first 3 months of treatment. The client should be taught to promptly report signs and symptoms of infection, such as a sore throat and fever. Clients having a sore throat and fever should have an immediate white blood cell count and differential performed, and the drug must be withheld until the results are obtained. Although propylthiouracil and methimazole are considered teratogenic and can lead to congenital hyperthyroidism (goiter) in the neonate, these medications still represent the treatment of choice. The client should be regulated on the lowest possible dose. Hyperthyroidism is associated with preterm labour and a low-birth-weight infant. The client should not breastfeed because medications such as propylthiouracil and methimazole are secreted in breast milk.

Several drugs are used as adjuncts in the therapy of thyroid storm. During hyperthyroid states, beta-adrenergic blocking drugs such as propranolol (Inderal), esmolol (Brevibloc), or metoprolol (Lopressor) are given to block the effects of the thyroid hormones on sympathetic receptors in the heart. The actions include a decrease in heart rate and strength of contraction, thereby decreasing myocardial oxygen demands. These effects occur quickly, whereas the actions of antithyroid drugs take longer to occur.

IV corticosteroids such as hydrocortisone (Solu-Cortef) or dexamethasone (Dexasone) may be ordered to treat acute hyperthyroid states. Corticosteroids block the conversion of T_4 to T_3 in peripheral tissues. In addition, severe hyperthyroid states create high levels of stress that deplete adrenal corticosteroids in the body, and administration of replacement doses is necessary.

Nursing Considerations

The role of the nurse in antithyroid therapy involves careful monitoring of the client's condition and providing education as it relates to the prescribed treatment. Assess the client for signs of hypothyroidism, such as weight gain, hypotension, bradycardia, fatigue, depression, sensitivity to cold environments, hair loss, and dry skin. Assess for complications and adverse effects specific to the antithyroid medication prescribed for the client.

For clients who are receiving propylthiouracil (PTU), monitor white blood cell count periodically because PTU may cause agranulocytosis, which puts the client at risk for infection. Assess for signs of jaundice and monitor liver enzymes because PTU is metabolized by the liver. Carefully monitor bleeding times for clients who are receiving anticoagulants because PTU causes an increase in bleeding.

Methimazole can be given PO, and the risk of adverse effects is lower than with PTU. Assess for blood dyscrasias such as agranulocytosis and jaundice. These adverse effects usually disappear when the drug is discontinued.

Radioactive iodine (I-131) is used to permanently decrease thyroid function by destroying part of the gland (ablation). Monitor thyroid function tests because this medication often requires adjustments to achieve a therapeutic dose that causes a euthyroid state. Inform the client about signs and symptoms of hypothyroidism. Because the client emits radiation after receiving this drug, contact with children and pregnant women should be avoided for the week following administration; close contact with others should be limited for a few days.

I-131 is contraindicated in clients who are pregnant or breastfeeding. Women who are receiving this agent should take precautions to avoid pregnancy. If a woman suspects that she is pregnant, she should contact her healthcare provider immediately. Women who will be receiving this treatment should stop breastfeeding for the duration of therapy and discuss alternative feeding methods with their healthcare provider.

Client education as it relates to antithyroid agents should include goals; reasons for obtaining baseline data such as vital signs and liver, renal, and cardiac function tests; and possible drug side effects. Include the following points when teaching clients about antithyroid agents:

- Keep all scheduled laboratory visits for testing.
- Do not breastfeed.
- Practise reliable contraception and notify the healthcare provider if pregnancy is planned or suspected.
- Immediately report nervousness, palpitations, and heat intolerance because these may indicate that the dose is too low.
- Immediately report excess fatigue, slow speech, hoarseness, and slow pulse because these may indicate that the dose is too high.
- Inform the healthcare provider if you are taking any of the following medications because they are contraindicated with antithyroid agents: aminophylline, heparin, and digoxin.

NCLEX Success Tips

Consider the nursing assessments related to hyperthyroidism vs. hypothyroidism. Understand the various diagnostic testings that accompany issues with the thyroid gland. Consider the location of the thyroid and the potential impact of a thyroidectomy: A, B, Cs.

Consider the effects of cardiac medications as a client moves from a hyperthyroid state to a normal thyroid state; dosages may need to be adjusted, or the client may experience side effects.

PROTOTYPE DRUG	Propylthiouracil (PTU)

Actions and Uses: Propylthiouracil decreases thyroid hormone levels in hyperthyroid states that are caused by the overproduction of thyroid hormone. It is also used to establish the normal thyroid state prior to surgery or radioactive iodine treatment and for palliative control of toxic nodular goiter. Propylthiouracil is not effective in treating thyroiditis because this condition is due to the over-release, not overproduction, of thyroid hormone.

Propylthiouracil inhibits the first step in the synthesis of thyroid hormone and suppresses the peripheral conversion of T_4 to T_3. It does not affect thyroid hormone that has already been synthesized, so therapeutic response may be delayed by 3 to 12 weeks until existing supplies of thyroid hormone have been depleted.

Pharmacokinetics: Propylthiouracil is administered PO and rapidly absorbed. It is concentrated by the thyroid gland during distribution, crosses the placenta, is secreted in breast milk, and is 60% to 80% protein bound. Onset of action is about 30 minutes. It is primarily metabolized by the liver, but therapeutic effect may take up to 3 weeks, and the kidneys excrete the drug. Half-life is 1 to 2 hours, and peak action is within 1 to 1.5 hours.

Administration Alerts:

- The use of propylthiouracil is contraindicated if the client has a hypersensitivity to the drug.
- Although contraindicated during pregnancy, the drug occasionally must be administered to women who experience a thyrotoxic crisis during pregnancy, and it is preferred over methimazole because less of the drug crosses the placenta.
- Propylthiouracil should be used with caution during active infection, lactation, and bone marrow depression. Because propylthiouracil can cause liver impairment, caution should be used when treating clients with pre-existing hepatic disease.

Adverse Effects and Interactions: Approximately 15% to 20% of clients taking this drug will experience leukopenia, which is normally asymptomatic. Serious hypersensitivity reactions are rare but may be serious and include agranulocytosis, aplastic anemia, thrombocytopenia, rash, urticaria, and glomerulonephritis. Arthralgias and joint swelling occur in 5% of clients. CNS effects include headache, vertigo, neuritis, and paresthesias. Propylthiouracil can also cause hypothyroidism and goiter at high doses.

Propylthiouracil increases the actions of anticoagulants, which creates an increased risk for bleeding. Iodine-containing drugs (amiodarone, potassium iodide, sodium iodide, radioactive iodine) and thyroid hormones can antagonize the effectiveness of this drug. Altered serum levels of metoprolol, propranolol, and digoxin can occur as the client moves from a hyperthyroid to a normal thyroid state. Cross-hypersensitivity occurs in about 50% of clients who have experienced a hypersensitivity reaction to methimazole, the other major antithyroid medication. Propylthiouracil should not be used with carbamazepine or clozapine (Clozaril) because this may increase the risk of agranulocytosis.

CHAPTER 29

Understanding the Chapter

Key Concepts Summary

The numbered key concepts provide a succinct summary of the important points from the corresponding numbered section within the chapter. If any of these points are not clear, refer to the numbered section within the chapter for review.

29.1 Thyroid hormones contain iodine and stimulate the basal metabolic rate of nearly all tissues.

29.2 An accurate diagnosis of thyroid hormone dysfunction is based on the client's symptoms and the results of diagnostic tests.

29.3 Hypothyroidism, or thyroid deficiency, can occur as a congenital or acquired disorder.

29.4 Hypothyroidism is treated by replacement therapy with thyroid hormone.

29.5 Hyperthyroidism, or Graves' disease, is an autoimmune disorder accompanied by ophthalmopathy and goiter.

29.6 Hyperthyroidism is treated with surgery or drugs that reduce the production of thyroid hormone.

Chapter 29 Scenario

Helen is a 42-year-old mother of three children who works full time in a department store. She has been feeling extremely tired and has been gaining weight, and she says that she feels cold all the time. Acting on her feelings that something might be wrong, she visits her healthcare provider. Her vital signs at that time are as follows: blood pressure 94/60 mm Hg, heart rate 58 beats/minute, temperature 36.3°C. Her weight has increased 13.6 kg since she was last seen 6 months ago. She confirms that her appetite has decreased. After completing a physical examination, the healthcare provider orders some laboratory tests, including T_3, T_4, and TSH.

Critical Thinking Questions

1. Based on the client's symptoms, what test results would you anticipate?

2. The healthcare provider orders levothyroxine (Synthroid) 200 μg PO daily for Helen. What will you teach Helen about this drug and when to take it?

3. Helen asks you if she will need to be on the medication for very long. How will you answer her?

4. What symptoms should Helen report to the healthcare provider while she is taking the Synthroid?

See Answers to Critical Thinking Questions in Appendix B.

NCLEX Practice Questions

1 A client on replacement therapy with levothyroxine (Synthroid) reports feeling nervous and is having occasional palpitations and tremors. The nurse recognizes that these symptoms may indicate which effect is occurring?

a. The client is still experiencing hypothyroidism and the dose may need to be increased.

b. The client now has normal thyroid function and the levothyroxine is no longer needed.

c. The client has developed diabetes and needs further evaluation.

d. The client is experiencing symptoms of hyperthyroidism and the drug dosage may need to be decreased.

2 Which of the following assessment findings would the nurse expect to observe in an adult client experiencing therapeutic effects from levothyroxine (Synthroid)? Select all that apply.

a. Constipation and weight gain

b. Decreased blinking and exophthalmos

c. Decreased reports of fatigue

d. Decreased blood cholesterol levels

e. Pulse rate between 60 and 100 beats/minute

3 A client will be treated with propylthiouracil (PTU) for hyperthyroidism. While the client is taking this drug, which symptoms will the nurse teach the client to report to the healthcare provider?

a. Sore throat, low-grade fever, chills

b. Increase in appetite and caloric intake

c. Tinnitus, altered taste, thickened saliva

d. Insomnia, nightmares, night sweats

4 Which assessment finding would cause the nurse to withhold the regularly scheduled dose of levothyroxine?

a. A 1 kg (2.2 lb) weight gain

b. A blood pressure reading of 100/70 mm Hg

c. A pulse rate of 110 beats/minute

d. A temperature of 37.9°C

5 A client is taking a solution of 5% iodine and 10% potassium iodide (Lugol's solution) prior to a thyroidectomy. The client asks why iodine solution is used since iodine is needed to make thyroid hormone. What would the nurse's best answer be?

a. "The symptoms you were having indicate that you were not receiving enough iodine."

b. "High levels of iodine can temporarily reduce the amount of thyroid hormone your body makes and secretes."

c. "High levels of iodine are always used prior to thyroidectomy to make up for the loss of iodine when the thyroid is removed."

d. "The high levels of iodine help prevent diabetes from developing."

See Answers to NCLEX Practice Questions in Appendix A.

PROTOTYPE DRUGS

Glucocorticoids
  Pr *Hydrocorti-
    sone (Cortef,
    Solu-Cortef)*
**Corticosteroids for
Non-endocrine
Conditions**

Mineralocorticoids
  *Fludrocortisone
  (Florinef)*

Antiadrenal Drugs

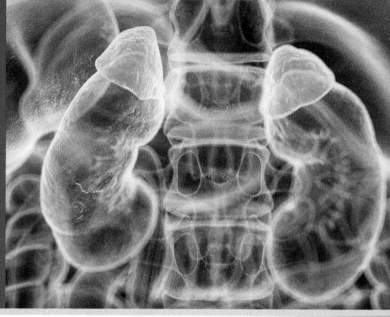

Sciepro/Science Photo Library/Getty Images

CHAPTER

30 Corticosteroids and Pharmacotherapy of Adrenal Disorders

LEARNING OUTCOMES

After reading this chapter, the student should be able to:

1. Identify the functions of the three classes of hormones secreted by the adrenal gland.
2. Diagram the negative feedback regulation of corticosteroid secretion.
3. Identify common properties of the corticosteroid medications.
4. Describe the potential adverse effects of long-term corticosteroid therapy.
5. Compare and contrast the pharmacotherapy of acute and chronic adrenocortical insufficiency.
6. Explain how corticosteroids affect the inflammatory and immune responses.
7. Recognize non-endocrine disorders that respond to corticosteroid therapy.
8. Describe indications for pharmacotherapy with mineralocorticoids.
9. Explain the pharmacotherapy of Cushing's syndrome.
10. Describe the nurse's role in the pharmacological management of adrenal disorders.
11. For each of the classes shown in the Prototype Drugs list, identify the prototype and representative drugs and explain the mechanism(s) of drug action, primary indications, contraindications, significant drug interactions, pregnancy category, and important adverse effects.
12. Apply the nursing process to the care of clients who are receiving pharmacotherapy with corticosteroids and mineralocorticoids.

CHAPTER OUTLINE

▶ Physiology of the Adrenal Gland

▶ Overview of Corticosteroid Pharmacotherapy

▶ Adverse Effects of Corticosteroids

▶ Replacement Therapy with Corticosteroids

▶ Corticosteroids in Inflammation

▶ Mineralocorticoids in Adrenal Insufficiency

▶ Pharmacotherapy of Cushing's Syndrome

Although small in size, the adrenal glands secrete hormones that affect every body tissue. Adrenal disorders range from excess hormone secretion to deficient hormone secretion. The specific pharmacotherapy depends on which portion of the adrenal gland is responsible for the abnormal secretion.

This chapter examines the pharmacological properties of corticosteroids that make them so important to pharmacotherapy.

Physiology of the Adrenal Gland

30.1 The adrenal glands secrete gonadocorticoids, mineralocorticoids, and corticosteroids.

Weighing only 5.5 grams, each pyramid-shaped adrenal gland that sits atop each kidney is divided into two major portions: an inner medulla and an outer cortex. The secretions from these two portions have very different functions.

The adrenal medulla secretes 75% to 80% epinephrine, with the remainder of the secretion being norepinephrine. Adrenal release of epinephrine is triggered by activation of the sympathetic division of the autonomic nervous system.

The adrenal cortex secretes three essential classes of steroid hormones: mineralocorticoids, glucocorticoids, and gonadocorticoids. Collectively, the mineralocorticoids and glucocorticoids are called corticosteroids or adrenocortical hormones. Although the terms *corticosteroid* and *glucocorticoid* are sometimes used interchangeably in clinical practice, the term *corticosteroid* technically refers to a hormone or drug that has both glucocorticoid and mineralocorticoid activity. The hormones secreted by the adrenal gland are illustrated in Figure 30.1.

Mineralocorticoids

Aldosterone accounts for more than 95% of the **mineralocorticoids** secreted by the adrenal glands. The primary functions of aldosterone are to conserve sodium and water and to promote the excretion of potassium by the renal tubule, thus regulating plasma volume.

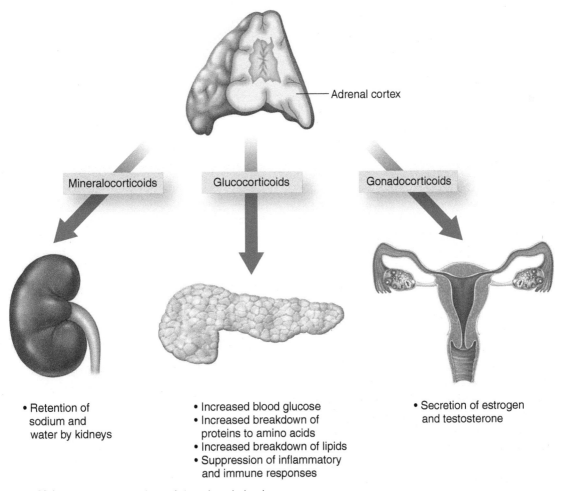

— Adrenal cortex

Mineralocorticoids

Glucocorticoids

Gonadocorticoids

- Retention of sodium and water by kidneys

- Increased blood glucose
- Increased breakdown of proteins to amino acids
- Increased breakdown of lipids
- Suppression of inflammatory and immune responses

- Secretion of estrogen and testosterone

Figure 30.1 Hormonal secretions of the adrenal gland.

Glucocorticoids

More than 30 different **glucocorticoids** are secreted from the adrenal cortex. Cortisol, also called hydrocortisone, is secreted in the highest amount and is the most important pharmacologically. The liver converts hydrocortisone into cortisone, an active metabolite that is also available as a drug. Corticosterone is an additional steroid secreted by the adrenal cortex.

Glucocorticoids prepare the body for long-term stress and affect the metabolism of nearly every cell. The effects of glucocorticoids are diverse and include the following:

* Increase the level of blood glucose (hyperglycemic effect) by inhibiting insulin secretion and promoting gluconeogenesis, which is the synthesis of carbohydrates from lipid and protein sources. This decreases glucose use by tissues and promotes the storage of glycogen in the liver.

* Increase the breakdown of proteins to amino acids. Amino acids are then converted to glucose and glycogen in the liver, resulting in protein depletion.

* Increase the breakdown of lipids (lipolysis). The fatty acids are then used as energy sources.

* Suppress the inflammatory and immune responses.

* Increase the sensitivity of vascular smooth muscle to the actions of norepinephrine and angiotensin II, thus modifying smooth muscle tone.

* Influence the central nervous system (CNS) by affecting mood and maintaining normal nerve excitability.

* Increase the breakdown of bony matrix, resulting in bone demineralization.

* Promote bronchodilation by making bronchial smooth muscle more responsive to sympathetic nervous system activation.

* Stabilize mast cells, inhibiting the release of inflammatory mediators.

As this list confirms, the glucocorticoids are essential hormones for maintaining homeostasis. When given as medications, some of the physiological actions of glucocorticoids are considered therapeutic effects, whereas others are considered adverse effects. Unfortunately, it is impossible to totally separate therapeutic effects from adverse effects when drugs with such widespread actions are used in pharmacotherapy.

The physiological levels of glucocorticoids vary based on circadian rhythm. The lowest serum levels occur during early sleep. Secretion rises during the night, with levels peaking at awakening and declining during the day, depending on the needs of the body. Stress can cause a rapid increase in glucocorticoid levels; when faced with internal inflammatory or stressful conditions, the secretion of glucocorticoids can increase to 10 times the baseline level.

Regulation of glucocorticoid levels begins with corticotropin-releasing factor (CRF), secreted by the hypothalamus. CRF travels to the pituitary where it causes the release of **adrenocorticotropic hormone (ACTH)**. ACTH then travels via the blood to reach the adrenal cortex, causing it to release glucocorticoids. When the serum level of cortisol rises, it provides negative feedback to the hypothalamus and pituitary to shut off further release of glucocorticoids.

Gonadocorticoids

The **gonadocorticoids**, or sex hormones, secreted by the adrenal cortex are mostly androgens, although small amounts of estrogens are also produced. The amounts of adrenal sex hormones are far less than the levels secreted by the testes or ovaries during the reproductive years. Though their amount is small, the adrenal gonadocorticoids contribute to the onset of puberty and are the primary source of endogenous estrogen in postmenopausal women (see Chapter 31). Tumours of the adrenal cortex (pheochromocytoma) can cause hypersecretion of gonadocorticoids, resulting in hirsutism and masculinization, signs that are more noticeable in women than in men.

Overview of Corticosteroid Pharmacotherapy

30.2 Corticosteroids are widely used, and all drugs in the class have very similar indications, actions, and adverse effects.

Corticosteroids are some of the most widely prescribed medications because they are useful in treating conditions that affect nearly every body system (see Table 30.1 for a list of select glucocorticoids). Furthermore, some of their indications are for diseases common to all age groups and for diseases that occur frequently in the population. Some are available over the counter (OTC).

Corticosteroids can be classified in many different ways. One method is based on pathophysiology, such as grouping corticosteroids used for the treatment of inflammation, allergies, or neoplasias. Another method is to group the drugs by body system, such as corticosteroids used for skin conditions, immune disorders, or lung diseases. A third method is to look at corticosteroid use based on the drugs' pharmacological actions, as listed in Table 30.2. In clinical practice, all methods are used.

Regardless of the method of classification, several general statements can be made about the corticosteroid medications:

* All act by the same mechanism.

* All have the same basic adverse effects, which are dose dependent.

TABLE 30.1 Select Glucocorticoids

Drug	Route and Adult Dose
Short Acting	
cortisone **Pr** hydrocortisone (Cortef, Solu-Cortef)	Topical, as directed by healthcare provider PO, 20-240 mg/day; IM/IV, start with 100-500 mg/dose at intervals of 2, 4, or 6 hours
Intermediate Acting	
methylprednisolone (Medrol)	PO, 4-48 mg/day in 1 to 4 divided doses initially; IM, 4-120 mg single dose; IV, 10-40 mg over a period of several minutes; intralesional, 20-60 mg
prednisolone (PediaPred) prednisone (see Chapter 42, page 499, for the Prototype Drug box)	PO, 5–60 mg qd PO, 5–60 mg qd
triamcinolone (Kenalog)	Topical, as directed by healthcare provider
Long Acting	
betamethasone (Celestone) dexamethasone (Dexasone)	Topical, as directed by healthcare provider PO/IM/IV, 0.75 to 9 mg/day in divided doses every 6 to 12 hours; intraarticular, intralesional or soft tissue, 0.4 to 6 mg/day

TABLE 30.2 Actions and Indications for Corticosteroids

Pharmacological Action	Indications
Reduce cell reproduction	Lymphomas and other neoplasms
Reduce joint inflammation	Rheumatoid arthritis, osteoarthritis, bursitis, tendonitis
Reduce lung inflammation	Asthma, chronic obstructive pulmonary disease (COPD)
Reduce skin inflammation	Dermatitis, psoriasis
Supply exogenous corticosteroids	Replacement therapy
Suppress allergic response	Allergic rhinitis; anaphylaxis
Suppress gastrointestinal (GI) inflammation	Inflammatory bowel disease
Suppress general inflammatory response	Systemic lupus erythematosus
Suppress immune response	Prophylaxis of transplant rejection Autoimmune hemolytic anemia
Suppress ocular inflammation	Conjunctivitis

- Indications and adverse effects vary by the dose, length of use, and route of administration.

- They are well absorbed when administered orally or parenterally, and they are widely distributed to all body tissues. Topical administration (intra-articular, inhalation, skin products, and ocular drops) results in systemic absorption, although at a slow rate.

- Most are highly bound to plasma proteins.

- All are metabolized by the liver and excreted by the kidneys.

- All have the potential to cross the placenta (pregnancy category C) and are secreted in breast milk. Their use should be avoided during pregnancy and lactation.

More than 20 corticosteroids are available as medications, and the choice of a particular drug depends primarily on the pharmacokinetic properties of the drug. The duration of action, which is sometimes used to classify these drugs, ranges from short to long acting. Some, such as hydrocortisone (Cortef), also have mineralocorticoid activity and may cause sodium and fluid retention; others, such as prednisone, have no such effect. Some corticosteroids are available by only one route, such as topical for dermal conditions or intranasal for allergic rhinitis.

Adverse Effects of Corticosteroids

30.3 Long-term therapy with corticosteroids has the potential to cause serious adverse effects in multiple body systems.

Low-dose or brief-duration regimens of corticosteroids produce few adverse effects. On the other hand, high doses taken for prolonged periods offer a significant risk for serious adverse effects. These adverse effects of corticosteroid therapy are well documented and can affect nearly any body system. The following list includes the most significant adverse events that result from long-term corticosteroid therapy:

- *Immune response.* Suppression of the immune and inflammatory responses increases clients' susceptibility to infections. Latent infections, such as herpesvirus or tuberculosis, may be reactivated during corticosteroid therapy. In addition, the anti-inflammatory actions of the corticosteroids may mask the signs of an existing infection.

- *Peptic ulcers.* Prolonged corticosteroid use is associated with the development of peptic ulcers, especially when these drugs are combined with nonsteroidal anti-inflammatory drugs (NSAIDs). Both classes of drugs reduce prostaglandin synthesis in the gastric mucosa, which normally provides protection from the high acidity in the stomach. Use of proton pump inhibitors may reduce the incidence of peptic ulcers in these clients

- *Osteoporosis.* Corticosteroids inhibit calcium absorption, suppress bone formation, and accelerate bone resorption—all actions that weaken the bony matrix. Up to 50% of clients on long-term corticosteroid therapy will sustain a fracture due to osteoporosis. Treatment with a bisphosphonate may reduce the incidence of fractures in these clients

- *Behavioural changes.* By an unknown mechanism, corticosteroids can induce psychological changes. These may be minor, such as nervousness or moodiness, or may involve hallucinations and increased suicidal tendencies.

- *Eye changes.* Cataracts and open-angle glaucoma are frequent adverse events of long-term corticosteroid therapy.

- *Metabolic changes.* Corticosteroids have a hyperglycemic action that raises serum glucose and can cause glucose intolerance, especially in clients with diabetes. Mobilization of lipids may cause hyperlipidemia and abnormal fat deposits. Electrolyte changes include hypocalcemia, hypokalemia, and hypernatremia. Fluid retention, weight gain, hypertension, and edema are other possible effects.

- *Myopathy.* Muscle wasting induced by corticosteroids may cause weakness and fatigue. The myopathy may involve ocular or respiratory muscles.

NCLEX Success Tip

Emergency treatment for acute adrenal insufficiency (Addisonian crisis) is intravenous (IV) infusion of hydrocortisone and saline solution. The client is usually given a dose containing hydrocortisone 100 mg IV in normal saline every 6 hours until blood pressure returns to normal.

Corticosteroids interact with many drugs. Their hyperglycemic effects may decrease the effectiveness of antidiabetic drugs. Combining glucocorticoids with other ulcerogenic drugs such as aspirin and other NSAIDs markedly increases the risk for peptic ulcer disease. Administration with certain diuretics may lead to hypocalcemia and hypokalemia.

An important goal during long-term corticosteroid therapy is to prevent the development of serious adverse effects. The following strategies are often used to minimize the incidence of serious adverse effects:

- Doses are kept to the lowest amount that will achieve the therapeutic goal. In some cases, concurrent drug therapy with a non-corticosteroid may be implemented to produce additive therapeutic effects, while keeping the corticosteroid dose low. Careful monitoring of the effectiveness of the drug is necessary.

- Corticosteroids may be administered every other day (alternate-day dosing) to minimize adrenal atrophy. This prevents constant, negative feedback on the pituitary and forces the client's adrenal glands to secrete endogenous corticosteroids every other day.

- For acute conditions, clients are administered large doses of corticosteroids for a few days and then the drug dose is gradually decreased until discontinued. This prevents the severe symptoms of adrenal atrophy from developing.

- Whenever possible, corticosteroids should be administered locally by inhalation, intra-articular injections, or topical applications to the skin, eyes, or ears to diminish the extent of systemic effects. Local administration rarely produces systemic adverse effects.

Replacement Therapy with Corticosteroids

30.4 Adrenocortical insufficiency is treated by administering physiological levels of corticosteroids.

Lack of adequate secretion by the adrenal cortex, or **adrenocortical insufficiency**, involves a lack of both glucocorticoids and mineralocorticoids. When pathology of the adrenal glands is the cause of the hyposecretion, it is called primary adrenocortical insufficiency, or **Addison's disease**. The most common cause of primary adrenocortical insufficiency is the autoimmune destruction of both adrenal glands. Hemorrhage, infections, or metastases in the adrenal glands are other potential causes. Addison's disease is rare and includes a deficiency of both glucocorticoids and mineralocorticoids.

Secondary adrenocortical insufficiency occurs when the adrenal glands are normal, but they are not receiving adequate stimulation due to lack of sufficient ACTH from the pituitary. Low serum levels of both ACTH and cortisol are diagnostic of secondary adrenocortical insufficiency because this indicates that the adrenal gland is not receiving ACTH stimulation. Secondary adrenocortical insufficiency is much more common than primary adrenocortical insufficiency and can occur when corticosteroids are suddenly withdrawn during pharmacotherapy. Symptoms of primary and secondary adrenocortical insufficiency are the same because both conditions are characterized by inadequate corticosteroid secretion.

The onset of chronic adrenocortical insufficiency may take several months or even years before an accurate diagnosis is made. Symptoms include hypoglycemia, fatigue, muscle weakness, hypotension, increased skin pigmentation, and gastrointestinal (GI) disturbances such as anorexia, vomiting, and diarrhea. Replacement therapy with corticosteroids is indicated. The goal of replacement therapy is to achieve the same physiological level of hormones in the blood that would be present if the adrenal glands were

functioning properly. Clients who require replacement therapy usually must take corticosteroids for their entire lifetime, and concurrent therapy with a mineralocorticoid such as fludrocortisone (Florinef) is necessary.

Acute adrenocortical insufficiency has a sudden onset and usually occurs when corticosteroids are abruptly withdrawn from a client who has been on long-term therapy. This is because constant, high amounts of corticosteroid medications provide continuous negative feedback to the hypothalamus and pituitary, shutting down the secretion of ACTH. Without stimulation by ACTH, the adrenal cortex shrinks and stops secreting endogenous corticosteroids, a condition known as **adrenal atrophy**. If the corticosteroid medication is abruptly withdrawn, the shrunken adrenal glands will not be able to secrete sufficient corticosteroids, and symptoms of **adrenal crisis** will appear. Symptoms of this condition include nausea, vomiting, lethargy, confusion, myalgia, arthralgia, fever, asthenia, acute abdominal pain, hypotension, seizures, renal failure, and coma. Immediate administration of IV hydrocortisone is essential because shock may quickly result if symptoms remain untreated. To prevent adrenal crisis, corticosteroids should be discontinued gradually.

The most frequently prescribed corticosteroids for treating adrenal insufficiency are hydrocortisone, prednisone, and dexamethasone (Dexasone). Doses of these drugs are individualized to the specific amount of replacement therapy needed by the client, and doses will need to be increased during periods of high stress. Hydrocortisone and dexamethasone can be administered by the intramuscular (IM) or IV routes for acute disease or by the oral (PO) route for maintenance doses. Prednisone is administered by the PO route. Because dexamethasone and prednisone have little or no mineralocorticoid activity, concurrent fludrocortisone therapy is necessary. Hydrocortisone has some intrinsic mineralocorticoid activity; therefore, concurrent administration of fludrocortisone may not be necessary.

PROTOTYPE DRUG | **Hydrocortisone (Cortef)**

Actions and Uses: Structurally identical to the natural hormone cortisol, hydrocortisone is a synthetic corticosteroid that is the drug of choice for treating adrenocortical insufficiency. When used for replacement therapy, it is given at physiological doses. Once proper dosing is achieved, the drug's therapeutic effects should mimic those of endogenous corticosteroids. Hydrocortisone is also available for the treatment of inflammation, allergic disorders, and many other conditions. Intra-articular injections may be given to decrease severe inflammation in affected joints.

Hydrocortisone is available in six different formulations. Hydrocortisone base (Aeroseb-HC, Alphaderm, Cetacort, others) and hydrocortisone acetate (Anusol HC, Cortaid, Cortef Acetate) are available as oral preparations, creams, and ointments. Hydrocortisone cypionate (Cortef Fluid) is an oral suspension. Hydrocortisone sodium phosphate (Hydrocortone Phosphate) and hydrocortisone sodium succinate (A-Hydrocort, Solu-Cortef) are for parenteral use only. Hydrocortisone valerate (Westcort) is only for topical applications.

Pharmacokinetics: Hydrocortisone is well absorbed after oral administration. It is widely distributed, crosses the placenta, and enters breast milk. It is metabolized by the liver. Its half-life in plasma is 1.5 to 2 hours and in tissue is 8 to 12 hours. Adrenal suppression lasts 1.5 days.

Administration Alerts:

- Administer exactly as prescribed and at the same time every day.
- Administer oral formulations with food.
- Hydrocortisone is pregnancy category C.

Adverse Effects and Interactions: When used at physiological doses for replacement therapy, adverse effects of hydrocortisone should not be evident. The client and nurse must be vigilant, however, in observing for signs of Cushing's syndrome, which can develop with overtreatment. If taken for longer than 2 weeks, hydrocortisone should be discontinued gradually. Hydrocortisone possesses some mineralocorticoid activity, so sodium and fluid retention may be noted. A wide range of CNS effects have been reported, including insomnia, anxiety, headache, vertigo, confusion, and depression. Cardiovascular effects may include hypertension and tachycardia. Long-term therapy may result in peptic ulcer disease.

Hydrocortisone interacts with many drugs; for example, barbiturates, phenytoin (Dilantin), and rifampin (Rifadin, Rofact) may increase hepatic metabolism, thus decreasing hydrocortisone levels. Estrogens potentiate the effects of hydrocortisone. NSAIDs compound ulcerogenic effects. Cholestyramine (Questran, Olestyr) and colestipol (Colestid) decrease hydrocortisone absorption. Diuretics and amphotericin B (Fungizone) exacerbate hypokalemia. Anticholinesterase agents may produce severe weakness. Hydrocortisone may cause a decrease in immune response to vaccines and toxoids.

Use with caution with herbal supplements, such as aloe and buckthorn (a laxative), which may create a potassium deficiency with chronic use or abuse.

Corticosteroids in Inflammation
30.5 Corticosteroids are frequently used to suppress the inflammatory and immune responses.

One of the most important physiological effects of corticosteroids is their natural ability to dampen the immune response and inhibit the synthesis of inflammatory mediators. When used to treat conditions characterized by hyperactive body defences, the anti-inflammatory effects of the corticosteroids are therapeutic. When the drugs are administered as replacement therapy, however, suppression of the immune response can result in an increased incidence of infections.

Part of the reason for the effectiveness of the corticosteroids in reducing inflammation and the immune response is that they act by multiple mechanisms. These mechanisms include the following:

- Decreased numbers of circulating lymphocytes, eosinophils, monocytes, and basophils
- Inhibited movement of macrophages and leukocytes to areas of inflammation

- Decreased production of inflammatory cytokines, including histamine, bradykinin, interferons, interleukins, and granulocyte-macrophage colony-stimulating factor
- Decreased formation of prostaglandins

It is important to note that the doses necessary to treat inflammatory and other non-endocrine diseases are much higher than those used to treat adrenocortical insufficiency. For example, a daily maintenance dose of prednisone for a client with Addison's disease is 7.5 mg/day. This amount approximates what would normally be secreted by the adrenal gland. Daily doses of prednisone for non-endocrine disorders are 5 to 30 mg for transplant prophylaxis; 80 mg for chronic lymphocytic leukemia; 40 to 60 mg for Crohn's disease; and 20 to 300 mg for systemic lupus erythematosus. At these high doses, the adverse effects of corticosteroids will quickly manifest, and the adrenal gland will begin to atrophy in only 2 to 4 weeks. Interventions should be planned to prevent anticipated adverse effects.

Arthritis
Arthritis is one of the most common diseases affecting older adults. Rheumatoid arthritis (RA) is a chronic autoimmune disease that causes inflammation of joints and is characterized by disfigurement and inflammation of multiple joints. Osteoarthritis is also a progressive joint disease, but it occurs with more advanced age and is characterized by less inflammation than RA. Both types of arthritis are treated with NSAIDs early in the course of the disease. Corticosteroids are administered when inflammation becomes severe, with therapy being limited to 1 to 2 weeks, or until the pain and inflammation subside. If the pain and inflammation are localized to one or two joints, intra-articular injections may be used. Corticosteroids offer only symptomatic treatment and do not alter the course of either type of arthritis. Arthritis pharmacotherapy is discussed in Chapter 61.

Inflammatory Bowel Disease
Inflammatory bowel disease (IBD) is characterized by ulceration in the distal portion of the small intestine (Crohn's disease) or in the large intestine (ulcerative colitis). Various drugs, including the 5-aminosalicylic acid drugs, are used to control inflammation, cramping, and diarrhea. Exacerbations are treated with corticosteroids for brief time periods. Budesonide (Entocort, Pulmicort, Rhinocort) is a corticosteroid that has a delayed release and remains in the intestine to treat the inflammation locally, without causing significant systemic effects. IBD pharmacotherapy is discussed in Chapter 35.

Asthma
Asthma is characterized by chronic inflammation that causes bronchoconstriction in the respiratory passages. Inhaled corticosteroids are preferred drugs for the prevention of asthmatic attacks and the management of chronic asthma. The inhaled agents produce few systemic adverse effects. Oral corticosteroids are used for the short-term management of acute asthma exacerbations. Asthma pharmacotherapy is discussed in Chapter 38.

Allergies
Allergic rhinitis is inflammation of the nasal mucosa caused by exposure to allergens. Corticosteroids are applied directly to the

nasal mucosa to prevent symptoms of allergic rhinitis. They have largely replaced antihistamines as drugs of choice for this condition. When administered intranasally, the corticosteroids do not exhibit systemic adverse effects. For acute allergies, corticosteroids may be administered parenterally. Because their onset of action is slow, however, they are always administered concurrently with other drugs, such as epinephrine, for this indication. The pharmacotherapy of allergic rhinitis is discussed in Chapter 42.

Transplant Rejection Prophylaxis

Successful tissue transplantation requires the use of immunosuppressant drugs; otherwise, the client's immune system would reject the transplant. One or more immunosuppressants are administered at the time of transplantation and are continued for several months following surgery. Corticosteroids are part of most therapeutic regimens to prevent transplant rejection. They may be used for several weeks or maintained for 3 to 6 months following surgery. The prophylaxis of transplant rejection is discussed in Chapter 41.

Dermatological Conditions

Topical corticosteroids are the most effective therapy for treating the inflammation and itching of dermatitis. These corticosteroids are specially formulated to penetrate deep into the skin layers. Topical corticosteroids such as betamethasone (Celestone) and hydrocortisone acetate are also the primary, initial treatment for psoriasis. High-potency corticosteroids are used for 1 to 2 weeks, followed by moderate- to low-potency corticosteroids for maintenance therapy. The pharmacotherapy of dermatological diseases is discussed in Chapter 62.

Neoplasms

Corticosteroids such as prednisone and dexamethasone are used as adjuncts in the treatment of certain neoplasms, especially acute childhood leukemias and Hodgkin's disease. They are always used in combination with other antineoplastics. The pharmacotherapy of cancer is discussed in Chapter 60.

Edema

Corticosteroids are occasionally used to treat disorders characterized by edema. They have been used for many years to reduce intracranial edema associated with trauma, tumours, and cerebral ischemia. These hormones tend to stabilize capillary membranes. Their effectiveness in treating edema is controversial.

Mineralocorticoids in Adrenal Insufficiency

30.6 Clients with adrenal insufficiency often require replacement therapy with mineralocorticoids.

Aldosterone is the primary hormone that regulates sodium and potassium balance in the body. Regulation of aldosterone secretion is through activation of the renin-angiotensin-aldosterone system. When plasma volume falls, the kidney secretes renin, which results in the production of angiotensin II. Angiotensin II then promotes aldosterone secretion, which in turn acts on the renal tubules to promote sodium and water retention and increased excretion of potassium.

Lack of adequate aldosterone secretion, or **hypoaldosteronism**, may be caused by a number of disorders. The three broad categories of hypoaldosteronism are as follows:

* *Decreased stimulation of the adrenal cortex.* Beta blockers, NSAIDs, and calcium channel blockers may reduce renin serum levels and suppress the stimulation of aldosterone secretion. Angiotensin-converting enzyme (ACE) inhibitors block the formation of angiotensin II, which is the normal signal for aldosterone secretion.

* *Hyposecretion of aldosterone.* Low aldosterone secretion may result from primary adrenal insufficiency (Addison's disease), which is usually a deficiency in the secretion of both glucocorticoids and mineralocorticoids. Heparin can also suppress aldosterone synthesis and secretion.

* *Aldosterone resistance.* The renal tubules may become resistant to the actions of aldosterone. Aldosterone resistance occurs during diseases of the renal tubules and may also result from therapy with spironolactone (Aldactone) or progestins.

Whenever possible, the cause of hypoaldosteronism is identified and treated. In some cases, replacement therapy with fludrocortisone is necessary.

Excessive secretion of aldosterone, or **hyperaldosteronism**, is usually caused by a benign tumour of the adrenal gland. Also known as Conn's syndrome, symptoms include hypertension caused by fluid retention and muscle weakness due to hypokalemia. Surgical excision of the adrenal tumor is the treatment of choice for most clients; however, pharmacotherapy with spironolactone may benefit clients who are at high surgical risk. Spironolactone is a potassium-sparing diuretic that blocks the actions of aldosterone in the renal tubule.

Pharmacotherapy of Cushing's Syndrome

30.7 Antiadrenal drugs may be administered to lower serum corticosteroid levels in clients with Cushing's syndrome.

Cushing's syndrome has a high mortality rate, and the therapeutic goal is to identify and treat the cause of the excess glucocorticoid secretion. If the cause is overtreatment with glucocorticoid drugs, a gradual reduction in dose is sufficient to reverse the syndrome. When the cause of the hypersecretion is an adrenal tumour or perhaps an ectopic tumour secreting ACTH, surgical removal is indicated. Clients with severe disease will receive drug therapy to quickly lower serum glucocorticoid levels. Combination therapy with aminoglutethimide (Cytadren) and metyrapone (Metopirone) is sometimes used. Aminoglutethimide suppresses adrenal function within 3 to 5 days; however, therapy is usually limited to 3 months because of its ineffectiveness over time. The antifungal drug ketoconazole (Nizoral) has been found to be a safer therapy for long-term use. Most antiadrenal agents inhibit the metabolic conversion of cholesterol to adrenal corticosteroids. They are not curative; their use is temporary until the tumour can be removed or otherwise treated with radiation or antineoplastics.

Nursing Considerations

The role of the nurse in antiadrenal therapy for Cushing's syndrome involves careful monitoring of the client's condition and providing education as it relates to the prescribed drug treatment. Assess and monitor laboratory values, including platelet count, bilirubin, and prothrombin. Assess for jaundice, bruising, and bleeding because antiadrenal therapy may cause leukopenia and thrombocytopenia. Monitor for orthostatic hypotension because the drugs cause decreased aldosterone production. Monitor for dizziness and assist with ambulation. Caution the client to change positions slowly. Ketoconazole administered at high levels is an effective corticosteroid inhibitor. This medication is metabolized in the liver; therefore, hepatic function must be assessed prior to administration and monitored during therapy. Ketoconazole is contraindicated in those with liver dysfunction and in those who abuse alcohol. Obtain a thorough history to assess for alcohol intake or possible HIV infection because these medications are contraindicated in these clients.

Client education as it relates to antiadrenal drugs should include goals, reasons for obtaining baseline data such as vital signs and the existence of underlying hematological disorders, and possible drug side effects. Include the following points when teaching clients about antiadrenal drugs:

- Immediately report unusual bleeding, change in colour of stool or urine, or yellowing of eyes or skin.
- Monitor temperature and report fever.
- Change positions slowly to avoid dizziness.
- Take medication with fruit juice or water to enhance absorption.

CONNECTIONS Lifespan Considerations

◀ Treatment of Cushing's Syndrome during Pregnancy

Aminoglutethimide is contraindicated during pregnancy. In animal studies, the drug has been shown to prevent fetal implantation and increase the potential for fetal death. Also, in pregnant animals the drug causes an unusual condition known as pseudohermaphroditism, in which an individual has the internal reproductive organs of only one sex but exhibits both male and female external genitalia.

Ketoconazole, in high doses, has also been shown to be teratogenic and embryotoxic in animals.

- Avoid alcohol use.
- Practise reliable contraception and notify the healthcare provider if pregnancy is planned or suspected.
- Keep all scheduled appointments and laboratory visits for testing.
- Practise relaxation techniques because increased stress may cause adverse effects of the drug.

NCLEX Success Tip

Consider the source and manifestations of too much vs. too little corticosteroid (whether endogenous or exogenous) and what the related nursing interventions are. Recall the effect on blood glucose levels, fluid, and electrolyte status. Be aware of the postoperative interventions required following the removal of an endocrine gland, for example monitoring calcium after thyroid surgery, or closely checking blood pressure after adrenal gland surgery.

NURSING PROCESS FOCUS

Clients Receiving Systemic Glucocorticoid Therapy

Assessment	Potential Nursing Diagnoses/Identified Patterns
Prior to administration: • Obtain complete health history, including allergies, drug history, and possible drug interactions. • Obtain complete physical examination, focusing on presenting symptoms. • Determine the reason the medication is being administered. • Obtain laboratory studies (long-term therapy), including serum sodium and potassium levels, hematocrit and hemoglobin levels, blood glucose level, and blood urea nitrogen (BUN).	• Risk for injury related to side effects of drug therapy • Risk for infection related to immunosuppression • Need for knowledge regarding drug therapy and adverse effects • Risk for altered body image related to side effects of drug therapy • Risk for fluid and electrolyte imbalance • Risk for unstable blood glucose level • Risk for impaired wound healing

Planning: Client Goals and Expected Outcomes

The client will:

- Demonstrate an understanding of the drug's action by accurately describing drug side effects and precautions
- Exhibit a decrease in the symptoms for which the drug is being given
- Exhibit no symptoms of infection
- Adhere to the treatment plan

Implementation

Interventions (Rationales)	Client Education/Discharge Planning
• Monitor vital signs. (Blood pressure may increase because of increased blood volume and potential vasoconstriction effect.)	• Instruct client to report dizziness, palpitations, or headaches
• Monitor for infection. Protect client from potential infections. (Glucocorticoids increase susceptibility to infections by suppressing the immune response.)	Instruct client to: • Avoid people with infection • Report fever, cough, sore throat, joint pain, increased weakness, and malaise • Consult with the healthcare provider before getting any immunizations
• Monitor client's adherence with drug treatment. (Sudden discontinuation of these agents can precipitate an adrenal crisis.)	Instruct client: • To never suddenly stop taking the medication • In proper use of self-administering tapering dose pack • To take oral medications with food
• Monitor for symptoms of Cushing's syndrome such as moon face, "buffalo hump" contour of shoulders, weight gain, muscle wasting, and increased deposits of fat in the trunk. (Symptoms may indicate excessive use of glucocorticoids.)	Instruct client: • To weigh self daily • That initial weight gain is expected; provide the client with weight gain parameters that warrant reporting • That there are multiple side effects of therapy and that changes in health status should be reported
• Monitor blood glucose levels. (Glucocorticoids cause an increase in gluconeogenesis and reduce glucose use.)	Instruct client to: • Report symptoms of hyperglycemia such as excessive thirst, copious urination, and insatiable appetite • Adjust insulin dose based on blood glucose level, as directed by the healthcare provider
• Monitor skin and mucous membranes for lacerations, abrasions, or breaks in integrity. (Glucocorticoids impair wound healing.)	Instruct client to: • Examine skin daily for cuts and scrapes and to cover any injuries with sterile bandages • Watch for symptoms of skin infection such as redness, swelling, and drainage • Notify the healthcare provider of any non-healing wound or symptoms of infection
• Monitor GI status for peptic ulcer development. (Glucocorticoids decrease gastric mucus production and predispose the client to peptic ulcers.)	• Instruct client to report GI side effects such as heartburn, abdominal pain, or tarry stools.
• Monitor serum electrolytes. (Glucocorticoids cause hypernatremia and hypokalemia.)	Instruct client to: • Consume a diet high in protein, calcium, and potassium but low in fat and concentrated simple carbohydrates • Keep all laboratory appointments
• Monitor changes in musculoskeletal system. (Glucocorticoids decrease bone density and strength and cause muscle atrophy and weakness.)	Instruct client: • To participate in exercise or physical activity to help maintain bone and muscle strength • That the drug may cause weakness in bones and muscles and to avoid strenuous activity that may cause injury
• Monitor emotional stability. (Glucocorticoids may produce mood and behaviour changes such as depression or feeling of invulnerability.)	• Instruct client that mood changes may be expected and to report mental status changes to the healthcare provider

Evaluation of Outcome Criteria

Evaluate effectiveness of drug therapy by confirming that client goals and expected outcomes have been met (see "Planning").

See Table 30.2 (page 349) for a list of drugs to which these nursing actions apply.

CHAPTER

30 Understanding the Chapter

Key Concepts Summary

The numbered key concepts provide a succinct summary of the important points from the corresponding numbered section within the chapter. If any of these points are not clear, refer to the numbered section within the chapter for review.

30.1 The adrenal glands secrete gonadocorticoids, mineralocorticoids, and corticosteroids.

30.2 Corticosteroids are widely used, and all drugs in the class have very similar indications, actions, and adverse effects.

30.3 Long-term therapy with corticosteroids has the potential to cause serious adverse effects in multiple body systems.

30.4 Adrenocortical insufficiency is treated by administering physiological levels of corticosteroids.

30.5 Corticosteroids are frequently used to suppress the inflammatory and immune responses.

30.6 Clients with adrenal insufficiency often require replacement therapy with mineralocorticoids.

30.7 Antiadrenal drugs may be administered to lower serum corticosteroid levels in clients with Cushing's syndrome.

Chapter 30 Scenario

Charlie Harness is a 61-year-old man, newly diagnosed this year with early chronic obstructive pulmonary disease (COPD) secondary to bouts of chronic bronchitis. Charlie had been a cigarette smoker since age 15 but proudly tells everyone that he "quit cold turkey 5 years ago and hasn't touched one since!" He was surprised by the diagnosis of COPD, even though he had been having increasingly long bouts of bronchitis and had noticed that he seemed more out of breath after each one. Charlie's father died at age 52 "from some kind of lung problem," which Charlie thinks might have been caused by smoking. Charlie has come to his healthcare provider today because of increasing shortness of breath. He relates this to "allergy season," when he feels his bronchitis flare and, with it, experiences increasing dyspnea. His physical examination reveals that Charlie is experiencing mild to moderate shortness of breath, pausing for a breath after two or three sentences. His pulse is 108 beats/minute, respiratory rate is 28 breaths/minute, and blood pressure is 150/80 mm Hg, and he is afebrile. A pulse oximeter reading is 94%, and you note that Charlie's past readings have been between 94% and 97%. His breath sounds reveal a prolonged expiratory phase and are

distant. He has inspiratory wheezing, and he tells you that he frequently coughs up small amounts of beige-white mucus. He denies abdominal distention or tenderness. His healthcare provider gives Charlie a prescription for an antibiotic and refill prescriptions for his bronchodilator and budesonide (Pulmicort) inhalers. Charlie is to return in 2 days for reassessment. He has recently discovered information about steroids and expresses some concern about the information he has read. He is considering not taking his budesonide inhaler anymore and asks you what he should do.

Critical Thinking Questions

1. Create a list of questions you would ask Charlie to determine if he is experiencing any adverse effects from the corticosteroids.

2. What would you tell this client related to abruptly discontinuing this medication? Why?

3. Charlie asks you if there are any precautions that he should take related to his budesonide. How would you respond?

See Answers to Critical Thinking Questions in Appendix B.

NCLEX Practice Questions

1 A client has been ordered methylprednisolone (Medrol Dosepak) for treatment of a significant poison ivy rash. The nurse will teach the client to report which adverse effects to the healthcare provider? Select all that apply.

a. Edema

b. Tinnitus

c. Eye pain or vision changes

d. Dizziness upon standing

e. Abdominal pain

2 A client has been taking a thiazide diuretic for treatment of hypertension and has been prescribed hydrocortisone (Cortef) for a significant allergic reaction to shellfish. Which symptom should be immediately reported to the provider?

a. Irregular heart rate and rhythm

b. Delayed wound healing

c. Weight gain of 1 to 1.4 kg (2 to 3 lb) in 1 week

d. Elevated serum lipid levels

3 An older adult client with chronic bronchitis has been receiving low-dose therapy with dexamethasone for several months to reduce the inflammation occurring secondary to the bronchitis. Which instructions should this client receive to reduce the risk of osteoporosis related to dexamethasone use? Select all that apply.

a. Perform weight-bearing exercises at least three to four times weekly.

b. Increase dietary intake of calcium- and vitamin D–rich fooperds.

c. Remain sedentary except during periods of exercise.

d. Increase fluid intake, including carbonated sodas, but avoid alcohol.

e. Request a prescription for a bisphosphonate drug from the provider.

4 A client with adrenocortical insufficiency has started therapy with fludrocortisone (Florinef). Which important intervention related to this drug therapy should the nurse teach the client?

a. "Report any abdominal pain or changes in your stool colour."

b. "Return monthly for laboratory work to assess blood lipid levels."

c. "Report any unusual changes in your mood."

d. "Weigh yourself daily, ideally at the same time each day."

5 A client who has been taking dexamethasone for rheumatoid arthritis was unable to take the drug for several days due to an intestinal virus. The client seeks treatment in the emergency department for complaints of severe nausea, vomiting, lethargy, fever, and hypotension. What drug would the nurse anticipate will be given to this client?

a. Fludrocortisone (Florinef)

b. Ketoconazole (Nizoral)

c. Hydrocortisone (Solu-Cortef)

d. Metyrapone (Metopirone)

See Answers to NCLEX Practice Questions in Appendix A.

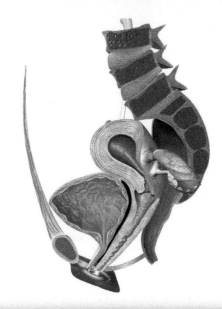

PROTOTYPE DRUGS

ORAL CONTRACEPTIVES
Estrogen-progestin combinations
Pr *ethinyl estradiol with norethindrone (Ortho-Novum 1/35)*
Progestin-only agents

HORMONE REPLACEMENT THERAPY
Estrogens and estrogen-progestin combinations
Pr *conjugated estrogens (Premarin)*

DRUGS FOR DYSFUNCTIONAL UTERINE BLEEDING
Progestins
Pr *medroxyprogesterone (Provera, Medroxy)*

UTERINE STIMULANTS AND RELAXANTS
Oxytocics *(stimulants)*
Pr *oxytocin (Pitocin)*
Ergot alkaloids
Prostaglandins
Tocolytics *(relaxants)*
Beta2-adrenergic agonists
Other tocolytics

science stuff/Alamy Stock Photo

31

Pharmacotherapy of Disorders of the Female Reproductive System

LEARNING OUTCOMES

After reading this chapter, the student should be able to:

1. Describe the roles of the hypothalamus, pituitary, and ovaries in maintaining female reproductive function.
2. Explain the mechanisms by which estrogens and progestins prevent conception.
3. Describe the nurse's role in the pharmacological management of clients who are taking oral contraceptives.
4. Compare and contrast the options available for long-term contraception.
5. Explain how drugs may be used to provide emergency contraception and to terminate early pregnancy.
6. Describe the role of drug therapy in the treatment of menopausal and postmenopausal symptoms.
7. Discuss the uses of progestins in the therapy of dysfunctional uterine bleeding.
8. Compare and contrast the use of uterine stimulants and relaxants in the treatment of antepartum and postpartum clients.
9. Explain how drug therapy may be used to treat female infertility.
10. For each of the drug classes listed in Prototype Drugs, identify a representative drug and explain its mechanism of action, therapeutic effects, and important adverse effects.
11. Describe and explain, based on pharmacological principles, the rationale for nursing assessment, planning, and interventions for clients with conditions of the female reproductive system.
12. Use the nursing process to care for clients who are receiving drug therapy for disorders and conditions of the female reproductive system.

CHAPTER OUTLINE

▸ Hypothalamic and Pituitary Regulation of Female Reproductive Function

▸ Ovarian Control of Female Reproductive Function

▸ Contraception
  ▸ Estrogens and Progestins as Oral Contraceptives
  ▸ Drugs for Long-Term Contraception and Newer Contraceptive Delivery Methods
  ▸ Emergency Contraception and Pharmacological Abortion

▸ Menopause
  ▸ Hormone Replacement Therapy

Hormones from the pituitary gland and gonads provide for the growth and maintenance of the female reproductive organs. Endogenous hormones can be supplemented with natural or synthetic hormones to achieve a variety of therapeutic goals, ranging from replacement therapy, to prevention of pregnancy, to milk production. This chapter examines drugs used to treat disorders and conditions associated with the female reproductive system.

Hypothalamic and Pituitary Regulation of Female Reproductive Function

31.1 Female reproductive function is controlled by GnRH from the hypothalamus and by FSH and LH from the pituitary.

Regulation of the female reproductive system is achieved by hormones from the hypothalamus, pituitary gland, and ovary. The hypothalamus secretes **gonadotropin-releasing hormone (GnRH)**, which travels a short distance to the pituitary to stimulate the secretion of **follicle-stimulating hormone (FSH)** and **luteinizing hormone (LH)**. Both of these pituitary hormones act on the ovary and cause immature ovarian follicles to begin developing. The rising and falling levels of pituitary hormones create two interrelated cycles that occur on a periodic, monthly basis: the ovarian and uterine cycles. The hormonal changes that occur during the ovarian and uterine cycles are illustrated in Figure 31.1.

Under the influence of FSH and LH, several ovarian follicles begin the maturation process each month during a woman's reproductive years. On approximately day 14 of the ovarian cycle, a surge of LH secretion causes one follicle to expel its oocyte, a process called **ovulation**. The ruptured follicle, minus its oocyte, remains in the ovary and is transformed into the hormone-secreting **corpus luteum**. The oocyte, on the other hand, begins its journey through the fallopian tube and eventually reaches the uterus. If conception does not occur, the outer lining of the uterus degenerates and is shed during menstruation.

Ovarian Control of Female Reproductive Function

31.2 Estrogens are secreted by ovarian follicles and are responsible for the secondary sex characteristics of the female. Progestins are secreted by the corpus luteum and prepare the endometrium for implantation.

As ovarian follicles mature, they secrete the female sex hormones **estrogen** and **progesterone**. Estrogen is actually a generic term for three different hormones: estradiol, estrone, and estriol. Estrogen is responsible for the maturation of the female reproductive organs and for the appearance of the secondary sex characteristics. In addition, estrogen has numerous metabolic effects on non-reproductive tissues, including the brain, kidneys, blood vessels, and skin. For example, estrogen helps to maintain low blood cholesterol levels and facilitates calcium uptake by bones to help maintain proper bone density (see Chapter 61). When women enter menopause at about age 50 to 55, the ovaries stop secreting estrogen.

In the last half of the ovarian cycle, the corpus luteum secretes a class of hormones called progestins, the most abundant of which is progesterone. In combination with estrogen, progesterone promotes breast development and regulates the monthly changes of the uterine cycle. Under the influence of estrogen and progesterone, the uterine endometrium becomes vascular and thickens in preparation for receiving a fertilized egg. High progesterone and estrogen levels in the final third of the uterine cycle provide negative feedback to shut off GnRH, FSH, and LH secretion. This negative feedback loop is illustrated in Figure 31.2. Without stimulation from FSH and LH, estrogen and progesterone levels fall sharply, the endometrium is shed, and menstrual bleeding begins.

CONTRACEPTION

Oral contraceptives are drugs used to prevent pregnancy. Most oral contraceptives are a combination of estrogens and progestins. In small doses, they prevent fertilization by inhibiting ovulation. Select oral contraceptives are shown in Table 31.1.

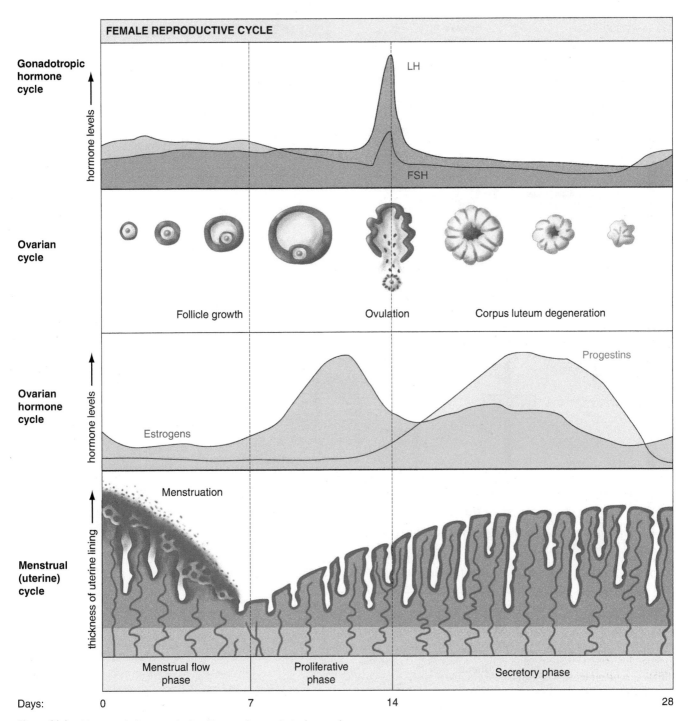

FEMALE REPRODUCTIVE CYCLE

Gonadotropic hormone cycle

hormone levels

LH

FSH

Ovarian cycle

Follicle growth

Ovulation

Corpus luteum degeneration

Ovarian hormone cycle

hormone levels

Estrogens

Progestins

Menstrual (uterine) cycle

thickness of uterine lining

Menstruation

Menstrual flow phase

Proliferative phase

Secretory phase

Days: 0   7   14   28

Figure 31.1 Hormonal changes during the ovarian and uterine cycles.
Pearson Education.

Selection of a contraceptive is based on effectiveness, safety, and personal choice. The decision to engage in sexual activity is one of the most important decisions in life; the choice affects not just the partners, but may affect generations to follow. A couple who is engaging in intercourse on a regular basis without contraceptive protection has a 90% probability of conceiving a child over the course of a year. Therefore, the voluntary choice to use contraceptive measures is a critical decision faced by most women in the childbearing years.

Prior to the 1960s, the three primary methods of avoiding pregnancy were total abstinence, abstinence during periods of greatest fertility (rhythm or calendar method), and withdrawal prior to ejaculation (coitus interruptus). The discovery of oral contraceptives and the development of novel long-term contraceptives have given couples more effective choices for birth control. Many options are now available, each of which has specific advantages and disadvantages.

Women make personal birth control decisions based on several factors. The effectiveness for preventing pregnancy and the safety of the medication or device are the highest priorities. Other factors, however, may be of personal concern. Women who engage in intercourse frequently or who are likely to forget to take their

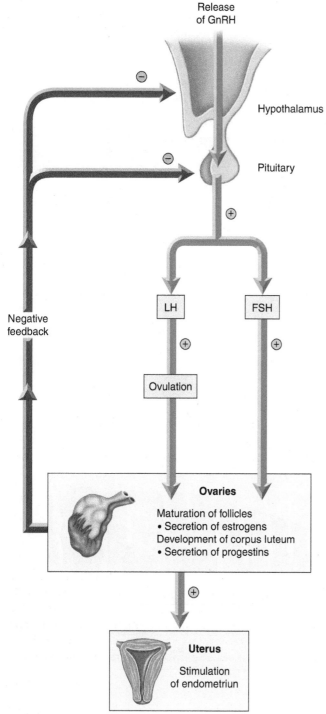

Figure 31.2   Negative feedback control of the female reproductive hormones

TABLE 31.1	Select Oral Contraceptives		
Trade Name	**Type**	**Estrogen**	**Progestin**
Alesse	Monophasic	Ethinyl estra-diol; 20 μg	Levonorgestrel; 0.1 mg
Marvelon	Monophasic	Ethinyl estra-diol; 30 μg	Desogestrel; 0.15 mg
Loestrin 1.5/30 Fe	Monophasic	Ethinyl estra-diol; 30 μg	Norethindrone; 1.5 mg
Ortho-Cyclen	Monophasic	Ethinyl estra-diol; 35 μg	Norgestimate; 0.25 mg
Yasmin	Monophasic	Ethinyl estra-diol; 30 μg	Drospirenone; 3 mg
Ortho-Novum 10/11	Biphasic	Ethinyl estra-diol; 35 μg	Norethindrone; 0.5 mg (phase 1)
		Ethinyl estra-diol; 35 μg	Norethindrone; 1.0 mg (phase 2)
Ortho-Novum 7/7/7	Triphasic	Ethinyl estra-diol; 35 μg	Norethindrone; 0.5 mg (phase 1)
		Ethinyl estra-diol; 35 μg	Norethindrone; 0.75 mg (phase 2)
		Ethinyl estra-diol; 35 μg	Norethindrone; 1.0 mg (phase 3)
Ortho Tri-Cyclen	Triphasic	Ethinyl estra-diol; 35 μg	Norgestimate; 0.18 mg (day 1-7)
		Ethinyl estra-diol; 35 μg	Norgestimate; 0.215 mg (day 8-14)
		Ethinyl estra-diol; 35 μg	Norgestimate; 0.25 mg (day 15-21)
Ortho Try-Cyclen Lo	Triphasic	Ethinyl estra-diol; 25 μg	Norgestimate dose follows the same dosage schedule as regular Ortho Tri-Cyclen
Micronor	Progestin only	None	Norethindrone; 0.35 mg
Nor-QD	Progestin only	None	Norethindrone; 0.35 mg
Ovrette	Progestin only	None	Norgestrel; 0.075 mg

medication may prefer the convenience of the long-acting contraceptives. For clients who have a history of thromboembolic disorders, barrier protection or the use of progestin-only types of contraceptives are safer options. Factors that influence their decisions include the following:

- Effectiveness of the chosen method
- Adverse effects and safety
- Age
- Frequency of intercourse
- Ease of use and the ability to adhere to the required regimen
- Pre-existing medical conditions
- Cultural beliefs and practices

Women who seek to prevent conception need to discuss the available options with their healthcare provider. Final decisions on choosing a contraceptive should be made voluntarily, with full knowledge of its advantages and disadvantages, effectiveness, adverse effects, contraindications, and potential long-term risks. When the desire to have children in the future no longer exists, sterilization of either the male or the female is the most common and effective option for birth control. Whatever

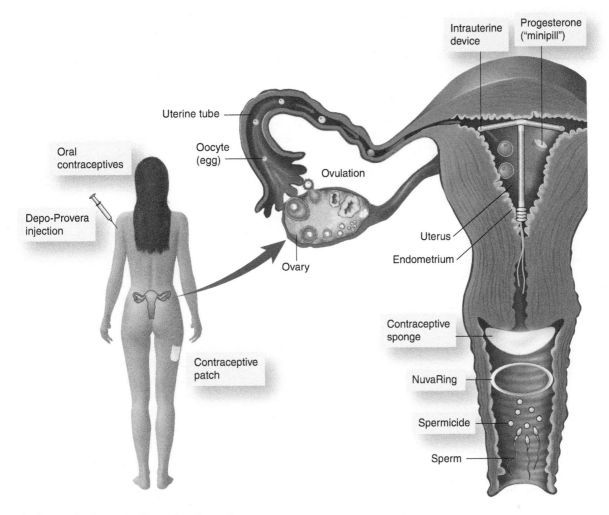

Figure 31.3 Mechanisms of actions of contraceptives.

the choice of birth control, personal motivation must be taken into consideration because it is important that the woman be consistent in using the chosen method if pregnancy is to be prevented. See Figure 31.3 for mechanisms of actions of contraceptives.

Estrogens and Progestins as Oral Contraceptives

31.3 Low doses of estrogens and progestins prevent conception by blocking ovulation. The adverse effects of combined oral contraceptives are uncommon but may be serious in some women.

The most widespread pharmacological use of the female sex hormones is to prevent pregnancy. When used appropriately, oral contraceptives are nearly 100% effective. Most oral contraceptives contain a combination of estrogen and progestin; a few preparations contain only progestin. The most common estrogen used for contraception is ethinyl estradiol, and the most common progestin is norethindrone.

A large number of oral contraceptive preparations are available, differing in dose and type of estrogen and progestin. Selection of a specific formulation is individualized to each client and is determined by which drug gives the best contraceptive protection with the fewest side effects. Daily doses of estrogen in oral contraceptives have declined from 150 μg, 40 years ago, to about 35 μg in modern formulations. This reduction has resulted in a decrease in estrogen-related adverse effects.

Typically, drug administration of an oral contraceptive begins on day 5 of the ovarian cycle and continues for 21 days. During the other 7 days of the month, the client takes a placebo. While the placebo serves no pharmacological purpose, it does encourage the client to take the pills on a daily basis. Some of these placebos contain iron, which replaces iron lost from menstrual bleeding. If a daily dose is missed, two pills taken the following day usually provide adequate contraception. If more than one day is missed, the client should observe other contraceptive precautions, such as using condoms, until the oral contraceptive doses can be resumed at the beginning of the next monthly cycle. Figure 31.4 shows a typical monthly oral contraceptive packet with the 28 pills.

The estrogen-progestin oral contraceptives act by providing negative feedback to the pituitary to shut down the secretion of

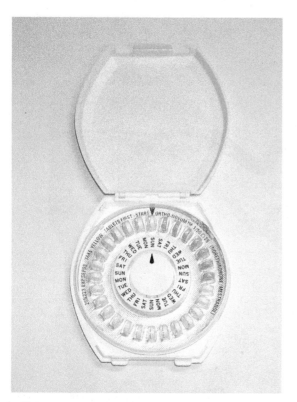

Figure 31.4 An oral contraceptive packet showing the daily doses and the different formulation taken in the last 7 days of the 28-day cycle.

LH and FSH. Without the influence of these pituitary hormones, the ovarian follicle cannot mature and ovulation is prevented. The estrogen-progestin agents also reduce the likelihood of implantation by making the uterine endometrium less favourable to receive an embryo. In addition to their contraceptive function, these agents are sometimes prescribed to promote timely and regular monthly cycles and to reduce the incidence of dysmenorrhea.

The three types of estrogen-progestin formulations are monophasic, biphasic, and triphasic. The most common is monophasic, which delivers a constant amount of estrogen and progestin throughout the menstrual cycle. In biphasic agents, the amount of estrogen in each pill remains constant, but the amount of progestin is increased toward the end of the menstrual cycle to better nourish the uterine lining. In triphasic formulations, the amount of estrogen remains the same, while the amount of progestin varies in three distinct phases during the 28-day cycle.

The progestin-only oral contraceptives, sometimes called minipills, prevent pregnancy primarily by producing thick, viscous mucus at the entrance to the uterus that discourages penetration by sperm. They also tend to inhibit implantation of a fertilized egg. Minipills are less effective than estrogen-progestin combinations, having a failure rate of 1% to 4%. Their use also results in a higher incidence of menstrual irregularities such as amenorrhea, prolonged bleeding, and breakthrough spotting. They are generally reserved for clients who are at high risk for side effects from estrogen. It is important for all kinds of birth control, estrogen with progesterone and progesterone only, to be taken at the same time each day to get 24-hour coverage. However, with the progesterone-only tablets it is extremely important that they are taken at the same time because effectiveness is not related to hormone regulation but rather to the amount of mucus produced that creates a barrier for sperm penetration.

Several long-term formulations of oral contraceptives are available. A deep intramuscular (IM) injection of medroxyprogesterone (Depo-Provera) provides 3 months of contraceptive protection. Ortho Evra is a transdermal patch containing ethinyl estradiol and norelgestromin that is worn on the skin. The patch is changed every 7 days for the first 3 weeks, followed by no patch during week 4. NuvaRing is a small ring containing estrogen and progestin that is inserted into the vagina to provide 3 weeks of contraceptive protection. The ring is removed during week 4, and a new ring is inserted during the first week of the next menstrual cycle. Mirena consists of a polyethylene cylinder that is placed in the uterus and releases levonorgestrel. This drug acts locally to prevent conception over 5 years. The efficacy of these long-term formulations is similar to that of oral contraceptives. They offer a major advantage for women who are likely to forget their daily pill or who prefer greater ease of use.

The "extended regimen" oral contraceptives are newer contraceptive drugs. Seasonale consists of tablets containing levonorgestrel and ethinyl estradiol that are taken for 84 consecutive days, followed by 7 inert tablets (without hormones). This allows for continuous contraceptive protection while extending the time between menses; only four periods are experienced per year. Seasonique is similar, but instead of inert tablets for 7 days the client takes low-dose estrogen tablets. Seasonique is claimed by the manufacturer to have a lower incidence of bloating and breakthrough bleeding.

Although oral contraceptives are safe for the large majority of women, there are some potentially serious adverse effects (Table 31.2). As with other medications, the higher the dose of estrogen or progesterone, the more likely the risk of side effects. With oral contraceptives, however, some side effects are more prominent at *lower* doses. Therefore, physicians try to prescribe the oral contraceptive with the lowest dose of hormones that will achieve the therapeutic goal of pregnancy prevention with minimal side effects.

Numerous drug-drug interactions are possible with estrogen and with progesterone. Several anticonvulsants and antibiotics can reduce the effectiveness of oral contraceptives, thus increasing a woman's risk for pregnancy. Because oral contraceptives can reduce the effectiveness of warfarin (Coumadin), insulin, and certain oral antihyperglycemic agents, dosage adjustment may be necessary.

The risk for cancer following long-term oral contraceptive use has been studied extensively. Because some studies have shown a small increase in breast cancer incidence, oral contraceptives are contraindicated in clients with known or suspected breast cancer. The incidences of endometrial cancer and ovarian cancer, however, are significantly reduced after long-term oral contraceptive administration. It is likely that the relationship between the long-term use of these drugs and cancer will continue to be a controversial and frequently researched topic.

NCLEX Success Tips

Use of oral contraceptives does not increase the risk for developing ovarian cancer but may actually be protective.

The nurse should teach clients that using oral contraceptive does not increase the risk of developing ovarian cancer. On the contrary, studies suggest that ovarian and endometrial cancers are reduced in women using oral contraceptives.

TABLE 31.2 Adverse Effects Associated with Oral Contraceptives (OCs)

Adverse Effect	Prevention
Breast milk reduction	Some studies suggest that OCs may reduce the quantity of breast milk. They should not be taken until 6 weeks postpartum.
Cancer	Women who test positive for human papillomavirus (HPV) have an increased risk for cervical cancer. These patients should have regular checkups. Because estrogens promote the growth of certain types of breast cancer, patients with a history of this cancer should not take OCs.
Glucose elevation	OCs may cause slight increases in blood glucose. Patients with diabetes should monitor their serum glucose carefully during OC therapy.
Hypertension	Risk is increased with age, dose, and length of therapy. Blood pressure should be monitored periodically and antihypertensives prescribed as needed.
Increased appetite, weight gain, fatigue, depression, acne, hirsutism	These are common effects that are often caused by high amounts of progestin. The dose of progestin may need to be lowered.
Lupus exacerbation	Symptoms of systemic lupus erythematosus may worsen in some patients. A progestin-only OC may be an option for these patients.
Menstrual irregularities	Amenorrhea or hypermenorrhea is often caused by low amounts of progestin. The dose of progestin may need to be increased. Breakthrough bleeding and spotting are common with the low-dose OCs. The patient may need a higher dose product.
Migraines	Estrogen may decrease or increase the incidence of migraines. Because migraines are a risk factor for stroke, patients with migraines should seek advice from their healthcare provider.
Nausea, edema, breast tenderness	These are common effects that are often caused by high amounts of estrogen. The dose of estrogen may need to be lowered.
Teratogenicity	Estrogens are pregnancy category X. Patients should be advised to discontinue OCs if pregnancy is confirmed.
Thromboembolic disorders	Estrogens promote blood clotting. OCs should not be prescribed for patients with a history of thromboembolic disorders, strokes, or coronary artery disease, or for those who are heavy smokers.

Nursing Considerations

The role of the nurse in oral contraceptive therapy involves careful monitoring of the client's condition and providing education as it relates to the prescribed drug treatment. Oral contraception is the most effective form of birth control, and there are many products available. Oral contraception is contraindicated for women with a history of stroke, myocardial infarction (MI), coronary artery disease (CAD), thromboembolic disorders, or estrogen-dependent tumours because of increases in estrogen levels and risk of thrombus formation. Assess for pregnancy before initiating oral contraceptive therapy. Obtain a complete health history, including personal and family history of breast cancer, liver tumours, and hemorrhagic disorders because these conditions are contraindications to the use of oral contraceptives. Risks and adverse effects are greater for women who smoke and are older than 35 years of age. Oral contraceptives should be used with caution in clients with hypertension, deep vein thrombosis, cardiac or renal disease, liver dysfunction, diabetes, gallbladder disease, and a history of depression.

Blood pressure should be monitored, as oral contraceptives can cause mild to moderate hypertension. Monitor for symptoms of thrombophlebitis, such as pain, redness, and tenderness of the calves. Oral contraceptives can mimic certain symptoms of pregnancy, including breast tenderness, nausea, bloating, and chloasma. Reassure the client that these side effects do not indicate pregnancy. Oral contraceptives may increase the risk for certain types of breast cancer; therefore, teach clients how to perform breast self-examinations and provide information on the routine scheduling of mammograms appropriate for their age group.

NCLEX Success Tips

A common side effect of oral contraceptives is decreased menstrual flow. Other adverse effects include breast tenderness, irritability, nausea, headaches, cyclic weight gain, and increased vaginal yeast infections. More serious adverse effects include hypertension, myocardial infarction, and thrombophlebitis. The nurse should instruct the client that decreased menstrual flow is normal.

Oral contraceptives are contraindicated for clients with a history of thrombophlebitis because a serious side effect of oral contraceptives is thrombus formation. Other contraindications include stroke and liver disease. Oral contraceptives are used cautiously in clients with hypertension or diabetes.

Menorrhagia is typically reduced through the use of oral contraceptives.

Oral contraceptives containing estrogen are not advised for women who are breastfeeding because the hormones decrease the production of breast milk. Women who are not breastfeeding may use oral contraceptive agents.

Although breastfeeding is not considered an effective form of contraception, breastfeeding usually delays the return of both ovulation and menstruation. The length of the delay varies with the duration of lactation and the frequency of breastfeeding.

Oral contraceptive agents inhibit ovulation by suppressing follicle-stimulating hormone and luteinizing hormone and have no effect on cervical mucus.

Client education as it relates to oral contraceptives should include goals, reasons for baseline assessment of vital signs and cardiovascular status, and possible drug side effects. Include the following points when teaching the client about oral contraceptives:

- Take medications as directed by the healthcare provider.
- Follow instructions for missed doses.
- Immediately report calf pain or redness, dyspnea, and chest pain.
- Monitor blood pressure regularly and report elevations.
- Avoid smoking.
- Perform monthly self-examination of breasts.
- Seek professional help if symptoms of depression occur.

NCLEX Success Tips

Women who take oral contraceptives are at higher risk for thromboembolic conditions. Severe calf pain needs to be investigated as a potential sign of deep vein thrombosis.

Absolute contraindications to oral contraceptives include prolonged immobilization or surgery to the leg and age of more than 35 years when a cigarette smoker, especially in those women who smoke more than 20 cigarettes per day. Oral contraceptives also interact with many antiepileptic drugs, including phenytoin (Dilantin), causing a reduction in the therapeutic dose and an alteration in the seizure threshold.

It is not necessary to monitor basal body temperature because ovulation does not occur when the medication is taken properly.

See Nursing Process Focus: Clients Receiving Oral Contraceptive Therapy for specific teaching points.

NCLEX Success Tips

Before starting a client on oral contraceptives, the nurse needs to assess the client for signs and symptoms of hypertension. Clients who have hypertension, thrombophlebitis, obesity, or a family history of cerebral or cardiovascular accident are poor candidates for oral contraceptives. In addition, women who smoke, who are older than 40 years of age, or who have a history of pulmonary disease should be advised to use a different method.

Iron-deficiency anemia is a common disorder in young women. Using oral contraceptives decreases the amount of menstrual flow and decreases the amount of iron lost through menses, providing a beneficial effect when used by clients with anemia.

PROTOTYPE DRUG	**Ethinyl Estradiol with Norethindrone (Ortho-Novum 1/35)**

Actions and Uses: Ortho-Novum is typical of the monophasic oral contraceptives, containing fixed amounts of estrogen (0.035 mg) and progesterone (1 mg) for 21 days followed by placebo tablets for 7 days. It is nearly 100% effective at preventing conception. Ortho-Novum is also available in a biphasic preparation. All preparations prevent ovulation by negative feedback control targeted at the hypothalamic-pituitary axis. When the right combination of estrogens and progestins is present in the bloodstream, the release of FSH and LH is inhibited, thus preventing ovulation. Non-contraceptive benefits of Ortho-Novum include improvement in menstrual cycle regularity and decreased incidence of dysmenorrhea.

Pharmacokinetics: Estradiol is well absorbed after oral administration. It is widely distributed, crosses the placenta, and enters breast milk. It is metabolized by the liver. Its half-life is unknown.

Administration Alerts:
- Tablets must be taken exactly as directed.
- If a dose is missed, take it as soon as remembered, or take two tablets the next day.
- Ethinyl estradiol with norethindrone is pregnancy category X.

NCLEX Success Tip

If a client forgets to take her oral contraceptive pill, she should take it as soon as she remembers. If a whole day has passed, take two pills on one day to get back on schedule.

Adverse Effects and Interactions: Common side effects include edema, unexplained loss of vision, diplopia, intolerance to contact lenses, gallbladder disease, nausea, abdominal cramps, changes in urinary function, dysmenorrhea, breast fullness, fatigue, skin rash, acne, headache, weight gain, mid-cycle breakthrough bleeding, vaginal candidiasis, photosensitivity, and changes in urinary patterns. Cardiovascular side effects may include hypertension and thromboembolic disorders.

Ethinyl estradiol interacts with many drugs. For example, rifampin (Rifadin, Rofact), some antibiotics, barbiturates, anticonvulsants, and antifungals decrease the efficacy of oral contraceptives, so increased risk for breakthrough bleeding and increased risk for pregnancy may occur. Ortho-Novum may also decrease the effects of oral anticoagulants.

NCLEX Success Tips

An alternative or additional method of birth control must be used when the client reports to the nurse that she is on oxcarbazepine (Trileptal; an antiepileptic) because this medication reduces the effectiveness of oral contraceptives.

Antibiotics may decrease the effectiveness of oral contraceptives. The client should be instructed to continue the contraceptives and use a barrier backup method until the next menstrual cycle. The client should not stop taking her oral contraceptives while receiving antibiotics.

Use with caution with herbal supplements. For example, breakthrough bleeding has been reported with concurrent use of St. John's wort.

NURSING PROCESS FOCUS

Clients Receiving Oral Contraceptive Therapy

Assessment	Potential Nursing Diagnoses/Identified Patterns
Prior to administration: - Obtain health history, including cigarette smoking and personal and family history of breast cancer. - Obtain drug history to determine possible drug interactions and allergies. - Assess cardiovascular status including hypertension, history of MI, cerebrovascular accident (CVA), and thromboembolic disease. - Determine if client is pregnant or lactating.	- Risk for fluid and electrolyte imbalance - Need for knowledge regarding drug therapy and adverse effects - Need for knowledge regarding importance of adherence to dosing schedule and management of a missed dose

---

Planning: Client Goals and Expected Outcomes

The client will:

- Report effective birth control
- Demonstrate an understanding of the drug's action by accurately describing drug side effects and precautions
- Take medication exactly as ordered to prevent pregnancy
- Immediately report effects such as symptoms of thrombophlebitis, difficulty breathing, visual disturbances, and severe headache

---

Implementation

Interventions (Rationales)	Client Education/Discharge Planning
• Monitor for the development of breast or other estrogen-dependent tumours. (Estrogen may cause tumour growth or proliferation.) • Monitor for thrombophlebitis or other thromboembolic disease. (Estrogen predisposes to thromboembolic disorders by increasing levels of clotting factors.) • Monitor for cardiac disorders and hypertension. (These drugs increase blood levels of angiotensin and aldosterone, which increases blood pressure.) • Encourage client not to smoke. (Smoking increases risk of thromboembolic disease.) • Monitor blood and urine glucose levels. (These drugs increase serum glucose levels.) • Monitor client's knowledge level of proper administration. (Incorrect use may lead to pregnancy.) • Encourage compliance with follow-up treatment. (Follow-up is necessary to avoid serious adverse effects.)	• Instruct client to immediately report if first-degree relative is diagnosed with any estrogen-dependent tumour • Instruct client to immediately report pain in calves, limited movement in legs, dyspnea, sudden severe chest pain, headache, seizures, anxiety, or fear Instruct client to: • Report immediately signs of possible cardiac problems such as chest pain, dyspnea, edema, tachycardia or bradycardia, and palpitations • Monitor blood pressure regularly • Report symptoms of hypertension such as headache, flushing, fatigue, dizziness, palpitations, tachycardia, and nosebleeds Instruct client to: • Be aware that the combination of oral contraceptives and smoking greatly increases risk for cardiovascular disease, especially MI • Be aware that the risk increases with age (>35 years) and with number of cigarettes smoked (15 or more/day) • Instruct client to monitor urine and blood glucose regularly and contact healthcare provider if hyperglycemia or hypoglycemia occurs Instruct client to: • Discontinue medication and notify healthcare provider if significant bleeding occurs at mid-cycle • Take missed dose as soon as remembered or take two tablets the next day. Use an alternate form of contraception for the remainder of the cycle. If three consecutive tablets are missed, begin a new compact of tablets, starting 7 days after last tablet was taken • Contact healthcare provider if two consecutive periods are missed, as pregnancy may have occurred Instruct client to: • Schedule annual Pap tests • Perform breast self-exams monthly and obtain routine mammograms as recommended by the healthcare provider

---

Evaluation of Outcome Criteria

Evaluate the effectiveness of drug therapy by confirming that client goals and expected outcomes have been met (see "Planning").

See Table 31.1 (page 360) for a list of drugs to which these nursing actions apply.

Drugs for Long-Term Contraception and Newer Contraceptive Delivery Methods

31.4 Long-acting contraceptives and novel delivery methods offer women additional birth control choices.

Delivery methods have been developed that are able to provide effective contraceptive protection for periods lasting from weeks to years. The long-acting drugs and novel delivery systems were developed to offer ease of use and improve adherence. They vary in efficacy, reversibility, and discreteness of use. It is important for nurses and clients to understand that the long-acting methods are not more effective than the daily oral contraceptives and that they have the same types of contraindications and adverse effects. These long-acting contraceptives deliver medications by patches, vaginal inserts, injections, subdermal implants, and intrauterine devices.

Transdermal Delivery Method

Transdermal hormonal contraception is a safe, effective, and easy-to-use birth control method. Approved in 2001, Ortho Evra is a topical patch worn on the skin of the buttock, arm, or trunk that contains ethinyl estradiol and norelgestromin. The patch slowly releases the hormones, which penetrate the skin and are distributed throughout the body. The patch is changed every 7 days for the first 3 weeks, followed by a patch-free week 4 (days 22 to 28). The patch may be worn during bathing, exercise, and other daily activities. Should the patch fall off, which occurs in about 5% of the applications, it should be replaced as soon as possible. Forgetting to replace or change the patch will result in a rapid loss of contraceptive protection. After the patch is removed, hormone levels return to normal within 3 days. The serum estrogen levels of clients who use the patch are 60% higher compared to those of clients who take combination oral contraceptives.

The most frequently reported adverse effects of the Ortho Evra patch include headache, vomiting, nausea, breast discomfort, breakthrough bleeding, and dysmenorrhea. Long-term effects and contraindications are the same as those for oral contraceptives. Some research suggests that clients using the patch have an increased risk of venous thromboembolism (VTE) compared to women taking oral contraceptives. To reduce postpartum risk for VTE, 3 to 6 weeks should elapse between delivery and use of the transdermal patch. Used patches still contain significant levels of hormones and must be discarded in a waste container away from children and pets. They should not be flushed down the toilet because residual estrogen can pollute wastewater, lakes, and streams.

Vaginal Delivery Method

The NuvaRing, illustrated in Figure 31.5, is a flexible, soft vaginal ring impregnated with a low-dose, sustained-release, combined hormonal contraceptive. It is approximately 2 to 3 inches in diameter and contains ethinyl estradiol and etonogestrel. The ring is inserted into the vagina once a month to provide 3 weeks of contraceptive protection. The ring slowly releases the hormones, which are absorbed across the vaginal mucosa into the blood and distributed throughout the body. The contraceptive action is systemic in nature and not localized to the vagina. The ring is removed at the end of week 3, and a new ring is inserted a week later during the first week of the next menstrual cycle. If forgotten and left in place for more than 3 weeks, contraceptive action will be lost.

The main adverse effects of NuvaRing are similar to those of combination oral contraceptives. Women sometimes discontinue using the vaginal delivery method due to discomfort of the device during intercourse. Women who are experiencing uterine prolapse must monitor the ring frequently because it may fall out.

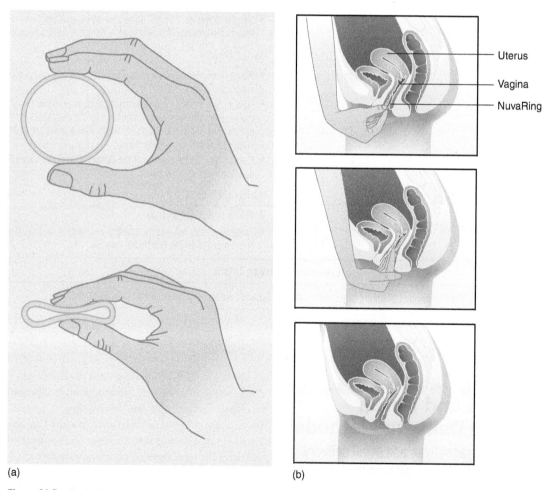

(a)   (b)

Figure 31.5 Vaginal medication administration: (a) the NuvaRing contraceptive; (b) proper insertion of the NuvaRing.

Adverse effects include nausea, bloating, headaches, breast tenderness, and breakthrough bleeding. If the ring is expelled from the vagina, it may be rinsed with water and replaced. Local effects may include vaginal irritation, sensation of a foreign body, and vaginitis. The NuvaRing should be discarded in a waste container away from children and not flushed down the toilet.

Depot Injection Methods

A single deep IM injection of 150 mg of Depo-Provera provides 3 months of contraceptive protection. The same drug may be injected subcutaneously (Depo-SubQ Provera) with the same duration of action and effectiveness. Medroxyprogesterone suppresses ovulation, inhibits sperm from reaching the egg by thickening the cervical mucus, and prevents a fertilized egg from implanting in the uterus. Neither of the depot delivery methods contains estrogen. The drug is usually given on days 1 through 5 of the menstrual cycle to postpartum women who are not breastfeeding. Breastfeeding women should wait until week 6 postpartum to take the drug. The dose is repeated every 3 months for as long as contraception is desired. The depot injection methods are very effective at preventing pregnancy.

Once injected the actions of the drug cannot be reversed, and fertility may not be restored for up to 12 months after discontinuation. The most common adverse effects are menstrual disturbances, headache, acne, injection-site reactions, weight gain, and decreased libido. This drug carries a black box warning that long-term use causes significant loss of bone mineral density. This drug is pregnancy category X. Medroxyprogesterone is also approved to treat inoperable endometrial and renal carcinomas and menstrual disturbances.

Intrauterine Devices

Two intrauterine devices (IUDs) are available. These devices, Paragard (a copper IUD) and Mirena, are all designed in a T shape and have been in use for many years. They are safe, inexpensive, and reliable methods of contraception. They offer a major advantage for women who are likely to forget a daily pill or who prefer greater ease of use. The IUD is not felt by the woman or her partner during intercourse, and it can be removed at any time. Fertility returns quickly after removal of the device. Despite these advantages, only 2% of women who use birth control use IUDs.

The oldest product, Paragard, also known as Copper T380A, is a plastic device that is partially covered with copper. It is inserted into the uterus, where the copper triggers a spermicidal-like reaction in the body that slows sperm motility and prevents the sperm from reaching the ovum. If fertilization does occur, implantation is not likely to happen because the copper causes endometrial changes to make the lining less favourable. Unlike the hormonal methods, Paragard has no effect on ovulation. It can be left in place for up to 10 years, and the main adverse effects are bleeding between menses, dysmenorrhea, and expulsion of the device. Paragard is an important non-hormonal option for clients who have contraindications to using estrogen or progesterone.

Mirena is an intrauterine system consisting of a polyethylene reservoir that contains levonorgestrel, which is slowly released. Contraception results from a thickening of the endometrium and increased cervical mucus that slows down sperm motility. Mirena decreases menstrual pain and lowers blood loss. This drug acts locally to prevent conception for up to 5 years. The effectiveness of Mirena is similar to that of oral contraceptives. This device may be removed at any time, and fertility returns quickly. The most common adverse effects of this IUD are uterine and vaginal bleeding alterations, amenorrhea, intermenstrual bleeding and spotting, abdominal or pelvic pain, and ovarian cysts.

Spermicides

Spermicides are drugs that kill sperm. They come in a variety of creams, foams, jellies, and suppositories that immobilize or destroy sperm when inserted into the vagina prior to intercourse. Two spermicides used in contraceptive products are nonoxynol-9 and octoxynol-9. Spermicides are available over the counter (OTC).

To be effective, spermicides must be applied high into the vagina, as close to the cervix as possible, approximately 20 minutes before intercourse. Most spermicides have a duration of action of only 1 hour and must be reapplied if coitus extends beyond this time.

The contraceptive sponge (Today Sponge), which is illustrated in Figure 31.6, is a soft absorbent sponge impregnated with nonoxynol-9. The sponge is moistened with water to activate the spermicides and inserted into the vagina to cover the cervix. The sponge releases the drug slowly and may provide up to 24 hours of contraceptive protection. It is left in place for 6 hours after intercourse but must be removed by 30 hours after insertion. The sponge delivery system has the same effectiveness as spermicidal gels, creams, and suppositories. Adverse effects include local irritation and vaginal dryness.

Clients should be informed that spermicides have low levels of effectiveness when used alone and therefore should be used in conjunction with barrier methods such as condoms and diaphragms. Research has also determined that nonoxynol-9 does not offer any protection against chlamydia, gonorrhea, or human immunodeficiency virus (HIV), as previously thought. In fact, frequent use of spermicides disrupts the vaginal epithelium and may actually increase the risk of HIV transmission from an infected partner. This drug also disrupts the anal mucosa, possibly

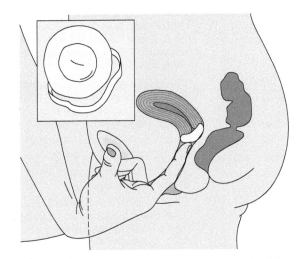

Figure 31.6 The contraceptive sponge is moistened well with water and inserted into the vagina with the concave portion positioned over the cervix.

increasing the risk of HIV transmission, and should not be used for anal intercourse. Patients must be instructed to take added precautions to prevent such transmissions.

Emergency Contraception and Pharmacological Abortion

31.5 Drugs for emergency contraception may be administered within 72 hours of unprotected sex to prevent implantation of the fertilized egg. Other agents may be given to stimulate uterine contractions to expel the implanted embryo.

Emergency contraception is the prevention of implantation following unprotected intercourse. Pharmacological abortion is the removal of an embryo by the use of drugs, after implantation has occurred. The treatment goal is to provide effective, immediate prevention or termination of pregnancy. Agents used for these purposes are listed in Table 31.3.

More than half of pregnancies in North America are unplanned. Some of these occur due to the inconsistent use or failure of contraceptive devices; even oral contraceptives have a failure rate of 0.3% to 1%. Emergency contraception following unprotected intercourse offers a means of protecting against unwanted pregnancies. The goal is to prevent implantation of a fertilized ovum.

Emergency contraception can be accomplished pharmacologically by the administration of various doses and combinations of estrogen and progestins. These drugs should be administered as soon as possible after unprotected intercourse; if taken more than 72 hours later, they become less effective. After 7 days, they are no longer effective. When used this way, these drugs act by preventing ovulation or implantation; they do not induce abortion. Taking 0.75 mg of levonorgestrel in two doses, 12 hours apart, has been shown to prevent conception. A combination of ethinyl estradiol and levonorgestrel is also effective, although nausea and vomiting are common and an antiemetic drug may be indicated to reduce these unpleasant side effects.

Once the ovum has been fertilized, several pharmacological choices are available to terminate the pregnancy. A single dose of mifepristone (Mifegymiso) followed 36 to 48 hours later by a single dose of misoprostol (Cytotec) is a frequently used treatment. Mifepristone is a synthetic steroid that blocks progesterone receptors in the uterus. If given within 3 days of intercourse, mifepristone alone is almost 100% effective at preventing pregnancy. Given up to 9 weeks after conception, mifepristone aborts the implanted embryo. Misoprostol is a prostaglandin that causes uterine contractions, thus increasing the effectiveness of the pharmacological abortion.

Although mifepristone-misoprostol should never be substituted for effective means of contraception, such as oral contraceptives, these medications do offer women a safer alternative to surgical abortion. The primary adverse effect is cramping that occurs soon after taking misoprostol. The most serious adverse effect is prolonged bleeding, which may continue for 1 to 2 weeks after dosing.

A few other agents may be used to promote pharmacological abortion. Methotrexate, an antineoplastic agent, combined with intravaginal misoprostol usually induces abortion within 24 hours. The prostaglandins carboprost (Hemabate) and dinoprostone (Cervidil, Prepidil, Prostin E$_2$) induce strong uterine contractions that can expel an implanted embryo up to the second trimester.

TABLE 31.3   Agents for Emergency Contraception and Pharmacological Abortion

Drug	Route and Adult Dose
Agents for Emergency Contraception	
ethinyl estradiol (Estinyl, Feminor)	Orally (PO), 5 mg/day for 5 consecutive days beginning within 72 hours of intercourse
ethinyl estradiol and levonorgestrel (Preven)	PO, 1 tablet (0.25 mg levonorgestrel and 0.05 mg ethinyl estradiol) taken as soon as possible but within 72 hours of unprotected intercourse, followed by 2 pills 12 hours later
levonorgestrel	PO, 2 tablets within 72 hours of unprotected intercourse, 2 tablets 12 hours later
Agents for Pharmacological Abortion	
carboprost (Hemabate)	IM, initial: 250 μg (1 mL) repeated at 1.5- to 3.5-hour intervals if indicated by uterine response; dosage may be increased to 500 μg (2 mL) if uterine contractility is inadequate after several doses of 250 μg (1 mL); not to exceed total dose of 12 mg or continuous administration for more than 2 days
dinoprostone (Cervidil, Prepidil, Prostin E$_2$)	Intravaginal, insert suppository (1 suppository = 20 mg) high in vagina, repeat every 2 to 5 hours until abortion occurs or membranes rupture (max total dose 240 mg)
methotrexate with misoprostol	IM, methotrexate (50 mg/m^2) followed 5 days later by intravaginal 800 μg of misoprostol
mifepristone (Mifegymiso) with misoprostol	PO, day 1: 200 mg of mifepristone; day 2 or 3 (if abortion has not occurred): 800 μg misoprostol buccally 24 to 48 hours after mifepristone administration (dose is administered as two 200 μg tablets in each cheek pouch held in place for 30 minutes) Alternative option: 200 mg mifepristone PO followed by 800 μg misoprostol vaginally 24 to 48 hours later

MENOPAUSE

Menopause is characterized by a progressive decrease in estrogen secretion by the ovaries, resulting in the permanent cessation of menses. Menopause is neither a disease nor a disorder but is a natural consequence of aging that is often accompanied by a number of unpleasant symptoms. Some of these symptoms respond well to pharmacotherapy.

Hormone Replacement Therapy

31.6 Estrogen-progestin combinations are used for hormone replacement therapy during and after menopause; however, their long-term use may have serious adverse effects.

Over the past 30 years, healthcare providers have commonly prescribed hormone replacement therapy to treat unpleasant

TABLE 31.4 Potential Consequences of Estrogen Loss Related to Menopause

Stage	Symptoms/Conditions
Early menopause	Mood disturbances, depression, irritability
	Insomnia
	Hot flashes
	Irregular menstrual cycles
	Headaches
Mid-menopause	Vaginal atrophy, increased infections, painful intercourse
	Skin atrophy
	Stress urinary incontinence
	Sexual disinterest
Postmenopause	Cardiovascular disease
	Osteoporosis
	Alzheimer's-like dementia
	Colon cancer

symptoms of menopause and to prevent the long-term consequences of estrogen loss listed in Table 31.4. Select estrogens and progestins and their dosages are shown in Table 31.5.

Hormone replacement therapy (HRT) refers to replacement of both estrogen and progesterone, whereas **estrogen replacement therapy (ERT)** refers to the replacement of estrogen alone. In 2002, the results of a large clinical study by the Women's Health Initiative (WHI) regarding the effects of HRT and ERT were analyzed. Data from the WHI research suggest that clients receiving HRT experienced a small, though significant, increased risk for serious adverse effects such as CAD,

TABLE 31.5 Select Estrogens and Progestins

Drug	Route and Adult Dose
Estrogens	
estradiol (Estraderm, Estrace)	PO, 1–2 mg every day (qd)
estradiol cypionate (Depo-estradiol)	IM, 1–5 mg every 3 to 4 weeks
estradiol valerate (Delestrogen)	IM, 10–20 mg every 4 weeks
Pr estrogen, conjugated (Premarin)	PO, 0.3–1.25 mg qd for 21 days each month
estropipate (Ogen)	PO, 0.75–6 mg qd for 21 days each month
ethinyl estradiol (Estinyl, Feminone)	PO, 0.02–0.05 mg qd for 21 days each month
Progestins	
Pr medroxyprogesterone (Provera, Medroxy)	PO, 5–10 mg qd on days 1–12 of menstrual cycle
norethindrone acetate (Norlutate)	PO, 2.5-10 mg/day for 5 to 10 days
progesterone micronized (Prometrium)	PO, 400 mg at bedtime for 10 days
Estrogen-Progestin Combinations	
Pr conjugated estrogens (Premarin)	PO, 0.625 mg/day continuously or in 25-day cycles
ethinyl estradiol/norethindrone acetate (FemHRT)	PO, 5 µg (1 tablet) qd

stroke, breast cancer, dementia, and VTE. The risks were higher in women older than age 60; women aged 50 to 59 actually experienced a slight *decrease* in cardiovascular side effects. Women taking estrogen-progestin combination HRT experienced a decreased risk for hip fractures and colorectal cancer. The potential adverse effects documented in the WHI study, and others, were significant enough to suggest that the potential benefits of long-term HRT may not outweigh the risks for many women. However, the results of this study remain controversial.

Women in the WHI study who took estrogen alone (Premarin) experienced a slightly increased risk for stroke and other thromboembolic disorders, but no increased risk for breast cancer, heart disease, or MI. Estrogen has been shown to prevent osteoporosis and reduce the incidence of fractures. The use of estrogen alone (ERT) is considered appropriate only for women who have had hysterectomies since it increases the risk for uterine cancer.

Although there is consensus that HRT does offer relief from immediate, distressing menopausal symptoms, as of 2008 it was recommended that women *not* undergo HRT to prevent coronary heart disease. In addition, although HRT appears to prevent osteoporotic bone fractures, women are encouraged to discuss alternatives with their healthcare provider. Undoubtedly, research will continue to provide valuable information on the long-term effects of HRT. Until then, the choice of HRT to treat menopausal symptoms remains a highly individualized one, between the client and her healthcare provider.

In addition to their use in treating menopausal symptoms, estrogens are used for female hypogonadism, primary ovarian failure, and as replacement therapy following surgical removal of the ovaries, usually combined with a progestin. The purpose of the progestin is to counteract some of the adverse effects of estrogen on the uterus. When used alone, estrogen increases the risk for uterine cancer.

High doses of estrogens are used to treat prostate and breast cancer. Prostate cancer is usually dependent on androgens for growth; administration of estrogens suppresses androgen secretion. As an antineoplastic hormone, estrogen is rarely used alone. It is one of many agents used in combination for the chemotherapy of cancer.

Nursing Considerations

For the use of estrogen-containing products as oral contraceptives, refer to Nursing Process Focus: Clients Receiving Oral Contraceptive Therapy (page 364).

The role of the nurse in HRT involves careful monitoring of the client's condition and providing education as it relates to the prescribed drug treatment. Conjugated estrogens are contraindicated for use in breast cancer (except in clients who are being treated for metastatic disease) and any suspected estrogen-dependent cancer. These conditions put the client at a higher risk for developing another cancer. Assess for pregnancy; conjugated estrogen is contraindicated in pregnancy and for use in women who intend to become pregnant in the immediate future because it can cause fetal harm. Assess for a history of thromboembolic disease because of potential side effects of the drug. Obtain a complete health history, including family history of breast and genital cancer. Cautious use of estrogen therapy must be exercised in a client who has a first-degree relative with a history of breast or genital cancer. Estrogen monotherapy places the woman at higher risk for cancer of the female reproductive organs. Obtain a history of CAD, hypertension, cerebrovascular disease, fibrocystic breast disease, breast nodules, and abnormal mammograms. Because of the risk for thromboembolism, monitor the client closely for signs and symptoms of thrombus or embolus, such as pain in the calves, limited movement in the legs, dyspnea, sudden severe chest pain, or anxiety. Encourage the client to report signs of depression, decreased libido, headache, fatigue, and weight gain. Because controversy surrounds the long-term use of these drugs as HRT, it is imperative for women to be aware of current research and discuss treatment alternatives with their healthcare provider before beginning pharmacotherapy. When using these drugs to treat male clients, inform them that secondary female characteristics, such as a higher voice, sparse body hair, and increased breast size, may develop. Inform the client that impotence may also occur.

Client education as it relates to HRT should include goals, reasons for obtaining baseline data such as vital signs and the existence of underlying cardiovascular disorders, and possible drug side effects. Include the following points when teaching clients about HRT:

- Immediately report calf tenderness, chest pain, or dyspnea.
- Take with food if gastrointestinal (GI) upset occurs.
- Schedule an annual Pap test and breast examination.
- Perform monthly self-examinations of breasts.
- Do not take other prescribed drugs, OTC medications, herbal remedies, or dietary supplements without notifying the healthcare provider.

See Nursing Process Focus: Clients Receiving Hormone Replacement Therapy for specific teaching points.

PROTOTYPE DRUG | Conjugated Estrogens (Premarin)

Actions and Uses: Premarin contains a mixture of different estrogens. It exerts several positive metabolic effects, including an increase in bone density and a reduction in low-density lipoprotein (LDL) cholesterol. It may also lower the risk of CAD and colon cancer in some clients. When used as postmenopausal HRT, estrogen is typically combined with a progestin. Conjugated estrogens may be administered by the IM or intravenous (IV) route for abnormal uterine bleeding due to hormonal imbalance.

Administration Alerts:
- Use a calibrated dosage applicator for administration of vaginal cream.
- For IM or IV administration of conjugated estrogens, reconstitute by first removing approximately 5 mL of air from the dry powder vial and then slowly injecting the diluent into the vial, aiming it at the side of the vial. Gently agitate to dissolve; do not shake.
- Administer IV push slowly, at a rate of 5 mg/minute.
- Premarin is pregnancy category X.

Pharmacokinetics: Premarin is well absorbed after oral administration. It is widely distributed, crosses the placenta, and enters breast milk. It is metabolized by the liver. Its half-life is unknown.

Adverse Effects and Interactions: Adverse effects of Premarin include nausea, fluid retention, edema, breast tenderness, abdominal cramps and bloating, acute pancreatitis, appetite changes, skin eruptions, mental depression, decreased libido, headache, fatigue, nervousness, and weight gain. Effects are dose dependent. Estrogens, when used alone, have been associated with a higher risk for uterine cancer. Although adding a progestin may exert a protective

NURSING PROCESS FOCUS

Clients Receiving Hormone Replacement Therapy

Assessment	Potential Nursing Diagnoses/Identified Patterns
Prior to administration: • Obtain complete health history, including personal or familial history of breast cancer, gallbladder disease, diabetes mellitus, and liver or kidney disease. • Obtain drug history to determine possible drug interactions and allergies. • Assess cardiovascular status, including hypertension and history of MI, CVA, and thromboembolic disease. • Determine if client is pregnant or lactating.	• Risk for fluid excess related to side effect of drug • Need for knowledge regarding drug therapy and possible adverse effects such as thrombophlebitis and pulmonary or cerebral embolism • Need for knowledge regarding importance of adherence to dosing schedule and management of a missed dose

Planning: Client Goals and Expected Outcomes

The client will:

- Report relief from symptoms of menopause
- Demonstrate an understanding of the drug's action by accurately describing drug side effects and precautions
- Immediately report such effects as symptoms of thrombophlebitis, difficulty breathing, visual disturbances, severe headache, and seizure activity

---

Implementation

Interventions (Rationales)	Client Education/Discharge Planning
• Monitor for thromboembolic disease. (Estrogen increases risk for thromboembolism.) • Monitor for abnormal uterine bleeding. (If undiagnosed tumour is present, these drugs can increase its size and cause uterine bleeding.) • Monitor breast health. (Estrogens promote the growth of certain breast cancers.) • Monitor for vision changes. (These drugs may worsen myopia or astigmatism and cause intolerance of contact lenses.) • Encourage client not to smoke. (Smoking increases risk of cardiovascular disease.) • Encourage client to avoid caffeine. (Estrogens and caffeine may lead to increased central nervous system stimulation.) • Monitor glucose levels. (Estrogens may increase blood glucose levels.) • Monitor for seizure activity. (Estrogen-induced fluid retention may increase risk of seizures.) • Monitor client's understanding and proper self-administration. (Improper administration may increase incidence of adverse effects.)	• Instruct client to report shortness of breath, feeling of heaviness, chest pain, severe headache, warmth, or swelling in affected part, usually the legs or pelvis • Instruct client to report excessive uterine bleeding or bleeding that occurs between menstruations • Instruct client to have regular breast exams, perform monthly breast self-exams, and obtain routine mammograms, as recommended by healthcare provider Instruct client to: • Obtain regular eye exams during HRT • Report changes in vision • Report any difficulty in wearing contact lenses • Instruct client to avoid smoking and participate in smoking cessation programs, if necessary Instruct client to: • Restrict caffeine consumption • Recognize common foods that contain caffeine: coffee, tea, carbonated beverages, chocolate, certain OTC medications • Report unusual nervousness, anxiety, and insomnia Instruct client to: • Monitor blood and urine glucose frequently, if diabetic • Report any consistent changes in blood glucose • Instruct client to be alert for possibility of seizures, even at night, and report any seizure-type symptoms Instruct client to: • Administer proper dose, form, and frequency of medication • Take with food to decrease GI irritation • Take daily dose at bedtime to decrease occurrence of side effects • Document menstruation and any problems that occur

---

Evaluation of Outcome Criteria

Evaluate the effectiveness of drug therapy by confirming that client goals and expected outcomes have been met (see "Planning").

See Table 31.5 (page 369), under the heading "Estrogens," for a list of drugs to which these nursing actions apply.

---

effect by lowering the risk for uterine cancer, recent studies suggest that the progestin may increase the risk for breast cancer following long-term use. The risk for adverse effects increases in clients over age 35 years.

Drug interactions include a decreased effect of tamoxifen (Nolvadex), enhanced corticosteroid effects, and decreased effects of anticoagulants, especially warfarin. The effects of estrogen may be decreased if taken with barbiturates or rifampin, and there is a possible increased effect of tricyclic antidepressants if taken with estrogens.

Use with caution with herbal supplements. For example, red clover and black cohosh may interfere with estrogen therapy. Effects of estrogen may be enhanced if combined with ginseng.

UTERINE ABNORMALITIES

Dysfunctional uterine bleeding is a condition in which hemorrhage occurs on a non-cyclic basis or in abnormal amounts. It

is the health problem most frequently reported by women and a common reason for hysterectomy. Progestins are the drugs of choice for treating uterine abnormalities.

Pharmacotherapy with Progestins

31.7 Progestins are prescribed for dysfunctional uterine bleeding. High doses of progestins are also used as antineoplastics.

Secreted by the corpus luteum, the function of endogenous progesterone is to prepare the uterus for implantation of the embryo and pregnancy. If implantation does not occur, levels of progesterone fall dramatically and menses begins. If pregnancy occurs, the ovary will continue to secrete progesterone to maintain a healthy endometrium until the placenta develops sufficiently to

Special Considerations

Estrogen Use and Psychosocial Issues

Because undesirable side effects may occur with estrogen use, communicate these prior to implementation of drug therapy. The nurse can explore the client's reaction to these potential risks. An assessment of the client's emotional support system should also be made before initiating drug therapy. Hirsutism, loss of hair, or a deepening of the voice can occur in the female client. The male client may develop secondary female characteristics such as a higher voice, lack of body hair, and increased breast size. Impotence may also develop and is viewed as a concern by most men.

Clients should be taught that these adverse effects are reversible and may subside with adjustment of dosage or discontinuation of estrogen therapy. This knowledge may allow both male and female clients to remain compliant when adverse effects occur. During therapy, clients may need emotional support to assist in dealing with these body image issues. The nurse can encourage this support, discuss these issues with family members, and refer clients for counselling. For the female client, the nurse can refer to an esthetician for hair removal or wig fitting. The male client and his sexual partner may need a referral to deal with issues surrounding impotence and its effect on their relationship.

Natural Therapies

Chaste Berry for Premenstrual Syndrome and Menopause

The chaste tree (*Vitex agnus-castus*) is a shrub common to riverbanks in the southern Mediterranean region. The dried berries have been used for thousands of years, with recorded references dating to the time of Hippocrates.

Chaste berries contain a number of active substances that increase dopamine action and also affect the pituitary gland. Inhibition of FSH release leads to effects similar to progesterone. Extracts have a physiological effect on premenstrual syndrome (PMS), as well as on the unpleasant symptoms of menopause. Many women who take the herbal remedy report reduction in PMS symptoms such as bloating, breast fullness, headache, irritability, mood swings, and anger. There is better regulation of the menstrual cycle and less bleeding. When used during menopause, it may help to reverse vaginal changes and diminished libido. It is reported to decrease prolactin levels and milk production in lactating women. Adverse effects are minor and include GI upset, rash, and headaches.

begin producing the hormone. Whereas the function of estrogen is to cause proliferation of the endometrium, progesterone limits and stabilizes endometrial growth.

Dysfunctional uterine bleeding can have a number of causes, including early abortion, pelvic neoplasms, thyroid disorders, pregnancy, and infection. Types of dysfunctional uterine bleeding include the following:

- Amenorrhea: absence of menstruation
- Oligomenorrhea: infrequent menstruation
- Menorrhagia: prolonged or excessive menstruation
- Breakthrough bleeding: hemorrhage between menstrual periods
- Postmenopausal bleeding: hemorrhage following menopause

Dysfunctional uterine bleeding is often caused by a hormonal imbalance between estrogen and progesterone. Although estrogen increases the thickness of the endometrium, bleeding occurs sporadically unless balanced by an adequate amount of progesterone secretion. Administration of a progestin in a pattern starting 5 days after the onset of menses and continuing for the next 20 days can sometimes help to re-establish a normal, monthly cyclic pattern. Oral contraceptives may also be prescribed for this disorder.

In cases of heavy bleeding, high doses of conjugated estrogens may be administered for 3 weeks prior to adding medroxyprogesterone for the last 10 days of therapy. Treatment with nonsteroidal anti-inflammatory drugs (NSAIDs) sometimes helps to reduce bleeding and ease painful menstrual flow. If aggressive hormonal therapy fails to stop the heavy bleeding, dilation and curettage (D&C) may be necessary.

Progestins are occasionally prescribed for the treatment of metastatic endometrial carcinoma. In these cases, they are used for palliation, usually in combination with other antineoplastics. Select progestins and their dosages are shown in Table 31.5 (page 369).

Nursing Considerations

The role of the nurse in progestin therapy involves careful monitoring of the client's condition and providing education as it relates to the prescribed drug treatment. Before administering progesterone, obtain baseline data, including blood pressure, weight, and pulse. Laboratory tests including complete blood count (CBC), liver function, serum glucose, and an electrolyte profile should be obtained. Progestin is contraindicated for use in clients with a personal or close family history of breast or genital malignancies, thromboembolic disorders, impaired liver function, and undiagnosed vaginal bleeding. It is also contraindicated in pregnancy or lactation. Clients with allergies to peanuts should avoid the use of Prometrium because the oral capsules contain peanut oil. Progestin must be used with caution in women with a history of depression, anemia, diabetes, asthma, seizure disorders, cardiac or kidney disorders, migraine headaches, previous ectopic pregnancies, history of sexually transmitted infections, unresolved abnormal Pap tests, or previous pelvic surgeries.

Monitor the client for side effects of these hormones. Susceptible clients may experience acute intermittent porphyria as a reaction to progesterone, so assess the client for severe, colicky abdominal pain; vomiting; distention; diarrhea; and constipation. Common side effects of progesterone include breakthrough bleeding, nausea, abdominal cramps, dizziness, edema, and weight gain. Monitor also for amenorrhea; sudden, severe headache; and signs of pulmonary embolism such as sudden severe chest pain and dyspnea. Report such symptoms to the healthcare provider immediately. Because progesterone can cause photosensitivity and phototoxicity, monitor for pruritus, sensitivity to light, acne, rash, and alopecia. Phototoxic reactions cause serious sunburn within 5 to 18 hours of sun exposure.

Client education as it relates to progestins should include goals, reasons for assessing cardiovascular status, and possible side effects. See Nursing Process Focus: Clients Receiving Progestin Therapy for specific teaching points.

NURSING PROCESS FOCUS

Clients Receiving Progestin Therapy

Assessment	Potential Nursing Diagnoses/Identified Patterns
Prior to administration: • Obtain complete health history, including personal and familial history of breast, endometrial, or renal cancer; liver or kidney disease; dysfunctional uterine bleeding; and endometrial hyperplasia. • Obtain drug history to determine possible drug interactions and allergies. • Assess cardiovascular status including history of thromboembolic disease.	• Risk for fluid excess related to side effect of drug • Need for knowledge regarding drug therapy and adverse effects • Need for knowledge regarding importance of adherence to dosing schedule

Planning: Client Goals and Expected Outcomes

The client will:

• Report relief from dysfunctional uterine bleeding or amenorrhea
• Demonstrate an understanding of the drug's action by accurately describing drug side effects and precautions
• Immediately report effects such as signs of embolism; sudden, severe headache; edema; vision changes; and phototoxicity

Implementation

Interventions (Rationales)	Client Education/Discharge Planning
• Monitor lab tests, including liver function, blood glucose, and sodium and chloride levels. (Progestins can affect electrolyte balance and liver function.) • Monitor for vision changes. (Progestins may cause retinal emboli or cerebrovascular thrombosis.) • Monitor for fluid imbalance. (Progestins cause fluid retention and weight gain.) • Monitor for integumentary effects of medication. (Progestins have multiple effects on the skin and associated structures.)	• Instruct client to obtain periodic lab tests and to monitor glucose levels closely if diabetic • Instruct client to report unexplained partial or complete loss of vision, ptosis, or diplopia • Instruct client to monitor for edema or weight gain by weighing self weekly and recording, especially clients who have asthma, seizure disorders, cardiac or kidney impairment, or migraines Instruct client to: • Report itching, photosensitivity, acne, rash, and hair overgrowth or loss • Avoid exposure to ultraviolet light and prolonged periods of time in the sun • Use sunscreen (>SPF 12) when outdoors • Recognize that these changes are temporary and will improve upon discontinuation of this medication

Evaluation of Outcome Criteria

Evaluate the effectiveness of drug therapy by confirming that client goals and expected outcomes have been met (see "Planning").

See Table 31.5 (page 369), under the heading "Progestins," for a list of drugs to which these nursing actions apply.

PROTOTYPE DRUG | **Medroxyprogesterone (Provera, Medroxy)**

Actions and Uses: Medroxyprogesterone is a synthetic progestin with a prolonged duration of action. Like its natural counterpart, the primary target tissue for medroxyprogesterone is the endometrium of the uterus. It inhibits the effect of estrogen on the uterus, thus restoring normal hormonal balance. Applications include dysfunctional uterine bleeding and secondary amenorrhea. Medroxyprogesterone may also be given IM for the palliation of metastatic uterine or renal carcinoma.

Pharmacokinetics: Medroxyprogesterone is well absorbed after oral administration. It is widely distributed and enters breast milk. It is metabolized by the liver. Its half-life is about 14.5 hours.

Administration Alerts:
• Give PO with meals to avoid gastric distress.

• Observe IM sites for abscess: presence of lump and discoloration of tissue.

• Medroxyprogesterone is pregnancy category X.

Adverse Effects and Interactions: The most common side effects are breakthrough bleeding and breast tenderness. Weight gain, depression, hypertension, nausea, vomiting, dysmenorrheal, and vaginal candidiasis may also occur. The most serious side effects relate to increased risk for thromboembolic disease.

Serum levels of medroxyprogesterone are decreased by aminoglutethimide (Cytadren), barbiturates, primidone, rifampin, rifabutin (Mycobutin), and topiramate (Topamax).

Use with caution with herbal supplements. For example, St. John's wort may cause intermenstrual bleeding and loss of efficacy.

LABOUR AND BREASTFEEDING

Oxytocics are agents that stimulate uterine contractions to promote the induction of labour. **Tocolytics** are used to inhibit uterine contractions during premature labour. These agents are shown in Table 31.6.

Pharmacological Management of Uterine Contractions

31.8 Oxytocics are drugs that stimulate uterine contractions and induce labour. Tocolytics slow uterine contractions to delay labour.

The most widely used oxytocic is the natural hormone oxytocin, which is secreted by the posterior portion of the pituitary gland. The target organs for oxytocin are the uterus and the breast. It is secreted in increasingly larger amounts as the growing fetus distends the uterus. As blood levels of oxytocin rise, the uterus is stimulated to contract, thus promoting labour and the delivery of the baby and the placenta. As pregnancy progresses, the number of oxytocin receptors in the uterus increases, making the uterus more sensitive to the effects of the hormone. Parenteral oxytocin may be given to initiate labour. Doses in an IV infusion are increased gradually, every 15 to 60 minutes, until a normal labour pattern is established. After delivery, an IV infusion of oxytocin may be given to control postpartum uterine bleeding by temporarily impeding blood flow to this organ.

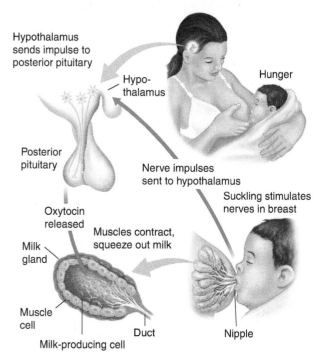

Figure 31.7 Oxytocin and breastfeeding.

In postpartum clients, oxytocin is released in response to suckling, causing milk to be ejected (let down) from the mammary glands. Oxytocin does not increase the volume of milk production. This function is provided by the pituitary hormone prolactin, which increases the synthesis of milk. The actions of oxytocin during breastfeeding are illustrated in Figure 31.7. When given for milk letdown, oxytocin is given intranasally several minutes before breastfeeding or pumping is anticipated.

Several prostaglandins are also used as uterine stimulants. Unlike most hormones that travel through the blood to affect distant tissues, **prostaglandins** are local hormones that act directly at the site where they are secreted. Although the body makes dozens of different prostaglandins, only a few have clinical use. Dinoprostone, prostaglandin E_2, is used to initiate labour, to prepare the cervix for labour, or to expel a fetus that has died. Mifepristone, a synthetic analogue of prostaglandin E_1, is used for emergency contraception and for pharmacological abortion, as described earlier in this chapter. Carboprost, 15-methyl prostaglandin F_2 alpha, can induce pharmacological abortion and may be indicated to control postpartum bleeding.

Tocolytics are uterine relaxants prescribed to *inhibit* the uterine contractions experienced during premature labour. Suppressing labour allows additional time for the fetus to develop and may permit the pregnancy to reach normal term. Premature birth is a leading cause of infant death. Typically, the mother is hooked up to a monitor with a sensor that records uterine contractions, and this information is used to determine the doses and timing of tocolytic medications.

Two $beta_2$-adrenergic agonists are used as uterine relaxants. Ritodrine (Yutopar) may be given by the oral or IV route to suppress labour contractions. It is more effective when administered before labour intensifies, and its use normally results in only a 1- to 2-day prolongation of pregnancy. Terbutaline is another $beta_2$-adrenergic agonist that may be used for uterine relaxation, although it is

TABLE 31.6 Uterine Stimulants and Relaxants

Drug	Route and Adult Dose
Stimulants (Oxytocics)	
Pr oxytocin (Pitocin)	Induction or stimulation of labour: IV, start with 0.5-1 milliunits/minute; gradually increase dose in increments of 1 to 2 milliunits/minute every 30 to 60 minutes until desired contraction pattern is established Postpartum uterine bleeding: IV, 10-40 units added to running infusion
Ergot Alkaloids	
ergonovine (Ergotrate Maleate)	IM/IV, 0.2 mg; may repeat dose in 2-4 hours if needed (max 5 total doses)
methylergonovine (Methergine)	PO, 0.2 mg 3-4 times daily in the puerperium for up to 7 days (max duration 1 week)
Prostaglandins	
carboprost (Hemabate)	IM, initial 250 µg (1 mL) repeated at 1.5- to 3.5-hour intervals if indicated by uterine response (max total dose is 2 mg [8 doses])
dinoprostone (Cervidil, Prepidil, Prostin E₂)	Intravaginal, 10 mg
misoprostol (Cytotec)	PO, 400-600 µg as a single dose
Relaxants (Tocolytics)	
Beta₂-Adrenergic Agonists	
ritodrine (Yutopar)	Dosing for relaxants varies considerably
Other Tocolytics	
magnesium sulfate (see Chapter 37, p. 444, for the Prototype Drug box)	
nifedipine (Adalat) (see Chapter 51, p. 640, for the Prototype Drug box)	

not approved for this purpose. The benefits of tocolytics must be carefully weighed against their potential adverse effects, which include tachycardia in both the mother and the fetus.

Nursing Considerations

The role of the nurse in uterine stimulant therapy involves careful monitoring of both the client and the fetus and providing education as it relates to the administered drug. The healthcare provider must evaluate the client for fetal presentation, especially for the presence of cephalopelvic disproportion.

To safely administer oxytocin, the fetus must be viable and vaginal delivery must be possible. If invasive cervical cancer, active herpes genitalis, or cord prolapse exists, oxytocin is contraindicated. Oxytocin is also contraindicated in clients with a history of previous uterine or cervical surgery, including cesarean section. This drug is not used if the client is a grand multipara, is older than 35 years of age, or has a history of uterine sepsis or traumatic birth. Previous sensitivity or allergic reaction to an ergot derivative contraindicates the use of oxytocin. Dinoprostone use is contraindicated in clients with active cardiac, pulmonary, renal, or hepatic disease. These medications must be used cautiously with vasoconstrictive drugs.

Monitor the client for side effects of these hormone-based medications. Because oxytocin increases the frequency and force of uterine contractions, the client in labour must be assessed frequently for elevations in blood pressure, heart rate, and fetal heart rate. The infusion must be discontinued if fetal distress is detected in order to prevent fetal anoxia. The nurse should administer oxygen and have the client change position to improve fetal oxygenation. Hypertensive crisis may occur if local or regional anesthesia is used in combination with oxytocin.

Uterine hyperstimulation is characterized by contractions that are less than 2 minutes apart, with force greater than 50 mm Hg or that last longer than 90 seconds. Oxytocin should be discontinued immediately if hyperstimulation occurs. Monitor fluid balance because prolonged IV infusion of oxytocin may cause water intoxication. Symptoms of water intoxication must be assessed and reported immediately and include drowsiness, listlessness, headache, confusion, anuria, and weight gain. Side effects of oxytocin include anxiety, maternal dyspnea, hypotension or hypertension, nausea, vomiting, neonatal jaundice, and maternal or fetal dysrhythmias.

See Nursing Process Focus: Clients Receiving Oxytocin for specific teaching points regarding this prototype drug.

NURSING PROCESS FOCUS

Clients Receiving Oxytocin

Assessment	Potential Nursing Diagnoses/Identified Patterns
Prior to administration: • Obtain complete health history, including past and present gynecological and obstetric history. • Obtain drug history to determine possible drug interactions and allergies.	• Risk for fluid excess related to the similarity of oxytocin to antidiuretic hormone (ADH) • Need for knowledge regarding drug therapy and possible adverse effects such as thrombophlebitis and pulmonary or cerebral embolism • Need for knowledge regarding importance of adherence to dosing schedule and management of a missed dose • Risk for injury to fetus related to strong uterine contractions

Planning: Client Goals and Expected Outcomes

The client will:

• Report increase in force and frequency of uterine contractions and/or letdown of milk for breastfeeding
• Demonstrate an understanding of the drug's action by accurately describing drug side effects and precautions
• Immediately report effects such as listlessness, headache, confusion, anuria, hypotension, nausea, vomiting, and weight gain

Implementation

Interventions (Rationales)	Client Education/Discharge Planning
• Monitor fetal heart rate. (Increase in force and frequency of uterine contractions may cause fetal distress.) • Monitor maternal status, including blood pressure; pulse; and frequency, duration, and intensity of contractions. • Monitor fluid balance. (Prolonged IV infusion may cause water intoxication.) • Monitor for postpartum/postabortion hemorrhage. (Oxytocin can be used to control postpartum bleeding.) • Monitor lactation status. (Oxytocin causes milk ejection within minutes after administration.)	• Instruct client about the purpose and importance of fetal monitoring. • Instruct client about the importance of monitoring maternal status. • Instruct client to report drowsiness, listlessness, headache, confusion, anuria, weight gain. Instruct client: • About the importance of being monitored frequently after delivery or after abortion • To report severe vaginal bleeding or increase in lochia Instruct client: • That oxytocin does not increase milk production • To monitor for decreased breast pain, redness, hardness, if taking oxytocin to decrease breast engorgement

Evaluation of Outcome Criteria

Evaluate the effectiveness of drug therapy by confirming that client goals and expected outcomes have been met (see "Planning").

PROTOTYPE DRUG   Oxytocin (Pitocin)

Actions and Uses: Oxytocin is a natural hormone secreted by the posterior pituitary that is a drug of choice for inducing labour. Oxytocin is given by several different routes depending on its intended action. Given by IV infusion antepartum, oxytocin induces labour by increasing the frequency and force of contractions of uterine smooth muscle. It is timed to the final stage of pregnancy, after the cervix is dilated, membranes have ruptured, and presentation of the fetus has occurred. Oxytocin may also be administered postpartum to reduce hemorrhage after expulsion of the placenta and to aid in returning normal muscular tone to the uterus. A second route of administration is intranasally to promote the ejection of milk from the mammary glands. Milk letdown occurs within minutes after applying spray or drops to the nostril during breastfeeding.

Pharmacokinetics: Oxytocin is well absorbed and widely distributed. It is rapidly metabolized by the liver. Its half-life is 3 to 9 minutes.

Administration Alerts:

- Dilute 10 U oxytocin in 1000 mL IV fluid prior to administration. For postpartum administration, up to 40 U may be added to 1000 mL of IV fluid.
- Incidence of allergic reactions is higher when given by IM or IV injection, rather than IV infusion.
- Oxytocin is pregnancy category C.

Adverse Effects and Interactions: When given IV, vital signs of the fetus and client are monitored continuously to avoid complications in the fetus, such as dysrhythmias or intracranial hemorrhage. Serious complications in the client may include uterine rupture, seizures, or coma. The risk of uterine rupture increases in women who have delivered five or more children. Although experience has shown the use of oxytocin to be quite safe, labour should be induced by this drug only when there are demonstrated risks to the mother or fetus in continuing the pregnancy.

Oxytocin interacts with several drugs. For example, vasoconstrictors used concurrently with oxytocin cause severe hypertension.

Use with caution with herbal supplements. For example, ephedra or ma huang used with oxytocin may lead to hypertension.

FEMALE INFERTILITY

Infertility is defined as the inability to become pregnant after at least 1 year of frequent, unprotected intercourse. Infertility is a common disorder, with as many as 25% of couples experiencing difficulty in conceiving children at some point during their reproductive lifetimes. It is estimated that females contribute to approximately 60% of the infertility disorders. Agents used to treat infertility are shown in Table 31.7.

Pharmacotherapy of Female Fertility

31.9 Medications may be administered to stimulate ovulation in order to increase female fertility.

Causes of female infertility are varied and include lack of ovulation, pelvic infection, and physical obstruction of the fallopian

TABLE 31.7   Agents for Female Infertility

Drug	Mechanism
bromocriptine mesylate	Reduces high prolactin levels
clomiphene (Clomid, Serophene)	Promotes follicle maturation and ovulation
danazol (Cyclomen)	Controls endometriosis
Human FSH (purified from the urine of postmenopausal women)	
urofollitropin (Bravelle)	Promotes follicle maturation and ovulation
Recombinant FSH	
follitropin alfa (Gonal-f)	Promotes follicle maturation and ovulation
follitropin beta (Follistim)	
GnRH and GnRH Analogues	
cetrorelix (Cetrotide)	
leuprolide (Lupron, Lupron Depot)	Promotes follicle maturation and ovulation or control of endometriosis
nafarelin (Synarel)	
ganirelix (Orgalutran)	
gonadorelin (Lutrepulse)	
goserelin (Zoladex)	
human chorionic gonadotropin (A.P.L., Chorex, Choron 10, Profasi HP, Pregnyl)	Promotes follicle maturation and ovulation
human menopausal gonadotropin (Pergonal, Humegon, Repronex)	Promotes follicle maturation and ovulation

tubes. Extensive testing is often necessary to determine the exact cause of the infertility. For women whose infertility has been determined to have an endocrine etiology, pharmacotherapy may be of value. Endocrine disruption of reproductive function can occur at the level of the hypothalamus, pituitary, or ovary, and pharmacotherapy is targeted to the specific cause of the dysfunction.

Lack of regular ovulation is a cause of infertility that can be successfully treated with drug therapy. Clomiphene (Clomid, Serophene) is a drug of choice for female infertility that acts as an antiestrogen. Clomiphene stimulates the release of LH, resulting in the maturation of more ovarian follicles than would normally occur. The rise in LH level is sufficient to induce ovulation in about 90% of treated clients. The pregnancy rate of clients taking clomiphene is high, and twins occur in about 5% of treated clients. Therapy is usually begun with a low dose of 50 mg for 5 days, following menses. If ovulation does not occur, the dose is increased to 100 mg for 5 days, then to 150 mg. If ovulation still is not induced, human chorionic gonadotropin (hCG) is added to the treatment. Made by the placenta during pregnancy, hCG is similar to LH and can mimic the LH surge that normally causes ovulation. The use of clomiphene assumes that the pituitary gland is able to respond by secreting LH and that the ovaries are responsive to LH. If either of these assumptions is false, other treatment options should be considered.

If the endocrine disruption is at the pituitary level, therapy with human menopausal gonadotropin (hMG) or gonadotropin-releasing hormone (GnRH) may be indicated. These therapies are generally indicated only after clomiphene has failed to induce ovulation. hMG is a combination of FSH and LH extracted from the urine of postmenopausal women, who secrete large amounts of these hormones. Also called menotropins, hMG acts on the ovaries to increase follicle maturation and results in a 25% incidence of multiple pregnancies. Successful therapy with hMG assumes that the ovaries are responsive to LH and FSH. Newer formulations use recombinant DNA technology to synthesize gonadotropins containing nearly pure FSH, rather than extracting the FSH-LH mixture from urine.

Given IV, gonadorelin (Lutrepulse) is a synthetic analogue of GnRH that is prescribed for clients who are unresponsive to clomiphene. GnRH analogues take over the function of the hypothalamus and attempt to restart normal hormonal rhythms. Other medications used to stimulate ovulation are bromocriptine and hCG.

Endometriosis, a common cause of infertility, is characterized by the presence of endometrial tissue in non-uterine locations such as the pelvis and ovaries. Being responsive to hormonal stimuli, this abnormal tissue can cause pain, dysfunctional bleeding, and dysmenorrhea. Leuprolide (Lupron, Eligard) is a GnRH agonist that produces an initial release of LH and FSH, followed by suppression due to the negative feedback effect on the pituitary. Many women experience relief from the symptoms of endometriosis after 3 to 6 months of leuprolide therapy, and the benefits may extend well beyond the treatment period. Leuprolide is also indicated for the palliative therapy of prostate cancer. As an alternative choice, danazol is an anabolic steroid that suppresses FSH production, which in turn shuts down both ectopic and normal endometrial activity. Whereas leuprolide is only given by the parenteral route, danazol is given orally.

CHAPTER
31 Understanding the Chapter

Key Concepts Summary

The numbered key concepts provide a succinct summary of the important points from the corresponding numbered section within the chapter. If any of these points are not clear, refer to the numbered section within the chapter for review.

31.1 Female reproductive function is controlled by GnRH from the hypothalamus and by FSH and LH from the pituitary.

31.2 Estrogens are secreted by ovarian follicles and are responsible for the secondary sex characteristics of the female. Progestins are secreted by the corpus luteum and prepare the endometrium for implantation.

31.3 Low doses of estrogens and progestins prevent conception by blocking ovulation. The adverse effects of combined oral contraceptives are uncommon but may be serious in some women.

31.4 Long-acting contraceptives and novel delivery methods offer women additional birth control choices.

31.5 Drugs for emergency contraception may be administered within 72 hours of unprotected sex to prevent implantation of the fertilized egg. Other agents may be given to stimulate uterine contractions to expel the implanted embryo.

31.6 Estrogen-progestin combinations are used for hormone replacement therapy during and after menopause; however, their long-term use may have serious adverse effects.

31.7 Progestins are prescribed for dysfunctional uterine bleeding. High doses of progestins are also used as antineoplastics.

31.8 Oxytocics are drugs that stimulate uterine contractions and induce labour. Tocolytics slow uterine contractions to delay labour.

31.9 Medications may be administered to stimulate ovulation in order to increase female fertility.

Chapter 31 Scenario

Eileen John is 46 years old and exhibiting signs of menopause. She reports a change in her menstrual cycle regularity. For the past year, her periods have occurred between 6 and 8 weeks apart and have lasted for only 2 to 3 days. Previously, she experienced her periods approximately every 28 days, and they lasted from 4 to 5 days. She reports to the nurse that she is now feeling easily fatigued and has more mood swings, occasional headaches, hot flashes, insomnia, bouts of depression, and irritability. She is also concerned about her loss of libido. She admits to smoking half a pack of cigarettes a day and drinking several cups of coffee during work hours. She has a family history of hypertension, cardiac disease, and diabetes, but she has never been diagnosed with any of these disorders.

A complete history and physical examination, along with a vaginal examination and a Pap test, are performed.

Critical Thinking Questions

1. Do you think that Eileen is a candidate for hormone replacement therapy? Why or why not?
2. Create a list of some treatment options for Eileen.
3. Eileen asks about the precautions related to suggested treatment options. How would you respond?

See Answers to Critical Thinking Questions in Appendix B.

NCLEX Practice Questions

1 A 52-year-old client experiencing symptoms of menopause is interested in taking hormone replacement therapy (HRT) with conjugated estrogen (Premarin). Which conditions may be a contraindication for HRT for this client? Select all that apply.
   a. History of type 2 diabetes mellitus
   b. History of deep venous thrombosis
   c. History of breast cancer with "lumpectomy" treatment
   d. History of hyperlipidemia, controlled by drug therapy
   e. History of two Caesarean sections

2 A nurse is evaluating the effect of an oxytocin infusion in a labouring woman. Which of the following indicates that the drug is exerting therapeutic effects?
   a. Hemorrhage is controlled.
   b. Contractions are sustained at 60 seconds long.
   c. Contractions are occurring every 4 minutes and lasting 20 seconds.
   d. Milk letdown has begun in preparation of breastfeeding.

3 Which instruction about clomiphene (Clomid) will a nurse provide to a woman with infertility?
   a. "The drug will be taken for a year and then re-evaluated for an increased dose."
   b. "After you are pregnant, the drug will be continued for the first 3 months of pregnancy to guard against miscarriage."
   c. "You may stay on this indefinitely until pregnancy occurs. There are few adverse effects."
   d. "If pregnancy does not occur within six cycles, other options for treatment will be explored."

4 A 48-year-old client has received a prescription for medroxyprogesterone (Provera) for treatment of dysfunctional uterine bleeding. Because of related adverse effects, the nurse will teach the client to monitor and report which symptoms?
   a. Insomnia or difficulty falling asleep
   b. Excessive mouth, eye, or vaginal dryness
   c. Joint pain or pain on ambulation
   d. Breakthrough spotting between menstrual periods

5 A client informs the healthcare provider that she has been trying to become pregnant for more than 2 years and has not used any form of contraception. The healthcare provider has prescribed clomiphene (Clomid) 50 mg/day for 5 days. The nurse should instruct the client to begin taking the drug on the
   a. First day of the menstrual cycle
   b. Fifth day of the menstrual cycle
   c. Fifth day after ovulation
   d. Last day of the menstrual cycle

See Answers to NCLEX Practice Questions in Appendix A.

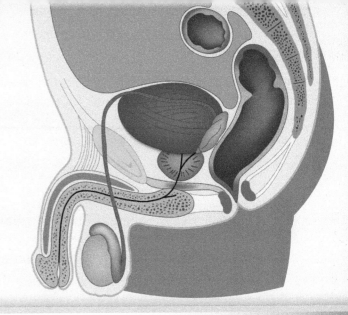

alexeyblogoodf/Fotolia

CHAPTER

32

Pharmacotherapy of Disorders of the Male Reproductive System

LEARNING OUTCOMES

After reading this chapter, the student should be able to:

1. Identify drug classes used for treating disorders of the male reproductive system.
2. Explain the therapeutic action of each class of drug in relation to the pathophysiology of the disorder being treated.
3. Explain the role of androgens in the treatment of male hypogonadism.
4. Describe the misuse and dangers associated with the use of anabolic steroids to enhance athletic performance.
5. Discuss the use of androgens as antineoplastic agents.
6. Explain the limited role of drugs in the therapy of male infertility.
7. Describe the role of drug therapy in the treatment of erectile dysfunction.
8. Describe the role of drug therapy in the treatment of benign prostatic hyperplasia (BPH).
9. For each of the drug classes listed in Prototype Drugs, identify a representative drug and explain its mechanism of action, therapeutic effects, and important adverse effects.
10. Describe and explain, based on pharmacological principles, the rationale for nursing assessment, planning, and interventions for clients who are receiving pharmacological therapy for disorders and conditions of the male reproductive system.
11. Use the nursing process to care for clients who are receiving drug therapy for disorders and conditions of the male reproductive system.

CHAPTER OUTLINE

▶ Hypothalamic and Pituitary Regulation of Male Reproductive Function

▶ Male Hypogonadism

  ▶ Pharmacotherapy with Androgens

▶ Male Sexual Dysfunction

▶ Male Infertility

  ▶ Pharmacotherapy of Male Infertility

▶ Erectile Dysfunction

  ▶ Pharmacotherapy of Erectile Dysfunction

▶ Benign Prostatic Hyperplasia

  ▶ Pharmacotherapy of Benign Prostatic Hyperplasia

Male reproductive function is regulated by a small number of hormones from the hypothalamus, pituitary, and gonads. Because hormonal secretion in the male is regular throughout the adult lifespan, pharmacological treatment of reproductive disorders in the male is less complex, and more limited, than in the female. This chapter examines drugs used to treat disorders and conditions of the male reproductive system.

Hypothalamic and Pituitary Regulation of Male Reproductive Function

32.1 FSH and LH from the pituitary regulate the secretion of testosterone, the primary hormone contributing to the growth, health, and maintenance of the male reproductive system.

The same pituitary hormones that control reproductive function in the female (Chapter 31) also affect the male. Although the name *follicle-stimulating hormone (FSH)* applies to its target in the female ovary, this same hormone regulates sperm production in the male. In males, luteinizing hormone (LH), sometimes called interstitial cell-stimulating hormone (ICSH), regulates the production of testosterone.

Although they are secreted in small amounts by the adrenal glands in females, **androgens** are considered male sex hormones. The testes secrete testosterone, the primary androgen responsible for maturation of the male sex organs and the secondary sex characteristics of the male. Unlike the cyclical secretion of estrogen and progesterone in the female, the secretion of testosterone is relatively constant in the adult male. Should the level of testosterone in the blood rise above normal, negative feedback is provided to the pituitary to shut off the secretion of LH and FSH. The relationship between the hypothalamus, pituitary, and male reproductive hormones is illustrated in Figure 32.1.

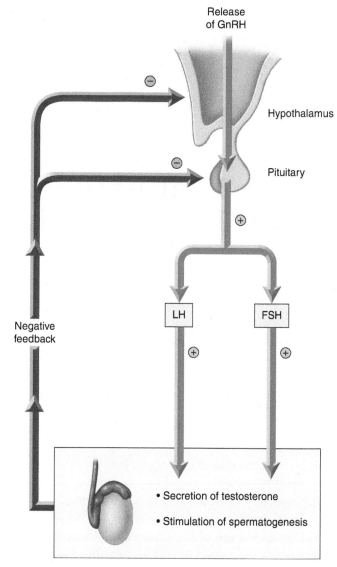

Figure 32.1 Hormonal control of the male reproductive hormones.

Like estrogen, testosterone has metabolic effects in tissues outside the reproductive system. Of particular note is its ability to build muscle mass, which contributes to the differences in muscle strength and body composition between males and females.

MALE HYPOGONADISM

Androgens include testosterone and related hormones that control many aspects of male reproductive function. Therapeutically, they are used to treat hypogonadism and certain cancers. These agents are listed in Table 32.1.

TABLE 32.1 Select Androgens

danazol (Danocrine)

fluoxymesterone (Halotestin)

methyltestosterone (Android, Testred)

nandrolone phenylpropionate (Durabolin, Hybolin)

testolactone (Teslac)

Pr testosterone (Andro 100, Histerone, Testoderm)

testosterone cypionate (Depotest, Andro-Cyp, Depo-Testosterone)

testosterone enanthate (Andro LA, Delatest, Delatestryl)

Pharmacotherapy with Androgens

32.2 Androgens are used to treat hypogonadism in males and breast cancer in females. Anabolic steroids are frequently abused by athletes and can result in serious adverse effects with long-term use.

Lack of sufficient testosterone secretion by the testes can result in male **hypogonadism**. Insufficient testosterone secretion may be caused by disorders of the pituitary or the testes. Deficiency in FSH and LH secretion by the pituitary will result in a lack of stimulus to the testes to produce androgens. Lack of FSH and LH secretion may have a number of causes, including Cushing's syndrome, thyroid disorders, estrogen-secreting tumours, and therapy with gonadotropin-releasing hormone (GnRH) agonists such as leuprolide. Hypogonadism may be congenital or acquired later in life.

Hypogonadism may also occur in clients with normal pituitary function if the testes are diseased or otherwise unresponsive to FSH and LH. Conditions that may cause testicular failure include mumps, testicular trauma or inflammation, and certain autoimmune disorders.

Symptoms of male hypogonadism include diminished appearance of the secondary male sex characteristics: sparse axillary, facial, and pubic hair; increase in subcutaneous fat; and small testicular size. In adult males, lack of testosterone can lead to erectile dysfunction, low sperm counts, and decreased **libido** (interest in intercourse). Nonspecific complaints may include fatigue, depression, and reduced muscle mass. In young males, lack of sufficient testosterone secretion may lead to delayed puberty.

Pharmacotherapy for male hypogonadism includes replacement therapy with testosterone or other androgens. Androgen therapy promotes normal gonadal development and often restores normal reproductive function. Secondary male sex characteristics reappear, a condition called masculinization or **virilization**.

Testosterone is available in a number of different formulations. Testosterone cypionate and testosterone enanthate are slowly absorbed after IM injections, which are given every 2 to 4 weeks. Testosterone pellets are implanted subcutaneously (SC) and last for 3 to 6 months. Several skin patch products are available, and these release testosterone over a 24-hour period. Testoderm patches are applied to the scrotal area, whereas Testoderm TTS and Androderm patches are applied to the arm, back,

or upper buttocks. Two gel systems are available as Testim and Androgel and are applied to the shoulders, upper arm, or abdomen. The alcohol-based gels dry quickly, and the testosterone is absorbed into the skin and released slowly to the blood. Buccal tablets adhere to the buccal mucosa in the small depression in the mouth where the gum meets the upper lip above the incisor teeth, and from there the drug is released and absorbed directly into the bloodstream over a 12-hour period.

Androgens have important physiological effects outside the reproductive system. Testosterone promotes the synthesis of erythropoietin, which explains why males usually have a slightly higher hematocrit than females. Testosterone has a profound anabolic effect on skeletal muscle, which is the rationale for giving this drug to debilitated clients who have muscle wasting disease.

Anabolic steroids are testosterone-like compounds with hormonal activity that are taken inappropriately by athletes who hope to build muscle mass and strength, thereby obtaining a competitive edge. When taken in large doses for prolonged periods, anabolic steroids can produce significant adverse effects, some of which may persist for months after discontinuation of the drug. These agents tend to raise cholesterol levels and may cause low sperm counts and impotence in men. In female athletes, menstrual irregularities are likely, with an obvious increase in masculine appearance. Permanent liver damage may result. Behavioural changes include aggression and psychological dependence. The use of anabolic steroids to improve athletic performance is illegal and strongly discouraged by healthcare providers and athletic associations. Most androgens are classified as Schedule III drugs due to their abuse potential.

High doses of androgens are occasionally used as a palliative measure to treat certain types of breast cancer, in combination with other antineoplastics. Because most prostate carcinomas are testosterone dependent, androgens should not be prescribed for older males unless the possibility of prostate cancer has been ruled out. Clients with prostate carcinoma are sometimes given a GnRH agonist such as leuprolide to reduce circulating testosterone levels.

NCLEX Success Tips

Clients with unilateral testicular cancer who undergo unilateral orchiectomy should not experience impotence if the other testis is normal.

The remaining testicle undergoes hyperplasia and produces enough testosterone to maintain sexual drive, libido, and secondary sexual characteristics, and testosterone levels will return to normal.

Sperm banking before unilateral orchiectomy or radiotherapy is commonly recommended because radiation or chemotherapy can affect fertility.

PROTOTYPE DRUG	Testosterone Base (Andriol, Androderm, AndroGel, Testim)

Actions and Uses: The primary therapeutic use of testosterone is for the treatment of hypogonadism in males by promoting virilization, including enlargement of the sexual organs, growth of facial hair, and a deepening of the voice. In adult males, testosterone administration will increase libido and restore masculine characteristics that may be deficient. Testosterone base acts by stimulating RNA synthesis and protein metabolism. High doses may suppress spermatogenesis.

Pharmacokinetics: Testosterone is well absorbed after buccal, transdermal, or IM administration. It is widely distributed, crosses the placenta, and enters breast milk. Testosterone is metabolized by the liver. Its half-life in plasma is less than 2 hours.

Administration Alerts:

- Place patch on hair-free, dry skin of the abdomen, back, thigh, upper arm, or as directed.
- Change patch site within an anatomical region every 24 hours and rotate to a different anatomical region every 7 days.
- Give IM injection into gluteal muscles.
- Testosterone is pregnancy category X.

Adverse Effects and Interactions: An obvious side effect of testosterone therapy is virilization, which is usually only of concern when the drug is taken by female clients. Increased libido may also occur. Salt and water are often retained, causing edema, and a diuretic may be indicated. Liver damage is rare, although it is a potentially serious adverse effect with some of the orally administered androgens. Acne and skin irritation is common during therapy.

Testosterone base interacts with several drugs. For example, when taken concurrently with oral anticoagulants, testosterone base may potentiate hypoprothrombinemia.

Use with caution with herbal supplements. Insulin requirements may decrease, and the risk of hepatotoxicity may increase when used with echinacea.

Nursing Considerations

The role of the nurse in androgen therapy involves careful monitoring of the client's condition and providing education as it relates to the prescribed drug regimen. Conduct a physical assessment for evidence of decreased hormone production, such as decreased or absent body hair, small testes, impaired sexual functioning, or delayed signs of puberty. Also assess the

CONNECTIONS | **Special Considerations**

◀ Androgen Abuse by Athletes

A serious problem with androgens is their abuse by athletes. The drugs have been used and abused to increase weight, muscle mass, and muscle strength. What began as a movement by weightlifters to enhance muscle mass in the early 1960s has progressed to most competitive sports and all age groups. Teen use has been increasing, and not just among athletes; some report taking the drugs simply to look better.

Anabolic steroids may be taken orally or IM. The oral forms are absorbed rapidly; they are sometimes preferred since they are excreted quickly and thus are less likely to be detected on drug screening. The IM injections may be water or oil based, with the oil forms having a prolonged duration and being more detectable. Most professional sport associations in Canada prohibit the use of androgens for these purposes, and any athlete proven to use them is banned from participation. Further encouraging their use is the fact that the serious effects of anabolic steroids are long term but not readily observable.

client's emotional status, as depression and mood swings may be symptoms of decreased hormone secretion. Monitor laboratory results, especially liver enzymes, if the client has a history of anabolic steroid use. Contraindications to androgen therapy include prostatic or male breast cancer, renal disease, cardiac and liver dysfunction, hypercalcemia, benign prostatic hyperplasia (BPH), and hypertension. Androgens must be used cautiously in prepubertal males and older adults, and in acute intermittent porphyria. Monitor for side effects such as acne, skin irritation, edema, and increased libido in male clients who are taking androgens. Some adverse reactions found to occur in females as a result of androgen use include deepening of the voice, increased acne or oily skin, increased hair growth, enlarged clitoris, and irregular menses.

Client education as it relates to androgen therapy should include goals; reasons for obtaining baseline data such as vital signs and tests for cardiac, liver, and renal function; and possible side effects. See Nursing Process Focus: Clients Receiving Androgen Therapy for specific teaching points.

NURSING PROCESS FOCUS

Clients Receiving Androgen Therapy

Assessment	Potential Nursing Diagnoses/Identified Patterns
Prior to administration: • Obtain complete health history, including male breast or prostatic cancer; BPH; cardiac, kidney, or liver disease; diabetes; and hypercalcemia. • Obtain lab results, including renal function tests, blood urea nitrogen (BUN), creatinine, and prostate-specific antigen (PSA). • Obtain drug history to determine possible drug interactions and allergies.	• Risk for sexual dysfunction related to effects of drug therapy or decreased hormone function • Risk for sleep disturbances related to effects of drug therapy • Need for knowledge regarding drug therapy and adverse effects • Risk for altered body image related to side effects of drug therapy

Planning: Client Goals and Expected Outcomes

The client will:

- Demonstrate improvement of the underlying condition for which testosterone was ordered
- Demonstrate an understanding of the drug's action by accurately describing drug side effects and precautions and the importance of follow-up care

Implementation	
Interventions (Rationales)	**Client Education/Discharge Planning**
• Monitor serum cholesterol levels. (Elevated cholesterol levels secondary to testosterone administration may increase client's risk of cardiovascular disease.)	Instruct client to: • Have cholesterol levels measured periodically during therapy • Implement changes that may lower risk of hypercholesterolemia: decrease fat in the diet, increase exercise, decrease consumption of red meat
• Monitor calcium levels. (Testosterone can cause hypercalcemia.) • Monitor bone growth in children and adolescents. (Premature epiphyseal closing may occur, leading to growth retardation.) • Monitor input, output, and client weight. (Testosterone can cause retention of salt and water, leading to edema.)	Instruct client to: • Have calcium levels checked during therapy • Recognize and report symptoms of increased serum calcium, including deep bone and flank pain, anorexia, nausea/vomiting, thirst, constipation, lethargy, and psychoses • Instruct pediatric caregiver to have bone age determinations on the child every 6 months. • Instruct client to check weight twice weekly and report increases, particularly if accompanied by dependent edema.
• Monitor blood glucose, especially in diabetics. (Testosterone therapy may change glucose tolerance.)	Instruct client to: • Monitor blood glucose daily and report significant changes to the healthcare provider • Recognize that adjustments may need to be made in hypoglycemic medications and diet
• Monitor proper self-administration.	Instruct client to: • Mark calendar so medication can be taken/given at appropriate intervals • Apply transdermal patch to dry, clean scrotal skin that has been dry-shaved and do not use chemical depilatories • Notify female partner of transdermal patch; there is a chance of absorbing testosterone, resulting in mild virilization • Avoid showering or swimming for at least 1 hour after gel application

Evaluation of Outcome Criteria
Evaluate the effectiveness of drug therapy by confirming that client goals and expected outcomes have been met (see "Planning").

See Table 32.1 (page 381) for a list of drugs to which these nursing actions apply.

MALE SEXUAL DYSFUNCTION

Approximately 50% of males will experience some form of sexual dysfunction during their adult life. The primary types of male dysfunction disorders may be classified as follows:

• Diminished libido: lack of interest in sexual activity

• Erectile dysfunction (ED): inability to obtain or maintain an erection

• Ejaculation disorder: premature, delayed, or retrograde ejaculation

• Infertility: inability to conceive a child

Certain causes of male sexual dysfunction are treatable, either medically or surgically, or can be improved to the degree that a couple can achieve successful conception or maintain a satisfactory sexual lifestyle. For example, therapy with testosterone can rapidly increase libido in clients who have insufficient serum testosterone levels or hypogonadism. Many men with ED can now be successfully treated with medications.

A large number of drugs can cause or worsen male sexual dysfunction, as listed in Table 32.2. In most cases, the dysfunction is dose related and is much less evident when a single drug is taken at low doses. However, taking multiple drugs that have the potential to cause sexual adverse effects may result in additive sexual dysfunction. The two most common drug classes that cause sexual dysfunction are antihypertensives and antidepressants. Because sexual adverse effects are a potential cause of nonadherence, nurses should ask specific questions about changes in sexual function when their clients are taking these drugs.

Many comorbid medical conditions are associated with sexual dysfunction. Conditions that result in general debility, such as pain, muscle weakness, shortness of breath, or stroke, may cause dysfunction. Diabetes and hypertension are the two chronic medical conditions most frequently associated with male sexual dysfunction. Clients who present with psychological conditions such as anxiety and depression have a high incidence of sexual dysfunction. Other factors associated with ED include obesity and cigarette smoking. Combining multiple risk factors—for example, a man who has diabetes, is obese, takes antihypertensive drugs, and smokes—will result in a high risk for sexual dysfunction.

Nurses play a key role in treating male sexual dysfunction by obtaining a thorough medical history and by recognizing factors that contribute to the disorder. Should clients experience unacceptable sexual adverse effects from their medications, alternative drugs can usually be substituted. Encouraging clients to receive treatment for anxiety, depression, and other comorbid conditions sometimes helps to improve the sexual dysfunction. All men at

TABLE 32.2 Drugs That May Cause or Worsen Male Sexual Dysfunction

Drug/Drug Class	Sexual Adverse Effect(s)
Antihypertensives	
alpha-adrenergic blockers (e.g., prazosin)	Retrograde ejaculation, priapism
angiotensin-converting enzyme (ACE) inhibitors (e.g., lisinopril)	ED
beta-adrenergic blockers (e.g., propranolol)	Diminished libido, ED
methyldopa	Diminished libido, ED
spironolactone	Diminished libido, ED
thiazide diuretics	ED
Nervous System Drugs	
carbamazepine	ED
haloperidol	Inhibited ejaculation, priapism
lithium carbonate	ED
phenothiazines (e.g., chlorpromazine)	Diminished libido, ED, inhibited ejaculation, priapism
selective serotonin reuptake inhibitors (e.g., fluoxetine)	Anorgasmy, inhibited ejaculation, diminished libido
trazodone	Priapism
tricyclic antidepressants (e.g., imipramine)	Diminished libido, ED, inhibited ejaculation
Other Drugs	
alcohol	ED
anabolic steroids	Infertility
antineoplastics (e.g., cyclophosphamide)	Infertility
cimetidine	Diminished libido, ED, gynecomastia
digoxin	ED
finasteride	ED
methotrexate	Infertility

risk for ED should be encouraged to maintain optimum weight, stop smoking, and limit their alcohol use.

MALE INFERTILITY

It is estimated that 30% to 40% of couples' infertility is caused by difficulties with the male reproductive system. Male infertility may have a psychological cause, which must be ruled out before pharmacotherapy is considered.

Pharmacotherapy of Male Infertility

32.3 Male infertility is difficult to treat pharmacologically; medications include hCG, menotropins, testolactone, and antiestrogens.

Like female infertility, male infertility may have a number of complex causes. **Oligospermia**, the presence of less than 20 million sperm per millilitre of ejaculate, is considered abnormal. **Azoospermia**, the complete absence of sperm in ejaculate, may indicate an obstruction of the vas deferens or ejaculatory duct, which can be corrected surgically. Infections such as mumps, chronic tuberculosis, and sexually transmitted infections can contribute to infertility. The possibility of ED must be considered and treated as discussed in Section 32.4. Infertility may occur with or without signs of hypogonadism.

The goal of endocrine pharmacotherapy of male infertility is to increase sperm production. Therapy often begins with IM injections of human chorionic gonadotropin (hCG), three times per week over 1 year. Although secreted by the placenta, the effects of hCG in the male are identical to those of LH: increasing testosterone secretion and stimulating spermatogenesis. Sperm counts are conducted periodically to assess therapeutic progress. If hCG is unsuccessful, therapy with menotropins may be attempted. Menotropins consist of a mixture of purified FSH and LH. For infertile clients who exhibit signs of hypogonadism, testosterone therapy also may be indicated.

Other pharmacological approaches to treating male infertility have been attempted. Antiestrogens such as tamoxifen and clomiphene have been used to block the negative feedback of estrogen (from the adrenal glands) to the pituitary and hypothalamus, thus increasing the levels of FSH and LH. Testolactone, an aromatase inhibitor, has been administered to block the metabolic conversion of testosterone to estrogen. Various nutritional supplements, such as zinc to improve sperm production, L-arginine to improve sperm motility, and vitamins C and E as antioxidants to reduce reactive intermediates, have been tested. Unfortunately, these and other attempts have not been conclusively shown to have any positive effect on male infertility.

Drug therapy for infertility is not as successful for males as it is for females because only about 5% of infertile males have a disorder with an endocrine etiology. Many years of therapy may be required. Because of the expense and the large number of injections needed, other means of conception may be explored, such as in vitro fertilization or intrauterine insemination.

ERECTILE DYSFUNCTION

Erectile dysfunction, or **impotence**, is a common disorder in men. The defining characteristic of this condition is the consistent inability either to obtain an erection or to sustain an erection long enough to achieve successful intercourse.

Pharmacotherapy of Erectile Dysfunction

32.4 Erectile dysfunction is a common disorder that may be successfully treated with sildenafil and other agents, which inhibit the enzyme phosphodiesterase-5.

The incidence of ED increases with advancing age, although it may occur in a male adult of any age. Certain diseases, most notably atherosclerosis, diabetes, stroke, and hypertension, are associated with a higher incidence of the condition. Psychogenic causes may include depression, fatigue, guilt, or fear of sexual failure. A number of common drugs, including thiazide diuretics, phenothiazines, serotonin reuptake inhibitors, tricyclic antidepressants (TCAs), propranolol, and diazepam, cause impotence as a side effect in some men. Loss of libido may be due to low testosterone secretion.

Penile erection has both neuromuscular and vascular components. Autonomic nerves dilate arterioles that lead to the major erectile tissues of the penis, called the **corpora cavernosa** (singular: corpus cavernosum). The corpora have vascular spaces that fill with blood to cause rigidity. The vasoconstriction of veins draining blood from the corpora allows the penis to remain rigid long enough for successful penetration. After ejaculation, the veins dilate, blood leaves the corpora, and the penis quickly loses its rigidity. Organic causes of ED may include damage to the nerves or blood vessels involved in the erection reflex.

The marketing of sildenafil, an inhibitor of the enzyme phosphodiesterase-5, has revolutionized the medical therapy of ED. When sildenafil was approved as the first pharmacological treatment for ED in 1998, it set a record for pharmaceutical sales for any new drug. Prior to the discovery of sildenafil, rigid or inflatable penile prostheses were implanted into the corpora. As an alternative to prostheses, drugs such as alprostadil (Muse, Caverject) or the combination of papaverine and phentolamine were injected directly into the corpora cavernosa just prior to intercourse. Injections caused pain in many clients and reduced the spontaneity associated with pleasurable intercourse. These alternative therapies are rare today, though they may be used for clients in whom sildenafil is contraindicated.

The nurse should be aware that sildenafil does not cause an erection; it merely enhances the erection caused by physical contact or other sexual stimuli. In addition, sildenafil is not as effective at promoting erections in men who do not have ED. Despite considerable research interest, no effects of sildenafil have been shown on female sexual function, and this drug is not approved for use by women.

Another phosphodiesterase-5 inhibitor, vardenafil, acts by the same mechanism as sildenafil but has a faster onset and slightly longer duration of action. The two drugs exhibit similar types of side effects. Tadalafil is a third phosphodiesterase-5 inhibitor that acts within 30 minutes and is reported to have a prolonged duration lasting from 24 to 36 hours.

Nursing Considerations

The role of the nurse in pharmacotherapy with ED agents involves careful monitoring of the client's condition and providing education as it relates to the prescribed drug regimen. Obtain a complete physical examination, including history of impaired sexual function, cardiovascular disease, and presence of emotional disturbances. Obtain and monitor results of laboratory tests related to liver function. Sildenafil and vardenafil are contraindicated with the use of organic nitrates and nitroglycerin because they potentiate the effect of nitrates, leading to severe hypotension. Nitrates are also found in recreational drugs, including amyl nitrate and nitrite, commonly called "poppers." Coadministration of vardenafil and alpha-adrenergic blockers can also lead to profound hypotension. These agents are contraindicated in clients with severe cardiovascular disease and in the presence of anatomical deformities of the penis.

Use cautiously in the client with hepatic dysfunction because these drugs are metabolized in the liver and drug accumulation

may lead to toxicity. Clients with cirrhosis or severe decreased liver function should start with lower doses. Clients with leukemia, sickle cell anemia, multiple myeloma, ulcer, or retinitis pigmentosa should also use sildenafil cautiously.

Monitor for side effects of the drug. Monitor for vision changes such as blurred vision, being unable to differentiate between green and blue, objects having a blue tinge, and photophobia. Also observe safety precautions until it is known whether sensory-perceptual alterations will occur, so that falls and other accidents can be avoided. The client should be monitored for presence of headache, dizziness, flushing, rash, nasal congestion, diarrhea, dyspepsia, urinary tract infection (UTI), chest pain, and indigestion.

Client education as it relates to ED agents should include goals, reasons for obtaining baseline data such as vital signs and tests for liver and cardiac function, and possible side effects. For clients receiving sildenafil or vardenafil, the following are important teaching points:

- Do not take more than one dose in a 24-hour period.
- Have vital signs, including blood pressure, checked routinely.
- Take sildenafil 1 hour prior to sexual activity and vardenafil 25 to 40 minutes prior to sexual activity.
- If taking nitrates or alpha blockers, do not use ED agents.
- Do not share medication.
- Do not take more than the recommended dose, as this increases the risk for side effects.

NCLEX Practice Tips

The client should notify the nurse promptly if he experiences sudden or decreased vision loss in one or both eyes. Sildenafil should not be taken more than once per day.

Sildenafil offers no protection against sexually transmitted diseases. Sildenafil has no effect in the absence of sexual stimulation.

Sildenafil may potentiate the hypotensive effect of tamsulosin, an alpha blocker, resulting in symptomatic hypotension in some clients. The medications should not be taken together.

PROTOTYPE DRUG | **Sildenafil (Viagra)**

Actions and Uses: Sildenafil acts by relaxing smooth muscle in the corpus cavernosum, thus allowing increased blood flow into the penis. The increased blood flow results in a firmer and longer-lasting erection in about 70% of men taking the drug. The onset of action is relatively rapid, less than 1 hour, and its effects last 2 to 4 hours. Sildenafil blocks the enzyme phosphodiesterase-5.

Pharmacokinetics: Sildenafil is rapidly absorbed after oral administration. It is widely distributed, but little enters semen. Sildenafil is 96% plasma protein bound. It is mostly metabolized by the liver. It is mostly excreted in feces, with a small amount excreted in urine. Half-life is 4 hours.

Administration Alerts:
- Avoid administration of sildenafil with meals, especially high-fat meals, because absorption is decreased.
- Avoid grapefruit juice when administering sildenafil.

Adverse Effects and Interactions: The most serious adverse effect, hypotension, occurs in clients who are concurrently taking organic nitrates for angina. Common side effects include headache, dizziness, flushing, rash, nasal congestion, diarrhea, dyspepsia, UTI, chest pain, and indigestion. Priapism, a sustained erection lasting longer than 6 hours, has been reported with sildenafil use and may lead to permanent damage to penile tissues.

Sildenafil interacts with many drugs. Cimetidine, erythromycin, and ketoconazole will increase serum levels of sildenafil and necessitate lower drug doses. Protease inhibitors will cause increased sildenafil levels, which may lead to toxicity. Rifampin may decrease sildenafil levels, leading to decreased effectiveness.

BENIGN PROSTATIC HYPERPLASIA

Benign prostatic hyperplasia (BPH), an abnormal enlargement of the prostate, is the most common benign neoplasm in men. The exact cause of BPH is unknown, but it exists to some degree in all older men. It is present in 70% of men by age 60 and in 90% by age 80. Other than age, the risk factors for BPH include a family history of the disorder, smoking, heavy alcohol consumption, hypertension, diabetes, a diet high in meats and fats, and African ancestry. BPH is not considered to be a precursor to prostate carcinoma, although it is well known that many men with BPH eventually experience prostate cancer.

The characteristic feature of BPH is an enlargement of the prostate gland that decreases the outflow of urine by obstructing the urethra, causing difficult urination. The pathogenesis of BPH involves two components: static and dynamic. The static factors are caused by the physical enlargement of the prostate gland due to the overgrowth of the epithelial cells. The gland can double or triple in size with aging, creating a blockage of urine outflow at the neck of the bladder. The dynamic factors occur due to excessive numbers of alpha$_1$-adrenergic receptors located in stromal tissue in the neck of the urinary bladder and in the prostate gland. When activated, these receptors compress the urethra and provide resistance to urine outflow from the bladder. The two mechanisms of disease, static and dynamic, have led to two different classes of drugs for treating the symptoms of BPH. These mechanisms are shown in Figure 32.2.

Certain frequently used medications may worsen symptoms of BPH. Alpha-adrenergic drugs, which include decongestants such as pseudoephedrine and phenylephrine, activate alpha$_1$-adrenergic receptors in the bladder neck, restricting urine flow. Drugs with anticholinergic effects, such as antihistamines, TCAs,

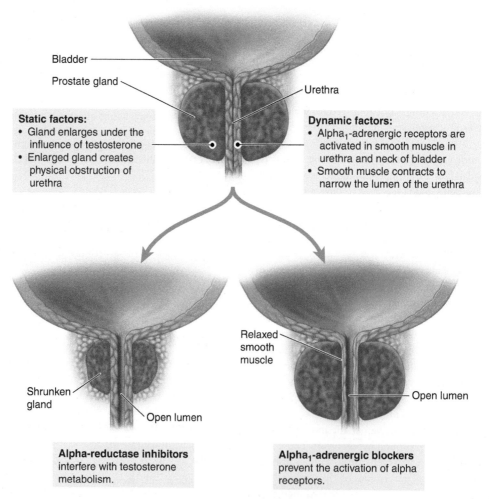

Figure 32.2 Mechanism of action of antiprostatic drugs.

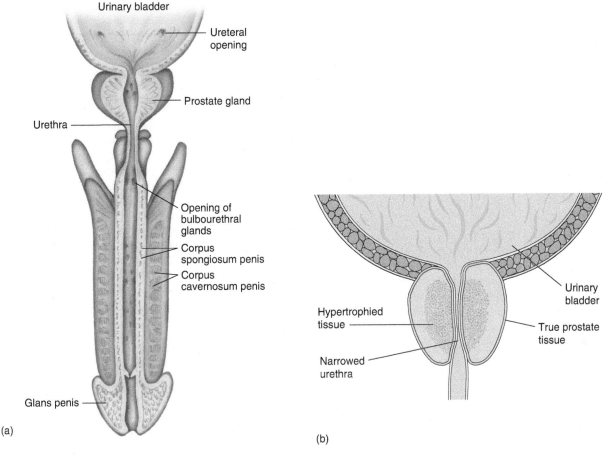

Figure 32.3 Benign prostatic hyperplasia: (a) normal prostate and penis; (b) benign prostatic hyperplasia.
Pearson Education.

or phenothiazines, may worsen the associated urinary retention. Testosterone and other anabolic steroids may increase prostate enlargement, which contributes to the physical obstruction of the urethra. Drugs that worsen symptoms of BPH should be avoided in older men.

There is no clear correlation between the symptoms experienced by clients and the size of the prostate. Some men may have minimal enlargement and experience moderate symptoms, whereas others may have extremely enlarged glands and be asymptomatic. This is because the smooth muscle in the urinary bladder has the ability to compensate for the obstruction by contracting with greater force to eject the urine stream. Over time, the bladder is no longer able to compensate and symptoms of BPH, such as increased urinary frequency (usually with small amounts of urine), increased urgency to urinate, post-void leakage, excessive nighttime urination (nocturia), decreased force of the urine stream, and a sensation that the bladder did not completely empty, manifest.

Some clients do not seek medical attention until complications caused by the long-standing obstruction at the neck of the urinary bladder arise. Serious complications include recurrent urinary infections, incontinence, gross hematuria, bladder stones, and chronic renal failure. BPH is illustrated in Figure 32.3.

Only a few drugs are available for the pharmacotherapy of BPH. Early in the course of the disease, drug therapy may be of benefit. These agents are listed in Table 32.3.

Pharmacotherapy of Benign Prostatic Hyperplasia

32.5 In its early stages, benign prostatic hyperplasia may be treated successfully with drug therapy, including finasteride and alpha$_1$-adrenergic blockers.

Although most of the symptoms of BPH are caused by static pressure of the enlarged prostate on the urethra, approximately 40% of the pressure has a functional component caused by increased smooth muscle tone in the region. Alpha$_1$-adrenergic receptors are located in smooth muscle cells in the neck of the urinary bladder and in the prostate gland. The role of these receptors in normal physiology is not completely understood. When activated, however, the alpha$_1$-adrenergic receptors provide resistance to urine outflow from the bladder and inhibit the micturition reflex.

TABLE 32.3 Agents for Benign Prostatic Hyperplasia

Drug	Route and Adult Dose
Alpha-Adrenergic Blockers	
doxazosin (Cardura) (see Chapter 51, page 646, for the Prototype Drug box)	PO, 1–8 mg qd
prazosin (Minipress)	PO, 1 mg qid or bid
tamsulosin (Flomax)	PO, 0.4 mg qd (max 0.8 mg/day)
terazosin (Hytrin)	PO, start with 1 mg at bedtime, then 1–5 mg/day (max 20 mg/day)
5-Alpha-Reductase Inhibitors	
dutasteride (Avodart)	0.5 mg/day
Pr finasteride (Proscar)	PO, 5 mg qd

Only a few drugs are available to treat benign enlargement of the prostate. Although the drugs have limited efficacy, they have some value in treating mild disease, as an alternative to surgery. Because pharmacotherapy alleviates the symptoms but does not cure the disease, these medications must be taken the remainder of the client's life or until surgery is indicated. The most common drug for BPH is finasteride, a 5-alpha-reductase inhibitor.

Although primarily used for hypertension, several alpha$_1$-adrenergic blockers have been approved for BPH. The selective alpha$_1$ blockers relax smooth muscle in the prostate gland, bladder neck, and urethra, thus easing the urinary obstruction. Doxazosin and terazosin are of particular value to clients who have both hypertension and BPH; these two disorders occur concurrently in about 25% of men over age 60. A third alpha$_1$ blocker, tamsulosin, has no effect on blood pressure, and its only indication is BPH. Drugs in this class improve urine flow and reduce other bothersome symptoms of BPH within 1 to 2 weeks after starting therapy. Primary adverse effects include headache, fatigue, and dizziness. Doxazosin and terazosin are not associated with an increased risk for sexual dysfunction, but ejaculatory dysfunction has been reported with tamsulosin. Reflex tachycardia due to stimulation of baroreceptors is common with alpha blockers. Additional information on the alpha blockers is presented in Chapter 51.

Nursing Considerations

The role of the nurse in drug therapy with antiprostatic agents involves careful monitoring of the client's condition and providing education as it relates to the prescribed drug regimen. Obtain a complete physical examination, including history of cardiovascular disease and sexual dysfunction. Also assess changes in urinary elimination, including urinary retention, nocturia, dribbling, difficulty starting urinary stream, frequency, and urgency. If the client is prescribed alpha blockers for treatment of prostatic hypertrophy, the client's vital signs, especially blood pressure and heart rate, should be assessed. The client may experience hypotension with the first few doses, and orthostatic hypotension may persist throughout treatment. The first-dose phenomenon, especially syncope, can occur. Monitor the client for evidence of orthostatic hypotension, dizziness, and gastrointestinal disturbances. Older adults are especially prone to the hypotensive and hypothermic effects related to vasodilation caused by these drugs. Alpha

blockers should be used cautiously in clients with asthma or heart failure because they cause bradycardia and bronchoconstriction.

Exercise caution in clients with decreased hepatic function because the drugs are metabolized in the liver. Clients with obstructive uropathy should use finasteride cautiously. Monitor the emotional status of clients who are taking alpha blockers, as depression is a common side effect. Inform the client that it may take 6 to 12 months of treatment before the drug relieves symptoms of BPH. Improvement will last only as long as the medication is continued.

Monitor for side effects of the antiprostatic agent. Side effects include impotence, decreased volume of ejaculate, and decreased libido. Inform the client to report these occurrences to the healthcare provider.

Client education related to antiprostatic agents should include goals, reasons for obtaining baseline data such as vital signs and tests for cardiac and renal function, and possible side effects. For clients who are receiving an alpha blocker, the following are important teaching points:

- Report increased difficulty with urinary voiding.
- Report significant side effects.
- Take medication at bedtime, and take the first dose immediately before getting into bed.
- Always arise slowly, avoiding sudden posture changes.

PROTOTYPE DRUG | **Finasteride (Proscar)**

Actions and Uses: Finasteride acts by inhibiting 5-alpha-reductase, the enzyme responsible for converting testosterone to one of its metabolites, 5-alpha-dihydrotestosterone. This metabolite causes proliferation of prostate cells and promotes enlargement of the gland. Because it inhibits the metabolism of testosterone, finasteride is sometimes called an antiandrogen. Finasteride promotes shrinkage of an enlarged prostate and subsequently helps to restore urinary function. It is most effective in clients with larger prostates. This drug is also marketed as Propecia, which is prescribed to promote hair regrowth in clients with male pattern baldness. Doses of finasteride are five times higher when prescribed for BPH than when prescribed for baldness.

Pharmacokinetics: Finasteride is well absorbed after oral administration. It is widely distributed, crosses the blood-brain barrier, and enters prostate tissue. Finasteride is 90% plasma protein bound. It is mostly metabolized by the liver. The drug is mostly excreted in feces, with a lesser amount excreted in urine. Half-life is 6 hours.

Administration Alerts:

- Tablets may be crushed for oral administration.

- The pregnant nurse or a nurse planning to get pregnant should avoid handling crushed medication, as it may be absorbed through the skin and cause harm to a male fetus.

Adverse Effects and Interactions: Finasteride causes various types of sexual dysfunction, including impotence, diminished libido, and ejaculatory dysfunction, in up to 16% of clients.

No clinically significant drug interactions have been established. Use with caution with herbal supplements. For example, saw palmetto may potentiate the effects of finasteride.

NURSING PROCESS FOCUS

Clients Receiving Finasteride (Proscar)

Assessment	Potential Nursing Diagnoses/Identified Patterns
Prior to administration: • Obtain complete health history, including liver disease and altered urinary functioning. • Obtain drug history to determine possible drug interactions and allergies. • Determine if client has a female partner who is pregnant or who is planning to become pregnant.	• Risk for sexual dysfunction related to effects of drug therapy or decreased hormone production • Nonadherence related to side effects of drug therapy • Need for knowledge regarding drug therapy and adverse effects

Planning: Client Goals and Expected Outcomes

The client will:

- Experience a decreased size of enlarged prostate gland
- Demonstrate an understanding of the drug's action by accurately describing drug side effects and precautions and the importance of follow-up care

Implementation

Interventions (Rationales)	Client Education/Discharge Planning
• Monitor urinary function. (Finasteride may interfere with PSA test results.) • Monitor female partner for pregnancy. (Finasteride is teratogenic to the male fetus.) • Monitor client's commitment to the medication regimen. (Maximum therapeutic effects may take several months.) • Monitor for adverse reactions.	Instruct client to: • Schedule a digital rectal exam and PSA test periodically during therapy • Recognize and report symptoms of BPH: urinary retention, hesitancy, difficulty starting stream, decreased diameter of stream, nocturia, dribbling, frequency • Avoid all fluids in evenings, especially caffeine-containing fluids and alcohol, to avoid nocturia • Drink adequate fluids early in day to decrease chances of kidney stones and UTI Instruct client and/or female partner to: • Avoid semen of man using finasteride • Avoid touching crushed tablets of finasteride to prevent transdermal absorption and the transfer of medication through the placenta to fetus • Use a reliable barrier contraceptive during therapy Instruct client and/or female partner to: • Continue medication even if there is no decrease in symptoms for 6 to 12 months, or no increase in hair growth for 3 months • Recognize that lifelong therapy may be necessary to control symptoms of BPH • Instruct client and/or female partner to report impotence, decreased volume of ejaculate, or decreased libido

Evaluation of Outcome Criteria

Evaluate the effectiveness of drug therapy by confirming that client goals and expected outcomes have been met (see "Planning").

32   Understanding the Chapter

Key Concepts Summary

The numbered key concepts provide a succinct summary of the important points from the corresponding numbered section within the chapter. If any of these points are not clear, refer to the numbered section within the chapter for review.

32.1 FSH and LH from the pituitary regulate the secretion of testosterone, the primary hormone contributing to the growth, health, and maintenance of the male reproductive system.

32.2 Androgens are used to treat hypogonadism in males and breast cancer in females. Anabolic steroids are frequently abused by athletes and can result in serious adverse effects with long-term use.

32.3 Male infertility is difficult to treat pharmacologically; medications include hCG, menotropins, testolactone, and antiestrogens.

32.4 Erectile dysfunction is a common disorder that may be successfully treated with sildenafil and other agents, which inhibit the enzyme phosphodiesterase-5.

32.5 In its early stages, benign prostatic hyperplasia may be treated successfully with drug therapy, including finasteride and alpha$_1$-adrenergic blockers.

Chapter 32 Scenario

One year after his divorce, Mike, a 54-year-old Caucasian male, began dating and soon met Dana. The couple found that they had a lot in common and enjoyed each other's company. As the relationship grew, the couple became more intimate and sexually involved. However, the emotional scars from Mike's previous marriage were painful and affected him deeply.

After the divorce, Mike was depressed and had low self-esteem. The condition required short-term hospitalization, and he now follows up with a psychiatrist on an outpatient basis. He has been taking antidepressants and was recently prescribed tadalafil (Cialis) for a diagnosis of ED. Mike also has a past history of hypertension and is taking nifedipine (Procardia).

Critical Thinking Questions

1. What factors in Mike's life and health history do you think are contributing to the diagnosis of ED?

2. If you were the nurse, what client education instructions would you provide to Mike regarding administration of tadalafil (Cialis) along with nifedipine (Procardia)?

3. After considering both options, Mike would rather be prescribed sildenafil (Viagra) instead of tadalafil (Cialis). What should the healthcare provider discuss with Mike about this request?

See Answers to Critical Thinking Questions in Appendix B.

NCLEX Practice Questions

1 An adult client has been receiving testosterone (Testoderm) for the treatment of primary hypogonadism. Which laboratory test would the nurse monitor to determine that this drug therapy is effective?

a. Red blood cell count

b. Sperm count

c. FSH

d. LH

2 A client with erectile dysfunction is being evaluated for pharmacotherapy. Which question should the nurse ask prior to initiating therapy with sildenafil (Viagra)?

a. "Are you currently taking medications for angina?"

b. "Do you have a history of diabetes?"

c. "Have you ever had an allergic reaction to penicillin products?"

d. "Have you ever been treated for gastric ulcers?"

3 A nurse is teaching a client who has received a prescription testosterone gel (AndroGel) for treatment of symptoms related to low androgen levels. Which instructions should the nurse give the client? Select all that apply.

a. "Apply the gel to the scrotal and perineal area daily."

b. "Avoid exposing women to the gel or to areas of skin where the gel has been applied."

c. "Report any weight gain over 2 kg (5 lb) in 1 week's time."

d. "Avoid showering or swimming for at least 12 to 14 hours after applying the gel."

e. "Maintain a low-fat diet and return periodically for blood lipid laboratory studies."

4 A nurse is counselling a client about the goal of therapy with sildenafil (Viagra). What will the nurse teach the client about the drug's effects?

a. It should always result in a penile erection within 10 minutes.

b. It is not effective if sexual dysfunction is psychological in nature.

c. It will result in less intense feelings with prolonged use.

d. It may heighten sexual response in female partners.

5 A nurse is teaching the client about the use of finasteride (Proscar). Which of the following are necessary facts about this medication? Select all that apply.

a. Finasteride promotes shrinkage of an enlarged prostate and helps restore urinary function.

b. The drug should not be handled by women who may be pregnant.

c. Finasteride affects both near and far vision in older adult males.

d. It may take 6 to 12 months before the benefits of finasteride are achieved.

e. The drug may cause significant dizziness, which can be avoided by making position changes slowly.

See Answers to NCLEX Practice Questions in Appendix A.

Pharmacology of Alterations in the Gastrointestinal System

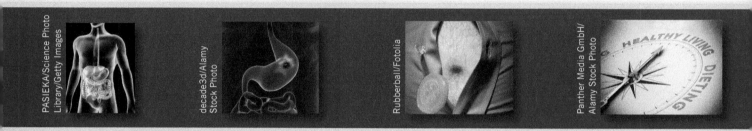

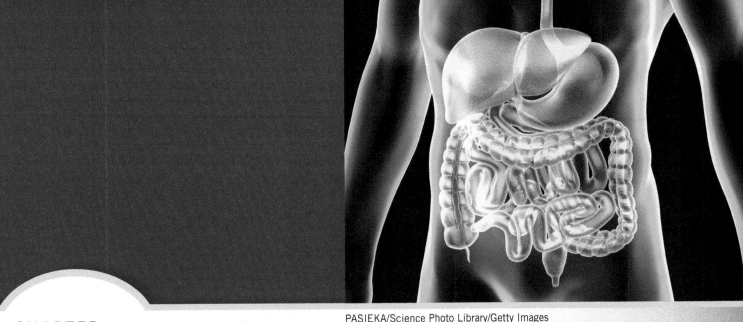

CHAPTER 33

Brief Review of the Gastrointestinal System

LEARNING OUTCOMES

After reading this chapter, the student should be able to:

1. Describe the major anatomical structures of the digestive system.
2. Outline the steps in the process of digestion.
3. Describe the primary functions of the stomach.
4. Analyze how the anatomical structures of the small intestine promote the absorption of nutrients and drugs.
5. Describe the primary structures and functions of the large intestine.
6. Describe the functions of the liver and their relevance to drug therapy.
7. Explain the hepatic portal system and its importance to drug therapy.
8. Explain the nervous control of digestion.
9. Explain the enzymatic breakdown of nutrients by the digestive system.

CHAPTER OUTLINE

▸ The Function of the Digestive System

▸ Physiology of the Upper Gastrointestinal Tract

▸ Physiology of the Lower Gastrointestinal Tract

▸ The Large Intestine

▸ Physiology of the Accessory Organs of Digestion

▸ Regulation of Digestive Processes

▸ Nutrient Categories and Metabolism

Very little of the food we eat is directly available to body cells. Food must be broken down, absorbed, and chemically modified before it is in a form that is useful to cells. The digestive system performs these functions and many more. This chapter focuses on the aspects of digestion and physiology that are applicable to pharmacotherapy. For a complete review of the digestive system, the student should refer to an anatomy and physiology textbook.

The Function of the Digestive System

33.1 The function of the digestive system is to extract nutrients from food to fuel metabolic processes in the body.

The **digestive system** consists of two basic anatomical divisions: the alimentary canal and the accessory organs. The **alimentary canal**, or gastrointestinal (GI) tract, is a long, continuous, hollow tube that extends from the mouth to the anus. The **accessory organs of digestion** include the salivary glands, liver, gallbladder, and pancreas. The major structures of the digestive system are illustrated in Figure 33.1.

The overall function of the digestive system is to extract nutrients from food so that they may be used to fuel the metabolic processes in the body. Because food is a complex substance, multiple steps are necessary before cells can use its components. These steps are ingestion, propulsion, digestion, absorption, and defecation.

Ingestion is taking food into the body by mouth. In some clients, ingestion bypasses the mouth and delivers nutrients directly into the stomach or small intestine via a feeding tube.

Substances are propelled along the GI tract by **peristalsis**, which is the rhythmic contractions of layers of smooth muscle. The speed at which substances move through the GI tract is critical to the absorption of drugs, nutrients, and water and for the removal of wastes. If peristalsis is too fast, substances will not have sufficient contact with the GI mucosa to be absorbed. In addition, the large intestine will not have enough time to absorb water, and diarrhea may result. Abnormally slow transit may result in constipation or even obstructions in the small or large intestine.

Digestion is the mechanical and chemical breakdown of food into a form that may be absorbed into the systemic circulation. To chemically break down ingested food, a large number of enzymes and other substances are required. Digestive enzymes are secreted by the salivary glands, stomach, small intestine, and pancreas. The liver makes bile, which is stored in the gallbladder until it is needed for lipid digestion.

Absorption is the movement of nutrients and other substances from the alimentary canal to the circulation. The inner lining of the alimentary canal, called the mucosa layer, provides a surface area for the various acids, bases, and enzymes to break down food. In many parts of the alimentary canal, the mucosa is folded and contains deep grooves and pits. The small intestine is lined with tiny projections called villi and microvilli that provide a huge surface area for the absorption of nutrients and medications.

Not all components of ingested food are useful to the human body or can be digested. The elimination of indigestible substances from the body is called **defecation**.

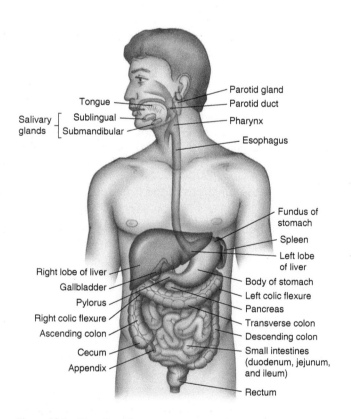

Figure 33.1 The digestive system.

Physiology of the Upper Gastrointestinal Tract

33.2 The upper gastrointestinal tract is responsible for mechanical and chemical digestion.

The upper GI tract consists of the mouth, pharynx, esophagus, and stomach. From a pharmacological perspective, the most important regions of the upper GI tract are the buccal and sublingual areas of the mouth and the stomach.

The epithelial mucosa of the buccal and sublingual regions is very thin, being only 40 to 50 cells in thickness. The mucosal layer, along with the salivary glands, secretes mucus, which lubricates and moistens the oral cavity. The mucus also serves as a liquid medium for drug administration inside the mouth. The oral mucosa in the sublingual region is relatively permeable, and drugs are absorbed rapidly. The buccal region is less permeable, and drug absorption is slower. The buccal region, however, has less salivary flow and drugs can be retained longer, making it better suited for sustained-release delivery systems.

The pharynx and esophagus serve as passageways for ingested food and liquids. Obstruction of these areas, or a loss of the swallowing reflex, precludes the administration of oral drugs. Little absorption occurs across the pharyngeal or esophageal mucosa because drugs travel quickly through these regions of the alimentary canal.

Food passes from the esophagus to the stomach by travelling through the lower esophageal (cardiac) sphincter. This ring of smooth muscle usually prevents the stomach contents from moving backwards, a condition known as gastroesophageal reflux. The stomach has both mechanical and chemical functions. The muscular squeezing of the stomach churns and mixes the food, breaking it down mechanically to a semi-solid known as **chyme**. Strong peristaltic contractions push the chyme toward the pylorus, where it encounters a second ring of smooth muscle called the pyloric sphincter. Located at the entrance to the small intestine, this sphincter regulates the flow of substances leaving the stomach. Chyme moves in "spurts" through the sphincter into the small intestine. Large pieces of food are refluxed back into the body of the stomach, where they are subjected to more churning to reduce them in size to about 2 mm so that they may pass through the sphincter.

The stomach also secretes substances that promote the processes of chemical digestion. Gastric glands extending deep into the mucosa of the stomach contain several cell types that are critical to digestion and that are important to the pharmacotherapy of digestive disorders:

- **Chief cells** secrete pepsinogen, an inactive form of the enzyme pepsin that chemically breaks down proteins.

- **Parietal cells** secrete 1 to 3 litres of hydrochloric acid each day. This strong acid helps to break down food, activates pepsinogen, and kills microbes that may have been ingested. Parietal cells also secrete intrinsic factor, which is essential for the absorption of vitamin B_{12}.

- **Enteroendocrine cells** secrete hormones that modify the digestive processes. In the stomach, the most important secretion is gastrin, which stimulates acid production by the parietal cells.

The combined secretion of the chief and parietal cells, known as gastric juice, is the most acidic fluid in the body, having a pH of 1.5 to 3.5. A number of natural defences protect the stomach mucosa against this extremely acidic fluid. Certain cells that line the surface of the stomach secrete a thick, mucous layer and bicarbonate ion to neutralize the acid. These form such an effective protective layer that the pH at the mucosal surface is nearly neutral. On reaching the duodenum, the stomach contents are further neutralized by bicarbonate from pancreatic and biliary secretions.

The pharmacological importance of the stomach lies in its capacity to absorb drugs. For most oral drugs, the stomach is not the primary site of absorption because the drug does not stay long in the organ. Stomach acidity (pH 1 to 2) can either assist in the absorption process or destroy the drug entirely. Drugs that are weak acids tend to be absorbed in the stomach. Protein drugs are destroyed by pepsin in the stomach before they are absorbed or have a chance to reach the small intestine.

Physiology of the Lower Gastrointestinal Tract

33.3 The small intestine is the longest portion of the alimentary canal and is the primary organ for absorption.

The lower GI tract consists of the small and large intestines. With its many folds and finger-like projections of villi and microvilli, the small intestine is highly specialized for absorption. The lining of each villus is composed of a single layer of epithelial cells and contains blood capillaries. Essentially, only a single cell separates a nutrient or drug molecule from the intestinal lumen of the body's circulatory system.

The first 25 centimetres (10 inches) of the small intestine, known as the duodenum, is the site where chyme mixes with bile from the gallbladder and digestive enzymes from the pancreas. Bile and pancreatic juice enter through an opening in the duodenum known as the duodenal papilla. The duodenum is sometimes considered part of the upper GI tract because of its proximity to the stomach. Peptic ulcer, the most common disorder of the duodenum, is discussed in Chapter 34.

The remainder of the small intestine consists of the jejunum and ileum. Because of its length and enormous absorptive surface, the first 1 to 2 metres of the jejunum is the site of the majority of nutrient and drug absorption. As the jejunum becomes the ileum, the diameter of the intestinal lumen diminishes and the villi become fewer in number. The terminal ileum is a primary site for the absorption of vitamin B_{12}, long-chain fatty acids, and fat-soluble vitamins. The ileum empties its contents into the large intestine through the ileocecal valve. Travel time for chyme through the entire small intestine varies from 3 to 6 hours.

The mucosa of the small intestine secretes intestinal juice, which is a mixture of mucus, digestive enzymes, and hormones.

The mucus has an alkaline pH, which neutralizes the acidity from the stomach. The small intestine also secretes cholecystokinin, a hormone that promotes pancreatic enzyme secretion and secretin, which stimulates bicarbonate production to make the small intestine more alkaline.

The Large Intestine

33.4 The large intestine contains host flora and is a major site of water reabsorption.

The large intestine, or colon, receives chyme from the ileum in a fluid state. The large intestine does not secrete digestive enzymes, nor does it have enteroendocrine cells to secrete hormones. With few exceptions, little reabsorption of nutrients occurs during the 12- to 24-hour journey through the colon. The large intestine does secrete a large amount of mucus, which helps to lubricate the fecal matter. The major functions of the colon are to reabsorb water and electrolytes from the waste material and to excrete the remaining fecal material from the body.

The colon harbours a substantial amount of bacteria and fungi, called the host flora, which serve a useful purpose by synthesizing B-complex vitamins and vitamin K. Disruption of the normal host flora can lead to diarrhea.

From a pharmacological perspective, the large intestine may be the site of therapeutic or adverse drug effects. A large number of drugs cause either diarrhea or constipation. These effects are usually self-limiting and can be prevented or managed through nursing interventions. When bowel patterns are significantly disrupted, drugs may be given to slow the activity (antidiarrheals) or increase the activity (laxatives) of the large intestine.

Of additional pharmacological importance are the drugs given by the rectal route. The mucosa of the rectum provides an excellent and rapid absorptive surface for drugs. It is a route of particular importance in children and in clients who are unable to take oral medications due to nausea, vomiting, or other pathology that prevents oral administration. The onset of action is usually slower than the oral route, and drug action is limited by the length of time that the client can retain the drug without defecation.

Physiology of the Accessory Organs of Digestion

33.5 The liver is the most important accessory digestive organ.

The accessory organs of digestion include the teeth, tongue, salivary glands, pancreas, gallbladder, and liver. Of these, the pancreas and liver have the most pharmacological importance. The endocrine functions of the pancreas, which include the secretion of insulin and glucagon, are discussed in Chapter 28.

The liver is one of the most important organs in pharmacology. Along with the kidneys, any drug that reaches the circulation, regardless of its route of administration, will pass through the liver. The overall function of the liver is to filter and process the nutrients and drugs delivered to it. Substances may be stored, chemically altered, or removed from the blood before they reach the general circulation. The following are some of the primary functions of the liver:

- *Regulation.* Stabilizes the serum levels of glucose, triglycerides, and cholesterol
- *Protection.* Removes toxic substances and waste products such as ammonia
- *Synthesis.* Synthesizes bile, plasma proteins, and certain clotting factors
- *Storage.* Stores iron and fat-soluble vitamins

When most drugs reach the liver, they are metabolized to less toxic substances that are excreted by the kidney more easily. The cytochrome P450 enzyme system in liver cells is especially active at metabolizing drugs. In a few cases, the liver changes the drug to a more active form. It is important to note that the handling of drugs and toxic substances by the liver can damage hepatocytes and impair their functions. This is especially true if the hepatocytes are chronically exposed to harmful substances such as alcohol. Hepatic impairment is a relatively common adverse effect of certain drugs. Whereas drug-induced hepatic impairment is often transient and asymptomatic, some drugs can cause severe, permanent, and even fatal liver damage.

The unique structure of the vascular system serving the liver is important to digestion as well as to pharmacology. The liver receives both oxygenated and deoxygenated blood. The **hepatic portal system**, shown in Figure 33.2, is a network of venous vessels that collects blood draining from the stomach, small intestine, and most of the large intestine. This blood is extremely rich in nutrients because it contains substances absorbed during digestion. It is important to know that this blood is delivered to the liver via the hepatic portal vein before it reaches the arterial circulation. The liver then can remove, store, excrete, or perform metabolic functions on these substances before they are sent into the inferior vena cava to reach other organs.

The hepatic portal system serves as an important homeostatic mechanism, allowing a relatively stable composition of blood to circulate through the body. In terms of drug therapy, nearly all oral medications enter the hepatic portal vein for processing by the liver before they reach their target tissue. In some cases, the liver inactivates a substantial percentage of the drug before it reaches the inferior vena cava, a phenomenon called the **first-pass effect**. Drugs that have a significant first-pass effect may be given by other routes, such as intramuscular, intravenous, subcutaneous, or topical. Although a drug will still eventually reach the liver by these routes, it will have an opportunity to also reach its target tissue. Note that the venous systems serving the head and the lower rectum are not parts of the hepatic portal system. Therefore, drugs that are given by the buccal, sublingual, or rectal routes bypass the first-pass effect of the liver.

As the liver makes bile, the bile is sent to the gallbladder where it is stored. When lipids enter the small intestine, the gallbladder contracts and sends its contents into the duodenum. The bile salts emulsify the lipids, making them easier to digest enzymatically. When bile salts reach the terminal portion of the ileum, 95% are reabsorbed into the hepatic portal circulation by a process called **enterohepatic recirculation**. This process has direct implications to pharmacotherapy. Certain drugs, including digoxin (Lanoxin,

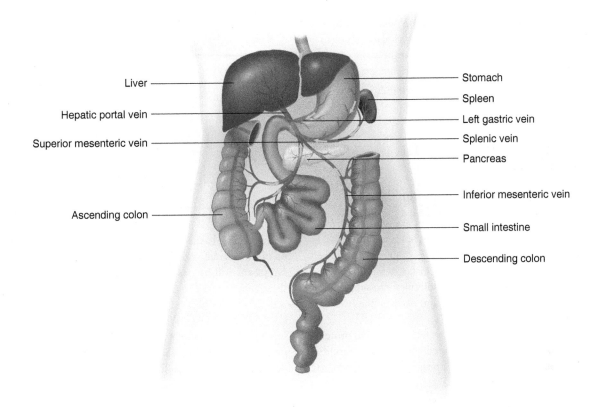

Figure 33.2 Hepatic portal circulation.

Toloxin), morphine, and estrogens, are eliminated in the bile and are reabsorbed by enterohepatic recirculation. Enterohepatic recirculation recycles the drug multiple times and can significantly extend a drug's half-life. Interactions can occur if one drug interferes with the enterohepatic recycling of another drug. Preventing this recycling can speed the elimination of a drug and reduce its therapeutic effectiveness. An example of such an interaction is when cholestyramine (Questran) interferes with the recycling of lorazepam (Ativan) and increases the clearance of lorazepam from the body.

The pancreas is an essential accessory digestive organ, secreting about a quart of pancreatic fluid into the duodenum each day. This fluid is alkaline (pH 7.5 to 8.8) and contains digestive enzymes to chemically break down carbohydrates, lipids, proteins, and nucleic acids. From a pharmacological perspective, the pancreas is relatively protected from drugs, and there are only a few therapies for pancreatic digestive disorders.

Regulation of Digestive Processes

33.6 Digestion is regulated by numerous hormonal and nervous factors.

Digestion is controlled through a large number of hormonal and nervous factors that influence the speed of peristalsis and the amount of saliva, mucus, acid, and enzyme secretions. Various

negative feedback loops help to regulate these activities so that digestion is a smooth, continuous process. Disruption of normal homeostatic mechanisms can cause cramping, due to excessive peristalsis, or peptic ulcers, due to the overproduction of gastric acid.

The nervous control of digestion is provided at several levels. Chapter 12 discusses the role of the autonomic nervous system (ANS) in controlling the contraction of smooth muscle and glandular secretion. Activation of the parasympathetic nervous system stimulates the digestive processes by increasing peristalsis, salivation, and digestive gland secretion. The sympathetic nervous system has the opposite effects, with beta$_2$-adrenergic receptors in the intestinal wall and alpha$_1$-adrenergic receptors in the salivary glands. Drugs that affect the ANS often affect the digestive processes.

The GI tract is also regulated by local reflexes called the **enteric nervous system (ENS)**. This system consists of a vast network of neurons in the submucosa of the alimentary canal that has sensory and motor functions. Chemoreceptors and stretch receptors sense the presence and amount of food in the GI tract and respond accordingly by changing motility without sending signals to the ANS.

The GI tract functions at an automatic level; no conscious thought is required as the system goes about its daily tasks of secretion and digestion. The central nervous system (CNS), however, can greatly influence the activity of digestive functions. For example, merely thinking of food can evoke powerful images. These may be positive, such as perhaps thinking of a steak sizzling on the grill or bread baking in the oven, and increase salivation and peristalsis. Images may also be negative and evoke feelings of nausea and vomiting at the sight of food. Mental health conditions such as depression, anxiety, excessive stress, and bipolar disorder can affect the appetite and digestive processes.

Nutrient Categories and Metabolism

33.7 The chemical breakdown of food is accomplished by digestive enzymes.

The three basic nutrients are carbohydrates, lipids, and proteins. In food, these nutrients are large molecules that cannot be absorbed across the mucosa of the alimentary canal. Chemical digestion must break down these complex food molecules into simpler substances so that they can be absorbed and used by the body for metabolic processes.

The breakdown of complex carbohydrates, lipids, and proteins requires digestive enzymes to be delivered when food is present at various parts of the alimentary canal, primarily the stomach and small intestine. These enzymes and their locations are listed in Table 33.1. Clients who secrete insufficient quantities of digestive enzymes may be administered these substances as drugs.

TABLE 33.1 Major Digestive Enzymes

Nutrient	Enzyme	Source
Proteins and polypeptides	Pepsin	Gastric glands
	Trypsin, chymotrypsin, carboxypeptidase	Pancreatic juice
	Aminopeptidase	Small intestine
Lipids	Pancreatic lipase	Pancreatic juice
Carbohydrates and starches	Salivary amylase	Saliva
	Pancreatic amylase	Pancreatic juice
	Maltase, sucrase, lactase	Small intestine

In addition to the three basic nutrients, the body requires a host of other vitamins and minerals for proper metabolism. Deficiency symptoms will be observed if a client has insufficient intake of these substances. The pharmacotherapy of vitamins and minerals is discussed in Chapter 37.

The intake of various nutrients in sufficient amounts is necessary to maintain good health and to allow the body to heal during periods of illness or injury. The intake of sufficient amounts of proteins, carbohydrates, fats, vitamins, and minerals can often be achieved by eating a well-balanced diet of foods and fluids. When this does not occur, enteral or parenteral therapy may be indicated, as discussed in Chapter 37.

CHAPTER

33 Understanding the Chapter

Key Concepts Summary

The numbered key concepts provide a succinct summary of the important points from the corresponding numbered section within the chapter. If any of these points are not clear, refer to the numbered section within the chapter for review.

33.1 The function of the digestive system is to extract nutrients from food to fuel metabolic processes in the body.

33.2 The upper gastrointestinal tract is responsible for mechanical and chemical digestion.

33.3 The small intestine is the longest portion of the alimentary canal and is the primary organ for absorption.

33.4 The large intestine contains host flora and is a major site of water reabsorption.

33.5 The liver is the most important accessory digestive organ.

33.6 Digestion is regulated by numerous hormonal and nervous factors.

33.7 The chemical breakdown of food is accomplished by digestive enzymes.

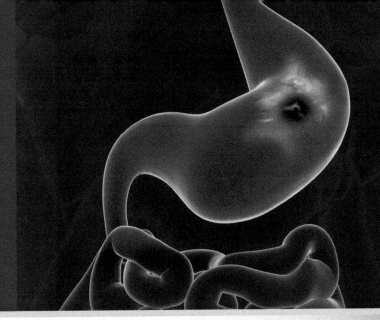

decade3d/Alamy Stock Photo

CHAPTER 34
Pharmacotherapy of Peptic Ulcer Disease

LEARNING OUTCOMES

After reading this chapter, the student should be able to:

1. Identify drug classes used to treat peptic ulcer disease.

2. Explain the therapeutic action of each drug class in relation to the pathophysiology of peptic ulcer disease.

3. Explain why two or more antibiotics are used concurrently in the treatment of *Helicobacter pylori*.

4. Describe the nurse's role in the pharmacological management of clients who are receiving drugs for peptic ulcer disease.

5. For each of the drug classes listed in Prototype Drugs, identify a representative drug and explain its mechanism of action, therapeutic effects, and important adverse effects.

6. Describe and explain, based on pharmacological principles, the rationale for nursing assessment, planning, and interventions for clients with peptic ulcer disease.

7. Use the nursing process to care for clients who are receiving drug therapy for peptic ulcer disease.

CHAPTER OUTLINE

▸ Acid Production by the Stomach

▸ Pathogenesis of Peptic Ulcer Disease

▸ Pathogenesis of Gastroesophageal Reflux Disease

▸ Pharmacotherapy of Peptic Ulcer Disease

▸ H₂-Receptor Antagonists

  ▸ Pharmacotherapy with H₂-Receptor Antagonists

▸ Proton Pump Inhibitors

  ▸ Pharmacotherapy with Proton Pump Inhibitors

▸ Antacids

  ▸ Pharmacotherapy with Antacids

▸ Antibiotics

  ▸ Pharmacotherapy with Combination Antibiotic Therapy

▸ Miscellaneous Drugs for Peptic Ulcer Disease

CONNECTIONS — Special Considerations

◀ Peptic Ulcer Disease

- About 5% to 10% of the world's population suffers at least once from peptic ulcers.
- The *Helicobacter pylori* bacterium is the most common cause of PUD.
- Among the 20% to 40% of Canadians who harbour *H. pylori*, most have no symptoms and only about 15% will develop a peptic ulcer.
- Foods and substances that reduce gastric acidity may help to relieve the pain.
- Milk may provide temporary relief until its digestion increases acid production.
- Smoking and foods that contain caffeine, such as coffee, tea, and soft drinks, may stimulate gastric acid production and worsen pain.
- OTC drugs are available to help reduce gastric acidity and promote comfort.
- Pharmacotherapy with prescription drugs is often required to eliminate *H. pylori* and promote healing.

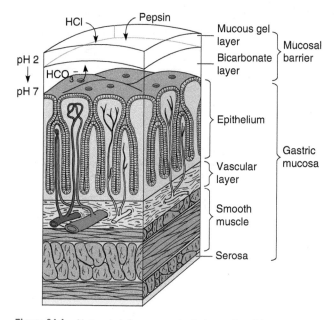

Figure 34.1 Natural defences against stomach acid.

Acid-related diseases of the upper gastrointestinal (GI) tract are some of the most common medical conditions. Drugs for these disorders are available over the counter (OTC), and many clients attempt self-treatment before seeking assistance from their healthcare provider. However, signs and symptoms of acid-related conditions of the upper GI tract may indicate more serious disease. This chapter examines the pharmacotherapy of two common disorders of the upper digestive system: peptic ulcer disease (PUD) and gastroesophageal reflux disease (GERD).

Acid Production by the Stomach

34.1 The stomach secretes enzymes and acid that accelerate the process of chemical digestion.

Food passes from the esophagus to the stomach by travelling through the cardiac (lower esophageal) sphincter. This ring of smooth muscle usually prevents the stomach contents from moving back up the esophagus, a condition known as **esophageal reflux**. A second ring of smooth muscle, the pyloric sphincter, is located at the entrance to the small intestine. This sphincter regulates the flow of substances leaving the stomach.

The stomach thoroughly mixes ingested food and secretes substances that promote the process of chemical digestion. Gastric glands extending deep into the **mucosa** of the stomach contain several cell types critical to digestion and the pharmacotherapy of digestive disorders. **Chief cells** secrete pepsinogen, an inactive form of the enzyme pepsin that chemically breaks down proteins. **Parietal cells** secrete

1 to 3 litres of hydrochloric acid each day. This strong acid helps to break down food, activates pepsinogen, and kills microbes that may have been ingested. Parietal cells also secrete **intrinsic factor**, which is essential for the absorption of vitamin B_{12} (see Chapter 37).

The combined secretions of the chief cells and parietal cells form gastric juice, which is the most acidic fluid in the body, having a pH of 1.5 to 3.5. A number of natural defences protect the stomach mucosa against this extremely acidic fluid. Certain cells lining the surface of the stomach secrete a thick, protective mucous layer and bicarbonate (HCO_3^-) ions to neutralize the acid. These form such an effective protective layer that the pH at the mucosal surface is nearly neutral. Once they reach the duodenum, the stomach contents are further neutralized by bicarbonate from pancreatic and biliary secretions. These natural defences are shown in Figure 34.1.

Pathogenesis of Peptic Ulcer Disease

34.2 Peptic ulcer disease (PUD) is caused by an erosion of the mucosal layer of the stomach or duodenum. Gastric ulcers are more commonly associated with cancer and require longer follow-up.

An ulcer is an erosion of the mucosal layer of the GI tract, usually associated with acute inflammation. Although ulcers may occur in any portion of the **alimentary canal**, the duodenum is the most common site. A **peptic ulcer** is a lesion located in either the stomach (gastric ulcer) or the small intestine (duodenal ulcer). Peptic ulcer disease (PUD) is associated with the following risk factors:

- Close family history of peptic ulcer disease
- Blood group O
- Smoking tobacco
- Beverages and food that contain caffeine
- Drugs, particularly glucocorticoids, acetylsalicylic acid (ASA [Aspirin]), and nonsteroidal anti-inflammatory drugs (NSAIDs)
- Excessive psychological stress
- Infection with *Helicobacter pylori*

The primary cause of PUD is infection by the gram-negative bacterium **Helicobacter pylori**. In non-infected clients, duodenal ulcers are commonly caused by drug therapy with NSAIDs. Secondary factors that contribute to the ulcer and its subsequent inflammation include hypersecretion of gastric acid and hyposecretion of adequate mucus for protection. Figure 34.2 illustrates the mechanism of peptic ulcer formation.

NSAIDs promote ulcer formation and inflammation both topically and systemically. Topically, NSAIDs cause direct cellular damage to GI mucosal cells. Systemically, NSAIDs interfere with prostaglandin synthesis via the enzyme cyclooxygenase (COX) in the stomach, which normally aids in the production of mucus and bicarbonate. NSAIDs decrease gastric blood flow and slow cellular repair. NSAIDs are also weak acids that are nonionized in gastric acid and able to diffuse across the mucous barrier into the gastric epithelial cells, which leads to further cellular damage.

Risk factors for NSAID-induced PUD include long-term use of NSAIDs, advanced age, history of ulcers, concomitant use of corticosteroids or anticoagulants, and alcohol use and cigarette smoking. In addition, *H. pylori* infection and NSAIDs act synergistically to promote ulcers. The combination poses a 3.5-fold greater risk of ulcers than either factor alone.

Zollinger-Ellison syndrome (ZES) is a less common cause of PUD. It is caused by a gastrinoma, a tumour of the pancreas or duodenum that secretes large amounts of the hormone gastrin. Because gastrin is the hormonal signal for increasing hydrochloric acid secretion, the huge amounts of acid easily overcome the protective defences, leading to multiple gastric and duodenal ulcers. Peptic ulcers are persistent, difficult to treat, and slow to heal. Symptoms of ZES are the same as those of PUD. The acid also irritates the GI tract, resulting in diarrhea. Treatment involves aggressive acid suppression with drugs.

Ulceration in the distal small intestine is known as Crohn's disease, and erosions in the large intestine are called ulcerative colitis. These diseases,together categorized as inflammatory bowel disease (IBD), are discussed in Chapter 35.

The characteristic symptom of a duodenal ulcer is a gnawing or burning, upper abdominal pain that occurs 1 to 3 hours after a meal. The pain disappears upon ingestion of food, and nighttime pain, nausea, and vomiting are uncommon. If the erosion progresses deeper into the mucosa, bleeding occurs and may be evident as either bright red blood in vomit or black, tarry stools. Many duodenal ulcers heal spontaneously, although they frequently recur after months of remission. Long-term medical follow-up is usually not necessary.

Gastric ulcers are less common than the duodenal type and have different symptoms. Although relieved by food, pain may continue even after a meal. Loss of appetite, known as anorexia, as well as weight loss and vomiting are more common. Remissions may be infrequent or absent. Medical follow-up of gastric ulcers should continue for several years because a small percentage of the erosions become cancerous. The most severe ulcers may penetrate through the wall of the stomach and cause death. Whereas duodenal ulcers occur most frequently in the 30- to 50-year age group, gastric ulcers are more common after age 60.

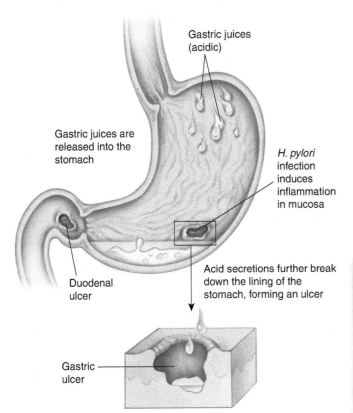

Gastric juices (acidic)

Gastric juices are released into the stomach

H. pylori infection induces inflammation in mucosa

Duodenal ulcer

Acid secretions further break down the lining of the stomach, forming an ulcer

Gastric ulcer

Figure 34.2   Mechanism of peptic ulcer formation.
Pearson Education.

Pathogenesis of Gastroesophageal Reflux Disease

34.3 Gastroesophageal reflux disease (GERD) is caused by acidic stomach contents entering the esophagus. GERD and PUD are treated with similar medications.

Gastroesophageal reflux disease (GERD) results when acidic stomach contents enter the esophagus. Although most often considered a disease of people older than age 40, GERD can also occur in infants. The prevalence of the disease is increasing among both children and adults.

In adults, the cause of GERD is usually transient weakening or relaxation of the lower esophageal sphincter (LES), a specialized muscle segment at the end of the esophagus. The sphincter may no longer close tightly, allowing movement of gastric contents upward into the esophagus when the stomach contracts. The acidic gastric contents cause an intense burning (heartburn) and, in some cases, injury to the esophagus. In addition, the pathogenesis of GERD involves decreased salivary secretions and diminished esophageal motility. The pathophysiology of GERD is shown in Figure 34.3.

Symptoms of GERD include heartburn, dysphagia, dyspepsia, chest pain, nausea, and belching. Symptoms worsen after large meals or exercise, or when in a reclining or recumbent position. There is growing evidence that clients with GERD may also present with symptoms such as chronic cough, wheezing, bronchitis,

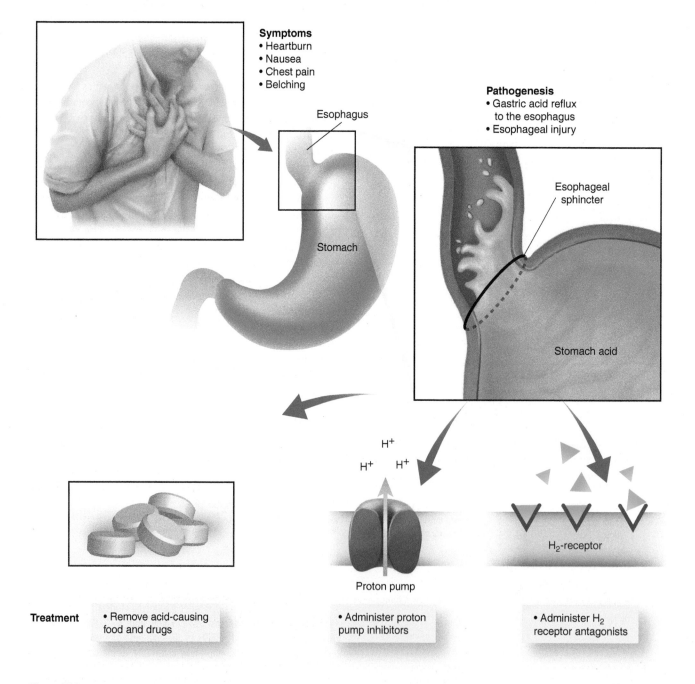

Figure 34.3 The pathophysiology and treatment of gastroesophageal reflux disease (GERD).

sore throat, or hoarseness. GERD is a chronic condition with alternating periods of exacerbation and remission.

A large number of substances and conditions can worsen GERD symptoms. These include caffeine, alcohol, citrus fruits, tomato-based products, onions, carbonated beverages, spicy food, chocolate, smoking, pregnancy, and obesity. Certain medications may also contribute to or worsen GERD. They include nitrates, benzodiazepines, anticholinergics, beta blockers, alpha blockers, estrogen, progesterone, iron, calcium channel blockers, NSAIDs, tricyclic antidepressants, opioids, levodopa-carbidopa (Sinemet), bisphosphonates, and some chemotherapy drugs.

Left untreated, GERD can lead to complications such as esophagitis, esophageal ulcers, or strictures. Approximately 10% of clients who are diagnosed with GERD will develop **Barrett's esophagus**, a condition that is associated with an increased risk for esophageal cancer. Warning signs and symptoms of GERD that suggest a more complicated disease may include unexplained weight loss, early satiety, anemia, vomiting, initial onset of symptoms after age 50, and prolonged anorexia or dysphagia. Clients who are experiencing these symptoms should notify their healthcare provider.

If GERD is associated with obesity, losing weight may eliminate the symptoms. Other lifestyle changes that can improve GERD symptoms include elevating the head of the bed, avoiding fatty or acidic foods, eating smaller meals at least 3 hours before sleep, and eliminating tobacco and alcohol use. Because clients often self-treat this disorder with OTC drugs, a good medication history may give clues to the presence of GERD. Also, clients should be informed that some medications can provoke GERD, and reviewing their medication history may prove helpful. Because drugs provide only symptomatic relief, surgery may become necessary to eliminate the cause of persistent GERD.

An emerging theory suggests that GERD may be a premalignant condition and that chronic acid suppression leads to an increase in esophageal malignancy. This theory is not universally accepted, however, and acid suppression currently remains the mainstay in the treatment of GERD. The presence of GERD does not warrant testing for *H. pylori* infection. Large studies have shown that neither the presence nor the absence of *H. pylori* has any influence on the development of GERD.

Pharmacotherapy of Peptic Ulcer Disease

34.4 Peptic ulcer disease is best treated by a combination of lifestyle changes and pharmacotherapy.

Before initiating pharmacotherapy, clients are usually advised to change lifestyle factors that contribute to PUD or GERD. For example, eliminating tobacco and alcohol use, and perhaps reducing stress, may cause an ulcer to go into remission.

For clients who require pharmacotherapy, a wide variety of both prescription and OTC drugs are available. These drugs fall into four primary classes, plus one miscellaneous group:

- H₂-receptor antagonists
- Proton pump inhibitors
- Antacids
- Antibiotics
- Miscellaneous drugs

CONNECTIONS Natural Therapies

◀ Ginger's Tonic Effects on the GI Tract

The use of ginger (*Zingiber officinale*) for medicinal purposes dates back to antiquity in India and China. The active ingredients of ginger, and those that create its spicy flavour and pungent odour, are located in its roots (rhizomes). It is sometimes standardized according to its active substances, gingerols and shogaols. It is sold in pharmacies as dried ginger root powder, at a dose of 250 to 1000 mg, and it is readily available at most grocery stores for home cooking. Ginger is one of the best studied herbs, and it appears to be useful for a number of digestive-related conditions. Perhaps its widest use is for treating nausea, including that caused from motion sickness, pregnancy morning sickness, and postoperative procedures. It has been shown to stimulate appetite, promote gastric secretions, and increase peristalsis. Its effects appear to be from direct action on the GI tract rather than on the central nervous system (CNS). Ginger has no toxicity when used at recommended doses. Overdoses may lead to CNS depression, inhibition of platelet aggregation, and cardiotonic effects.

The goals of pharmacotherapy are to provide immediate relief from symptoms, promote healing of the ulcer, and prevent future recurrence of the disease. The choice of medication depends on the source of the disease (infectious versus inflammatory), the severity of symptoms, and the convenience of OTC versus prescription drugs. The mechanisms of action of the four major drug classes for PUD are shown in Figure 34.4.

H₂-RECEPTOR ANTAGONISTS

The discovery of the H₂-receptor antagonists in the 1970s marked a major breakthrough in the treatment of PUD. Since then, they have become available OTC and are often drugs of choice in the treatment of peptic ulcer disease. These agents are listed in Table 34.1.

NCLEX Success Tips

Cimetidine (Tagamet) interferes with the metabolism of theophylline and may cause theophylline toxicity.

When given by rapid intravenous (IV) infusion, cimetidine may cause profound hypotension and other cardiotoxic effects.

Cimetidine is prescribed by some surgeons to reduce the level of acid in the stomach contents, altering the pH to reduce the risk of complications should aspiration of vomitus occur.

Cimetidine is a histamine receptor antagonist that decreases the quantity of gastric secretions. It may be used in hiatal hernia therapy to prevent or treat the esophagitis and heartburn associated with reflux.

Pharmacotherapy with H₂-Receptor Antagonists

34.5 H₂-receptor blockers slow acid secretion by the stomach and are often drugs of choice in treating PUD and GERD.

Histamine has two types of receptors: H₁ and H₂. Activation of H₁ receptors produces the classic symptoms of allergy, whereas the H₂ receptors are responsible for increasing acid secretion in the stomach.

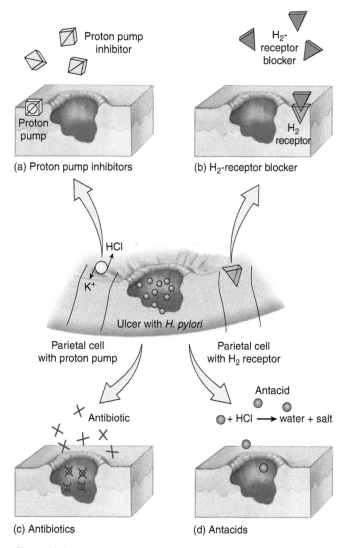

Figure 34.4 Mechanisms of action of antiulcer drugs.

Cimetidine, the first **H₂-receptor antagonist**, and other drugs in this class are quite effective at suppressing the volume and acidity of stomach acid. These drugs are used to treat the symptoms of both PUD and GERD, and several agents in this class are available OTC for the treatment of heartburn. Side effects of the H₂-receptor blockers are minor and rarely cause discontinuation of therapy.

Nursing Considerations

The role of the nurse in H₂-receptor antagonist therapy involves careful monitoring of the client's condition and providing education

TABLE 34.1	H₂-Receptor Antagonists
Drug	**Route and Adult Dose**
cimetidine (Tagamet)	Ulcer treatment: Orally (PO), 300 mg four times daily or 800 mg at bedtime or 400 mg twice daily (bid); ulcer prophylaxis: PO, 400 mg at bedtime; GERD: 400 mg four times daily or 800 mg bid
famotidine (Pepcid)	GERD: PO, 20 mg bid; ulcer treatment, 150 mg bid; ulcer prophylaxis, 150 mg qd
nizatidine (Axid)	PO, GERD: PO, 150 mg bid; ulcer treatment: 150 mg bid; ulcer prophylaxis, 150 mg qd
Pr ranitidine (Zantac)	GERD: 150 mg bid; ulcer treatment: PO, 150 mg bid or 300 mg once daily (qd); ulcer prophylaxis: 150 mg at bedtime

as it relates to the prescribed drug regimen. Because some H₂-receptor blockers are available without prescription, assess the client's use of OTC formulations to avoid duplication of doses. If using OTC formulations, clients should be advised to seek medical attention if symptoms persist or recur. Persistent pain or heartburn may be symptoms of more serious disease that requires medical treatment. Drugs in this class are usually well tolerated. Cimetidine is used less frequently than other H₂-receptor antagonists because of numerous drug-drug interactions (it inhibits hepatic drug-metabolizing enzymes) and because it must be taken up to four times a day. Safety during pregnancy and lactation for drugs in this class has not been established (pregnancy category B).

IV preparations of H₂-receptor antagonists are occasionally used. Because dysrhythmias and hypotension have occurred with IV cimetidine, ranitidine (Zantac) or famotidine (Pepcid) is used if the IV route is necessary.

CNS side effects such as dizziness, drowsiness, confusion, and headache are more likely to occur in elderly clients. Assess for kidney and liver function. These drugs are mainly excreted via the kidneys. Clients with diminished kidney function require smaller dosages and are more likely to experience adverse effects due to the accumulation of the drug in the blood. Although rare, these medications can cause hepatotoxicity. Long-term use of H₂-receptor antagonists may lead to vitamin B₁₂ deficiency because they decrease absorption of the vitamin. Iron supplements may be needed, as this mineral is best absorbed in an acidic environment. Monitor complete blood count (CBC) for possible anemia with long-term use.

Client education as it relates to H₂-receptor antagonists should include goals, reasons for obtaining baseline data such as vital signs and tests for cardiac and renal disorders, and possible side effects. See Nursing Process Focus: Clients Receiving H₂-Receptor Antagonist Therapy for specific teaching points.

NURSING PROCESS FOCUS

Clients Receiving H₂-Receptor Antagonist Therapy

Assessment	Potential Nursing Diagnoses/Identified Patterns
Prior to administration: • Obtain a complete health history, including allergies, drug history, and possible drug interactions. • Assess client for signs of GI bleeding. • Obtain baseline vital signs. • Assess level of consciousness. • Obtain results of CBC and liver and renal function tests.	• Risk for falls related to adverse effect of drug • Need for knowledge regarding drug therapy • Acute pain related to gastric irritation from ineffective drug therapy • Nutrition imbalance related to adverse effects of drug

---

Planning: Client Goals and Expected Outcomes

The client will:

- Report episodes of drowsiness or dizziness
- Report recurrence of abdominal pain or discomfort during drug therapy
- Accurately describe the drug's intended effects, side effects, and precautions

---

Implementation

Interventions (Rationales)	Client Education/Discharge Planning
• Monitor use of OTC drugs to avoid drug interactions, especially with cimetidine therapy. • Monitor level of abdominal pain or discomfort to assess effectiveness of drug therapy. • Monitor client's use of alcohol. (Alcohol can increase gastric irritation.) • Discuss possible drug interactions. (Antacids can decrease the effectiveness of other drugs taken concurrently.) • Institute effective safety measures regarding falls. (Drugs may cause drowsiness or dizziness.) • Explain need for lifestyle changes. (Smoking and certain foods increase gastric acid secretion.) • Observe client for signs of GI bleeding.	• Instruct client to consult with healthcare provider before taking other medications or herbal products • Advise client that pain relief may not occur for several days after beginning therapy • Instruct client to avoid alcohol use • Instruct client to take H$_2$-receptor antagonists and other medications at least 1 hour before antacids • Instruct client to avoid driving or performing hazardous activities until drug effects are known Encourage client to: • Stop smoking; provide information on smoke cessation programs • Avoid alcohol and foods that cause stomach discomfort • Instruct client to immediately report episodes of blood in stool or vomitus or increase in abdominal discomfort

---

Evaluation of Outcome Criteria

Evaluate the effectiveness of drug therapy by confirming that client goals and expected outcomes have been met (see "Planning").

See Table 34.1 for a list of drugs to which these nursing actions apply.

NCLEX Success Tips

The nurse should instruct clients with peptic ulcer to avoid acetylsalicylic acid (as it's a gastric irritant) to prevent further erosion of the stomach lining.

Clients with peptic ulcer should eat small, frequent meals rather than three large ones. Antacids and ranitidine prevent acid accumulation in the stomach and should be taken even after symptoms subside.

Caffeine should be avoided in clients with peptic ulcer because it increases acid production in the stomach.

H$_2$-receptor antagonists, such as ranitidine, reduce gastric acid secretion. Antisecretories, or proton-pump inhibitors, such as omeprazole (Losec), help ulcers heal quickly, in 4 to 8 weeks.

Cytoprotective drugs, such as sucralfate, protect the ulcer surface against acid, bile, and pepsin. Antacids reduce acid concentration and help reduce symptoms.

Antacids such as magnesium hydroxide (Milk of Magnesia) provide short-term relief for gastric ulcers and reflux but do not exert effects in the small intestine.

Additional treatment for duodenal ulcers includes avoidance of irritants such as alcohol, caffeine, and tobacco. Clients should avoid foods that aggravate their symptoms, which commonly include foods that are highly spiced.

Stress management is an important tool in ulcer treatment because stress increases release of cortisol, which can cause ulcers.

Ranitidine blocks secretion of hydrochloric acid. Clients who take only one daily dose of ranitidine are usually advised to take it at bedtime to inhibit nocturnal secretion of acid. Clients who take the drug twice per day are advised to take it in the morning and at bedtime. It is not necessary to take the drug before meals. The client should take the drug regularly, not just when pain occurs.

PROTOTYPE DRUG   Ranitidine (Zantac)

Actions and Uses: Ranitidine acts by blocking H$_2$ receptors in the stomach to decrease acid production. It has a higher potency than cimetidine, which allows it to be administered once daily, usually at bedtime. Adequate healing of the ulcer takes approximately 4 to 8 weeks, although those at high risk for PUD may continue on drug maintenance for prolonged periods to prevent recurrence. Gastric ulcers heal more slowly than duodenal ulcers, and thus require longer therapy. IV and intramuscular (IM) forms are available for the treatment of stress-induced bleeding in acute situations.

Pharmacokinetics: Ranitidine has a duration of action of 8 to 12 hours. Oral drug is metabolized in the liver on first pass. About 50% is absorbed, and 30% is excreted unchanged in the urine. The half-life is 1.7 to 3 hours.

Administration Alert:

- Ranitidine may cause an increase in serum creatinine, aspartate aminotransferase (AST), alanine aminotransferase (ALT), alkaline phosphatase, and total bilirubin.

- Ranitidine is pregnancy category B.

Adverse Effects and Interactions: Ranitidine does not cross the blood-brain barrier to any appreciable extent, so the confusion and CNS depression observed with cimetidine are not expected with ranitidine. Although rare, severe reductions in the number of red and white blood cells and platelets are possible;

therefore, periodic blood counts may be performed. High doses may result in impotence or a loss of libido in men.

Although ranitidine has fewer drug-drug interactions than cimetidine, it interacts with several drugs. For example, ranitidine may reduce the absorption of cefpodoxime, ketoconazole (Nizoral), and itraconazole (Sporanox).

PROTON PUMP INHIBITORS

Proton pump inhibitors act by blocking the enzyme responsible for the secretion of hydrochloric acid in the stomach. They are widely used in the short-term therapy of peptic ulcer disease. These agents are listed in Table 34.2.

Pharmacotherapy with Proton Pump Inhibitors

34.6 Proton pump inhibitors block the enzyme H^+, K^+-ATPase and are effective at reducing gastric acid secretion.

Proton pump inhibitors are relatively new drugs that have become widely used for the treatment of PUD and GERD. Drugs in this class reduce acid secretion in the stomach by binding irreversibly to the enzyme H^+, K^+-ATPase. In the parietal cells of the stomach, **H^+, K^+-ATPase** acts as a pump to release acid (also called hydrogen ions [H^+] or protons) onto the surface of the GI mucosa. The proton pump inhibitors reduce acid secretion to a greater extent than the H_2-receptor antagonists and have a longer duration of action. All agents in this class have similar efficacy and side effects. The side effects of proton pump inhibitors are generally infrequent and minor. The newer agents esomeprazole (Nexium) and pantoprazole (Pantoloc, Tecta) offer the convenience of once-a-day dosing.

Nursing Considerations

The role of the nurse in proton pump inhibitor therapy involves careful monitoring of the client's condition and providing education

◀ H_2-Receptor Antagonists and Vitamin B_{12} in Older Adults

H_2-receptor blockers decrease the secretion of hydrochloric acid in the stomach. However, gastric acid is essential for releasing vitamin B_{12} from food, in which it is bound in a protein matrix. By affecting stomach acidity, these drugs can affect the absorption of this essential vitamin.

H_2-receptor blockers are frequently prescribed for older adults, who are more likely to have pre-existing lower vitamin B_{12} reserves or even deficiencies. With aging, the ability to produce adequate amounts of hydrochloric acid, intrinsic factor, and digestive enzymes progressively diminishes. These losses can lead to lower absorption rates, depletion of reserves, and eventual B_{12} deficiency. The nurse must educate older adults who are taking these drugs on the importance of including plenty of foods rich in vitamin B_{12} in their diets, including red meat, poultry, fish, and eggs.

TABLE 34.2   Proton Pump Inhibitors

Drug	Route and Adult Dose
esomeprazole (Nexium)	PO, 20–40 mg qd
lansoprazole (Prevacid)	PO, 15–60 mg qd
Pr omeprazole (Losec)	PO, 10–40 mg qd
pantoprazole (Pantoloc, Tecta)	PO, 20–40 mg qd
rabeprazole (Pariet)	PO, 10–20 mg qd

as it relates to the prescribed drug regimen. Proton pump inhibitors are usually well tolerated for short-term use. With long-term use, liver function should be periodically monitored, as should serum gastrin because oversecretion of gastrin occurs with constant acid suppression. Generally, proton pump inhibitors are not used during pregnancy and lactation; they range from pregnancy categories B (rabeprazole [Pariet]) to C (omeprazole and lansoprazole [Prevacid]). The nurse should assess for drug-drug interactions. Proton pump inhibitors will affect the absorption of medications, vitamins, and minerals that need an acidic environment in the stomach. The nurse should obtain the client's history of smoking because smoking increases stomach acid production.

These drugs should be taken 30 minutes prior to eating, usually before breakfast. Proton pump inhibitors are unstable in an acidic environment and are enteric coated to be absorbed in the small intestine. These drugs may be administered at the same time as antacids. Proton pump inhibitors are usually administered in combination with clarithromycin for the treatment of *H. pylori*.

The nurse should monitor for adverse effects such as diarrhea, headache, and dizziness. Proton pump inhibitors are a relatively new class of drug; therefore, the long-term effects have not been fully determined.

Client education as it relates to proton pump inhibitors should include goals; reasons for obtaining baseline data such as vital signs, diagnostic procedures, and laboratory tests; and possible side effects. Following are important points to include when teaching clients regarding proton pump inhibitors:

- Take medication before meals.
- Inform the healthcare provider of significant diarrhea.
- Do not crush, break, or chew the medication.
- Avoid smoking, alcohol, and foods that cause gastric discomfort.
- Report GI bleeding, abdominal pain, and heartburn.
- Eat foods with beneficial bacteria, such as yogurt, or take *Acidophilus* to replace "friendly" bacteria.
- Sleep with head elevated 30 degrees. A foam wedge under the top end of the mattress or risers under the top end of the bed frame may be used to keep the head elevated.

PROTOTYPE DRUG   Omeprazole (Losec)

Actions and Uses: Omeprazole was the first proton pump inhibitor to be approved for peptic ulcer disease. It reduces acid secretion in the stomach by binding irreversibly to the enzyme H^+, K^+-ATPase. Although this agent can take 2 hours to reach therapeutic levels, its effects may last 72 hours. It is used for the short-term therapy (4 to 8 weeks) of peptic ulcers and GERD. Most clients are symptom-free after 2 weeks of therapy. It is used for longer periods in clients who have chronic hypersecretion of gastric acid, a condition known as Zollinger-Ellison syndrome. It is the most effective drug for this syndrome. Omeprazole is only available in oral form.

Pharmacokinetics: Omeprazole is rapidly absorbed and 95% protein bound. It is metabolized by the liver and is excreted by the kidneys. The half-life is 30 minutes to 1 hour.

Administration Alerts:

* Administer before meals.
* Tablets should not be chewed, divided, or crushed.
* Drug may be administered with antacids.
* Omeprazole is pregnancy category C.

Adverse Effects and Interactions: Adverse effects are generally minor and include headache, nausea, diarrhea, rash, and abdominal pain. The main concern with proton pump inhibitors is that long-term use has been associated with an increased risk for gastric cancer in laboratory animals. Because of this possibility, therapy is generally limited to 2 months.

Omeprazole interacts with several drugs. For example, concurrent use of diazepam (Valium), phenytoin (Dilantin), and CNS depressants will cause increased blood levels of these drugs. Concurrent use of warfarin (Coumadin) may increase the likelihood of bleeding.

ANTACIDS

Antacids are alkaline substances that have been used to neutralize stomach acid for hundreds of years. These agents, listed in Table 34.3, are readily available as OTC drugs.

Pharmacotherapy with Antacids

34.7 Antacids are effective at neutralizing stomach acid and are inexpensive OTC therapy for PUD and GERD.

Prior to the development of H₂-receptor antagonists and proton pump inhibitors, antacids were the mainstay of peptic ulcer and GERD pharmacotherapy. Indeed, many clients still use these inexpensive and readily available OTC drugs. However, antacids are no longer recommended as the sole drug class for peptic ulcer disease.

Antacids are alkaline, inorganic compounds of aluminum, magnesium, sodium, or calcium. The most common are combinations of aluminum hydroxide (Amphojel) and magnesium hydroxide, which are bases capable of rapidly neutralizing stomach acid. Chewable tablets and liquid formulations are available. Simethicone (Ovol, Phazyme) is sometimes added to antacid preparations because it reduces gas bubbles that cause bloating and discomfort. A few products combine antacids and H₂-receptor blockers into a single tablet; for example, Pepcid Complete contains calcium carbonate, magnesium hydroxide, and famotidine.

Unless taken in extremely large amounts, antacids are very safe. Antacids that contain sodium, calcium, or magnesium can result in absorption of these minerals into the general circulation. This absorption is generally not a problem unless the client is on a sodium-restricted diet or has other conditions such as diminished renal function that could result in accumulation of these minerals. In fact, some manufacturers advertise their antacid products as calcium supplements. Clients should follow the label instructions carefully and not take more than the recommended dosage.

All of the antacids are equally effective at neutralizing acid and reducing symptoms of heartburn when given in therapeutic doses. Each type has certain disadvantages that may preclude their use:

* *Sodium.* Antacids that contain sodium should not be taken by clients on sodium-restricted diets or by those with hypertension, heart failure, or renal impairment because they may promote fluid retention.
* *Magnesium.* Absorption of magnesium from high doses of magnesium-containing antacids can cause symptoms of hypermagnesemia (fatigue, hypotension, and dysrhythmias). Magnesium also acts as a laxative when it reaches the large intestine.
* *Calcium.* Antacids that contain calcium can cause constipation and may cause or aggravate kidney stones. When absorbed, hypercalcemia is possible, and renal failure may occur at very high doses. Administering calcium carbonate antacids with milk or any items with vitamin D can cause **milk-alkali syndrome** to occur. Early symptoms are the same as those of hypercalcemia and include headache, urinary frequency, anorexia, nausea, and fatigue. Milk-alkali syndrome may result in permanent renal damage if the drug is continued at high doses.
* *Aluminum.* Aluminum antacids are not absorbed to any great extent, but they can cause constipation. The constipation effect

TABLE 34.3 Antacids

Drug	Route and Adult Dose
Pr aluminum hydroxide (Amphojel)	PO, 600 mg three times a day (tid) or four times a day (qid)
calcium carbonate (Caltrate, Tums)	PO, 1–2 g bid–tid
calcium carbonate with magnesium hydroxide (Mylanta, Rolaids)	PO, 2–4 capsules or tablets as needed (PRN) (max 12 tablets/day)
magnesium hydroxide (Milk of Magnesia)	PO, 2.4–4.8 g (30–60 mL)/day in 1 or more divided doses
magnesium hydroxide and aluminum hydroxide (Almagel, Diovol, Gelusil, Maalox)	PO, 2–4 tablets PRN (max 16 tablets/day)
magnesium hydroxide and aluminum hydroxide with simethicone (Mylanta, Maalox Plus, others)	PO, 10–20 mL PRN (max 120 mL/day) or 2–4 tablets PRN (max 24 tablets/day)
sodium bicarbonate (Alka-Seltzer) (see Chapter 53, page 677, for the Prototype Drug box)	PO, 0.3–2.0 g qd–qid or ½ tsp of powder in glass of water

is balanced when aluminum is combined with magnesium salts. Aluminum carbonate and aluminum hydroxide may interfere with dietary phosphate absorption to cause hypophosphatemia.

- *Bicarbonate.* Being a base, antacids that contain bicarbonate may provoke metabolic alkalosis (e.g., fatigue, mental status changes, muscle twitching, depressed respiratory rate) in clients at risk. Bicarbonate combines with gastric acid to form carbon dioxide, which causes bloating and belching.

Drug interactions with antacids occur by several mechanisms. Because antacids increase stomach pH, they affect the solubility and absorption of many oral drugs. Drugs that are weak acids are non-ionized in the acidic environment of the stomach and are thus readily absorbed. If an antacid is given concurrently with a weak acid, the pH of the stomach will rise and result in a more ionized drug that is less readily absorbed. On the other hand, a drug that is a weak base is absorbed in a more alkaline medium. In other words, when taken with antacids, acidic drugs may have less therapeutic effect, and basic drugs may exhibit a greater effect. Examples of acidic drugs include NSAIDs, sulfonylureas, salicylates, warfarin, barbiturates, isoniazid (Isotamine), and digoxin (Lanoxin, Toloxin). Basic drugs include morphine sulfate, antihistamines, tricyclic antidepressants, amphetamines, and quinidine (Quinate).

Enteric-coated or delayed-release drugs are designed to dissolve when they reach the alkaline environment in the small intestine. By raising the pH of the stomach, antacids may "fool" enteric-coated tablets into dissolving early and releasing their contents into the stomach. The drug may either irritate the stomach lining, causing nausea or vomiting, or be inactivated.

Drug interactions may also occur if the antacid physically binds to other drugs. For example, certain antacids form chemical complexes with tetracyclines, preventing the antibiotic from being absorbed. Digoxin is another drug whose absorption is affected by binding to antacids.

A third mechanism of drug interaction is due to the effects of antacids on urine pH. Making the urine pH more alkaline increases the excretion of acidic drugs such as acetylsalicylic acid and inhibits the excretion of basic drugs such as amphetamines.

Because antacids are widely used OTC by clients for self-treatment, nurses must emphasize that these drugs be used only as directed on the label due to the potential for adverse effects. To decrease the potential for antacid-drug interactions, nurses should advise that other medications be taken at least 1 hour before or 2 hours after giving an antacid.

Nursing Considerations

The role of the nurse in antacid therapy involves careful monitoring of the client's condition and providing education as it relates to the prescribed drug regimen. Antacids are for occasional use only, and clients should seek medical attention if symptoms persist or recur. The nurse should obtain a medical history, including the use of OTC and prescription drugs. The nurse should assess the client for signs of renal insufficiency; magnesium-containing antacids should be used with caution in these clients. Hypermagnesemia may occur because the kidneys are unable to excrete excess magnesium.

When used according to label directions, antacids have few side effects. Magnesium- and aluminum-based products may cause diarrhea, and those with calcium may cause constipation.

Client education as it relates to antacids should include goals, reasons for obtaining baseline data, and possible side effects. The following are important points the nurse should include when teaching clients regarding antacids:

- Clients with renal failure should avoid magnesium-based antacids.
- Clients with heart failure or hypertension should be advised to avoid sodium-based antacids.
- Take antacids at least 2 hours before or 2 hours after other oral medications. Antacids directly affect the acidity of the stomach and may interfere with drug absorption.
- Note the number and consistency of stools since antacids may alter bowel activity.
- Medication may make stools appear white.
- Shake liquid preparations thoroughly before dispensing.

PROTOTYPE DRUG	Aluminum Hydroxide (Amphojel)

Actions and Uses: Aluminum hydroxide is an inorganic agent used alone or in combination with other antacids such as magnesium hydroxide. Unlike calcium-based antacids that can be absorbed and cause systemic effects, aluminum compounds have minimal absorption. Their primary action is to neutralize stomach acid by raising the pH of the stomach contents. Unlike H_2-receptor antagonists and proton pump inhibitors, aluminum antacids do not reduce the volume of acid secretion. They are most effectively used in combination with other antiulcer agents for the symptomatic relief of heartburn due to PUD or GERD.

Pharmacokinetics: Aluminum hydroxide has an onset of action of 20 to 40 minutes. The duration of action is 2 hours when taken with food and 3 hours when taken 1 to 2 hours after food. It has an unknown half-life, is minimally absorbed, and is mostly excreted in the feces.

Administration Alerts:

- Aluminum antacids should be administered at least 2 hours before or after other drugs because drug absorption could be affected.
- There is no specific treatment for overdose.
- Aluminum hydroxide is pregnancy category C.

Adverse Effects and Interactions: When given in high doses, aluminum compounds may interfere with phosphate metabolism and cause constipation. They are often combined with magnesium compounds, which counteract the constipation. Like many other antacids, aluminum compounds should not be taken with other medications, as they may interfere with their absorption. Sodium polystyrene sulfonate (Kayexalate) may cause systemic alkalosis. Excessive or chronic use may lead to hypophosphatemia.

ANTIBIOTICS

The gram-negative bacterium *H. pylori* is associated with 90% of all duodenal ulcers and 75% of all gastric ulcers. It is also strongly associated with gastric cancer. To more rapidly and completely eliminate peptic ulcers, several antibiotics are used to eradicate this bacterium.

Pharmacotherapy with Combination Antibiotic Therapy

34.8 Combinations of antibiotics are administered to eliminate *H. pylori,* the cause of many peptic ulcers.

H. pylori has adapted well as a human pathogen by devising ways to neutralize the high acidity surrounding it and by making chemicals called adhesins that allow it to stick tightly to the GI mucosa. *H. pylori* infections can remain active for life if not treated appropriately. Elimination of this organism causes ulcers to heal more rapidly and to remain in remission longer. The following antibiotics are commonly used for this purpose:

- Amoxicillin (Amoxil)
- Clarithromycin (Biaxin)
- Metronidazole (Flagyl)
- Tetracycline
- Bismuth subsalicylate (Pepto-Bismol)

Two or more antibiotics are given concurrently to increase the effectiveness of therapy and to lower the potential for bacterial resistance. The antibiotics are also combined with a proton pump inhibitor or an H_2-receptor antagonist. Bismuth compounds are sometimes added to the antibiotic regimen. Although technically not antibiotics, bismuth compounds inhibit bacterial growth and prevent *H. pylori* from adhering to the gastric mucosa. Antibiotic therapy generally continues for 7 to 14 days. Additional information on antibacterial agents can be found in Chapter 44.

MISCELLANEOUS DRUGS FOR PEPTIC ULCER DISEASE

34.9 Several miscellaneous drugs, including sucralfate, misoprostol, and metoclopramide, are also beneficial in treating PUD.

Several additional drugs are beneficial in treating peptic ulcer disease. Sucralfate consists of sucrose (a sugar) plus aluminum hydroxide (an antacid). The drug produces a thick, gel-like substance that coats the ulcer, protecting it against further erosion and promoting healing. It does not affect the secretion of gastric acid. Little of the drug is absorbed from the GI tract. Other than constipation, side effects are minimal.

Misoprostol (Cytotec) is a prostaglandin-like substance that acts by inhibiting gastric acid secretion and stimulating the production of protective mucus. Its primary use is for the prevention of peptic ulcers in clients who are taking high doses of NSAIDs or glucocorticoids. Diarrhea and abdominal cramping are relatively common. Classified as a pregnancy category X drug, misoprostol is contraindicated in clients who are pregnant. In fact, misoprostol is sometimes used to terminate pregnancies, as discussed in Chapter 31.

NCLEX Success Tips

Misoprostol is used to protect the stomach's lining when a client has a peptic ulcer. Misoprostol does not affect the cardiac or respiratory systems.

Misoprostol is a synthetic prostaglandin E_1 analogue that will replace gastric prostaglandins depleted by steroid therapy and thereby prevent the development of gastritis or peptic ulcer disease. Omeprazole is a proton pump inhibitor that will decrease gastric acidity; over-the-counter antacids may help to decrease acidity. Diphenhydramine (Benadryl) is an antihistamine, which will not help.

Metoclopramide (Metonia, Maxeran) is occasionally used for the short-term therapy (4 to 12 weeks) of symptomatic GERD or PUD in clients who fail to respond to first-line agents. It is more commonly prescribed to treat nausea and vomiting associated with surgery or cancer chemotherapy. Metoclopramide is available by the PO, IM, or IV route. It causes muscles in the upper intestine to contract, resulting in faster emptying of the stomach. It also decreases esophageal relaxation and blocks food from entering the esophagus, which is of benefit in clients with GERD.

CNS adverse effects such as drowsiness, fatigue, confusion, and insomnia may occur in a significant number of clients.

NCLEX Success Tips

Metoclopramide (Metonia) can cause sedation. Alcohol and other central nervous system depressants add to this sedation. A client who is taking this drug should be cautioned to avoid driving or performing other hazardous activities for a few hours after taking the drug. Clients may take antacids, antihypertensives, and anticoagulants while on metoclopramide.

Clients taking metoclopramide should be instructed to report any involuntary movements of the face, eyes, or extremities because adverse effects of the drug include extrapyramidal reactions and parkinsonism-like reactions. Other common adverse effects include diarrhea (not constipation) and nausea.

CHAPTER

34

Understanding the Chapter

Key Concepts Summary

The numbered key concepts provide a succinct summary of the important points from the corresponding numbered section within the chapter. If any of these points are not clear, refer to the numbered section within the chapter for review.

34.1 The stomach secretes enzymes and acid that accelerate the process of chemical digestion.

34.2 Peptic ulcer disease (PUD) is caused by an erosion of the mucosal layer of the stomach or duodenum. Gastric ulcers are more commonly associated with cancer and require longer follow-up.

34.3 Gastroesophageal reflux disease (GERD) is caused by acidic stomach contents entering the esophagus. GERD and PUD are treated with similar medications.

34.4 Peptic ulcer disease is best treated by a combination of lifestyle changes and pharmacotherapy.

34.5 H_2-receptor blockers slow acid secretion by the stomach and are often drugs of choice in treating PUD and GERD.

34.6 Proton pump inhibitors block the enzyme H^+,K^+-ATPase and are effective at reducing gastric acid secretion.

34.7 Antacids are effective at neutralizing stomach acid and are inexpensive OTC therapy for PUD and GERD.

34.8 Combinations of antibiotics are administered to eliminate *H. pylori,* the cause of many peptic ulcers.

34.9 Several miscellaneous drugs, including sucralfate, misoprostol, and metoclopramide, are also beneficial in treating PUD.

Chapter 34 Scenario

Hugh Marshall is a 71-year-old man who has been taking ibuprofen (Motrin) for a shoulder injury and assumed that this was the cause of his stomach pain. He is a one-pack-per-day smoker and drinks one glass of wine every night with dinner. His medical history includes hypertension, for which he takes a combination diuretic and angiotensin-converting enzyme (ACE) inhibitor. He stopped taking his ibuprofen, but the stomach pain did not subside. Because of worsening symptoms, an endoscopy was performed, which confirmed the presence of *H. pylori*. He is worried about taking antibiotics because he has been allergic to penicillin in the past.

Critical Thinking Questions

1. Based on the scenario, what risk factors for PUD does Hugh have?

2. How would you, as the nurse, describe the recommended treatment for *H. pylori*–induced PUD to him?

3. Why would you be concerned about this client with a history of hypertension using NSAIDs?

See Answers to Critical Thinking Questions in Appendix B.

NCLEX Practice Questions

1 The client has developed severe diarrhea following 4 days of self-administered antacid preparation. The nurse suspects that the diarrhea may have been caused by which type of antacid?

   a. Aluminum compounds

   b. Magnesium compounds

   c. Calcium compounds

   d. Sodium compounds

2 Omeprazole (Losec) is prescribed for a client with gastroesophageal reflux disease. The nurse will monitor for a reduction in which symptom to determine if the drug therapy is effective? Select all that apply.

   a. Dysphagia

   b. Dyspepsia

   c. Appetite

d. Nausea

e. Belching

3 A nurse is scheduling her client's daily medication. When would be the most appropriate time for the client to receive proton pump inhibitors?

a. At night

b. After fasting at least 2 hours

c. About half an hour before a meal

d. About 2 to 3 hours after eating

4 A client who has duodenal ulcers is receiving long-term therapy with ranitidine (Zantac). The nurse includes in the care plan that the client should be monitored for which adverse effects?

a. Photophobia and skin irritations

b. Neutropenia and thrombocytopenia

c. Dyspnea and productive coughing

d. Urinary hesitation and fluid retention

5 A nurse is caring for a client with gastroesophageal reflux disease should question the order for which drug?

a. H$_2$-receptor antagonists

b. Proton pump inhibitors

c. Antibiotics

d. Antacids

See Answers to NCLEX Practice Questions in Appendix A.

PROTOTYPE DRUGS

**DRUGS FOR CONSTIPA-
TION: LAXATIVES**
Bulk-forming agents
Pr *psyllium mucilloid
(Metamucil, Psyllium)*
Stool softeners/surfactants
Stimulants
Saline and osmotic agents
Miscellaneous agents

**DRUGS FOR DIARRHEA:
ANTIDIARRHEALS**
Opioids
Pr *diphenoxylate with atro-
pine (Lomotil)*
Miscellaneous agents

**DRUGS FOR NAUSEA
AND VOMITING**
Anticholinergics
Antihistamines
Benzodiazepines
Cannabinoids
Glucocorticoids
Phenothiazines and
phenothiazine-like agents
Pr *prochlorperazine
(Stemetil)*
Serotonin receptor
antagonists

**DRUGS FOR
PANCREATITIS**
Pr *pancrelipase
(Lipancreatin, Pancrease)*

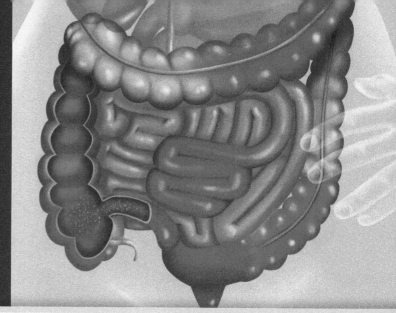

CHAPTER 35

Pharmacotherapy of Bowel Disorders and Other Gastrointestinal Alterations

LEARNING OUTCOMES

After reading this chapter, the student should be able to:

1. Identify drug classes used for treating bowel disorders, nausea, vomiting, and pancreatitis.

2. Explain the therapeutic action of each class of drugs used to treat bowel disorders, nausea, vomiting, and pancreatitis in relation to the pathophysiology of these conditions.

3. Discuss the role of the nurse regarding the non-pharmacological management of constipation.

4. Compare and contrast the types of drugs used to treat inflammatory bowel disease and irritable bowel syndrome.

5. Describe the nurse's role in the pharmacological management of clients who are receiving drugs for the management of bowel disorders, nausea, vomiting, and pancreatitis.

6. For each of the drug classes listed in Prototype Drugs, identify a representative drug and explain its mechanism of action, therapeutic effects, and important adverse effects.

7. Describe and explain, based on pharmacological principles, the rationale for nursing assessment, planning, and interventions for clients with bowel disorders, nausea, vomiting, and pancreatitis.

8. Use the nursing process to care for clients receiving drug therapy for bowel disorders, nausea, vomiting, and pancreatitis.

CHAPTER OUTLINE

▶ Constipation
  ▶ Pathophysiology of Constipation
  ▶ Pharmacotherapy with Laxatives
▶ Diarrhea
  ▶ Pathophysiology of Diarrhea
  ▶ Pharmacotherapy with Antidiarrheals
▶ Nausea and Vomiting
  ▶ Pathophysiology of Nausea and Vomiting
  ▶ Pharmacotherapy with Antiemetics
▶ Inflammatory Bowel Disease
▶ Irritable Bowel Syndrome
▶ Pancreatitis
  ▶ Pharmacotherapy of Pancreatitis

Bowel disorders, nausea, and vomiting are among the most common complaints for which clients seek medical consultation. These nonspecific symptoms may be caused by any number of infectious, metabolic, inflammatory, neoplastic, or neuropsychological disorders. In addition, nausea, vomiting, constipation, and diarrhea are the most common side effects of oral medications. Symptoms often resolve without the need for pharmacotherapy. When severe or prolonged, however, bowel disorders, nausea, and vomiting may lead to serious consequences unless drug therapy is initiated. Pancreatitis is a less common and more serious disorder that requires pharmacotherapy. This chapter examines the pharmacotherapy of these conditions associated with the gastrointestinal (GI) tract.

CONSTIPATION

Constipation is identified by a decrease in the frequency and number of bowel movements. Stools may become dry, hard, and difficult to evacuate from the rectum.

Pathophysiology of Constipation

35.1 Constipation, the infrequent passage of hard, small stools, is a common disorder caused by slow motility of material through the large intestine.

As waste material travels through the large intestine, water is reabsorbed. Reabsorption of the proper amount of water results in stools of a normal, soft consistency. If the waste material remains in the colon for an extended period, however, too much water will be reabsorbed, leading to small, hard stools. Constipation may cause abdominal distention and discomfort, and flatulence.

The etiology of constipation may be related to a lack of exercise, insufficient food intake (especially insoluble **dietary fibre**), diminished fluid intake, or a medication regimen that includes drugs that reduce intestinal motility. Lifestyle modifications that incorporate positive dietary changes and physical activity should be considered before drugs are used. Foods that can cause constipation include alcoholic beverages, products with a high content of refined white flour, dairy products, and chocolate. The normal frequency of bowel movements varies widely among individuals, from two to three per day to as few as one per week.

Occasional constipation is common and does not require drug therapy. Chronic constipation experienced as infrequent and painful bowel movements, accompanied by severe straining, may justify initiation of treatment. In its most severe form, constipation can lead to a fecal impaction and complete obstruction of the bowel. Constipation occurs more frequently in older adults because fecal transit

time through the colon slows with aging; this population also exercises less and has a higher frequency of chronic disorders that cause constipation. Laxatives are drugs that promote bowel movements. Many are available over the counter (OTC) for the self-treatment of simple constipation. Laxatives are identified in Table 35.1.

NCLEX Success Tips

Medications for constipation that are considered safe during pregnancy include compounds that produce bulk, such as psyllium (Metamucil).

Docusate (Colace, Soflax), bisacodyl (Dulcolax), and magnesium hydroxide (Milk of Magnesia) can also be used.

Mineral oil prevents the absorption of vitamins and minerals within the GI tract.

Magnesium is normally excreted by the kidneys. When the kidneys fail, magnesium can accumulate and cause severe neurological problems.

Stool softener should be withheld if the client reports loose stools.

Stool softeners taken daily promote absorption of liquid into the stool, creating a softer mass. They may be taken on a daily basis without developing a dependence. Dependence is an adverse effect of daily laxative use.

Enemas used daily or on a frequent basis can also lead to dependence of the bowel on an external source of stimulation.

TABLE 35.1   Laxatives and Cathartics

Drug	Route and Adult Dose
Bulk-Forming Agents	
Pr psyllium mucilloid (Metamucil, Psyllium)	Orally (PO), 2.5 to 30 g per day (qd) in divided doses
Saline and Osmotic Agents	
magnesium hydroxide (Milk of Magnesia)	PO, 15-60 mL in divided doses
polyethylene glycol (Lax-A-Day, Peg3350, Pegalax, Relaxa)	PO, 17 g (1 heaping tablespoon) dissolved in 120-240 mL (4-8 oz) water qd
sodium biphosphate (Fleet Enema)	Rectal, contents of one 4.5 oz enema as a single dose
Stimulants	
bisacodyl (Dulcolax)	PO, 5-15 mg qd either on a scheduled basis or PRN
castor oil	PO, 15–60 mL qd PRN
Stool Softeners/Surfactants	
docusate (Colace, Soflax)	PO, 50–500 mg qd
Miscellaneous Agents	
mineral oil	PO, 45 mL twice a day (bid)

Pharmacotherapy with Laxatives

35.2 Laxatives are drugs given to promote emptying of the large intestine by stimulating peristalsis, lubricating the fecal mass, or adding more bulk to the colon contents.

Laxatives are drugs that promote evacuation of the large bowel, or **defecation**. **Cathartic** implies a stronger and more complete bowel emptying. A variety of prescription and OTC formulations are available, including tablets, liquids, and suppositories, to treat existing constipation or to prevent this disorder.

Prophylactic laxative pharmacotherapy is appropriate postoperatively. Such treatment is indicated to preclude straining or bearing down during defecation—a situation that has the potential to precipitate increased intra-abdominal and intraocular pressure and blood pressure. Drugs, in conjunction with enemas, are often given to cleanse the bowel prior to diagnostic or surgical procedures of the colon or genitourinary tract. Cathartics are usually the drug of choice preceding diagnostic procedures of the colon, such as colonoscopy and barium enema.

Laxatives have several important indications. These may be divided into prophylaxis of constipation and treatment of constipation:

Prophylaxis

- Clients who have had a myocardial infarction (MI) or those with rectal pathology who should not be straining
- Clients who are receiving drug therapies and have constipation as a known adverse effect
- Clients who are bedridden or otherwise unable to exercise
- Clients who are pregnant
- Elderly clients with weak abdominal or perineal muscles

Treatment

- Relieve simple, chronic constipation
- Accelerate the removal of ingested toxic substances after overdose or poisoning
- Accelerate the removal of dead parasites after antihelminthic drug therapy
- Cleanse the bowel prior to diagnostic or surgical procedures of the colon or genitourinary tract, including colonoscopy or barium enema

The most common adverse effects of laxatives include abdominal distention and cramping. Diarrhea may result from excessive use. When cleansing the bowel prior to a colonoscopy or purging the bowel of toxic substances or parasites, forceful, frequent bowel movements are expected outcomes. Care must be taken to rule out acute abdominal pathology such as bowel obstruction prior to administration, because the drugs will increase colon pressure and possibly cause bowel perforation.

When taken in prescribed amounts, laxatives have few side effects. These drugs are often classified into four primary groups and a miscellaneous category:

- Bulk-forming agents absorb water, thus adding size to the fecal mass. They are often taken prophylactically to prevent constipation.
- Stool softeners (surfactants) reduce surface tension by causing more water and fat to be absorbed into the stool. They are often used in clients who have undergone recent surgery.
- Stimulants irritate the bowel to increase peristalsis; they may cause cramping in clients.
- Osmotic laxatives such as saline are not absorbed in the intestine; they pull water into the fecal mass to create a more watery stool.
- Miscellaneous agents include mineral oil, which acts within the intestine by lubricating the stool and the colon mucosa.

Nursing Considerations

The role of the nurse in laxative therapy involves careful monitoring of the client's condition and providing education as it relates to the prescribed drug. Prior to pharmacotherapy with laxatives, the nurse must assess the abdomen for distention and bowel sounds. If there is absence of bowel sounds, peristalsis must be restored prior to laxative therapy. Assess bowel patterns. A client with a sudden, unexplained change in bowel patterns should be evaluated, as this change could indicate a serious condition such as colon cancer. Also assess for esophageal obstruction, intestinal obstruction, fecal impaction, and undiagnosed abdominal pain. Laxatives are contraindicated in all of these conditions due to the risk for causing bowel perforation. If diarrhea occurs, laxative use should be discontinued. There are many products to prevent and treat constipation. Because most are OTC medications, there is a risk for misuse and overuse.

Bulk-forming laxatives are pregnancy category C and should be used with caution during pregnancy and lactation. Because fibre absorbs water and expands to provide "bulk," these agents must be taken with plenty of water. These laxatives will not be effective unless taken with one to two glasses of water. Assess the client's ability to swallow, as obstruction can occur if the product does not clear the esophagus or if a stricture exists. Bulk-forming products may take 24 to 48 hours to be effective and may be taken on a regular basis to prevent constipation.

Stool softeners are generally prescribed for clients who have experienced a sudden change in lifestyle that puts them at risk for constipation, such as a surgery, injury, or conditions such as MI where straining during defecation should be avoided. They are contraindicated during pregnancy and lactation (pregnancy category C). Assess for the development of diarrhea and cramping; if diarrhea develops, the medication should be withheld. Docusate is contraindicated in clients with abdominal pain accompanied by nausea and vomiting, with fecal impaction, and with intestinal obstruction or perforation. Docusate sodium should not be given to clients who are on sodium restriction. Docusate potassium should not be given to clients with renal impairment. Docusate increases systemic absorption of mineral oil, so these two medications should not be given concurrently. Docusate should not be taken with certain herbal products such as senna, cascara, rhubarb, and aloe, as it will increase their absorption and the risk for liver toxicity.

Stimulant laxatives act as irritants to the bowel and increase peristalsis. They are the quickest acting and most likely to cause diarrhea and cramping. Bowel rupture could occur if obstruction is present. Stimulant laxatives are not used during pregnancy and lactation (pregnancy category C). Because of their rapid and potent effects, the nurse must pay particular attention to responding to the client's need to use a bedpan or quickly get to the bathroom. These products are also used as a "bowel prep" prior to bowel exams or surgeries, sometimes in combination with osmotic laxatives and enemas. As the client will be nothing by mouth (NPO) prior to the procedure, it is important to assess for signs of dehydration and changes in vital signs. It may be necessary to initiate intravenous (IV) fluids. Herbal stimulant laxatives, such as cascara and senna, are common components of OTC weight loss products, and clients taking them may experience rebound, severe constipation if these medications are abruptly withdrawn.

Saline or osmotic laxatives pull water into the GI tract. Most are pregnancy category B. Dehydration may result when these medications are taken frequently or in excess if the client has inadequate fluid intake. Osmotic laxatives are highly potent, work within hours, and are often a part of bowel prep.

Lactulose relieves constipation by increasing stool water content and acidity. Lactulose is a disaccharide that reaches the colon mostly unchanged, increasing osmotic pressure and water content. In the colon, bacteria act on lactulose to produce lactic acid and draw ammonia ions from the bloodstream. The acidification of colonic contents helps to increase stool volume and frequency. Reducing the dose usually controls abdominal cramping and diarrhea should they occur. Lactulose should not be taken within 2 hours of another medication because the desired effect of the other medication may be reduced. Lactulose should not be used in the presence of abdominal pain, nausea, fever, or vomiting. It is contraindicated in patients requiring a low galactose diet and is pregnancy category B.

NCLEX Success Tips

In cirrhosis, the liver fails to convert ammonia to urea. Ammonia then builds up in the blood and is carried to the brain, causing cerebral dysfunction. When this occurs, the client will often have a decreased level of consciousness and appear confused. Constipation also leads to increased ammonia production.

Lactulose, a hyperosmotic laxative, is administered to promote ammonia excretion in the stool by acidifying the colon contents, which retards diffusion of nonionic ammonia from the colon to the blood while promoting its migration from the blood to the colon, and thus improve cerebral function. Because level of consciousness (LOC) is an accurate indicator of cerebral function, the nurse can evaluate the effectiveness of lactulose by monitoring the client's LOC.

The expected effect of lactulose is for the client to have 2 to 3 soft stools per day to help reduce the pH and serum ammonia levels, which will prevent hepatic encephalopathy.

The taste of lactulose is a problem for some clients. Mixing it with fruit juice, water, or milk can make it more palatable. Lactulose should not be given with antacids, which may inhibit its action. Lactulose should not be taken with a laxative because increased stooling is an adverse effect of the drug and would be potentiated by using a laxative. Lactulose comes in the form of syrup for oral or rectal administration.

Client education as it relates to these medications should include goals, reasons for obtaining baseline data such as vital signs and abdominal assessment, and possible side effects. The following are other important points to include when teaching clients regarding laxatives:

- Follow label instructions carefully, and do not take more than the recommended dose.
- If changes in bowel patterns persist or become more severe, seek medical attention.
- Take bulk-forming agents at a different time than other medications to ensure proper absorption.

See Nursing Process Focus: Clients Receiving Laxative Therapy for additional teaching points.

PROTOTYPE DRUG	Psyllium Mucilloid (Metamucil, Psyllium)

Actions and Uses: Psyllium is derived from the seeds of the plantain plant. Like other bulk-forming laxatives, psyllium is an insoluble fibre that is indigestible and not absorbed from the GI tract. When taken with a sufficient quantity of water, psyllium swells and increases the size of the fecal mass. The larger the fecal mass, the more the defecation reflex will be stimulated, thus promoting the passage of stool. Several doses of psyllium may be needed to produce a therapeutic effect. Frequent use of psyllium may effect a small reduction in blood cholesterol level.

Pharmacokinetics: Psyllium is not absorbed and has an onset of action of 12 to 24 hours.

Administration Alerts:

- Mix with 250 mL of water, fruit juice, or milk, and administer immediately.
- Follow each dose with an additional 250 mL of liquid.
- Observe elderly clients closely for possible aspiration.
- Psyllium is pregnancy category C.

Adverse Effects and Interactions: Psyllium rarely produces side effects. It generally causes less cramping than the stimulant-type laxatives and results in a more natural bowel movement. If taken with insufficient water, it may cause obstructions in the esophagus or intestine. Psyllium should not be administered to clients who have undiagnosed abdominal pain.

Psyllium may decrease the absorption and effects of warfarin, digoxin, nitrofurantoin, antibiotics, and salicylates.

DIARRHEA

Diarrhea is an increase in the frequency and fluidity of bowel movements. Diarrhea is not a disease; it is a symptom of an underlying disorder.

Pathophysiology of Diarrhea

35.3 Diarrhea is an increase in the fluidity of feces that occurs when the colon fails to reabsorb enough water.

The small intestine receives about 9 L of fluid, or **chyme**, daily. Most is reabsorbed, such that only about 1 L reaches the colon. Travel through the colon results in even more reabsorption, and

NURSING PROCESS FOCUS

Clients Receiving Laxative Therapy

Assessment	Potential Nursing Diagnoses/Identified Patterns
Prior to administration: • Obtain complete health history, including allergies, drug history, and possible drug interactions. • Assess bowel elimination pattern. • Assess bowel sounds.	• Risk for injury (intestinal obstruction) related to adverse effects from drug therapy • Constipation • Fluid and electrolyte imbalance

Planning: Client Goals and Expected Outcomes

The client will:

• Report relief from constipation
• Demonstrate an understanding of the drug's action by accurately describing drug side effects and precautions
• Immediately report effects such as nausea, vomiting, diarrhea, abdominal pain, and lack of bowel movement

Implementation

Interventions (Rationales)	Client Education/Discharge Planning
• Monitor frequency, volume, and consistency of bowel movements. (Changes in bowel habits can indicate a serious condition.) • Monitor client's ability to swallow. (Bulk laxatives can swell and cause obstruction in the esophagus.) • Monitor client's fluid intake. (Esophageal or intestinal obstruction may result if the client does not take adequate amounts of fluid with the medication.)	Advise client to: • Discontinue laxative use if diarrhea occurs • Notify the healthcare provider if constipation continues • Take medication as prescribed • Increase fluids and dietary fibre, such as whole grains, fibrous fruits, and vegetables • Expect results from medication within 2 to 3 days after initial dose • Instruct client to discontinue medication and notify the healthcare provider if having difficulty swallowing Instruct client to: • Drink six 250-mL glasses of fluid per day • Mix medication in 250 mL of liquid

Evaluation of Outcome Criteria

Evaluate the effectiveness of drug therapy by confirming that client goals and expected outcomes have been met (see "Planning").

See Table 35.1 for a list of drugs to which these nursing actions apply.

---

only about 100 mL remains to form stools. Should the small or large intestines fail to reabsorb sufficient fluids, diarrhea may occur.

Like constipation, occasional diarrhea is a common disorder that does not warrant drug therapy. When prolonged or severe, especially in children, diarrhea can result in significant loss of body fluids, and pharmacotherapy is indicated. Prolonged diarrhea may lead to acid-base or electrolyte disorders (see Chapter 53).

Common causes of diarrhea include the following:

• *Infection.* Viral and bacterial infections are the most common cause of diarrhea. Intestinal protozoans and helminths are less common causes. The most frequently encountered diarrhea-producing organisms are *Campylobacter, Salmonella, Cryptosporidium, Giardia, Shigella, Escherichia coli* (traveller's diarrhea), and *Staphylococcus.*

• *Drugs.* Antibiotics often cause diarrhea by killing normal intestinal flora, thereby allowing an overgrowth of opportunistic pathogenic organisms. Laxatives, magnesium antacids, digoxin

(Lanoxin, Toloxin), orlistat (Xenical), and nonsteroidal anti-inflammatory drugs (NSAIDs) are also common causes.

• *Inflammation.* Ulcerative colitis, Crohn's disease, and irritable bowel syndrome (IBS) cause inflammation of the bowel mucosa, leading to periods of intense diarrhea.

• *Foods.* Various foods can cause diarrhea, such as dairy products in lactose-intolerant clients, foods with capsaicin (hot pepper), and chronic alcohol ingestion.

• *Malabsorption.* Diseases of the small intestine and pancreas can cause insufficient absorption of foods and fluid.

It is vital to assess and treat the cause of the diarrhea. Assessing the client's recent travels, dietary habits, immune system competence, and recent drug history may provide information about the cause of the diarrhea. Critically ill clients with a reduced immune response who are exposed to many antibiotics may have diarrhea related to pseudomembranous colitis, a condition that may lead to shock and death.

TABLE 35.2   Antidiarrheals

Drug	Route and Adult Dose
Opioids	
belladonna with opium	Rectal, 1 suppository bid to four times a day (qid) PRN
Pr diphenoxylate with atropine (Lomotil)	PO, 5 mg (2 tabs) tid-qid until control achieved (max 20 mg/day); dosing is based on diphenoxylate content
loperamide (Imodium)	PO, 4 mg as a single dose, then 2 mg after each diarrhea episode (max 16 mg/day)
Miscellaneous Agents	
bismuth subsalicylate (Pepto-Bismol)	PO, 2 tabs or 30 mL regular strength after each diarrhea episode (max 4.2 g/day)
attapulgite (Kaopectate)	PO (give after each bowel movement), 1200-1500 mg/day (max 8400 mg/day)

Ulceration in the distal portion of the small intestine, called **Crohn's disease**, and erosions in the large intestine, called **ulcerative colitis**, are common causes of diarrhea. Together these diseases are categorized as inflammatory bowel disease and are treated with anti-inflammatory medications. Particularly severe cases of inflammatory bowel disease may require immunosuppressant drugs such as cyclosporine or methotrexate.

Irritable bowel syndrome (IBS), also known as spastic colon or mucous colitis, is a common disorder of the lower GI tract. Symptoms include abdominal pain, bloating, excessive gas, and colicky cramping. Bowel habits are frequently affected, with diarrhea alternating with constipation, and there may be mucus in the stool. IBS is considered a functional bowel disorder, meaning that the normal operation of the digestive tract is impaired without the presence of detectable organic disease. It is not a precursor of more serious disease. Stress is often a precipitating factor along with dietary factors. Treatment is supportive, with drug therapy targeted at symptomatic treatment.

For occasional, mild cases of diarrhea, OTC products are effective at returning elimination patterns to normal. For chronic or severe cases, the opioids are the most efficacious of the antidiarrheal agents. The antidiarrheals are listed in Table 35.2.

Pharmacotherapy with Antidiarrheals

35.4 For simple diarrhea, OTC medications are effective. Opioids are the most effective drugs for controlling severe diarrhea.

Pharmacotherapy related to diarrhea depends on the severity of the condition and identifiable causal factors. If the cause is an infectious disease, an antibiotic or antiparasitic drug is indicated. Should the cause be inflammatory in nature, anti-inflammatory drugs are warranted. When the cause appears to be due to a side effect of pharmacotherapy, the healthcare provider may discontinue the offending medication, lower the dose, or substitute an alternative drug.

The most effective drugs for the symptomatic treatment of diarrhea are the opioids. They slow peristalsis in the colon with only a slight risk of dependence. The most common opioid antidiarrheals are codeine and diphenoxylate with atropine (Lomotil). Diphenoxylate is a Schedule V agent that acts directly on the intestine to slow peristalsis, thereby allowing for more fluid and electrolyte absorption in the large intestine. The opioids cause central nervous system (CNS) depression at high doses and are generally reserved for more severe cases due to the potential for dependence.

OTC drugs for diarrhea act by a number of different mechanisms. Loperamide (Imodium) is an analogue of meperidine (Demerol), although it has no narcotic effects and is not classified as a controlled substance. Low-dose loperamide is available OTC; higher doses are available by prescription. Other OTC treatments include bismuth subsalicylate (Pepto-Bismol), which acts to bind and absorb toxins. The psyllium and pectin preparations may also slow diarrhea since they tend to absorb large amounts of fluid and form bulkier stools. Intestinal flora modifiers are supplements that help to correct the altered GI flora; a good source of healthy bacteria is yogurt with active cultures.

Nursing Considerations

The role of the nurse in antidiarrheal therapy involves careful monitoring of the client's condition and providing education as it relates to the prescribed drug regimen. Antidiarrheal drugs should be given for symptomatic relief of diarrhea while the underlying cause is treated. Because diarrhea can cause a loss of fluid and electrolytes, hydration status and serum potassium, magnesium, and bicarbonate should be assessed. Assess for blood in the stool. The nurse needs to be especially observant of infants, children, and older adults because diarrhea can quickly lead to dehydration and electrolyte imbalance in these clients. Because antidiarrheals are excreted in the liver and kidneys, hepatic and renal function should be assessed.

Antidiarrheals are generally not used during pregnancy and lactation. They should not be used in conditions where constipation should be avoided, such as pseudomembranous colitis or severe ulcerative colitis, because the drugs could worsen or mask these conditions. Toxic megacolon has occurred in clients with ulcerative colitis who are taking loperamide. Because drowsiness may occur with opioids, assess the client's ability to get out of bed safely. Antidiarrheals are contraindicated in clients with severe dehydration, electrolyte imbalance, liver and renal disorders, and glaucoma. Opioid antidiarrheals should be used with caution in clients with a history of drug abuse. Adverse reactions occur more frequently in children, especially those with Down syndrome.

Client education as it relates to these drugs should include goals, reasons for obtaining baseline data such as vital signs and abdominal assessment, and possible side effects. The following are other important points to include when teaching clients regarding antidiarrheals:

- Seek medical care for diarrhea that does not resolve within 2 days, or if a fever develops or dehydration occurs. (Infants, children, and older adults are at greatest risk and may need medical attention sooner.)
- Discontinue medication once frequent or watery stools have stopped.
- Seek medical care if the presence of blood is found in the stool.

See Nursing Process Focus: Clients Receiving Antidiarrheal Therapy for additional teaching points.

CONNECTIONS | Special Considerations

◀ Cultural Remedies for Diarrhea

Because diarrhea is an age-old malady that affects all populations, different cultures have adopted tried-and-true symptomatic remedies for the condition. One preparation, used by people in many regions of the world, is cornstarch (a heaping teaspoonful) in a glass of tepid water. For centuries, mothers have boiled rice and given the diluted rice water to babies with diarrhea. The rationale behind these two therapies is that they work by absorbing excess water in the intestines, thus stopping the diarrhea. Although a rationale was not related in earlier times, people of many cultures found that eating grated apple that had turned brown alleviated symptoms. This apparently evolved into what is known today as the ABCs of diarrhea treatment: apples, bananas (just barely ripe), and carrots. The underlying principle is that the pectin present in these foods oxidizes, producing the same ingredient found in many OTC diarrhea medicines. Packets of oral rehydration salts (ORS) that include sodium, potassium, and glucose to be mixed in water (245 mOsm/L) are recommended by the World Health Organization (WHO) for home management of diarrhea. Current recommendations can be found on the WHO's website.

PROTOTYPE DRUG | Diphenoxylate with Atropine (Lomotil)

Actions and Uses: The primary antidiarrheal ingredient in Lomotil is diphenoxylate. Like other opioids, diphenoxylate slows peristalsis, allowing time for additional water reabsorption from the colon and formation of more solid stools. It acts within 45 to 60 minutes. It is effective for moderate to severe diarrhea, but it is not recommended for children. The atropine in Lomotil is not added for its anticholinergic effect but to discourage clients from taking too much of the drug.

Pharmacokinetics: Diphenoxylate is well absorbed, enters breast milk, and is mostly metabolized by the liver. It has a half-life of 2.5 hours.

Administration Alert:

- Diphenoxylate is pregnancy category C.

Adverse Effects and Interactions: Unlike most opioids, diphenoxylate has no analgesic properties and has an extremely low potential for abuse. Some clients experience dizziness or drowsiness, and care should be taken not to drive or operate machinery until the effects of the drug are known.

Diphenoxylate with atropine interacts with several other drugs. For example, other CNS depressants, including alcohol, will add to its CNS depressant effect. At higher doses, the anticholinergic effects of atropine may be observed, which include drowsiness, dry mouth, and tachycardia. When taken with monoamine oxidase (MAO) inhibitors, diphenoxylate may cause hypertensive crisis.

CONNECTIONS | Natural Therapies

◀ Probiotics for Diarrhea

Lactobacillus acidophilus is a probiotic bacterium normally found in the human alimentary canal and the vagina. It is considered to be protective, inhibiting the growth of potentially pathogenic species such as *Escherichia coli, Candida albicans, Helicobacter pylori,* and *Gardnerella vaginalis.* One mechanism used by *L. acidophilus* to limit the growth of other bacterial species is the generation of hydrogen peroxide, which is toxic to most cells.

The primary use of *L. acidophilus* is to restore the normal flora of the intestine after diarrhea, particularly from antibiotic therapy. This probiotic may also help to restore normal microflora in the vagina, although the evidence for this effect is not conclusive. *L. acidophilus* may be obtained by drinking *L. acidophilus* milk or by eating yogurt or kefir containing live (or active) cultures. Those who wish to obtain *L. acidophilus* from yogurt should read labels carefully because not all products contain active cultures; frozen yogurt contains no active cultures. Supplements include capsules, tablets, and granules. Doses are not standardized, and tablet doses range from 50 to 500 mg.

CONNECTIONS | Lifespan Considerations

◀ Management of Diarrhea

- Infants, children, and older adults with diarrhea are at risk for rapidly occurring dehydration and electrolyte imbalance.
- Rehydration and electrolyte replacement are important components of treatment.
- Antidiarrheals are not generally used during pregnancy and lactation.
- Clients of all ages should be advised to seek medical care if diarrhea does not resolve within 2 days or if fever or dehydration occurs.
- Elderly clients are at increased risk for falls related to the drowsiness that may occur with dehydration and opioid antidiarrheals.

NURSING PROCESS FOCUS

Clients Receiving Antidiarrheal Therapy

Assessment	Potential Nursing Diagnoses/Identified Patterns
Prior to administration: • Obtain complete health history, including allergies, drug history, and possible drug interactions. • Assess sodium, chloride, and potassium levels. • Evaluate results of stool culture. • Assess for presence of dehydration. • Obtain vital signs and electrocardiogram (ECG).	• Risk for fluid volume: deficit related to fluid loss from diarrhea • Risk for injury (falls) related to drowsiness, a side effect of drug therapy

---

Planning: Client Goals and Expected Outcomes

The client will:

- Report relief of diarrhea
- Demonstrate an understanding of the drug's action by accurately describing drug side effects and precautions
- Immediately report effects such as persistent diarrhea, constipation, abdominal pain, blood in stool, confusion, dizziness, or fever

---

Implementation

Interventions (Rationales)	Client Education/Discharge Planning
• Monitor frequency, volume, and consistency of stools. (This will determine the effectiveness of drug therapy.) • Minimize the risk of dehydration and electrolyte imbalance. (These may occur secondary to diarrhea.) • Prevent accidental overdosage. • Monitor for dry mouth. (This is a side effect of the medications.) • Initiate safety measures to prevent falls. (These medications may cause drowsiness.) • Monitor electrolyte levels.	Advise client to: • Record the frequency of stools • Note if any blood is present in stools • Report immediately any abdominal pain or abdominal distention • Instruct client to increase fluid intake and drink electrolyte-enriched fluids • Instruct client to include foods that will minimize diarrhea, such as yogurt, bland foods, and foods high in pectin (apples, bananas, and citrus fruits) • Advise client who is using liquid preparations to use the dropper included to measure medication dosage. Do not use household measurements • Advise client to suck on ice or sour candy or to chew gum to relieve sensation of dry mouth Advise client to: • Refrain from driving or performing hazardous activities until the effects of drug are known • Abstain from using alcohol and other CNS depressants Advise client to: • Keep all laboratory appointments • Report weakness and muscle cramping

---

Evaluation of Outcome Criteria

Evaluate the effectiveness of drug therapy by confirming that client goals and expected outcomes have been met (see "Planning").

See Table 35.2 for a list of drugs to which these nursing actions apply.

CONNECTIONS ▸ **Special Considerations**

◀ Treatment for Watery Diarrhea in Infants and Children

- Oral rehydration solutions should be used routinely for watery diarrhea and dehydration.
- Feeding should be continued through rehydration to maintain nutrition.
- Antimotility drugs (e.g., loperamide and diphenoxylate with atropine [Lomotil]) should not be used due to safety considerations.
- Acetorphan (not yet available in Canada) is a safe and effective antisecretory drug that can be used routinely.
- Bismuth subsalicylate is an effective and generally safe antisecretory drug; it should not be given in the presence of chickenpox or influenza because of the danger of Reye's syndrome.
- Kaolin-pectin, fibre, and activated charcoal should not be used.
- Some *Lactobacillus* species may be used to modify intestinal flora.
- Folic acid and vitamin A are indicated only in cases of overt deficiency.
- Antibiotics should be used sparingly except in cases of severe bacterial diarrhea.
- Zinc therapy may be useful in malnourished children.

Source: Recommendations of the Canadian Paediatric Society's Nutrition Committee, February 2006, http://www.cps.ca/.

NAUSEA AND VOMITING

Nausea is an unpleasant, subjective sensation that usually occurs in the midepigastrium and is accompanied by weakness, diaphoresis, and hyperproduction of saliva. It is sometimes accompanied by dizziness. Intense nausea often leads to vomiting, or **emesis**, in which the stomach contents are forced upward into the esophagus and out the mouth.

Pathophysiology of Nausea and Vomiting

35.5 Vomiting is a defence mechanism used by the body to rid itself of toxic substances. Nausea is an uncomfortable feeling that may precede vomiting.

Vomiting is a defence mechanism used by the body to rid itself of toxic substances. Vomiting is a reflex primarily controlled by a portion of the medulla of the brain known as the **vomiting centre**, which receives sensory signals from the digestive tract, the inner ear, and the cerebral cortex. Interestingly, the vomiting centre is not protected by the blood-brain barrier, as is the vast majority of the brain. These neurons can directly sense the presence of toxic substances in the blood. Once the vomiting reflex is triggered, wavelike contractions of the stomach quickly propel its contents up and out of the body.

Nausea and vomiting are common symptoms associated with a wide variety of conditions such as GI infections, food poisoning, stress, nervousness, emotional imbalances, changes in body position (motion sickness), and extreme pain. Other conditions that promote nausea and vomiting are general anesthetic agents, migraine headache, trauma to the head or abdominal organs, inner ear disorders, and diabetes. Psychological factors play a significant role, as clients often become nauseated during periods of extreme stress or when confronted with unpleasant sights, smells, or sounds.

The nausea and vomiting experienced by many women during the first trimester of pregnancy is referred to as morning sickness. Should this become acute, with continual vomiting, this condition may lead to hyperemesis gravidarum, a situation in which the health and safety of the mother and developing baby can become severely compromised. Pharmacotherapy is initiated only after other antinausea measures have been ineffective.

Many drugs, by their chemical nature, bring about nausea or vomiting as a side effect. The most extreme example of this occurs with the antineoplastic drugs, most of which cause intense nausea and vomiting.

The foremost problem secondary to nausea and vomiting is dehydration. When large amounts of fluids are vomited, water in the plasma moves from the blood to other body tissues, resulting in dehydration. Because the contents lost from the stomach are strongly acidic, vomiting may cause a change in the pH of the blood, resulting in metabolic alkalosis. With excessive loss, severe acid-base disturbances can lead to vascular collapse that results in death if medical intervention is not initiated. Dehydration is exceptionally dangerous for infants, small children, and older adults and is evidenced by dry mouth, sticky saliva, and reduced urine output with urine that is dark yellow-orange to brown.

Nausea and vomiting may be prevented or alleviated with natural remedies or by the use of drugs from several different classes. The treatment goal for nausea or vomiting is removal of the cause, when feasible.

Drugs from at least seven different classes are used to prevent nausea and vomiting. Many of these act by inhibiting dopamine or serotonin receptors in the brain. The antiemetics are shown in Table 35.3.

Pharmacotherapy with Antiemetics

35.6 Symptomatic treatment of nausea and vomiting includes drugs from many different classes, including phenolthiazines, antihistamines, cannabinoids, corticosteroids, benzodiazepines, and serotonin receptor antagonists.

A large number of **antiemetics** are available to treat nausea and vomiting, and selection of a particular agent depends on the experience of the healthcare provider and the cause of the nausea. For example, nausea due to motion sickness is effectively treated with anticholinergics or antihistamines. Nausea and vomiting associated with antineoplastic agents is often

TABLE 35.3   Select Antiemetics

Drug	Route and Adult Dose
Anticholinergics	
scopolamine (Buscopan, Hyoscine, Transderm-V)	Patch, apply 1 patch to hairless area behind the ear at least 4 hours prior to exposure and every 3 days as needed; SC, 0.6-1 mg tid-qid; PO, 10-20 mg/day
Antihistamines	
dimenhydrinate (Gravol)	PO, 50–100 mg q4–6h (max 400 mg/day)
diphenhydramine (Benadryl) (see Chapter 42, page 504, for the Prototype Drug box)	PO, 25–50 mg tid–qid (max 300 mg/day)
hydroxyzine (Atarax)	IM, 25-100 mg/dose
Cannabinoids	
cannabidiol (Sativex)	Buccal, 1 spray every 4 hours (q4h) PRN (max 4 sprays per day)
Glucocorticoids	
dexamethasone (Dexasone)	PO, 0.25–4 mg bid–qid
methylprednisolone (Solu-Medrol)	PO, 4–48 mg/day in divided doses IV, 40–250 mg q4–6h
Phenothiazines and Phenothiazine-Like Agents	
metoclopramide (Metonia, Maxeran)	PO, 2 mg/kg 1 hour prior to chemotherapy
perphenazine	PO, 8–16 mg bid–qid
Pr prochlorperazine (Stemetil)	PO, 5–10 mg tid or qid (max 40 mg/day)
promethazine (Histanil, Phenergan)	PO/IM/IV/rectal, 12.5 to 25 mg every 4 to 6 hours PRN
Serotonin Receptor Antagonists	
dolasetron (Anzemet)	PO, 100 mg 1 hour prior to chemotherapy
granisetron	IV, 10 µg/kg 30 minutes prior to chemotherapy
ondansetron (Zofran)	PO, 4-8 mg tid PRN

treated with the phenothiazines, glucocorticoids, or serotonin receptor blockers. Aprepitant (Emend) is the first of a new class of antiemetic, the neurokinin receptor antagonists, used to prevent nausea and vomiting after antineoplastic therapy. To prevent loss of the medication due to vomiting, many antiemetics are administered through the IM, IV, or suppository routes.

Clients who are receiving antineoplastic drugs may receive three or more antiemetics to reduce the nausea and vomiting from chemotherapy. In fact, therapy with antineoplastic drugs is one of the most common reasons why antiemetic drugs are prescribed.

Motion sickness is a disorder that affects a portion of the inner ear known as the **vestibular apparatus** that is associated with significant nausea. The most common drug used for motion sickness is scopolamine, which is usually administered as a transdermal patch. Antihistamines such as dimenhydrinate

(Gravol) and meclizine are also effective but may cause significant drowsiness in some clients. Drugs used to treat motion sickness are most effective when taken 20 to 60 minutes before travel is expected.

On some occasions, it is desirable to *stimulate* the vomiting reflex with drugs called **emetics**. Indications for emetics include ingestion of poisons and overdoses of oral drugs. Ipecac syrup, given orally, or apomorphine (Apokyn), given subcutaneously (SC), will induce vomiting in about 15 minutes.

Nursing Considerations

The role of the nurse in antiemetic therapy involves careful monitoring of the client's condition and providing education as it relates to the prescribed drug regimen. Assess symptoms that precipitated the vomiting or that are occurring concurrently. If a client becomes sedated and continues to vomit, a nasogastric tube insertion with suction may be indicated. Antiemetics are contraindicated in clients who are hypersensitive to the drugs, have bone marrow depression, are comatose, or experience vomiting of unknown cause. These drugs are used with caution in clients with breast cancer. Client safety is a concern, as drowsiness is a frequent side effect of antiemetics. Clients may be at risk for falls because of medication side effects and sensation of weakness from vomiting. Orthostatic hypotension is a side effect of some antiemetics.

Drugs used to stimulate emesis should be used only in emergency situations under the direction of a healthcare provider. They are used only when the client is alert, because of the risk for aspiration. When the client is comatose, a gastric lavage tube is placed and attached to suction to empty gastric contents.

Client education as it relates to antiemetics should include goals, reasons for obtaining baseline data such as vital signs and abdominal assessment, and possible side effects. The following are important points to include when teaching clients regarding antiemetics:

- Use assistance to get out of bed until effects of the medication are known.
- Avoid driving and performing hazardous tasks.
- If blood is vomited or if the vomiting is associated with severe abdominal pain, notify the healthcare provider immediately.
- Do not use OTC antiemetics for prolonged periods; vomiting may be a symptom of a serious disorder that requires medical attention.
- Before inducing vomiting with an OTC emetic, check with the healthcare provider; some poisons and caustic chemicals should not be vomited.

PROTOTYPE DRUG | **Prochlorperazine (Stemetil)**

Actions and Uses: Prochlorperazine is a phenothiazine, a class of drug usually prescribed for psychoses (see Chapter 19). The phenothiazines are the largest group of drugs prescribed for severe nausea and vomiting, and prochlorperazine is the most frequently prescribed antiemetic in its class. Prochlorperazine acts by blocking dopamine receptors in the brain, which inhibits signals to the vomiting centre in the medulla.

Pharmacokinetics: Prochlorperazine is frequently given intramuscularly (IM) or rectally, whereby absorption is more consistent than when given orally. It is widely distributed and is about 90% protein bound. It is highly metabolized by the liver. Its half-life is unknown.

Administration Alerts:

- Administer oral dosage 2 hours before or after antacids and antidiarrheals.
- Prochlorperazine is pregnancy category C.

Adverse Effects and Interactions: Prochlorperazine produces dose-related anticholinergic side effects such as dry mouth, sedation, constipation, orthostatic hypotension, and tachycardia. When used for prolonged periods at higher doses, extrapyramidal symptoms resembling those of Parkinson's disease are a serious concern.

Prochlorperazine interacts with alcohol to increase central nervous system (CNS) depression. Antacids and antidiarrheals inhibit absorption of prochlorperazine. When taken with phenobarbital (Phenobarb), metabolism of prochlorperazine is increased.

INFLAMMATORY BOWEL DISEASE

35.7 Inflammatory bowel disease is treated with immunosuppressants and anti-inflammatory drugs.

Inflammatory bowel disease (IBD) is characterized by the presence of ulcers in the intestinal tract. Crohn's disease or Crohn's lesions typically appear in the distal region of the small intestine (terminal **ileum**), although they can affect any region of the GI tract from the mouth to the anus. Crohn's lesions usually are discontinuous: affected areas of the intestinal mucosa alternate with normal areas. The mucosal erosions characteristic of ulcerative colitis begin in the rectum and progress in an uninterrupted manner throughout the rest of the large intestine. Approximately 233 000 Canadians live with IBD: 129 000 with Crohn's disease and 10 000 with ulcerative colitis. More than 10 200 new cases are diagnosed each year: 5700 cases of Crohn's disease and 4500 cases of ulcerative colitis. Canada has among the highest reported prevalence (number of people) and incidence (number of new cases per year) rates of IBD in the world. Currently, the prevalence of IBD in Canada is nearly 0.7%, which equates to more than 1 in 150 Canadians.

The etiology of IBD remains largely unknown. Several genes involved with immune responses are associated with the disorder. It is hypothesized that these defective genes cause hyperactivity of T-cell responses to normal flora in the terminal ileum and colon. These hyperactive responses result in chronic intestinal inflammation.

In addition to genetic susceptibility, certain environmental triggers exacerbate symptoms of IBD. The best studied trigger for Crohn's disease is smoking. Infections, the use of NSAIDs, and a high level of stress are additional environmental factors that have been identified. Less well known are triggers for ulcerative colitis; in many clients, triggers cannot be identified. It is known that symptoms of ulcerative colitis tend to peak between ages 15 and 30 and again between ages 50 and 70.

Symptoms of IBD range from mild to acute, and the condition is characterized by alternating periods of remission and exacerbation. The most common clinical presentation of ulcerative colitis is abdominal cramping with frequent bowel movements. Severe disease may lead to weight loss, bloody diarrhea, high fever, and dehydration. The client with Crohn's disease also is seen abdominal pain, cramping, and diarrhea, which may have been present for years before seeking treatment. Symptoms of Crohn's disease are often similar to those of ulcerative colitis. Clients with IBD have an increased risk for acquiring GI cancer.

The expected outcomes for the pharmacotherapy of IBD are as follows:

- Reduce the acute symptoms of active disease by induction therapy and place the disease in remission.
- Keep the disease in remission with maintenance therapy.
- Change the natural course or progression of the disease.

Multiple medications are used to treat IBD, and pharmacotherapy is conducted in a stepwise manner, starting with the safest and best established medications for the disorder. The first step of IBD treatment is usually with 5-aminosalicylic acid (5-ASA) agents that include sulfasalazine (Salazopurin), olsalazine (Dipentum), balsalazide (Colazal), and mesalamine (Asacol, Pentasa, Salofalk). These drugs act rapidly and exhibit a higher safety profile than the second-line agents. While effective at initially reducing symptoms, the 5-ASA medications are not as effective at maintaining remission.

When IBD symptoms are more intense or when clients have not responded well to the 5-ASA drugs, oral corticosteroids such as prednisone are used. Because of their potentially serious long-term adverse effects, however, they are prescribed for the shortest length of time needed to send the disease into remission. In hospitalized clients, IV corticosteroids may be used to put IBD into remission. For a detailed discussion of corticosteroid therapy, refer to Chapter 30.

IRRITABLE BOWEL SYNDROME

35.8 Irritable bowel syndrome is treated with dietary management, symptomatic therapy, and drugs that regulate intestinal motility.

As discussed earlier in the chapter, irritable bowel syndrome (IBS), also known as spastic colon or mucous colitis, is a common disorder of the lower GI tract characterized by symptoms that include abdominal pain, visible bloating, excessive gas, and colicky cramping. Bowel habits are altered, with diarrhea alternating with constipation, and there may be mucus in the stool. Pain is usually relieved by defecation, although the client usually feels as if the evacuation is incomplete. Symptoms of IBS are likely caused by altered GI motility, increased peristalsis, and increased pain sensitivity of the GI tract.

The diagnosis of IBS is sometimes one of exclusion, ruling out other diseases such as colon cancer, ulcerative colitis, intestinal infections, Crohn's disease, and diverticulitis. It is not a precursor of more serious disease, and symptoms such as bleeding, anorexia, weight loss, or fever are not usually experienced by clients with IBS. IBS is considered a functional bowel disorder, meaning that the normal operation of the digestive tract is impaired without the presence of detectable organic disease. A diagnosis of IBS requires that the client has experienced recurrent abdominal pain or discomfort for at least 3 days per month during the previous 3 months that is associated with two or more of the following:

- Relieved by defecation
- Onset associated with a change in stool frequency
- Onset associated with a change in stool form or appearance

Treatment of IBS is supportive, with drug therapy targeted at symptomatic treatment depending on whether constipation or diarrhea is the predominant symptom. There is no single treatment that is effective for all, or even most, clients.

Lifestyle Changes, Diet, and Aggravating Medications

Stress is not a cause of IBS, but it can influence the condition. Attempts should be made to identify stressors and develop positive coping strategies. Psychotherapy, relaxation techniques, and hypnosis may benefit some clients. Food-specific triggers are not always apparent. However, the client should keep a food diary in an attempt to recognize and avoid foods that appear to worsen the condition. Dietary restriction of caffeine, wheat, or lactose-based products may be attempted. Foods that cause bloating and flatulence such as beans, cabbage, and peas should be avoided.

Part of a medical history for IBS should include drugs that may be contributing to the symptoms of IBS. Common drugs that may cause constipation include NSAIDs, calcium channel blockers, anticholinergics, and opioids. Diarrhea may result from the use of laxatives, magnesium-containing antacids, or antibiotics. Sometimes a change in medication can help to reduce IBS symptoms.

Dietary Fibre and Laxatives

Constipation, diarrhea, cramping, painful bowel movements, and rectal urgency occur frequently in clients with IBS. Because constipation and diarrhea often alternate, pharmacotherapy can be challenging. Fibre supplementation with non-prescription bulk laxatives such as psyllium has long been recommended as a treatment for IBS and can help to regulate bowel movements to bring relief to some clients. Unfortunately, increased fibre intake will worsen the symptoms in some clients. Loperamide, an antidiarrheal, is effective at relieving symptoms of diarrhea in clients with IBS.

Antidepressant Therapy

For many years the tricyclic antidepressants such as amitriptyline (Elavil), desipramine, and doxepin (Sinequan) have been used to treat clients with IBS who have pain as a major symptom. Studies on the effectiveness of these drugs in reducing pain and diarrhea in clients with IBS are conflicting, but they may be indicated for those who have depression as a comorbid condition. Selective serotonin reuptake inhibitors (SSRIs) such as paroxetine (Paxil) have also been studied, but results suggest that their effectiveness at treating IBS is mild at best. While antidepressants may relieve pain for some clients, they are not first-line drugs for IBS.

Drug-Specific Therapies

Alosetron (Lotronex) is a serotonin (5-HT$_3$) antagonist approved for diarrhea-predominant IBS in women.

Drugs that are used to treat IBS do not alter the course of the disease and in some cases may actually worsen the symptoms. Research has not demonstrated that these drugs are any more effective than non-pharmacological treatments such as IBS support groups, relaxation therapy, or dietary changes. There is no prototype drug for this condition. Drugs that provide symptomatic relief for some clients include alosetron, antispasmodic drugs (dicyclomine [Bentylol] and hyoscyamine [Levsin]), linaclotide (Constella), and lubiprostone (Amitiza).

PANCREATITIS

The pancreas secretes essential digestive enzymes. The enzymatic portion of pancreatic juice contains carboxypeptidase, chymotrypsin, and trypsin, which are converted to their active forms once they reach the small intestine. Three other pancreatic enzymes—lipase, amylase, and nuclease—are secreted in their active form but require the presence of bile for optimum activity. Because lack of secretion can result in malabsorption disorders, replacement therapy is sometimes required.

Pancreatitis results when amylase and lipase remain in the pancreas rather than being released into the **duodenum**. The enzymes escape into the surrounding tissue, causing inflammation in the pancreas, or pancreatitis. Pancreatitis can be either acute or chronic.

Pharmacotherapy of Pancreatitis

35.9 Pancreatitis results when pancreatic enzymes are trapped in the pancreas and are not released into the duodenum. Pharmacotherapy includes replacement enzymes and supportive drugs for pain relief and gastric acid reduction.

Acute pancreatitis usually occurs in middle-aged adults and is often associated with gallstones in women and alcoholism in men. Symptoms of acute pancreatitis present suddenly, often after eating a fatty meal or consuming excessive amounts of alcohol. The most common symptom is a continuous, severe pain in the epigastric area that often radiates to the back. Laboratory reports may reveal elevated serum amylase and lipase as well as hypocalcemia. Most clients recover from the illness and regain normal pancreatic function. Some clients have recurrent attacks and progress to chronic pancreatitis.

Many clients with acute pancreatitis require only bedrest and withholding of food and fluids by mouth for a few days for the symptoms to subside. For clients with acute pain, meperidine brings effective relief. To reduce or neutralize gastric secretions, H$_2$ blockers, such as cimetidine (Tagamet), or proton pump inhibitors, such as omeprazole (Losec), may be prescribed. To decrease the amount of pancreatic enzymes secreted, carbonic anhydrase inhibitors, such as acetazolamide (Diamox), or antispasmodics, such as dicyclomine, may be prescribed. In particularly severe cases, IV fluids and total parenteral nutrition may be necessary.

Most cases of chronic pancreatitis are associated with alcoholism. Alcohol is thought to promote the formation of insoluble proteins that occlude the pancreatic duct. Pancreatic juice is prevented from flowing into the duodenum and remains in the pancreas to damage cells and cause inflammation. Other causes include spasms of the hepatopancreatic sphincter and strictures or stones in the pancreatic duct system. Symptoms include chronic epigastric or left upper quadrant pain, anorexia, nausea, vomiting, and weight loss. **Steatorrhea**, the passing of bulky, foul-smelling, fatty stools, occurs late in the course of the disease.

Drugs prescribed for the treatment of acute pancreatitis may also be prescribed in cases of chronic pancreatitis. In addition, the client with chronic pancreatitis may require insulin and is likely to need anti-emetics and a pancreatic enzyme supplement such as pancrelipase or pancreatin to digest fats, proteins, and complex carbohydrates because chronic pancreatitis eventually leads to pancreatic insufficiency.

Nursing Considerations

The role of the nurse in pancreatic enzyme replacement therapy involves careful monitoring of the client's condition and providing education as it relates to the prescribed drug regimen. Assessment of the client with acute or chronic pancreatitis should include a complete assessment, physical examination, health history, psychosocial history, and lifestyle history. Obtain information about alcohol use and other drugs, tobacco use, and dietary habits. Spicy foods, gas-forming foods, cola drinks, coffee, and tea stimulate gastric and pancreatic secretions; assess the client for intake of these foods.

Assess and monitor the presence, amount, and type of pain as well as breathing patterns, which may be rapid and shallow due to pain. Assess the symmetry of the chest wall and the movement of the chest and diaphragm since the client with pancreatitis is at risk for atelectasis and can develop pleural effusion as a result of ineffective breathing patterns. Monitor blood gases, as hypoventilation can result in hypercapnia. The client may have other abnormal findings such as elevated serum and urinary amylase, and elevated serum bilirubin. Monitor the client's nutritional status and hydration status, which may be impaired due to nausea and vomiting. Assess for signs of infection. Contraindications include a history of allergy to pork protein or enzymes because the drug has a porcine (pork) origin. Safety in pregnancy and lactation has not been established.

Client education as it relates to pancreatic enzymes should include goals, reasons for obtaining baseline data such as vital signs and tests for cardiac and renal disorders, and possible side effects. Explain the importance of bedrest and a calm environment in decreasing metabolic rate, pain, and pancreatic secretions. The following are other important points to include when teaching clients regarding pancreatic enzyme replacement:

- Eliminate all alcohol, smoking, spicy foods, gas-forming foods, cola drinks, coffee, and tea.
- Restrict fat intake and eat smaller and more frequent meals.
- Take pancreatic enzymes with meals or snacks.
- Weigh self and report significant changes to the healthcare provider.
- Report pain and seek relief before it becomes intense.
- Report episodes of nausea and vomiting.
- Sitting up, leaning forward, or curling in a fetal position may help to decrease pain.
- Observe stools for colour, frequency, and consistency and report abnormalities.

◀ Psychosocial and Community Impacts of Alcohol-Related Pancreatitis

Clients with acute pancreatitis are most often middle aged; those with chronic pancreatitis are most often in their 50s or 60s. Clients whose pancreatitis is associated with gallstones may receive a different type and amount of support from significant others, from the community, and even from nurses compared with those who have pancreatitis associated with alcoholism. Nurses need to examine their feelings and attitudes related to alcoholism in general and to clients with alcoholism-associated pancreatitis in particular and will need to adopt attitudes to help the client attain treatment goals.

Clients who abuse alcohol often need referral to community agencies to manage their addiction and/or to remain in recovery. Family members may also need referral to community agencies for help in dealing with altered family processes due to the client's drinking and any role they may have played in enabling the client to abuse alcohol.

PROTOTYPE DRUG **Pancrelipase (Lipancreatin, Pancrease)**

Actions and Uses: Pancrelipase contains lipase, protease, and amylase of porcine origin. This agent facilitates the breakdown and conversion of lipids into glycerol and fatty acids, starches into dextrin and sugars, and proteins into peptides. It is used as replacement therapy for clients with insufficient pancreatic exocrine secretions.

Pancrelipase is available in powder, tablet, and delayed-release capsule formulations. On an equal-weight basis, pancrelipase is more potent than pancreatin, with 12 times the lipolytic activity. It also contains at least four times as much trypsin and amylase.

NCLEX Success Tip

Digestion begins in the mouth. Pancrelipase needs to be swallowed whole in order to reach the stomach before digestion begins and cannot be crushed, chewed, or held in the mouth. In order for the medication to be effective, it must be taken before meals or snacks. The medication needs to be stored in a dry place but does not require refrigeration.

Pharmacokinetics: Pancrelipase is given orally and acts locally in the GI tract. It is not absorbed and is excreted in the feces.

Administration Alerts:
- Do not crush or open enteric-coated tablets.
- Powder forms may be sprinkled on food.
- Give the drug with meals or 1 to 2 hours before meals, or as directed by the healthcare provider.
- Pancrelipase is pregnancy category C.

Adverse Effects and Interactions: Side effects of pancrelipase are uncommon since the enzymes are not absorbed. The most common side effects are GI symptoms of nausea, vomiting, and diarrhea. The drug can cause metabolic symptoms of hyperuricosuria.

Pancrelipase interacts with iron, which may result in decreased absorption of iron.

CHAPTER 35 Understanding the Chapter

Key Concepts Summary

The numbered key concepts provide a succinct summary of the important points from the corresponding numbered section within the chapter. If any of these points are not clear, refer to the numbered section within the chapter for review.

35.1 Constipation, the infrequent passage of hard, small stools, is a common disorder caused by slow motility of material through the large intestine.

35.2 Laxatives are drugs given to promote emptying of the large intestine by stimulating peristalsis, lubricating the fecal mass, or adding more bulk to the colon contents.

35.3 Diarrhea is an increase in the fluidity of feces that occurs when the colon fails to reabsorb enough water.

35.4 For simple diarrhea, OTC medications are effective. Opioids are the most effective drugs for controlling severe diarrhea.

35.5 Vomiting is a defence mechanism used by the body to rid itself of toxic substances. Nausea is an uncomfortable feeling that may precede vomiting.

35.6 Symptomatic treatment of nausea and vomiting includes drugs from many different classes, including phenolthiazines, antihistamines, cannabinoids, corticosteroids, benzodiazepines, and serotonin receptor antagonists.

35.7 Inflammatory bowel disease is treated with immunosuppressants and anti-inflammatory drugs.

35.8 Irritable bowel syndrome is treated with dietary management, symptomatic therapy, and drugs that regulate intestinal motility.

35.9 Pancreatitis results when pancreatic enzymes are trapped in the pancreas and are not released into the duodenum. Pharmacotherapy includes replacement enzymes and supportive drugs for pain relief and gastric acid reduction.

Chapter 35 Scenario

Kerry O'Grady is a 20-year-old university student who is studying to be a middle school teacher. She was diagnosed with IBS at the end of her first year of university after enduring multiple bouts of abdominal cramping, diarrhea, constipation, gas, and bloating. She thought these symptoms were caused by the stress of her first year of university because her symptoms eased over the summer break. Now the IBS has returned and diarrhea occurs more often than constipation. Some days she finds that she is unable to sit through an entire class without having to leave for the washroom. She is increasingly worried about her grades, and she is sure that the stress is not helping her condition either.

The doctor in the Student Health Services office has prescribed several weeks of dicyclomine (Bentylol) to be followed by loperamide (Imodium) after the diarrhea has slowed from the dicyclomine.

Critical Thinking Questions

1. How will the dicyclomine (Bentylol) and loperamide (Imodium) help to treat Kerry's symptoms?

2. Considering the adverse effects of dicyclomine and loperamide, what should you as the nurse teach Kerry about her university course schedule?

3. What other non-drug measures might Kerry try to ease her symptoms?

See Answers to Critical Thinking Questions in Appendix B.

NCLEX Practice Questions

1 A client is taking diphenoxylate with atropine (Lomotil). What does the nurse assess when monitoring for therapeutic effects?

   a. Reduction of abdominal cramping

   b. Minimal passage of flatus

   c. Decrease in loose, watery stools

   d. Increased bowel sounds

2 Ondansetron (Zofran) has been ordered prior to chemotherapy for a client receiving treatment for lymphoma. Prior to administering this drug, the nurse will review the client's past medical history for which condition?

   a. Allergy to soy and/or soy products

   b. History of chronic constipation

   c. Glaucoma

   d. Cardiac dysrhythmias

3 A nurse should question the order for pancrelipase (Pancreaze) for which client?

   a. A client with an allergy to pork products

   b. A client with hypertension

   c. A client with coronary artery disease

   d. A client with hypersensitivity to iodine products

4 A healthcare provider orders magnesium hydroxide (Milk of Magnesia) for a client with constipation, secondary to postoperative opioid use. Before administering the drug, the nurse will assess

   a. Blood pressure

   b. Dosage of the opioid drug prescribed

   c. The client's ability to ambulate to the bathroom

   d. Bowel sounds

5 A client asks the nurse about using an over-the-counter drug bismuth subsalicylate (Pepto-Bismol) to treat a daughter's diarrhea. On which of the following factors will the nurse base her recommendation? Select all that apply.

   a. Cause of diarrhea

   b. Normal activity level

   c. Age

   d. Weight

   e. School schedule

See Answers to NCLEX Practice Questions in Appendix A.

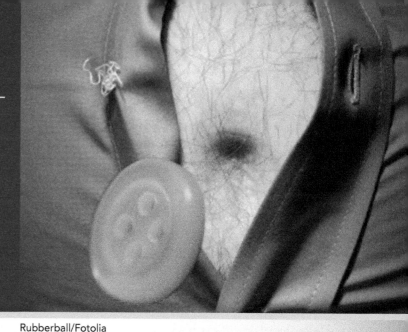

PROTOTYPE DRUGS

Pr *orlistat (Xenical)* **Anorexiants**	**Adjuncts to Obesity Therapy**

CHAPTER 36

Pharmacotherapy of Obesity and Weight Management

LEARNING OUTCOMES

After reading this chapter, the student should be able to:

1. Identify genetic and lifestyle factors that contribute to obesity.
2. Explain how energy imbalances can cause weight gain or loss.
3. Describe the role of the hypothalamus in regulating appetite.
4. Describe how obesity is measured.
5. Outline the major components of a successful weight management program.
6. Identify several weight loss agents that were removed from the market due to their adverse effects.
7. Describe the nurse's role in the pharmacological management of obesity.
8. For each of the drug classes listed in Prototype Drugs, identify the prototype and representative drugs and explain the mechanism(s) of drug action, primary indications, contraindications, significant drug interactions, pregnancy category, and important adverse effects.
9. Apply the nursing process to care for clients who are receiving antiobesity therapy.

CHAPTER OUTLINE

▶ Etiology of Obesity

▶ Measurement of Obesity

▶ Non-pharmacological Therapies for Obesity

▶ Pharmacotherapy with Drugs for Weight Loss

The Canadian Institute for Health information (www.cihi.ca) reports that 1 in 4 Canadians are obese. The cost of obesity to Canada's healthcare system stems from the comorbidities associated with obesity, such as diabetes and hypertension. Frequent visits to the hospital, the cost of medications, and treating long-term complications such as blindness (retinopathy from diabetes), dialysis (diabetes), and cerebrovascular accident (hypertension) compound the cost of health care. Missed workdays due to illness add to the overall economic burden. Some patients choose to undergo bariatric surgery, gastric balloons, and stomach ligation; all of these surgeries are extremely costly and often performed outside Canada. Once patients return to Canada, the Canadian healthcare system is responsible for the cost of potential complications from bariatric surgeries. The estimated total cost of all these factors is roughly $7 billion. Additional money is spent on attempts to lose weight. In the majority of cases, people experience little long-term success in sustaining their weight loss. Obesity is closely associated with increased health risks that include premature death, hypertension, hyperlipidemia, diabetes mellitus, heart disease, sleep apnea, osteoarthritis, and some cancers. This chapter examines the etiology, pathogenesis, and treatment of obesity.

Etiology of Obesity

36.1 Genetic and lifestyle factors contribute to the etiology of obesity.

Despite considerable research, the specific causes of obesity have not been identified. The etiology is likely a complex combination of genetic, lifestyle, and physiological factors. In a few cases, weight gain can be attributed to medical conditions, the most common being hypothyroidism. Certain rare disorders of the hypothalamus can also cause overeating. Drugs such as corticosteroids are clearly causes of weight gain.

Studies of family histories and twins support a strong genetic component to obesity. Researchers have identified a few genetic mutations that lead to obesity, although these are rare and do not contribute significantly to the extent of obesity currently observed in the population. Although a family history does not cause a person to be obese, it predisposes that person to weight gain. The predisposition is best overcome by preventing weight gain. This is particularly important in identifying children at risk for adult obesity and implementing interventions aimed at prevention.

Lifestyle factors play a key role in the development of obesity, the two most obvious factors being diet and physical activity. The fundamental shift in obesity levels in the past 3 decades has likely been due to high-fat, calorie-dense diets combined with sedentary lifestyles.

There are many theories on the relationship between specific dietary practices and obesity. Often these are fuelled by fad diets rather than research. While it is certainly true that the body metabolizes and stores carbohydrates, lipids, and proteins differently, no specific dietary nutrient limitation has been clearly demonstrated to prevent obesity or to result in more sustainable weight loss.

Despite the ongoing debate on the "best" diet, the fact remains that body weight is most likely determined by energy (calorie) balance. Simply stated, if the number of calories consumed equals the number of calories expended, the person will maintain (balance) body weight at the current level. Changes in weight occur when there is an energy imbalance.

Therefore, to lose weight one has to expend more calories than one consumes. In terms of weight loss or gain, the source of the calories—carbohydrates, proteins, or lipids—probably does not matter. Of course, the source is important in terms of overall health and wellness. Indeed, there remains considerable debate in the medical community as to which of the energy sources (carbohydrate, protein, or lipid) contributes the most to adult obesity.

The second half of the energy equation is energy expenditure. Physical activity expends calories and can result in either prevention of weight gain or a faster loss of weight. The most successful diet plans always combine a reduction in calories with an increase in physical activity.

Hunger occurs when the hypothalamus recognizes the levels of certain chemicals (glucose) or hormones (insulin) in the blood. Hunger is a normal physiological response that drives people to seek nourishment. Appetite is somewhat different from hunger. **Appetite** is a psychological response that drives food intake based on associations and memory. For example, people often eat not because they are experiencing hunger, but because it is a particular time of day or they find the act of eating pleasurable or social.

Measurement of Obesity

36.2 Obesity is measured by using the body mass index and waist circumference.

Obesity is defined by several different measures. In simple terms, obesity is being more than 20% above the ideal weight. The ideal weight fluctuates depending on the person's gender, height, and general build.

NCLEX Success Tips

The greatest determinant of childhood obesity is environmental factors, which include parental diet choices and influence. Children of obese parents are inclined to obesity based on the food served in the family home.

The most important factor predisposing to the development of type 2 diabetes mellitus is obesity. Insulin resistance increases with obesity. Obesity is a risk factor for osteoarthritis because it places increased stress on the joints.

The most commonly accepted measurement of obesity is the **body mass index (BMI)**. BMI is determined by dividing body weight (in kilograms) by the square of height (in metres). In adults, a BMI of 25 kg/m^2 indicates that the person is overweight. Obesity is defined by a BMI of 30 kg/m^2. BMI measurement is not accurate in athletes due to the higher proportion of muscle to fat in these persons.

NCLEX Success Tip

The most accurate way to determine whether an adolescent has a problem with obesity is to calculate the body mass index (BMI), which indicates a relationship between height and weight.

Another clinical measure of obesity is waist circumference, as measured by a simple tape measure. Waist circumference values of 80 cm (32 in.) for women and 94 cm (37 in.) for men are associated with increased health risk. Waist measurements greater than 88 cm for women and 102 cm for men have the greatest health risks. Waist circumference correlates well with BMI and also provides an estimate of abdominal (visceral) fat, which is more strongly associated with health risk than is fat stored in other regions of the body.

Non-pharmacological Therapies for Obesity

36.3 Non-pharmacological treatment of obesity should be attempted prior to initiating pharmacotherapy.

Prior to the initiation of drug therapy, the healthcare provider and client must first attempt to achieve weight management through non-pharmacological means. This involves making three major lifestyle changes, to diet, exercise, and behaviour modification. To obtain successful, sustained weight loss, lifestyle changes can be physically and emotionally demanding for a client who is obese.

Choosing a sustainable diet is often the biggest hurdle for clients. Although it may have taken decades or longer to become obese, no one wants it to take decades to lose weight. Weight loss schemes and fad diets that claim rapid weight loss while making few changes in dietary habits provide strong attractions to clients with obesity who are desperate to lose weight. The nurse should assist clients in setting realistic goals and steer them away from fad diets that may be unhealthy as well as unsuccessful. Severe restriction of any of the food groups—proteins, carbohydrates, or lipids—is not necessary or recommended by nutritionists. Examining the client's diet and reducing the normal intake to 1000 to 1200 kcal/day for women and 1200 to 1600 kcal/day for men is usually sufficient, although small, progressive steps will be needed to achieve these values in clients who are accustomed to consuming two to six times the recommended daily calorie values. Weight loss of 0.5 to 1 kg (1 to 2 lb.) per week is usually a realistic goal and is physically safe.

Exercise is an essential component of any weight management program. However, many clients with obesity have other chronic health problems that could affect an exercise program, the most common being diabetes, hypertension, and heart disease. The client should receive a thorough medical workup to be certain that there are no physical contraindications to starting an exercise program. The client who is obese should begin with very modest exercise goals and proceed to more challenging physical activity under the guidance of a healthcare provider. Exercise should be combined with calorie restriction because increased physical activity by itself is not an efficient method for losing weight.

Behaviour modification is another essential component of successful weight management programs. The client likely became obese due to poor eating habits and behaviours, which must be changed for the remainder of the person's life. For extremely obese clients, the weight loss program will extend for 1 year or longer; therefore, support groups should be encouraged. Breaking learned habits of eating is challenging, and relapses always occur. Support groups can provide valuable help in adjusting to new lifestyle patterns.

Surgery is an option for clients with extreme obesity who have a BMI over 40 kg/m^2 and who have been unsuccessful in conventional weight loss programs. Surgery involves either restricting the size of the stomach or bypassing it altogether. Restriction operations remove part of the stomach or place a band around it. This creates a smaller, pouchlike stomach that fills rapidly to give a feeling of fullness. The restriction operations result in weight loss because less food can be consumed. Bypass operations create a small stomach pouch and attach a portion of the jejunum to the pouch, essentially bypassing most of the stomach and duodenum. Bypass operations lead to weight loss because the lowered food intake is combined with malabsorption. Most clients who have obesity surgery experience significant weight loss: 50% to 75% of their excess weight within 1 year. Some do not lose weight, however, and 10% to 20% experience complications such as bleeding or require additional surgery due to stomal stenosis, which is narrowing of the connection between the stomach and intestines.

Pharmacotherapy with Drugs for Weight Loss

36.4 Drugs used for weight management affect appetite or the absorption of fats.

Despite the public's desire for effective drugs to induce weight loss, there are few such drugs on the market. The approved agents are used for the treatment of obesity, although they produce only modest effects.

Obesity may be defined as being more than 20% above the ideal body weight for one's height and age. Because of the prevalence of obesity in society and the difficulty most clients experience when following weight reduction plans for extended periods of time, drug manufacturers have long sought to develop safe drugs that induce weight loss. The quest for the "magic weight loss pill," however, has been disappointing. Indeed, many of the popular weight loss products have been discontinued due to health concerns. In the 1970s, amphetamine and dextroamphetamine (Dexedrine) were widely prescribed as **anorexiants** to reduce appetite; however, these drugs are addictive and are rarely prescribed for this purpose today. In the 1990s, the combination of fenfluramine and phentermine (Fen-Phen) was widely prescribed until fenfluramine was removed from the market for causing heart valve defects.

Attempts to produce drugs that promote safer weight loss by blocking lipid absorption resulted in orlistat (Xenical). Orlistat blocks the absorption of about 30% of dietary fat in the gastrointestinal (GI) tract by inhibiting GI lipases that are required for the systemic absorption of dietary triglycerides. Because orlistat may decrease absorption of other substances, including fat-soluble vitamins and some drugs, vitamin supplements and monitoring are often required. GI side effects such as flatus, oily fecal spotting, and abdominal discomfort can be avoided by restricting fat intake. GI side effects often diminish after 4 weeks of therapy. When combined with a reduced-calorie diet and moderate exercise, orlistat produces a gradual weight loss of about 10% of initial body weight over a period of 1 year.

Weight loss drugs are prescribed for clients with a BMI of at least 30 kg/m^2 or greater, or with a BMI of 27 kg/m^2 or greater when other risk factors for disease such as hypertension, hyperlipidemia, or diabetes exist.

Nursing Considerations

The role of the nurse in weight loss therapy involves careful monitoring of the client's condition and providing education as it relates to the prescribed drug regimen. With weight loss drugs, encourage lifestyle changes that will have a greater effect on weight reduction in the long term. Drugs for weight loss have limited effectiveness, and some have serious side effects.

Amphetamine and other stimulant-type anorexiants can be dangerous due to cardiovascular side effects such as hypertension, tachycardia, and dysrhythmias and due to their potential for dependence. Use of these drugs must be closely monitored. These drugs should not be used during pregnancy or lactation.

Orlistat is contraindicated in pregnancy and lactation (pregnancy category X), malabsorption syndrome, cholestasis, and obesity due to organic causes. Blood glucose levels should be monitored in clients with diabetes mellitus. Orlistat is used with caution in clients with frequent diarrhea and those with known deficiencies of fat-soluble vitamins. A fat-soluble vitamin supplement should be taken at least 2 hours before or after a dose of orlistat. Clients should be advised to take orlistat during or immediately following a meal containing fat.

Client education as it relates to these drugs should include goals, reasons for obtaining baseline data such as vital signs, and possible side effects. The following are important points to include when teaching clients regarding weight loss drugs:

- Lifestyle modifications are necessary for sustained weight loss to occur; the client should be encouraged to seek support groups for long-term weight management.
- Maintain close medical follow-up with amphetamine medications.
- Do not take any OTC or herbal medications without the healthcare provider's approval.
- Advise clients who are taking orlistat of the following:
  - Take a multivitamin each day.
  - Dose may be omitted if there is no fat present in the meal or if the meal is skipped.
  - Excessive flatus and fecal leakage may occur when a high-fat meal is consumed.

PROTOTYPE DRUG | **Orlistat (Xenical)**

Actions and Uses: Orlistat is only used in adults in order to assist in weight loss or to reduce the risk of regaining already lost weight in individuals who are obese. This medication must be used together with a reduced-calorie diet and improved exercise in order to obtain maximum benefit. Xenical produces its action by blocking fatty food absorption through the intestines.

Pharmacokinetics: Orlistat (Xenical) inhibits gastric and pancreatic lipases and, when these are blocked, triglycerides from the diet are not hydrolyzed and are therefore unabsorbable through the gastro-intestinal tract. Xenical primarily produces only a local action in the intestines and is taken orally; only trace amounts are absorbed into the blood stream. Excretion of the drug is mainly through the faeces.

Administration Alerts:
- Must not be taken by pregnant women as weight loss is not recommended in pregnancy.
- Should not be given to patients with gall bladder disease or chronic malabsorption syndrome, or history of eating disorders.
- Should not be given to clients under 18 years of age.
- Consider administering multivitamins to patients on orlistat (Vitamins A, D, E, K).

Adverse Effects and Interactions: Many gastro-intestinal side effects such as nausea, vomiting, flatulence, diarrhea, gas bloating, stomach pain, rectal pain, and loss of appetite have been reported in patients taking Xenical. Patients should report any adverse effects to their health care practitioner, including blood in urine, confusion, drowsiness, or mood changes. Xenical may also reduce the absorption of other oral medications administered at same time.

36 Understanding the Chapter

Key Concepts Summary

The numbered key concepts provide a succinct summary of the important points from the corresponding numbered section within the chapter. If any of these points are not clear, refer to the numbered section within the chapter for review.

36.1 Genetic and lifestyle factors contribute to the etiology of obesity.

36.2 Obesity is measured by using the body mass index and waist circumference.

36.3 Non-pharmacological treatment of obesity should be attempted prior to initiating pharmacotherapy.

36.4 Drugs used for weight management affect appetite or the absorption of fats.

Chapter 36 Scenario

Rosemary, a 55-year-old female, has just had her annual physical examination with the nurse practitioner. She was shocked to learn that she has gained just under 13.6 kg since her office visit 2 years ago, 7.7 kg in the last year alone. She went through menopause 2 years ago and thought that some of the mild edema and resulting weight gain she previously experienced around the time of her menses was over. Rosemary has always been under or at normal weight except for at the last office visit. At that time she was going through a personally stressful period and was not concerned about the weight gain. She works in an office as a financial manager, spending most of her day at her desk. Although she tries to get outside for a lunchtime walk, on most days there is just too much to do in the office.

The rest of her physical examination was unremarkable except for a borderline hypertensive reading on her blood pressure of 138/82 mm Hg. Her height is 1.6 metres, and she now weighs 79.5 kg. She states that she "watches what she eats" and normally eats three meals per day: a hurried breakfast of "something from the local fast-food place" on the drive to work, a sandwich at her desk or "whatever the rest of the office is ordering for takeout" for lunch, and a "regular dinner" at home

each night with her husband. On the evenings when her husband is not home for dinner, Rosemary picks up something at the local supermarket from the prepared food aisle. She also enjoys a glass of wine with dinner. When the nurse and Rosemary add up the approximate number of calories Rosemary consumes, the average total is more than 2000 per day. Rosemary is upset and asks the nurse about weight loss strategies.

Critical Thinking Questions

1. Rosemary asks about diet pills because her mother used to take them on occasion. What would you tell her about the availability of these drugs today?

2. Rosemary was prescribed orlistat (Xenical) by her GP, what does Rosemary need to know about orlistat before deciding to take it? What teaching does she need about taking orlistat?

3. What factors have contributed to Rosemary's weight gain over the past 2 years? What general health teaching would be appropriate for Rosemary to aid her in her weight reduction?

See Answers to Critical Thinking Questions in Appendix B.

NCLEX Practice Questions

1 A client has been started on orlistat (Xenical). The nurse will teach this client to take the medication

a. Once in the morning

b. When a feeling of hunger is noticed

c. Before daily exercise

d. Just prior to each meal containing fats

2 A nurse would instruct a client taking orlistat (Xenical) to do which of the following?

a. Drink at least 2 to 3 litres of diet soda per day.

b. Always wear sunscreen when outdoors or when exposed to direct sunlight.

c. Rise slowly from a sitting or supine position.

d. Take a daily vitamin supplement containing fat-soluble vitamins.

3 A nurse is instructing a client taking orlistat (Xenical) about adverse effects of the medication. Which symptoms indicate the presence of an expected adverse effect?

a. Flatus with discharge and oily stool

b. Heartburn and dyspepsia

c. Constipation with fecal impaction

d. Nausea with projectile vomiting

4 Which of the following measures is used to assess the presence of obesity? Select all that apply.

a. Body weight

b. Body mass index

c. Waist circumference

d. Treadmill test

e. Buoyancy analysis

See Answers to NCLEX Practice Questions in Appendix A.

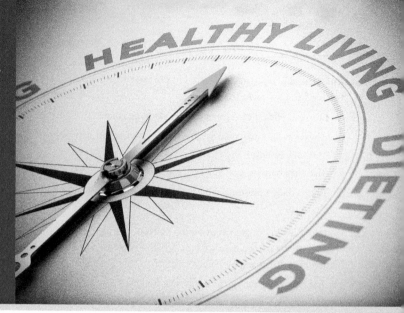

Panther Media GmbH/Alamy Stock Photo

PROTOTYPE DRUGS

VITAMINS
Lipid soluble
    Pr *vitamin A*
Water soluble
    Pr *folic acid*

MINERALS
Macrominerals

Pr *magnesium sulfate (Epsom Salts)*
Microminerals

NUTRITIONAL SUPPLEMENTS
Enteral nutrition
Parenteral nutrition

CHAPTER

37 Pharmacotherapy of Nutritional Disorders

LEARNING OUTCOMES

After reading this chapter, the student should be able to:

1. Identify drug classes used for treating nutritional disorders.

2. Explain the therapeutic action of common vitamins and minerals and conditions for which they may be beneficial.

3. Compare and contrast the properties of water-soluble and fat-soluble vitamins.

4. Compare and contrast the properties of macrominerals and trace minerals.

5. Compare and contrast enteral and parenteral methods of providing nutrition.

6. Identify differences among oligomeric, polymeric, modular, and specialized formulations for enteral nutrition.

7. For each of the drug classes listed in Prototype Drugs, identify a representative drug and explain its mechanism of action, therapeutic effects, and important adverse effects.

8. Describe and explain, based on pharmacological principles, the rationale for nursing assessment, planning, and interventions for clients with nutritional disorders.

9. Use the nursing process to care for clients who are receiving pharmacotherapy for nutritional disorders.

CHAPTER OUTLINE

▶ Vitamins

  ▶ Role of Vitamins in Maintaining Health

  ▶ Classification of Vitamins

  ▶ Recommended Dietary Reference Intakes

  ▶ Indications for Vitamin Pharmacotherapy

▶ Lipid-Soluble Vitamins

  ▶ Pharmacotherapy with Lipid-Soluble Vitamins

▶ Water-Soluble Vitamins

  ▶ Pharmacotherapy with Water-Soluble Vitamins

▶ Minerals

  ▶ Pharmacotherapy with Minerals

The nutritional supplement business is a multibillion-dollar industry. Although clever marketing often leads clients to believe that vitamin and dietary supplements are essential to maintain health, most people obtain all necessary nutrients through a balanced diet. Once the body has obtained the amounts of vitamins, minerals, and nutrients it needs to carry on metabolism, the excess is simply excreted or stored. In certain conditions, however, dietary supplementation is necessary and will benefit the client's health. This chapter focuses on these conditions and explores the role of vitamins, minerals, and nutritional supplements in pharmacology.

VITAMINS

Vitamins are essential substances needed in very small amounts to maintain homeostasis. Clients with a low or unbalanced dietary intake, those who are pregnant, or those experiencing a chronic disease may benefit from vitamin therapy.

CONNECTIONS Lifespan Considerations

◀ Vitamins, Minerals, and Other Nutrients

- Vitamin and mineral requirements change across the lifespan.
- Infants, children, and clients who are pregnant or lactating have different nutritional needs than the average adult.
- Administration of folic acid during pregnancy has been found to reduce birth defects in the nervous system of the baby.
- Heavy menstrual periods may result in significant iron loss.
- Perimenopausal women and older adults may benefit from calcium and vitamin D supplements to prevent osteoporosis.
- Adults over age 50 years absorb less vitamin B_{12} from food and may require fortified foods or a supplement.

Role of Vitamins in Maintaining Health

37.1 Vitamins are organic substances that are needed in small amounts to promote growth and maintain health. Deficiency of a vitamin will result in disease.

Vitamins are naturally occurring organic substances that are critical for metabolism as well as regulation of cell function and human growth and development. They contain carbon, are found in living organisms such as plants and animals, and function primarily as catalysts that speed up biochemical processes. Vitamins must be taken into the body from the external environment, usually through the diet, and are not manufactured by the body with the exception of vitamin D. Lack of sufficient amounts of vitamins results in symptoms of deficiency. People must consume vitamin supplements when their diet is lacking in these necessary nutrients or when they have health conditions that cause vitamin deficiencies. Most people have no need for vitamins as long as they eat a well-balanced diet. Vitamins can be destroyed by heat, sunlight, exposure to moisture and air, mould, and oxidation. Although a healthy diet is the best way to maintain adequate vitamin and mineral intake, individual supplements are available as an additional way to meet the minimum daily requirements for some people. However, it is important to remember that vitamin and mineral products should supplement a healthy balanced diet; they are not substitutes for good nutrition.

Since the discovery of thiamine in 1911, more than a dozen vitamins have been identified. Because scientists did not know the chemical structures of the vitamins when they were discovered, they assigned letters and numbers such as A, B_{12}, and C. These names are still widely used today.

An important characteristic of vitamins, with the exception of vitamin D, is that human cells cannot synthesize them. Vitamins, or their precursors known as **provitamins**, must be supplied in the diet. A second important characteristic is that if the vitamin is not present in adequate amounts, the body's metabolism will be disrupted and disease will result. Furthermore, the symptoms of the deficiency can be reversed by the administration of the missing vitamin.

Vitamins serve diverse and important roles. For example, the B complex vitamins are coenzymes essential to many metabolic pathways. Vitamin A is a precursor of retinal, a pigment needed for vision. Calcium metabolism is regulated by a hormone that is derived from vitamin D. Without vitamin K, abnormal prothrombin is produced and blood clotting is affected.

Classification of Vitamins

37.2 Vitamins are classified as lipid soluble (A, D, E, and K) or water soluble (C and B complex).

Vitamins are divided into two basic groups: those that dissolve in water (water soluble) and those that dissolve in lipids (fat soluble). Vitamin C and the B complex vitamins are the primary **water-soluble vitamins**. This group of vitamins is stored briefly in the body and then excreted in the urine. The body's supply of water-soluble vitamins must be replenished on a daily basis. One exception is vitamin B_{12}, which is stored in the liver. In contrast, **fat-soluble vitamins** are stored in the liver and fatty tissue of the human body and need only intermittent renewal. Because they are stored and not readily excreted, the possibility of toxicity from overdosing is greater with the fat-soluble group, which includes vitamins A, D, E, and K.

The difference in solubility affects the way the vitamins are absorbed by the gastrointestinal (GI) tract and stored in the body.

The water-soluble vitamins are absorbed with water in the digestive tract and readily dissolve in blood and body fluids. When excess water-soluble vitamins are absorbed, they cannot be stored for later use and are simply excreted in the urine. Because they are not stored to any significant degree, they must be ingested daily; otherwise, deficiencies will quickly develop.

Fat-soluble vitamins, on the other hand, cannot be absorbed in sufficient quantity in the small intestine unless they are ingested with lipids. These vitamins can be stored in large quantities in the liver and adipose tissue. Should the client not ingest sufficient amounts, fat-soluble vitamins are removed from storage depots in the body, as needed. Unfortunately, storage may lead to dangerously high levels of these vitamins if they are taken in excessive amounts.

Recommended Dietary Reference Intakes

37.3 Failure to meet the recommended dietary reference intake (DRI) for vitamins may result in deficiency disorders.

Scientists in Canada and the United States have been working together to establish nutrient recommendations based on the latest scientific research. These recommendations for the dietary intake of vitamins and other nutrients are called the **dietary reference intakes (DRIs)**. The DRI values represent the *average* amount of vitamin or other nutrient needed daily to prevent a deficiency in a healthy adult. The DRIs are revised periodically to reflect the latest scientific research. Current DRIs for vitamins are shown in Table 37.1.

TABLE 37.1 Vitamins

Vitamin	Function	RDI		Common Cause of Deficiency
		Men	**Women**	
A	Visual pigments, epithelial cells	900 µg (3000 IU)	700 µg (2333 IU)	Prolonged dietary deprivation, particularly when rice is the main food source; pancreatic disease; cirrhosis
B complex				
biotin	Coenzyme in metabolic reactions	30 µg	30 µg	Deficiencies are rare
cyanocobalamin, B_{12}	Coenzyme in nucleic acid metabolism	2.4 µg	2.4 µg	Lack of intrinsic factor; inadequate intake of foods of animal origin
folate, B_9	Coenzyme in amino acid and nucleic acid metabolism	400 µg	400 µg	Pregnancy (note that the RDI increases to 1000 µg during pregnancy); alcoholism; cancer; oral contraceptive use
niacin, B_3	Coenzyme in metabolic reactions	16 mg	14 mg	Prolonged dietary deprivation, particularly when corn (maize) or millet is the main food source; chronic diarrhea; liver disease; alcoholism
pantothenic acid, B_5	Coenzyme in metabolic reactions	5 mg	5 mg	Deficiencies are rare
pyridoxine, B_6	Coenzyme in amino acid metabolism	1.3 mg	1.3 mg	Alcoholism; oral contraceptive use; malabsorption diseases
riboflavin, B_2	Coenzyme in metabolic reactions	1.3 mg	1.1 mg	Inadequate consumption of milk or animal products; chronic diarrhea; liver disease; alcoholism
thiamine, B_1	Coenzyme in metabolic reactions	1.2 mg	1.1 mg	Prolonged dietary deprivation, particularly when rice is the main food source; hyperthyroidism; pregnancy; liver disease; alcoholism
C (ascorbic acid)	Coenzyme and antioxidant	90 mg	75 mg	Inadequate intake of fruits and vegetables; pregnancy; chronic inflammatory disease; burns; diarrhea; alcoholism

TABLE 37.1   Vitamins (continued)

D	Calcium and phosphate metabolism	5–15 µg*(200–600 IU)	5–15 µg*(200–600 IU)	Low dietary intake; inadequate exposure to sunlight *Several sources now recommend 25 µg (1000 IU)/day.
E	Antioxidant	15 mg	15 mg	Premature birth; malabsorption diseases
K	Cofactor in blood clotting	120 µg	95 µg	Newborns; liver disease; long-term parenteral nutrition; certain drugs such as cephalosporins and salicylates

NCLEX Success Tips

Intestinal bacteria synthesize such nutritional substances as vitamin K, thiamine, riboflavin, vitamin B_{12}, folic acid, biotin, and nicotinic acid. Antibiotic therapy may interfere with synthesis of these substances, including vitamin K.

Deficiencies of vitamin C results in a small-cell microcytic anemia. Broccoli, citrus fruits (such as oranges), and tomatoes are good sources of vitamin C.

Folate and vitamin B_{12} deficiencies result in a large-cell macrocytic anemia.

Good sources of vitamin B_{12} include meats and dairy products.

Three or more servings of dairy products meet the calcium requirement.

Spinach contains oxalates, which decrease the availability of calcium.

Vitamin A supplements can lead to anorexia, irritability, hair loss, and damage to the fetus.

Common food sources of vitamin A include dairy products, liver, egg yolks, fruits, and vegetables.

Pregnant women should avoid megadoses of vitamin A because fetal malformations may occur.

Vitamin E is a powerful antioxidant that helps to prevent oxidation of the cell membrane.

Vitamin, mineral, or herbal supplements should never substitute for a balanced diet. Furthermore, although the label on a vitamin supplement may indicate that it contains 100% of the DRI for a particular vitamin, the body may absorb as little as 10% to 15% of the amount ingested. With the exception of vitamins A and D, it is not harmful for most clients to consume two to three times the recommended level.

Health Canada, under the Food and Drugs Act, regulates labelling of food products. To help consumers select foods based on nutritional requirements, standardized Nutrition Facts tables are mandatory on most food products. As shown in Figure 37.1, the Nutrition Facts table lists the amount of calories and 13 core nutrients per serving of the product as well as the "% Daily Value" based on DRIs.

Nutrition Facts
Per 125 mL (87 g)

Amount	% Daily Value
Calories 80	
Fat 0.5 g	1 %
Saturated 0 g + Trans 0 g	0 %
Cholesterol 0 mg	
Sodium 0 mg	0 %
Carbohydrate 18 g	6 %
Fibre 2 g	8 %
Sugars 2 g	
Protein 3 g	

Vitamin A	2%	Vitamin C	10 %
Calcium	0%	Iron	2 %

Figure 37.1 Nutrition Facts table.

Indications for Vitamin Pharmacotherapy

37.4 Vitamin therapy is indicated for conditions such as poor nutritional intake, pregnancy, and chronic disease states.

Most clients who eat a normal, balanced diet are able to obtain all the necessary nutrients they need without vitamin supplementation. Indeed, megavitamin therapy is not only expensive, but also harmful to health if taken for prolonged periods. **Hypervitaminosis**, or toxic levels of vitamins, has been reported for vitamins A, C, D, E, B_6, niacin, and folic acid. In North America, syndromes of vitamin excess may actually be more common than those of vitamin deficiency.

Vitamin deficiencies follow certain patterns. The following are general characteristics of vitamin deficiency disorders:

* Clients more commonly present with multiple vitamin deficiencies than with a single vitamin deficiency.

* Symptoms of deficiency are nonspecific and often do not appear until the deficiency has been present for a prolonged period.

* Deficiencies in North Americans are most often the result of poverty, fad diets, chronic alcohol or drug abuse, or prolonged parenteral feeding.

Certain clients and conditions require higher levels of vitamins. Infancy and childhood are times of potential deficiency due to the high growth demands placed on the body. In addition, requirements for all nutrients are increased during pregnancy and lactation. With normal aging, the absorption of food diminishes and the quantity of ingested food is often reduced, leading to a higher risk of vitamin deficiencies in elderly clients. Vitamin deficiencies in clients with chronic liver and kidney disease are well documented.

Certain drugs affect vitamin metabolism. Alcohol is known for its ability to inhibit the absorption of thiamine and folic acid: alcohol abuse is the most common cause of thiamine deficiency in North America. Folic acid levels may be reduced in clients who are taking phenothiazines, oral contraceptives, phenytoin (Dilantin), or barbiturates. Vitamin D deficiency can be caused by therapy with certain anticonvulsants. Inhibition of vitamin B_{12} absorption has been reported with a number of drugs, including trifluoperazine, alcohol, and oral contraceptives. The nurse must be aware of these drug interactions and recommend vitamin therapy when appropriate.

LIPID-SOLUBLE VITAMINS

The lipid-soluble vitamins are abundant in both plant and animal foods and are relatively stable during cooking.

Pharmacotherapy with Lipid-Soluble Vitamins

37.5 Deficiencies of vitamins A, D, E, or K are indications for pharmacotherapy with lipid-soluble vitamins.

Lipid-soluble vitamins are absorbed from the intestine with dietary lipids and are stored primarily in the liver. When consumed in high amounts, these vitamins can accumulate to toxic levels and produce hypervitaminosis. Because these are over-the-counter (OTC) agents, clients must be strongly advised to carefully follow the instructions of the healthcare provider, or the label directions, for proper dosage. It is not unusual to find some OTC preparations that contain 200% to 400% of the DRI. Lipid-soluble vitamins for treating nutritional deficiency are listed in Table 37.2.

Vitamin A, also known as retinol, is obtained from foods that contain **carotenes**, which are precursors to vitamin A that are converted to retinol in the wall of the small intestine following absorption. The most abundant and biologically active carotene is beta-carotene. During metabolism, each molecule of beta-carotene yields two molecules of vitamin A. Good sources of dietary vitamin A include yellow and dark leafy vegetables, butter, eggs, whole milk, and liver.

Vitamin D is actually a group of chemicals that share similar activity. Vitamin D_2, also known as **ergocalciferol**, is obtained from fortified milk, margarine, and other dairy products. Vitamin D_3 is formed in the skin by a chemical reaction that requires ultraviolet radiation. The pharmacology of the D vitamins and a Prototype Drug for the active form of vitamin D are detailed in Chapter 61.

Vitamin E consists of about eight chemicals, called **tocopherols**, that have similar activity. Alpha-tocopherol comprises 90% of the tocopherols and is the only one of pharmacological importance. Dosage is sometimes reported as milligrams of alpha-tocopherol equivalents (TE). Vitamin E is found in plant seed oils, whole-grain cereals, eggs, and certain organ meats such as liver, pancreas, and heart. It is considered a primary antioxidant, preventing the formation of free radicals that damage cell membranes and cellular structures. Deficiency in adults has been observed only with severe malabsorption disorders; however, deficiency in premature neonates may lead to hemolytic anemia. Clients may self-administer vitamin E because it is thought to be useful in preventing heart disease and increasing sexual prowess. Unlike most other vitamins, therapeutic doses of vitamin E have not been clearly established, although supplements available OTC suggest doses of 100 to 400 units per day. In addition to oral and IM preparations, a topical form is available to treat dry, cracked skin.

Vitamin K is also a mixture of several chemicals. Vitamin K_1 is found in plant sources, particularly green leafy vegetables, tomatoes, cauliflower, egg yolks, liver, and cheese. Vitamin K_2 is synthesized by microbial flora in the colon. Deficiency states, caused by inadequate intake or by antibiotic destruction of normal intestinal flora, may result in delayed hemostasis. The body does not have large stores of vitamin K, and a deficiency may occur in only 1 to 2 weeks. Certain clotting factors (II, VII, IX, and X) are dependent on vitamin K for their biosynthesis. Vitamin K is used as a treatment for clients with clotting disorders and is the antidote for warfarin (Coumadin) overdose. It is also given to infants at birth to promote blood clotting. Administration of vitamin K completely reverses deficiency symptoms.

NCLEX Success Tips

Because green leafy vegetables are high in vitamin K, they are not recommended for clients receiving warfarin.

At birth, vitamin K-dependent blood-clotting factors are significantly decreased, and there is a transitory deficiency in blood coagulation during the second and fifth days of life. As a preventive measure, 0.5 to 1 mg of vitamin K is administered to the newborn during the first day of life to aid in blood clotting.

Vitamin K (phytonadione) helps with clotting factors. The newborn has no flora in the colon to develop clotting factors.

Vitamin K is given to the newborn to help stimulate clotting factors within the newborn body. The injection is given once and should be given prior to any invasive procedure that may cause bleeding.

Vitamin K is the antidote for warfarin excess.

Broad-spectrum antibiotics that destroy aerobic and anaerobic bacteria also destroy the normal flora of the GI tract, which are responsible for absorbing water and certain nutrients (such as vitamin K). Destruction of the GI flora, in turn, leads to diarrhea.

Vitamin B_6, folate, and vitamin B_{12} have been shown to reduce homocysteine levels.

For vitamin K synthesis in the intestines to begin, food and normal intestinal flora are needed. However, at birth, the neonate's intestines are sterile. Therefore, vitamin K is administered via injection to prevent a vitamin K deficiency that may result in a bleeding tendency. When administered, vitamin K promotes formation in the liver of clotting factors II, VII, IX, and X.

Vitamins B_6, B_{12}, and iron are important in the production of red blood cells. Therefore, the nurse should question the client specifically about food intake that contains these vitamins and minerals. Vitamin C helps iron absorption and plays a small role in red blood cell production.

Bran can interfere and decrease the absorption of digoxin (Lanoxin, Toloxin) resulting in unexpectedly low serum concentration levels.

The nurse should ask the client about alcohol use because heavy alcohol use causes fluid excretion, resulting in heavy losses of calcium in urine. If the client uses antacids containing aluminum or magnesium, a net loss of calcium can occur. If the client has a high-fibre diet, the fibre can bind up some of the dietary calcium.

TABLE 37.2   Lipid-Soluble Vitamins for Treating Nutritional Disorders

Drug	Route and Adult Dose
Pr vitamin A	Orally (PO), 500 000 IU/day for 3 days, followed by 50 000 IU/day for 2 weeks, then 10 000–20 000 IU/day for 2 months
	Intramuscular (IM), only indicated when oral administration is not feasible or when absorption is insufficient (malabsorption syndrome)
vitamin D: calcitriol (Calcijex, Rocaltrol)	PO, start with 0.25 μg/day; may increase dose by 0.25 μg/day at 2-4 week intervals (max 0.5-1 μg/day); discontinue use immediately for hyperkalemia
vitamin E: tocopherol (Aquasol E, Pro E)	PO, 60–75 IU/day
vitamin K: phytonadione (AquaMEPHYTON)	PO/subcutaneous (SC)/IM, 2.5–10 mg (up to 25 mg), may be repeated after 6–8 hours if needed

Nursing Considerations

The role of the nurse in drug therapy with fat-soluble vitamins involves careful monitoring of the client's condition and providing education as it relates to the prescribed drug regimen. The nurse is responsible for assessing, counselling, and monitoring clients who are taking fat-soluble vitamins. Because these vitamins are available OTC, clients consider them relatively harmless. The nurse should teach clients that excessive vitamin intake can be harmful.

For all fat-soluble vitamins, the nurse should begin with assessment for deficiency. The symptoms of inadequate supply or storage of fat-soluble vitamins are dependent on the specific nutrient. For example, clients who are deficient in vitamin A frequently report problems with night vision, skin lesions, or mucous membrane dysfunction. A baseline visual acuity exam should be performed. In severe vitamin D deficiency, clients experience skeletal abnormalities, such as rickets in children and osteomalacia in adults. The nurse should assess laboratory tests for serum levels of calcium, phosphorus, magnesium, alkaline phosphatase, and creatinine to determine electrolyte and mineral balance. An insufficient level of vitamin E has no obvious effects, but the vitamin is believed to protect cellular components from oxidation. Bleeding tendencies are characteristic of vitamin K deficiency. Clients should be assessed for impaired liver function, because fat-soluble vitamins are stored in the liver, and for malabsorption disorders that could prevent the absorption of the vitamins.

The nurse should also assess the client's dietary intake. Clients should be instructed about foods that may supply the necessary fat-soluble vitamins essential for good health. When performing dietary counselling, it is critical that the nurse consider the socioeconomic status and culture of the client when recommending foods that may be used to treat deficiency. The nurse should suggest foods that the client can afford and would eat.

Fat-soluble vitamins stored in the liver can accumulate to toxic levels, causing accidental hypervitaminosis. Chronic overdose will affect many organs, including the liver. Excessive vitamin A intake during pregnancy can result in severe birth defects. Intravenous infusion of vitamin K is only used in emergency situations because it may cause bronchospasm and respiratory or cardiac arrest. Large doses of vitamin E appear to be non-toxic; however, the nurse should monitor clients who are concurrently taking warfarin for increased risk for bleeding.

Client education as it relates to fat-soluble vitamins should include goals, reasons for obtaining baseline data such as laboratory tests for liver function and complete blood count (CBC), and possible side effects. The following are important points the nurse should include when teaching clients about fat-soluble vitamins:

- Take vitamins only as prescribed or as directed on the label. Do not double the dosage.
- Discontinue using the vitamin and notify the healthcare provider immediately if toxicity symptoms occur.
- Consult the healthcare provider before taking OTC drugs; they might contain additional fat-soluble vitamins and lead to toxicity.
- Include vitamin-rich foods in your diet to decrease the need for vitamin supplements.

PROTOTYPE DRUG	Vitamin A

Actions and Uses: Vitamin A is essential for general growth and development, particularly of the bones, teeth, and epithelial membranes. It is necessary for proper wound healing, essential for the biosynthesis of steroids, and is one of the pigments required

NURSING PROCESS FOCUS

Clients Receiving Vitamin A

Assessment	Potential Nursing Diagnoses/Identified Patterns
Prior to administration: - Obtain complete health history, including allergies, drug history, and possible drug interactions. - Obtain complete physical examination. - Assess for the presence or history of vitamin A deficiency, such as inadequate dietary intake, malabsorption diseases, and impaired liver function. - Obtain baseline vision acuity examination. - Assess integrity of skin and mucous membranes. - Obtain the following laboratory studies: serum vitamin A level, CBC, liver function profile, and serum protein/albumin levels.	- Nutritional deficiency - Disturbed sensory perception related to vitamin A deficiency - Risk for impaired skin integrity - Deficient knowledge regarding drug therapy

Planning: Client Goals and Expected Outcomes

The client will:

- Exhibit improvement in serum vitamin A level
- Demonstrate an understanding of the drug's action by accurately describing drug side effects and precautions
- Immediately report side effects such as increased nausea, vomiting, headache, loss of hair, lethargy, and malaise

Implementation	
Interventions (Rationales)	**Client Education/Discharge Planning**
• Monitor client's diet to determine intake of vitamin A foods. (Deficiency state may be caused by poor dietary habits.) • Periodically monitor visual acuity. (Vitamin A may cause miosis, papilledema, and nystagmus.) • Monitor for symptoms of vitamin A toxicity. (Storage of excess vitamin A can lead to hypervitaminosis.) • Monitor for signs of intracranial pressure. (Vitamin A may cause increased intracranial pressure if taken in large doses.) • Assess for use of mineral oil. (Mineral oil inhibits the absorption of vitamin A.) • Monitor for drug interactions with oral contraceptives. (Concurrent use of vitamin A and oral contraceptives can cause toxic levels of vitamin A.)	Instruct client to: • Maintain a dietary log for 48 hours • Eat foods rich in vitamin A, such as egg yolks, butter, milk, liver, dark leafy vegetables, and orange fruits and vegetables • Advise client to report any changes in vision Instruct client to: • Watch for signs and symptoms of vitamin A overdose such as nausea, vomiting, anorexia, dry skin and lips, headache, and loss of hair • Immediately stop taking medication if signs of toxicity are noted Instruct client to: • Follow dosage directions given by the healthcare provider or on the label • Immediately report any changes in neurological status such as increased sleepiness, headaches, lethargy, and malaise • Advise client to avoid laxatives that contain mineral oil Instruct client to: • Adhere to medication schedule and avoid double doses of the vitamin • Keep appointments for follow-up laboratory studies if taking oral contraceptives

Evaluation of Outcome Criteria

Evaluate the effectiveness of drug therapy by confirming that client goals and expected outcomes have been met (see "Planning").

for night vision. Vitamin A is indicated in deficiency states and during periods of increased need such as pregnancy, lactation, or debilitated states. Night blindness and slow wound healing can be effectively treated with as little as 30 000 IU of vitamin A given daily over a week. It is also prescribed for GI disorders when absorption in the small intestine is diminished or absent. Topical forms are available for acne, psoriasis, and other skin disorders. Doses of vitamin A are sometimes measured in retinoid equivalents (RE). In severe deficiency states, up to 500 000 IU may be given per day for 3 days, gradually tapering off to 10 000 to 20 000 IU/day.

Pharmacokinetics: Vitamin A is metabolized in the liver and GI tract and is excreted in urine and feces. It has a variable half-life.

Administration Alerts:
• Vitamin A is pregnancy category A at low doses.
• Vitamin A is pregnancy category X at doses above the DRI.

Adverse Effects and Interactions: Adverse effects are not observed with low doses of vitamin A. Acute ingestion produces serious central nervous system (CNS) toxicity, including headache, irritability, drowsiness, delirium, and possible coma. Long-term ingestion of high amounts causes drying and scaling of the skin, alopecia, fatigue, anorexia, vomiting, and leukopenia.

People taking vitamin A should avoid taking mineral oil and cholestyramine, as both may decrease the absorption of vitamin A.

WATER-SOLUBLE VITAMINS

The water-soluble vitamins consist of the B complex vitamins and vitamin C.

CONNECTIONS **Special Considerations**

◀ **Vitamin Supplements and Client Communication**

In the current culture, many people take vitamin supplements. Product advertising promotes vitamin supplements as a means to maintain optimal health. If taken in recommended dosages, vitamin toxicity is not a concern in healthy people; however, some vitamin supplements should be taken with caution, as they can interact with prescribed medications. Some food products are fortified with vitamins or minerals. For example, certain manufacturers claim that their cereals and juices have 100% of the DRI for particular vitamins and minerals. People who take supplements may not consider these fortified foods as vitamin sources, and accidental overdosage can result.

Healthcare providers should adopt a non-judgmental attitude that promotes trust and honest communication with the client. In this way, the client will be open about the use of vitamin and nutritional supplements. Acceptance and understanding are necessary to assist clients to take vitamins in a responsible way that does not compromise clinical drug treatment.

Pharmacotherapy with Water-Soluble Vitamins

37.6 Deficiencies of vitamin C, thiamine, niacin, riboflavin, folic acid, cyanocobalamin, or pyridoxine are indications for pharmacotherapy with water-soluble vitamins.

The B complex group is composed of 12 different vitamins that are grouped together because they were originally derived from

TABLE 37.3 Water-Soluble Vitamins for Treating Nutritional Disorders

Drug	Route and Adult Dose
vitamin B_1: thiamine (Betaxin)	PO, 5–30 mg/day IV/IM, 50–100 mg three times a day (tid)
vitamin B_2: riboflavin	PO, 100 mg once (qd) or twice per day (bid)
vitamin B_3: niacin (Niaspan, Niodan)	PO, 50 mg bid or 100 mg qd
vitamin B_6: pyridoxine	PO/IM/IV, 2.5–20 mg/day for 3 weeks, then may reduce to 2.5–5 mg/day
Pr vitamin B_9: folic acid	PO/IM/SC/IV, ≤ 1 mg/day
vitamin B_{12}: cyanocobalamin	PO, 1000–2000 µg/day for 1–2 weeks; maintenance dose is 1000 µg/day IM/deep SC, 100–1000 µg/month
vitamin C: ascorbic acid (Activa C, Apo-C, Bio-C, others)	PO/IV/IM/SC, 150–500 mg/day in 1 to 2 doses

yeast and foods that counteracted the disease beriberi. They have very different chemical structures and serve different metabolic functions. The B vitamins are known by their chemical name as well as their vitamin number. For example, vitamin B_{12} is also called cyanocobalamin. Water-soluble vitamins for treating nutritional deficiencies are given in Table 37.3.

NCLEX Success Tips

Clients who take sulfasalazine (Salazopurin) are susceptible to developing impaired folic acid absorption. Common clinical manifestations of a folic acid deficiency are gastrointestinal disturbances, such as anorexia, nausea, vomiting, and a smooth, beefy red tongue. The client should be encouraged to eat food high in folic acid, such as green leafy vegetables, meat, fish, legumes, and whole grains.

Isoniazid (Isotamine) competes for the available vitamin B_6 in the body and leaves the client at risk for developing neuropathies related to vitamin deficiency. Supplemental vitamin B_6 is routinely prescribed to address this issue.

Vitamin B_1, or thiamine, is a precursor of an enzyme responsible for several steps in the oxidation of carbohydrates. It is abundant in both plant and animal products, especially whole-grain foods, dried beans, and peanuts. Because of its abundance, thiamine deficiency in North America is not common, except in alcoholics and in clients with chronic liver disease. Thiamine deficiency, or **beriberi**, is characterized by neurological signs such as paresthesia, neuralgia, and progressive loss of feeling and reflexes. Chronic deficiency can result in heart failure. Severe deficiencies may require parenteral thiamine up to 100 mg/day. With pharmacotherapy, symptoms can be completely reversed in the early stages of the disease; however, permanent disability can result in clients with prolonged deficiency.

Numbness and tingling in the hands and feet are symptoms of peripheralpolyneuritis, which results from inadequate intake of vitamin B_1 (thiamine) secondary to prolonged and excessive alcohol intake. Treatment includes reducing alcohol intake and correcting nutritional deficiencies through diet and vitamin supplements.

Thiamine specifically prevents the development of Wernicke's encephalopathy, a reversible amnestic disorder caused by a diet deficient in thiamine secondary to poor nutritional intake that commonly accompanies chronic alcoholism. It is characterized by nystagmus, ataxia, and mental status changes. Because clients with chronic alcoholism would rather drink alcohol than eat, clients are depleted of vitamins and nutrients.

Vitamin B_2, or riboflavin, is a component of coenzymes that participate in a number of different oxidation-reduction reactions. Riboflavin is

abundantly found in plant and animal products, including wheat germ, eggs, cheese, fish, nuts, and green leafy vegetables. Like thiamine, deficiency of riboflavin is most commonly observed in alcoholics. Signs of deficiency include corneal vascularization and anemia, as well as skin abnormalities such as dermatitis and cheilosis. Most symptoms are resolved by administering 25 to 100 mg/day until improvement is noted.

Vitamin B_3, or niacin, is a key component of nicotinamide adenine dinucleotide and nicotinamide adenine dinucleotide phosphate, two coenzymes that are essential for oxidative metabolism. Niacin is synthesized from the amino acid tryptophan and is widely distributed in both animal and plant foods, including beans, wheat germ, meats, nuts, and whole-grain breads. Niacin deficiency, or **pellagra**, is most commonly seen in alcoholics and in areas of the world where corn is the primary food source. Early symptoms include fatigue, anorexia, and drying of the skin. Advanced symptoms include three classic signs: dermatitis, diarrhea, and dementia. Deficiency is treated with niacin at dosages ranging from 10 to 25 mg/day. When used to treat hyperlipidemia, niacin is given as nicotinic acid and doses are much higher—up to 3 g/day (see Chapter 49).

Vitamin B_6, or pyridoxine, consists of several closely related compounds, including pyridoxine itself, pyridoxal, and pyridoxamine. Vitamin B_6 is essential for the synthesis of heme and is a primary coenzyme involved in the metabolism of amino acids. It is also needed for the synthesis of the neurotransmitter gamma-aminobutyric acid (GABA). Deficiency states can be the result of alcoholism, uremia, hypothyroidism, or heart failure. Certain drugs can cause vitamin B_6 deficiency, including isoniazid, cycloserine (Seromycin), hydralazine (Apresoline), oral contraceptives, and pyrazinamide (Tebrazid). Clients receiving these drugs may routinely receive B_6 supplements. Deficiency symptoms include skin abnormalities, cheilosis, fatigue, and irritability. Symptoms reverse after administration of about 10 to 20 mg/day for several weeks.

Vitamin B_9, more commonly known as folate or folic acid, is metabolized to tetrahydrofolate, which is essential for normal DNA synthesis and for erythropoiesis. Folic acid is widely distributed in plant products, especially green leafy vegetables and citrus fruits.

Vitamin B_{12}, or cyanocobalamin, is folate of a cobalt-containing vitamin that is a required coenzyme for a number of metabolic pathways. It also has important roles in cell replication, erythrocyte maturation, and myelin synthesis. Sources include lean meat, seafood, liver, and milk. Deficiency of vitamin B_{12} results in **pernicious (megaloblastic) anemia**.

Vitamin C, or ascorbic acid, is the most commonly purchased OTC vitamin. It is a potent antioxidant and serves many functions, including collagen synthesis, tissue healing, and maintenance of bone, teeth, and epithelial tissue. Many consumers purchase the vitamin for its ability to prevent the common cold, a function that has not been definitively proven. Deficiency of vitamin C, or **scurvy**, is caused by diets deficient in fruits and vegetables.

Alcoholics, cigarette smokers, cancer clients, and those with renal failure are at highest risk of vitamin C deficiency. Symptoms include fatigue, bleeding gums and other hemorrhages, gingivitis, and poor wound healing. Symptoms can normally be reversed by the administration of 300 to 1000 mg/day of vitamin C for several weeks.

Ascorbic acid (vitamin C) increases iron absorption. Taking iron with a food rich in ascorbic acid, such as orange juice, increases absorption. Milk delays iron absorption. It is best to give iron on an empty stomach to increase absorption.

Nursing Considerations

The role of the nurse in water-soluble vitamin therapy involves careful monitoring of the client's condition and providing education as it relates to the prescribed drug regimen. Water-soluble vitamins are used for multiple reasons in health care. The nurse should determine the reason for the specific vitamin therapy being prescribed and assess for the presence or absence of the associated symptoms.

Thiamine (Betaxin) is often administered to hospitalized clients who have severe liver disease. If thiamine deficiency is not corrected in these clients, irreversible brain damage may occur. There are no known adverse effects from oral administration of thiamine, and parenteral administration rarely causes any type of adverse effect. Niacin (Niaspan, Niodan) may be administered in the treatment of niacin deficiency or as an adjunct in cholesterol-lowering therapy. Pyridoxine deficiency is associated with poor nutritional status, chronic debilitating diseases, and alcohol abuse. Both niacin and pyridoxine may cause severe flushing. The nurse should inform the client that this is an expected reaction and will not cause permanent harm. Most clients tolerate therapy with B vitamins with few adverse effects.

CONNECTIONS | Natural Therapies

◀ Vitamin C and the Common Cold

Although there is a great deal of anecdotal evidence that vitamin C helps to fend off a cold, the claims are unsubstantiated; however, vitamin C may be useful as an immune stimulator and modulator in some circumstances. Several studies have shown that vitamin C can significantly reduce the duration and severity of colds in some people and reduce the incidence of colds in others. It is thought that this is due, at least in part, to the antihistamine activity of vitamin C. The best results were obtained with doses of 2 g/day (or greater). Preliminary evidence also suggests that vitamin C can be useful in improving respiratory infections.

NURSING PROCESS FOCUS

Clients Receiving Folic Acid

Assessment	Potential Nursing Diagnoses/Identified Patterns
Prior to administration: • Obtain complete health history, including allergies, drug history, and possible drug interactions. • Obtain a complete physical examination, with special attention to symptoms related to anemic states such as pallor, fatigue, weakness, tachycardia, and shortness of breath. • Obtain the following laboratory studies: folic acid levels, hemoglobin, hematocrit, and reticulocyte counts. • Obtain CBC to determine the type of anemia present. (Folic acid is not beneficial in normocytic anemia, refractory anemia, and aplastic anemia.)	• Nutritional deficiency • Deficient knowledge regarding drug therapy

Planning: Client Goals and Expected Outcomes

The client will:

• Exhibit improvement in serum folic acid level
• Demonstrate an understanding of the drug's action by accurately describing drug side effects and precautions
• Immediately report side effects such as continued weakness and fatigue

Implementation

Interventions (Rationales)	Client Education/Discharge Planning
• Monitor client's dietary intake of folic acid–containing foods. (Deficiency state may be caused by poor dietary habits.) • Encourage client to conserve energy. (Anemia, caused by folic acid deficiency, may lead to weakness and fatigue.) • Encourage client to take medication appropriately.	Instruct client to: • Eat foods high in folic acid such as vegetables, fruits, and organ meats • Consult with the healthcare provider concerning amount of folic acid that should be in the diet Advise client to: • Rest when tired and not to overexert • Plan activities to avoid fatigue Instruct client to: • Avoid use of alcohol because it increases folic acid requirements • Take only the amount of the drug prescribed

Evaluation of Outcome Criteria

Evaluate the effectiveness of drug therapy by confirming that client goals and expected outcomes have been met (see "Planning").

Vitamin C, readily available as an OTC nutritional supplement, may cause diarrhea, nausea, vomiting, abdominal pain, and hyperuricemia in high doses. Clients with a history of kidney stones should be cautioned against using vitamin C unless directed by a healthcare provider because excessive intake may promote renal calculi formation. Clients who are taking vitamin C should be advised to increase fluid intake. Most clients are able to take vitamin C without experiencing serious side effects.

Client education as it relates to water-soluble vitamins should include goals, reasons for obtaining baseline data such as CBC and laboratory tests for liver function, and possible side effects. The following are the important points the nurse should include when teaching clients about water-soluble vitamins:

- Niacin and pyridoxine may cause a feeling of warmth and flushing of skin, but this will diminish with continued therapy.
- Include vitamin-rich foods (whole grains, fresh vegetables, fresh fruits, lean meats, and dairy products) in the diet to decrease the need for vitamin supplements.
- Water-soluble vitamins are not stored in the body and must be replenished daily.
- Take vitamins only as prescribed or as directed on the label. Do not double the dosage.

PROTOTYPE DRUG	Folic Acid

Actions and Uses: Folic acid is administered to reverse symptoms of deficiency, which most commonly occurs in clients with inadequate intake, such as with chronic alcohol abuse. Because this vitamin is destroyed by high temperatures, people who overcook their food may experience folate deficiency. Pregnancy markedly increases the need for dietary folic acid; folic acid is given during pregnancy to promote normal fetal growth.

Because insufficient vitamin B_{12} creates a lack of activated folic acid, deficiency symptoms resemble those of vitamin B_{12} deficiency. The megaloblastic anemia observed in folate-deficient clients, however, does not include the severe nervous system symptoms seen in clients with B_{12} deficiency. Administration of 1 mg/day of oral folic acid often reverses the deficiency symptoms within 5 to 7 days.

Pharmacokinetics: Folic acid is well absorbed and widely distributed. It peaks in 30 to 60 minutes. It is metabolized in the liver to its active metabolite, dihydrofolate reductase. Excess folic acid is excreted by the kidneys.

Administration Alert:

- Folic acid is pregnancy category A.

Adverse Effects and Interactions: Side effects during folic acid therapy are uncommon. Clients may feel flushed following IV injections. Allergies to folic acid are possible.

Folic acid interacts with many drugs. For example, phenytoin, trimethoprim-sulfisoxazole (Bactrim, Septra), and other medications may interfere with the absorption of folic acid. Chloramphenicol (Chlormycetin) may antagonize effects of folate therapy. Oral contraceptives, alcohol, barbiturates, methotrexate, and primidone may cause folate deficiency.

MINERALS

Minerals are inorganic substances that are needed in small amounts to maintain homeostasis. Minerals are classified as macrominerals or microminerals; the macrominerals must be ingested in larger amounts. A normal, balanced diet will provide the proper amounts of the required minerals for most clients. The primary minerals used in pharmacotherapy are shown in Table 37.4.

TABLE 37.4 Minerals for Treating Nutritional Disorders

Drug	Route and Adult Dose
sodium bicarbonate (see Chapter 53, page 677, for the Prototype Drug box)	PO, 0.3–2.0 g every day to four times a day (qd–qid), or 1 tsp of powder in glass of water
	PO, 10–100 mEq/hour in divided doses
potassium chloride (K-Dur, Slow K) (see Chapter 53, page 675, for the Prototype Drug box)	PO/IV, 40–80 mEq/day
Calcium Salts	
calcium carbonate (Caltrate, Os-Cal, Tums)	PO, 1–2 g twice a day (bid)–tid
calcium chloride (Calciject, Calcitrans, others)	IV, 0.5–1.0 g qd–every 3 days (q3d)
calcium citrate (Citracal)	PO, 1–2 g bid–tid
calcium phosphate tribasic	PO, 1–2 g bid–tid
calcium gluconate (Calciforte) (see Chapter 61, page 784, for the Prototype Drug box)	PO, 1–2 g bid–qid
calcium lactate	PO, 325 mg–1.3 g tid with meals

(continued)

TABLE 37.4   Minerals for Treating Nutritional Disorders (*continued*)

Iron Salts

ferrous fumarate (Palafer)	PO, 200 mg tid–qid
ferrous gluconate (Apo-Ferrous Gluconate)	PO, 325–600 mg qid, may be gradually increased to 650 mg qid as needed and tolerated
ferrous sulfate (Apo-Ferrous Sulfate) (see Chapter 57, page 736, for the Prototype Drug box)	PO, 750–1500 mg qd in 1 to 3 divided doses
iron dextran (Dextran)	IM/IV, dose is individualized and determined from a table of correlations between client's weight and hemoglobin per package insert (max 100 mg [2 mL] of iron dextran within 24 hours)
iron sucrose injection (Venofer)	IV, 1 mL (20 mg) injected in dialysis line at rate of 1 mL/minute up to 5 mL (100 mg), or infuse 100 mg in normal saline (NS) over 15 minutes one to three times/week

Magnesium

magnesium chloride (Magnolex)	PO, 270–400 mg qd
magnesium oxide	PO, 400–1200 mg/day in divided doses
Pr magnesium sulfate (Epsom Salts)	IV/IM, 0.5–3.0 g qd

Phosphorous

monobasic potassium phosphate	PO, 1 g qid
monobasic potassium and sodium phosphates	PO, 250 mg qid (max 2 g phosphorous/day)
potassium phosphate	PO, 1.45 g qid
	IV, 10 mmol phosphorous/day
potassium and sodium phosphates	PO, 250 mg phosphorous qid

Zinc

zinc acetate (Zincum Aceticum)	PO, 50 mg tid
zinc gluconate	PO, 20–100 mg (20 mg lozenges may be taken to a max of six lozenges/day)
zinc sulfate	PO, 15–220 mg qd

Pharmacotherapy with Minerals

37.7 Minerals are inorganic substances that are needed in very small amounts to maintain normal body metabolism.

Minerals are essential substances that constitute about 4% of the body weight and serve many diverse functions. Some are present primarily as essential ions or electrolytes in body fluids; others are bound to organic molecules such as hemoglobin, phospholipids, or metabolic enzymes. Those minerals that function as critical electrolytes in the body, most notably sodium and potassium, are covered in more detail in Chapter 53. Sodium chloride and potassium chloride are featured as Prototype Drugs in that chapter.

Because minerals are needed in very small amounts for human metabolism, a normal balanced diet will supply the necessary quantities for most clients. Like vitamins, excess amounts of minerals can lead to toxicity, and clients should be advised not to exceed recommended doses. Mineral supplements, however, are indicated for certain disorders. Iron-deficiency anemia is the most common nutritional deficiency in the world and is a common indication for iron supplements. Women at high risk for osteoporosis are advised to consume extra calcium, either in their diet or as a dietary supplement.

Certain drugs affect normal mineral metabolism. Clients who are taking loop or thiazide diuretics can have significant potassium loss. Corticosteroids and oral contraceptives are among several classes of drug that can promote sodium retention. The uptake of iodine by the thyroid gland can be impaired by certain oral hypoglycemics and lithium carbonate (Carbolith, Lithane). Oral contraceptives have been reported to lower the plasma levels of zinc and to increase those of copper. Changes to mineral intake may be required when these drugs are used.

Pharmacotherapy with Macrominerals

37.8 Pharmacotherapy with macrominerals includes agents containing calcium, magnesium, potassium, or phosphorous.

Macrominerals (major minerals) are inorganic substances that must be obtained daily from dietary sources in amounts of 100 mg or higher. The macrominerals include calcium, chlorine, magnesium, phosphorous, potassium, sodium, and sulphur. As bone salts, calcium and phosphorous comprise approximately 75% of the total mineral content in the body. Recommended DRIs have been established for each of the macrominerals except sulphur, as listed in Table 37.5.

Calcium is essential for nerve conduction, muscular contraction, and hemostasis. Much of the body's calcium is bound in the bony matrix of the skeleton. Hypocalcemia occurs when serum calcium falls below 4.5 mEq/L and may be caused by inadequate intake of calcium-containing foods, lack of vitamin D, chronic diarrhea, or decreased secretion of parathyroid hormone.

TABLE 37.5 Macrominerals

Mineral	DRI	Function
calcium	1000–1200 mg	Forms bone matrix; regulates nerve conduction and muscle contraction
chloride	1800–2300 mg	Major anion in body fluids; part of gastric acid secretion
iron	men: 8 mg women: 8–18 mg	Prevention of iron-deficiency anemia
magnesium	men: 400–420 mg women: 310–320 mg	Cofactor for many enzymes; necessary for normal nerve conduction and muscle contraction
phosphorous	700 mg	Forms bone matrix; part of adenosine triphosphate (ATP) and nucleic acids
potassium	4700 g	Necessary for normal nerve conduction and muscle contraction; principal cation in intracellular fluid; essential for acid-base and electrolyte balance
sodium	1200–1500 mg	Necessary for normal nerve conduction and muscle contraction; principal cation in extracellular fluid; essential for acid-base and electrolyte balance
sulphur	Not established	Component of proteins, B vitamins, and other critical molecules

Symptoms of hypocalcemia involve the nervous and muscular systems. The client often becomes irritable and restless, and muscular twitches, cramps, spasms, and cardiac abnormalities are common. Long-term hypocalcemia may lead to fractures. Pharmacotherapy includes calcium compounds, which are available in many oral formulations, including calcium carbonate, calcium citrate, calcium gluconate, and calcium lactate. In severe cases, IV preparations are administered. Calcium gluconate is featured as a Prototype Drug in Chapter 61. Phosphorous is an essential mineral that is often bound to calcium in the form of calcium phosphate in bones. In addition to its role in bone formation, phosphorous is a component of ATP and nucleic acids. Phosphate (PO_4^{-2}) is an important buffer in the blood. Because of its close relationship to phosphate, phosphorous balance is normally considered the same as phosphate balance. Symptoms of hypophosphatemia include weakness, muscle tremor, anorexia, weak pulse, and bleeding abnormalities. When serum phosphorous falls below 1.5 mEq/L, phosphate therapy is usually administered. Sodium phosphate and potassium phosphate are available for phosphorous deficiencies.

Magnesium is the second most abundant intracellular cation. Like potassium, it is necessary for proper neuromuscular function. Magnesium serves a metabolic role in activating certain enzymes in the breakdown of carbohydrates and proteins. Hypomagnesemia is generally asymptomatic until serum magnesium falls below 1.0 mEq/L. Because it produces few symptoms in its early stages, it is sometimes described as the most common undiagnosed electrolyte abnormality. Clients may experience general weakness, dysrhythmias, hypertension, loss of deep tendon reflexes, and respiratory depression. These symptoms are sometimes mistaken for hypokalemia. Pharmacotherapy with magnesium sulfate can quickly reverse symptoms of hypomagnesemia. Magnesium sulfate is a CNS depressant and is sometimes given to either prevent or terminate seizures associated with eclampsia. Magnesium salts have additional applications as cathartics and antacids (magnesium citrate, magnesium hydroxide, and magnesium oxide) and as analgesics (magnesium salicylate).

Nursing Considerations

The role of the nurse in macromineral therapy involves careful monitoring of the client's condition and providing education as it relates to the prescribed drug regimen. Macrominerals are used for multiple reasons in health care. The nurse should determine the reason for the specific macromineral therapy being prescribed and assess for the presence or absence of the associated symptoms.

Although minerals cause no harm in small amounts, larger doses can cause life-threatening adverse effects. Calcium is one of the most common minerals in use. To prevent and treat osteoporosis, it is recommended that adult women take 1200 mg/day of calcium. Common side effects include mild GI distress and constipation. Prolonged therapy with calcium may increase the risk for hypercalcemia, especially in clients with decreased liver and renal function. Symptoms of hypercalcemia include nausea, vomiting, constipation, frequent urination, lethargy, and depression. Since calcium interacts with many drugs, such as glucocorticoids, thiazide diuretics, and tetracyclines, the client should inform the healthcare provider when using calcium supplements. The client should also be advised to avoid zinc-rich foods such as legumes, nuts, sprouts, and soy that impair calcium absorption.

Phosphorous is a mineral sometimes used as a dietary supplement. Clients who are on a sodium- or potassium-restricted diet should not use phosphorous supplements. Most adverse effects of excess phosphate are mild and include GI distress, diarrhea, and dizziness. The client should stop taking phosphorous at the first sign of seizure activity, as excess phosphorous can promote seizures. Antacids should be avoided because they may decrease serum phosphorous levels.

Magnesium sulfate is given to correct hypomagnesemia, evacuate the bowel in preparation for diagnostic examinations, and treat seizures associated with eclampsia of pregnancy. The medication is given orally to replace magnesium and by the IM or IV routes to prevent or terminate eclamptic seizures. When given IV, it is important for the nurse to assess the neurological status of the client because overdose can lead to reduced reflexes and muscle weakness. The nurse should monitor for changes in level of consciousness, deep tendon reflexes, thirst, and confusion. Because of its effects on muscles and the heart, magnesium sulfate is contraindicated in clients with myocardial damage, heart block, and recent cardiac arrest. It has a laxative effect when given orally, so it should not be given to clients with abdominal pain, nausea, vomiting, or intestinal obstruction. Magnesium sulfate should be used with caution in clients with impaired kidney function and those on cardiac glycosides.

NCLEX Success Tips

The nurse should anticipate administering 10 mL of 10% by IV push over 3 to 5 minutes as a calcium gluconate antidote for magnesium toxicity.

Typical signs of hypermagnesemia include decreased deep tendon reflexes, sweating or a flushing of the skin, oliguria, decreased respirations, and lethargy progressing to coma as the toxicity increases. The nurse should check the client's patellar, biceps, and radial reflexes regularly during magnesium sulfate therapy.

Magnesium is normally excreted by the kidneys. When the kidneys fail, magnesium can accumulate and cause severe neurological problems.

Magnesium hydroxide can lead to magnesium toxicity in clients with chronic renal failure.

Client education as it relates to macromineral therapy should include goals, reasons for obtaining baseline data such as CBC and laboratory tests for liver function, and possible side effects. The following are the important points the nurse should include when teaching clients about minerals:

- Take minerals only as prescribed or as directed on the label. Overdose may lead to toxicity.
- Discontinue using the medication and notify the healthcare provider immediately if toxicity symptoms occur.
- Consult the healthcare provider before taking OTC drugs; they might contain additional minerals and lead to toxicity.

- Eat a well-balanced diet to eliminate or reduce the need for mineral supplements.

PROTOTYPE DRUG   **Magnesium Sulfate**

Actions and Uses: Severe hypomagnesemia can be rapidly reversed by the administration of IM or IV magnesium sulfate. Hypomagnesemia has a number of causes, including loss of body fluids due to diarrhea, diuretics, and nasogastric suctioning; and prolonged parenteral feeding with magnesium-free solutions. Oral forms of magnesium sulfate are used as cathartics when complete evacuation of the colon is desired. Its action as a CNS depressant has led to its occasional use as an anticonvulsant.

Pharmacokinetics: Magnesium sulfate is well absorbed, widely distributed, and excreted mainly by the kidneys. Its onset of action is 1 to 2 hours. It has an unknown half-life.

NURSING PROCESS FOCUS

Clients Receiving Magnesium Sulfate

Assessment	Potential Nursing Diagnoses/Identified Patterns
Prior to administration: - Obtain complete health history, including allergies, drug history, and possible drug interactions. - Obtain complete physical examination with special attention to respiratory status and deep tendon reflexes. - Assess for the presence or history of malnutrition, hypomagnesia, seizure activity, pre-eclampsia, and kidney disease. - Obtain serum magnesium level and renal profile.	- Deficient knowledge regarding drug therapy - Risk for injury related to disease conditions and adverse effects of drug

Planning: Client Goals and Expected Outcomes

The client will:
- Exhibit improvement in serum magnesium level
- Accurately describe the drug's intended effects, side effects, and precautions
- Immediately report side effects such as lowered pulse, dizziness, difficulty breathing, and weakness

Implementation

Interventions (Rationales)	Client Education/Discharge Planning
- Assess magnesium level to determine deficiency. (The therapeutic range is very narrow; toxic levels may develop quickly.) - Monitor vital signs frequently throughout IV infusion. (Magnesium sulfate depresses respirations, pulse rate, and rhythm.) - Report urine output of <100 mL/hour to the healthcare provider. (Clients who have impaired renal function will have decreased renal clearance, leading to toxicity.) - Observe newborns for signs and symptoms of magnesium toxicity if the mother received magnesium sulfate during labour. (The neonate may have received some amount of magnesium that could cause skeletal muscle and cardiac muscle depression.)	- Instruct client that magnesium sulfate should be taken only on the advice of a healthcare provider - Instruct client to report any difficulty breathing, low pulse rate, or dizziness - Instruct client to report any problems with urination or edema - Advise labouring mothers who are receiving magnesium sulfate that the newborn will be monitored closely after birth

Evaluation of Outcome Criteria

Evaluate the effectiveness of drug therapy by confirming that client goals and expected outcomes have been met (see "Planning").

Administration Alerts:

- Continuously monitor client during IV infusion for early signs of decreased cardiac function.
- Monitor serum magnesium levels every 6 hours during parenteral infusion.
- When giving IV infusion, give required dose over 4 hours.
- Magnesium sulfate is pregnancy category A.

Adverse Effects and Interactions: IV infusions of magnesium sulfate require careful observation to avoid toxicity. Early signs of magnesium overdose include flushing of the skin, sedation, confusion, intense thirst, and muscle weakness. Extreme levels cause neuromuscular blockade with resultant respiratory paralysis and heart block and may cause circulatory collapse, complete heart block, and respiratory failure. Plasma magnesium levels should be monitored frequently. Clients who are receiving CNS depressants may experience increased sedation. Because of these potentially fatal adverse effects, the use of magnesium sulfate is restricted to severe magnesium deficiency. Mild to moderate hypomagnesemia is treated with oral forms of magnesium such as magnesium gluconate or magnesium hydroxide.

Administration of neuromuscular blocking agents with magnesium sulfate may increase respiratory depression and apnea.

Pharmacotherapy with Microminerals

37.9 Pharmacotherapy with microminerals includes agents containing iron, iodine, fluorine, or zinc.

The nine **microminerals**, commonly called trace minerals, are required daily in amounts of 20 mg or less. The fact that they are needed in such small amounts does not diminish their role in human health; deficiencies in some of the trace minerals can result in profound illness. The functions of some of the trace minerals, such as iron and iodine, are well established; the roles of others are less completely understood. The DRI for each of the microminerals is shown in Table 37.6.

Iron is an essential micromineral most commonly associated with hemoglobin. Excellent sources of dietary iron include meat, shellfish, nuts, and legumes. Excess iron in the body results in hemochromatosis, whereas lack of iron results in iron-deficiency anemia. The pharmacology of iron supplements is presented in Chapter 57, where ferrous sulfate (Fer-In-Sol) is featured as a Prototype Drug (page 736).

Iodine is a trace mineral needed to synthesize thyroid hormone. The most common source of dietary iodine is iodized salt. When dietary intake of iodine is low, hypothyroidism occurs and enlargement of the thyroid gland (goiter) results. At high concentrations, iodine suppresses thyroid function. Lugol's solution, a mixture containing 5% elemental iodine and 10% potassium iodide, is given to hyperthyroid clients prior to thyroidectomy or during a thyrotoxic crisis. Sodium iodide acts by rapidly suppressing the secretion of thyroid hormone and is indicated for clients who are having an acute thyroid crisis. Radioactive iodine (I-131) is given to destroy overactive thyroid glands. Pharmacotherapeutic uses of iodine as a

TABLE 37.6 Microminerals

Trace Mineral	DRI	Function
chromium	0.05–2.0 mg	Potentiates insulin and promotes normal protein, fat, and carbohydrate
cobalt	0.1 µg	Cofactor for vitamin B$_{12}$ and several oxidative enzymes
copper	1.5–3.0 mg	Cofactor for hemoglobin synthesis
fluorine	1.5–4.0 mg	Influences tooth structure and has possible effects on growth
iodine	150 µg	Component of thyroid hormones
iron	men: 10–12 mg women: 10–15 mg	Component of hemoglobin and some enzymes of oxidative phosphorylation
manganese	2–5 mg	Cofactor in some enzymes of lipid, carbohydrate, and protein metabolism
molybdenum	75–250 mg	Cofactor for certain enzymes
selenium	men: 50–70 µg women: 50–55 µg	Antioxidant cofactor for certain enzymes
zinc	12–15 mg	Cofactor of certain enzymes, including carbonic anhydrase; needed for proper protein structure, normal growth, and wound healing

drug extend beyond the treatment of thyroid disease. Iodine is an effective topical antiseptic that can be found in creams, tinctures, and solutions. Iodine molecules such as iothalamate and diatrizoate are very dense and serve as diagnostic contrast agents in radiological procedures of the urinary and cardiovascular systems. The role of potassium iodide in protecting the thyroid gland during acute radiation exposure is discussed in Chapter 29.

Fluorine is a trace mineral found abundantly in nature and is best known for its effects on bones and teeth. Research has validated that adding fluoride to the water supply in very small amounts (1 part per billion) can reduce the incidence of dental caries. This effect is more pronounced in children, as fluoride is incorporated into the enamel of growing teeth. Concentrated fluoride solutions can also be applied topically by dental professionals. Sodium fluoride and stannous fluoride are components of most toothpastes and oral rinses. Because high amounts of fluoride can be quite toxic, the use of fluoride-containing products should be closely monitored in children.

Zinc is a component of at least 100 enzymes, including alcohol dehydrogenase, carbonic anhydrase, and alkaline phosphatase. This trace mineral has a regulatory function in enzymes that control nucleic acid synthesis and has been implicated in wound healing, male fertility, bone formation, and cell-mediated immunity. Zinc sulfate, zinc acetate, and zinc gluconate are available to prevent and treat deficiency states. In addition, lozenges containing zinc are available OTC for treating sore throats and symptoms of the common cold.

NUTRITIONAL SUPPLEMENTS

The nurse will encounter a large number of clients who are undernourished. Major goals in resolving nutritional deficiencies are to identify the specific type of deficiency and supply the missing nutrient. Nutritional supplements may be needed for short-term therapy or for the remainder of the client's life.

Etiology of Undernutrition

37.10 Undernutrition may be caused by low dietary intake, malabsorption disorders, fad diets, or wasting disorders such as cancer or AIDS.

When the client is taking in or absorbing fewer nutrients than required for normal body growth and maintenance, **undernutrition** occurs. Successful pharmacotherapy relies on the skills of the nurse in identifying the symptoms and causes of the client's undernutrition.

Causes of undernutrition range from the simple to the complex and include the following:

- Aging
- HIV/AIDS
- Alcoholism
- Burns
- Cancer
- Chronic inflammatory bowel disease
- Chronic neurological disease such as progressive dysphagia and multiple sclerosis
- Eating disorders
- Gastrointestinal disorders
- Short bowel syndrome
- Surgery
- Trauma

The most obvious cause of undernutrition is low dietary intake, although reasons for the inadequate intake must be assessed. Clients may have no resources to purchase food and may be suffering from starvation. Clinical depression leads many clients to shun food. Elderly clients may have poor-fitting dentures or difficulty chewing or swallowing after a stroke. In terminal disease, clients may be comatose or otherwise unable to take food orally. Although the etiologies differ, clients with insufficient intake will exhibit a similar pattern of general weakness, muscle wasting, and loss of subcutaneous fat.

When the undernutrition is caused by lack of one specific nutrient, vitamin, or mineral, the disorder is more difficult to diagnose. Clients may be on a fad diet that lacks only protein or only fat. Certain digestive disorders may lead to malabsorption of specific nutrients or vitamins. Clients may simply avoid certain foods such as green leafy vegetables, dairy products, or meat products, which can lead to specific nutritional deficiencies. Proper pharmacotherapy requires the expert knowledge and assessment skills of the nurse so that the correct treatment can be administered.

Enteral Nutrition

37.11 Enteral nutrition, provided orally or through a feeding tube, is a means of meeting a client's complete nutritional needs.

A large number of nutritional supplements are available. A common method of classifying these agents is by their route of administration. When products are administered via the GI tract, either orally or through a feeding tube, this is classified as **enteral nutrition**. Administration by means of IV infusion is called **parenteral nutrition**.

When the client's condition permits, enteral nutrition is best provided by oral consumption. Oral feeding allows natural digestive processes to occur and requires less intense nursing care. It does, however, rely on client adherence since it is not feasible for the healthcare provider to observe the client at every meal.

Tube feeding, or enteral tube alimentation, is necessary when the client has difficulty swallowing or is otherwise unable to take meals orally. Various tube feeding routes are possible, including nasogastric, nasoduodenal, nasojejunal, gastrostomy, or jejunostomy. An advantage of tube feeding is that the nurse can precisely measure and record the amount of enteral nutrition the client is receiving.

The particular enteral product is chosen to address the specific nutritional needs of the client. Because of the wide diversity in their formulas, it is difficult to categorize enteral products, and several different methods are used. A simple method is to classify enteral products as oligomeric, polymeric, modular, or specialized formulations.

Oligomeric formulations are agents that contain varying amounts of free amino acids and peptide combinations. Indications include partial bowel obstruction, irritable bowel syndrome, radiation enteritis, bowel fistulas, and short bowel syndrome. Sample products include Vivonex T.E.N. and Tolerex.

Polymeric formulations are the most common enteral preparations. These products contain various mixtures of proteins, carbohydrates, and lipids. Indications include general undernutrition, although the client must have a fully functioning GI tract. Sample products include Isosource, Resource, and Ensure-Plus.

Modular formulations contain a single nutrient, protein, lipid, or carbohydrate. Indications include a single nutrient deficiency. They may be added to other formulations to provide more specific nutrient needs. Sample products include ProMod, Polycose, Resource GlutaSolve, and MCT Oil.

Specialized formulations are products that contain a specific nutrient combination for a particular condition. Indications include a specific disease state such as hepatic failure or renal failure, or a specific genetic enzyme deficiency. Sample products include Citrotein, Pulmocare, and Suplena.

Clients sometimes exhibit GI intolerance to enteral nutrition, usually expressed as vomiting, nausea, or diarrhea. Therapy is often started slowly, with small quantities, so that side effects can be assessed. The nurse must observe for drug interactions that occasionally occur when drugs are given along with enteral nutrition.

Enteral feedings can be delivered by bolus, intermittent drip or infusion, continuous infusion, or cyclic intermittent infusion.

Bolus feedings were the first method introduced and typically deliver 250 to 400 mL of formula every 4 to 6 hours via a syringe or funnel. This method takes about 15 minutes to complete and may not be well tolerated due to the large volume of solution introduced in such a short period. The bolus method can also cause nausea, vomiting, abdominal cramping, and diarrhea, and there is a greater risk for aspiration. It is used with medically stable or ambulatory clients who have adequate absorptive capacity to tolerate the larger volume of fluid.

Intermittent feedings are administered every 3 to 6 hours and take about 30 to 60 minutes to infuse. They can be delivered either by gravity drip or by feeding pump infusion, with 300 to 400 mL of solution administered at each feeding. These feedings commonly use a feeding bag and are considered an inexpensive method of administering enteral nutrition to the client.

Continuous infusion feedings are often prescribed for critically ill clients or those with duodenal or jejunal entry feeding tubes. This type of feeding is often delivered by an infusion pump at a slow rate over a 16- to 24-hour period. Continual enteral feeding methods result in the client meeting his or her nutritional goals much quicker. Furthermore, the continuous method of delivery is more successful because it helps to prevent complications such as dumping syndrome and avoids the need for frequent irrigation of the tube. **Dumping syndrome** is the result of a sudden influx of feeding into the GI tract and the creation of a high osmotic gradient within the small intestine. This in turn causes a sudden shift of fluid from the vascular compartment to the intestinal lumen. Plasma volume decreases, causing vasomotor responses such as an increased pulse rate, decreased blood pressure, pallor, sweating, weakness, and dizziness. The increased intestinal fluid results in distention and produces a feeling of fullness, abdominal cramping, nausea, vomiting, and diarrhea.

Cyclic feedings are commonly infused over 8 to 16 hours daily (day or night). Infusions during the daytime hours are recommended for clients who are restless during sleep or who have a greater risk for aspiration. Nighttime infusion allows clients more freedom during the day and is frequently used for ambulatory clients.

Total Parenteral Nutrition

37.12 Total parenteral nutrition (TPN) is a means of supplying nutrition to clients via a peripheral vein (short term) or central vein (long term).

Parenteral nutrition is often used for clients who are unable to eat or tolerate any form of enteral nutrition. It is frequently given to clients with severe GI disorders such as diseases of the small bowel (Crohn's disease, fistulas, adhesions, postoperative ileus), necrotizing pancreatitis, hyperemesis gravidarum (maternity clients), and pediatric clients with congenital anomalies or prolonged diarrhea. It is also used for clients with demonstrated undernutrition (less than 50% of the metabolic needs met for more than 7 days) as well as for clients with AIDS, cancer chemotherapy- or radiation-induced enteritis, burns, severe trauma, or anorexia.

Parenteral nutrition is also referred to as **total parenteral nutrition (TPN)** or hyperalimentation and is administered solely by the IV route. It can be delivered via a peripheral line or a central line, depending on the hypertonicity of the solution. TPN can provide all of the calories, glucose, protein, fats, minerals, and trace elements needed by the body to sustain growth and to promote weight gain as well as wound healing. A **partial parenteral nutrition** solution is one that lacks an essential element, usually fats or lipids.

Peripheral vein total parenteral nutrition is used when a central venous line cannot be accessed or when it is not appropriate for the client. These situations may include clients in whom the subclavian vein is inaccessible due to scar tissue from repeated IV line punctures or in clients with extensive trauma, severe burns, or cancer in the region of the upper torso or chest. These clients may be relatively healthy with only a slight nutritional deficit that cannot be met with enteral therapy. Peripheral parenteral nutrition (PPN) is considered a temporary measure until a central line can be placed, and the solution administered is usually lower in osmolality than the solution delivered through a central line. PPN is advantageous because there are fewer risks associated with the catheter placement, care of the infusion site is simpler, and the complications associated with hyperosmolar solutions can be avoided.

Problems associated with PPN include the need for several large peripheral veins, because the catheter site is routinely rotated to prevent infection. The vein must also be able to accommodate the larger-sized venous catheter. PPN is associated with a high risk for phlebitis and is therefore reserved for clients with robust veins. Peripherally inserted central catheters (PICC lines) are often inserted in clients for home therapy with peripheral vein total parenteral nutrition.

Central vein total parenteral nutrition is the administration of the solution through a central vein such as the subclavian or the internal jugular vein. Because of the hypertonicity of the parenteral solution, the catheter tip must always be positioned in the superior vena cava so that the solution can be immediately diluted to a more tolerable concentration. The central vein total parenteral nutrition solution usually consists of crystalline amino acids, dextrose, and lipid emulsions with the addition of vitamins, minerals, trace elements, essential electrolytes, and water.

Central vein total parenteral nutrition is used in clients with limited peripheral access or in clients whose nutritional needs cannot be met by peripheral vein total parenteral nutrition formulas. It is usually considered the access of choice for long-term parenteral therapy and is always administered using an infusion pump in order to precisely monitor the amount of solution given.

TPN solutions may be modified daily based on the client's laboratory results, the underlying disorder, the rate of metabolism, and other factors. Like the enteral products, the basic components include carbohydrates, lipids, amino acids (proteins), electrolytes, minerals, and vitamins.

Carbohydrates

Carbohydrates and lipids are the primary sources of calories for the client on TPN. Dextrose is the most common carbohydrate source because it is inexpensive and readily available from cornstarch, beet, or cane sugar. The DRI of carbohydrates for adult clients ranges from 25 to 35 kcal/kg. When administered through a central line, the concentration of dextrose in the TPN solution usually comprises 25% to 35% of the overall solution.

When dextrose is administered as the primary calorie source (without lipids added), hyperglycemia can occur. Because insulin is required for dextrose use, a combination of dextrose and lipids may help to reduce the risk for hyperglycemia and the client's need for supplemental insulin injections. Dextrose increases the metabolic rate and the production of carbon dioxide, which may increase the demands placed on the client's respiratory system. The addition of lipids will also decrease this risk. Abruptly stopping the TPN solution can result in hypoglycemia due to the continued release of endogenous insulin. This problem can be avoided by substituting a dextrose 10% solution until the new TPN solution bag is available or by gradually tapering the solution over a 24-hour period when discontinuing parenteral therapy.

Lipids

Unlike amino acids and concentrated dextrose solutions, fat emulsions are isotonic, which means that they can be infused through either a peripheral or a central line. They are often a requirement for clients who are receiving TPN therapy for longer than 5 days. Lipid preparations that are currently available are produced from either safflower oil (Liposyn) or soybean oil (Intralipid). The principal fatty acids used in these preparations are linoleic, linolenic, oleic, palmitic, and stearic acids.

Fat emulsions can be hazardous for clients with liver disease, pulmonary disease, anemia, or blood coagulation disorders, with the most common adverse effect being hyperlipidemia. Fat emboli and death can occur when lipids are administered to premature, preterm, or low-birth-weight infants.

Amino Acids

Amino acids are needed by the body to promote the production of proteins, to conserve lean body mass, and to help promote wound healing. The DRI for infants and children ranges from 1.4 to 2.5 g/kg/day, whereas adults require 0.8 to 1 g/kg/day. Essential amino acids cannot be produced by the body, whereas non-essential amino acids can be synthesized from a nitrogen source, such as ammonium salts or urea. Amino acids must be closely monitored in clients with renal failure, because the blood urea nitrogen (BUN) level can become elevated. For the client with liver failure, the administration of amino acids may result in hepatic coma due to the liver's inability to process nitrogen.

Electrolytes and Minerals

Electrolytes, including sodium, potassium, magnesium, calcium, phosphorus, chloride, and acetate, can be added to the TPN formula as salts. Specific electrolyte amounts are ordered daily by the healthcare provider, based on pre-existing deficiencies and the client's current medical condition. To prevent interactions between specific elements and crystallization of the solution, the pharmacist should add the electrolytes.

Trace mineral mixtures typically contain copper, chromium, manganese, selenium, and zinc and are commercially available to meet the specific nutritional needs of the client. Trace minerals are metabolic cofactors that are essential for the proper functioning of several enzyme systems.

Although it is routine to monitor serum electrolyte levels, serum levels of the trace minerals are generally not monitored. Trace mineral administration should be decreased or withheld in clients who have a limited capacity to excrete them. For example, selenium and chromium should not be used in clients with renal impairment, whereas copper and manganese should be withheld in clients with severe hepatic disease.

Vitamins

Vitamins are essential components of the TPN regimen. Most commercially prepared vitamin formulas can be given on alternate days in order to meet the client's need for both fat-soluble vitamins and water-soluble vitamins, and they can be added to the existing TPN solution. Vitamin K is usually administered weekly by SC or IM injection.

NURSING PROCESS FOCUS

Clients Receiving Total Parenteral Nutrition

Assessment	Potential Nursing Diagnoses/Identified Patterns
Prior to administration: • Obtain complete health history, including allergies, drug history, and possible drug interactions. • Obtain complete physical examination. • Assess for the presence or history of nutritional deficit such as inadequate oral intake, GI disease, and increased metabolic need. • Obtain the following laboratory studies: total protein/albumin levels, creatinine/BUN, CBC, electrolytes, lipid profile, and serum iron levels.	• Nutritional deficiency • Knowledge regarding drug therapy may be inadequate • Risk for infection • Risk for fluid imbalance

Planning: Client Goals and Expected Outcomes

The client will:

• Exhibit improvement or stabilization of nutritional status
• Accurately describe the drug's intended effects, side effects, and precautions
• Immediately report side effects such as symptoms of hypoglycemia or hyperglycemia, fever, chills, cough, or malaise

---

Implementation

Interventions (Rationales)	Client Education/Discharge Planning
• Monitor vital signs, observing for signs of infection such as elevated temperature. (Bacteria may grow in high-glucose and high-protein solutions.) • Take extraordinary precautions to prevent infection. • Use strict aseptic technique with IV tubing, dressing changes, and TPN solution. • Refrigerate solution until 30 minutes before using. • Comply with healthcare facility protocol for tubing and filter changes. • Monitor blood glucose levels. Observe for signs of hyperglycemia or hypoglycemia and administer insulin as directed. (Blood glucose levels may be affected if TPN is turned off, the rate is reduced, or excess levels of insulin are added to the solution.) • Monitor for signs of fluid overload. (TPN is a hypertonic solution and can create intravascular shifting of extracellular fluid.) • Monitor renal status, including intake and output ratio, daily weight, and laboratory studies such as serum creatinine and BUN. • Maintain accurate infusion rate with infusion pump. • Make rate changes gradually and never discontinue TPN abruptly. • Increase or decrease flow rate by no more than 10% to prevent fluctuation in blood glucose levels.	• Instruct client to report fever, chills, soreness of or drainage at the infusion site, cough, and malaise • Instruct client that the infusion site is at high risk for infection, and stress the need for sterile dressings and aseptic technique with solutions and tubing Instruct client to report symptoms of: • Hyperglycemia (excessive thirst, copious urination, and insatiable hunger) • Hypoglycemia (nervousness, irritability, and dizziness) • Instruct client to report shortness of breath, heart palpitations, swelling, or decreased urine output Instruct client to: • Weigh self daily • Monitor intake and output • Report sudden increases in weight or decreased urinary output • Keep all appointments for follow-up care and laboratory testing Instruct client: • About the importance of maintaining the prescribed rate of infusion • To never stop the TPN solution abruptly unless instructed by the healthcare provider

Evaluation of Outcome Criteria

Evaluate the effectiveness of drug therapy by confirming that client goals and expected outcomes have been met (see "Planning").

CHAPTER

37

Understanding the Chapter

Key Concepts Summary

The numbered key concepts provide a succinct summary of the important points from the corresponding numbered section within the chapter. If any of these points are not clear, refer to the numbered section within the chapter for review.

37.1 Vitamins are organic substances that are needed in small amounts to promote growth and maintain health. Deficiency of a vitamin will result in disease.

37.2 Vitamins are classified as lipid soluble (A, D, E, and K) or water soluble (C and B complex).

37.3 Failure to meet the recommended dietary reference intake (DRI) for vitamins may result in deficiency disorders.

37.4 Vitamin therapy is indicated for conditions such as poor nutritional intake, pregnancy, and chronic disease states.

37.5 Deficiencies of vitamins A, D, E, or K are indications for pharmacotherapy with lipid-soluble vitamins.

37.6 Deficiencies of vitamin C, thiamine, niacin, riboflavin, folic acid, cyanocobalamin, or pyridoxine are indications for pharmacotherapy with water-soluble vitamins.

37.7 Minerals are inorganic substances that are needed in very small amounts to maintain normal body metabolism.

37.8 Pharmacotherapy with macrominerals includes agents containing calcium, magnesium, potassium, or phosphorous.

37.9 Pharmacotherapy with microminerals includes agents containing iron, iodine, fluorine, or zinc.

37.10 Undernutrition may be caused by low dietary intake, malabsorption disorders, fad diets, or wasting disorders such as cancer or AIDS.

37.11 Enteral nutrition, provided orally or through a feeding tube, is a means of meeting a client's complete nutritional needs.

37.12 Total parenteral nutrition (TPN) is a means of supplying nutrition to clients via a peripheral vein (short term) or central vein (long term).

Chapter 37 Scenario

Charlene Garrett is a 32-year-old mother of a 1-year-old girl. She returned to work part time 3 months ago as a special education instructor working with a group of preschoolers with special needs. Her husband watches their daughter two evenings a week so that Charlene can resume her work toward a master's degree in special education at the local university.

Lately Charlene has begun feeling more stressed and tired. It is almost the end of the semester and papers are due; the holidays arrive in another month, and both sides of the family will be coming to visit; and Charlene and her husband have delayed celebrating the baby's birthday this month so that the families can enjoy the celebration when they visit.

Charlene lives next door and asks you, a nurse, about vitamin therapy to help her through this stressful period and to increase her energy level. She tells you that she still has some prenatal vitamins and wonders if she should take them.

Critical Thinking Questions

1. What other assessment data might you want to gather from Charlene before recommending vitamin therapy?

2. Should Charlene take the prenatal vitamins? Why or why not?

3. What other recommendations would you give to Charlene regarding vitamin therapy?

See Answers to Critical Thinking Questions in Appendix B.

NCLEX Practice Questions

1 A healthcare provider has ordered oral vitamin A supplements for a client. The serum level of vitamin A may be increased if the client is also taking

   a. Vitamins D and E

   b. Oral contraceptives

   c. Mineral oil

   d. Antibiotics

2 Pyridoxine (vitamin B_6) may cause antagonistic drug effects for a client taking

   a. Isoniazid (Isotamine)

   b. Oral contraceptives

   c. Hydralazine (Apresoline)

   d. Anti-parkinsonism drugs

3 The nurse would suspect a calcium deficiency in a client exhibiting

   a. Night blindness

   b. Anemia

   c. Muscle cramping and spasms

   d. Bleeding abnormalities

4 To meet his nutritional goals, a client is placed on enteral feedings via a nasogastric (NG) tube. Which intervention should the nurse perform in order to ensure that the client is maintaining a proper fluid balance?

   a. Weigh the client every other day.

   b. Maintain a strict record of intake and output, and flush the nasogastric tube once per day.

   c. Provide free water in addition to that used for irrigating the tube.

   d. Assess the skin around the tube insertion site for any drainage or irritation.

5 The nurse is making rounds at the beginning of the shift and notes that a client's total parenteral nutrition bag is empty. Which solution should the nurse hang until the total parenteral nutrition solution can be properly prepared and delivered to the nursing unit?

   a. 5% dextrose in water (D_5W)

   b. 5% dextrose in Ringer's lactate (D_5RL)

   c. 5% dextrose in 0.9% sodium chloride (D_5NS)

   d. 10% dextrose in water ($D_{10}W$)

See Answers to NCLEX Practice Questions in Appendix A.

Pharmacology of Alterations in the Respiratory System

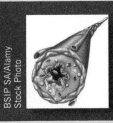

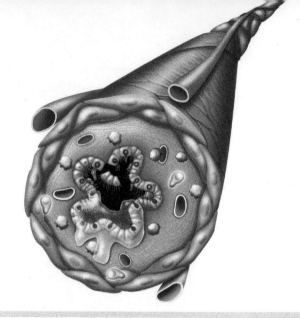

BSIP SA/Alamy Stock Photo

CHAPTER 38

Pharmacotherapy of Asthma, Common Cold, and Other Pulmonary Disorders

LEARNING OUTCOMES

After reading this chapter, the student should be able to:

1. List drug classes used for treating pulmonary disorders and discuss differences among their mechanisms of action.
2. Compare the advantages and disadvantages of using the inhalation route of drug administration for pulmonary drugs.
3. Describe the types of devices used to deliver aerosol therapies via the inhalation route.
4. Explain how drugs that modify the autonomic nervous system can be used to modify airflow in the bronchial tree.
5. Describe how drugs can be used to relieve the common symptoms of asthma, chronic bronchitis, and emphysema based on their underlying pathophysiology.
6. Describe the nurse's role in the pharmacological and non-pharmacological treatment of pulmonary disorders.
7. For each of the drug classes listed in Prototype Drugs, identify a representative drug and explain its mechanism of action, therapeutic effects, and important adverse effects.
8. Describe and explain, based on pharmacological principles, the rationale for nursing assessment, planning, and interventions for clients with pulmonary disorders.
9. Use the nursing process to care for clients who are receiving drug therapy for pulmonary disorders.

CHAPTER OUTLINE

▸ Physiology of the Respiratory System

▸ Bronchiolar Smooth Muscle

▸ Administration of Pulmonary Drugs via Inhalation

▸ Asthma
  ▸ Pathophysiology of Asthma

▸ Beta-Adrenergic Agonists
  ▸ Treating Asthma with Beta-Adrenergic Agonists

▸ Methylxanthines and Anticholinergics
  ▸ Treating Asthma with Methylxanthines and Anticholinergics

▸ Glucocorticoids
  ▸ Pharmacotherapy of Asthma with Glucocorticoids

The respiratory system is one of the most important organ systems—a mere 5 to 6 minutes without breathing may result in death. When functioning properly, the respiratory system provides the body with the oxygen critical for all cells to carry on normal activities. Measurement of the rate and depth of respiration and listening to chest sounds with a stethoscope provide the nurse with valuable clues as to what may be happening internally. The respiratory system also provides a means by which the body can rid itself of excess acids and bases, a topic that is covered in Chapter 53. This chapter examines drugs used in the pharmacotherapy of asthma, the common cold, and chronic obstructive pulmonary disease.

Physiology of the Respiratory System

38.1 The physiology of the respiratory system involves two main processes. Ventilation moves air into and out of the lungs and perfusion allows for gas exchange across capillaries.

The primary function of the respiratory system is to bring oxygen (O_2) into the body and to remove carbon dioxide (CO_2) from it. The process by which gases are exchanged is called **respiration**. The basic structures of the respiratory system are shown in Figure 38.1.

Ventilation is the process of moving air into and out of the lungs. As the diaphragm contracts and lowers in position, it creates a negative pressure that draws air into the lungs, and inspiration occurs. During expiration, the diaphragm relaxes and air leaves the lung passively, with no energy expenditure required. Ventilation is a purely mechanical process that occurs approximately 12 to 18 times per minute in adults, a rate determined by neurons in the brainstem. This rate may be modified by a number of factors, including emotions, fever, stress, the pH of the blood, and certain medications.

Air entering the respiratory system travels through the nose, pharynx, and trachea into the bronchi, which divide into progressively smaller passages called bronchioles. The bronchial tree ends in dilated sacs called alveoli, which have no smooth muscle but are abundantly rich in capillaries. The extremely thin membrane of the alveoli separates the airway from the pulmonary capillaries, allowing gases to readily move between the internal environment of the blood and the inspired air. As oxygen crosses this membrane, it is exchanged for carbon dioxide, a cellular waste product that travels from the blood to the air. The lung is richly supplied with blood. Blood flow through the lung is called **perfusion**. The process of gas exchange is shown in Figure 38.1.

Bronchiolar Smooth Muscle

38.2 Bronchioles are lined with smooth muscle that controls the amount of air entering the lungs. Dilation and constriction of the airways are controlled by the autonomic nervous system.

Bronchioles are muscular, elastic structures whose internal diameter, or lumen, varies with the specific needs of the body. Changes in the diameter of the bronchiolar lumen are made possible by smooth muscle controlled by the autonomic nervous system. During the fight-or-flight response, beta$_2$-adrenergic receptors of the sympathetic nervous system are stimulated, the bronchiolar smooth muscle relaxes, and bronchodilation occurs. This allows more air to enter the alveoli, thus increasing the oxygen supply to the body during periods of stress or exercise. Sympathetic nervous system activation also increases the rate and depth of breathing. Drugs that stimulate beta$_2$-adrenergic receptors to cause bronchodilation are some of the most common drugs for treating pulmonary disorders.

When nerves from the parasympathetic nervous system are activated, bronchiolar smooth muscle contracts and the airway diameter narrows, resulting in bronchoconstriction. Bronchoconstriction increases airway resistance, causing breathing to be more

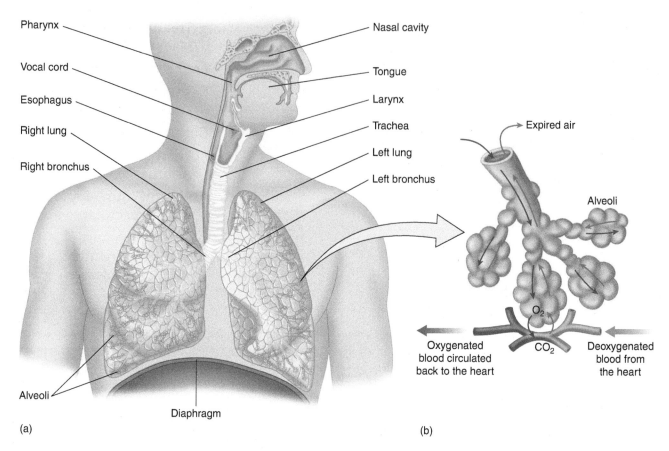

(a)

(b)

Figure 38.1 The respiratory system.

laboured and the client to become short of breath. Parasympathetic stimulation also has the effect of slowing the rate and depth of respiration.

Administration of Pulmonary Drugs via Inhalation

38.3 Inhalation is a common route of administration for pulmonary drugs because it delivers drugs directly to the site of action. Nebulizers, MDIs, and DPIs are devices used for aerosol therapies.

The respiratory system offers a rapid and efficient mechanism for delivering drugs. The enormous surface area of the bronchioles and alveoli and the rich blood supply to these areas results in an almost instantaneous onset of action for inhaled substances.

Pulmonary drugs are delivered to the respiratory system by aerosol therapy. An **aerosol** is a suspension of minute liquid droplets or fine solid particles suspended in a gas. Aerosol therapy can give immediate relief for **bronchospasm**, a condition during which the bronchiolar smooth muscle contracts, leaving the client gasping for breath. Drugs may also be given to loosen viscous mucus in the bronchial tree. The major advantage of

aerosol therapy is that it delivers the drugs to their immediate site of action, thus reducing systemic side effects. To produce the same therapeutic action, an oral drug would have to be given at higher doses, and it would be distributed to all body tissues.

It should be clearly understood that agents delivered by inhalation can produce systemic effects due to absorption. For example, anesthetics such as nitrous oxide and halothane (Fluothane) are delivered via the inhalation route and are rapidly distributed to cause central nervous system (CNS) depression (see Chapter 24). Solvents such as paint thinners and glues are sometimes intentionally inhaled and can cause serious adverse effects on the nervous system, or even death. The nurse must always monitor for systemic effects from inhalation drugs.

Several devices are used to deliver drugs via the inhalation route. **Nebulizers** are small machines that vaporize a liquid medication into a fine mist that can be inhaled using a face mask or handheld device. If the drug is a solid, it may be administered using a **dry powder inhaler (DPI)**. A DPI is a small device that is activated by the process of inhalation to deliver a fine powder directly to the bronchial tree. Turbohalers and rotahalers are types of DPIs. **Metered dose inhalers (MDIs)** are a third type of device commonly used to deliver respiratory drugs. MDIs use a propellant to deliver a measured dose of drug to the lungs during each breath. The client times the inhalation to the puffs of drug emitted from the MDI.

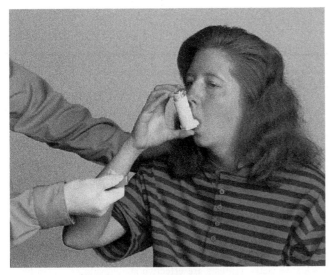

(a) Metered dose inhaler

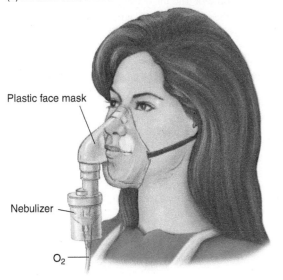

(b) Nebulizer with attached face mask

Figure 38.2 Devices used to deliver respiratory drugs.
Source: Pearson Education.

There are disadvantages to administering aerosol therapy. The precise dose received by the client is difficult to measure because it depends on the client's breathing pattern and the correct use of the aerosol device. Even under optimal conditions, only 10% to 50% of the drug actually reaches the bronchial tree. A spacer can improve drug distribution to the lungs: see http://asthma.ca/adults/treatment/spacers.php. The nurse must carefully instruct clients on the correct use of these devices. To reduce the oral absorption of inhaled medicines, clients should rinse their mouth thoroughly following drug use. Two devices used to deliver respiratory drugs are shown in Figure 38.2.

ASTHMA

Asthma is a chronic disease with both inflammatory and bronchospasm components. Drugs may be given to decrease the frequency of asthma attacks or to terminate attacks in progress.

Pathophysiology of Asthma

38.4 Asthma is a chronic disease that has both inflammation and bronchospasm components. Treatment should focus on the reduction of inflammation. Environmental control can help to reduce inflammation and prevent asthma attacks.

Asthma is one of the most common chronic conditions in Canada, affecting more than 2.2 million Canadians. The disease is characterized by acute bronchospasm, causing intense breathlessness, coughing, and gasping for air. Along with bronchoconstriction, the acute inflammatory response is initiated, stimulating mucus secretion and edema in the airways. These conditions are illustrated in Figure 38.3. Status asthmaticus is a severe, prolonged form of asthma unresponsive to drug treatment that may lead to respiratory failure. Typical causes of asthma attacks are listed in Table 38.1.

Although the exact cause of asthma is unknown, it is believed to be the result of chronic airway inflammation. Controlling environmental factors that contribute to inflammation and asthma, such as dust mites and animal fur, may help to slow disease progression and prevent asthma attacks. Because asthma has both a bronchoconstriction component and an inflammation component,

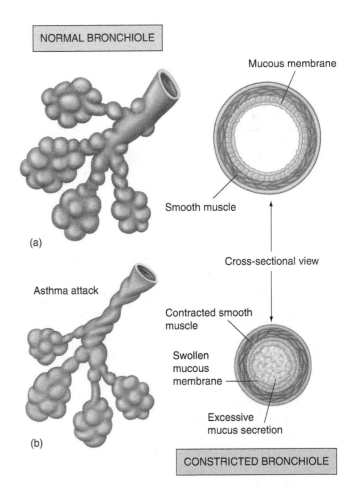

Figure 38.3 Changes in bronchioles during an asthma attack: (a) normal bronchiole; (b) constricted bronchiole.

TABLE 38.1   Common Causes of Asthma

Cause	Sources
Air pollutants	Tobacco smoke
	Ozone
	Nitrous and sulfur oxides
	Fumes from cleaning fluids or solvents
	Burning leaves
Allergens	Pollen from trees, grasses, and weeds
	Animal dander
	Household dust and dust mites
	Mould
Chemicals and food	Drugs, including acetylsalicylic acid (ASA [Aspirin]), ibuprofen (Advil, Motrin), and beta blockers
	Sulfite preservatives
	Food and condiments, including nuts, monosodium glutamate, shellfish, and dairy products
Respiratory infections	Bacterial, fungal, and viral
Stress	Emotional stress/anxiety
	Exercise in dry, cold climates

pharmacotherapy of the disease focuses on one or both of these mechanisms. The goals of drug therapy are twofold: to terminate bronchospasm during an acute asthma attack and to reduce the frequency of acute asthma attacks and prevent further airway damage. Different medications are usually needed to achieve each of these goals. A summary of the various classes of drugs used to treat respiratory diseases is illustrated in Figure 38.4.

According to the Canadian Asthma Consensus Guidelines that were endorsed in 2003, the five fundamental aspects of asthma care are as follows:

1. Achieve acceptable control of the disease.

2. Treatment of asthma should focus on managing inflammation; inhaled glucocorticoids are the first-line anti-inflammatory therapy.

3. Control the environment.

4. A written action plan for guided self-management should be provided for all clients.

5. If acceptable control is not obtained, other drugs can be used in addition to moderate doses of corticosteroid.

BETA-ADRENERGIC AGONISTS

Selective beta$_2$ agonists are effective at relieving acute bronchospasm. They are some of the most frequently prescribed agents for the pharmacotherapy of asthma and other pulmonary diseases. These drugs are listed in Table 38.2.

NCLEX Success Tips

Salbutamol (Ventolin) is a rapidly acting bronchodilator and is the first-line medication in "rescue" inhalers that reverses airway narrowing in acute asthma attacks.

Salbutamol, a beta$_2$-adrenergic agonist that causes dilation of the bronchioles, is prescribed to prevent and treat wheezing, difficulty breathing, and chest tightness caused by lung diseases such as asthma and chronic obstructive pulmonary disease (COPD). It's given by nebulization or metered-dose inhalation and may be given as often as every 30 to 60 minutes until relief is accomplished. It opens and relaxes the airways, allowing a greater exchange of air, which is reflected as a higher peak expiratory flow rate.

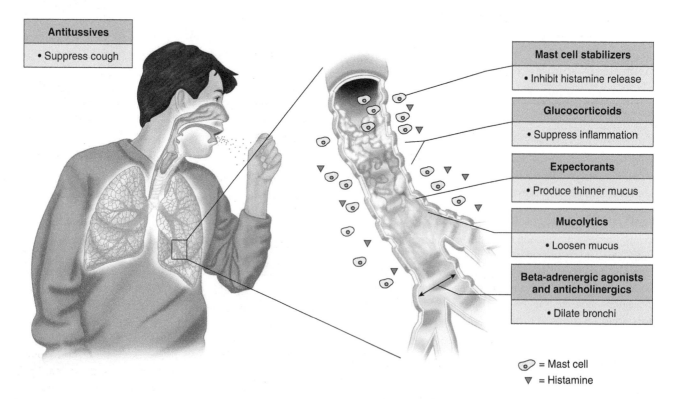

Figure 38.4 Drugs used to treat respiratory disorders.

Irritability, nervousness, tachycardia, insomnia, and anxiety are common side effects of beta-adrenergic agonist bronchodilators that result from sympathetic nervous system stimulation. The expected therapeutic effect of a bronchodilator is decreased dyspnea and slower breathing.

Fluticasone (Flovent) and salmeterol (Serevent) is a combination drug used as a prophylactic agent to help prevent bronchial asthma attacks. The fluticasone is an inhaled corticosteroid that reduces inflammation. The salmeterol is a long-acting beta agonist that reduces bronchospasms. The drug must be taken on a consistent basis, twice per day, over a long period of time to be effective.

Salmeterol is a beta$_2$ agonist, a maintenance drug that the asthmatic client uses twice daily, every 12 hours. Salmeterol can be used to prevent exercise-induced bronchospasms, but it should be taken 30 to 60 minutes before exercise. If the client is taking salmeterol twice daily, it should not be used in additional doses before exercise; twice daily is the maximum dosage. Indications for salmeterol include only asthma and bronchospasm induced by chronic obstructive pulmonary disease.

If the client is ordered a bronchodilator and another inhaled medication, the bronchodilator should be administered first to dilate the airways and to enhance the effectiveness of the second medication.

Advair Diskus is a combination of steroid and bronchodilator used in the treatment of chronic asthma and chronic obstructive airway disease. The medication is intended to be used daily. It is not a rescue inhaler, and additional doses do not improve respiratory function. Evaluation of effectiveness includes improvement in respiratory status and the ability to perform activities of daily living/quality of life activities such as walking and playing. Side effects of the medication include an increase in cough and sputum production.

Beta blockers are contraindicated in a client who's wheezing because it's a beta$_2$-adrenergic antagonist.

Signs and symptoms of salbutamol toxicity that the nurse should instruct the parents to watch for include tachycardia, restlessness, nausea, vomiting, and dizziness.

NCLEX Success Tip

When using inhalers, clients should first shake the inhaler to activate the MDI and then breathe out through the mouth. Next, the client should activate the MDI while inhaling, hold the breath for 5 to 10 seconds, and then exhale normally.

TABLE 38.2 Bronchodilators Used for Asthma

Drug	Route and Adult Dose
Beta-Adrenergic Agonists	
formoterol (Foradil, Oxeze Turbuhaler)	DPI, 12 μg inhalation capsule every 12 hours (q12h)
metaproterenol (Alupent, Orciprenaline)	MDI, 2–3 inhalations every 3–4 hours (q3–4h) (max 12 inhalations/day)
salbutamol (Ventolin)	MDI, 1-2 inhalations tid-qid/day (max 8 inhalations/day); also available as a nebulizer solution, 2.5 mg tid-qid PRN
Pr salmeterol (Serevent)	MDI/DPI, 1 inhalation twice a day (bid)
Methylxanthines	
aminophylline	PO, 0.25–0.75 mg/kg/hour divided qid
theophylline (Uniphyl, Theolair)	PO, 0.4–0.6 mg/kg/hour divided tid–qid
Anticholinergics	
Pr ipratropium (Atrovent)	MDI, 2 inhalations qid (max 12 inhalations/day)

Treating Asthma with Beta-Adrenergic Agonists

38.5 Beta-adrenergic agonists are the most effective drugs for relieving acute bronchospasm. These agents act by activating beta$_2$ receptors in bronchial smooth muscle to cause bronchodilation.

Beta-adrenergic agonists (sympathomimetics) are drugs of choice in the treatment of acute bronchoconstriction. Sympathomimetics selective for beta$_2$ receptors in the lung have largely replaced the older, non-selective agents such as epinephrine because they produce fewer cardiac side effects. Sympathomimetics act by relaxing bronchial smooth muscle; the resulting bronchodilation lowers airway resistance and makes breathing easier for the client.

A practical method used to classify beta-adrenergic agonists for asthma is by their duration of action. The ultrashort-acting drugs, including isoproterenol (Isuprel), produce bronchodilation immediately, but their effects last only 2 to 3 hours. Short-acting agents, such as metaproterenol (Alupent, Orciprenaline), terbutaline (Bricanyl), and pirbuterol (Maxair), also act quickly but last for 5 to 6 hours. Intermediate-acting sympathomimetics, such as salbutamol, last for about 8 hours. The longest acting agent, salmeterol, has effects that last for as long as 12 hours. The ultrashort-, short-, and intermediate-acting drugs act quickly enough to terminate acute asthmatic episodes. The onset of action for salmeterol is too long for it to be indicated for acute asthma attack termination. Formoterol (Foradil, Oxeze Turbuhaler) is the newest beta$_2$-adrenergic agonist, combining a very rapid onset of action (1 to 3 minutes) with a 12-hour duration.

Inhaled beta-adrenergic agonists produce little systemic toxicity because only small amounts of the drugs are absorbed. When given orally, a longer duration of action is achieved, but systemic side effects such as tachycardia are experienced more frequently; these drugs are sometimes contraindicated for clients with dysrhythmias. Tolerance may develop to the therapeutic effects of the beta-adrenergic agonists; therefore, the client must be instructed to seek medical attention should the drugs become less effective with continued use.

Nursing Considerations

The role of the nurse in asthma therapy with beta-adrenergic agonists involves careful monitoring of the client's condition and providing education as it relates to the prescribed drug regimen. Experiencing breathing difficulties can be distressing and greatly affect a client's quality of life. Controlling asthma is vital to a person's ability to perform normal activities of daily living. When beta-adrenergic agonists are used as bronchodilators, they help to reduce respiratory distress.

Assess the client's adherence to medication and the presence of side effects. Assess for the presence or history of bradycardia, dysrhythmias, myocardial infarction (MI), hypothyroidism, decreased renal function, diabetes mellitus, glaucoma, benign prostatic hyperplasia, and tuberculosis. Beta-adrenergic agonists should not be used if the client has a history of dysrhythmia or MI. Drugs in this class may cause many undesirable side effects. For clients who are using isoproterenol (Isuprel), rebound bronchospasm may occur when the effects of the drug wear off.

Instruct the client on the use of the inhaler, and observe its use. Instruct the client to hold his or her breath for 10 seconds after inhaling the medication and wait for 2 full minutes before the second inhalation.

Client education as it relates to beta-adrenergic agonists should include goals, reasons for obtaining baseline data such as vital signs and tests for cardiac and renal function, and possible side effects. The following are important points to include when teaching clients regarding beta-adrenergic agonists:

- Limit the use of products that contain caffeine.
- Immediately report difficulty breathing, heart palpitations, tremor, vomiting, nervousness, and vision changes.

| PROTOTYPE DRUG | **Salmeterol (Serevent Diskhaler Disk)** |

Actions and Uses: Salmeterol acts by selectively binding to beta$_2$-adrenergic receptors in bronchial smooth muscle to cause bronchodilation. When taken 30 to 60 minutes prior to physical activity, it has been shown to prevent exercise-induced bronchospasm. Its 12-hour duration of action is longer than that of many other bronchodilators, thus making it ideal for asthma maintenance therapy. Because salmeterol takes 15 to 25 minutes to act, it is not indicated for the termination of acute bronchospasm.

Pharmacokinetics: There is minimal systemic absorption of salmeterol following inhalation. It has a half-life of 3 to 4 hours.

Administration Alerts:
- Proper use of the DPI is important for effective delivery of drug. Observe and instruct the client in proper use.
- Salmeterol is pregnancy category C.

Adverse Effects and Interactions: Serious adverse effects from salmeterol are uncommon. Like other beta agonists, some clients experience headaches, nervousness, and restlessness. Because of its potential to cause tachycardia, clients with heart disease should be monitored regularly. Excessive use of salmeterol (more than three times per week) for asthma attacks, waking with symptoms, or regular dyspnea are signs of uncontrolled asthma that requires adjustment of medications.

Concurrent use of beta blockers will antagonize the effects of salmeterol.

METHYLXANTHINES AND ANTICHOLINERGICS

Although beta agonists are drugs of choice for treating acute bronchospasm, drugs in the methylxanthine and anticholinergic classes are alternatives for the treatment of asthma. The methylxanthines are older, established drugs. Only one anticholinergic is in widespread use. These agents are listed in Table 38.2.

Treating Asthma with Methylxanthines and Anticholinergics

38.6 Methylxanthines and anticholinergics are bronchodilators occasionally used as alternatives to the beta agonists in asthma therapy.

The **methylxanthines**, such as theophylline (Uniphyl, Theolair) and aminophylline, comprise a group of bronchodilators that are chemically related to caffeine. Theophylline has a narrow margin of safety and interacts with a large number of other drugs. Side effects such as nausea, vomiting, and CNS stimulation are relatively common, and dysrhythmias may be observed at high doses. Because of their chemical similarities, clients should avoid caffeine-containing foods and beverages when taking methylxanthines. These agents are given by the PO or intravenous (IV) route. Having been largely replaced by safer and more effective drugs, the current use of theophylline is primarily for the long-term, oral prophylaxis of persistent asthma.

NCLEX Success Tip

Methylxanthines such as theophylline are highly potent bronchodilators used to relieve asthma symptoms. The bronchodilation will result in decreased wheezing.

Blocking the parasympathetic nervous system produces similar effects to stimulation of the sympathetic nervous system. It is predictable then that anticholinergic drugs would cause bronchodilation and have potential use in the pharmacotherapy of asthma and other pulmonary diseases. Ipratropium (Atrovent) is the most common anticholinergic prescribed for asthma and COPD pharmacotherapy. It has a slower onset of action than most beta agonists and produces less intense bronchodilation. Anticholinergic side effects that are associated with drugs in this class are much milder when the drugs are administered by inhalation rather than systemically.

Nursing Considerations

The role of the nurse in asthma therapy with methylxanthines and anticholinergics involves careful monitoring of the client's condition and providing education as it relates to the prescribed drug regimen. Assess respiration rate before and after the first dose from an MDI because the first dose may precipitate bronchospasm. Monitor vital signs and intake and output throughout therapy, as these drugs cause diuresis. Elderly clients who are using methylxanthines should be monitored carefully for toxicity, as these clients may exhibit increased sensitivity due to decreased hepatic metabolism.

Methylxanthines may cause dysrhythmias, nausea, vomiting, and irritation of the upper respiratory tract, which may result in cough, drying of mucous membranes, and a bitter taste. To help with dry mouth and bitterness, clients can rinse their mouths frequently or use sugarless, hard candy.

NCLEX Success Tip

Theophylline and other methylxanthine agents make the central respiratory centre more sensitive to carbon dioxide and stimulate the respiratory drive. Inhibition of phosphodiesterase is the drug's mechanism of action in treating asthma and other reversible obstructive airway diseases—not COPD.

Anticholinergic bronchodilators should be used cautiously in elderly men with benign prostatic hypertrophy and in all clients with glaucoma. The complete nursing process applied to clients receiving anticholinergics is presented in Nursing Process Focus: Clients Receiving Anticholinergic Therapy in Chapter 14, page 148.

Client education as it relates to methylxanthines should include goals, reasons for obtaining baseline data such as vital signs and tests for cardiac and renal function, and possible side effects. Instruct the client to immediately report the following: inability to urinate or have a bowel movement, severe headache, heart palpitations, difficulty breathing, changes in vision, and eye pain.

For additional nursing considerations, see Nursing Process Focus: Clients Receiving Bronchodilators.

NURSING PROCESS FOCUS

Clients Receiving Bronchodilators

Assessment	Potential Nursing Diagnoses/Identified Patterns
Prior to administration: • Obtain complete health history, including allergies, drug history, and possible drug reactions. • Assess for symptoms related to respiratory insufficiency such as dyspnea, orthopnea, cyanosis, nasal flaring, wheezing, and weakness. • Obtain vital signs. • Auscultate bilateral breath sounds for air movement and adventitious sounds (rales, rhonchi, wheezes). • Assess pulmonary function with pulse oximeter, peak expiratory flow meter, and/or arterial blood gases to establish baseline.	• Need for knowledge regarding drug therapy, adverse effects, and importance of adherence to treatment • Need for knowledge about management of asthma attacks • Need for knowledge of environmental modifications to reduce inflammation and disease progression • Anxiety related to difficulty breathing • Activity intolerance related to ineffective drug therapy • Disturbed sleep pattern related to side effects of drugs

Planning: Client Goals and Expected Outcomes

The client will:

• Exhibit adequate oxygenation as evidenced by improved lung sounds and pulmonary function values
• Report a reduction in subjective symptoms of respiratory deficiency
• Demonstrate an understanding of the drug by accurately describing the drug's purpose, action, side effects, and precautions
• Report at least 6 hours of uninterrupted sleep

Implementation

Interventions (Rationales)	Client Education/Discharge Planning
• Monitor vital signs, including pulse, blood pressure, and respiratory rate. • Monitor pulmonary function with pulse oximeter, peak expiratory flow meter, and/or arterial blood gases. (Monitoring is necessary to assess drug effectiveness.) • Monitor the client's ability to use inhaler. (Proper use ensures correct dosage.) • Observe for side effects specific to the medication used. • Maintain an environment free of respiratory contaminants such as dust, dry air, flowers, and smoke. (These substances may exacerbate bronchial constriction.) • Maintain adequate dietary intake of essential nutrients and vitamins. (Dyspnea interferes with proper nutrition.) • Ensure client maintains adequate hydration of 3 to 4 L per day (to liquefy pulmonary secretions). • Provide emotional and psychosocial support during periods of shortness of breath. • Monitor client adherence. (Maintaining therapeutic drug levels is essential to effective therapy.)	Instruct client to: • Use medication as directed even if asymptomatic • Report difficulty with breathing • Instruct client to report symptoms of deteriorating respiratory status such as increased dyspnea, breathlessness with speech, and/or orthopnea Instruct client: • In proper use of metered dose inhaler • To strictly use the medication as prescribed; do not "double up" on doses • To rinse mouth thoroughly following use • Instruct client regarding side effects and to report specific drug side effects Instruct client to: • Avoid respiratory irritants • Maintain "clean air environment" • Stop smoking and avoid secondhand smoke, if applicable Instruct client to: • Maintain nutrition with foods high in essential nutrients • Consume small, frequent meals to prevent fatigue • Consume 3 to 4 L of fluid per day if not contraindicated • Avoid caffeine (increases CNS irritability) • Instruct client in relaxation techniques and controlled breathing techniques • Inform the client of the importance of ongoing medication compliance and follow-up

Evaluation of Outcome Criteria

Evaluate the effectiveness of drug therapy by confirming that client goals and expected outcomes have been met (see "Planning").

See Table 38.2 (page 457) for a list of drugs to which these nursing actions apply.

CONNECTIONS ◀ Special Considerations

◀ Asthma Management in Schools

Approximately 10% of children have asthma. Researchers suggest that asthma is one of the most common causes of school absenteeism. In a typical class of 30 children or youth, 2 students suffer from asthma attacks each year while at school. Children cannot learn while experiencing wheezing, coughing, and shortness of breath.

Assisting schools to develop asthma management programs has become the focus of several federal agencies and dozens of professional and client advocacy groups. Many schools are adopting asthma management plans as part of a coordinated school health program. Schools with these programs have established "asthma-friendly" policies, such as allowing students to carry and administer quick-relief asthma medications. In addition, the schools routinely maintain a copy of the student's asthma action plan from the caregiver or healthcare provider.

The role of the school nurse is to review the plan, determine the student's specific needs, and ensure that the student has immediate access to quick-relief asthma medication. The optimal plan for each student is determined case by case, with input from the student, parents, healthcare provider, and school nurse. Typically, older students are permitted to carry the inhaler and to self-administer as needed. The nurse often keeps a backup supply of the student's medication. For younger children, a supervised health assistant may be delegated to administer the medication.

PROTOTYPE DRUG | Ipratropium (Atrovent)

Actions and Uses: Ipratropium is an anticholinergic (muscarinic antagonist) that causes bronchodilation by blocking cholinergic receptors in bronchial smooth muscle. It is administered via inhalation and can relieve acute bronchospasm within minutes after administration. Effects may peak in 1 to 2 hours and continue for up to 6 hours. Ipratropium is less effective than the beta$_2$ agonists but is sometimes combined with beta agonists or glucocorticoids for its additive effects. It is also prescribed for chronic bronchitis and for the symptomatic relief of nasal congestion.

Pharmacokinetics: There is minimal systemic absorption of ipratropium following inhalation. It has a half-life of 2 hours.

Administration Alerts:

- Proper use of the MDI is important for effective delivery of the drug. Observe and instruct the client in proper use.
- Avoid contact with eyes.
- Ipratropium is pregnancy category B.

Adverse Effects and Interactions: Because it is not readily absorbed from the lungs, ipratropium produces few systemic side effects. Irritation of the upper respiratory tract may result in cough, drying of the nasal mucosa, or hoarseness. It produces a bitter taste, which may be relieved by rinsing the mouth after use.

NCLEX Success Tip

Ipratropium is a bronchodilator, and its anticholinergic effects can aggravate urine retention.

GLUCOCORTICOIDS

Inhaled glucocorticoids are used for the long-term prevention of asthma attacks. Oral glucocorticoids may be used for the short-term management of acute asthma. The glucocorticoids are listed in Table 38.3.

Pharmacotherapy of Asthma with Glucocorticoids

38.7 Inhaled glucocorticoids are first-line therapy for asthma. They reduce inflammation and provide long-term prophylaxis of attacks. Oral glucocorticoids are also available.

Glucocorticoids are first-line therapy for the pharmacotherapy of asthma. When inhaled on a daily schedule, these hormones suppress airway inflammation without major side effects and help

TABLE 38.3   Anti-Inflammatory Drugs Used for Asthma

Drug	Route and Adult Dose
Glucocorticoids	
Pr beclomethasone (QVAR)	MDI, 50-400 μg bid (max 400 μg bid)
budesonide (Pulmicort)	DPI, 400 to 2400 μg/day in 2–4 divided doses
fluticasone (Flovent) (see Chapter 42, page 506, for the Prototype Drug box)	MDI 100–500 μg bid
methylprednisolone (Medrol, Depo-Medrol, Solu-Medrol)	PO, 4–48 mg every day (qd); intramuscularly (IM)/IV, 10–40 mg, repeated if needed
prednisone (see Chapter 42, page 499, for the Prototype Drug box)	PO, 5–60 mg qd
Mast Cell Stabilizers	
cromolyn	MDI, 1 inhalation qid
nedocromil (Tilade)	MDI, 2 inhalations qid 14 mg/day
Leukotriene Modifiers	
montelukast (Singulair)	PO, 10 mg qd in evening
zafirlukast (Accolate)	PO, 20 mg bid 1 hour before or 2 hours after meals

to prevent acute asthma attacks. Clients should be informed that inhaled glucocorticoids must be taken daily to produce their therapeutic effect and that these drugs are not effective at terminating episodes in progress. For some clients with mild, persistent asthma who do not wish to take inhaled steroid therapy daily, an as-needed treatment strategy may be acceptable provided that it is accompanied by education and an action plan with clear instructions about how and when to increase medication use. Nevertheless, daily inhaled steroid treatment remains the preferred evidence-based therapy for asthma.

For severe, persistent asthma that is unresponsive to other treatments, oral glucocorticoids may be prescribed. If taken for longer than 10 days, oral glucocorticoids can produce significant adverse effects, including adrenal gland atrophy, peptic ulcers, and hyperglycemia. Other uses and adverse effects of glucocorticoids are presented in Chapter 30.

Nursing Considerations

The role of the nurse in asthma pharmacotherapy with glucocorticoids involves careful monitoring of the client's condition and providing education as it relates to the prescribed treatment. Assess the client for the presence or history of asthma, seasonal rhinitis, hypertension, heart disease, and blood clots. Monitor the client's vital signs and body weight, and assess for signs and symptoms of infection. The steroid inhalers should be used cautiously in clients with hypertension, gastrointestinal (GI) disease, congestive heart failure, or thromboembolic disease.

Because the primary purpose of inhaled glucocorticoids is to *prevent* respiratory distress, the client should be advised that this medication should not be used during an acute asthma attack. Excessive use of a short-acting bronchodilator (more than three times per week) for acute asthma attacks, waking with symptoms, or regular dyspnea are signs of uncontrolled asthma that require adjustment of the glucocorticoid dosage. In addition, the client should be alert for signs and symptoms of simple infections, as glucocorticoids inhibit the inflammatory response and can mask the signs of infection. The client should be advised to rinse the mouth after using steroid inhalers because the drugs may promote fungal infections of the mouth and throat. Glucocorticoids also increase blood glucose levels and should be closely monitored in individuals with diabetes mellitus.

Client education as it relates to glucocorticoids should include goals, reasons for obtaining baseline data such as vital signs and tests for cardiac and renal function, and possible side effects. The following are the important points to include when teaching clients regarding glucocorticoids:

- Monitor temperature and blood pressure daily and report elevation to the healthcare provider.

- If diabetic, monitor blood glucose level closely and report unexplained or consistent elevations.

- Report occurrence of tarry stools, edema, dizziness, or difficulty breathing.

- Do not use these medications to terminate acute asthma attacks. Discuss with the healthcare provider the appropriate medication to stop attacks.

PROTOTYPE DRUG | **Beclomethasone (QVAR)**

Actions and Uses: Beclomethasone is a glucocorticoid available through aerosol inhalation (MDI) for asthma or as a nasal spray for allergic rhinitis. For asthma, two inhalations, two to three times per day, usually provide adequate prophylaxis. Beclomethasone acts by reducing inflammation, thus decreasing the frequency of asthma attacks. It is not a bronchodilator and should not be used to terminate asthma attacks in progress.

Pharmacokinetics: There is minimal systemic absorption of beclomethasone when inhaled. It has a half-life of 1.5 hours.

Administration Alerts:

- Do not use if the client is experiencing an acute asthma attack.
- Oral inhalation products and nasal spray products are not to be used interchangeably.
- Beclomethasone is pregnancy category C.

Adverse Effects and Interactions: Inhaled beclomethasone produces few systemic side effects. Because small amounts may be swallowed with each dose, the client should be observed for signs of glucocorticoid toxicity when taking the drug for prolonged periods. Local effects may include hoarseness of the voice. Like all glucocorticoids, the anti-inflammatory properties of beclomethasone can mask signs of infection, and the drug is contraindicated if active infection is present. A large percentage of clients who take beclomethasone on a long-term basis will develop candidiasis, a fungal infection in the throat, due to the constant deposits of drug in the oral cavity.

MAST CELL STABILIZERS

Two mast cell stabilizers serve limited though important roles in the prophylaxis of asthma. The mast cell stabilizers act by inhibiting the release of histamine from mast cells. These drugs are listed in Table 38.3.

Treating Asthma with Mast Cell Stabilizers

38.8 Cromolyn, a mast cell stabilizer, is a safe drug used for the prophylaxis of asthma, but it is ineffective at relieving acute bronchospasm.

Cromolyn is classified as mast cell stabilizers because its action serves to inhibit mast cells from releasing histamine and other chemical mediators of inflammation. By reducing inflammation, it is able to prevent asthma attacks. As with the glucocorticoids, clients must be informed that this agent should be taken on a daily basis and that it is not effective at terminating acute attacks. Maximum therapeutic benefit may take several weeks. Cromolyn is pregnancy category B.

Cromolyn was the first mast stabilizer discovered. When administered via an MDI or a nebulizer, this drug is a safe alternative to glucocorticoids. An intranasal form of cromolyn is used in the treatment of seasonal allergies. Side effects include stinging or burning of the nasal mucosa, irritation of the throat, and nasal congestion. Although not common, bronchospasm and anaphylaxis have been reported. Because of its short half-life (80 minutes), it must be inhaled four to six times per day.

LEUKOTRIENE MODIFIERS

The leukotriene modifiers are newer drugs, approved in the 1990s, that are used to reduce inflammation and ease bronchoconstriction. They modify the action of leukotrienes, which are mediators of the inflammatory response in asthmatic clients. These drugs are listed in Table 38.3.

Treating Asthma with Leukotriene Modifiers

38.9 The leukotriene modifiers, whose primary use is in asthma prophylaxis, act by reducing the inflammatory component of asthma.

Leukotrienes are mediators of the immune response that promote airway edema, inflammation, and bronchoconstriction. Zileuton (Zyflo) acts by blocking lipoxygenase, the enzyme that converts arachidonic acid into leukotrienes. The remaining two agents in this class, zafirlukast (Accolate) and montelukast (Singulair), act by blocking leukotriene receptors.

The leukotriene modifiers are approved for the prophylaxis of chronic asthma. They are not bronchodilators and are ineffective in terminating acute asthma attacks. They are all given orally. Because zileuton is taken four times a day, it offers less client convenience than montelukast or zafirlukast, which are taken every 12 hours. Zileuton has a more rapid onset of action (2 hours) than the other two leukotriene modifiers, which take as long as 1 week to obtain therapeutic benefit.

Few serious adverse effects are associated with the leukotriene modifiers. Headache, cough, nasal congestion, or GI upset may occur. Clients older than age 55 must be monitored carefully for signs of infection because these clients have been found to experience an increased frequency of infections when taking leukotriene modifiers. These agents may be contraindicated in clients with significant hepatic dysfunction or chronic alcoholism because they are extensively metabolized by the liver.

COMMON COLD

The common cold is a viral infection of the upper respiratory tract that produces a characteristic array of annoying symptoms. It is fortunate that the disorder is self-limiting because there is no cure or effective prevention for colds. Therapies used to relieve symptoms may include the same classes of drugs used for allergic

rhinitis (Chapter 42), such as antihistamines, decongestants, and additional drugs such as those that suppress cough and loosen bronchial secretions.

Pharmacotherapy with Antitussives

38.10 Antitussives are effective at relieving cough due to the common cold. Opioids are used for severe cough. Non-opioids such as dextromethorphan are used for mild or moderate cough.

Antitussives are drugs used to dampen the cough reflex. They are of value in treating coughs due to allergies or the common cold.

Cough is a natural reflex mechanism that serves to forcibly remove excess secretions and foreign material from the respiratory system. In diseases such as emphysema and bronchitis, or when liquids have been aspirated into the bronchi, it is not desirable to suppress the normal cough reflex. Dry, hacking, non-productive cough, however, can be quite irritating to the membranes of the throat and can deprive a client of much needed rest. It is this type of situation in which therapy with antitussives may be warranted. Antitussives are classified as opioids or non-opioids and are listed in Table 38.4.

Opioids, the most efficacious antitussives, act by raising the cough threshold in the CNS. Codeine and hydrocodone (Hydocan) are the most frequently used opioid antitussives. Doses needed to suppress the cough reflex are very low, so there is minimal potential for dependence. Most opioid cough mixtures are classified as Schedule III, IV, or V drugs and are reserved for more serious cough conditions. Although not common, overdose from opioid cough remedies may result in significant respiratory depression.

TABLE 38.4   Agents for the Common Cold and Removal of Excessive Bronchial Mucus

Drug	Route and Adult Dose
Antitussives: Opioids	
codeine	PO, 10–20 mg q4–6h as needed (PRN) (max 120 mg/24 hours)
hydrocodone bitartrate (Hycodan, others)	PO, 5 mL every 4–6 hours PRN (max 30 mL/24 hours)
Antitussives: Non-Opioids	
Pr dextromethorphan (Koffex DM)	PO, 10–20 mg every 4 hours (q4h) or 30 mg every 6–8 hours (q6–8h) (max 120 mg/day)
Expectorants	
guaifenesin (Benylin, Balminil)	PO, 200–400 mg q4h (max 2.4 g/day)
Mucolytics	
acetylcysteine (Mucomyst)	MDI, 1–10 mL of 20% solution q4–6h or 2–20 mL of 10% solution q4–6h

TABLE 38.5 Opioid Combination Drugs for Severe Cold Symptoms

Trade Name	Opioid	Non-Opioid Ingredients
Ambenyl Cough Syrup	codeine	bromodiphenhydramine
Calcidrine Syrup	codeine	calcium iodide
Codamine Syrup	hydrocodone	phenylpropanolamine
Codiclear DH Syrup	hydrocodone	guaifenesin
Codimal DH	hydrocodone	phenylephrine, pyrilamine
Hycodan	hydrocodone	homatropine
Hycomine Compound	hydrocodone	phenylephrine, chlorpheniramine, acetaminophen
Hycotuss Expectorant	hydrocodone	guaifenesin
Novahistine DH	codeine	pseudoephedrine, chlorpheniramine
Phenergan with Codeine	codeine	promethazine
Robitussin A-C	codeine	guaifenesin
Tega-Tussin Syrup	hydrocodone	phenylephrine, chlorpheniramine
Triaminic Expectorant DH	hydrocodone	phenylpropanolamine, pyrilamine, pheniramine, guaifenesin
Tussionex	hydrocodone	chlorpheniramine

Care must be taken when using these medications in clients who have asthma or allergies since bronchoconstriction may occur. Opioids may be combined with other agents such as antihistamines, decongestants, and non-opioid antitussives in the therapy of severe cold or flu symptoms. Some of these combinations are shown in Table 38.5.

The most frequently used non-opioid antitussive is dextromethorphan (Koffex DM). At low doses, this drug is available in over-the-counter (OTC) cold and flu medications. Higher doses are available by prescription to treat more severe cough. Dextromethorphan is chemically similar to the opioids and also acts in the CNS to raise the cough threshold. Although not as efficacious as codeine, there is no risk for dependence with dextromethorphan.

Benzonatate is a non-opioid antitussive that acts by a different mechanism. Chemically related to the local anesthetic tetracaine, benzonatate suppresses the cough reflex by anesthetizing stretch receptors in the lungs. If chewed, the drug can cause the side effect of numbing the mouth and pharynx. Side effects are uncommon but may include sedation, nausea, headache, and dizziness.

Nursing Considerations

The role of the nurse in antitussive therapy involves careful monitoring of the client's condition and providing education as it relates to the prescribed drug regimen. The nursing care related to clients who are receiving antitussive drugs is dependent on the agent used. For all antitussive drugs, assess the client for the presence or history of persistent non-productive cough, respiratory distress, shortness of breath, and productive cough.

When codeine or other opioids are prescribed, the client should be monitored for drowsiness. Because cough is a protective mechanism used to clear the lungs of microbes, antitussive drugs should be used in moderation and only to treat cough when it interferes with activities of daily living, rest, or sleep. Extreme caution should be used when administering antitussive drugs to individuals with chronic lung conditions, as normal respiratory function is already impaired. Because cough may be a symptom of other serious pulmonary conditions, antitussive drugs should be used for only 3 days, unless otherwise approved by the healthcare provider.

Client education as it relates to antitussives includes goals, reasons for obtaining baseline data such as vital signs and tests for cardiac and renal function, and possible side effects. The following are the specific points to include when teaching clients regarding antitussives:

- Avoid driving and performing hazardous activities while taking opioid antitussives.
- Avoid use of alcohol, which can cause increased CNS depression.
- Immediately report the following: coughing up green- or yellow-tinged secretions, difficulty breathing, excessive drowsiness, constipation, and nausea or vomiting.
- Store opioid antitussives away from children.

PROTOTYPE DRUG Dextromethorphan (Koffex DM)

Actions and Uses: Dextromethorphan is a drug included in most cold and flu preparations. It is available in a large variety of formulations, including tablets, liquid-filled capsules, lozenges, and liquids. Like codeine, it acts in the medulla, though it lacks the analgesic and euphoric effects of the opioids and does not produce dependence. Clients whose cough is not relieved by dextromethorphan after several days of therapy should see their healthcare provider.

Pharmacokinetics: Dextromethorphan is rapidly absorbed from the GI tract, with an onset of action usually within 15 to 30 minutes. It crosses the blood-brain barrier and placenta and enters breast milk. Dextromethorphan and its active metabolite, dextrorphan, are excreted in urine. Its half-life is unknown.

Administration Alerts:
- Avoid pulmonary irritants, such as smoking and other fumes, as these agents may decrease drug effectiveness.
- Dextromethorphan is pregnancy category C.

Adverse Effects and Interactions: Side effects due to dextromethorphan are rare. Dizziness, drowsiness, and GI upset occur in some clients.

Drug interactions with dextromethorphan include a high risk for excitation, hypotension, and hyperpyrexia when used concurrently with monoamine oxidase inhibitors. Concurrent use with alcohol may result in increased CNS depression.

Pharmacotherapy with Expectorants and Mucolytics

38.11 Expectorants promote mucus secretion, making the mucus thinner and easier to remove by cough. Mucolytics are agents used to break down thick bronchial secretions.

Certain drugs are available to control excess mucus production. Expectorants increase bronchial secretions, and mucolytics help to loosen thick bronchial secretions. These agents are listed in Table 38.4.

Expectorants are drugs that increase bronchial secretions. They act by reducing the thickness, or viscosity, of bronchial secretions, thus increasing mucus flow so that the mucus can more easily be removed by coughing. The most effective OTC expectorant is guaifenesin (Benylin, Balminil). Like dextromethorphan, guaifenesin produces few adverse effects and is a common ingredient in many OTC cold and flu preparations. Higher doses of guaifenesin are available by prescription.

Mucolytics are drugs used to break down the chemical structure of mucus molecules. Mucolytics cause thick, viscous bronchial secretions to become thinner and more able to be removed by coughing. Acetylcysteine (Mucomyst), one of the few mucolytics available, is delivered by the inhalation route and is not available OTC. It is used in clients who have cystic fibrosis, chronic bronchitis, or other diseases that produce large amounts of thick bronchial secretions. Another mucolytic, dornase alfa (Pulmozyme), is used to break down DNA molecules in thick bronchial mucus, causing it to become less viscous.

CHRONIC OBSTRUCTIVE PULMONARY DISEASE

Chronic obstructive pulmonary disease (COPD) is a generic term used to describe several pulmonary conditions characterized by cough, mucus production, and impaired gas exchange. Drugs may be used to bring symptomatic relief, but they do not cure the disorders.

Pharmacotherapy of COPD

38.12 Chronic obstructive pulmonary disease (COPD) is a progressive disorder treated with multiple pulmonary drugs. Bronchodilators, expectorants, mucolytics, antibiotics, and oxygen may offer symptomatic relief.

COPD is a major cause of death and disability. The three specific COPD conditions are asthma, chronic bronchitis, and emphysema. Chronic bronchitis and emphysema are strongly associated with smoking tobacco products and, secondarily, with breathing air pollutants. In **chronic bronchitis**, excess mucus is produced in the bronchial tree due to inflammation and irritation from tobacco smoke or pollutants. The airway becomes partially obstructed with mucus, thus resulting in the classic signs of dyspnea and coughing. An early sign of bronchitis is often a productive cough that occurs upon awakening. Wheezing and decreased exercise tolerance are additional clinical signs. Because microbes enjoy the mucus-rich environment, pulmonary infections are common. Gas exchange may be impaired.

COPD is progressive, with the terminal stage being **emphysema**. After years of chronic inflammation, the bronchioles lose their elasticity and the alveoli dilate to maximum size. The bronchioles collapse during exhalation, which restricts airflow and traps air in the lungs. The client suffers extreme dyspnea from even the slightest physical activity.

Clients with COPD may receive a number of pulmonary drugs for symptomatic relief. The goals of pharmacotherapy are to treat infections, control cough, and relieve bronchospasm. Most clients receive bronchodilators such as anticholinergics, beta$_2$ agonists, or inhaled glucocorticoids. Mucolytics and expectorants are sometimes used to reduce the viscosity of the bronchial mucus and to aid in its removal. Oxygen therapy assists breathing in emphysema clients. Antibiotics may be prescribed for clients who experience multiple bouts of pulmonary infection.

Clients should be taught to avoid taking any drugs that have beta-antagonist activity or otherwise cause bronchoconstriction. Respiratory depressants such as opioids and barbiturates should be avoided. It is important to note that none of the pharmacotherapies offer a cure for COPD; they only treat the symptoms of a progressively worsening disease. The most important teaching point for the nurse is to strongly encourage smoking cessation in these clients.

CONNECTIONS ‹ Special Considerations

◀ Respiratory Distress Syndrome

Respiratory distress syndrome (RDS) is a condition, primarily occurring in premature babies, in which the lungs do not produce surfactant. Surfactant forms a thin layer on the inner surface of the alveoli to raise the surface tension. This prevents the alveolus from collapsing during expiration. If birth occurs before the pneumocytes in the lung are mature enough to secrete surfactant, the alveoli collapse and RDS results.

Surfactant medications can be delivered to the newborn either as prophylactic therapy or as rescue therapy after symptoms develop. The two surfactant agents used for RDS are colfosceril and beractant (Survanta). These drugs are administered intratracheally every 4 to 6 hours, until the client's condition improves.

CHAPTER

38 Understanding the Chapter

Key Concepts Summary

The numbered key concepts provide a succinct summary of the important points from the corresponding numbered section within the chapter. If any of these points are not clear, refer to the numbered section within the chapter for review.

38.1 The physiology of the respiratory system involves two main processes. Ventilation moves air into and out of the lungs and perfusion allows for gas exchange across capillaries.

38.2 Bronchioles are lined with smooth muscle that controls the amount of air entering the lungs. Dilation and constriction of the airways are controlled by the autonomic nervous system.

38.3 Inhalation is a common route of administration for pulmonary drugs because it delivers drugs directly to the site of action. Nebulizers, MDIs, and DPIs are devices used for aerosol therapies.

38.4 Asthma is a chronic disease that has both inflammation and bronchospasm components. Treatment should focus on the reduction of inflammation. Environmental control can help to reduce inflammation and prevent asthma attacks.

38.5 Beta-adrenergic agonists are the most effective drugs for relieving acute bronchospasm. These agents act by activating $beta_2$ receptors in bronchial smooth muscle to cause bronchodilation.

38.6 Methylxanthines and anticholinergics are bronchodilators occasionally used as alternatives to the beta agonists in asthma therapy.

38.7 Inhaled glucocorticoids are first-line therapy for asthma. They reduce inflammation and provide long-term prophylaxis of attacks. Oral glucocorticoids are also available.

38.8 Cromolyn, a mast cell stabilizer, is a safe drug used for the prophylaxis of asthma, but it is ineffective at relieving acute bronchospasm.

38.9 The leukotriene modifiers, whose primary use is in asthma prophylaxis, act by reducing the inflammatory component of asthma.

38.10 Antitussives are effective at relieving cough due to the common cold. Opioids are used for severe cough. Nonopioids such as dextromethorphan are used for mild or moderate cough.

38.11 Expectorants promote mucus secretion, making the mucus thinner and easier to remove by cough. Mucolytics are agents used to break down thick bronchial secretions.

38.12 Chronic obstructive pulmonary disease (COPD) is a progressive disorder treated with multiple pulmonary drugs. Bronchodilators, expectorants, mucolytics, antibiotics, and oxygen may offer symptomatic relief.

Chapter 38 Scenario

Nathan is a 12-year-old boy with a history of asthma, diagnosed 2 years ago. He is outgoing and active and participates in a swim club and a basketball team, but he has had a difficult time adjusting to the limitations of his asthma. He has learned to control acute attacks by using an salbutamol (Ventolin) metered dose inhaler, and because his asthma is often triggered by exercise, he has also been using a budesonide (Pulmicort) inhaler and taking montelukast (Singulair).

After competing in a swim meet at the local indoor pool, Nathan began experiencing respiratory distress. He alerted his coach, who retrieved the salbutamol inhaler from Nathan's backpack. After two inhalations, Nathan was still in distress and the rescue squad was called.

On admission to the emergency department, Nathan is in obvious distress with pulse oximeter readings of 90% to 91%. He has nasal flaring, bilateral wheezing is heard in his lung fields, his pulse rate is 122 beats/minute, and he is orthopneic. While treatment is started, the nurse asks him questions that he can nod or shake his head to answer. He shakes his head "no" when asked if he used his budesonide inhaler today and shrugs when asked about his last dose of montelukast.

Critical Thinking Questions

1. Considering his history, medications, and the location where Nathan's asthma attack occurred, what might explain his acute attack?

2. What medications would you anticipate will be prescribed to treat Nathan's acute asthmatic attack and why?

3. What changes might be made to Nathan's medications? What teaching will Nathan and his family need prior to discharge?

See Answers to Critical Thinking Questions in Appendix B.

NCLEX Practice Questions

1 A client with asthma asks which of the prescribed medications should be used in the event of an acute episode of bronchospasm. The nurse will instruct the client to use

a. Salbutamol, a beta agonist bronchodilator, by inhalation

b. Beclomethasone, a glucocorticoid anti-inflammatory drug, by inhalation

c. Ipratropium, an anticholinergic bronchodilator, by inhalation

d. Zafirlukast, a leukotriene modifier, by mouth

2 A client is prescribed beclomethasone (QVAR), a glucocorticoid inhaler. Education by the nurse will include the instruction

a. "Check your heart rate, because this may cause tachycardia."

b. "Limit your coffee intake while on this drug."

c. "Rinse your mouth out well after each use."

d. "You may feel shaky and nervous after using this drug."

3 The nurse should inform the client who is prescribed a nebulizer treatment with salbutamol (Ventolin) that a common adverse effect is

a. An increased heart rate with palpitations

b. A predisposition to infection

c. Sedation

d. Temporary dyspnea

4 The nurse should monitor a client who is taking beclomethasone (QVAR) for evidence of (select all that apply)

a. Infection

b. Hyperglycemia

c. Urinary retention

d. Tachycardia

e. Photophobia

5 Despite repeated demonstrations of proper inhaler use by the nurse, a client is unable to demonstrate proper technique in using the training inhaler. The client is becoming frustrated. What is the best action for the nurse to take?

a. Encourage the client to keep practising just a little longer.

b. Notify the healthcare provider that the client is incompetent.

c. Provide a spacer for use with the MDI inhaler.

d. Switch to an oral form of a beta agonist.

See Answers to NCLEX Practice Questions in Appendix A.

UNIT 9

Pharmacology of Alterations in Body Defences

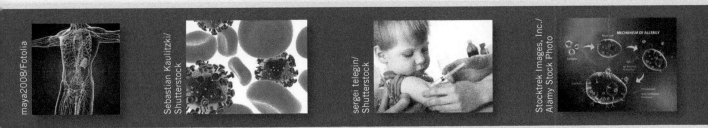

maya2008/Fotolia

Sebastian Kaulitzki/ Shutterstock

sergei telegin/ Shutterstock

Stocktrek Images, Inc./ Alamy Stock Photo

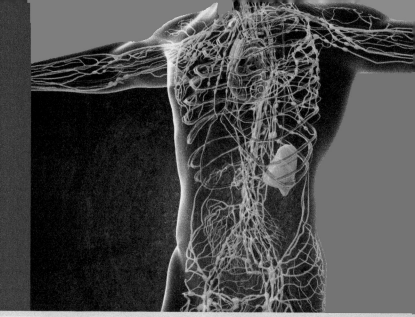

CHAPTER
39

Brief Review of Body Defences and the Immune System

LEARNING OUTCOMES

After reading this chapter, the student should be able to:

1. Identify the major components of the lymphatic system.
2. Describe the components of the nonspecific body defence system and their functions.
3. Compare and contrast specific and nonspecific body defences.
4. Identify the signs and symptoms of inflammation.
5. Outline the basic steps in the acute inflammatory response.
6. Explain the role of histamine and other chemical mediators in the inflammatory response.
7. Compare and contrast the humoral and cell-mediated immune responses.

CHAPTER OUTLINE

▸ The Lymphatic System

▸ Innate (Nonspecific) Body Defences

▸ Inflammation

▸ Chemical Mediators of Inflammation

▸ Specific (Adaptive) Body Defences

▸ Humoral Immune Response

▸ Cell-Mediated Immune Response

adaptive defences, 471

antibodies, 472

antigen, 471

B cell, 472

complement system, 470

cytokines, 473

histamine, 471

immunity, 469

inflammation, 470

innate body defences, 469

interferons (IFNs), 470

lymph nodes, 469

lymphatic system, 469

phagocytes, 470

plasma cells, 472

T cells, 473

The Lymphatic System

39.1 The lymphatic system is the primary organ system that protects the body from invasion by foreign agents.

The components of the lymphatic system provide the body with **immunity**, which is the ability to resist injury and infections. The **lymphatic system** comprises a network of cells, vessels, and tissues that provide immune surveillance. This monitoring function begins when fluid leaves the capillaries due to the osmotic forces and high pressure in the capillaries. This fluid, known as lymph, enters blind-ended lymphatic vessels and slowly travels on its journey through the lymphatic system. As much as 3 litres of fluid per day travel through the highly branched lymphatic vessel network to eventually return to the cardiovascular circulation.

Lymphatic vessels carry more than escaped fluid. Viruses, bacteria, cellular debris, and even cancer cells can enter these vessels. Should these pathogens or cancer cells be permitted to return to the bloodstream, an infection (or cancer) could quickly spread throughout the body with potentially disastrous consequences. Fortunately, before these pathogens can return to the general circulation, they must pass through dozens of **lymph nodes**, which are the principal lymphoid organs in the body. Lymph nodes are solid, spherical bodies that are packed with macrophages and lymphocytes, which are cells specialized to recognize anything that is "non-self" or foreign to the body. Recognition of these foreign agents activates the immune response, which neutralizes or removes the pathogens before they can reach the general circulation. Each lymph node serves as a mini-filter, removing up to 99% of the foreign agents entering the node. Should a pathogen be clever enough to escape surveillance in a lymph node, it is then faced with passing through dozens, and sometimes hundreds, more lymph nodes in the lymphatic system.

In addition to lymph vessels and nodes, lymphoid tissues line connective tissue at every potential portal of entrance into the body, including the gastrointestinal (GI) tract, respiratory tract, and genitourinary tract. Lymphoid tissue contains lymphocytes, which "patrol" the region for potential injury or exposure to microbes. Other large collections of lymphoid tissue include the tonsils, spleen, and thymus. These are considered organs of the lymphatic system.

Although the lymphatic system can be divided into individual structures and components for ease of study, it is best to think of it as an integrated whole. The various components of this system are in continuous communication and work together as a single unit to accomplish effective immune surveillance. A malfunction in any one single component may alter the effectiveness of the entire lymphatic system.

Innate (Nonspecific) Body Defences

39.2 Innate body defences are the body's first line of defence against pathogens.

Innate body defences are those that are present even before an infection has occurred and that provide the first line of protection from pathogens. These are sometimes referred to as nonspecific defences because they are unable to distinguish one type of threat from another; the body's response is the same regardless of the particular pathogen. A summary of nonspecific body defences is given in Table 39.1. A useful way to

TABLE 39.1 Summary of Nonspecific Body Defences

Component	Functions
Physical Barriers	
Skin	Forms a mechanical barrier to prevent pathogens and other harmful substances from entering the body. Surface contains keratin, which is resistant to water and acid.
Mucous membranes	Line the portals of entry to inhibit the entry of pathogens. Mucus inhibits microbial growth. Cilia in the respiratory tract and saliva in the mouth discourage pathogen entry.
Cellular Barriers	
Phagocytes	Ingest antigens. Specific types include neutrophils, eosinophils, and monocytes, which differentiate into macrophages. Also include dendritic cells that reside deep in the skin, in lymph nodes, and in the inner lining of the respiratory and digestive tracts.
Natural killer (NK) cells	Directly attack virus-infected and cancer cells by releasing substances that are toxic to the antigen.
Interferons	Proteins secreted by cells infected by viruses. They protect uninfected cells and also stimulate the activity of phagocytes and NK cells; used as medications to treat certain types of cancer.
Process Barriers	
Complement	Promotes inflammation and phagocytosis; lyses microbes.
Fever	Systemic response that increases body temperature to activate body defences; inhibits the growth of some microbes.
Inflammation	Limits the spread of infection and releases substances that attract phagocytes; initiates repair of the injured area.

categorize the innate defences is to consider them as types of barriers:

- Physical barriers: skin and mucous membranes
- Cellular barriers: phagocytes, natural killer cells, and dendritic cells
- Process barriers: complement, fever, and inflammation.

Physical Barriers

The skin and mucous membranes are considered the first line of defence against pathogen invasion. The intact skin is a formidable physical barrier to pathogens. The cells of the epidermis are packed tightly together, which discourages penetration by microbes. The outer layer of skin cells is continually shed, along with any microbes that may be clinging to them. The accessory structures of the skin secrete sebum (oil), sweat, and antimicrobial peptides that discourage microbial growth on the surface. The skin is also colonized with a variety of bacteria and fungi that are normally harmless to the host. This microbiota (flora) competes with pathogens for space and nutrients, thus creating an unfavourable growth environment for harmful organisms. However, should the skin become broken or compromised by needlesticks or catheters, some species of normal flora may become pathogenic.

The body cavities that open to the outside environment are lined with a mucosal epithelium that not only provides a physical barrier, but also contains proteins, lysozymes, and other substances that discourage pathogen growth. The respiratory tract secretes a sticky mucus that traps microbes. The stomach and genitourinary tracts provide an acidic environment that kills many microbes. Like the skin, the mucosa of the mouth, colon, and vagina have a normal population of flora, which discourages pathogen growth by competing for space and nutrients.

Cellular Barriers

Once physical barriers are breached, **phagocytes** are the primary cells of innate immunity. The primary job of phagocytes is to engulf pathogens and other foreign substances that enter the body. Once engulfed, the phagocytes destroy the microbe in vesicles called lysosomes, which contain powerful destructive enzymes. As expected, phagocytes are found in large numbers in the blood, in lymphatic tissues, and in locations where pathogens have the highest likelihood of entering. For example, the deeper layers of the epidermis contain specialized phagocytes called dendritic cells, which are able to remove pathogens that penetrate the superficial layers. Phagocytes have the ability to migrate to distant sites when an infection is detected, a process called chemotaxis.

Phagocytes have proteins on their surface that allow them to recognize cells and cellular components that are "non-self." When recognized as "non-self," the pathogen is internalized and destroyed within the phagocyte. Pieces of the microbe are sometimes displayed on the plasma membrane of the phagocyte, which serves to activate other components of the immune response. Not all pathogens can be engulfed by phagocytosis. Some, such as Mycobacterium tuberculosis, are not only resistant to phagocytosis, but also can multiply while residing inside macrophages.

Cancer cells or virus-infected cells attract a different type of innate cellular response: natural killer (NK) cells. Found in most

lymphoid organs, NK cells are not phagocytic, but they do release toxins that kill cancer cells or virus-infected cells. NK cells also secrete chemicals that enhance inflammation and modulate the adaptive immune response.

Interferons (IFNs) are antimicrobial proteins that are crucial components of the innate body defence system. Released by infected macrophages and lymphocytes, IFNs protect uninfected cells from the pathogen. IFNs have been isolated and are now available as medications for the treatment of immune disorders.

Process Barriers

Processes associated with innate defences are complement activation, fever, and inflammation. The **complement system** is a cluster of 20 plasma proteins that combine in a specific sequence and order when an infection occurs. Activation of complement attracts phagocytes to the infection site, attacks and breaks down the cell walls of pathogens, and stimulates the inflammatory process.

Other key processes of the nonspecific defence system are fever and inflammation. Fever accelerates body defences and associated repair processes by raising the temperature of the body. When excessive, however, fever can harm the body and must be treated with drugs known as antipyretics (see Chapter 42). From a pharmacological perspective, one of the most important nonspecific defences is inflammation. Because of its significance, inflammation is presented separately in Sections 39.3 and 39.4.

Inflammation

39.3 Inflammation is a nonspecific defence mechanism that neutralizes or destroys foreign substances and microbes.

Inflammation occurs in response to many different stimuli, including physical injury, exposure to toxic chemicals, extreme heat, invading microorganisms, or death of cells. Inflammation is considered a nonspecific defence mechanism because it proceeds in the same manner regardless of the cause.

The central purposes of inflammation are to contain the injury, destroy the pathogen, and initiate repair of the area. The repair of the injured area can proceed at a faster pace by neutralizing the foreign agent and removing cellular debris and dead cells. Signs of inflammation include swelling, pain, warmth, and redness of the affected area.

Inflammation may be classified as acute or chronic. During acute inflammation, such as that caused by minor physical injury, 8 to 10 days are normally needed for the symptoms to resolve and for repair to begin. If the body cannot neutralize the damaging agent, inflammation may continue for long periods and become chronic. In chronic autoimmune disorders such as lupus and rheumatoid arthritis (RA), inflammation may persist for years, with symptoms becoming progressively worse over time. Other disorders such as seasonal allergy arise at predictable times during each year, and inflammation may produce only minor, annoying symptoms.

Chemical Mediators of Inflammation

39.4 Inflammation proceeds with the release of chemical mediators.

During inflammation, pathogens, chemicals, or physical trauma cause the damaged tissue to release chemical mediators that act as alarms to notify the surrounding area of the injury. Chemical mediators of inflammation include histamine, leukotrienes, bradykinin, complement, and prostaglandins. These inflammatory mediators, which are listed in Table 39.2, are sometimes called pro-inflammatory substances. Some of the inflammatory mediators are important targets for anti-inflammatory drugs. For example, acetylsalicylic acid (ASA [Aspirin]) and ibuprofen (Advil, Motrin) are prostaglandin inhibitors that are effective at treating fever, pain, and inflammation.

The rapid release of the chemical mediators of inflammation on a large scale throughout the body is responsible for anaphylaxis, a life-threatening allergic response that may result in shock and death. A number of chemicals, insect stings, foods, and some therapeutic drugs can cause this widespread release of histamine from mast cells if the person has an allergy to these substances.

Histamine is a key chemical mediator of inflammation. It is stored primarily within mast cells located in tissue spaces under epithelial membranes such as the skin, bronchial tree, and digestive tract and along blood vessels. Mast cells detect foreign agents or injury and respond by releasing histamine, which initiates the inflammatory response within seconds. In addition to its role in inflammation, histamine also directly stimulates pain receptors and is a primary agent responsible for the symptoms of seasonal allergies.

When released at an injury site, histamine dilates nearby blood vessels, causing the capillaries to become more permeable. Plasma, complement proteins, and phagocytes can then enter the area to neutralize microbes or their toxins. The affected area may become congested with blood, which can lead to significant swelling and pain. Figure 39.1 illustrates the fundamental steps in acute inflammation.

Histamine interacts with two different receptors to elicit an inflammatory response. H_1 receptors are present in the smooth muscle of the vascular system, the respiratory passages, and the digestive tract. Stimulation of these receptors results in itching, pain, edema, vasodilation, bronchoconstriction, and the characteristic symptoms of inflammation and allergy. In contrast, H_2 receptors are present primarily in the stomach, and their stimulation results in the secretion of large amounts of hydrochloric acid.

Drugs that act as specific antagonists for H_1 and H_2 receptors are in widespread therapeutic use. H_1-receptor antagonists, which are used to treat allergies and inflammation, are discussed in Chapter 42. H_2-receptor antagonists are used to treat peptic ulcersand are discussed in Chapter 34.

TABLE 39.2	Chemical Mediators of Inflammation
Mediator	**Description**
Bradykinin	Protein present in an inactive form in plasma and mast cells; increases vascular permeability and causes pain; effects are similar to those of histamine; broken down by angiotensin-converting enzyme (ACE).
Complement	Series of at least 20 proteins that combine in a cascade fashion to neutralize or destroy an antigen; stimulates histamine release by mast cells; causes cell lysis.
C-reactive protein	Occurs as an early response to acute inflammation; activates complement; used as a biomarker to gauge the extent of inflammation.
Histamine	Stored and released by mast cells; causes vasodilation, smooth muscle constriction, tissue swelling, and itching.
Leukotrienes	Lipids stored and released by mast cells; effects are similar to those of histamine; synthesized from arachidonic acid; responsible for some symptoms of asthma and allergies.
Prostaglandins	Lipid present in most tissues and stored and released by mast cells; increase capillary permeability, attract white blood cells to the site of inflammation, cause pain, and induce fever; aspirin inhibits their synthesis; some are available as medications.
Tumour necrosis factor (TNF)	A cytokine that promotes inflammation and the programmed death of cells (apoptosis).

Specific (Adaptive) Body Defences

39.5 The specific body defences include the humoral and cell-mediated immune systems.

The body also has the ability to mount a third line of defence that is specific to certain threats. For example, a specific defence may act against only a single species of bacteria and be ineffective against all others. These are known as **adaptive defences** or, more commonly, the immune response. The primary cell of the immune response is the lymphocyte.

Microbes and foreign substances that elicit an immune response are called **antigens**. Foreign proteins, such as those present on the surfaces of pollen grains, bacteria, non-human cells, and viruses, are the strongest antigens. Typically, only a small fragment or piece of a foreign protein is required to activate the immune system. It is estimated that the immune system is able to recognize and react to more than a billion different antigens.

The immune response is extremely complex. The following are several important aspects of the immune response:

1. *Specificity.* Each aspect of the immune response recognizes only particular pathogens and not others. Recognition of the antigen is dependent on the immune cells interacting with specific foreign proteins. Once an immune response is mounted, it generally affects only the one specific antigen that was recognized.

2. *Systemic.* Despite being specific to a particular antigen, the immune response is systemic. Therefore, antigens that exist in remote regions beyond the initial site of infection will be neutralized.

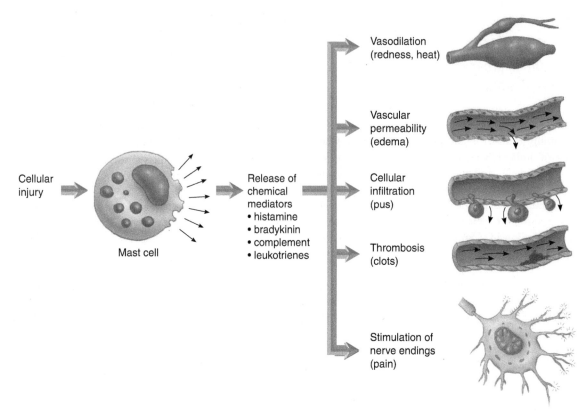

Figure 39.1   Steps in acute inflammation.

3. *Memory.* After an antigen interaction occurs, cells of the adaptive immune system remember the immune response. This is different from the components of nonspecific defences, which have no memory. Upon subsequent exposures to the same antigen, the body is able to mount a stronger and more rapid response.

The basic steps of the immune response involve recognition of the antigen, communication and coordination with other defence cells, and destruction or suppression of the antigen. A large number of chemical messengers and complex interactions are involved in the immune response, many of which have yet to be discovered. The two primary divisions of the immune response are antibody-mediated (humoral) immunity and cell-mediated immunity.

Humoral Immune Response

39.6 The humoral immune response is mediated by B lymphocytes and includes the secretion of antibodies.

The humoral immune response is triggered when an antigen encounters a B lymphocyte, more simply known as a **B cell**. The activated B cell divides to form millions of identical copies of itself in a process known as clonal division. Most cells in this clone are called **plasma cells**, whose primary function is to secrete antibodies specific to the antigen that initiated the challenge. Each plasma cell is capable of manufacturing antibodies at an astounding rate: as many as 2000 antibodies each second.

Circulating through body fluids are **antibodies**, also known as immunoglobulins (Ig), which physically interact with antigens to neutralize or mark them for destruction by other cells of the immune response. The activation of complement, with subsequent inflammation and enhanced phagocytosis, is a major defence mechanism resulting from the formation of antigen-antibody complexes. Peak production of antibodies occurs about 10 days after an initial antigen challenge. The important functions of antibodies are illustrated in Figure 39.2.

After the antigen challenge, memory B cells are formed that will remember the specific antigen-antibody interaction. Should the body be exposed to the same antigen in the future, the humoral immune system will manufacture even higher levels of antibodies in a shorter period, approximately 2 to 3 days. For some antigens, such as those for measles, mumps, or chickenpox, memory can be retained for an entire lifetime. Vaccines are sometimes administered to produce these memory cells in advance of exposure to the antigen, so that when the body is exposed to the actual organism it can mount a fast and effective response (see Chapter 41).

It is important to remember that the body contains millions of different B cells, each programmed to react to a specific antigen. These B cells, in turn, are able to construct millions of different types of antibodies, each specific to a particular antigen. The body is pre-programmed with the genetic information to defend against millions of different antigens. Although it is unlikely that an individual will ever be infected with all of the different antigens during a lifetime, the body is waiting for the challenge.

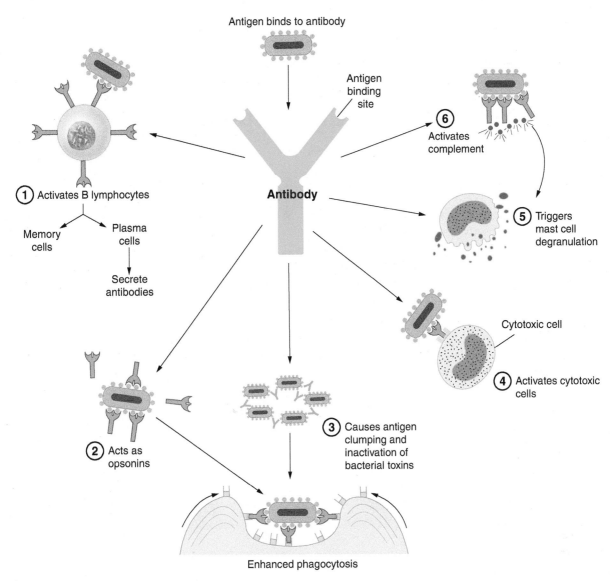

Antigen binds to antibody

Antigen binding site

Antibody

① Activates B lymphocytes

Memory cells

Plasma cells

Secrete antibodies

② Acts as opsonins

③ Causes antigen clumping and inactivation of bacterial toxins

④ Activates cytotoxic cells

Cytotoxic cell

⑤ Triggers mast cell degranulation

⑥ Activates complement

Enhanced phagocytosis

Figure 39.2 Functions of antibodies.

From *Human Physiology: An Integrated Approach* (5th ed.), by D. U. Silverthorn, 2013. Printed and electronically reproduced by permission. Upper Saddle River, NJ: Pearson Education, Inc.

Cell-Mediated Immune Response

39.7 The cell-mediated immune response is mediated by T lymphocytes and includes the secretion of cytokines.

A second branch of the immune response involves T lymphocytes, or **T cells**. Two major types of T cells are called helper T cells and cytotoxic T cells. These cells are named after a protein receptor on their plasma membrane. The helper T cells have a CD4 receptor, and the cytotoxic T cells have a CD8 receptor. The helper (CD4) T cells are particularly important because they are responsible for activating most other immune cells, including B cells and other types of T cells. The cytotoxic (CD8) T cells travel throughout the body, directly killing certain bacteria, parasites, virus-infected cells, and cancer cells.

T cells rapidly form clones after they are activated or sensitized following an encounter with their specific antigen. Unlike B cells, however, T cells do not produce antibodies. Instead, activated T cells produce huge amounts of **cytokines**, which are hormone-like proteins that regulate the intensity and duration of the immune response and mediate cell-to-cell communication. Some cytokines kill foreign organisms directly, whereas others induce inflammation or enhance the killing power of macrophages. Specific cytokines released by activated T cells include interleukins, interferon gamma, tumour necrosis factor (TNF), and perforin. Some cytokines are used therapeutically to stimulate the immune system. Small amounts of cytokines are also secreted by certain macrophages, B lymphocytes, mast cells, endothelial cells, and the stromal cells of the spleen, thymus, and bone marrow.

Like B cells, some sensitized T cells become memory cells. If the client encounters the same antigen in the future, the memory T cells assist in mounting a more rapid immune response.

CHAPTER

39

Understanding the Chapter

Key Concepts Summary

The numbered key concepts provide a succinct summary of the important points from the corresponding numbered section within the chapter. If any of these points are not clear, refer to the numbered section within the chapter for review.

39.1 The lymphatic system is the primary organ system that protects the body from invasion by foreign agents.

39.2 Innate body defences are the body's first line of defence against pathogens.

39.3 Inflammation is a nonspecific defence mechanism that neutralizes or destroys foreign substances and microbes.

39.4 Inflammation proceeds with the release of chemical mediators.

39.5 The specific body defences include the humoral and cell-mediated immune systems.

39.6 The humoral immune response is mediated by B lymphocytes and includes the secretion of antibodies.

39.7 The cell-mediated immune response is mediated by T lymphocytes and includes the secretion of cytokines.

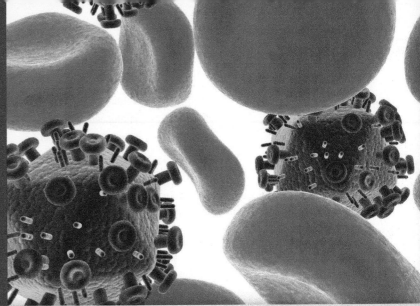

Sebastian Kaulitzki/Shutterstock

CHAPTER

40

Pharmacotherapy with Immunostimulants and Immunosuppressants

LEARNING OUTCOMES

After reading this chapter, the student should be able to:

1. Compare and contrast the therapeutic applications of the immunostimulants and immunosuppressants.

2. Describe the roles of interferons, interleukins, and other cytokines in modulating the immune response.

3. Explain why therapy with immunosuppressant medications is necessary following organ transplants.

4. Identify the classes of drugs used as immunosuppressants.

5. For each of the drug classes listed in Prototype Drugs, identify a representative drug and explain its mechanism of action, therapeutic effects, and important adverse effects.

6. Apply the nursing process to care for clients who are receiving immunostimulants and immunosuppressants.

CHAPTER OUTLINE

▶ Immunomodulators

▶ Pharmacotherapy with Biological Response Modifiers

▶ Immunosuppressants

  ▶ Immunosuppressants to Prevent Transplant Rejection

  ▶ Corticosteroids as Immunosuppressants

KEY TERMS

biological response
modifiers, 477

calcineurin, 480

cytokines, 477

immunomodulator, 476

immunostimulants, 476

immunosuppressants, 476

interferons (IFNs), 477

interleukins (ILs), 477

monoclonal antibody, 480

polyclonal antibody, 480

transplant rejection, 480

The immune system and other body defences are truly formidable deterrents to invading microorganisms. A healthy defence system can protect the body from life-threatening infections caused by thousands of different species of organisms, often over an entire lifetime. In addition, body defences can protect against internal invaders such as cancer cells. There are certain circumstances, however, when drugs may be necessary to modulate the body's defences. This chapter examines pharmacotherapy with agents that either stimulate or suppress immune function.

Immunomodulators

40.1 Immunomodulators are substances that either enhance or suppress the ability of the body to fight infection and disease.

Body defences are composed of a complex system of cells, tissues, and processes designed with a single goal: to protect the body from invasion by foreign substances, or antigens, that may cause harm. Some of these defences are specific to a single species of microbe, whereas others are nonspecific and provide the same response or protection regardless of the invading pathogen. The student should review the components of body defences in Chapter 39 before proceeding.

Immunomodulator is a general term referring to any drug or therapy that affects body defences. An overview of the immunomodulators is given in Figure 40.1. Two basic types of immunomodulators are used for pharmacotherapy:

- **Immunostimulants** are drugs that increase the ability of the immune system to fight infection and disease (see Table 40.1 for common immunostimulants). In most cases, these drugs are used to treat clients with cancer. The use of immunostimulants to treat cancer is called immunotherapy. Some immunostimulants are also used to treat hepatitis. The use of colony-stimulating factors (CSFs) to treat neutropenia is presented in Chapter 57, and the application of vaccines to boost the immune response is presented in Chapter 41.

- **Immunosuppressants** are drugs that diminish the ability of the immune system to fight infection and disease. Immunosuppressants are used to prevent transplant rejection and to dampen hyperactive immune responses, such as those that may occur during exacerbations of systemic lupus erythematosus or rheumatoid arthritis (RA).

NCLEX Success Tip

Intravesical instillation of BCG commonly causes hematuria. Other common adverse effects of BCG include urinary frequency and dysuria.

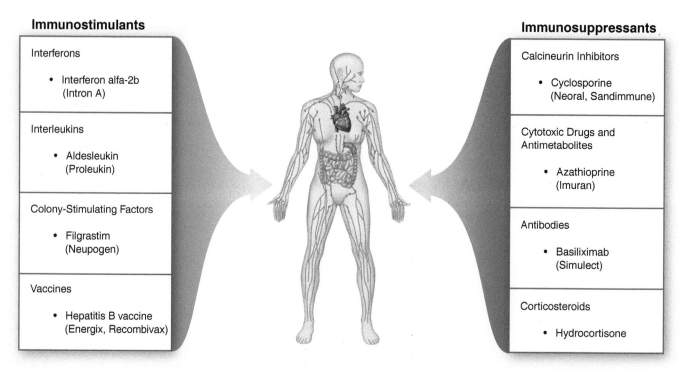

Figure 40.1 Overview of immunomodulators.

TABLE 40.1   Immunostimulants

Drug	Route and Adult Dose
aldesleukin (Proleukin): interleukin 2	Intravenous (IV), 600 000 IU/kg (0.037 mg/kg) every 8 hours (q8h) by a 15-minute IV infusion for a total of 14 doses
bacillus Calmette-Guérin (BCG) vaccine	Interdermal, 0.1 mL
Pr interferon alfa-2 (Intron A)	Intramuscular/subcutaneous (IM/SC), 2 million U/m^2 three times/week
interferon beta-1a (Avonex, Rebif)	IM, 30 µg every week (qwk)
interferon beta-1b (Betaseron)	SC, 0.25 mg (8 million IU) every other day (qod)
oprelvekin (Neumega): interleukin 11	SC, 50 µg/kg once daily starting 6–24 hours after completing chemotherapy and continuing until platelet count is ≥50 000 cells/µL or up to 21 days
peginterferon alfa-2a (Pegasys)	SC, 180 µg once weekly for 48 weeks

Pharmacotherapy with Biological Response Modifiers

40.2 Interferons are biological response modifiers that have antiviral and antineoplastic activity.

When challenged by specific antigens, certain macrophages, B and T lymphocytes, mast cells, endothelial cells, and stromal cells of the spleen, thymus, and bone marrow secrete **cytokines** that help to defend against the invading organism. These natural cytokines have been identified and, through recombinant DNA technology, large enough quantities can be made available to treat certain disorders. A handful of immunostimulants, sometimes called **biological response modifiers**, have been approved to boost certain functions of the immune system.

Interferons (IFNs) are cytokines secreted by lymphocytes and macrophages that have been infected with a virus. After secretion, interferons attach to uninfected cells and signal them to secrete antiviral proteins. Part of the nonspecific defence system, interferons slow the spread of viral infections and enhance the activity of existing leukocytes. The actions of interferons include modulation of immune functions, such as increasing phagocytosis and enhancing the cytotoxic activity of T cells. The two major classes of interferon that have clinical utility are alpha and beta. The alpha class has the widest therapeutic application (when used as medications, the spelling is changed to alfa). Indications for interferon alpha therapy include hairy cell leukemia, AIDS-related Kaposi's sarcoma, chronic myelogenous leukemia (alfa-2a), and chronic hepatitis B or C (alfa-2b). Interferon beta is primarily reserved for the treatment of severe multiple sclerosis.

Interleukins (ILs) are another class of cytokines synthesized by lymphocytes, monocytes, macrophages, and certain other cells that enhance the capabilities of the immune system. At least 20 different interleukins have been identified, though only a few are available as medications. The interleukins have widespread effects on immune function, including stimulation of T-cell function, stimulation of B-cell and plasma cell production, and promotion of inflammation. Interleukin 2, derived from helper T lymphocytes, causes proliferation of T lymphocytes and activated B lymphocytes. It is available as aldesleukin (Proleukin), which is approved for the treatment of metastatic renal carcinoma. Interleukin 11, derived from bone marrow cells, is a growth factor with multiple hematopoietic effects. It is marketed as oprelvekin (Neumega) for its ability to stimulate platelet production in immunosuppressed clients (see Chapter 57).

In addition to interferons and interleukins, a few additional biological response modifiers are available to enhance the immune system. Bacillus Calmette-Guérin (BCG) vaccine is an attenuated strain of *Mycobacterium bovis* used for the pharmacotherapy of certain types of bladder cancer.

Nursing Considerations

The role of the nurse in immunostimulant therapy involves careful monitoring of the client's condition and providing education as it relates to the prescribed drug regimen. Immunostimulants are powerful drugs that not only affect target cells, but also may seriously affect other body systems. Prior to starting a client on these drugs, a thorough assessment, including a complete health history and present signs and symptoms, should be performed because these drugs have serious side effects. The nurse should assess for the presence or history of the following diseases or disorders: chronic hepatitis, hairy cell leukemia, malignant melanoma, condyloma acuminata, AIDS-related Kaposi's sarcoma, and renal disorders including cancer. Assessment of infections and cancer verifies the need for these drugs. Immunostimulants are contraindicated for clients with renal or liver disease and in pregnancy. Also before beginning therapy, laboratory tests, including a complete blood count (CBC), electrolytes, renal function, and liver enzymes, should be obtained to provide baseline data. Vital signs and body weight should be measured at the initial assessment and throughout the treatment regimen to monitor progress. As with any drug, the nurse should check for allergies and drug interactions.

Interferon alfa-2b should be used with caution in clients with hepatitis other than hepatitis C, leukopenia, and pulmonary disease. Interferon alfa-2a should be used with caution in clients with cardiac disease, herpes zoster, and recent exposure to chickenpox.

The client should be kept well hydrated during pharmacotherapy. Use of immunostimulants can lead to the development of encephalopathy; therefore, the nurse should assess for changes in mental status. The nurse should be especially vigilant for signs and symptoms of depression and suicidal ideation. Additional nursing interventions may be needed depending on the medication given. When interferon alfa-2b is administered, it may promote development of leukemia because of bone marrow suppression. Periodic blood tests should be obtained to exclude the possibility of leukemia development.

Assessment of a client's pregnancy status prior to beginning interferon beta-1b (Betaseron) therapy and throughout therapy should be done, as this drug may cause spontaneous abortion. The nurse should instruct the client to use reliable birth control while taking this drug. During the use of interleukin 2, the client should be instructed not to use corticosteroids because these hormones reduce the drug's antitumor effectiveness. Liver, endocrine, or neurological adverse effects that occur during therapy may be permanent.

Because immunostimulants act on fast-growing cells, such as those in the lining of the stomach, nausea and stomatitis are common side effects. The nurse should provide small, frequent feedings and use non–alcohol-based mouthwash to treat mouth ulcers. Clients who are taking immunostimulants should immediately report any of the following side effects: hematuria, petechiae, tarry stools, bruising, fever, sore throat, jaundice, dark-coloured urine, clay-coloured stools, feelings of sadness, and nervousness.

See Nursing Process Focus: Clients Receiving Immunostimulant Therapy for specific teaching points.

PROTOTYPE DRUG	Interferon Alfa-2 (Intron A)

Actions and Uses: Interferon alfa-2 is a biological response modifier that is available as interferon alfa-2b (Intron A). Interferon alfa-2b is a natural protein that is produced by human lymphocytes 4 to 6 hours after viral stimulation. Indications include hairy cell leukemia, hepatitis C, and malignant melanoma. An unlabelled use is for AIDS-related Kaposi's sarcoma. Interferon alfa-2b affects cancer cells by two mechanisms. First, it enhances or stimulates the immune system to remove antigens. Second, the drug suppresses the growth of cancer cells. As expected from its origin, interferon alfa-2 also has antiviral activity.

NURSING PROCESS FOCUS

Clients Receiving Immunostimulant Therapy

Assessment	Potential Nursing Diagnoses/Identified Patterns
• Obtain health history, including medical conditions, allergies, drug history, and possible drug interactions. • Obtain laboratory work: CBC, electrolytes, and liver enzymes. • Obtain weight and vital signs, especially blood pressure. • Assess mental alertness.	• Safety from physical injury related to side effects of drug • Alterations in comfort and nutrition (gastrointestinal [GI] upset may occur related to side effects of drug) • Risk for infection related to bone marrow suppression secondary to drug • Need for knowledge regarding drug therapy and adverse effects

Planning: Client Goals and Expected Outcomes

The client will:

• Experience increased immune system function
• Demonstrate an understanding of the drug's action by accurately describing drug side effects and precautions
• Immediately report effects such as fever, chills, sore throat, unusual bleeding, chest pain, palpitations, dizziness, and change in mental status
• Demonstrate the ability to self-administer IM or SC injection

Implementation

Interventions (Rationales)	Client Education/Discharge Planning
• Monitor for leukopenia, neutropenia, thrombocytopenia, anemia, increased liver enzymes (due to possible bone marrow suppression and liver damage). • Ensure that the drug is properly administered. • Monitor vital signs. (Loss of vascular tone leading to extravasation of plasma proteins and fluids into extravascular spaces may cause hypotension and dysrhythmias.) • Monitor for common side effects such as muscle aches, fever, weight loss, anorexia, nausea and vomiting, and arthralgia (due to high doses of medications). • Monitor blood glucose levels. (Blood glucose may increase in clients with pancreatitis.) • Monitor for changes in mental status. Drugs may cause depression, confusion, fatigue, visual disturbances, and numbness. (Alpha interferons cause or aggravate neuropsychiatric disorders.)	Instruct client to: • Comply with all ordered laboratory tests • Immediately report any unusual bleeding or jaundice • Avoid crowds and people with infections • Avoid activities that can cause bleeding or impairment of skin integrity • Instruct client in proper technique for self-administration of IM or SC injection Instruct client to: • Monitor blood pressure and pulse every day and report any reading outside normal limits • Report any palpitations immediately Instruct client to: • Take medication at bedtime to reduce side effects • Use frequent mouth care and small frequent feedings to reduce GI disturbances • Take acetaminophen (Tylenol) for flu-like symptoms • Instruct client to have blood glucose checked at regular intervals • Client should report any mental changes, particularly depression or thoughts of suicide

Evaluation of Outcome Criteria

Evaluate the effectiveness of drug therapy by confirming that client goals and expected outcomes have been met (see "Planning").

See Table 40.1 (page 477) for a list of drugs to which these nursing actions apply.

Pharmacokinetics: Interferon alfa-2 is administered by the SC or IM route. It is metabolized in the liver and kidney and excreted in urine. The half-life is 5 hours.

Administration Alerts:

- The drug should be administered under the careful guidance of a qualified healthcare provider.
- SC administration is recommended for clients at risk for bleeding (platelet count less than 50×10^9/L).
- Interferon alfa-2 is pregnancy category C.

Adverse Effects and Interactions: Like with many immunostimulants, the most common side effect is a flu-like syndrome of fever, chills, dizziness, and fatigue that usually diminishes as therapy progresses. Nausea, vomiting, diarrhea, and anorexia are relatively common. With prolonged therapy, more serious toxicity such as immunosuppression, hepatotoxicity, and neurotoxicity may be observed.

Interferon alfa-2 interacts with many drugs; for example, it may increase theophylline (Theolair, Uniphyl) levels. There is additive myelosuppression with antineoplastics. Zidovudine (Retrovir) may increase hematological toxicity.

IMMUNOSUPPRESSANTS

Drugs used to inhibit the immune response are called immunosuppressants. They are used for clients who are receiving transplanted tissues or organs. These agents are shown in Table 40.2.

TABLE 40.2 Immunosuppressants

Drug	Route and Adult Dose (Maximum Dose Where Indicated)	Adverse Effects
Antibodies		
antithymocyte globulin (Atgam, Thymoglobulin)	IV (Atgam), 10–20 mg/kg qd for 8–14 days IV: (Thymoglobulin): 1.5 mg/kg daily infused over 4–6 hours for 7–14 days	*Local reactions at the injection site (pain, erythema, myalgia), influenza-like symptoms (malaise, fever, chills), headache, dizziness*
basiliximab (Simulect)	Acute renal transplant rejection prophylaxis: IV, 20 mg within 2 hours prior to transplant surgery followed by a second 20 mg dose 4 days after transplantation; second dose should be withheld if complications occur	Anaphylaxis, hypertension, infections (may occur in many different body systems), thrombocytopenia, leukopenia, renal impairment (basiliximab), antithymocyte globulin
Cytotoxic Drugs and Antimetabolites		
anakinra (Kineret)	SC, 100 mg (0.67 mL) once daily	*Injection-site reactions, urinary tract infection, headache, nausea, diarrhea, sinusitis, arthralgia, flu-like symptoms* Leukopenia, infections, malignancy, anaphylaxis
azathioprine (Imuran)	Orally (PO)/IV, 3–5 mg/kg/day initially; may be able to reduce to 1–3 mg/kg/day	*Nausea, vomiting, anorexia* Severe nausea and vomiting, bone marrow suppression, thrombocytopenia, serious infections, malignancy, hepatotoxicity
belatacept (Nulojix)	IV, 5–10 mg/kg using enclosed silicone-free disposable syringe; dose is given at day 0 then end of week 2, week 4, week 8, and week 12; maintenance phase is 5 mg/kg every 4 weeks (plus or minus 3 days) beginning at the end of week 16 following transplantation	*Anemia, diarrhea, urinary tract infection, peripheral edema, hypertension, pyrexia, cough, nausea, leukopenia* Post-transplant lymphproliferative disorder, progressive multifocal leukoencephalopathy, serious infections, malignancies
cyclophosphamide (Procytox)	IV, start with 40–50 mg/kg (1500 to 1800 mg/m²) administered as 10 to 20 mg/kg/day over 2–5 days; maintenance dose is 10–15 mg/kg (350–550 mg/m²) every 7–10 days or 3–5 mg/kg (110 to 185 mg/m²) twice weekly PO, start with 1–5 mg/kg/day; maintenance dose is 1–5 mg/kg/day	*Nausea, vomiting, anorexia, neutropenia, alopecia* Anaphylaxis, leukopenia, pulmonary emboli, interstitial pulmonary fibrosis, toxic epidermal necrolysis, Stevens–Johnson syndrome, hemorrhagic cystitis, oligospermia
etanercept (Enbrel)	SC, 50 mg once/week	*Injection-site reactions (pain, erythema, myalgia), abdominal pain, vomiting, headache* Infections, pancytopenia, leukopenia, anemia, myocardial infarction (MI), heart failure, malignancy
methotrexate	PO/IM/IV, 15–30 mg/day for 5 days; repeat every 12 weeks for three courses	*Headache, glossitis, gingivitis, mild leukopenia, nausea, alopecia* Ulcerative stomatitis, myelosuppression, aplastic anemia, hepatic cirrhosis, nephrotoxicity, sudden death, pulmonary fibrosis, or pneumonia
mycophenolate (CellCept, Myfortic)	PO/IV, 720 mg-1.5 g twice a day (bid) in combination with corticosteroids and cyclosporine; start within 24 hours of transplant	*Peripheral edema, diarrhea, headache, tremor, dyspepsia, abdominal pain* Urinary tract infection, leukopenia, anemia, thrombocytopenia, sepsis, hypertension
thalidomide (Thalomid)	PO, 100–300 mg/day (max 400 mg/day) for at least 2 weeks	*Rash, mild leukopenia, fever, dizziness, diarrhea, malaise, drowsiness* Toxic epidermal necrolysis, birth defects (pregnancy category X), orthostatic hypotension, neutropenia, peripheral neuropathy

(continued)

TABLE 40.2 Immunosuppressants (continued)

Drug	Route and Adult Dose (Maximum Dose Where Indicated)	Adverse Effects
Calcineurin Inhibitors		
cyclosporine (Neoral, Sandimmune)	Transplants: PO, 5–10 mg/kg/day Autoimmune disorders: PO, 1.25–2.5 mg/kg/day (max 4 mg/day)	*Hirsutism, tremor, nausea, vomiting* Hypertension, MI, nephrotoxicity, hyperkalemia, seizures, paresthesia, hepatotoxicity
tacrolimus (Prograf, Advagraf)	PO, 0.1–0.15 mg/kg/day in two divided doses every 12 hours; give first PO dose 8–12 hours after discontinuing IV therapy IV, 0.03–0.05 mg/kg/day as continuous infusion	*Oliguria, nausea, constipation, diarrhea, headache, abdominal pain, insomnia, peripheral edema, fever* Infections, hypertension, nephrotoxicity, neurotoxicity (tremors, paresthesia, psychosis), hyperkalemia, anemia, hyperglycemia, malignancy, thrombocytopenia, seizures
Kinase Inhibitors (Rapamycins)		
everolimus (Afinitor)	PO, 10 mg once daily	Leukopenia, anemia, thrombocytopenia, sepsis, secondary infections, malignancy, anaphylaxis, interstitial lung disease or pneumonia, birth defects
sirolimus (Rapamune)	PO, 6–15 mg loading dose immediately after the transplant, then 2–5 mg/day maintenance dose	
temsirolimus (Torisel)	IV, 25 mg once weekly infused over 30–60 minutes	

Note: Italics indicate common adverse effects. <u>Underline</u> indicates serious adverse effects.

CONNECTIONS | Natural Therapies

◀ Echinacea for Boosting the Immune System

Echinacea purpurea, or purple coneflower, is a popular medicinal botanical. Native to central Canada and the Midwestern United States, the flowers, leaves, and stems of this plant are harvested and dried. Preparations include dried powder, tincture, fluid extracts, and teas. No single ingredient seems to be responsible for the herb's activity; a large number of active chemicals have been identified from the extracts.

Echinacea was used by Aboriginal peoples to treat various wounds and injuries. Echinacea is purported to boost the immune system by increasing phagocytosis and inhibiting the bacterial enzyme hyaluronidase. Some substances in echinacea might have antiviral activity, although this has yet to be confirmed by research; therefore, the herb is sometimes taken to treat the common cold and influenza. In general, it is used as a supportive treatment for any disease involving inflammation and to enhance the immune system. Side effects are rare; however, it may interfere with drugs that have immunosuppressant effects.

Immunosuppressants to Prevent Transplant Rejection

40.3 Immunosuppressants are used to prevent transplant rejection and for the treatment of autoimmune disorders.

The immune response is normally viewed as a life saver, protecting individuals from a host of pathogens in the environment. For those who are receiving organ or tissue transplants, however, the immune response is the enemy. Transplanted organs always contain some antigens that trigger the immune response. This response, called **transplant rejection**, is often acute; antibodies sometimes destroy the transplanted tissue within a few days. The cell-mediated system responds more slowly to the transplant, attacking it about 2 weeks after surgery. Even if the organ survives

these attacks, rejection of the transplant may occur months or even years after surgery.

Immunosuppressants are drugs given to dampen the immune response. Transplantation would be impossible without the use of effective immunosuppressant drugs. In addition, these agents may be prescribed for severe cases of RA or other inflammatory diseases. Although the mechanisms of action of the immunosuppressant drugs differ, most are toxic to bone marrow and produce significant adverse effects. Due to the suppressed immune system, infections are common and the client must be protected from situations in which exposure to pathogens is likely. Certain tumours such as lymphomas occur more frequently in transplant recipients than in the general population because their immune systems are suppressed by immunosuppressive drugs.

Drugs used to dampen the immune response include glucocorticoids, antimetabolites, antibodies, and calcineurin inhibitors. The glucocorticoids are potent inhibitors of inflammation that are discussed in detail in Chapters 30 and 42. Antimetabolites such as sirolimus (Rapamune) and azathioprine (Imuran) inhibit aspects of lymphocyte replication. **Monoclonal** and **polyclonal antibodies** such as basiliximab (Simulect) and muromonab-CD3 interact with specific antigens on the surface of lymphocytes to destroy them. By binding to the intracellular messenger **calcineurin**, cyclosporine (Sandimmune, Neoral) and tacrolimus (Prograf, Advagraf) disrupt T-cell function. Because the primary indication for some of these immunosuppressants is to treat specific cancers, the student should also refer to Chapter 60.

Nursing Considerations

The role of the nurse in immunosuppressant therapy involves careful monitoring of the client's condition and providing education as it relates to the prescribed drug regimen. When providing care for clients who are taking immunosuppressants, an assessment should be done to determine the presence or history of organ transplant or grafting and to verify the need for these drugs. A client with leukemia, metastatic cancer, active infection, or renal or liver disease could be made worse by taking immunosuppressants, so they are contraindicated. They are also contraindicated in pregnancy. These drugs should be used with caution in clients who have pancreatic or bowel dysfunction, hyperkalemia, hypertension, and infection. The nurse should obtain vital signs and laboratory testing, including CBC, electrolytes, and liver profile, to provide baseline data and reveal any abnormalities.

Many immunosuppressants act on T lymphocytes, suppressing the normal cell-mediated immune reaction. Due to their effect on the immune system, a superimposed infection may occur, causing an increase in the white blood cell (WBC) count. Monitor vital signs, especially temperature, and laboratory results for indications

of infection. The degree of bone marrow suppression (thrombocytopenia and leukopenia) must be carefully monitored, as these adverse effects may be life-threatening.

It is important that clients immediately report the following signs and symptoms: alopecia, increased pigmentation, arthralgia, respiratory distress, edema, nausea, vomiting, paresthesia, fever, blood in the urine, black stools, and feelings of sadness. Clients who are taking azathioprine should be informed and monitored for the development of secondary malignancies.

See Nursing Process Focus: Clients Receiving Immunosuppressant Therapy for specific teaching points.

NURSING PROCESS FOCUS

Clients Receiving Immunosuppressant Therapy

Assessment	Potential Nursing Diagnoses/Identified Patterns
• Obtain health history, including allergies, drug history, and possible drug interactions. • Assess for presence of metastatic cancer, active infection, renal or liver disease, and pregnancy. • Assess skin integrity; specifically look for lesions and skin colour. • Obtain laboratory work: CBC, electrolytes, and liver enzymes. • Obtain vital signs, especially temperature and blood pressure.	• Risk for infection related to depressed immune response secondary to drug • Risk for injury related to thrombocytopenia secondary to drug

Planning: Client Goals and Expected Outcomes

The client will:

• Experience no symptoms of organ or allograft rejection

• Immediately report elevated temperature, unusual bleeding, sore throat, mouth ulcers, and fatigue to the healthcare provider

• Demonstrate an understanding of the drug's action by accurately describing drug side effects and precautions

Implementation

Interventions (Rationales)	Client Education/Discharge Planning
• Assess renal function. (Drugs cause nephrotoxicity in many clients due to physiological changes in the kidneys such as microcalcifications and interstitial fibrosis.) • Monitor liver function. (There is an increased risk for liver toxicity.) • Watch for signs and symptoms of infection, including elevated temperature. (There is an increased risk for infection due to immune suppression.) • Monitor vital signs, especially temperature and blood pressure. (Drugs may cause hypertension, especially in clients with kidney transplants.) • Monitor for the following possible side effects: hirsutism, leukopenia, gingival hyperplasia, gynecomastia, sinusitis, and hyperkalemia. • Monitor client for avoidance of drinking grapefruit juice. (This will increase cyclosporine levels by up to 70%.) • Assess nutritional status. (Drugs may cause weight gain.)	Advise client to: • Keep accurate record of urine output • Report significant reduction in urine flow • Instruct client as to the importance of regular laboratory testing Instruct client to: • Use thorough, frequent handwashing • Avoid crowds and people with infections Teach client to: • Monitor blood pressure and temperature, ensuring proper use of home equipment • Keep all appointments with the healthcare provider Advise client to: • See a dentist on a regular basis • Comply with regular laboratory assessments (CBC, electrolytes, and hormone levels) Instruct client to • Completely avoid drinking grapefruit juice • Take medication with food to decrease GI upset • Instruct client regarding a healthy diet that avoids excessive fats and sugars

Evaluation of Outcome Criteria

Evaluate the effectiveness of drug therapy by confirming that client goals and expected outcomes have been met (see "Planning").

See Table 40.2 (pages 479–480) for a list of drugs to which these nursing actions apply.

PROTOTYPE DRUG | **Cyclosporine (Neoral, Sandimmune)**

Actions and Uses: Cyclosporine is a complex chemical obtained from a soil fungus. Its primary mechanism of action is to inhibit helper T cells. Unlike some of the more cytotoxic immunosuppressants, it is less toxic to bone marrow cells. When prescribed for transplant recipients, it is primarily used in combination with high doses of a glucocorticoid such as prednisone. Cyclosporine is given by the oral (PO) route for prevention of transplant rejection, RA, and severe psoriasis. An IV form is available for transplant rejection and for severe cases of ulcerative colitis or Crohn's disease. An ophthalmic solution is used to increase tear production for clients with conjunctivitis.

Administration Alerts:

- Neoral (microemulsion) and Sandimmune are not bioequivalent and cannot be used interchangeably without the supervision of a healthcare provider.
- Cyclosporine is pregnancy category C.

Pharmacokinetics: The drug is administered by the PO or IV route. Cyclosporine PO undergoes significant first-pass metabolism with about 10% to 60% absorption. Cyclosporine is 90% to 98% protein bound. It is widely distributed, crosses the placenta, and enters breast milk. It is extensively metabolized in the liver with small amounts excreted in bile and urine. Half-life is approximately 19 hours.

Adverse Effects and Interactions: The primary adverse effect of cyclosporine occurs in the kidney, with up to 75% of clients experiencing a reduction in urine flow. Other common side effects are tremor, hypertension, and elevated hepatic enzymes. Although infections are common during cyclosporine therapy, they are fewer than with some of the other immunosuppressants. Periodic blood counts are necessary to be certain that WBCs do not fall below $4000/mm^3$ or platelets below $75\,000/mm^3$.

Drugs that decrease cyclosporine levels include phenytoin (Dilantin), phenobarbital (Phenobarb), carbamazepine (Tegretol), and rifampin (Rifadin, Rofact). Drugs that increase cyclosporine levels include antifungal drugs and macrolide antibiotics. Grapefruit juice can raise cyclosporine levels by up to 70%.

Use with caution with herbal supplements; for example, the immune-stimulating effects of astragalus and echinacea may interfere with immunosuppressants.

NCLEX Success Tips

Because liquid cyclosporine has a very unpleasant taste, diluting it with chocolate milk or orange juice will lessen the strong taste and help the child take the medication as ordered.

It is not acceptable to miss a dose because the drug's effectiveness is based on therapeutic blood levels, and skipping a dose could lower the level.

Cyclosporine should not be given by nasogastric tube because it adheres to the plastic tube and, thus, all of the drug may not be administered.

Taking the medication over a period of time could negatively affect the blood level.

Hyperacute rejection isn't treatable; the only way to stop this reaction is to remove the transplanted organ or tissue. Although cyclosporine is used to treat acute transplant rejection, it doesn't halt hyperacute rejection.

Corticosteroids as Immunosuppressants

40.4 Corticosteroids are widely used as immunosuppressants but have significant long-term adverse effects.

The corticosteroids, or glucocorticoids, are potent inhibitors of inflammation and are discussed in detail in Chapters 30 and 42. They are often the drugs of choice for the short-term therapy of severe inflammation.

In addition to their anti-inflammatory effects, corticosteroids affect nearly every aspect of the immune response. They intervene at multiple steps in the immune response, including antigen presentation, production of cytokines, and the proliferation of lymphocytes.

- *Lymphocyte effect.* A single dose of corticosteroid reduces circulating lymphocyte counts within a few hours. This inhibits the ability of the body to react to an antigen challenge.
- *Monocyte effect.* Corticosteroids quickly deplete the body of monocytes and macrophages. Macrophages are responsible for presenting antigens to lymphocytes.
- *Neutrophil effect.* Corticosteroids cause neutrophils to move from the bone marrow into the general circulation, resulting in increased numbers of circulating neutrophils. The drug then prevents the neutrophils from migrating out of the circulation to sites of inflammation.
- *Other effects.* Corticosteroids block the production of prostaglandins and ILs. This results in T cells being unable to react to antigens and proliferate.

Two common drugs in this class, prednisone and methylprednisolone (Medrol), have been widely used to prevent transplant rejection since the 1960s. When used for a few weeks, the corticosteroids are safe and effective immunosuppressants. The long-term adverse effects of corticosteroids, however, are serious and include osteoporosis, cataract formation, mental status changes, fluid and salt retention, hypertension, hyperglycemia, obesity, and adrenal atrophy. Because of their long-term effects, healthcare providers have begun to look at the possibility of eliminating corticosteroids from the transplant regimen. Some regimens call for the initial use of corticosteroids, with their gradual withdrawal at some point, usually within 3 to 6 months following the transplant. The issue remains unresolved and is an area of active research.

CHAPTER

40 Understanding the Chapter

Key Concepts Summary

The numbered key concepts provide a succinct summary of the important points from the corresponding numbered section within the chapter. If any of these points are not clear, refer to the numbered section within the chapter for review.

40.1 Immunomodulators are substances that either enhance or suppress the ability of the body to fight infection and disease.

40.2 Interferons are biological response modifiers that have antiviral and antineoplastic activity.

40.3 Immunosuppressants are used to prevent transplant rejection and for the treatment of autoimmune disorders.

40.4 Corticosteroids are widely used as immunosuppressants but have significant long-term adverse effects.

Chapter 40 Scenario

Carol Banks is a 42-year-old woman who has been diagnosed with hepatitis C and who is being seen by her healthcare provider at an office visit. She reports having right upper quadrant pain, fatigue, anorexia, nausea, and vomiting. She has been feeling progressively worse for the past year but has not sought medical care for her symptoms until now. She has lost 5.4 kg (12 lb.) over the past 6 months.

Before her diagnosis, Carol was hospitalized to receive IV fluids for dehydration and to be evaluated further. Once in the hospital, a full hepatitis panel found that she is positive for hepatitis C virus (HCV).

During the initial interview with Carol at the hospital, she disclosed that she had been addicted to illegal IV drugs for 15 years and had been an alcohol abuser for 20 years. However, Carol claimed that she had abstained from substance abuse for the past 5 years. She resides

with her husband and three children and is employed as a clerk in a local retail convenience store.

As part of the treatment for Carol's hepatitis she was prescribed interferon alfa-2b (Intron A). She was taught to self-administer (subcutaneously) the standard dose of IFN, 3 million units, given three times weekly.

Critical Thinking Questions

1. Discuss the rationale for the use of interferon alfa-2b (Intron A) in the treatment of hepatitis C.
2. What adverse effects is Carol experiencing with this drug therapy? How can the nurse assist Carol to cope with the related adverse effects?
3. Identify the client education that Carol will need concerning her drug therapy.

See Answers to Critical Thinking Questions in Appendix B.

NCLEX Practice Questions

1 The nurse is monitoring the laboratory findings of a client who is taking interferon alfa-2b (Intron A). Which findings would indicate that the client is experiencing common adverse effects?

a. Flu-like symptoms of fever, chills, fatigue, and weight loss
b. Depression with thoughts of suicide
c. Edema, hypotension, and tachycardia
d. Fluid volume overload, hypertension, renal insufficiency

2 A client is receiving basiliximab (Simulect) and cyclosporine (Sandimmune) after a kidney transplant to prevent transplant rejection. The client develops a high fever and chills, with a

temperature of (39.4°C). The nurse interprets that the client is most likely experiencing

a. Capillary leak syndrome
b. A significant infection related to immunosuppression
c. Graft-versus-host rejection
d. Androgen-insensitivity syndrome

3 The nurse who for a client receiving cyclosporine (Sandimmune) will discontinue the medication immediately and call the provider if which of the following occurs?

a. Red blood cell count above 8.5 million/mm^3
b. White blood cell count below 4000/mm^3

c. Platelet count above 100 000/mm^3

d. Serum creatinine level less than 1.0 mg/100 mL

4 Azathioprine (Imuran) is prescribed to a client who had a renal transplant. The nurse reviews the client's medical record. Which of the following factors would make the nurse question the medication order?

a. Benign prostatic hyperplasia

b. Cataracts

c. Varicella zoster

d. Rheumatoid arthritis

5 The nurse is instructing a client who is receiving tacrolimus (Prograf) following a liver transplant. Which point should be included in the teaching plan?

a. Take a "baby" strength aspirin every day.

b. Increase physical activity to avoid weight gain.

c. Record radial pulse rate every morning in a journal.

d. Avoid raw fruits and vegetables and eat only fully cooked meats.

See Answers to NCLEX Practice Questions in Appendix A.

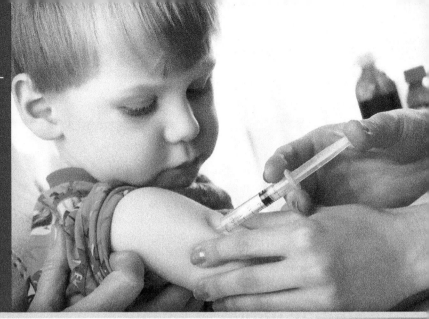

PROTOTYPE DRUGS

ACTIVE IMMUNITY	PASSIVE IMMUNITY
Pr *Hepatitis B vaccine (Engerix-B, Recombivax HB)*	*Rh$_o$(D) Immune Globulin (WinRho)*

CHAPTER 41

Pharmacotherapy of Immune System Modulation and Immunization

LEARNING OUTCOMES

After reading this chapter, the student should be able to:

1. Compare and contrast active and passive immunity.
2. Explain the immune response that leads to the development of active immunity.
3. Prepare a table listing the types of vaccines, their indications, and their schedules.
4. Explain why it is important to administer childhood vaccines at specific ages.
5. Identify contraindications for vaccine administration.
6. Explain the rationale for administering antibodies to establish passive immunity.
7. Apply the nursing process to care for clients who are receiving immunizing agents.

CHAPTER OUTLINE

▸ Administration of Vaccines and the Immune System

▸ Types of Vaccines

Vaccinations have become one of the most important medical interventions for the prevention of serious infectious disease. Routine vaccinations for polio, pertussis, diphtheria, tetanus, and measles are estimated to prevent 3 million deaths annually. This chapter examines the role of vaccines in promoting the health of both children and adults and the potential adverse effects of these drugs.

Administration of Vaccines and the Immune System

41.1 Vaccines are used to activate the immune system for the purpose of disease prevention.

Vaccines are used to activate the immune system for the purpose of disease prevention.

An immune response occurs when an antigen is recognized by the B or T lymphocytes.

Lymphocytes attack antigens by binding to them through certain receptor proteins on their surface. Sometimes they recognize a toxin or secretion produced by the organism. Scientists have used this knowledge to create vaccines, which are biological products that prevent disease. Vaccines consist of suspensions of one of the following:

- Microbes that have been killed
- Microbes that are alive but weakened (**attenuated**) so that they are unable to produce disease
- Bacterial toxins, called **toxoids**, that have been modified to destroy their hazardous properties

Antigens are microbes and foreign substances that elicit an immune response. Most microbes, non-human proteins, bacterial or plant toxins, and normal cells that become damaged or cancerous are considered antigens. After the first exposure to an antigen, sufficient time is needed for the body to process the antigen and mount an effective response. It is during this time, known as the **incubation period**, that the symptoms of infection and tissue injury develop. During this first antigen exposure, memory B cells or T cells are formed. Should a second or subsequent exposure to the same antigen occur, the memory cells react quickly to produce a more rapid immune response with fewer (or no) symptoms of infection.

Edward Jenner was the first to use the term *vaccination*. **Vaccination** is the process of introducing foreign proteins or inactive cells (vaccines) into the body to trigger immune activation *before* the client is exposed to the real pathogen. As a result of the vaccination, memory B cells or T cells are formed. When later exposed to the real infectious organism, these cells will react quickly by producing large quantities of antibodies and cytokines that help to neutralize or destroy the antigen. Although some vaccinations are needed only once, most require follow-up doses, known as

boosters, to provide prolonged protection. The type of response induced by the real pathogen, or its vaccine, is called **active immunity**. During this response the body produces its own antibodies in response to exposure. The active immunity induced by vaccines closely resembles that caused by natural exposure to the antigen, including the generation of memory cells. The term **immunization** is considered equivalent to the term *vaccination*, and either one may be used to describe this process of disease prevention.

The effectiveness of most vaccines can be assessed by measuring the amount of antibodies produced after the vaccine has been administered, a quantity called *titre*. If the titre falls below a specified, protective level over time, a booster dose is indicated. Antibodies are a product of the humoral immune system. The cell-mediated immune system is also important in producing immunity, but its cellular responses are less readily measured.

Passive immunity occurs when preformed antibodies are transferred or "donated" from one person to another. For example, maternal antibodies cross the placenta and provide protection for the fetus and newborn. Other examples of passive immunity include the administration of immune globulin following exposure to hepatitis; antivenins for snakebites; and sera to treat botulism, tetanus, and rabies (see Table 41.1 for common immune globulin

TABLE 41.1 Immune Globulin Preparations

Drug	Route and Adult Dose
Cytomegalovirus immune globulin (CytoGam)	Intravenous (IV), 150 mg/kg within 72 hours of transplantation, then 100 mg/kg at 2, 4, 6, and 8 weeks post-transplant, then 50 mg/kg at 12 and 16 weeks post-transplant
Hepatitis B immune globulin (HyperHep B)	Intramuscular (IM), 0.06 mL/kg as soon as possible after exposure, preferably within 24 hours but no later then 7 days, repeat 28–30 days after exposure
Immune globulin intramuscular (Gamastan)	IM, 0.02–0.06 mL/kg as soon as possible after exposure if hepatitis B immune globulin is unavailable
Immune globulin intravenous (Gammagard, Iveegam)	IV, 100–200 mg/kg/month; IM, 1.2 mL/kg followed by 0.6 mL/kg every 2 to 4 weeks (q2–4wk)
Rabies immune globulin (Imogam, Hyperab)	IM (gluteal), 20 IU/kg
Rh₀(D) immune globulin (WinRho)	IM/IV, one vial or 300 μg at approximately 28 weeks, followed by one vial of minidose or 120 μg within 72 hours of delivery if infant is Rh positive
Tetanus immune globulin (HyperTet)	IM, 250 units

preparations). The drugs for passive immunity are administered when the client has already been exposed to a virulent pathogen, or when the client is at very high risk for exposure and there is not sufficient time to develop active immunity. Clients who are immunosuppressed may receive these agents to prevent infections. Because these drugs do not stimulate the client's immune system, no memory cells are produced and protective effects last only 2 to 3 weeks.

Most vaccines are administered with the goal of *preventing* illness. Common vaccines include those used to prevent clients from acquiring measles, influenza, diphtheria, polio, pertussis (whooping cough), tetanus, and hepatitis B. Recently, two vaccines have been added to the immunization schedule in Canada: one for human papillomavirus (HPV [Gardasil]) and another for chicken pox (varicella). HPV is believed to be the primary cause of cervical cancer. The highest incidence is in women aged 20 to 24 years. Anthrax vaccine has been used to immunize people who are at high risk for exposure to anthrax from a potential bioterrorism incident. In the case of infection by the human immunodeficiency virus (HIV), experimental HIV vaccines are given after infection has occurred for the purpose of enhancing the immune response, rather than preventing the disease. Unlike other vaccines, experimental vaccines for HIV have thus far been unable to prevent acquired immune deficiency syndrome (AIDS).

Types of Vaccines

41.2 Vaccination is the process of introducing foreign proteins or inactive cells (vaccines) into the body to trigger immune activation before the patient is exposed to the real pathogen.

All vaccines used for routine immunization are effective in preventing disease and have a low risk for serious adverse effects. The diseases, however, can have serious or even fatal consequences. Common side effects of vaccines include redness and discomfort at the site of injection and fever. Although severe reactions are uncommon, anaphylaxis is possible. Vaccinations are contraindicated for clients who have a weak immune system or who are currently experiencing symptoms such as diarrhea, vomiting, or fever.

Effective vaccines have been produced for a number of debilitating diseases, and their widespread use has prevented serious illness in millions of clients, particularly children. One disease, smallpox, has been completely eliminated from the planet through immunization, and others such as polio have diminished to extremely low levels. Immunization is not mandatory in Canada. Immunization is a shared responsibility between federal and provincial/territorial governments. Although some provinces have legislation that requires proof of immunization for school entrance, exceptions are permitted for reasons of conscience, religion, allergies, and medical conditions. Table 41.2 lists some common childhood vaccines and their schedules as recommended by the National Advisory Committee on Immunization (NACI). Nurses should be familiar with recommendations in their jurisdiction, as they may differ from those of the NACI.

Although vaccinations have proved a resounding success in children, many adults die of diseases that could be prevented by vaccination. Most mortality from vaccine-preventable disease in adults is from influenza and pneumococcal disease. Hepatitis B is the most important vaccine-preventable infectious occupational disease for healthcare workers. The risk of being infected is a consequence of the prevalence of virus carriers in the population receiving care, the frequency of exposure to blood and other body fluids, and the contagiousness of hepatitis B virus. All Canadian adults require maintenance of immunity to tetanus and diphtheria, preferably with combined (Td) toxoid and a single dose of acellular pertussis vaccine. A vaccine for HPV is newly available in Canada for pre-exposure use in young females to reduce risk for cervical cancer caused by HPV. HPV vaccine is administered in three doses over 6 months at 0, 2, and 6 months (Table 41.3 describes the adult immunization schedule). See the HPV vaccine immunization schedule for adults at the NACI website: http://www.phac-aspc.gc.ca/naci-ccni/acs-dcc/2015/hpv-vph_0215-eng.php

NCLEX Success Tips

Hepatitis B immune globulin (HyperHep B) is given as prophylactic therapy to individuals who have been exposed to hepatitis B. Interferon has been approved to treat hepatitis B.

Hepatitis B immune globulin at birth provides the infant with passive immunity against hepatitis B and serves as a prophylactic treatment.

RhoGAM is given to new mothers who are Rh-negative and not previously sensitized and who have given birth to an Rh-positive infant. RhoGAM must be given within 72 hours of the birth of the infant because antibody formation begins at that time.

The purpose of the RhoGAM is to provide passive antibody immunity and prevent Rh-positive sensitization with the next pregnancy.

The RhoGAM does not cross the placenta and destroy fetal Rh-positive cells.

Most Rh-negative clients also receive RhoGAM during the prenatal period at 28 weeks' gestation and then again after birth. The drug is given to Rh-negative mothers who have a negative Coombs test and give birth to Rh-positive neonates. If there is doubt about the fetus's blood type after pregnancy is terminated, the mother should receive the medication.

Giving $RH_0(D)$ immune globulin only at 28 weeks' gestation wouldn't prevent isoimmunization from occurring after placental separation, when fetal blood enters the maternal circulation. Giving $RH_0(D)$ immune globulin only within 72 hours after delivery wouldn't prevent isoimmunization caused by passage of fetal blood into the maternal circulation during gestation.

Giving $Rh_0(D)$ immune globulin within 24 hours after birth would be too soon because maternal sensitization occurs in approximately 72 hours.

Rh sensitization can be prevented by $Rh_0(D)$ immune globulin, which clears the maternal circulation of Rh-positive cells before sensitization can occur, thereby blocking maternal antibody production to Rh-positive cells. Administration of this drug will not prevent future Rh-positive fetuses, nor will it prevent future abortions.

Based on Public Health Agency of Canada, http://www.phac-aspc.gc.ca/.

Elderly clients, especially those with existing respiratory compromise, are good candidates for the pneumonia vaccine (Pneumovax, Prevnar). This vaccine provides immunity and prophylaxis against pneumococcal pneumonia or bacteremia in adults or children at risk. The nurse should encourage the client to take the vaccine. Taking the vaccine is not related to frequency of asthma attacks, and the vaccine is not contraindicated for clients with asthma.

Clients who have a chronic illness, have experienced a serious illness, reside in long-term care facilities, or are 65 years of age or older are encouraged to obtain pneumococcal and influenza vaccinations.

TABLE 41.2   National Advisory Committee on Immunization (NACI) Recommendations for Routine Childhood Vaccination in Canada

Vaccine [±]	Birth	2 mos	4 mos	6 mos	12 mos	15 mos	18 mos	23 mos	2 years	4 years	5 years	6 years	9 years	12 years	14 years	15 years	16 years	17 years
DTaP-IPV-Hib or DTaP-HB-IPV-Hib		[A] or [B] 1st dose	[A] or [B] 2nd dose	[A] or [B] 3rd dose	[A] or 4th dose Generally at 18 months of age													
DTaP-IPV or Tdap-IPV										[C]								
Tdap																[D]		
Rot		[E] 2 or 3 doses Complete series before 8 months																
Pneu-C-13		[F]			[F]													
Men-C-C		[G] According to P/T schedule			[G] Generally at 12 months													
Men-C-C or Men-C-ACYW														[H]				
MMR and Var					[I] + [J]			[I] + [J]										
								OR										
MMRV					[K]			[K] Generally at 4–6 years										
HB		[L] 3 doses																
								OR										
HB																[M] 2 or 3 doses		
HPV														[N] 2 or 3 doses				
								OR										
HPV																[Q] 3 doses		
Inf							[P] 1 or 2 doses Recommended annually							[P] 1 dose Recommended annually				

[±]   For abbreviations and brand names of vaccines refer to Contents of Immunizing Agents Available for Use in Canada in Part 1.

[A]   **Diphtheria toxoid- tetanus toxoid- acellular pertussis- inactivated polio-** *Haemophilus influenzae* **type b** (DTaP-IPV-Hib). For infants and children beginning primary immunization at 7 months of age and older, the number of doses of Hib vaccine required varies by age.

[B]   **Diphtheria toxoid- tetanus toxoid- acellular pertussis- hepatitis B- inactivated polio-** *Haemophilus influenzae* **type b** (DTaP-HB-IPV-Hib). Alternative schedules may be used: DTaP-HB-IPV-Hib at 2, 4 and 12-23 months of age with DTaP-IPV-Hib vaccine at 6 months of age; or DTaP-HB-IPV -Hib at 2, 4 and 6 months of age with DTaP-IPV-Hib vaccine at 12-23 months of age.

[C]   **Diphtheria toxoid- tetanus toxoid- acellular pertussis- inactivated polio** or **tetanus toxoid- reduced diphtheria toxoid- reduced acellular pertussis- inactivated polio.**

[D]   **Tetanus toxoid- reduced diphtheria toxoid- reduced acellular pertussis** (Tdap): 10 years after last dose of DTaP- or Tdap-containing vaccine.

[E]   **Rotavirus:** Rotavirus pentavalent vaccine - 3 doses, 4 to 10 weeks apart; Rotavirus monovalent vaccine - 2 doses, at least 4 weeks apart. Give the first dose starting at 6 weeks and before 15 weeks of age. Administer all doses before 8 months of age.

[F]   **Pneumococcal conjugate 13-valent** (Pneu-C-13): healthy infants beginning primary immunization at 2-6 months of age: 3 or 4 dose schedule. For a 3 dose schedule: 2, 4 months of age, followed by a booster dose at 12 months of age. For a 4 dose schedule: minimum of 8 weeks interval between doses beginning at 2 months of age, followed by a booster dose at 12-15 months of age. Healthy infants beginning primary immunization at 7-11 months of age: 2 doses, at least 8 weeks apart followed by a booster dose at 12-15 months of age, at least 8 weeks after the second dose. Children who have received age-appropriate pneumococcal vaccination with a pneumococcal conjugate vaccine but not Pneu-C-13 vaccine: 12-35 months of age - 1 dose; 36-59 months of age and of aboriginal origin or attend group child care - 1 dose; other healthy children 36-59 months of age - consider 1 dose.

[G]   **Meningococcal conjugate monovalent:** children 12-48 months of age: 1 dose routinely provided at 12 months of age, regardless of any doses given during the first year of life. Immunization may be considered for unimmunized children 5-11 years of age.

[H]   **Meningococcal conjugate monovalent** or **meningococcal conjugate quadrivalent:** early adolescence (around 12 years of age) - 1 dose, even if meningococcal conjugate vaccine received at a younger age. Vaccine chosen depends on local epidemiology and programmatic considerations.

TABLE 41.2 (continued)

L I ⎤ **Measles-mumps-rubella:** first dose at 12-15 months of age; second dose at 18 months of age or anytime thereafter, but should be given no later than around school entry.

⎡ J ⎤ **Varicella (chickenpox):** first dose at 12-15 months of age; second dose at 18 months of age or anytime thereafter, but should be given no later than around school entry.

⎡ K ⎤ **Measles-mumps-rubella-varicella:** first dose at 12-15 months of age; second dose at 18 months of age or anytime thereafter, but should be given no later than around school entry.

⎡ L ⎤ **Hepatitis B:** months 0, 1 and 6 (first dose = month 0) with at least 4 weeks between the first and second dose, at least 2 months between the second and third dose, and at least 4 months between the first and third dose. Alternatively, can be administered as DTaP-HB-IPV-Hib vaccine, with first dose at 2 months of age.

⎡ M ⎤ **Hepatitis B:** 9-17 years of age - months 0, 1 and 6 (first dose = month 0) with at least 4 weeks between the first and second dose, at least 2 months between the second and third dose, and at least 4 months between the first and third dose. 11-15 years of age - 2 doses; schedule depends on the product used.

⎡ N ⎤ **Human papillomavirus (HPV):** Girls, 9-14 years of age: HPV bivalent (HPV2) or HPV quadrivalent (HPV4) vaccine - months 0 and 6-12 (first dose = month 0). Alternatively, a 3 dose schedule may be used for HPV2 vaccine - months 0, 1 and 6 (first dose = month 0), for HPV4 vaccine - months 0, 2 and 6 (first dose = month 0), and HPV nonavalent (HPV9) vaccine - months 0, 2 and 6 (first dose = month 0). Boys, 9-14 years of age: HPV4 vaccine - months 0 and 6-12 (first dose = month 0). For a 2 dose schedule, the minimum interval between doses is 6 months. Alternatively, a 3 dose schedule may be used for HPV4 vaccine - months 0, 2 and 6 (first dose = month 0), and HPV9 vaccine - months 0, 2 and 6 (first dose = month 0)

⎡ O ⎤ **Human papillomavirus:** Girls, 15-17 years of age: HPV2 vaccine - months 0, 1 and 6 (first dose = month 0), HPV4 vaccine - months 0, 2 and 6 (first dose = month 0) or HPV9 vaccine - months 0, 2 and 6 (first dose = month 0). Boys, 15-17 years of age: HPV4 vaccine - months 0, 2 and 6 (first dose = month 0) or HPV9 vaccine - months 0, 2 and 6 (first dose = month 0). In individuals who received the first dose of HPV2 or HPV4 vaccine between 9-14 years of age, a 2 dose schedule can be used with the second dose administered at least 6 months after the first dose.

⎡ P ⎤ **Influenza:** recommended annually for anyone 6 months of age and older without contraindications. Children 6 months-less than 9 years of age, receiving influenza vaccine for the first time - 2 doses, at least 4 weeks apart. Children 6 months-8 years of age, previously immunized with influenza vaccine and children 9 years of age and older - 1 dose.

TABLE 41.3 Adult Immunization Schedule: Routine and Specific Risk Situations

Vaccine or Toxoid	Indication	Schedule
Tetanus and diphtheria given as Td; tetanus, diphtheria, and pertussis given as Tdap	Routine for all adults	Td booster every 10 years (doses 1 and 2 given 4–8 weeks apart and dose 3 given 6–12 months later; one of the doses should be given as Tdap for pertussis protection if not previously given)
Measles, mumps, and rubella given as MMR	Routine for adults who have no record or an unclear history of prior immunization	1 dose for adults born in or after 1970 without a history of measles or without evidence of immunity to rubella or mumps; second dose for select groups
Varicella	Routine for adults who have no record or an unclear history of prior immunization	Doses 1 and 2 at least 4 weeks apart for susceptible adults (no history of natural disease or seronegativity)
Influenza	Adults ≥65 years; adults <65 years at high risk for influenza-related complications and their household contacts; healthcare workers	Every autumn using current recommended vaccine formulation
Pneumococcal polysaccharide	Adults ≥65 years; adults <65 years who have conditions that put them at increased risk of pneumococcal disease	1 dose
Hepatitis A	Occupational risk; lifestyle; travel to areas with inadequate sanitation; post-exposure immunopro-phylaxis; adults with chronic liver disease	2 doses 6–12 months apart
Hepatitis B	Occupational risk; lifestyle; post-exposure immuno-prophylaxis; adults with chronic liver disease	3 doses at 0, 1, and 6 months
HPV	Pre-exposure use in young females/males to reduce risk for cervical cancer caused by HPV	3 doses at 0, 2, and 6 months
Bacillus Calmette-Guérin (BCG)	Rarely used; consider for high-risk exposure	1 dose
Poliomyelitis	Travel to endemic areas; other risk group	Primary series doses 1 and 2 given 4–8 weeks apart and dose 3 given 6–12 months later; 1 booster dose if >10 years since primary series
Meningococcal conjugate	Young adults	1 dose
Rabies, pre-exposure use	Occupational; high-risk travellers	3 doses at days 0, 7, and 21

HPV infection, or genital warts, can lead to dysplastic changes of the cervix, referred to as cervical intraepithelial neoplasia. The development of cervical cancer remains the largest threat of all condyloma-associated neoplasias. Infertility, pelvic inflammatory disease, and rectal cancer are not complications of genital warts.

Vaccines are preventative in nature and ideally given before exposure. Focusing on the benefits of cancer prevention is most appropriate, rather than discussing with parents the potential that their child may become sexually active without their knowledge. It is true that HPV is most common in adolescents and women in their late twenties, but parents still may not perceive that their child is at risk. Discussing the possibility of exposure through assault raises fears and does not focus on prevention.

PROTOTYPE DRUG | **Hepatitis B Vaccine (Recombivax, Engerix-B)**

Actions and Uses: Hepatitis B vaccine (Recombivax) is used to provide active immunity in individuals who are at risk for exposure to hepatitis B virus (HBV). It is indicated for infants born to HBV-positive mothers and those at high risk for exposure to HBV-infected blood, including nurses, physicians, dentists, dental hygienists, morticians, and paramedics. Because HBV infection is extremely difficult to treat, it is prudent for all healthcare workers to receive the HBV vaccine before beginning their clinical education, unless contraindicated. HBV vaccine does not provide protection against exposure to other (non-B) hepatitis viruses. HBV vaccine is produced by splicing the gene for HBV surface antigen into yeast and harvesting the protein product. It is prepared from recombinant yeast cultures rather than from human blood. Vaccination requires three IM injections; the second dose is given 1 month after the first, and the third dose is given 6 months after the first.

Pharmacokinetics: The pharmacokinetics of HBV vaccine are unknown. The onset of action is 2 weeks, with a peak in 6 months.

Administration Alerts:

- In adults, use the deltoid muscle for the injection site, unless contraindicated.

CONNECTIONS **Cultural Considerations**

◀ **Immunization**

Childhood immunizations have proven to be one of the most effective means of preventing and controlling the spread of infectious and communicable diseases, although hundreds of preschool-age children are not being immunized. In general, immunization levels are lower among Aboriginal peoples, immigrants, older adults, populations with low socioeconomic status, and some religious groups. According to International Circumpolar Surveillance (ICS), the incidence of invasive pneumococcal disease from 1999 to 2004 was higher among Aboriginals, at 38 per 100 000, than non-Aboriginals, at 9.6 per 100 000 (ICS, unpublished data, 2006). Limited access to preventive services; limited knowledge about vaccination; and attitudes and cultural beliefs about immunization, illness, and health care may contribute to these statistics.

Based on Public Health Agency of Canada, INK "http://www.phac-aspc.gc.ca/".

- Epinephrine (1:1000) should be immediately available to treat a possible anaphylactic reaction.

- Titres should be done a few months after the series is completed to confirm immunity.

- HBV vaccine is pregnancy category C.

Adverse Effects and Interactions: HBV vaccine is well tolerated, and few serious adverse reactions have been reported. Pain and inflammation at the injection site are the most common side effects. Some clients experience transient fever or fatigue. Hypersensitivity reactions such as urticaria or anaphylaxis are possible.

This vaccine is contraindicated in clients with hypersensitivity to yeast or HBV vaccine. The drug should be administered with caution in clients with fever or active infections or in those with compromised cardiopulmonary status.

CHAPTER

41 Understanding the Chapter

Key Concepts Summary

The numbered key concepts provide a succinct summary of the important points from the corresponding numbered section within the chapter. If any of these points are not clear, refer to the numbered section within the chapter for review.

41.1 Vaccines are used to activate the immune system for the purpose of disease prevention.

41.2 Vaccination is the process of introducing foreign proteins or inactive cells (vaccines) into the body to trigger immune activation before the patient is exposed to the real pathogen.

Chapter 41 Scenario

Mr. and Mrs. Abbott arrive in the office where you work with their 4-month-old infant, Samantha, for her checkup. She is scheduled to receive the following immunizations today: Tdap, *Haemophilus influenzae* type b (Hib), pneumococcal conjugate vaccine (PCV), and inactivated polio vaccine (IPV). Mrs. Abbott states, "I don't think these immunizations are necessary. Don't these shots usually make children sick?"

As first-time parents, Mr. and Mrs. Abbott are new to the experience of childhood immunizations and require careful teaching. While obtaining her history, you find that 4-month-old Samantha has been doing well and is in the 90th percentile for height and the 89th percentile for weight. She has achieved the developmental milestones for her age and is bright and interacts well with her environment.

Critical Thinking Questions

1. What information should be obtained from Mr. and Mrs. Abbott about Samantha's first response to immunization?

2. Why is it important to discuss the potential adverse effects of vaccines with Samantha's parents?

3. What educational information should be given to Mr. and Mrs. Abbott?

See Answers to Critical Thinking Questions in Appendix B.

NCLEX Practice Questions

1. Mary is a 4-month-old infant who is brought to the clinic for her first checkup. Her mother tells the nurse that the child has never been ill. Which factor would the nurse consider most significant in assessing the baby's likelihood of receiving immunizations?
   a. Allergies to previously administered medications
   b. Mother's preconceptions and reservations relating to vaccines
   c. Maternal and paternal allergies or reactions to vaccine administration
   d. Nurse's knowledge of the recommended pediatric immunization schedule

2. The nurse is preparing to administer an MMR vaccination to a 15-month-old child. What would cause the nurse to hold the injection and recheck this order with the provider?
   a. The mother tells the nurse that the family will be going to the beach for the next few weeks.
   b. The mother states that she was told she'd had a reaction to the injection when she was a child.
   c. The mother tells the nurse that her husband is having chemotherapy for Hodgkin's lymphoma.
   d. The mother tells the nurse that the child's older brother is home with a cold virus.

3. The nurse determines that her client understands the teaching given for required care following a tetanus toxoid injection when the client states,
   a. "I will keep my arm still for the next 24 hours to give the vaccine time to absorb."
   b. "I will limit my fluid intake for the next 8 hours in case I have nausea."
   c. "I will avoid crowds and people with viruses for the next 7 days."
   d. "I will take some acetaminophen (Tylenol) or ibuprofen (Advil) if my arm is sore."

4. The occupational health nurse will be administering hepatitis B vaccine to a new employee. Which assessment finding discovered by the nurse would necessitate withholding the injection? The client is
   a. A two-pack-per-day smoker
   b. Known to have transient hypertension
   c. Allergic to yeast and yeast products
   d. Frightened by needles and injections

5. A postpartum client received $Rh_o(D)$ immune globulin (RhoGAM) therapy after the delivery of an 8-lb baby boy. The nurse performs which important intervention during the course of this treatment?
   a. Monitoring the client for 20 minutes following the administration for a hypersensitivity reaction
   b. Evaluating the laboratory results for thrombocytopenia, anemia, and increased liver enzymes
   c. Providing the client with the information needed to maintain a low–saturated fat, low-cholesterol diet
   d. Instructing the client to use non-medicated sugar-free lozenges or hard candies to relieve a cough

See Answers to NCLEX Practice Questions in Appendix A.

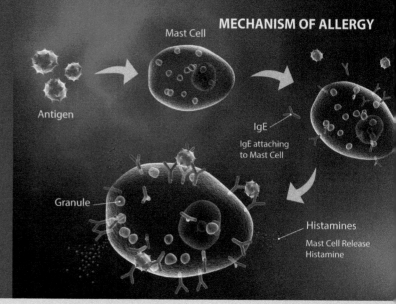

PROTOTYPE DRUGS

ANTI-INFLAMMATORY DRUGS
  Nonsteroidal anti-inflammatory drugs (NSAIDs)
    Pr *ibuprofen (Motrin, Advil)*
  Systemic glucocorticoids
    Pr *prednisone*

ANTIPYRETICS
    Pr *acetaminophen (Tylenol)*

ALLERGY DRUGS
  H_1-receptor antagonists (antihistamines)
    Pr *diphenhydramine (Allerdryl, Benadryl)*
    Pr *fexofenadine (Allegra)*
  Intranasal glucocorticoids
    Pr *fluticasone (Flonase)*
  Adrenergics

ANAPHYLAXIS DRUGS
    Pr *epinephrine (Adrenalin)*

MECHANISM OF ALLERGY

Mast Cell

Antigen

IgE

IgE attaching to Mast Cell

Granule

Histamines

Mast Cell Release Histamine

Stocktrek Images, Inc./Alamy Stock Photo

CHAPTER

42 Pharmacotherapy of Inflammation, Fever, and Allergies

LEARNING OUTCOMES

After reading this chapter, the student should be able to:

1. Explain the pathophysiology of inflammation and fever.

2. Explain the therapeutic action of drugs used for treating inflammation in relation to the acute inflammatory response and signs and symptoms of inflammation.

3. Differentiate between histamine H_1 and H_2 receptors.

4. Discuss the role of the nurse regarding the non-pharmacological management of clients who are receiving drugs for inflammation, fever, and allergies.

5. Describe the nurse's role in the pharmacological management of clients who are receiving drugs for inflammation, fever, and allergies.

6. For each of the drug classes listed in Prototype Drugs, identify a representative drug and explain its mechanism of action, therapeutic effects, and important adverse effects.

7. Describe and explain, based on pharmacological principles, the rationale for nursing assessment, planning, and interventions for clients with inflammation, fever, and allergies.

8. Use the nursing process to care for clients who are receiving drug therapy for inflammation, fever, and allergies.

CHAPTER OUTLINE

▶ The Function of Inflammation

▶ The Role of Histamine in Inflammation

▶ Histamine Receptors

▶ Nonsteroidal Anti-Inflammatory Drugs
  ▶ Treating Inflammation with NSAIDs

▶ Systemic Glucocorticoids
  ▶ Treating Acute or Severe Inflammation with Systemic Glucocorticoids

▶ Fever
  ▶ Treating Fever with Antipyretics

▶ Allergy
  ▶ Pharmacotherapy of Allergic Rhinitis

Inflammation is a nonspecific response to injury that destroys agents that could damage human tissue. Through the process of inflammation, a large number of potentially damaging chemicals and foreign agents may be neutralized. A large number of conditions, including physical trauma, burns, chemical injury, infections, hypersensitivity reactions, or tissue necrosis (death), can trigger inflammation. Although it is a natural defence mechanism, excessive inflammation causes symptoms that range from minor discomfort to severe, disabling pain, fever, and limitation of mobility.

The pain and redness of inflammation following minor abrasions and cuts is something that everyone has experienced. Although there is some discomfort from such scrapes, inflammation is a normal and expected part of our body's defence against injury. It is these sorts of conditions in which pharmacotherapy may be required.

Similarly, the allergy symptoms of nasal congestion, scratchy throat, and postnasal drip are familiar to millions of clients. Allergy symptoms may range from annoying to life-threatening and are common indications for drug therapy.

This chapter examines drugs used to diminish the inflammatory response and to reduce fever. Also discussed in this chapter are drugs that reduce allergic reactions and prevent their occurrence.

The Function of Inflammation

42.1 Inflammation is a natural, nonspecific response that limits the spread of invading microorganisms or injury. Acute inflammation occurs over several days, whereas chronic inflammation may continue for months or years.

The human body has developed many complex means to defend against injury and invading organisms. Inflammation is one of these defence mechanisms. **Inflammation** is a complex process that may occur in response to a large number of different stimuli, including physical injury, exposure to toxic chemicals, extreme heat, invading microorganisms, or death of cells. It is considered a nonspecific defence mechanism because the physiological processes of inflammation proceed in the same manner regardless of the cause. The specific immune defences of the body are presented in Chapter 39.

The central purpose of inflammation is to contain the injury or destroy the foreign agent. By neutralizing the foreign agent and removing cellular debris and dead cells, repair of the injured area can proceed at a faster pace. Signs of inflammation include swelling, pain, warmth, and redness of the affected area.

Inflammation may be classified as acute or chronic. During acute inflammation, such as that caused by minor physical injury, 8 to 10 days are normally needed for the symptoms to resolve and for repair to begin. If the body cannot contain or neutralize the damaging agent, inflammation may continue for prolonged periods and become chronic. In chronic autoimmune disorders such as lupus and rheumatoid arthritis, inflammation may persist for years, with symptoms becoming progressively worse over time. Other disorders such as seasonal allergy arise at predictable times during each year, and inflammation may produce only minor, annoying symptoms.

The pharmacotherapy of inflammation includes drugs that decrease the natural inflammatory response. Most anti-inflammatory drugs are nonspecific; this means that whether the inflammation is caused from injury or allergy, the drug will exhibit the same anti-inflammatory actions. A few anti-inflammatory drugs are specific to certain diseases, such as those used to treat gout (see Chapter 61). The following diseases have an inflammatory component and may benefit from anti-inflammatory drugs:

- Allergic rhinitis
- Anaphylaxis

- Ankylosing spondylitis
- Contact dermatitis
- Crohn's disease
- Glomerulonephritis
- Hashimoto's thyroiditis
- Peptic ulcers
- Rheumatoid arthritis
- Systemic lupus erythematosus
- Ulcerative colitis

The Role of Histamine in Inflammation

42.2 Histamine is a key chemical mediator in inflammation. Release of histamine produces vasodilation, allowing capillaries to become leaky, thus causing tissue swelling.

Whether the injury is due to pathogens, chemicals, or physical trauma, the damaged tissue releases a number of chemical mediators that act as "alarms" to notify the surrounding area of the injury. Chemical mediators of inflammation include **histamine**, **leukotrienes**, **bradykinin**, **complement**, and **prostaglandins**. Table 42.1 lists the sources and actions of these mediators.

Histamine is a key chemical mediator of inflammation. It is primarily stored within **mast cells** located in tissue spaces under epithelial membranes such as those of the skin, bronchial tree, digestive tract, and blood vessels. Mast cells detect foreign agents

TABLE 42.1   Chemical Mediators of Inflammation

Mediator	Description
Bradykinin	Present in an inactive form in plasma and also stored and released by mast cells; vasodilator that causes pain; effects are similar to those of histamine
Complement	Series of at least 20 proteins that combine in a cascade fashion to neutralize or destroy an antigen
Histamine	Stored and released by mast cells; causes dilation of blood vessels, smooth muscle constriction, tissue swelling, and itching
Leukotrienes	Stored and released by mast cells; effects are similar to those of histamine
Prostaglandins	Present in most tissues and stored and released by mast cells; increase capillary permeability, attract white blood cells to site of inflammation, and cause pain

or injury and respond by releasing histamine, which initiates the inflammatory response within seconds. In addition to its role in inflammation, histamine also directly stimulates pain receptors and produces symptoms of seasonal allergies.

When released at an injury site, histamine dilates nearby blood vessels, causing capillaries to become more permeable. Plasma and components such as complement proteins and phagocytes can then enter the area to neutralize foreign agents. The affected area may become congested with blood, a condition called **hyperemia**, which can lead to significant swelling and pain. Figure 42.1 illustrates the fundamental steps in acute inflammation.

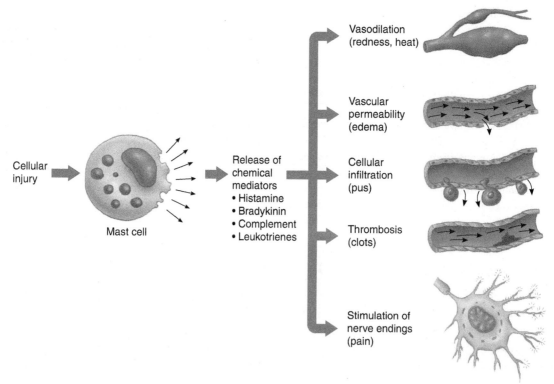

Figure 42.1   Steps in acute inflammation.
Source: Pearson Education

Rapid release of the chemical mediators of inflammation on a larger scale throughout the body is responsible for the distressing symptoms of **anaphylaxis**, a life-threatening allergic response that may result in shock and death. A number of chemicals, insect stings, foods, and some therapeutic drugs can elicit this widespread release of histamine from mast cells if the person has an allergy to these substances. The pharmacotherapy of anaphylaxis is presented in Chapter 58.

Histamine Receptors

42.3 Histamine can produce its effects by interacting with two different receptors. The classic antihistamines used for allergies block histamine H₁ receptors in vascular smooth muscle, in the bronchi, and on sensory nerves. The H₂-receptor antagonists are used to treat peptic ulcers.

There are at least two different receptors by which histamine can elicit a response. **H₁ receptors** are present in the smooth muscle of the vascular system, the bronchial tree, and the digestive tract. Stimulation of these receptors results in itching, pain, edema, vasodilation, and bronchoconstriction. In contrast, **H₂ receptors** are primarily present in the stomach, and their stimulation results in the secretion of large amounts of hydrochloric acid.

Drugs that act as specific antagonists for H₁ and H₂ receptors are in widespread therapeutic use. H₁-receptor antagonists, used to treat allergies and inflammation, are discussed later in this chapter. H₂-receptor antagonists are used to treat peptic ulcers and are discussed in Chapter 34.

NONSTEROIDAL ANTI-INFLAMMATORY DRUGS

Nonsteroidal anti-inflammatory drugs (NSAIDs) such as acetylsalicylic acid (ASA [Aspirin]) and ibuprofen (Motrin, Advil) have analgesic, antipyretic, and anti-inflammatory effects. They are drugs of choice in the treatment of mild to moderate inflammation. These agents are listed in Table 42.2.

NCLEX Success Tips

You should not use two NSAIDS together (be careful, as some NSAIDS are available over the counter and some are prescription only).

Once therapy is started, it takes hours or days for relief from pain to occur. However, it takes 3 to 4 weeks for the anti-inflammatory effects to occur, including reduction in swelling and less pain with movement.

Toxicity or GI bleeding may occur when NSAIDs are combined. The missed dose will need to be made up to maintain the serum level and to maintain therapeutic effectiveness of the drug.

CONNECTIONS | Lifespan Considerations

◀ NSAID Use

- NSAIDs should be used cautiously in elderly clients because of the potential for drug accumulation and increased bleeding.
- Use may be cautioned in pregnancy and lactation, depending on the specific drug.
- Use ibuprofen with caution in infants younger than 6 months, and use naproxen (Aleve, Naprosyn) with caution in children younger than 2 years.
- Acetylsalicylic acid (ASA) is contraindicated in children who have or are at risk of varicella or influenza infections because of the possibility of developing Reye's syndrome. **Reye's syndrome** is a rare, though potentially fatal, disorder characterized by an acute increase in intracranial pressure and massive accumulations of lipids in the liver.
- Clients should not breastfeed while taking COX-2 inhibitors, as they can be transmitted to the infant through breast milk.

TABLE 42.2   Select Nonsteroidal Anti-Inflammatory Drugs

Drug	Route and Adult Dose
acetylsalicylic acid (Aspirin) (see Chapter 23, page 266, for the Prototype Drug box)	Orally (PO), 350–650 mg every 4 hours (q4h) (max 4 g/day) for pain/fever PO, 81–325 mg/day for prevention of acute myocardial infarction or thrombosis
Selective COX-2 inhibitors	
celecoxib (Celebrex)	PO, 100–200 mg twice a day (bid) (max 400 mg/day)
Ibuprofen and Similar Agents	
diclofenac (Voltaren)	PO, 50 mg every 6–8 hours (max 100 mg/day)
diflunisal	PO, 250–500 mg bid (max 1500 mg/day)
etodolac	PO, 200–400 mg 3 times a day (tid)–qid (max 1200 mg/day)
flurbiprofen (Ansaid)	PO, 200–300 mg/day in 2–4 divided doses (max single dose 100 mg)
Pr ibuprofen (Motrin, Advil)	PO, 400–800 mg tid–qid (max 3200 mg/day)
ketoprofen	PO, 75 mg tid or 50 mg qid (max 300 mg/day)
nabumetone	PO, 1000 mg every day (qd) (max 2000 mg/day)
naproxen (Aleve, Naprosyn)	PO, 250–500 mg bid (max 1000 mg/day)
oxaprozin	PO, 600–1200 mg qd (max 1800 mg/day)
piroxicam	PO, 10–20 mg/day in 1–2 divided doses (max 20 mg/day)

Treating Inflammation with NSAIDs

42.4 Nonsteroidal anti-inflammatory drugs (NSAIDs) are the primary drugs for the treatment of simple inflammation. Newer selective COX-2 inhibitors cause less GI distress but have more cardiovascular risks and side effects.

Newer selective COX-2 inhibitors cause less GI distress but have more cardiovascular risks and side effects. Because of their high safety margin and availability as over-the-counter (OTC) drugs, the NSAIDs are first-line drugs for the treatment of mild to moderate inflammation. The NSAID class includes some of the most commonly used drugs in medicine, including ASA, ibuprofen, and the newer COX-2 inhibitors. All NSAIDs have approximately the same efficacy, although the side effect profiles vary among the different drugs. The NSAIDs also exhibit analgesic and antipyretic actions. Although acetaminophen (Tylenol) shares the analgesic and antipyretic properties of these other drugs, it has no anti-inflammatory action and is not considered an NSAID.

NSAIDs act by inhibiting the synthesis of prostaglandins. Prostaglandins are lipids that promote inflammation and are found in all tissues. The NSAIDs block inflammation by inhibiting **cyclooxygenase** (COX), the key enzyme in the biosynthesis of prostaglandins. There are two forms of COX, cyclooxygenase-1 (**COX-1**) and cyclooxygenase-2 (**COX-2**). COX-1 is present is all tissues and serves protective functions such as reducing gastric acid secretion, promoting renal blood flow, and regulating smooth muscle tone in blood vessels and the bronchial tree. COX-2, on the other hand, is present only after tissue injury and serves to promote inflammation. Therefore, two nearly identical enzymes serve very different functions. The two forms of cyclooxygenase are compared in Table 42.3.

First-generation NSAIDs, such as ASA and ibuprofen, block both COX-1 and COX-2. Although inflammation is reduced, the inhibition of COX-1 results in undesirable side effects such as bleeding, gastric upset, and reduced kidney function.

ASA binds to both COX-1 and COX-2 enzymes, changing their structure and preventing them from forming inflammatory prostaglandins. This inhibition of cyclooxygenase is particularly prolonged in platelets, where a single dose of ASA may cause total inhibition for the entire 8- to 11-day lifespan of the platelet. Because it is readily available, inexpensive, and effective, ASA is often a drug of first choice for treating mild inflammation.

Unfortunately, large doses of ASA are necessary to suppress severe inflammation, which results in a greater incidence of side effects than when the drug is used for pain or fever. The most common adverse effects observed during high-dose ASA therapy relate to the digestive system. By increasing gastric acid secretion and irritating the stomach lining, ASA may produce epigastric pain, heartburn, and even bleeding due to ulceration. Some ASA formulations are buffered or enteric coated to minimize gastrointestinal (GI) side effects. Because ASA also has a potent anticoagulant effect, the potential for bleeding must be carefully monitored. High doses may produce **salicylism**, a syndrome that includes symptoms such as tinnitus, dizziness, headache, and sweating.

Ibuprofen and a large number of ibuprofen-like drugs are first-generation NSAIDs developed as alternatives to ASA. Like ASA, they exhibit their effects through inhibition of both COX-1 and COX-2, although the inhibition by these drugs is reversible. Because they share the same mechanism of action, all drugs in this class have similar efficacy for treating pain, fever, and inflammation. However, the duration of action varies, and clients may respond better to one than another. The most common side effects of ibuprofen-like NSAIDs are nausea, vomiting, and GI upset (which can be reduced by administering these medications with food). These agents have the potential to cause gastric ulceration and bleeding; however, the incidence is less than that of ASA. There is some cross-hypersensitivity between ASA and other first-generation NSAIDs.

The newest and most controversial class of NSAIDs selectively inhibit COX-2. Inhibition of COX-2 produces the analgesic, anti-inflammatory, and antipyretic actions typical of older NSAIDs without adverse effects on the digestive system and blood coagulation. Therefore, these drugs became the drugs of choice for the treatment of moderate to severe inflammation. However, in 2004 rofecoxib (Vioxx) was withdrawn from the market because data showed that the risk for stroke and heart attack doubled in clients who used the drug for extended periods. Celecoxib (Celebrex) is the only drug in this class currently available in Canada. Celecoxib is also used to reduce the number of colorectal polyps in adults with familial adenomatous polyposis (FAP), who have an almost 100% risk for colon cancer.

Nursing Considerations

The role of the nurse in NSAID pharmacotherapy involves careful monitoring of the client's condition and providing education as it relates to the prescribed drug regimen. Assess for sensitivity to NSAIDs, bleeding disorders, peptic ulcer disease, anticoagulants (including herbals with anticoagulant effects), alcoholism, congestive heart failure, fluid retention, hypertension, and renal disease because NSAIDs may be contraindicated in such conditions. NSAIDs promote fluid retention, which may exacerbate hypertension and heart failure. Drugs in this class should not be administered to clients with liver dysfunction because NSAIDs are primarily metabolized in the liver. When the liver is not functioning effectively, metabolites may reach toxic levels and lead to hepatic failure.

Prior to initiation of NSAID therapy, obtain baseline kidney and liver function tests and a complete blood count (CBC). Monitor bleeding time with long-term administration. During therapy, assess for changes in pain (intensity, frequency, and type) and

TABLE 42.3	Forms of Cyclooxygenase	
	Cyclooxygenase-1	Cyclooxygenase-2
Location	Present in all tissues	Present at sites of tissue injury
Functions	Protects gastric mucosa, supports kidney function, promotes platelet aggregation	Mediates inflammation, sensitizes pain receptors, mediates fever in the brain
Inhibition by medications	Undesirable: increases risk for gastric bleeding and kidney failure	Desirable: results in suppression of inflammation

reduction in temperature and inflammation to determine effectiveness. Assess for GI bleeding, hepatitis, nephrotoxicity, hemolytic anemia, and salicylate toxicity. Other common side effects may include tinnitus, abdominal cramping, and heartburn.

Client education as it relates to NSAIDs should include goals, reasons for obtaining baseline data such as vital signs and laboratory tests, and possible side effects. The following are important points to include when teaching clients regarding NSAIDs:

- Do not give drugs containing ASA to children; Reye's syndrome is a life-threatening disorder.
- Take NSAIDs with food or milk to decrease gastric upset.
- Read labels of OTC drugs carefully, as many (e.g., medications for common cold) contain multiple ingredients, including NSAIDs.
- Avoid alcohol.
- Consult a healthcare provider before taking herbal products while taking NSAIDs.
- Optimal effects from NSAID therapy may not occur for 1 to 3 weeks.
- Report immediately signs of bleeding such as dark-coloured urine or stool, increased bruising, or gingival bleeding; unexplained fatigue; headache or dizziness; changes in hearing (especially ringing in the ears); swelling; itching; or skin rash.

PROTOTYPE DRUG | **Ibuprofen (Motrin, Advil)**

Actions and Uses: Ibuprofen is an older drug used to relieve mild to moderate pain, fever, and inflammation. Its action is due to inhibition of prostaglandin synthesis. Common indications include musculoskeletal disorders such as rheumatoid arthritis and osteoarthritis, mild to moderate pain, reduction of fever, and primary dysmenorrhea. It is available as tablets and as an oral suspension for children.

Administration Alerts:
- Give the drug on an empty stomach as tolerated. If nausea, vomiting, or abdominal pain occur, give with food.
- Ibuprofen is pregnancy category B.
- Ibuprofen is contraindicated during the third trimester since it can cause premature closure of the ductus arteriosus.

Pharmacokinetics: Ibuprofen is about 80% absorbed from the GI tract, with minimal distribution into breast milk. It is highly (99%) protein bound. It is mostly metabolized by the liver, and about 1% is excreted unchanged in urine. Half-life is 2 to 4 hours in adults and 1 to 2 hours in children.

Adverse Effects and Interactions: Side effects of ibuprofen are generally mild and include nausea, heartburn, epigastric pain, and dizziness. Ibuprofen can decrease platelet function. GI ulceration with occult or gross bleeding may occur, especially in clients who take high doses for prolonged periods or regularly consume alcohol. Clients with active peptic ulcers should not take ibuprofen.

Ibuprofen interacts with many other drugs and herbal products. It should be avoided when taking anticoagulants since it competes for plasma binding sites and may significantly increase risk for bleeding. ASA use can decrease the anti-inflammatory

---

action of ibuprofen. Ibuprofen may increase plasma levels of lithium (Carbolith, Lithane), causing lithium toxicity. The actions of certain diuretics may be diminished when they are taken concurrently with ibuprofen.

Use with caution with herbal supplements, such as feverfew, garlic, ginger, and ginkgo biloba, which may increase the risk for bleeding.

Ibuprofen is contraindicated in clients with significant renal or hepatic impairment and in those who have nasal polyps, angioedema, or bronchospasm due to ASA or other NSAIDs.

There is no specific treatment for overdose. Administration of an alkaline drug may increase the urinary excretion of ibuprofen.

SYSTEMIC GLUCOCORTICOIDS

Glucocorticoids have wide therapeutic application. One of their most useful properties is a potent anti-inflammatory action that can suppress severe cases of inflammation. Because of potentially serious adverse effects, however, systemic glucocorticoids are reserved for the short-term treatment of severe disease. These agents are listed in Table 42.4.

TABLE 42.4 Select PO Corticosteroids for Severe Inflammation

Drug	Route and Adult Dose
cortisone	PO, 20–300 mg/day in divided doses
dexamethasone (Dexasone)	PO, 0.25–4 mg bid–qid
hydrocortisone (Cortef) (see Chapter 30, page 350, for the Prototype Drug box)	PO, 15–240 mg every 12 hours
methylprednisolone (Depo-Medrol, Medrol, Solu-Medrol)	PO, 2–60 mg/day in 1–4 divided doses
prednisolone (Pediapred)	PO, 5–60 mg qd
Pr prednisone	PO, 5–60 mg qd

NCLEX Success Tips

Betamethasone (Celestone) therapy is indicated when the fetal lungs are immature. The fetus must be between 28 and 34 weeks' gestation and birth must be delayed for 24 to 48 hours for the drug to achieve a therapeutic effect.

Betamethasone (Dexasone) is a corticosteroid that induces the production of surfactant. The pulmonary maturation that results causes the fetal lungs to mature more rapidly than normal. Because the lungs are mature, the risk of respiratory distress in the neonate is lowered but not eliminated. Betamethasone also decreases the surface tension within the alveoli.

Dexamethasone (Dexasone) is commonly ordered to help reduce edema caused by brain tumours. Elevation in glucose level is a common adverse reaction to the drug. The nurse should notify the physician of the elevated fingerstick glucose level and ask about insulin therapy and whether the drug should be administered. The nurse shouldn't wait until the physician makes rounds to report the elevated glucose level; a delay in treatment could cause further elevation in the glucose level.

The nurse should instruct the client who is taking dexamethasone and furosemide (Lasix) to observe for signs and symptoms of hypokalemia, such as malaise, muscle weakness, vomiting, and a paralytic ileus, because both dexamethasone and furosemide deplete serum potassium.

A serious adverse effect of intravenous (IV) administration of methylprednisolone (Medrol) is hypertension, which occurs more frequently when the infusion is administered at too rapid a flow rate.

Adverse effects of methylprednisolone and other steroids include GI bleeding and wound infection. To help prevent GI bleeding, the physician is likely to order an antacid or a histamine$_2$-receptor antagonist such as famotidine.

Treating Acute or Severe Inflammation with Systemic Glucocorticoids

42.5 Systemic glucocorticoids are effective in treating acute or severe inflammation. Overtreatment with these drugs can cause a serious condition called Cushing's syndrome; therefore, therapy for inflammation is generally short term.

Glucocorticoids are natural hormones released by the adrenal cortex that have powerful effects on nearly every cell in the body. When used to treat inflammatory disorders, the drug doses are many times higher than those naturally present in the blood. The uses of glucocorticoids include the treatment of neoplasia (Chapter 60), asthma (Chapter 38), arthritis (Chapter 61), and corticosteroid deficiency (Chapter 30).

Glucocorticoids have the ability to suppress histamine release and inhibit the synthesis of prostaglandins by COX-2. In addition, they can inhibit the immune system by suppressing certain functions of phagocytes and lymphocytes. These multiple actions markedly reduce inflammation, making glucocorticoids the most effective medications available for the treatment of severe inflammatory disorders.

Unfortunately, the glucocorticoid drugs have a number of serious adverse effects that limit their therapeutic utility. These include suppression of the normal functions of the adrenal gland (adrenal insufficiency), hyperglycemia, mood changes, cataracts, peptic ulcers, electrolyte imbalances, and osteoporosis. Because of their effectiveness at reducing the signs and symptoms of inflammation, glucocorticoids can mask infections that may be present in the client. This combination of masking signs of infection and suppressing the immune response creates a potential for existing infections to grow rapidly and remain undetected. An active infection is usually a contraindication for glucocorticoid therapy.

Because the appearance of these adverse effects is a function of the dose and duration of therapy, treatment is often limited to the short-term control of acute disease. When longer therapy is indicated, doses are kept as low as possible and alternate-day therapy is sometimes implemented: the medication is taken every other day to encourage the client's adrenal gland to function on the days when no drug is given. During long-term therapy, the nurse must be alert for signs of overtreatment, a condition referred to as **Cushing's syndrome**. Because the body becomes accustomed to high doses of glucocorticoids, clients must discontinue glucocorticoids gradually; abrupt withdrawal can result in acute lack of adrenal function.

Nursing Considerations

The role of the nurse in systemic glucocorticoid therapy involves careful monitoring of the client's condition and providing education as it relates to the prescribed drug regimen. Before beginning therapy, the nurse should screen the client for existing infection. If infection is discovered prior to or during therapy, antibiotics may be required. Glucocorticoids should be used with great caution in clients with human immunodeficiency virus (HIV) or tuberculosis infections.

Prior to therapy, the nurse must also assess the client's metabolic status and fluid and electrolyte balance. Body weight and baseline laboratory data should be obtained, including CBC, serum glucose, and sodium and potassium levels. Clients with blood disorders should be observed for possible exacerbation because glucocorticoids promote red blood cell proliferation. These drugs also suppress osteoblast formation, so they should be administered with caution to clients with osteoporosis or other bone disorders. Clients with diabetes mellitus must be monitored carefully because glucocorticoids increase serum glucose. Clients with heart failure, hypertension, or renal disease must be monitored closely due to drug-induced sodium and fluid retention. Glucocorticoids can cross the placenta and affect the developing fetus, so they should be used in pregnancy only when benefits outweigh risks (pregnancy category C). Women who are receiving high-dose glucocorticoid therapy should be warned against breastfeeding.

The client should be monitored for development of Cushing's syndrome (adrenocortical excess). Signs include bruising and a characteristic pattern of fat deposits in the cheeks (moon face), shoulders (buffalo hump), and abdomen. Clients with existing mental or emotional disorders should be monitored closely: glucocorticoids may trigger mania in bipolar clients. Glucocorticoids may also exacerbate the symptoms of myasthenia gravis, contributing to the risk for respiratory failure.

Glucocorticoids promote the development of gastric ulcers by altering the protective mucous lining of the stomach. Local irritation may be reduced by administering oral doses with food or an antacid. However, the risk for GI bleeding remains, especially with long-term therapy, since changes in the stomach result from *systemic* drug action. Therefore, these drugs should always be administered with caution to clients who have a history of peptic ulcer disease. Glucocorticoids also promote capillary fragility; intramuscular (IM) injections should be administered deep into the muscle mass to avoid atrophy or abscesses.

Client education as it relates to glucocorticoids should include goals, reasons for obtaining baseline data such as blood tests and body weight, and possible side effects. The following are important points to include when teaching clients regarding glucocorticoids:

- Take the medication at the same time each day.
- Never abruptly discontinue taking the medication.
- Take with food to avoid gastric irritation.
- Guard against infection: avoid persons with infections and wash hands frequently.
- Weigh yourself daily and check ankles and legs for signs of swelling, because corticosteroids are know to cause fluid retention.
- Immediately report the following: difficulty breathing; heartburn; chest, abdominal, or joint/bone pain; nosebleed; bloody cough, vomit, urine, or stools; fever; chills; red streaks from wounds or any other sign of infection; increased thirst or urination; fruity breath odour (or significantly elevated daily serum glucose); falls or other accidents (deep lacerations may require antibiotic therapy); and mood swings.

See Nursing Process Focus: Clients Receiving Systemic Glucocorticoid Therapy in Chapter 30 for additional teaching points.

PROTOTYPE DRUG | **Prednisone**

Actions and Uses: Prednisone is a synthetic glucocorticoid. Its actions are the result of being metabolized to an active form, which is also available as a drug called prednisolone (Pediapred). When used for inflammation, duration of therapy is commonly limited to 4 to 10 days. Alternate-day dosing is used for longer-term therapy to allow the client's adrenal gland to function. Prednisone is occasionally used to prevent inflammation and reduce risk of bronchospasm in clients with asthma and for clients with certain cancers such as Hodgkin's disease, acute leukemia, and lymphomas.

Administration Alerts:

- IM injections should be administered deep into the muscle mass to avoid atrophy or abscesses.
- Do not use if a systemic infection is present.
- Drug should not be discontinued abruptly.
- Prednisone is pregnancy category C.

Pharmacokinetics: Prednisone is well absorbed after oral administration. It is widely distributed, crosses the placenta, and enters breast milk. Prednisone is converted to prednisolone in the liver and then is metabolized by the liver. Its half-life in plasma is about 3.5 hours. Adrenal suppression lasts 30 to 36 hours.

Adverse Effects and Interactions: When used for short-term therapy, prednisone has few serious adverse effects.

Long-term therapy may result in Cushing's syndrome, a condition that includes hyperglycemia, fat redistribution to the shoulders and face, muscle weakness, bruising, and bones that easily fracture. Because glucocorticoids can raise blood glucose levels, diabetic clients may require an adjustment in the doses of insulin or hypoglycedmic agents. Gastric ulcers may occur with long-term therapy, and an antiulcer medication may be prescribed prophylactically.

Prednisone interacts with many drugs. For example, barbiturates, phenytoin (Dilantin), and rifampin (Rifadin, Rofact) increase steroid metabolism. Concurrent use with amphotericin B (Fungizone) or diuretics increases potassium loss. Prednisone may inhibit antibody response to toxoids and vaccines.

Use with caution with herbal supplements, such as aloe and senna, which may increase potassium loss. Licorice may potentiate the effect of glucocorticoids.

FEVER

Like inflammation, fever is a natural mechanism in the body's defence system to remove foreign organisms. Many species of bacteria are killed by high fever. The goal of antipyretic therapy is to lower body temperature while treating the underlying cause of the fever, usually an infection. The NSAIDs and acetaminophen are generally safe, effective drugs for reducing fever.

Prolonged, high fever can become quite dangerous, especially in young children in whom fever can stimulate febrile seizures. In adults, excessively high fever can break down body tissues, reduce mental acuity, and lead to delirium or coma, particularly among elderly clients. In rare instances, an elevated fever may be fatal. Often the healthcare provider must determine whether the fever needs to be dealt with aggressively or allowed to run its course. Drugs used to treat fever are called **antipyretics**.

Treating Fever with Antipyretics

42.6 Acetaminophen and NSAIDs are the primary agents used to treat fever.

In most clients, fever is more of a discomfort than a life-threatening problem and can be controlled effectively by inexpensive OTC drugs. ASA, ibuprofen, and acetaminophen are all effective antipyretics. Many of these drugs are marketed for different age groups, including special, flavoured brands for infants and children. For fast delivery and effectiveness, drugs may come in various forms, including gels, caplets, enteric-coated tablets, and suspensions. ASA and acetaminophen are also available as suppositories. The antipyretics come in various dosages and concentrations, including extra strength.

Until the 1980s, ASA was the most common therapy for fever in children; however, ASA has been implicated in the development of Reye's syndrome. ASA and other salicylates are now contraindicated in children and teenagers with fever. Because of the potential for Reye's syndrome, some healthcare providers also advise against administering *any* NSAID to children or teens. Therefore, acetaminophen has become the antipyretic of choice to treat most fevers.

Nursing Considerations

The role of the nurse in antipyretic therapy involves careful monitoring of the client's condition and providing education as it relates to the prescribed drug regimen. Prior to administering an antipyretic, obtain the client's vital signs, especially temperature. Assess the client's developmental status, the origin of the fever, and associated symptoms to determine the appropriate formulation or route for the antipyretic. For example, clients who are vomiting should receive an antipyretic by suppository, and very young children are generally given flavoured elixirs.

Baseline laboratory data are necessary to assess the client's kidney and liver status; antipyretics may cause toxicity in clients with diminished organ function. Acetaminophen is contraindicated in clients with significant liver disease, including viral hepatitis and cirrhosis, and alcoholism because it is metabolized by the liver and can greatly increase the risk for hepatotoxicity. Acetaminophen also inhibits warfarin metabolism and may produce toxic accumulation of this drug and cause serious bleeding. NSAIDs may also be contraindicated with warfarin because they also promote bleeding.

Advise the client or caregiver that liquid forms of acetaminophen and ibuprofen come in different strengths; all children's liquid formulations are not the same. Children under 1 year should be given "infant drops" rather than "children's liquid." Acetaminophen is one of the substances most frequently implicated in poisonings of Canadian children younger than 6 years of age. Clients should be advised to consult the nurse regarding safe dosages. Inform the client that acetaminophen overdosage can cause hepatic failure.

See Nursing Process Focus: Clients Receiving Antipyretic Therapy for additional teaching points.

NURSING PROCESS FOCUS

Clients Receiving Antipyretic Therapy

Assessment	Potential Nursing Diagnoses/Identified Patterns
Prior to administration: • Obtain complete health history (mental and physical), including data on origin of fever, recent surgeries, and trauma. • Obtain vital signs; assess in context of client's baseline values. • Obtain client's complete medication history, including nicotine and alcohol consumption, to determine possible drug allergies and/or interactions.	• Discomfort • Hyperthermia • Risk for dehydration • Need for knowledge regarding drug therapy and adverse effects • Safety from injury related to side effects of drug therapy

Planning: Client Goals and Expected Outcomes

The client will:

• Experience a reduction in body temperature
• Demonstrate an understanding of the drug's action by accurately describing drug side effects and precautions

Implementation

Interventions (Rationales)	Client Education/Discharge Planning
• Assess for intolerance to ASA for possible cross-hypersensitivity to other NSAIDs or acetaminophen. • Monitor hepatic and renal function. (Antipyretics are metabolized in the liver and excreted by the kidneys.) • Use with caution in clients with a history of excessive alcohol consumption. (Alcohol increases the risk of liver damage associated with acetaminophen or NSAID administration.) • Use with caution in diabetics. Observe for signs of hypoglycemia that may occur with acetaminophen usage.	• Inform client to immediately report any difficulty breathing, itching, or skin rash Instruct client: • To report signs of liver toxicity: nausea, vomiting, anorexia, bleeding, severe upper or lower abdominal pain, heartburn, jaundice, or a change in the colour or character of stools • To adhere to laboratory testing regimen for serum blood tests as directed • Advise client to abstain from alcohol while taking this medication • Advise clients with diabetes mellitus that acetaminophen may cause low blood sugar and require adjustment of doses of insulin or oral hypoglycemic agents Instruct client to immediately report: • Excessive thirst • Large increase or decrease in urine output

Evaluation of Outcome Criteria

Evaluate the effectiveness of drug therapy by confirming that client goals and expected outcomes have been met (see "Planning").

See Table 42.2 for a list of the drugs to which these nursing actions apply. Acetaminophen is also covered in this Nursing Process Focus chart.

Cultural Considerations

◀ Ethnic Considerations in Acetaminophen Metabolism

Certain ethnic populations, including Asians, Africans, and Saudis, have higher rates of an enzyme deficiency that affects how their body metabolizes certain drugs. More than 200 million people worldwide are believed to have a hereditary deficiency of the enzyme glucose-6-phosphate dehydrogenase (G6PD). Clients with G6PD deficiency are at risk for developing hemolysis after ingestion of certain drugs, including acetaminophen. Conflicting data exist on whether therapeutic dosages of acetaminophen can cause hemolysis in these clients. However, because acetaminophen is one of the most common drugs ingested in intentional overdoses, healthcare providers should recommend that clients with G6PD deficiency avoid this drug.

PROTOTYPE DRUG	Acetaminophen (Tylenol)

Actions and Uses: Acetaminophen reduces fever by direct action at the level of the hypothalamus and causes dilation of peripheral blood vessels, enabling sweating and dissipation of heat. Acetaminophen and ASA have equal efficacy in relieving pain and reducing fever.

Acetaminophen has no anti-inflammatory action; therefore, it is not effective in treating arthritis or pain caused by tissue swelling following injury. The primary therapeutic usefulness of acetaminophen is for the treatment of fever in children and for relief of mild to moderate pain when aspirin is contraindicated.

Pharmacokinetics: Acetaminophen is well absorbed after oral administration. Rectal absorption varies. It is widely distributed in the body, crosses the placenta, and enters breast milk. It is almost completely metabolized in the liver. The metabolites are excreted in urine. The metabolites may also be toxic in overdose. Half-life is 1 to 3 hours.

Administration Alerts:

- Liquid forms are available in varying concentrations. For administration in children, the appropriate strength product must be used to avoid toxicity.
- Acetaminophen is pregnancy category B.

Adverse Effects and Interactions: Acetaminophen is quite safe, and adverse effects are uncommon at therapeutic doses. Unlike ASA, acetaminophen has no direct anti-inflammatory effect and does not affect blood coagulation or cause gastric irritation. It is not recommended in clients who are malnourished. In such cases, acute toxicity may result, leading to renal failure, which can be fatal. Other signs of acute toxicity include nausea, vomiting, chills, and abdominal discomfort.

Acetaminophen inhibits warfarin (Coumadin) metabolism, causing warfarin to accumulate to toxic levels. High-dose or long-term acetaminophen usage may result in elevated warfarin levels and bleeding. Ingestion of this drug with alcohol is not recommended due to the possibility of liver failure from hepatic necrosis.

The client should avoid taking herbs that have the potential for liver toxicity, including comfrey, coltsfoot, and chaparral.

Acetylcysteine (Mucomyst) is the antidote for acetaminophen overdose.

ALLERGY

Allergies are caused by a hyperresponse of body defences. Because histamine is released during an allergic response, many signs and symptoms of allergy are similar to those of inflammation. Allergies also involve mediators of the immune response.

Pharmacotherapy of Allergic Rhinitis

42.7 Allergic rhinitis is a disorder characterized by sneezing, watery eyes, and nasal congestion.

Allergic rhinitis, or hay fever, is a common disorder that afflicts millions of people annually. Symptoms resemble those of the common cold: tearing eyes, sneezing, nasal congestion, postnasal drip, and itching of the throat. The cause of all allergies is exposure to an antigen. An antigen may be defined as anything that is recognized as foreign by the body. Certain foods, industrial chemicals, drugs, pollen, animal proteins, and even latex gloves can be antigens. A more detailed discussion of the immune system and the pharmacotherapy of immune disorders is included in Chapters 39 and 40.

The exact cause of a client's allergic rhinitis is often difficult to pinpoint; however, common causes include pollen from weeds, grasses, and trees; moulds; dust mites; certain foods; and animal dander. Chemical fumes, tobacco smoke, or air pollutants such as ozone are non-allergenic factors that may worsen symptoms. While some clients experience symptoms at specific times of the year, when pollen and mould are at high levels in the environment, other clients are afflicted continuously throughout the year.

The fundamental symptomatic problem of allergic rhinitis is inflammation of the mucous membranes in the nose, throat, and airways. Chemical mediators such as histamine are released that initiate the distressing symptoms. The mechanism of allergic rhinitis is illustrated in Figure 42.2.

Drugs used to treat allergic rhinitis may be grouped into two basic categories: preventers and relievers. Preventers are used for prophylaxis and include antihistamines, glucocorticoids, and mast cell stabilizers. Relievers are used to provide immediate, though temporary, relief of acute allergy symptoms once they have occurred. Relievers include the oral and intranasal adrenergics that are used as nasal decongestants.

H₁-RECEPTOR ANTAGONISTS (ANTIHISTAMINES)

Antihistamines block the actions of histamine at the H_1 receptor. H_1-receptor antagonists are commonly called antihistamines. Because the term *antihistamine* is nonspecific and does not indicate which of the two histamine receptors are affected, H_1-receptor antagonist is a more accurate name. These drugs are widely used OTC for relief of allergy symptoms, motion sickness, and insomnia. These agents are listed in Table 42.5.

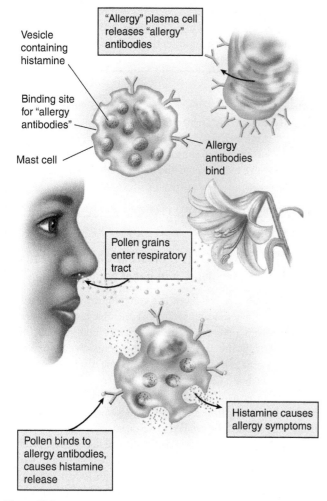

Vesicle containing histamine

"Allergy" plasma cell releases "allergy" antibodies

Binding site for "allergy antibodies"

Mast cell

Allergy antibodies bind

Pollen grains enter respiratory tract

Histamine causes allergy symptoms

Pollen binds to allergy antibodies, causes histamine release

Figure 42.2 Allergic rhinitis.

Treating Allergic Rhinitis with H₁-Receptor Antagonists

42.8 Antihistamines, or H₁-receptor antagonists, can provide relief from the symptoms of allergic rhinitis. Newer drugs in this class are non-sedating and offer the advantage of once-a-day dosage.

Although a large number of H_1-receptor antagonists are available for use, their efficacies, therapeutic uses, and side effects are quite similar. These drugs are classified by their generation and their ability to cause sedation, which can be a limiting side effect in some clients. The older, first-generation drugs have the potential to cause significant drowsiness, whereas the second-generation agents lack this effect in most clients. Care must be taken to avoid alcohol and other central nervous system (CNS) depressants when taking antihistamines because their sedating effects may be additive.

The most common therapeutic use of H_1-receptor antagonists is for the treatment of allergies. These medications provide symptomatic relief from the sneezing, runny nose, and itching of the eyes, nose, and throat characteristic of allergic rhinitis. H_1-receptor antagonists are used in OTC cold and sinus medicines, often in combination with other drugs such as decongestants and antitussives. Common OTC antihistamine combinations used to treat allergies are shown in Table 42.6.

Antihistamines are most effective when taken prophylactically to prevent allergic symptoms. Their effectiveness may diminish with long-term use. It should be noted that during severe allergic reactions such as anaphylaxis, histamine is just one of several chemical mediators released; therefore, H_1-receptor antagonists alone are not efficacious in treating these acute disorders.

Although most antihistamines are given orally, azelastine (Astelin) was the first to be available by the intranasal route. Azelastine is considered as safe and effective as the oral antihistamines. Although it is a first-generation agent, azelastine causes less drowsiness than others in its class because it is applied locally, and little systemic absorption occurs.

H_1-receptor antagonists are effective in treating a number of other disorders. Motion sickness responds well to these drugs. They are also some of the few drugs available to treat vertigo, a form of dizziness that causes significant nausea. Some of the older antihistamines are marketed as OTC sleep aids, taking advantage of their ability to cause drowsiness.

Nursing Considerations

First-Generation H₁-Receptor Antagonists The role of the nurse in drug therapy with first-generation H_1-receptor antagonists involves careful monitoring of the client's condition and providing education as it relates to the prescribed drug regimen. Before administering a first-generation antihistamine, obtain baseline vital signs, including electrocardiogram (ECG) in clients with a history of heart disease. First-generation H_1-receptor antagonists are contraindicated in clients with a history of dysrhythmias and heart failure. These drugs can cause vasodilation due to H_1 stimulation.

First-generation H_1-receptor antagonists may cause CNS depression, so they may be contraindicated in clients with a history of depression or sleep disorders, such as narcolepsy and sleep apnea.

TABLE 42.5 H₁-Receptor Antagonists

Drug	Route and Adult Dose
First-Generation Agents	
chlorpheniramine (Benylin)	PO, 2–4 mg tid–qid (max 24 mg/day)
cyproheptadine	PO, 4 mg tid or qid (max 0.5 mg/kg/day)
Pr diphenhydramine (Allerdryl, Benadryl)	PO, 25–50 mg tid–qid (max 300 mg/day)
promethazine (Phenergan, Histantil)	PO, 6.25–12.5 mg daily up to 3 times per day
Second-Generation Agents	
cetirizine (Reactine)	PO, 5–10 mg qd (max 10 mg/day)
desloratadine (Aerius)	PO, 5 mg qd (max 5 mg/day)
Pr fexofenadine (Allegra)	PO, 60 mg every 12 hours (max 120 mg/day)
loratadine (Claritin)	PO, 10 mg qd (max 10 mg/day)

TABLE 42.6 Select OTC Antihistamine Combinations Available for Allergic Rhinitis

Brand Name	Antihistamine	Decongestant	Analgesic
Actifed Cold and Allergy tablets	Triprolidine	Pseudoephedrine	–
Actifed Cold and Sinus caplets	Chlorpheniramine	Pseudoephedrine	Acetaminophen
Benadryl Allergy/Cold tablets	Diphenhydramine	Pseudoephedrine	Acetaminophen
Chlor-Trimeton Allergy/Decongestant tablets	Chlorpheniramine	Pseudoephedrine	–
Dimetapp Cold and Allergy chewable tablets	Brompheniramine	Phenylpropanolamine	–
Sinutab Sinus Allergy tablets	Chlorpheniramine	Pseudoephedrine	Acetaminophen
Sudafed Cold and Allergy tablets	Chlorpheniramine	Pseudoephedrine	–
Triaminic Cold/Allergy softchews	Chlorpheniramine	Pseudoephedrine	–
Tylenol Allergy Sinus Nighttime caplets	Diphenhydramine	Pseudoephedrine	Acetaminophen

Because the anticholinergic effects of H_1-receptor antagonists can place clients with narrow-angle glaucoma at risk for injury, they are contraindicated in these clients. Drugs in this class sometimes cause idiosyncratic CNS stimulation; therefore, they may be contraindicated in clients with seizure disorders. Idiosyncratic CNS stimulation, causing hyperactivity, is more common in children.

Elderly clients should be monitored for profound sedation and altered consciousness, which may contribute to falls or other injuries. Prior to initiation of therapy, assess for history of allergy and identify the presence of symptoms such as urticaria, angioedema, nausea, vomiting, motion sickness, and excess mucus production. The agents should be used with caution during pregnancy (pregnancy category C). H_1-receptor antagonists are secreted in breast milk and should not be used by clients who are breastfeeding.

Client education as it relates to first-generation H_1-receptor antagonists should include goals; reasons for obtaining baseline data such as vital signs, ECG, and laboratory blood work; and possible side effects.

See Nursing Process Focus: Clients Receiving Antihistamine Therapy for specific teaching points.

Second-Generation H_1-Receptor Antagonists The role of the nurse in drug therapy with second-generation H_1-receptor antagonists involves careful monitoring of the client's condition and providing education as it relates to the prescribed drug regimen. Prior to initiating therapy, assess for the presence or history of allergic rhinitis, conjunctivitis, urticaria, and atopic dermatitis. Baseline vital signs, including ECG in clients with a history of cardiac disease, should be obtained.

Second-generation H_1-receptor antagonists are generally contraindicated in clients with dysrhythmias because the drugs prolong the QT interval. Due to their anticholinergic effects on the respiratory system, these agents are contraindicated in clients with asthma and in clients who use nicotine. These drugs are metabolized by the liver and excreted by the kidneys; therefore, they are contraindicated in clients with severe liver or renal impairment. Loratadine (Claritin) is most effective when given on an empty stomach.

These drugs should be used with caution in clients with urinary retention due to their anticholinergic effects on the bladder. Anticholinergic activity also affects clients with open-angle glaucoma and hypertension; these clients must be monitored closely. Drugs in this classification are contraindicated in pregnant women in their third trimester due to the possibility of fetal malformation. These drugs should be used with caution in young children because the long-term effects of these drugs on growth and development have not been established.

Client education as it relates to second-generation H_1-receptor antagonists should include goals; reasons for obtaining baseline data such as vital signs, ECG, and laboratory blood work; and possible side effects.

See Nursing Process Focus: Clients Receiving Antihistamine Therapy for specific teaching points.

NURSING PROCESS FOCUS

Clients Receiving Antihistamine Therapy

Assessment	Potential Nursing Diagnoses/Identified Patterns
Prior to administration: • Obtain complete health history, including data on anaphylaxis, asthma, and cardiac disease, plus allergies, drug history, and possible drug interactions. • Obtain ECG and vital signs; assess in context of client's baseline values. • Assess respiratory status: breathing pattern. • Assess neurological status and level of consciousness (LOC).	• Presence of somnolence, agitation, or disturbed sleep • Altered breathing pattern • Ineffective airway clearance • Thirst • Need for knowledge regarding drug therapy and adverse effects • Safety from injury related to side effects of drug therapy

---

Planning: Client Goals and Expected Outcomes

The client will:

- Report relief from allergic symptoms such as congestion, itching, or postnasal drip
- Demonstrate an understanding of the drug's action by accurately describing drug side effects and precautions

---

Implementation

Interventions (Rationales)	Client Education/Discharge Planning
<ul><li>Auscultate breath sounds before administering. Use with caution in clients with asthma or chronic obstructive pulmonary disease (COPD). Keep resuscitative equipment accessible. (Anticholinergic effects of antihistamines may trigger paradoxical bronchospasm.)</li><li>Monitor vital signs (including ECG) before administering. Use with extreme caution in clients with a history of cardiovascular disease. (Anticholinergic effects can increase heart rate and lower blood pressure. Fatal dysrhythmias and cardiovascular collapse have been reported in some clients receiving antihistamines.)</li><li>Monitor thyroid function. Use with caution in clients with a history of hyperthyroidism. (Antihistamines exacerbate CNS-stimulating effects of hyperthyroidism and may trigger thyroid storm.)</li><li>Monitor for vision changes. Use with caution in clients with narrow-angle glaucoma. (Antihistamines can increase intraocular pressure and cause photosensitivity.)</li><li>Monitor neurological status, especially LOC. Use with caution in clients with a history of seizure disorder. (Antihistamines lower the seizure threshold. Older adults are at increased risk for serious sedation and other anticholinergic effects.)</li><li>Observe for signs of renal toxicity. Measure intake and output. Use with caution in clients with a history of kidney or urinary tract disease. (Antihistamines promote urinary retention.)</li><li>Use with caution in clients with diabetes mellitus. Monitor serum glucose levels with increased frequency (e.g., from daily to tid, before meals). (Antihistamines decrease serum glucose levels.)</li><li>Monitor for GI side effects. Use with caution in clients with a history of GI disorders, especially peptic ulcers or liver disease. (Antihistamines block H_1 receptors, altering the mucosal lining of the stomach. These drugs are metabolized in the liver, increasing the risk of hepatotoxicity.)</li><li>Monitor for side effects such as dry mouth; observe for signs of anticholinergic crisis.</li></ul>	<ul><li>Instruct client to immediately report wheezing or difficulty breathing.</li><li>Advise asthmatics to consult the nurse regarding the use of injectable epinephrine in emergency situations</li></ul>Instruct client to:<ul><li>Immediately report dizziness; palpitations; headache; or chest, arm, or back pain accompanied by nausea/vomiting and/or sweating</li><li>Monitor vital signs daily, ensuring proper use of home equipment</li><li>Instruct client to immediately report nervousness or restlessness, insomnia, fever, profuse sweating, thirst, and mood changes</li></ul>Instruct client to:<ul><li>Immediately report head or eye pain and visual changes</li><li>Wear dark glasses, use sunscreen, and avoid excessive sun exposure</li></ul>Instruct client to:<ul><li>Immediately report seizure activity, including any changes in character and pattern of seizures</li><li>Avoid driving or performing hazardous activities until effects of the drug are known</li><li>Instruct client to immediately report flank pain, difficulty urinating, reduced urine output, and changes in the appearance of urine (cloudy, with sediment, odour, etc.)</li></ul>Instruct client to:<ul><li>Immediately report symptoms of hypoglycemia</li><li>Consult the healthcare provider regarding timing of glucose monitoring and reportable results (e.g., "less than 4 mmol/L")</li></ul>Instruct client to:<ul><li>Immediately report nausea, vomiting, anorexia, bleeding, chest or abdominal pain, heartburn, jaundice, or a change in the colour or character of stools</li><li>Avoid substances that irritate the stomach such as spicy foods, alcoholic beverages, and nicotine; take drug with food to avoid stomach upset</li></ul>Instruct client to:<ul><li>Immediately report fever or flushing accompanied by difficulty swallowing ("cotton mouth"), blurred vision, and confusion</li><li>Avoid mixing OTC antihistamines; always consult the healthcare provider before taking any OTC drugs or herbal supplements</li><li>Suck on hard candy to relieve dry mouth, and to maintain adequate fluid intake</li></ul>

Evaluation of Outcome Criteria

Evaluate the effectiveness of drug therapy by confirming that client goals and expected outcomes have been met (see "Planning").

See Table 42.6 for a list of drugs to which these nursing actions apply.

PROTOTYPE DRUG **Diphenhydramine (Allerdryl, Benadryl)**

Actions and Uses: Diphenhydramine is a first-generation H_1-receptor antagonist that is a component of some OTC drugs. Its primary use is to treat minor symptoms of allergy and the common cold such as sneezing, runny nose, and tearing of the eyes. OTC preparations may combine diphenhydramine with an analgesic, decongestant, or expectorant. Diphenhydramine is also used as a topical agent to treat rashes, and an IM form is available for severe allergic reactions. Other indications for diphenhydramine include Parkinson's disease, motion sickness, and insomnia.

Pharmacokinetics: Diphenhydramine is well absorbed after oral administration. Due to first-pass metabolism, about 50% of an oral dose reaches systemic circulation. It is widely distributed, crosses the placenta, and enters breast milk. It is almost completely metabolized in the liver. Half-life is 4–7 hours (children), 7–12 hours (adults), and 9–18 hours (elderly).

Administration Alerts:

- There is an increased risk for anaphylactic shock when this drug is administered parenterally.
- When administering IV, inject at a rate of 25 mg/minute to reduce the risk of shock.
- When administering IM, inject deep into the muscle to minimize tissue irritation.
- Antihistamines may cause false-positive readings for allergy skin tests.
- Diphenhydramine is pregnancy category B.

Adverse Effects and Interactions: Older H_1-receptor antagonists such as diphenhydramine cause significant drowsiness, although this usually diminishes with long-term use. Occasionally a client will exhibit CNS stimulation and excitability rather than drowsiness. Anticholinergic effects such as dry mouth, tachycardia, and mild hypotension are seen in some clients. Diphenhydramine may cause photosensitivity.

Diphenhydramine interacts with multiple drugs, particularly CNS depressants (such as alcohol), which enhance sedation. Other OTC cold preparations may increase anticholinergic side effects.

PROTOTYPE DRUG | Fexofenadine (Allegra)

Actions and Uses: Fexofenadine is a second-generation H_1-receptor antagonist with efficacy equivalent to that of diphenhydramine. Its primary action is to block the effects of histamine at H_1 receptors. When taken prophylactically, it reduces the severity of nasal congestion, sneezing, and tearing of the eyes. Its long half-life of more than 14 hours offers the advantage of it being administered once or twice daily. Fexofenadine is available only in oral form. Allegra-D combines fexofenadine with pseudoephedrine, a decongestant.

Pharmacokinetics: Fexofenadine is well absorbed after oral administration. Distribution is unknown. It is excreted in urine (80%) and feces. Half-life is 14 hours.

Administration Alert:

- There is limited information available related to the use of fexofenadine in pregnancy. When a second generation antihistamine is needed, other agents are currently preferred.

Adverse Effects and Interactions: The major advantage of fexofenadine over first-generation antihistamines is that it causes less drowsiness. Although considered non-sedating, the drug can still cause drowsiness in some clients. Other side effects are usually minor and include headache and upset stomach.

No clinically significant drug interactions have been established. However, concurrent use with other antihistamines or CNS depressants may cause synergistic sedative effects.

TABLE 42.7 Intranasal Glucocorticoids

Drug	Route and Adult Dose
beclomethasone (Beconase AQ) (see Chapter 38, page 461, for the Prototype Drug box)	1–2 sprays in each nostril qd–bid (max 2 sprays in each nostril bid)
budesonide (Rhinocort)	1–2 sprays in each nostril qd–bid (max 4 sprays/day)
ciclesonide (Omnaris)	2 sprays in each nostril qd
flunisolide (Nasalide, Rhinalar)	2 sprays bid; may increase to tid if needed (max 8 sprays/day in each nostril
Pr fluticasone (Flonase)	2 sprays in each nostril qd (max 4 sprays/day in each nostril)
mometasone (Nasonex)	1–2 sprays in each nostril qd
triamcinolone (Nasacort AQ)	1–2 sprays in each nostril qd

INTRANASAL GLUCOCORTICOIDS

Glucocorticoids may be applied directly to the nasal mucosa to prevent symptoms of allergic rhinitis. They have begun to replace antihistamines as drugs of choice for the treatment of chronic allergic rhinitis. These drugs are listed in Table 42.7.

Treating Allergic Rhinitis with Intranasal Glucocorticoids

42.9 Intranasal glucocorticoids have become drugs of choice in treating allergic rhinitis due to their high efficacy and wide margin of safety.

Section 42.5 discusses the importance of the glucocorticoids in treating severe inflammation. As systemic drugs, their use is limited by serious side effects. Intranasal glucocorticoids, however, produce none of the potentially serious adverse effects that are observed when these hormones are given orally or parenterally. Because of their effectiveness and safety, the intranasal glucocorticoids have joined antihistamines as first-line drugs in the treatment of allergic rhinitis.

Intranasal glucocorticoids are administered with a metered-spray device that delivers a consistent dose of drug per spray. When administered properly, their action is limited to the nasal passages. The most frequently reported side effects are an intense burning sensation in the nose immediately after spraying and drying of the nasal mucosa.

Nursing Considerations

The role of the nurse in drug therapy with intranasal glucocorticoids involves careful monitoring of the client's condition and providing education as it relates to the prescribed drug regimen. Prior to administering glucocorticoid nasal spray, assess the nares for excoriation or bleeding. Broken mucous membranes allow direct access to the bloodstream, increasing the likelihood of systemic effects. The mouth and throat should be examined for signs of infection because glucocorticoids may slow the healing process and mask infections. Intranasal glucocorticoids are contraindicated in clients who demonstrate hypersensitivity to any of the ingredients, including preservatives, in the nasal spray.

Monitor the client for alterations in the nasal and oral mucosa and for signs of upper respiratory (especially oropharyngeal) infection. Signs and symptoms of GI distress should be monitored because swallowing large quantities of the drug may contribute to dyspepsia and systemic drug absorption. Monitor for signs of Cushing's syndrome.

Client education as it relates to intranasal glucocorticoids should include goals, reasons for obtaining baseline data such as vital signs and laboratory blood work, and possible side effects. Instruct the client in the correct use and care of the nasal spray device. Because these medications may take 2 to 4 weeks to be effective, the nurse must advise the client not to discontinue use prematurely. Clients may expect these drugs to act as quickly and effectively as decongestants. All clients, especially children, must be urged not to swallow excess amounts of the drug, which is likely to drain down the back of the throat following application. Swallowing large amounts of drug residue increases the risk for systemic side effects. Nasal decongestant sprays are sometimes prescribed with intranasal glucocorticoids for clients with chronic rhinitis. Decongestant sprays should be administered first to clear the nasal passages, allowing for adequate application of the glucocorticoid mist.

The following are other important points to include when teaching clients regarding intranasal glucocorticoids:

- Take the medication exactly as prescribed; additional dosing will not speed relief.

- Shake inhalers thoroughly before spraying.

- Gently clear the nose before spraying. Avoid clearing the nose immediately after spraying.

- Report nosebleeds and nasal burning or irritation that lasts more than a few doses.

- Following administration, spit out the postnasal medication residue.

- Use a humidifier, preservative-free nasal saline spray, or petroleum jelly to ease nasal dryness.

PROTOTYPE DRUG | **Fluticasone (Flonase)**

Actions and Uses: Fluticasone is typical of the intranasal glucocorticoids used to treat seasonal allergic rhinitis. Therapy usually begins with two sprays in each nostril, twice daily, and decreases to one dose per day. Fluticasone acts to decrease local inflammation in the nasal passages, thus decreasing nasal stuffiness.

Pharmacokinetics: Less than 2% of fluticasone is absorbed. Small amounts of all glucocorticoids administered intranasally are swallowed. Small amounts cross the placenta and enter breast milk. Fluticasone is rapidly metabolized in the liver. Half-life is 3 hours.

Administration Alerts:

- Directions for use provided by the manufacturer should be carefully followed by the client.

- Fluticasone is pregnancy category C.

Adverse Effects and Interactions: Side effects of fluticasone are rare. Small amounts of the intranasal glucocorticoids are sometimes swallowed, thus increasing the potential for systemic

TABLE 42.8 Sympathomimetics for Allergic Rhinitis	
Drug	**Route and Adult Dose**
oxymetazoline (Drixoral, Dristan)	Intranasal (0.05%), 2–3 sprays bid for up to 3–5 days
pseudoephedrine (Sudafed)	PO, 60 mg every 4–6 hours (q4–6h) (max 120 mg/day)
xylometazoline (Otrivin)	Intranasal (0.1%), one to two sprays bid (max three doses/day)

side effects. Nasal irritation and bleeding occur in a small number of clients. Concomitant use of a local nasal decongestant spray may increase the risk for irritation or bleeding.

Use with caution with herbal supplements, such as licorice, which may potentiate the effects of glucocorticoids.

ADRENERGICS

Adrenergics stimulate the sympathetic nervous system. They may be administered orally or intranasally to dry the nasal mucosa. The agents used for nasal congestion are listed in Table 42.8.

Treating Nasal Congestion with Adrenergics

42.10 Oral and intranasal adrenergics are used to alleviate the nasal congestion associated with allergic rhinitis and the common cold. Intranasal drugs are more efficacious but can be used only for 3 to 5 days due to rebound congestion.

As discussed in Chapter 14, adrenergics, or adrenergic agonists, are agents that stimulate the sympathetic branch of the autonomic nervous system. Adrenergics with alpha-adrenergic activity are effective at relieving the nasal congestion associated with allergic rhinitis when given by either the oral or the intranasal route. The intranasal preparations such as oxymetazoline (Drixoral, Dristan) are available OTC as sprays or drops and produce an effective response within minutes. Because of their local action, intranasal adrenergics produce few systemic effects. The most serious, limiting side effect of the intranasal preparations is **rebound congestion**. Prolonged use causes hypersecretion of mucus and worsening of nasal congestion once the drug effects wear off. This sometimes leads to a cycle of increased drug use as the condition worsens. Because of this rebound congestion, intranasal adrenergics should be used for no longer than 3 to 5 days.

When administered orally, adrenergics do not produce rebound congestion. Their onset of action by this route, however, is much slower than the intranasal route, and they are less effective at relieving severe congestion. The possibility of systemic side effects is also greater with the oral drugs. Potential side effects include hypertension and CNS stimulation that may lead to insomnia and anxiety. Pseudoephedrine (Sudafed) is the most common adrenergic (sympathomimetic) found in oral OTC cold and allergy medicines.

◀ Drugs in the Community: Pseudoephedrine and Drug Abuse

Pseudoephedrine is an effective and common decongestant. However, it is one of the ingredients that can be used to manufacture methamphetamine, an illegal and highly addictive CNS stimulant.

In an effort to decrease the in-home production of methamphetamine, the amount of OTC drugs that contain pseudoephedrine that can be purchased at any one time has been limited. Products containing pseudoephedrine that were once available OTC must now be requested. Also, some manufacturers have replaced pseudoephedrine with phenylephrine (Neo-Synephrine) as the active agent in OTC cold medications.

Because the adrenergics only relieve nasal congestion, they are often combined with antihistamines to control the sneezing and tearing of allergic rhinitis. It is interesting to note that some OTC drugs having the same basic name may contain different adrenergics. For example, Neo-Synephrine preparations with a 12-hour duration contain the drug oxymetazoline; Neo-Synephrine preparations that last 4 to 6 hours contain phenylephrine.

NCLEX Success Tips

Overuse of nasal spray containing pseudoephedrine can lead to rhinitis medicamentosa, which is a rebound effect causing increased swelling and congestion.

Adverse effects of pseudoephedrine are experienced primarily in the cardiovascular system and through sympathetic effects on the CNS. The most common CNS adverse effects include restlessness, dizziness, tension, anxiety, insomnia, and weakness. Common cardiovascular adverse effects include tachycardia, hypertension, palpitations, and arrhythmias.

Pseudoephedrine can increase blood pressure and increase urinary retention with an enlarged prostate and should be avoided.

Nursing Considerations

The role of the nurse in drug therapy with adrenergics for nasal congestion involves careful monitoring of the client's condition and providing education as it relates to the prescribed drug regimen. Assess for the presence or history of nasal congestion and assess the nares for signs of excoriation or bleeding. Before and during pharmacotherapy, assess vital signs, especially pulse and blood pressure. Oral adrenergics are contraindicated in clients with hypertension due to vasoconstriction caused by stimulation of alpha-adrenergic receptors on systemic blood vessels.

Alpha-adrenergic agonists should be used with caution in clients with prostatic enlargement since these drugs increase smooth muscle activity in the prostate gland and may diminish urinary outflow (see Chapter 14). Clients with thyroid disorders and diabetes mellitus are at risk because adrenergics can increase serum glucose and body metabolism.

These agents should be used with caution in clients with psychiatric disorders, due to an increased risk for agitation. The CNS depression effect of these drugs can seriously exacerbate symptoms of clinical depression.

Client education as it relates to adrenergics for nasal congestion should include goals, reasons for obtaining baseline data such as vital signs and tests for cardiac or metabolic disorders, and possible side effects. The following are important points to include when teaching clients regarding adrenergics:

- Limit use of intranasal preparations to 3 to 5 days to prevent rebound congestion.
- Avoid using other OTC cold or allergy preparations (especially those containing antihistamines) while taking adrenergics because these agents may cause excessive drowsiness.
- Follow the nurse's directions for the use and care of nasal spray dispensers and for proper inhalation technique.
- Report the following immediately: palpitations or chest pain, dizziness or fainting, fever, visual changes, excessively dry mouth, confusion, numbness or tingling in the face or limbs, severe headache, insomnia, restlessness or nervousness, nosebleeds, or persistent intranasal pain or irritation.

See Nursing Process Focus: Clients Receiving Adrenergic Therapy in Chapter 14 for more information.

ANAPHYLAXIS

Anaphylaxis is a potentially fatal condition in which body defences produce a hyperresponse to an antigen. Upon first exposure, the antigen produces no symptoms; however, the body responds by becoming highly sensitized to a subsequent exposure. During anaphylaxis, the body responds quickly, sometimes within minutes after exposure to the antigen, by releasing massive amounts of histamine and other mediators of the inflammatory response. Shortly after exposure to the antigen, the client may experience itching, hives, and a tightness in the throat or chest. Swelling occurs around the larynx, causing a non-productive cough and the voice to become hoarse. As anaphylaxis progresses, the client experiences a rapid fall in blood pressure and difficulty breathing due to bronchoconstriction. The hypotension causes a rebound speeding up of the heart called reflex tachycardia. Without medical intervention, anaphylaxis leads to a profound shock, which is often fatal. Figure 42.3 illustrates the symptoms of anaphylaxis.

Pharmacotherapy of Anaphylaxis

42.11 Anaphylaxis is a serious and often fatal allergic response that is treated with a large number of different drugs, including adrenergics, antihistamines, and glucocorticoids.

Pharmacotherapy of anaphylaxis is symptomatic and involves supporting the cardiovascular system and preventing further hyperresponse by body defences. Various medications are used to treat the symptoms of anaphylaxis depending on the severity of the symptoms. Oxygen is usually administered immediately. Adrenergics such as epinephrine can rapidly reverse hypotension. Antihistamines such as diphenhydramine may be administered IM or IV to prevent stimulation of H_1 receptors. A bronchodilator such as salbutamol (Ventolin) is sometimes administered by inhalation to relieve the acute shortness of breath caused by histamine. Systemic glucocorticoids such as hydrocortisone (Cortef) may be administered to dampen the inflammatory response. The pharmacotherapy of shock is presented in Chapter 58.

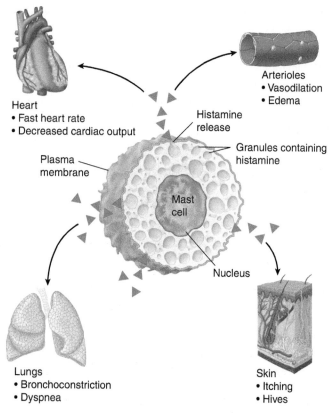

Heart
• Fast heart rate
• Decreased cardiac output

Plasma membrane

Arterioles
• Vasodilation
• Edema

Histamine release

Granules containing histamine

Mast cell

Nucleus

Lungs
• Bronchoconstriction
• Dyspnea

Skin
• Itching
• Hives

Figure 42.3 Symptoms of anaphylaxis.

Nursing Considerations

The role of the nurse in drug therapy with epinephrine involves careful monitoring of the client's condition and providing education as it relates to the drug. Epinephrine is generally administered as an emergency response to severe allergic reactions. Although epinephrine is contraindicated for clients with known hypersensitivity to this drug, in life-threatening situations there are no absolute contraindications to its use.

Epinephrine must be administered with caution to clients with cardiac disease or a history of cerebral atherosclerosis because epinephrine can cause a steep rise in blood pressure as a result of peripheral vascular constriction combined with cardiac stimulation; this rise in blood pressure can lead to intracranial bleeding, dysrhythmias, or pulmonary edema. Epinephrine must also be administered with caution to clients with hyperthyroidism; epinephrine exacerbates tachycardia.

Epinephrine is frequently administered in the emergency department setting; resuscitative equipment must be readily accessible. Parenteral epinephrine is irritating to tissues; therefore, IV sites must be closely monitored for signs of extravasation. Vital signs, including ECG, are monitored continuously during epinephrine infusions. Auscultate the chest before and after epinephrine injection to monitor improvement in bronchoconstriction (wheezing). Clients with a history of closed-angle glaucoma should be monitored for visual changes as a result of changes in intraocular pressure.

Clients with a history of recurrent anaphylaxis may be prescribed epinephrine to be self-administered intramuscularly via an automatic injectable device (EpiPen, Allerject). The nurse should instruct these clients regarding safe "pen" storage and disposal and the proper injection technique. Clients should be encouraged

to use the medication-free "trainer" pen to practise the technique. Advise the client to expect some medication to remain in the pen after injection and to report all episodes requiring pen usage to the healthcare provider.

Client education as it relates to epinephrine should include goals, reasons for obtaining baseline data such as vital signs and ECG, and possible side effects. The following are the important points to include when teaching clients regarding epinephrine:

• Seek emergency medical attention immediately if a single auto-injection of epinephrine fails to bring relief.

• Report burning, irritation, tenderness, swelling, or hardness at IV or IM injection sites.

• Immediately report changes in LOC, particularly feeling faint.

• Report any of the following: palpitations, chest pain, nausea, vomiting, sweating, weakness, dizziness, confusion, blurred vision, headache, anxiety, or sense of impending doom.

See Nursing Process Focus: Clients Receiving Adrenergic Therapy in Chapter 14 for more information.

PROTOTYPE DRUG   **Epinephrine (Adrenalin)**

Actions and Uses: Subcutaneous (SC) or IV epinephrine is a drug of choice for anaphylaxis because it can reverse many of the distressing symptoms within minutes. Epinephrine is a non-selective adrenergic agonist, stimulating both alpha- and beta-adrenergic receptors. Almost immediately after injection, blood pressure rises due to stimulation of alpha$_1$ receptors. Activation of beta$_2$ receptors in the bronchi opens the airways and relieves the client's shortness of breath. Cardiac output increases due to stimulation of beta$_1$ receptors in the heart.

Pharmacokinetics: Epinephrine is well absorbed after SC injection. It crosses the placenta and enters breast milk but does not cross the blood-brain barrier. Action is rapidly terminated by reuptake into neurons and metabolism.

NCLEX Success Tip

Symptoms of hives and redness at the bee sting site coupled with a progression of symptoms including respiratory difficulty and an impending feeling of doom indicate anaphylaxis. Emergency treatment of anaphylaxis is an injection of epinephrine.

Administration Alerts:

• Parenteral epinephrine is an irritant that may cause tissue damage if extravasation occurs.

• Epinephrine is pregnancy category C.

Adverse Effects and Interactions: When administered parenterally, epinephrine may cause serious adverse effects. Hypertension and dysrhythmias may occur rapidly; therefore, the client should be monitored continuously following injection.

Epinephrine interacts with many drugs. For example, it may increase hypertension with phenothiazines and oxytocin. There may be additive toxicities with other adrenergics. Monoamine oxidase (MAO) inhibitors, tricyclic antidepressants, and alpha- and beta-adrenergic agents potentiate the actions of epinephrine.

CHAPTER

42 Understanding the Chapter

Key Concepts Summary

The numbered key concepts provide a succinct summary of the important points from the corresponding numbered section within the chapter. If any of these points are not clear, refer to that numbered section within the chapter for review.

42.1 Inflammation is a natural, nonspecific response that limits the spread of invading microorganisms or injury. Acute inflammation occurs over several days, whereas chronic inflammation may continue for months or years.

42.2 Histamine is a key chemical mediator in inflammation. Release of histamine produces vasodilation, allowing capillaries to become leaky, thus causing tissue swelling.

42.3 Histamine can produce its effects by interacting with two different receptors. The classic antihistamines used for allergies block histamine H_1 receptors in vascular smooth muscle, in the bronchi, and on sensory nerves. The H_2-receptor antagonists are used to treat peptic ulcers.

42.4 Nonsteroidal anti-inflammatory drugs (NSAIDs) are the primary drugs for the treatment of simple inflammation. Newer selective COX-2 inhibitors cause less GI distress but have more cardiovascular risks and side effects.

42.5 Systemic glucocorticoids are effective in treating acute or severe inflammation. Overtreatment with these drugs can

cause a serious condition called Cushing's syndrome; therefore, therapy for inflammation is generally short term.

42.6 Acetaminophen and NSAIDs are the primary agents used to treat fever.

42.7 Allergic rhinitis is a disorder characterized by sneezing, watery eyes, and nasal congestion.

42.8 Antihistamines, or H_1-receptor antagonists, can provide relief from the symptoms of allergic rhinitis. Newer drugs in this class are non-sedating and offer the advantage of once-a-day dosage.

42.9 Intranasal glucocorticoids have become drugs of choice in treating allergic rhinitis due to their high efficacy and wide margin of safety.

42.10 Oral and intranasal adrenergics are used to alleviate the nasal congestion associated with allergic rhinitis and the common cold. Intranasal drugs are more efficacious but can be used only for 3 to 5 days due to rebound congestion.

42.11 Anaphylaxis is a serious and often fatal allergic response that is treated with a large number of different drugs, including adrenergics, antihistamines, and glucocorticoids.

Chapter 42 Scenario

Joycee Layne is a 17-year-old high school student in her senior year. She is an honours student, works hard to get good grades, and hates to miss school. For the past 3 days, she has not been feeling well. This morning her temperature is 39°C, and she has chills and a headache. Several of her friends at school have the flu. She has taken ibuprofen for fevers and menstrual cramps in the past, but Joycee cannot find any in the house as she gets ready to head off to school. Her parents have already left for work, and they trust her to check with you, the nurse who lives next door, before taking any medication. Joycee calls you to ask if it is okay to take the aspirin her mom uses for her arthritis so she can go to school? As the nurse, this presents an opportunity for you to teach Joycee about aspirin and her fever.

Critical Thinking Questions

1. Describe the pathophysiology of fever and inflammation.
2. Why is aspirin administered for fever?
3. Should Joycee take the aspirin? Why or why not?
4. What will you teach Joycee about aspirin and the flu-like symptoms she is having? What additional client teaching will she need?

See Answers to Critical Thinking Questions in Appendix B.

NCLEX Practice Questions

1 A 30-year-old client with depression has attempted suicide by overdosing on acetaminophen (Tylenol). The nurse in the emergency department anticipates that the client's treatment will consist of

   a. An intravenous infusion with normal saline to infuse at 1000 mL per hour

   b. The administration of acetylcysteine (Mucomyst) by intravenous infusion

   c. Preparation for cardioversion due to the impending arrhythmia

   d. The assessment of liver hepatic enzymes to determine hepatotoxicity

2 A client has a fever and is allergic to aspirin. Which medication does the nurse anticipate administering to reduce the client's fever?

   a. Ibuprofen (Motrin, Advil)

   b. Ketorolac (Toradol)

   c. Acetaminophen (Tylenol)

   d. Celecoxib (Celebrex)

3 An 80-year-old woman who is scheduled for a total knee replacement next month currently takes ibuprofen (Motrin, Advil) 600 mg three times per day. Which client teaching intervention is most important?

   a. Continue ibuprofen (Motrin, Advil) until surgery.

   b. Stop ibuprofen (Motrin, Advil) today.

   c. Decrease ibuprofen (Motrin, Advil) to two times per day.

   d. Stop ibuprofen (Motrin, Advil) 7 to 14 days before surgery.

4 The nurse should question the order of acetaminophen (Tylenol) for which of the following clients?

   a. A client with cirrhosis of the liver

   b. A client with chronic obstructive pulmonary disease

   c. A client with breast cancer

   d. A client who is taking warfarin (Coumadin)

5 A client takes aspirin (acetylsalicylic acid) daily for pain in the right knee. Which toxic effects may be present with aspirin overdosage? Select all that apply.

   a. Tinnitus

   b. Hyperventilation

   c. Gastrointestinal bleeding

   d. Decreased urinary output

   e. Peripheral neuropathy

See Answers to NCLEX Practice Questions in Appendix A.

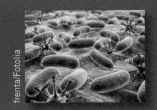

frenta/Fotolia

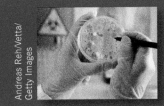

Andreas Reh/Vetta/
Getty Images

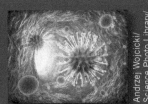

Andrzej Wojcicki/
Science Photo Library/
Brand X Pictures/Getty
Images

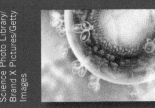

MedicalRF.com/
Getty Images

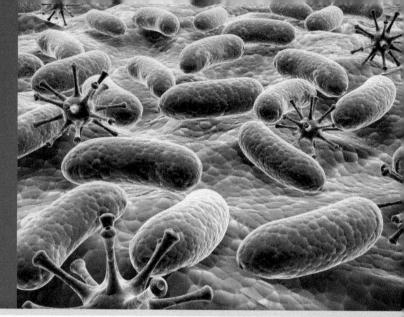
frenta/Fotolia

CHAPTER 43

Basic Principles of Anti-Infective Pharmacotherapy

LEARNING OUTCOMES

After reading this chapter, the student should be able to:

1. Explain the mechanisms by which pathogens infect the body.
2. Describe methods for classifying bacteria.
3. Explain the mechanisms by which anti-infective drugs act to kill pathogens or restrict their growth.
4. Describe the clinical significance of bacterial resistance.
5. Identify steps that the nurse can take to limit the development of resistance.
6. Describe the clinical rationale for selecting specific antibiotics.
7. Identify the role of the nurse in preventing, identifying, and treating adverse effects due to antibiotic therapy.
8. Explain how the client's immune status, history of allergic reactions, age, pregnancy status, genetics, or local tissue conditions influence anti-infective pharmacotherapy.
9. Explain the clinical importance of selecting the correct antibiotic for the individual client.
10. Describe the development of superinfections.

CHAPTER OUTLINE

▸ Pathogenicity and Virulence

▸ Describing and Classifying Bacteria

▸ Classification of Anti-Infectives

▸ Mechanisms of Action of Anti-Infectives

▸ Acquired Resistance

▸ Selection of Antibiotics

▸ Indications for and Selection of Specific Anti-Infectives

▸ Use of Anti-Infectives to Prevent Infections

▸ Host Factors That Affect Anti-Infective Selection

▸ Superinfections

acquired resistance, 517

aerobic, 514

anaerobic, 514

antibiotic, 514

anti-infective, 514

antimicrobial (antibacterial)
   resistance, 518

bacteriocidal, 515

bacteriostatic, 515

broad-spectrum antibiotic, 519

conjugation, 518

culture and sensitivity (C&S) testing, 519

endotoxins, 513

exotoxins, 513

gram negative, 514

gram positive, 513

health care–associated infections
   (HAIs), 518

host flora, 519

invasiveness, 513

microbial antagonism, 521

mutations, 518

narrow-spectrum antibiotic, 519

nosocomial infections, 518

pathogenicity, 513

pathogens, 513

peptidoglycan, 515

selective toxicity, 515

superinfections, 521

virulence, 513

The human body has adapted quite well to living in a world full of microorganisms (microbes). In the air, water, food, and soil, microbes have been essential components of life on the planet for billions of years. In some cases, these microorganisms coexist in intimate contact with human beings. Fortunately, of the millions of species of microbes, only a relative few are harmful to human health. The purpose of this chapter is to present the fundamental principles that apply to the pharmacotherapy of infectious diseases.

Pathogenicity and Virulence

43.1 Pathogens cause disease due to their ability to invade tissues or secrete toxins.

The first challenge in studying the pharmacotherapy of infectious disease is to understand the terminology that is used to describe the organisms and drugs. Microbes that are capable of causing human disease, or **pathogens**, include viruses, bacteria, fungi, unicellular organisms (protozoans), and multicellular animals (e.g., fleas, mites, and worms).

Some pathogens are extremely infectious and life threatening to humans, whereas others simply cause annoying symptoms or none at all. **Pathogenicity**, the ability of an organism to cause disease, depends on an organism's speed of reproduction and its skill in bypassing or overcoming body defences. Organisms that usually infect only when the body's immune system is suppressed are called *opportunistic pathogens*.

Virulence is a quantitative measure of an organism's pathogenicity. A highly virulent microbe is one that can produce disease when present in very small numbers. Virulent pathogens produce their devastating effects through two primary characteristics: invasiveness and toxicity.

Invasiveness is the ability of a pathogen to grow extremely rapidly and cause direct damage to surrounding tissues by their sheer numbers. Because a week or more may be needed to mount an immune response against the organism, this exponential growth can rapidly overwhelm body defences and disrupt normal cellular function. Some streptococci, staphylococci, and clostridia secrete hyaluronidase, an enzyme that digests the matrix between human cells, allowing the bacteria to penetrate anatomical barriers more easily. *Staphylococcus aureus* secretes the enzyme coagulase, causing fibrin to be deposited on its cells, thereby protecting it from phagocytes.

The second characteristic of virulence is the production of toxins, or toxicity. **Exotoxins** are proteins released by bacteria into surrounding tissues that have the ability to inactivate or kill host cells. *Clostridium botulinum*, the organism responsible for botulism, produces one of the most potent toxins known that binds to presynaptic motor neurons to prevent the release of acetylcholine. Symptoms of exotoxin-producing bacteria are usually caused by the toxin itself, not the bacteria. For example, clients experience food poisoning by ingesting food containing the toxins produced by the organisms; growth of the bacteria in the body is not required. Most exotoxins are water soluble and can readily enter the blood to cause systemic toxemia.

Endotoxins are harmful non-protein chemicals that are part of the outer layer of the normal cell wall of gram-negative bacteria. After the bacterial cell dies, endotoxins are liberated into the surrounding tissue and induce macrophages to release large amounts of cytokines, causing generalized inflammation, fever, and chills. Rapid decreases in the number of lymphocytes, leukocytes, and platelets may occur. The initial doses of antibiotic therapy may actually worsen symptoms by lysing bacteria and releasing larger amounts of endotoxins. Even very small amounts of some bacterial endotoxins may disrupt normal cellular activity and, in extreme cases, result in death.

Describing and Classifying Bacteria

43.2 Bacteria are described by their staining characteristics, shape, and ability to use oxygen.

Because of the enormous number of bacterial species, several descriptive systems have been developed to simplify their study. It is important for nurses to learn these classification schemes, because drugs that are effective against one organism in a class are likely to be effective against other pathogens in the same class. Common bacterial pathogens and the types of diseases they cause are shown in Table 43.1.

One of the simplest methods of classifying microbes is to examine them microscopically after a crystal violet Gram stain has been applied to the microbes. Some bacteria contain a thick cell wall composed of peptidoglycan and retain the violet colour after staining. These bacteria are called **gram positive** and include

TABLE 43.1 Common Bacterial Pathogens and Diseases

Name of Organism	Disease(s)	Description
Borrelia burgdorferi	Lyme disease	From tick bites
Chlamydia trachomatis	Venereal disease, endometriosis	Most common cause of sexually transmitted infections (STIs)
Escherichia coli	Traveller's diarrhea, urinary tract infection (UTI), bacteremia, endometriosis	Part of host flora in gastrointestinal (GI) tract
Haemophilus	Pneumonia, meningitis in children, bacteremia, otitis media, sinusitis	Some *Haemophilus* species are host flora in the upper respiratory tract
Klebsiella	Pneumonia, UTI	Usually infects immunosuppressed clients
Mycobacterium leprae	Leprosy	Most cases occur in immigrants from Africa or Asia
Mycobacterium tuberculosis	Tuberculosis	Incidence very high in clients infected with human immunodeficiency virus (HIV)
Mycoplasma pneumoniae	Pneumonia	Most common cause of pneumonia in clients ages 5–35 years
Neisseria gonorrhoeae	Gonorrhea and other STIs, endometriosis, neonatal eye infection	Some *Neisseria* species are normal host flora
Neisseria meningitidis	Meningitis in children	Some *Neisseria* species are normal host flora
Pneumococci	Pneumonia, otitis media, meningitis, bacteremia, endocarditis	Part of normal flora in upper respiratory tract
Proteus mirabilis	UTI, skin infections	Part of host flora in GI tract
Pseudomonas aeruginosa	UTI, skin infections, septicemia	Usually infects immunosuppressed clients
Rickettsia rickettsii	Rocky Mountain spotted fever	From tick bites
Salmonella enteritidis	Food poisoning	From infected animal products, raw eggs, undercooked meat or chicken
Salmonella typhi	Typhoid fever	From inadequately treated food or water supplies
Staphylococcus aureus	Pneumonia, food poisoning, impetigo, abscesses, bacteremia, endocarditis, toxic shock syndrome	Some *Staphylococcus* species are normal host flora
Streptococcus	Pharyngitis, pneumonia, skin infections, septicemia, endocarditis	Some *Streptococcus* species are normal host flora
Vibrio cholerae	Cholera	From inadequately treated food or water supplies

Staphylococcus, Streptococcus, and *Enterococcus.* Bacteria that have thinner cell walls will lose the violet stain and are called **gram negative**. Examples of gram-negative bacteria include *Bacteroides, Escherichia, Klebsiella, Pseudomonas,* and *Salmonella.* The distinction between gram-positive and gram-negative bacteria is a profound one that reflects important biochemical and physiological differences between the two groups. Many antibiotics are effective against only one of the two groups. For example, gram-negative bacteria are generally susceptible to the tetracycline class but are resistant to the sulfonamides. This generalization, however, quickly breaks down when resistant strains develop.

Bacteria are often described by their basic shape, which can be readily determined microscopically. Those with rod shapes are called bacilli, those that are spherical are called cocci, and those that are spiral are called spirilla. The shape, along with the Gram stain, helps pathologists to identify organisms that are isolated from infectious specimens.

A third factor used to categorize bacteria is their ability to use oxygen. Those that thrive in an oxygen-rich environment are called **aerobic**; those that grow optimally without oxygen are called **anaerobic**. Some organisms have the ability to change their metabolism and survive in either aerobic or anaerobic conditions, depending on their external environment. Antibiotics are often selective for either aerobes or anaerobes.

Classification of Anti-Infectives

43.3 Anti-infective drugs are classified by their susceptible organisms, chemical structures, and mechanisms of action.

Anti-infective is a general term that applies to any medication that is effective against pathogens. In its broadest sense, an anti-infective drug may be used to treat bacterial, fungal, viral, or parasitic infections. To distinguish among the various anti-infectives, these medications are classified as antibacterial, antifungal, antiviral, antiprotozoan, and antihelminthic based on the type of organism they treat.

The most frequent term used to describe an antibacterial drug is antibiotic. Technically, **antibiotic** refers to a natural substance produced by a microorganism that can kill other microorganisms. However, many of the newer drugs that are available to treat bacterial infections are now produced synthetically. In clinical practice, the terms *antibacterial* and *antibiotic* are used interchangeably to refer to any drug that is effective against bacteria. In this text, antibiotic and antibacterial are used interchangeably.

Classifying drugs only by their susceptible organism, such as an antibacterial, tells us nothing about the properties, actions, or adverse effects of a drug. With more than 300 antibacterials available, it is helpful to group these drugs into subclasses that share

TABLE 43.2 Classification of Anti-Infective Drugs

Mechanism of Action	Chemical Class	Examples
Inhibition of cell wall synthesis	Penicillins Cephalosporins Carbapenems Miscellaneous	penicillin G cefotaxime (Claforan) imipenem (Primaxin) isoniazid (Isotamine) vancomycin (Vancocin)
Inhibition of protein synthesis	Aminoglycosides Tetracyclines Macrolides Oxazolidinones	gentamicin (Garamycin) tetracycline erythromycin (Eryc) linezolid (Zyvox)
Disruption of plasma membrane	Azoles Polyenes	amphotericin B (Fungizone) fluconazole (Diflucan) nystatin
Inhibition of nucleic acid synthesis	Fluoroquinolones	ciprofloxacin (Cipro)
Inhibition of metabolic pathways	Sulfonamides	dapsone (Aczone) trimethoprim-sulfamethoxazole (Bactrim, Septra)

similar therapeutic properties. Two means of grouping are widely used: chemical classes and pharmacological classes.

Class names such as aminoglycosides, fluoroquinolone, and sulfonamides refer to the fundamental chemical structure shared by a group of anti-infectives. Anti-infectives that belong to the same chemical class have close structural similarities and usually share similar antibacterial properties and adverse effects. Although chemical names are sometimes long and difficult to pronounce, placing drugs into chemical classes will assist the student in mentally organizing these drugs into distinct therapeutic groups.

Pharmacological classes are used to group anti-infectives by their mechanism of action. Like chemical classes, placing an antibiotic into a pharmacological class allows the nurse to develop a mental framework on which to organize these medications and to predict similar actions and adverse effects. Examples of pharmacological classes grouped by their mechanisms of action with representative drugs are listed in Table 43.2. It is important that the nurse learn both the chemical class and the pharmacological class for each antibiotic because this will provide a deeper understanding of the drug's therapeutic action and potential adverse effects.

Mechanisms of Action of Anti-Infectives

43.4 Anti-infective drugs act by selectively targeting a pathogen's metabolism or life cycle.

Although the immune system provides elaborate defences against microbial invaders, there are times when the body defences become overwhelmed by an infection. Furthermore, there are times when acquiring an infection could be a serious health challenge for a client, and it is best to prevent it. Whether it is used for treating or preventing disease, the primary goal of anti-infective therapy is to assist the body in eliminating a pathogen. Drugs that

accomplish this goal by killing bacteria are called **bacteriocidal**. Some drugs do not kill pathogens but instead slow their growth, allowing natural body defences to eliminate the microorganisms. These growth-slowing drugs are called **bacteriostatic**.

Bacterial cells have distinct anatomical and physiological differences compared to human cells. Bacteria incorporate different chemicals into their membranes and use unique biochemical pathways and enzymes to manage their rapid growth. Even the more complex pathogens such as fungi and protozoans have different cell structures and use certain metabolic pathways not found in human cells. Antibiotics exert **selective toxicity** by targeting these unique differences between human and bacterial, fungal, and protozoan cells. Through this selective action, these pathogens can be killed, or their growth severely hampered, without any major effects on human cells. Of course, there are limits to this selective toxicity, depending on the specific antibiotic and the dose employed. Adverse effects can be expected from all anti-infectives. There are five major methods by which antibacterials exert their selective toxicity: inhibition of cell wall synthesis, inhibition of protein synthesis, disruption of the plasma cell membrane, inhibition of nucleic acid synthesis, and inhibition of metabolic pathways (antimetabolites). This is an oversimplification of antibacterial actions because some of these drugs act by multiple mechanisms and a few act by unknown mechanisms. Furthermore, as new drugs are developed they often act by new mechanisms and become the only medication in a class. Indeed, although the five major classes encompass the majority of anti-infectives, the "miscellaneous" group of anti-infectives has expanded into a large class (see Chapter 44).

Inhibition of Cell Wall Synthesis

Unlike human cells, bacteria have rigid cell walls that create a high osmotic pressure within the cells. The cell wall primarily consists of **peptidoglycan**, a strong, repeating network of carbohydrate and protein chains found only in bacteria and that contains sugars bound to peptides. Disruption of this wall causes the cell to absorb water and eventually lyse. The presence of a unique cell wall gives several means by which antibiotics may act. Fungi also have a unique cell wall that contains lipids that are not used in human cells.

The penicillins and cephalosporins bind to specific proteins that are essential to building the bacterial cell wall. Vancomycin (Vancocin) acts by preventing the formation of peptide chains that are used in the construction of the cell wall. Several drugs that are effective against *Mycobacterium tuberculosis*, including isoniazid (Isotamine), act by inhibiting the incorporation of mycolic acid, an important component of the cell wall of this mycobacterium.

Inhibition of Protein Synthesis

Both bacterial and human cells conduct protein synthesis, so this may seem an unlikely target for antibiotics. However, proteins are constructed on the surface of ribosomes, and these organelles have different structures in humans and bacteria. This difference in ribosomal structure accounts for the selective toxicity of certain antibiotics for bacterial cells.

The fact that protein synthesis occurs in several steps affords different mechanisms by which antibiotics may act. For example, the tetracyclines interfere with the transfer of ribonucleic acid (RNA), which carries the amino acids to the ribosome. The aminoglycosides change the shape of the ribosome so that protein synthesis is impeded.

Disruption of the Plasma Cell Membrane

A few antibacterial and antifungal medications act by interfering with the pathogen's plasma membrane. For example, when polymyxin B attaches to the phospholipids in bacterial plasma membranes, the permeability of the membrane changes and substances escape from the cell. The antifungal drug amphotericin B (Fungizone) shuts down the synthesis of ergosterol, a lipid essential to the integrity of fungal plasma membranes.

Inhibition of Nucleic Acid Synthesis

Although deoxyribonucleic acid (DNA) and RNA synthesis are complex processes that occur in both human and bacterial cells, the molecular structures of the various enzymes required for these processes differ considerably. The largest group of antibiotics that inhibits DNA synthesis is the fluoroquinolones. These drugs affect bacterial DNA gyrase, an enzyme that uncoils DNA during the replication process.

Inhibition of Metabolic Pathways (Antimetabolites)

Because they divide rapidly, bacterial cells need a steady supply of nutrients and metabolites. A few drugs structurally resemble these building blocks and "fool" the bacterial cell into using them for growth. The sulfonamide antibiotics resemble para-aminobenzoic acid, a precursor to folic acid. Folic acid, a B vitamin that is essential to human metabolism, is also essential to bacteria. When the bacteria attempt to use the sulfonamides, bacterial protein synthesis is blocked.

Other Mechanisms of Action

Anti-infectives act by a number of other miscellaneous mechanisms. The antifungal drug griseofulvin (Grifulvin) inhibits the formation of mitotic microtubules. Antiretrovirals such as zidovudine (Retrovir, AZT) block the synthesis of viral DNA by inhibiting the enzyme reverse transcriptase. Mebendazole (Vermox) kills parasitic worms by preventing their absorption of nutrients.

Many other possible mechanisms exist. As the understanding of bacterial physiology increases, it is likely that pharmacologists will develop anti-infectives with entirely new mechanisms of action. The primary mechanisms of action of antibacterial drugs are illustrated in Figure 43.1.

Acquired Resistance

43.5 Acquired resistance is a major clinical problem that is worsened by improper use of anti-infectives.

In the 1950s, healthcare providers called antibiotics "miracle drugs" and predicted that all infectious disease would one day be eliminated. It did not take long, however, to discover that these miracle drugs were rapidly becoming ineffective. How could a

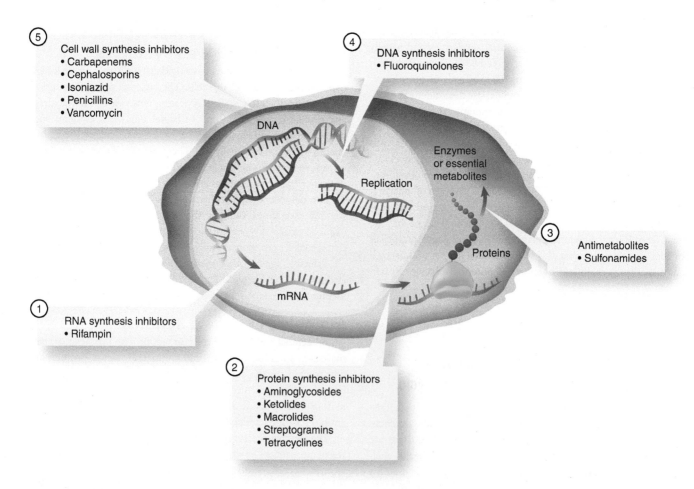

Figure 43.1 Mechanisms of action of antimicrobial drugs.

drug that once killed nearly 100% of a species of bacteria soon prove to be ineffective? The answer is acquired resistance.

Acquired resistance is the ability of an organism to become unresponsive over time to the effects of an anti-infective. Resistance can occur in bacteria, fungi, viruses, and protozoans. It is a major clinical problem that is growing in importance.

Mechanisms of Resistance

How can an organism become insensitive to a drug that kills other members of its species? Medicine has discovered a number of mechanisms by which pathogens acquire resistance (see Figure 43.2):

- *Destruction of the drug.* Organisms can produce an enzyme that destroys or deactivates the drug. For example, some bacteria are able to produce beta-lactamase, an enzyme that splits the active portion of the drug molecule. Organisms that produce beta-lactamase are resistant to many of the penicillin and cephalosporin antibiotics.

- *Prevention of drug entry into the pathogen.* Some antibiotics must enter the pathogen to cause their action. Some bacteria have developed enzymes that inactivate the drug as it crosses the cell wall. Others have changed the structure of the channels

or pores that the antibiotic normally uses to enter the cell. Resistance to penicillins and tetracyclines can occur by these methods.

- *Removal by resistance pumps.* Some bacteria have developed a system that rapidly pumps the antibiotic out of the bacterial cell before it can reach intracellular targets such as ribosomes. Resistant bacteria have developed several types of pumps, each of which is used to remove different antibiotics.

- *Alteration of the drug's target site.* Most antibiotics bind to a specific receptor that is located on the cell surface or inside the bacteria. Certain bacteria have changed the shape of these receptors, so they no longer bind the drug. This mechanism of resistance is common for the sulfonamides. For the macrolide antibiotics, mutations have resulted in changes to the structure of the bacterial ribosome, which is the receptor for macrolide binding.

- *Development of alternative metabolic pathways.* Some antibiotics act by depleting the pathogen of an essential substance necessary for growth. Some resistant organisms have survived antibiotic application by synthesizing larger amounts of the essential substance or by finding an alternative means of obtaining it from the environment.

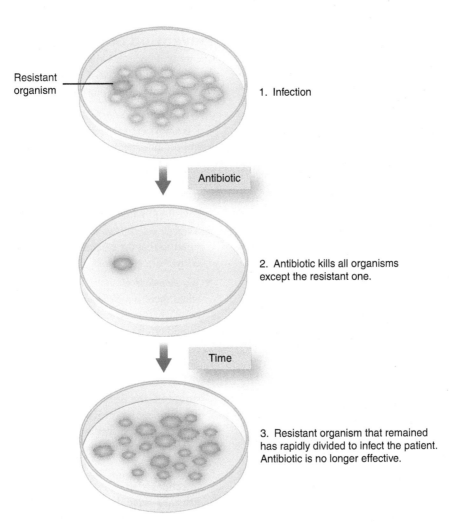

Figure 43.2 Acquired resistance.

How do bacteria change their physiology to become resistant to antibiotics? The answer lies in the nature of bacterial cell division. Microorganisms have the ability to replicate extremely rapidly. Under ideal conditions *Escherichia coli* can produce a million cells every 20 minutes, or 1×10^{21} cells in only 24 hours. During exponential division, bacteria make frequent errors, or **mutations**, while duplicating their genetic code. These mutations, which occur spontaneously and randomly, occasionally result in a change in physiology that gives a bacterial cell a reproductive advantage over its neighbours. For example, the mutated bacterium may be able to survive in harsher conditions, change the shape of its organelles, or perhaps grow faster than other bacterial cells.

It is possible for such a random mutation to confer drug resistance for a microorganism. Once the mutation produces a resistant strain, the microbes permanently lose sensitivity to that specific drug and often to other drugs in the same pharmacological and chemical class. Over several decades, these drug-resistant mutants may colonize a large segment of the human population, thus making the medication essentially useless as a first-line antibiotic.

Promotion of Resistance

The widespread and sometimes unwarranted use of antibiotics has promoted the development of drug-resistant bacterial strains. By killing strains of bacteria that are sensitive to the drug, the only bacteria remaining to replicate are those that acquired the mutations that made them insensitive to the effects of the antibiotic. These drug-resistant bacteria are then free to grow, unrestrained by their neighbours that are killed by the antibiotic. Soon the client develops an infection that is resistant to conventional drug therapy

After acquiring resistance, the mutated bacterium may pass its resistance gene to other bacteria through **conjugation**, which is the direct transfer of small pieces of circular DNA called plasmids. Through conjugation, it is quite possible for a bacterium that has never been exposed to the antibiotic to become resistant. Furthermore, because conjugation is not species specific, resistance genes may be passed from one species to a totally different species.

It is important to understand that the antibiotic itself does not cause changes in bacterial physiology, nor does the microorganism have a master plan to become resistant or to actively defeat the drug. The mutation occurs randomly—the result of accident and pure chance. The promotion and growth of the resistant strain, however, is not due to chance. The antibiotic kills the surrounding cells that are susceptible to the drug, leaving the mutated bacterium plenty of room to divide and infect. It should also be understood that it is the bacteria that become resistant, not the client.

The widespread and sometimes unwarranted use of antibiotics has led to a large number of resistant bacterial strains, referred to as **antimicrobial** (or **antibacterial**) **resistance**. At least 60% of *Staphylococcus aureus* infections are now resistant to penicillin, and resistant strains of *Enterococcus faecalis, Enterococcus faecium,* and *Pseudomonas aeruginosa* are becoming major clinical problems. The longer an antibiotic is used in the population and the more often it is prescribed, the larger the percentage of resistant strains. Infections acquired in a hospital or other healthcare setting, called **nosocomial infections**, are often resistant to common antibiotics.

The Canadian Integrated Program for Antimicrobial Resistance Surveillance (CIPARS) monitors trends in antimicrobial use and antimicrobial resistance in select bacterial organisms from human, animal, and food sources across Canada. Appropriate measures to contain the emergence and spread of resistant bacteria between animals, food, and people in Canada are identified. This information is used to develop evidence-based policies to control antimicrobial use in hospital, community, and agricultural settings and thus to prolong the effectiveness of antimicrobial drugs.

Healthcare providers can play an important role in delaying the emergence of resistance by restricting the use of antibiotics to those conditions deemed medically necessary. In most cases, antibiotics are given when there is clear evidence of bacterial infection. Some clients, however, receive antibiotics to *prevent* an infection, a practice called prophylactic use or chemoprophylaxis. Examples of clients who might receive prophylactic antibiotics include those who have a suppressed immune system; those who have experienced deep puncture wounds such as from dog bites; or those who have prosthetic heart valves, prior to receiving medical or dental surgery.

It is not uncommon for clients to stop taking an antibiotic once they begin to feel better. Discontinuing an antibiotic before all organisms have been killed promotes the emergence of resistant strains. Instruct the client that many organisms still remain, even after the symptoms disappear. The importance of taking the entire drug regimen must be stressed.

Prevention of Resistant Strains

Clients and their healthcare providers play important roles in delaying the emergence of resistance to antibiotics. The following are suggested ways to prevent resistance:

- *Prevent infections when possible.* Nurses must teach their clients that it is always easier to prevent an infection than to treat one. One important aspect of prevention is getting immunizations to protect against diseases such as influenza, tetanus, polio, measles, and hepatitis B. Prevention also includes proper care and hygiene of catheters, which are significant sources of microorganisms and provide portals of entry into the body.

- *Diagnose and treat the infection properly.* Infections should be cultured so that the offending organism can be identified and the correct drug chosen.

- *Use antimicrobials wisely.* Antibiotics should be prescribed only when there is a clear rationale for their use. The drugs should be taken for the full length of therapy, and the prescription should not be renewed if the infection has been eliminated or prevented. The more often an antibiotic is prescribed in the population, the larger will be the percentage of resistant strains.

- *Prevent transmission.* Nurses can contain infections and stop the spread of the disease in their work settings by using proper infection control procedures. In addition, nurses should teach their clients the methods of proper hygiene to prevent the transmission of infectious disease in the home and community settings.

Infections that are acquired in a healthcare setting, called **health care–associated infections (HAIs)** or nosocomial infections, are often resistant to common antibiotics. The most common site of HAIs is the urinary tract, followed by surgical wounds, the respiratory tract, and bacteremia.

There are four general sources of HAIs:

- *Client flora.* Bacteria normally residing on the skin and in the lung or genitourinary tract
- *Invasive devices.* Urinary catheters, vascular catheters, endotracheal tubes, and endoscopes
- *Medical personnel.* Infected healthcare workers or non-infectious carriers
- *Medical environment.* Contaminated instruments, air, food, or fluids

Many times, clients are at risk for HAIs caused by resistant organisms. Two types of resistant strains are especially important to pharmacotherapy: methicillin-resistant *Staphylococcus aureus* and vancomycin-resistant enterococci.

Methicillin-Resistant *Staphylococcus aureus* (MRSA) MRSA is a type of bacterium that is resistant to certain antibiotics such as methicillin, amoxicillin, and penicillin. At least 60% of *S. aureus* infections are now resistant to penicillin. The term *methicillin resistant* is still used for these infections despite the fact that methicillin was removed from the market many years ago.

MRSA infections are most frequently acquired in hospitals and long-term care facilities. These hospital-acquired infections (HA-MRSA) occur primarily in clients with weakened immune systems. MRSA infections that occur in non-hospitalized settings are called community-acquired infections (CA-MRSA). CA-MRSA infections occur in otherwise healthy people and are usually manifested as skin and soft tissue infections, such as pimples and boils. The strains that are responsible for HA-MRSA infections appear to be distinctly different from those that cause CA-MRSA infections; therefore, the pharmacotherapy of the two infections differs somewhat.

Therapeutic options for clients with serious MRSA infections are limited. In recent years, MRSA strains have developed resistance to most classes of antimicrobials, including fluoroquinolones, macrolides, aminoglycosides, tetracyclines, and clindamycin (Dalacin). In general, the HA-MRSA strains are resistant to more classes than the CA-MRSA infections. Until recently, vancomycin was the only antibiotic effective for treating serious MRSA infections. Unfortunately, MRSA strains that are also resistant to vancomycin have appeared. Several newer antibiotics, including linezolid (Zyvox), quinupristin-dalfopristin (Synercid), and daptomycin (Cubicin), are now available to treat multidrug-resistant strains of MRSA.

Vancomycin-Resistant Enterococci (VRE) Enterococci are normal inhabitants of the human gastrointestinal (GI) tract and the female genital tract. Enterococci are also frequently found in wounds and pressure ulcers in hospitalized clients or nursing home residents. Clients with compromised immune systems are at greatest risk. Because enterococci are hardy organisms, they can survive for prolonged periods on environmental surfaces, and healthcare workers using poor infection control techniques can easily spread them. More than 95% of VRE strains in the United States are *Enterococcus faecium*.

Like MRSA, VRE infections represent a major therapeutic challenge, and treatment options are limited. Strains that are resistant to the most commonly used classes of antibiotics have been isolated. Virtually all are resistant to high levels of ampicillin, which is the conventional treatment for enterococci infections. In the 1990s, vancomycin became the only antibiotic effective against multidrug-resistant VRE strains. Unfortunately, each year finds more VRE strains becoming resistant to vancomycin, and newer antibiotics must be used for these infections.

Selection of Antibiotics

43.6 Careful selection of the correct antibiotic is essential for effective pharmacotherapy and to limit adverse effects.

It is essential for the healthcare provider to select an antibiotic that will be effective against the specific pathogen that is causing the client's infection. Selecting an incorrect drug will delay proper treatment, giving the pathogens more time to invade or secrete toxins. For acute infections, treatment delays of just a few hours or days can lead to poorer client prognosis and even death. Prescribing ineffective antibiotics also promotes the development of resistance and may cause unnecessary adverse effects in the client.

For the correct antibiotic to be chosen, identification of the causative agent is necessary. Although gathering data on symptoms is important, many infections produce the same signs early in their course; therefore, more exact laboratory means of diagnosis are necessary.

Specimens such as urine, sputum, blood, or pus are examined in the laboratory for the purpose of isolating and identifying specific pathogens. After isolation, the microbe is exposed to different antibiotics in the laboratory to determine the most effective ones. This process of isolating the infectious organism and identifying the most effective antibiotic is called **culture and sensitivity (C&S) testing**. Other laboratory techniques include examination of the blood for specific antibodies, direct antigen detection, and DNA probe hybridization.

Ideally, the pathogen should be identified before anti-infective therapy is begun. However, laboratory testing and identification may take several days or, in the case of viruses, several weeks. Indeed, some pathogens cannot be cultured at all. If the infection is severe, therapy is often begun with a **broad-spectrum antibiotic**, which is one that is effective against a wide variety of different microbial species. After C&S testing is completed, the drug may be changed to a **narrow-spectrum antibiotic**, which is one that is effective against a smaller group of microbes or only the isolated species. In general, narrow-spectrum antibiotics have less effect on **host flora**, thus causing fewer adverse effects. Host flora are microorganisms that normally inhabit the human body.

Anti-infectives should not be prescribed for infections such as the common cold or for disorders for which antibiotics serve no therapeutic advantage. Antibiotics do not affect viral diseases such as the common cold, although many clients with this self-limiting disorder believe that these drugs will speed their recovery. Another example of anti-infective misuse is prescribing antibiotics to clients who have a cough due to chronic bronchitis. It should be understood, however, that healthcare providers may prescribe anti-infectives to prevent a secondary infection from developing. For example, an elderly client with a severe cold may develop a weakened immune response. Therefore, the healthcare provider may order an antibiotic not for the viral infection, but to prevent a secondary bacterial infection from developing.

Indications for and Selection of Specific Anti-Infectives

43.7 Depending on the pathogen, anti-infective therapy may be conducted with a single drug or a combination of drugs.

If C&S testing confirms that an infection is caused by only one species of microbe, antibiotic therapy is usually begun with a single drug. In some cases, combining two antibiotics may actually decrease each drug's effectiveness, a phenomenon known as *antagonism*. For example, giving a drug that slows bacterial growth may interfere with an antibiotic that depends on a high bacterial growth rate to produce its bacteriocidal effect. Use of multiple antibiotics can also promote the emergence of multidrug-resistant strains and produce unnecessary adverse effects.

In well-defined circumstances, combination therapy with multiple antibiotics is warranted. For example, multiple anti-infective drugs are indicated if different species of pathogens are causing the infection. Clients may present with a life-threatening infection of unknown etiology, and the healthcare provider may need to prescribe several antibiotics until the specific pathogens can be identified. In some cases, two antibiotics have been shown through clinical research to work synergistically, producing a greater kill rate than would be achieved by either antibiotic given alone. Examples of situations where multidrug therapy is clearly warranted are for the pharmacotherapy of tuberculosis and HIV–acquired immune deficiency syndrome (AIDS).

Use of Anti-Infectives to Prevent Infections

43.8 Anti-infectives may be administered to prevent infections.

In most cases, anti-infectives are given when there is clear evidence of infection. This is because healthcare providers have developed clear rationales for prescribing these drugs to discourage the emergence of resistant strains.

However, anti-infectives are administered to prevent infections in certain high-risk clients. In these cases, research has demonstrated that the benefits of infection prophylaxis outweigh the increased risk for adverse effects or the potential for producing resistant strains. Prophylactic anti-infectives are indicated for the following clinical situations:

- Antibiotics for clients with suppressed immune systems, including those with HIV-AIDS or profound neutropenia
- Antibiotics for clients with deep puncture wounds such as from dog bites
- Antibiotics for clients with prosthetic heart valves, prior to receiving medical or dental surgery, to prevent bacterial endocarditis

- Antibiotics for clients who are undergoing specific types of surgery, such as cardiovascular surgery, orthopedic surgery, and surgery of the alimentary canal, where it has been shown that antibiotic use decreases the risk of postoperative infections
- Antimalarial drugs for clients who are entering areas of the world where malaria is endemic
- Antitubercular drugs for close personal contacts of clients who have confirmed or suspected active tuberculosis
- Antiretrovirals to prevent the transmission of HIV to newborns when the mother is HIV positive
- Antiretrovirals for healthcare workers who have a confirmed exposure to HIV-contaminated body fluids

Prophylactic therapy with anti-infectives is usually conducted using specific protocols that designate the duration of therapy. For example, zidovudine is given to an HIV-positive pregnant client beginning by week 14 of pregnancy until birth, after which the drug is given to the neonate for 6 weeks.

Host Factors That Affect Anti-Infective Selection

43.9 Client factors such as host defences, local tissue conditions, history of allergic reactions, age, pregnancy status, and genetics influence the choice of anti-infective.

Client factors such as host defences, local tissue conditions, history of allergic reactions, age, pregnancy status, and genetics influence the choice of anti-infective. The most important factor in selecting an appropriate antibiotic is to be certain that the microbe is sensitive to the bacteriocidal or bacteriostatic effects of the drug. Once the appropriate drug has been chosen, the nurse must consider a number of host factors that have the potential to significantly influence the success of anti-infective therapy.

Host Defences

Remember that the primary goal of antibiotic therapy is to kill enough of the pathogen or slow its growth such that natural body defences can overcome the invading agents. An anti-infective is rarely able to eliminate a pathogen without help from a functioning immune system. Clients with weakened immune defences often require the administration of prophylactic antibiotics. Should an infection occur in these clients, anti-infective therapy is more aggressive and prolonged. Examples of clients who may require this type of antibiotic therapy include those with AIDS and those with neutropenia caused by immunosuppressive or antineoplastic medications.

Local Tissue Conditions

Anti-infectives must be able to reach the area of infection in sufficient concentrations to be effective; therefore, local conditions at the infection site are important to the success of pharmacotherapy. Infections of the central nervous system (CNS) are particularly difficult to treat because many medications are unable to cross the blood-brain barrier to reach the brain and associated tissues. Injury or inflammation at an infection site can cause tissues to become acidic or anaerobic and have poor circulation. Excessive pus formation or large hematomas can impede drugs from reaching their targets. Pathogens such as mycobacteria, salmonella, toxoplasma, and listeria can reside intracellularly and thus be resistant to antibacterial action.

Factors that hinder the drug from reaching microbes will limit therapeutic success, and adjustments in treatment may be necessary. Increasing the dosage or switching to a different route of drug administration may be indicated. Occasionally, it is necessary to switch to a different antibiotic that is more effective for conditions specific to the infection site.

Allergy History

Although not common, serious hypersensitivity reactions to antibiotics may be fatal. The penicillins are the class of antibacterials that have the highest incidence of allergic reactions: between 0.7% and 10% of all clients who receive these drugs exhibit some degree of hypersensitivity.

Client assessment must always include a thorough medication history. A previous acute allergic incident with a drug is highly predictive of future hypersensitivity to the same medication. Because the client may have been exposed to an antibiotic unknowingly, such as through food products or moulds, allergic reactions can occur without any apparent previous exposure. If severe allergy to a drug is established, it is best to avoid all drugs in the same chemical class.

Other Host Factors

Age, pregnancy status, and genetics are additional factors that influence anti-infective pharmacotherapy. Infants and older adults are less able to metabolize and excrete antibiotics; therefore, doses are generally decreased. Because of polypharmacy in older clients, this group is more likely to be taking multiple drugs that could interact with antibiotics.

Some antibiotics are readily secreted in breast milk or cross the placenta. For example, tetracyclines taken by the mother can cause teeth discoloration in the newborn, and aminoglycosides can affect hearing. Some anti-infectives are pregnancy category D,

such as minocycline (Minocin), doxycycline (Vibramycin), neomycin, and streptomycin. The benefits of antibiotic use in pregnant or lactating women must be carefully weighed against the potential risks to the fetus and neonate.

A genetic absence of certain enzymes can lead to an inability of a client to metabolize antibiotics to their inactive forms. For example, clients with a deficiency of the enzyme glucose-6-phosphate dehydrogenase should not receive sulfonamides, chloramphenicol (Chloromycetin), or nalidixic acid due to the possibility of erythrocyte rupture.

Superinfections

43.10 Superinfections can occur when an anti-infective antibiotic kills host flora.

Microorganisms that normally inhabit the human body, or host flora, are present on the surface of the skin and in the upper respiratory, genitourinary, and intestinal tracts. Some of these microbes serve useful purposes by producing natural antibacterial substances or by breaking down toxic agents. The various host flora are in competition with each other for physical space and nutrients. This **microbial antagonism** helps to protect the host from being overrun by pathogenic organisms.

Antibiotics are unable to distinguish between host flora and pathogenic organisms. When an antibiotic kills the host's normal flora, additional nutrients and space are available for pathogenic microorganisms to grow unchecked. These new, secondary infections caused by antibiotic use are called **superinfections**, or suprainfections. The appearance of a new infection while receiving anti-infective therapy is highly suspicious of a superinfection. Signs and symptoms of superinfection commonly include diarrhea, bladder pain, painful urination, or abnormal vaginal discharges.

Broad-spectrum antibiotics are more likely to cause superinfections because they kill many microbial species, which sometimes includes host flora. Organisms that commonly cause superinfections are *Clostridium albicans* in the vagina, streptococci in the oral cavity, and *Clostridium difficile* in the colon.

Understanding the Chapter

Key Concepts Summary

The numbered key concepts provide a succinct summary of the important points from the corresponding numbered section within the chapter. If any of these points are not clear, refer to the numbered section within the chapter for review.

43.1 Pathogens cause disease due to their ability to invade tissues or secrete toxins.

43.2 Bacteria are described by their staining characteristics, shape, and ability to use oxygen.

43.3 Anti-infective drugs are classified by their susceptible organisms, chemical structures, and mechanisms of action.

43.4 Anti-infective drugs act by selectively targeting a pathogen's metabolism or life cycle.

43.5 Acquired resistance is a major clinical problem that is worsened by improper use of anti-infectives.

43.6 Careful selection of the correct antibiotic is essential for effective pharmacotherapy and to limit adverse effects.

43.7 Depending on the pathogen, anti-infective therapy may be conducted with a single drug or a combination of drugs.

43.8 Anti-infectives may be administered to prevent infections.

43.9 Client factors such as host defences, local tissue conditions, history of allergic reactions, age, pregnancy status, and genetics influence the choice of anti-infective.

43.10 Superinfections can occur when an anti-infective antibiotic kills host flora.

PROTOTYPE DRUGS

PENICILLINS
    Pr *penicillin G potassium*

CEPHALOSPORINS
    Pr *cefotaxime (Claforan)*

TETRACYCLINES
    Pr *tetracycline*

MACROLIDES
    Pr *erythromycin (Eryc)*

AMINOGLYCOSIDES
    Pr *gentamicin (Garamycin)*

FLUOROQUINOLONES
    Pr *ciprofloxacin (Cipro)*

SULFONAMIDES
    Pr *trimethoprim-sulfa-methoxazole (Bactrim, Septra)*

MISCELLANEOUS ANTI-BACTERIALS
    Pr *vancomycin (Vancocin)*

ANTITUBERCULAR AGENTS
    Pr *isoniazid*
    Pr *dapsone*

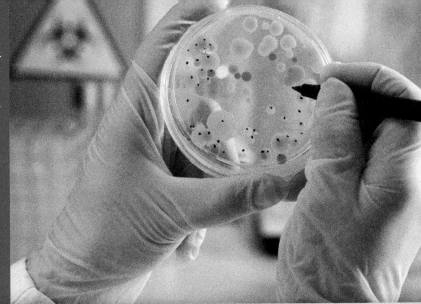

Andreas Reh/Vetta/Getty Images

CHAPTER 44

Pharmacotherapy of Bacterial Infections

LEARNING OUTCOMES

After reading this chapter, the student should be able to:

1. Identify drug classes used for treating bacterial infections.
2. Explain the therapeutic action of each class of anti-infective drug in relation to the pathophysiology of infection.
3. Identify the mechanism of development and symptoms of super-infections caused by anti-infective therapy.
4. Explain how the pharmacotherapy of tuberculosis differs from that of other infections.
5. Discuss the role of the nurse regarding the non-pharmacological management of bacterial infections, including prevention, promotion of healing, and client teaching.
6. Describe the nurse's role in the pharmacological management of clients who are receiving drugs for bacterial infections.
7. For each of the drug classes listed in Prototype Drugs, identify a representative drug and explain its mechanism of action, therapeutic effects, and important adverse effects.
8. Describe and explain, based on pharmacological principles, the rationale for nursing assessment, planning, and interventions for clients with bacterial infections.
9. Use the nursing process to care for clients who are receiving drug therapy for bacterial infections.

CHAPTER OUTLINE

▸ Antibacterial Agents
▸ Penicillins
  ▸ Pharmacotherapy with Penicillins
▸ Cephalosporins
  ▸ Pharmacotherapy with Cephalosporins
▸ Tetracyclines
  ▸ Pharmacotherapy with Tetracyclines
▸ Macrolides
  ▸ Pharmacotherapy with Macrolides
▸ Aminoglycosides
  ▸ Pharmacotherapy with Aminoglycosides
▸ Fluoroquinolones
  ▸ Pharmacotherapy with Fluoroquinolones

The discovery and development of the first anti-infective drugs in the mid-1900s was a milestone in the field of medicine. Humans no longer die in massive numbers from infectious organisms such as *Yersinia pestis*, which killed 25% of the known human population in the 14th century due to the bubonic plague. This chapter examines the penicillins, cephalosporins, and other antibiotic drugs that are used in the pharmacotherapy of bacterial infections.

ANTIBACTERIAL AGENTS

Antibacterial agents form a large number of chemical classes. Although drugs within a class have similarities in their mechanisms and spectrum of activity, each is slightly different and learning the differences among and therapeutic applications of antibacterial agents can be challenging. Basic nursing assessments and interventions apply to all antibiotic therapies; however, the plan of care should be individualized based on the client's condition, the infection, and the antibacterial agent prescribed.

PENICILLINS

Although not the first **anti-infective** discovered, penicillin was the first mass-produced **antibiotic**. Isolated from the fungus *Penicillium* in 1941, the drug quickly became a miracle product by preventing thousands of deaths from infections. Penicillins are indicated for the treatment of pneumonia; meningitis; skin, bone, and joint infections; stomach infections; blood and heart valve infections; gas gangrene; tetanus; anthrax; and sickle cell anemia in infants. The penicillins are listed in Table 44.1.

NCLEX Success Tips

Prior to administering penicillin, the nurse should determine whether the client is allergic to the medication. If the client isn't sure he or she is allergic, the nurse should hold off on administering the medication and notify the physician. Many clients can't act as their own advocates; they rely on nurses to protect their rights. If a client is allergic to penicillin, a nurse should alert the pharmacist and label the client's chart appropriately.

Ampicillin and other antibiotics can cause anaphylactic reaction if the client is allergic to it. To reverse anaphylactic shock, the nurse first should administer epinephrine, a potent bronchodilator, as ordered. The physician is likely to order additional medications, such as antihistamines and corticosteroids; if these medications do not relieve the respiratory compromise associated with anaphylaxis, the nurse should prepare to intubate the client. No antidote for penicillin exists.

TABLE 44.1 Penicillins

Drug	Route and Adult Dose
Narrow Spectrum/Pencillinase Sensitive	
penicillin G benzathine (Bicillin L-A)	Intramuscular (IM), 1.2–2.4 million units as a single dose
penicillin G procaine (Wycillin)	IM, 600 000–1.2 million units every day (qd)
penicillin V (Pen-VK)	Orally (PO), 125–500 mg every 6–8 hours
Narrow Spectrum/Penicillinase Resistant	
cloxacillin (Orbenin)	PO, 250–500 mg every 6 hours (q6h)
dicloxacillin (Diclocil)	PO, 125–500 mg four times a day (qid)
Broad Spectrum (Aminopenicillins)	
amoxicillin (Amoxil)	PO, 250–500 every 8–12 hours
amoxicillin-clavulanate (Clavulin)	PO, 250 or 500 mg tablet (each with 125 mg clavulanic acid) every 8–12 hours (q8–12h)
ampicillin	PO, 250–500 mg twice a day (bid)
Extended Spectrum	
carbenicillin	PO, 382–764 mg qid
piperacillin	IM/IV, 6–8 g/day (100–125 mg/kg/day) in divided doses every 6–12 hours
piperacillin and tazobactam (Tazocin)	IV, 3.375 g every 6 hours or 4.5 g every 6 to 8 hours (max 18 g/day)

Before giving cephalosporins, the nurse should notify the physician if the client is allergic to penicillin.

Penicillin should be given on an empty stomach.

Pharmacotherapy with Penicillins

44.1 Penicillins kill bacteria by disrupting the cell wall. Allergies occur most frequently with the penicillins.

Penicillins kill bacteria by disrupting their cell walls. Many bacterial cell walls contain a substance called **penicillin-binding protein**

◀ **Cultural Beliefs and Antibacterials**

People hold beliefs that affect their readiness to adopt prescription drugs and therapies. For example, some Aboriginal Canadians may choose to access a sweat lodge to restore health. Many Aboriginals believe that sweating helps to open clogged pores, stimulate the natural flow of sweat, and rid the body of wastes.

Many ethnic groups, including some Chinese, Africans, and Hispanics, believe that illness is caused by an imbalance in hot and cold. In a healthy individual, hot and cold are in balance; when an imbalance occurs, disease results. Illnesses are classified as either hot or cold. For example, sore throat and diarrhea are considered hot diseases; colds, upper respiratory infections, arthritis, and rheumatism are considered cold diseases. Treatment in such cultures is to restore the body's balance through the addition or subtraction of herbs, foods, or medications that are classified as either hot or cold. To treat a hot disease, medications or herbs considered cold are used. For example, penicillin is considered a hot medicine, but amoxicillin is less hot. Using acetaminophen with amoxicillin makes it cooler.

that serves as a receptor for penicillin. Penicillin weakens the cell wall and allows water to enter, thus killing the organism. Human cells do not contain cell walls; therefore, the actions of the penicillins are specific to bacterial cells.

The portion of the chemical structure of penicillin that is responsible for its antibacterial activity is the **beta-lactam ring**. Some bacteria secrete an enzyme, called **beta-lactamase**, or **penicillinase**, that splits the beta-lactam ring. This structural change causes these bacteria to become resistant to the effects of most penicillins. Since their discovery, large numbers of resistant bacterial strains have appeared that now limit the therapeutic usefulness of the penicillins. The action of penicillinase is illustrated in Figure 44.1.

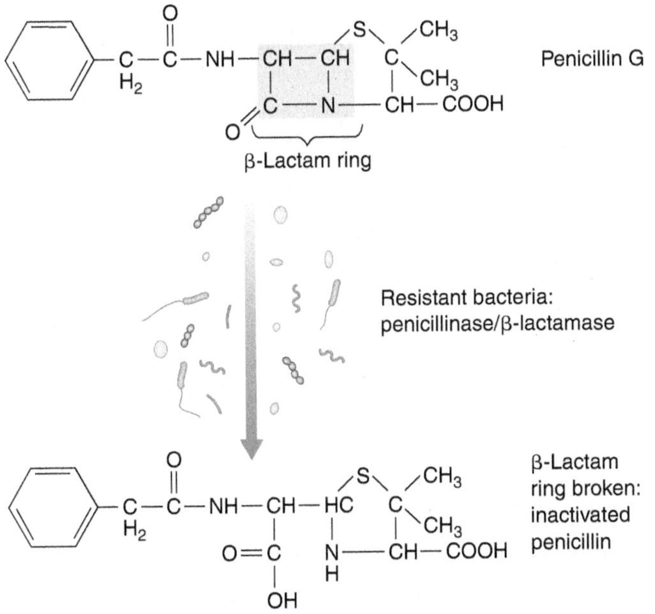

Figure 44.1 Action of penicillinase.

Chemical modifications to the original penicillin molecule produced drugs that offer several advantages. Oxacillin and cloxacillin (Orbenin) are effective against penicillinase-producing bacteria and are called penicillinase-resistant penicillins. The aminopenicillins, such as ampicillin and amoxicillin (Amoxil), are effective against a wider range of microorganisms and are called broad-spectrum penicillins. The extended-spectrum penicillins, such as carbenicillin and piperacillin, are effective against even more microbes, including *Pseudomonas, Enterobacter, Klebsiella,* and *Bacteroides fragilis.*

Although each drug in this class has certain unique properties, some generalizations can be made about the penicillins:

- Most are more effective against gram-positive bacteria, although a few have activity against gram-negative bacteria.
- Most have a narrow spectrum of antimicrobial activity.
- They are widely distributed to most body tissues, although only small amounts reach the cerebrospinal fluid (CSF).
- Nearly all are rapidly excreted by the kidneys.
- Most have short half-lives.

In general, the adverse effects of penicillins are minor; they are one of the safest classes of antibiotic. This has contributed to their widespread use for more than 50 years. Allergy to penicillin is the most common adverse effect. Common symptoms of penicillin allergy include rash and fever. Incidence of anaphylaxis ranges from 0.04% to 2%. Allergy to one penicillin increases the risk of allergy to other drugs in the same class.

Nursing Considerations

The role of the nurse in drug therapy with penicillins involves careful monitoring of the client's condition and providing education as it relates to the prescribed drug regimen. Since allergies occur more frequently with penicillins than with any other antibiotic class, it is essential to assess previous drug reactions to penicillin prior to administration. If the client has a history of severe penicillin allergic reaction, cephalosporins should be avoided due to risk for cross-sensitization. Specimens for culture and sensitivity should be obtained prior to the start of antibiotic therapy.

Vital signs, electrolytes, and renal function tests should be obtained prior to and during therapy. Because some penicillin preparations contain high levels of sodium and potassium salts, monitor the client for hyperkalemia and hypernatremia prior to and during therapy. Cardiac status should be monitored, including electrocardiogram (ECG) changes, due to the possibility of worsening an existing heart failure related to the increased sodium intake. In addition, the client should be monitored for indications of response to therapy, including reduced fever, normal white blood cell (WBC) count, absence of symptoms such as cough, and improved appetite.

After parenteral administration of penicillins, the client should be observed for 30 minutes for possible allergic reactions, especially with the first dose. Sensitivity may be immediate, accelerated, or delayed.

Clients with impaired renal function may require smaller doses because the majority of penicillin is excreted through the kidneys. Penicillins should be used with caution during lactation because the drug enters breast milk. Monitor for bleeding in those clients on anticoagulant therapy who are receiving high doses of parenteral carbenicillin or piperacillin because these drugs may interfere with platelet aggregation.

A small number of clients may develop a serious **superinfection** called antibiotic-associated pseudomembranous colitis (AAPMC). In this condition, the organism *Clostridium difficile* secretes a toxin that causes severe inflammation of the bowel wall, followed by necrosis. This results in a potentially life-threatening infection. Clients with this condition have two to five semi-solid or liquid stools per day. Antidiarrheal drugs should not be administered because these agents cause the toxin to be retained in the bowel. When AAPMC occurs, antibiotic therapy should be discontinued, and fluid and electrolyte replacement is essential.

As with other antibiotics, penicillins may cause other, less severe superinfections with symptoms such as abdominal cramping and diarrhea. Replacement of natural colon flora with probiotic supplements or cultured dairy products such as yogurt or buttermilk may help to alleviate symptoms. Superinfections in elderly, debilitated, or immunosuppressed clients may be serious and require immediate interventions.

Client education as it relates to penicillins should include goals, reasons for obtaining baseline data, and possible side effects. The following are important points to include when teaching clients regarding penicillins:

- Wear a MedicAlert bracelet if allergic to penicillins.
- Take penicillin V (Pen-VK), amoxicillin, and amoxicillin-clavulanate (Clavulin) with meals to decrease gastrointestinal (GI) distress. Take all other penicillins with a full glass of water, 1 hour before or 2 hours after meals to increase absorption.
- Oral penicillin G should be taken with water because acidic fruit juice can inactivate the drug's antibacterial activity.
- Do not discontinue the drug regimen before the complete prescription has been taken.
- Avoid use of penicillins while breastfeeding, unless the mother has consulted a healthcare provider (physician, pharmacist).
- Consult with the nurse about taking probiotic supplements or cultured dairy products during antibiotic therapy.
- Report significant side effects immediately, including severe abdominal or stomach cramps, abdominal tenderness, convulsions, decreased urine output, and severe watery or bloody diarrhea.

See Nursing Process Focus: Clients Receiving Antibacterial Therapy (page 537) for the nursing process applied to all antibacterials.

PROTOTYPE DRUG	Penicillin G Potassium

Actions and Uses: Similar to penicillin V, penicillin G is a drug of choice against streptococci, pneumococci, and staphylococci organisms that do not produce penicillinase. It is also a medication of choice for gonorrhea and syphilis caused by susceptible strains. Penicillin V is more acid stable; more than 70% is absorbed after an oral dose compared to the 15% to 30% from penicillin G. Because of its low oral absorption, penicillin G is often given by the IV or IM routes. Penicillinase-producing organisms inactivate both penicillin G and penicillin V.

Pharmacokinetics: Penicillin G is administered IM or IV. About 60% is protein bound. It is widely distributed, crosses the placenta, and enters breast milk. It is excreted mostly unchanged in urine. Half-life is 30 minutes.

Administration Alerts:

- After parenteral administration, observe for possible allergic reactions for 30 minutes, especially following the first dose.
- Do not mix penicillin and aminoglycosides in the same IV solution. Give IV medications 1 hour apart to prevent interactions.
- Penicillin G is pregnancy category B.

Adverse Effects and Interactions: Penicillin G has few side effects. Anaphylaxis is the most serious adverse effect.

Diarrhea, nausea, and vomiting are the most common adverse effects and can cause serious complications in certain populations such as children and older adults. Pain at the injection site may occur, and superinfections are possible. Since penicillin G is excreted extensively by the kidneys, renal disease can result in excessive accumulation of the drug.

Penicillin G may decrease the efficacy of oral contraceptives. Colestipol (Colestid) taken with this medication will decrease the absorption of penicillin. Potassium-sparing diuretics may cause hyperkalemia when administered with penicillin G potassium.

CEPHALOSPORINS

Isolated shortly after the penicillins, the four generations of cephalosporins comprise the largest antibiotic class. Like the penicillins, the cephalosporins contain a beta-lactam ring that is mostly responsible for their antimicrobial activity. The cephalosporins are bactericidal and act by attaching to penicillin-binding protein to inhibit cell wall synthesis. The cephalosporins are listed in Table 44.2.

Over decades of use, many bacterial strains have developed resistance to the cephalosporins. Like the penicillins, the primary mechanism of resistance is the secretion of beta-lactamase enzymes (sometimes called cephalosporinases). Although third-generation agents were initially unaffected by beta-lactamase, resistant strains that can inactivate drugs in this generation have been identified. None of the cephalosporins has significant activity against methicillin-resistant *Staphylococcus aureus* (MRSA) or penicillin-resistant *Streptococcus pneumoniae*.

In general, the cephalosporins are safe drugs with adverse effects similar to those of the penicillins. Allergic reactions are the most common adverse effect. Although cephalosporins are sometimes prescribed for clients who are allergic to penicillin, nurses must be aware that 5% to 10% of clients who are allergic to penicillin will also exhibit hypersensitivity to cephalosporins. Despite this small incidence of cross-allergy, the cephalosporins offer a reasonable alternative for clients who are unable to take penicillin. Cephalosporins are contraindicated, however, for clients who have experienced anaphylaxis following penicillin exposure.

In addition to allergy, rash and GI complaints are common adverse effects of cephalosporins. Nurses should continually assess for the presence of superinfections. Because cephalosporins are secreted in small amounts in breast milk, they should be used with caution in nursing mothers.

TABLE 44.2 Cephalosporins

Drug	Route and Adult Dose
First Generation	
cefadroxil	PO, 500 mg–1 g qd–bid (max 2 g/day)
cefazolin (Ancef)	IV/IM, 250 mg–2 g three times a day (tid) (max 12 g/day)
cephalexin (Keflex)	PO, 250–1000 mg every 6 hours (max 4 g/day)
Second Generation	
cefaclor (Ceclor)	PO, 250–500 mg tid
cefotetan (Cefotan)	IV/IM, 1–2 g q12h
cefoxitin	IV/IM, 1–2 g every 6–8 hours (q6–8h) (max 12 g/day)
cefprozil (Cefzil)	PO, 250–500 mg qd–bid
cefuroxime (Ceftin)	PO, 250–500 mg bid
Third Generation	
cefdinir (Omnicef)	PO, 300 mg bid or 600 mg qd
cefixime (Suprax)	PO, 400 mg qd
Pr cefotaxime (Claforan)	IV/IM, 1–2 g bid–tid (max 12 g/day)
ceftazidime (Fortaz)	IV/IM, 1–2 mg q8–12h, up to 2 g q6h (max 6 g/day)
ceftriaxone (Rocephin)	IV/IM, 1–2 g every 12–24 hours (q12–24h) (max 4 g/day)
Fourth Generation	
cefepime (Maxipime)	IV, 2 g every 8 hours

Nearly all cephalosporins are eliminated by the kidneys. Earlier-generation cephalosporins exhibited kidney toxicity, but this is diminished with the later-generation drugs in this class. Clients with pre-existing renal impairment or those who are concurrently receiving nephrotoxic drugs should be monitored carefully during therapy with any cephalosporin. Kidney function tests should be evaluated on a regular basis.

Other adverse effects are specific to particular cephalosporins. For example, cefotetan interferes with vitamin K metabolism and increases the risk for bleeding due to hypoprothrombinemia. Nurses must carefully monitor prothrombin time (PT) in clients who are taking these drugs, particularly those who are concurrently taking anticoagulants. Cefotetan (Cefotan) produces a disulfiram (Antabuse)-like reaction when taken concurrently with alcohol. Cephalosporins cause pain at IM injection sites, and thrombophlebitis can occur when given IV. More than half of the cephalosporins are only administered parenterally.

NCLEX Success Tips

When the surgeon prescribes an antibiotic to be given at a specific time related to the scheduled time of the surgical procedure, it is imperative that the nurse give antibiotic on time. Legally, the nurse considers 30 minutes on either side of the scheduled time to be acceptable for administering medications.

A client who has an allergy to penicillin may have a cross-sensitivity to cephalosporin, and the drug should be given with caution. The nurse should ask the client whether he or she has taken cephalosporin before. The nurse should inform the pharmacy of the client's allergy after asking the client about prior use of cephalosporin. The medication should not be administered until the nurse first inquires about the client's exposure to cephalosporin and then consults the pharmacist or physician.

The nurse should monitor the blood levels of antibiotics, WBC count, serum creatinine, and blood urea nitrogen (BUN) in clients with renal problems receiving ceftriaxone (Rocephin). The kidneys are responsible for filtering out the ceftriaxone sodium. Increased levels of these laboratory values should be reported to the physician immediately.

Pharmacotherapy with Cephalosporins

44.2 The cephalosporins are similar in structure and function to the penicillins and are one of the most widely prescribed anti-infective classes. Cross-sensitivity may exist with the penicillins in some clients.

More than 20 cephalosporins are available and classified by their "generation." First-generation cephalosporins contain a beta-lactam ring; bacteria producing beta-lactamase will usually be resistant to these agents. The second-generation cephalosporins are more potent, more resistant to beta-lactamase, and exhibit a broader spectrum than the first-generation drugs. The third-generation cephalosporins generally have a longer duration of action, have an even broader spectrum, and are resistant to beta-lactamase. Third-generation cephalosporins are sometimes the drugs of choice against infections by *Pseudomonas, Klebsiella, Neisseria, Salmonella, Proteus,* and *Haemophilus influenzae.* Newer, fourth-generation drugs are more effective against organisms that have developed resistance to earlier cephalosporins. Third- and fourth-generation agents are capable of entering the CSF to treat central nervous system (CNS) infections. There are not always clear distinctions among the generations.

The primary therapeutic use of the cephalosporins is for gram-negative infections and for clients who cannot tolerate the less expensive penicillins. Side effects are similar to those of the penicillins, with allergic reactions being the most common adverse effect. It is common for clients with a mild allergy to penicillin to be given a cephalosporin. Earlier-generation cephalosporins exhibited kidney toxicity, but this is diminished with the newer drugs.

Nursing Considerations

The role of the nurse in cephalosporin therapy involves careful monitoring of the client's condition and providing education as it relates to the prescribed drug regimen. The cephalosporins are generally the treatment of choice for clients with gram-negative infections. Assess the client for the presence or history of bleeding disorders because cephalosporins may reduce prothrombin levels through interference with vitamin K metabolism. Liver function should be assessed because liver function is important in vitamin K production. Renal function should be assessed because most cephalosporins are excreted by the kidney. Culture and sensitivity testing should be performed before and during therapy.

Due to elimination of cephalosporins through the kidneys, it is necessary to monitor intake and output, BUN, and serum creatinine. If the client is concurrently taking nonsteroidal anti-inflammatory drugs (NSAIDs), monitor blood coagulation studies because cephalosporins increase the effect of platelet inhibition.

Cephalosporins should be used with caution in pregnant or lactating clients, as they can be transferred to the fetus and infant. Doses should be adjusted appropriately in clients with impaired renal or hepatic function. Certain cephalosporins will cause a disulfiram-like reaction when alcoholic beverages are consumed. Typical reactions include severe vomiting, weakness, blurred vision, and profound hypotension.

Cephalosporins may predispose clients to **pseudomembranous colitis (PMC)**, especially if there is pre-existing GI pathology. Less severe superinfections may also occur. Eating cultured dairy products such as yogurt or kefir may suppress superinfections.

Client education as it relates to cephalosporins should include goals, reasons for obtaining baseline data, and possible side effects. The following are important points to include when teaching clients regarding cephalosporins:

- Avoid alcohol use while taking cephalosporins.
- Eat cultured dairy products to help discourage superinfections.
- Report significant side effects, including diarrhea, onset of flu-like symptoms, blistering or peeling of skin, seizures, decreased urine output, hearing loss, skin rash, breathing difficulty, and unusual tiredness or weakness.

See Nursing Process Focus: Clients Receiving Antibacterial Therapy (page 537) for the nursing process applied to all antibacterials.

PROTOTYPE DRUG | **Cefotaxime (Claforan)**

Actions and Uses: Cefotaxime is a third-generation cephalosporin with a broad spectrum of activity against gram-negative organisms. It is effective against many bacteria that have developed resistance to earlier-generation cephalosporins and to other classes of anti-infectives. Cefotaxime exhibits bactericidal activity by inhibiting cell wall synthesis. It is prescribed for serious infections of the lower respiratory tract, CNS, genitourinary system, bones, and joints. It may also be used for blood infections such as bacteremia or septicemia. Like many other cephalosporins, cefotaxime is not absorbed from the GI tract and must be given by the IM or IV route.

Pharmacokinetics: Cefotaxime is well absorbed after IM administration. It is widely distributed, crosses the placenta, enters breast milk, and enters CSF. It is partly metabolized by the liver. About 50% is excreted unchanged in urine. Half-life is about 1 hour.

Administration Alerts:
- IM injections should be administered deep into a large muscle mass to prevent injury to surrounding tissues.
- Cefotaxime is pregnancy category B.

Adverse Effects and Interactions: For most clients, cefotaxime and the other cephalosporins are safe medications. Hypersensitivity is the most common adverse effect, although symptoms may include only a minor rash and itching. Anaphylaxis is possible, so the nurse should be alert for this reaction. GI-related side

effects such as diarrhea, vomiting, and nausea may occur. Some clients experience considerable pain at the injection site.

Cefotaxime interacts with probenecid, causing decreased renal elimination of the drug. Alcohol interacts with cefotaxime to produce a disulfiram-like reaction. Cefotaxime interacts with NSAIDs to cause an increase in platelet inhibition.

TABLE 44.3	Tetracyclines
Drug	**Route and Adult Dose**
demeclocycline (Declomycin)	PO, 150 mg q6h or 300 mg q12h (max 2.4 g/day)
doxycycline (Vibramycin)	PO/IV, 100 mg bid on day 1, then 100 mg qd (max 200 mg/day)
minocycline (Minocin)	PO, 200 mg as one dose followed by 100 mg bid (max 400 mg/day)
Pr tetracycline	PO, 250–500 mg bid–qid (max 2 g/day)

TETRACYCLINES

The first tetracyclines were extracted from *Streptomyces* soil microorganisms in 1948. Tetracyclines exert a bacteriostatic effect by selectively inhibiting bacterial protein synthesis. The four tetracyclines are effective against a large number of different gram-negative and gram-positive organisms and have one of the broadest spectrums of any class of antibiotic. The tetracyclines are listed in Table 44.3.

NCLEX Success Tip

Tetracycline should not be administered to children younger than age 8 because it may cause enamel hypoplasia and permanent yellowish-grey to brownish tooth discoloration.

Pharmacotherapy with Tetracyclines

44.3 Tetracyclines have some of the broadest spectrums, but they are drugs of choice for relatively few diseases.

The widespread use of tetracyclines in the 1950s and 1960s resulted in a large number of resistant bacterial strains that now limit their therapeutic utility. They are drugs of choice for only a few diseases: Rocky Mountain spotted fever, typhus, cholera, Lyme disease, ulcers caused by *Helicobacter pylori*, and chlamydial infections. They are occasionally used for the treatment of acne vulgaris.

Tetracyclines exert a bacteriostatic effect by selectively inhibiting bacterial protein synthesis. Tetracyclines bind to the 30S bacterial ribosome, thereby preventing the addition of amino acids to the growing polypeptide chain. Resistance to tetracyclines develops when bacteria prevent tetracyclines from concentrating inside their cells, or when their ribosome shape is altered so that the antibiotic can no longer bind. In addition to having ribosomes with different structures, human cells lack the active transport system required for tetracyclines to enter their cells. At high doses, however, tetracyclines begin to exert toxicity on human cells.

All tetracyclines have the same spectrum of antimicrobial activity and similar adverse effects. Several have topical and parenteral formulations. They are sometimes classified by their duration of action as short acting, intermediate acting, or long acting.

Most PO tetracyclines should be taken on an empty stomach to maximize their absorption. Because gastric distress is relatively common with drugs in this class, clients will often take tetracyclines with food. However, these drugs bind metal ions such as calcium, magnesium, aluminium, and iron, and tetracyclines should not be taken with milk or iron supplements. Food, milk, or other dairy products can reduce drug absorption by 50% or more. Food does not interfere with absorption of the longer-acting drugs doxycycline (Vibramycin) and minocycline (Minocin).

Because most tetracyclines are incompletely absorbed, they remain in the GI tract in high concentrations, often killing normal flora in the colon. Tetracycline-induced diarrhea is common and could indicate toxic effects on normal flora or a bowel superinfection. The presence of diarrhea must be monitored carefully due to the possibility of pseudomembranous colitis (PMC). Caused by *Clostridium difficile*, this is a rare though potentially severe disorder resulting from therapy with tetracyclines and other classes of antibiotics.

When administered parenterally or in high doses, certain tetracyclines can cause hepatotoxicity, especially in clients with pre-existing liver disease. Some clients experience photosensitivity during therapy, making their skin especially susceptible to sunburn. Photosensitivity may appear as exaggerated sunburn within minutes to hours of exposure and is often accompanied by a tingling, burning sensation. Because of their broad spectrum, superinfections due to *Candida albicans* are relatively common. Women who are on oral contraceptives may be more susceptible to vaginal candidiasis. Tetracyclines are usually contraindicated in pregnant or lactating women and in children under the age of 8 years because these drugs cause yellow-brown teeth discoloration and may slow the overall growth rate in fetuses or children.

NCLEX Success Tip

Oral contraceptives may interact with other medications, and the effectiveness may be decreased if the client is prescribed ampicillin, tetracycline, or anticonvulsants, such as phenytoin (Dilantin).

Nursing Considerations

The role of the nurse in tetracycline therapy involves careful monitoring of the client's condition and providing education as it relates to the prescribed drug regimen. Assess the client for the presence or history of acne vulgaris, actinomycosis, anthrax, malaria, syphilis, urinary tract infection (UTI), rickettsial infection, and Lyme disease. This class of antibiotic can treat all of these disorders. Prior to administration, assess for a history of hypersensitivity to tetracyclines. If possible, culture and sensitivity results should be obtained before therapy is initiated. Laboratory tests, including complete blood count (CBC) and kidney and liver function studies, should be done. Monitor the client's body temperature, WBC count, and culture/sensitivity results to determine the effectiveness of the treatment as well as to observe for superinfections.

Tetracycline decreases the effectiveness of oral contraceptives, so female clients should use an alternate method of birth control while taking the medication. Tetracyclines should be used with caution in clients who have impaired kidney or liver function.

Oral and perineal hygiene care is extremely important to decrease the risk for superinfections due to *Candida*. Tetracyclines cause photosensitivity, which may lead to tingling and burning of the skin, similar to sunburn. Photosensitivity reaction may appear within a few minutes to hours after sun exposure and may persist for several days after pharmacotherapy is completed.

Client education as it relates to tetracyclines should include goals, reasons for obtaining baseline data such as tests for culture and sensitivity, and possible side effects. The following are important points to include when teaching clients regarding tetracyclines:

* Do not save medication because toxic effects may occur if it is taken past the expiration date.
* Do not take these medications with milk products, iron supplements, magnesium-containing laxatives, or antacids.
* Wait 1 to 3 hours after taking tetracyclines before taking antacids.
* Take tetracyclines at least 2 hours before or after taking lipid-lowering drugs such as colestipol and cholestyramine (Questran, Olestyr).
* Report significant side effects immediately, including increased photosensitivity of skin to sunlight, abdominal pain, loss of appetite, nausea and vomiting, visual changes, and yellowing of skin.

See Nursing Process Focus: Clients Receiving Antibacterial Therapy (page 537) for the nursing process applied to all antibacterials.

PROTOTYPE DRUG | Tetracycline

Actions and Uses: Tetracycline is effective against a broad range of gram-positive and gram-negative organisms, including chlamydiae, rickettsiae, and mycoplasma. Tetracycline is given orally, though it has a short half-life that may require administration four times per day. Topical and oral preparations are available for treating acne. An IM preparation is available; injections may cause local irritation and be extremely painful.

Pharmacokinetics: Tetracycline is mostly absorbed after PO administration. It is widely distributed, crosses the placenta, enters breast milk, and enters CSF. It is excreted unchanged in urine. Half-life is 6 to 12 hours.

Administration Alerts:
* Administer oral drug with a full glass of water to decrease esophageal and GI irritation.
* Administer antacids and tetracycline 1 to 3 hours apart.
* Administer antilipidemic agents at least 2 hours before or after tetracycline.
* Tetracycline is pregnancy category D.

Adverse Effects and Interactions: Being a **broad-spectrum antibiotic**, tetracycline has a tendency to affect vaginal, oral, and intestinal flora and cause superinfections. Tetracycline irritates the GI mucosa and may cause nausea, vomiting, epigastric burning, and diarrhea. Diarrhea may be severe enough to cause discontinuation of therapy. Other common side effects include discoloration of the teeth and photosensitivity.

Oral tetracycline interacts with milk products, iron supplements, magnesium-containing laxatives, and antacids. These products reduce the absorption and serum levels of tetracyclines. Tetracycline binds with certain lipid-lowering drugs (colestipol and cholestyramine), thereby decreasing the antibiotic's absorption. This drug decreases the effectiveness of oral contraceptives.

MACROLIDES

Erythromycin (Eryc), the first macrolide antibiotic, was isolated from *Streptomyces* in a soil sample in 1952. The macrolide antibiotics inhibit bacterial protein synthesis and may be either bactericidal or bacteriostatic depending on the dose and the target organism.

Pharmacotherapy with Macrolides

44.4 The macrolides are safe alternatives to penicillin for many diseases.

Macrolides are considered safe alternatives to penicillin, although they are drugs of first choice for relatively few diseases. Common uses of macrolides include the treatment of whooping cough, Legionnaire's disease, and infections by *Streptococcus*, *H. influenzae*, *Mycoplasma pneumoniae*, and *Chlamydia*. The macrolides are listed in Table 44.4.

The macrolides inhibit bacterial protein synthesis by binding to the 50S ribosomal subunit, thus preventing movement of the ribosome along the messenger RNA (mRNA). Macrolides do not bind to human ribosomes, thus offering a degree of selective toxicity. These drugs are usually bacteriostatic, though they may be bacteriocidal depending on the dose and the target organism.

The newer macrolides have longer half-lives and generally cause less GI irritation than erythromycin, which is the original drug from which macrolides were synthesized. Azithromycin (Zithromax) has an extended half-life such that it can be administered for only 5 days rather than the 10-day therapy required for most antibiotics. A single dose of azithromycin is effective against *N. gonorrhoeae*. The brief duration of therapy is thought to increase client adherence and to offset the added cost of azithromycin.

Like most of the older antibiotics, macrolide-resistant strains are becoming more common. Many organisms develop resistance to macrolides by pumping it out of the cell before the antibiotic has a chance to reach an effective concentration. In some cases, bacteria have modified the shape of their 50S ribosomal subunit so that it no longer binds the drug.

The macrolides are well tolerated and considered to be one of the safest antibiotic classes. The most common adverse effects are GI related and include nausea, vomiting, abdominal cramping, and diarrhea. These GI symptoms occur whether the drug is administered PO or IV. Taking the drug with food can significantly inhibit the absorption of azithromycin suspension. Thus these drugs should be taken on an empty stomach.

Many macrolides have an enteric coating, which serves two purposes. First, the coating allows the drug to dissolve in the small intestine rather than the stomach, causing less gastric irritation. Second, the macrolides are inactivated in gastric acid, and the enteric coating allows it to avoid destruction and reach the small intestine where they are readily absorbed in the alkaline environment.

Macrolides are metabolized and concentrated in the liver and excreted into bile. Because macrolides decrease the hepatic metabolism of other drugs, a number of drug-drug interactions are possible. When macrolides prevent the conversion of drugs to their less active form, the serum levels of these other drugs will increase and cause potential toxicity. For example, warfarin (Coumadin) is extensively metabolized to its inactive form in the liver. If given concurrently with erythromycin, the destruction of warfarin is diminished and greater amounts of "active" warfarin remain in the blood for longer periods. Because warfarin increases bleeding time, this could result in prolonged bleeding in a client. In general, doses of drugs that are metabolized in the liver should be reduced, or at least carefully monitored, if they are given concurrently with macrolides.

Nursing Considerations

The role of the nurse in macrolide therapy involves careful monitoring of the client's condition and providing education as it relates to the prescribed drug regimen. Assess for the presence of respiratory infection, GI tract infection, skin and soft tissue infections, otitis media, gonorrhea, non-gonococcal urethritis, and *H. pylori* treatment. Macrolides are indicated for the pharmacological treatment of these disorders. The client should be examined for history of cardiac disorders, as macrolides may exacerbate existing heart disease. Due to toxic effects on the liver, hepatic enzymes should be monitored with certain macrolides such as erythromycin estolate.

The client should be assessed for a history of hypersensitivity to macrolides. Rashes or other signs of hypersensitivity should be reported immediately. Culture and sensitivity testing should be performed before initiation of macrolide therapy.

Macrolides are contraindicated in clients with hepatic disease since the liver metabolizes these drugs. These agents should be used with caution in pregnant or breastfeeding women to avoid harm to the fetus or newborn.

Multiple drug-drug interactions occur with macrolides. Certain anesthetic agents (alfentanil [Alfenta]) and anticonvulsant drugs (carbamazepine [Tegretol]) may interact with macrolides to cause

TABLE 44.4   Macrolides

Drug	Route and Adult Dose
azithromycin (Zithromax)	PO, 500 mg for one dose, then 250 mg qd; IV, 500 mg qd for one or two doses, then 250 mg qd
clarithromycin (Biaxin)	PO, 250–500 mg every 12 hours, or 1000 mg (extended release) daily
Pr erythromycin (Eryc)	PO, base: 250–500 mg every 6–12 hours (max 4 g/day)
	IV, 15–20 mg/kg/day divided every 6 hours or 500 mg to 1 g every 6 hours (max 4 g/day)

serum drug levels to rise and result in toxicity. Macrolides should be used cautiously with clients who are receiving cyclosporine (Sandimmune, Neoral), and drug levels must be monitored due to the risk for nephrotoxicity. Clients who are receiving warfarin need to be monitored closely because macrolides may decrease warfarin metabolism and excretion. Coagulation studies, such as international normalized ratio (INR), need to be monitored more frequently, as dosage adjustments may be required. Clarithromycin (Biaxin) and zidovudine (AZT, Retrovir) must be administered at least 4 hours apart to avoid interaction, which results in a delayed time for peak concentration of zidovudine.

Client education as it relates to macrolides should include goals, reasons for obtaining baseline data such as culture and sensitivity tests, and possible side effects. The following are important points to include when teaching clients regarding macrolides:

- Do not discontinue the medication before the complete prescription has been taken.
- Do not take with or immediately before or after fruit juices.
- Notify the healthcare provider before taking other prescription or over-the-counter (OTC) medications or herbal products because macrolides interact with many substances.
- Report significant side effects immediately, including severe skin rash, itching, or hives; difficulty breathing or swallowing; yellowing of skin or eyes; dark urine; and pale stools.

See Nursing Process Focus: Clients Receiving Antibacterial Therapy (page 537) for the nursing process applied to all antibacterials.

PROTOTYPE DRUG | **Erythromycin (Eryc)**

Actions and Uses: Erythromycin is inactivated by stomach acid and is thus administered as coated tablets or capsules that are intended to dissolve in the small intestine. Its main application is for clients who are unable to tolerate penicillins or who may have a penicillin-resistant infection. It has a spectrum similar to that of the penicillins and is effective against most gram-positive bacteria. It is often a preferred drug for infections caused by *Bordetella pertussis* (whooping cough) and *Corynebacterium diphtheriae*.

NCLEX Success Tips

Ophthalmia neonatorum prophylaxis involves the instillation of 0.5% erythromycin or 1% tetracycline ointment into a neonate's eyes. This procedure is performed to prevent gonorrheal conjunctivitis. Currently, Canada and the United States mandate that this treatment be given within 1 hour after birth to decrease the risk of permanent eye damage and blindness.

The instillation of erythromycin into the neonate's eyes provides prophylaxis for ophthalmia neonatorum, or neonatal blindness caused by gonorrhea in the mother. Erythromycin is also effective in the prevention of infection and conjunctivitis from *chlamydia trachomatis*.

Pharmacokinetics: Absorption of erythromycin is variable. It is widely distributed, crosses the placenta, and enters breast milk. It is partly metabolized by the liver and is mostly excreted in bile with a small amount excreted unchanged in urine. Half-life is 1 to 2 hours.

Administration Alerts:

- Administer oral drug on an empty stomach with a full glass of water.
- For suspensions, shake the bottle thoroughly to ensure that the drug is well mixed.
- Do not give with or immediately before or after fruit juices.
- Erythromycin is pregnancy category B.

Adverse Effects and Interactions: The most common side effects of erythromycin are nausea, abdominal cramping, and vomiting, although these are rarely serious enough to cause discontinuation of therapy. Concurrent administration with food may be necessary to reduce these side effects. The most severe adverse effect is hepatotoxicity caused by the estolate form of the drug.

Anesthetic agents and anticonvulsant drugs may interact with erythromycin to cause serum drug levels to rise and result in toxicity. This drug interacts with cyclosporine, increasing the risk for nephrotoxicity. It may increase the effects of warfarin. Erythromycin may interact with medications that contain xanthine to cause an increase in theophylline levels.

AMINOGLYCOSIDES

The first aminoglycoside, streptomycin, was named after *Streptomyces griseus,* the soil organism from which it was isolated in 1942. Once widely used, streptomycin is now usually restricted to the treatment of tuberculosis (TB) due to the development of a large number of resistant strains. Although more toxic than other antibiotic classes, aminoglycosides have important therapeutic applications for the treatment of aerobic gram-negative bacteria, mycobacteria, and some protozoans. The aminoglycosides are listed in Table 44.5.

NCLEX Success Tip

Aminoglycosides have a high risk of ototoxicity, which is indicated by hearing loss and tinnitus. An aminoglycoside may cause nephrotoxicity and ototoxicity when given concomitantly with cisplatin.

NCLEX Success Tips

The most significant adverse reactions to gentamicin and other aminoglycosides are ototoxicity (indicated by vertigo, tinnitus, and hearing loss) and nephrotoxicity (indicated by urinary cells or casts, oliguria, proteinuria, and reduced creatinine clearance). These adverse reactions are most common in elderly and dehydrated clients, those with renal impairment, and those receiving concomitant therapy with another potentially ototoxic or nephrotoxic drug.

Irreversible deafness can develop if the onset of ototoxicity is not detected early.

TABLE 44.5 Aminoglycosides

Drug	Route and Adult Dose
Pr gentamicin (Garamycin)	IM/IV, 3–5 mg/kg/day in divided doses every 8 hours
streptomycin	IM, 15–30 mg/kg/day or 1–2 g/day
tobramycin	IM/IV, 1–2.5 mg/kg/dose every 8 to 12 hours (max 5 mg/kg/day)

Pharmacotherapy with Aminoglycosides

44.5 The aminoglycosides are narrow-spectrum drugs that have the potential to cause serious adverse effects such as ototoxicity, nephrotoxicity, and neuromuscular blockade.

Aminoglycosides are bactericidal and act by inhibiting bacterial protein synthesis and by causing the synthesis of abnormal proteins. They are normally reserved for serious systemic infections caused by aerobic gram-negative organisms, including *Escherichia coli, Serratia, Proteus, Klebsiella,* and *Pseudomonas.*

Most aminoglycosides are polar compounds that are poorly absorbed from the GI tract. Less than 1% of an oral dose is absorbed; therefore, aminoglycosides must be administered parenterally to treat systemic infections. Because aminoglycosides travel through the alimentary canal unchanged, they are occasionally given PO to sterilize the bowel prior to intestinal surgery. Tobramycin is available for opthalmic use. Paromomycin (Humatin) is given orally for the treatment of parasitic infections.

Due to their polar nature, aminoglycosides cannot enter most human cells. Although distributed to most body fluids, not enough of the drugs enter the CSF for them to treat CNS infections. However, aminoglycosides can cross the placenta. If taken late in pregnancy, streptomycin can cause hearing loss in the child. In addition, aminoglycosides concentrate in renal tissue, which leads to potential nephrotoxicity.

Resistance develops quickly when aminoglycosides are administered as monotherapy. Resistance occurs when a species acquires an ability to degrade the antibiotic. Once degraded by the bacterial enzymes, these drugs are unable to bind with the bacterial ribosome. Some resistance also occurs when **mutations** change the shape of the bacterial ribosome so that it no longer binds the aminoglycoside. The emergence of aminoglycoside-resistant strains of *Enterococcus faecalis* and *Enterococcus faecium* has become a serious clinical problem because there are few therapeutic alternatives to treat these infections. Once resistance develops to an aminoglycoside, the mutant strain is usually resistant to the other drugs in this class. An exception is amikacin (Amikin), which appears to have some activity against gentamicin (Garamycin)-resistant strains.

Several techniques have been used to increase the effectiveness of the aminoglycosides. Administering these drugs in one large dose per day rather than in smaller divided doses results in a greater bacteriocidal effect and fewer resistant microbes. A second technique is to administer aminoglycosides and penicillins concurrently (though not mixed in the same IV solution). The penicillin weakens the cell wall, allowing a greater amount of aminoglycoside to enter and reach its ribosomal targets.

Aminoglycosides are excreted almost exclusively by the kidneys. Because certain tissues bind the drugs very tightly, renal excretion may be prolonged up to 20 days after discontinuation of the drug. Although serum drug levels may fall below what is considered a minimally effective concentration, some antimicrobial activity continues during this time. This is known as a **post-antibiotic effect**.

The clinical applications of the aminoglycosides are limited by their potential to cause serious adverse effects. The degree and types of toxicity are similar for all drugs in this class. For example,

all aminoglycosides can impair both hearing and balance. Damage to sensory cells in the cochlea causes hearing loss. Balance is affected by damage to sensory cells in the vestibular apparatus of the inner ear. As much as 25% of clients who are taking aminoglycoside antibiotics may experience some ototoxicity. This effect is more prominent when the medications are used for longer than 10 days or when the client has pre-existing kidney impairment, causing high serum drug levels. The damage to sensory cells is cumulative; repeated doses of the drug can damage increasing numbers of cells. Because many older adults have some degree of pre-existing hearing impairment, permanent deafness may occur in this group. Signs of impending inner ear damage include high-pitched tinnitus, headache, nausea, vomiting, and vertigo. Signs of ototoxicity may continue for several weeks after the drugs are discontinued. If hearing and balance functions are not carefully monitored during therapy and proper interventions are not implemented, the ototoxicity may become irreversible.

One of the most serious adverse effects of aminoglycosides is their potential to cause nephrotoxicity. Aminoglycosides directly injure renal tubule cells, and this nephrotoxicity may be severe, affecting up to 26% of clients who are receiving these antibiotics. As expected, clients who are receiving higher doses for longer periods are most affected. Those with pre-existing renal impairment or those who are receiving concurrent therapy with other nephrotoxic drugs must be monitored carefully: regular evaluation of urinalysis, BUN, and serum creatinine results is essential. Serum drug concentrations should be obtained regularly, and doses should be adjusted accordingly to prevent permanent damage. If recognized early, renal damage caused by aminoglycosides is reversible. Impaired kidney function may cause drug serum levels to rise, thus increasing the risk or worsening of ototoxicity.

A less common though serious adverse effect of aminoglycosides is neuromuscular blockade. Aminoglycosides inhibit the release of acetylcholine at synapses. Giving other drugs that affect acetylcholine release, such as anesthetics or neuromuscular blockers, can result in profound apnea and prolonged muscle paralysis. Because they have fewer acetylcholine receptors, clients with myasthenia gravis are especially at risk. To avoid this problem, aminoglycosides may be discontinued prior to surgery. IV calcium salts have been found to reverse aminoglycoside-induced neuromuscular blockade.

Nursing Considerations

The role of the nurse in aminoglycoside therapy involves careful monitoring of the client's condition and providing education as it relates to the prescribed drug regimen. Assess the client for a history of previous allergic reaction to aminoglycosides. These anti-infectives are most noted for their toxic effects on the kidneys and vestibular apparatus; therefore, the client should be monitored for ototoxicity and nephrotoxicity during the course of therapy. Baseline audiometry, renal function, and vestibular function need to be assessed prior to the initial administration of aminoglycosides and throughout therapy. Hearing loss may occur after therapy has been completed. Baseline urinalysis is necessary prior to initiation and throughout therapy, as renal impairment may increase the risk of toxicity. With streptomycin therapy, caloric tests are assessed for baseline data and to monitor for vestibular toxicity.

Neuromuscular function may also be impaired in clients who are receiving aminoglycosides. Clients with neuromuscular diseases, such as myasthenia gravis and Parkinson's disease, may experience greater muscle weakness due to neuromuscular blockade caused by aminoglycosides. These antibiotics also should be used with caution in clients who are receiving anesthetics because an interaction may cause neuromuscular blockade.

These drugs should be used with caution in neonates, infants, and older adults. Infants may experience neuromuscular blockade from aminoglycosides due to their immature neurological system. Elderly clients are at a higher risk for nephrotoxicity and ototoxicity because of reduced renal function and may require lower doses. Clients should be instructed to increase fluid intake, unless otherwise contraindicated, to promote excretion of the medications. Superinfection is a side effect of aminoglycoside therapy, and the client should be monitored for diarrhea, vaginal discharge, stomatitis, and glossitis.

Client education as it relates to aminoglycosides should include goals, reasons for obtaining baseline data such as vestibular function tests, and possible side effects. The following are important points to include when teaching clients regarding aminoglycosides:

- Increase fluid intake.
- Immediately report significant side effects, including tinnitus, high-frequency hearing loss, persistent headache, nausea, and vertigo.

See Nursing Process Focus: Clients Receiving Antibacterial Therapy (page 537) for the nursing process applied to all antibacterials.

PROTOTYPE DRUG	Gentamicin (Garamycin)

Actions and Uses: Gentamicin is a broad-spectrum, bactericidal antibiotic usually prescribed for serious urinary, respiratory, neurological, or GI infections when less toxic antibiotics are contraindicated. It is often used in combination with other antibiotics or when drugs from other classes have proven ineffective. It is used parenterally, or as drops, for eye infections.

Administration Alerts:

- For IM administration, give deep into a large muscle.
- Use only IM and IV drug solutions that are clear and colourless or slightly yellow. Discard discoloured solutions or those that contain particulate matter.
- Gentamicin is pregnancy category D.

Pharmacokinetics: Gentamicin is well absorbed after IM administration. It is widely distributed, crosses the placenta, and enters breast milk. It is mostly excreted in urine. Half-life is 2 to 4 hours.

Adverse Effects and Interactions: As with other aminoglycosides, adverse effects from gentamicin may be severe. Ototoxicity can produce a loss of hearing or balance, which may become permanent with continued use. Frequent hearing tests should be conducted so that gentamicin may be discontinued if early signs of ototoxicity are detected.

Gentamicin is excreted unchanged, primarily by the kidneys. The nurse must be alert for signs of reduced kidney function, including proteinuria and elevated BUN and creatinine levels. Nephrotoxicity is of particular concern for clients with pre-existing kidney disease and may limit therapy. Resistance to gentamicin is increasing and some cross-resistance among aminoglycosides has been reported.

The risk for ototoxicity increases if the client is currently taking amphotericin B (Fungizone), furosemide (Lasix), acetylsalicylic acid (ASA [Aspirin]), bumetanide (Burinex), ethacrynic acid (Edecrin), cisplatin, or humatin.

Concurrent use with amphotericin B, capreomycin, cisplatin, polymyxin B, and vancomycin (Vancocin) increases the risk for nephrotoxicity.

FLUOROQUINOLONES

In the past decade, the fluoroquinolones have become an increasingly important class of antibiotic. The first drug in this class, nalidixic acid, was approved in 1962. Classified as a quinolone, the use of nalidixic acid was restricted to UTIs due to its narrow spectrum of activity and a high incidence of bacterial resistance. The development of fluorinated quinolones with a wider spectrum of activity began in the late 1980s and continues today. Four generations of fluoroquinolones are now available, classified by their microbiological activity. All fluoroquinolones have activity against gram-negative **pathogens**; the later-generation agents are significantly more effective against gram-positive agents. The fluoroquinolones are listed in Table 44.6.

Pharmacotherapy with Fluoroquinolones

44.6 The use of fluoroquinolones has expanded far beyond their initial role in treating urinary tract infections.

The fluoroquinolones are bactericidal and affect DNA synthesis by inhibiting two bacterial enzymes: DNA gyrase and topoisomerase IV. Agents in this class are infrequently first-line drugs, although they are extensively used as alternatives to other antibiotics. Clinical applications include infections of the respiratory, GI, and gynecological tracts and some skin and soft tissue infections. The most widely used drug in this class, ciprofloxacin (Cipro), is an agent of choice for post-exposure prophylaxis of *Bacillus anthracis*. A newer agent, moxifloxacin (Avelox), is highly effective against anaerobes. Recent studies suggest that some fluoroquinolones may be effective against *Mycobacterium tuberculosis*.

TABLE 44.6 Fluoroquinolones

Drug	Route and Adult Dose
Second Generation	
Pr ciprofloxacin (Cipro)	PO, 250–750 mg bid; IV, 400 mg q12h
norfloxacin (Noroxin)	PO, 400 mg bid
ofloxacin	PO, 200–400 mg bid
Third Generation	
levofloxacin (Levaquin)	PO/IV, 250–750 mg every 24 hours
Fourth Generation	
gemifloxacin (Factive)	PO, 320 mg qd
moxifloxacin (Avelox)	PO/IV, 400 mg qd

A major advantage of the fluoroquinolones is that they are well absorbed orally and may be administered either once or twice a day. They have a favourable safety profile, with nausea, vomiting, and diarrhea being the most common side effects. Although they may be taken with food, they should not be taken concurrently with multivitamins or mineral supplements since calcium, magnesium, iron, and zinc ions can reduce absorption of the antibiotic by as much as 90%.

The most serious adverse effects are dysrhythmias (gatifloxacin [Zymar] and moxifloxacin) and liver failure. CNS effects such as dizziness, headache, and sleep disturbances affect 1% to 8% of clients. Because animal studies have suggested that fluoroquinolones affect cartilage development, use in children must be monitored carefully. Use in pregnant or lactating clients should be avoided.

Along with doxycycline, streptomycin, and penicillin, several fluoroquinolones are indicated for pathogens that could potentially be used in a bioterrorism incident. As mentioned, ciprofloxacin is a drug of choice for post-exposure prophylaxis to *Bacillus anthracis*, the causative agent of anthrax. Ciprofloxacin is also indicated for post-exposure prophylaxis to other potential biological warfare pathogens such as *Yersinia pestis* (plague), *Francisella tularensis* (tularemia), and *Brucella melitensis* (brucellosis). Details on the pharmacotherapy of bioterrorism agents are presented in Chapter 64.

Fluoroquinolones are well absorbed orally and may be administered either once or twice a day, making them ideal for outpatient therapy. The serum levels of these drugs after PO administration are nearly equivalent to the levels achieved during IV administration. This allows for a rapid, smooth transition from IV therapy to oral therapy, potentially decreasing the length of the hospital stay. Like aminoglycosides, fluoroquinolones exhibit a post-antibiotic effect. Their bacteriocidal actions continue after serum levels fall to below minimum inhibitory concentrations.

Nursing Considerations

The role of the nurse in fluoroquinolone therapy involves careful monitoring of the client's condition and providing education as it relates to the prescribed drug regimen. Assess for allergic reactions to fluoroquinolones before beginning therapy. Because these agents may decrease leukocytes, the WBC count should be carefully monitored. When possible, culture and sensitivity testing should be performed before beginning therapy.

These drugs are contraindicated in clients with a history of hypersensitivity to fluoroquinolones. They should be used with caution in clients with epilepsy, cerebral arteriosclerosis, or alcoholism due to a potential drug interaction that increases the risk for CNS toxicity. Clients with liver and renal dysfunction should be monitored carefully due to the drug being metabolized by the liver and excreted by the kidneys.

Norfloxacin (Noroxin) should be taken on an empty stomach. Antacids and ferrous sulfate may decrease the absorption of fluoroquinolones, reducing antibiotic effectiveness. The fluoroquinolones should be administered at least 2 hours before these drugs. Coagulation studies (INR) need to be monitored frequently if these antibiotics are administered concurrently with warfarin due to interactions that can lead to increased anticoagulation effects.

Monitor urinary output and report quantities of less than 1000 mL in 24 hours to the healthcare provider. The client should be encouraged to drink eight or more glasses of water per day to decrease the risk of crystalluria, which irritates the kidneys. Advise the client to discontinue the drug and notify the healthcare provider if signs of hypersensitivity occur.

The nurse should inform the client that these drugs may cause dizziness and lightheadedness and to avoid driving or performing hazardous tasks during drug therapy. These agents should be used with caution during pregnancy and breastfeeding due to untoward effects caused by the passage of antimicrobials to the fetus and newborn. Safety for use by children under 18 years has not been established.

Clients who are receiving norfloxacin should be informed that photophobia is possible. Some fluoroquinolones, such as ciprofloxacin, may affect tendons, especially in children. The client should refrain from physical exercise if calf, ankle, or Achilles tendon pain occurs.

Client education as it relates to fluoroquinolones should include goals, reasons for obtaining baseline data such as laboratory work and culture and sensitivity tests, and possible side effects. The following are important points to include when teaching clients regarding fluoroquinolones:

- Wear sunglasses; avoid exposure to bright lights and direct sunlight when taking norfloxacin.
- Report the first signs of tendon pain or inflammation.
- Report the following side effects immediately: dizziness, restlessness, stomach distress, diarrhea, psychosis, confusion, and irregular or fast heart rate.

See Nursing Process Focus: Clients Receiving Antibacterial Therapy (page 537) for the nursing process applied to all antibacterials.

| **PROTOTYPE DRUG** | **Ciprofloxacin (Cipro)** |

Actions and Uses: Ciprofloxacin, a second-generation fluoroquinolone, was approved in 1987 and is the most widely used drug in this class. By inhibiting bacterial DNA gyrase, ciprofloxacin affects bacterial replication and DNA repair. It is more effective against gram-negative than gram-positive organisms. It is prescribed for respiratory infections, bone and joint infections, GI infections, ophthalmic infections, sinusitis, and prostatitis. The drug is rapidly absorbed after oral administration and is distributed to most body tissues. Oral and IV forms are available.

NCLEX Success Tips

Ciprofloxacin should not be taken with dairy products or other significant sources of calcium, such as collard greens, calcium supplements, calcium carbonate antacids, or calcium-fortified juice. Clients may take a missed dose as soon as they remember. However, if it is very close to the time of the next dose, the missed dose should be omitted. The client should not take a double dose.

To reduce the risk of crystalluria, the client should drink 2000 to 3000 mL of water per day. The client should not take an antacid before taking ciprofloxacin. An antacid decreases the absorption of the drug. The client may get light-headed from ciprofloxacin. If so, the client should not drive a motor vehicle and should contact the physician.

A black box warning for ciprofloxacin is that the medication may increase the anticoagulant effects of warfarin. The nurse should instruct the client to report increased bleeding and to monitor the prothrombin time (PT) and the international normalized ratio (INR) closely.

Ciprofloxacin may cause photosensitivity reactions; the nurse must advise the client to avoid excessive sunlight or artificial ultraviolet light during therapy.

Pharmacokinetics: Ciprofloxacin is well absorbed after PO administration. It may be given IV. It is widely distributed, crosses the placenta, and enters breast milk. It is partly metabolized by the liver. About 50% is excreted unchanged in urine. Half-life is 4 hours.

Administration Alerts:

- Administer at least 4 hours before antacids and ferrous sulfate (Fer-In-Sol).
- Ciprofloxacin is pregnancy category C.

Adverse Effects and Interactions: GI side effects may occur in as much as 20% of clients. Ciprofloxacin may be administered with food to diminish adverse GI effects. However, the client should not take this drug with antacids or mineral supplements since drug absorption will be diminished. Some clients report headache and dizziness. Caffeine should be restricted to avoid excessive nervousness, anxiety, and tachycardia.

Concurrent administration with warfarin may increase anticoagulant effects. This drug may increase theophylline levels 15% to 30%. Antacids, ferrous sulfate, and sucralfate decrease the absorption of ciprofloxacin.

SULFONAMIDES

The discovery of the sulfonamides in the 1930s heralded a new era in the treatment of infectious disease. With their wide spectrum of activity against both gram-positive and gram-negative bacteria, the sulfonamides significantly reduced mortality from susceptible microbes and earned its discoverer a Nobel Prize in medicine in 1938. Sulfonamides suppress bacterial growth by inhibiting the essential compound folic acid, which is responsible for cellular biosynthesis. Sulfonamides are active against a broad spectrum of microorganisms. The sulfonamides are listed in Table 44.7.

TABLE 44.7 Sulfonamides

Drug	Route and Adult Dose
sulfacetamide (Bleph-10)	Ophthalmic, one to three drops of 10% solution into lower conjunctival sac every 2–3 hours (q2–3h), may increase interval as client responds or use 1.5–2.5 cm of 10% ointment q6h and at bedtime
Pr trimethoprim-sulfamethoxazole (Bactrim, Septra)	SS (single strength): 400 mg sulfamethoxazole + 80 mg trimethoprim; DS (double strength): 800 mg sulfamethoxazole + 160 mg trimethoprim; dosing is 1 tablet bid

Pharmacotherapy with Sulfonamides

44.7 Once widely prescribed, resistance has limited the usefulness of sulfonamides to urinary tract infections and a few other specific infections.

Several factors have led to a significant decline in the use of sulfonamides. Their widespread use over several decades resulted in a substantial number of resistant strains. The development of the penicillins, cephalosporins, and macrolides gave healthcare providers a larger choice of agents, some of which exhibited an improved safety profile over the sulfonamides. Approval of the combination antibiotic trimethoprim-sulfamethoxazole (Bactrim, Septra) marked a resurgence in the use of sulfonamides in treating UTIs. Agents in this drug class are also given for *Pneumocystis carinii* pneumonia and *Shigella* infections of the small bowel.

Sulfonamides are classified by their absorption and excretion characteristics. Some, such as sulfisoxazole and sulfamethoxazole, are rapidly absorbed when given orally and excreted rapidly by the kidney. Others such as sulfasalazine (Salazopyrin) are poorly absorbed and remain in the alimentary canal to treat intestinal infections. A third group, including sulfadiazine, is used for topical infections.

In general, the sulfonamides are safe drugs; however, some adverse effects may be serious. Adverse effects include the formation of crystals in the urine, hypersensitivity reactions, nausea, and vomiting. Although not common, sulfonamides can produce potentially fatal blood abnormalities, such as aplastic anemia, acute hemolytic anemia, and agranulocytosis.

Nursing Considerations

The role of the nurse in sulfonamide therapy involves careful monitoring of the client's condition and providing education as it relates to the prescribed drug regimen. Assess for anemia and other hematological disorders because sulfonamides may cause hemolytic anemia and blood dyscrasias due to a genetically determined deficiency in some clients' red blood cells. Assess renal function, as sulfonamides may increase the risk for crystalluria. Culture and sensitivity results should be obtained before initiating sulfonamide therapy. CBC and urinalysis should be obtained during therapy.

Sulfonamides are contraindicated during pregnancy and lactation and for infants younger than 2 months of age due to the drug's ability to promote jaundice. Agents in this class must be used with caution in clients with renal impairment. Sulfonamides have a low solubility that may cause crystals to form in urine and obstruct the kidneys or ureters. Encourage increasing fluids to 3000 mL per day to achieve a urinary output of 1500 mL per 24 hours to decrease the possibility of crystalluria.

Cross-sensitivity exists with diuretics, such as acetazolamide (Diamox) and the thiazides, and with sulfonylurea antidiabetic agents. All of these agents should be avoided in clients with a history of hypersensitivity to sulfonamides because this can induce a skin abnormality called Stevens-Johnson syndrome. Instruct the client to stop taking the drug and contact a healthcare provider if rash occurs.

Client education as it relates to sulfonamides should include goals, reasons for obtaining baseline data such as laboratory work and culture and sensitivity tests, and possible side effects. The following are the important points to include when teaching clients regarding sulfonamides:

- Avoid exposure to direct sunlight; use sunscreen and protective clothing to decrease effects of photosensitivity.
- Take oral medications with a full glass of water.
- Increase fluid intake to 1500 to 3000 mL per day unless otherwise contraindicated.
- Immediately report significant side effects, including abdominal or stomach cramps or pain, blood in urine, confusion, difficulty breathing, and fever.

See Nursing Process Focus: Clients Receiving Antibacterial Therapy (page 537) for the nursing process applied to all antibacterials.

PROTOTYPE DRUG	Trimethoprim-Sulfamethoxazole (Bactrim, Septra)

Actions and Uses: The fixed combination of the sulfonamide sulfamethoxazole (SMZ) with the anti-infective trimethoprim (TMP) is most commonly used in the pharmacotherapy of UTIs. It is also approved for the treatment of *P. carinii* pneumonia, *Shigella* infections of the small bowel, and for acute episodes of chronic bronchitis.

Both SMZ and TMP are inhibitors of the bacterial metabolism of folic acid, or folate. Their action is synergistic: a greater bacterial kill is achieved by the fixed combination than would be achieved with either drug used separately. Because humans obtain the precursors of folate in their diets, these medications are selective for bacterial folate metabolism. Another advantage of the combination is that development of resistance is lower than that observed when either agent is used alone.

Pharmacokinetics: This combination is well absorbed after PO administration. It is partly metabolized by the liver. Less than 40% is excreted unchanged in urine. Half-life is 6 to 12 hours.

Administration Alerts:
- Administer oral drugs with a full glass of water.
- Trimethoprim-sulfamethoxazole is pregnancy category D.

Adverse Effects and Interactions: The most common side effect of TMP-SMZ involves skin rashes, which are characteristic of sulfonamides. Nausea and vomiting are not uncommon. This medication should be used cautiously in clients with pre-existing kidney disease since crystalluria, oliguria, and renal failure have been reported. Periodic laboratory evaluation of the blood is usually performed to identify early signs of agranulocytosis or thrombocytopenia.

TMP and SMZ may enhance the effects of oral anticoagulants. These drugs may also increase methotrexate toxicity.

MISCELLANEOUS ANTIBACTERIALS

44.8 A number of miscellaneous antibacterials have specific indications, distinct antibacterial mechanisms, and related nursing care.

Some anti-infectives cannot be grouped into classes, or the class is too small to warrant separate discussion. That is not to diminish their importance in medicine, as some of the miscellaneous anti-infectives are critical drugs in certain situations. The miscellaneous antibiotics are listed in Table 44.8.

NCLEX Success Tip
The most toxic reaction to chloramphenicol (Chloromycetin) is bone marrow suppression.

Clindamycin (Dalacin C) is effective against both gram-positive and gram-negative bacteria. Susceptible bacteria include *Fusobacterium* and *Clostridium perfringens*. It is sometimes the drug of choice for oral infections caused by bacteroides. It is considered to be appropriate treatment when less toxic alternatives are not effective options. It is contraindicated in clients with a history of hypersensitivity to clindamycin or lincomycin (Lincocin), regional enteritis, or ulcerative colitis. Clindamycin is limited in use because it is associated with PMC, the most severe adverse effect of this drug. The client should report significant side effects, including diarrhea, rashes, difficulty breathing, itching, and difficulty swallowing, to the healthcare provider immediately.

Quinupristin-dalfopristin (Synercid) is a combination drug that is the first in a new class of antibiotics called streptogramins. Streptogramins are reserved to treat infections caused by antibiotic-resistant gram-positive organisms. Quinupristin-dalfopristin is primarily indicated for treatment of vancomycin-resistant *E. faecium* infections and is contraindicated in clients with hypersensitivity to this drug. It is used cautiously in clients with renal or hepatic dysfunction. Hepatotoxicity is the most serious adverse effect of this drug. The client should report significant side effects—including irritation, pain, or burning at the IV infusion site; joint and muscle pain; rash; diarrhea; and vomiting—to the healthcare provider immediately.

Linezolid (Zyvoxam) is significant in being the first drug in a new class of antibiotics called the oxazolidinones. This drug is

TABLE 44.8 Select Miscellaneous Antibacterials

Drug	Route and Adult Dose
chloramphenicol (Chloromycetin)	IV, 50–100 mg/kg/day in divided doses every 6 hours (max 4 g/day)
clindamycin (Dalacin C)	PO, 150–450 mg qid
fosfomycin (Monurol)	PO, 3-g sachet dissolved in 3–4 oz of water as a single dose
methenamine (Mandelamine)	PO, 1 g qid
nitrofurantoin (Macrobid, Macrodantin)	PO, 50–100 mg qid; Macrobid 100 mg bid
quinupristin-dalfopristin (Synercid)	IV, 7.5 mg/kg infused over 60 minutes every 8 hours (q8h)
Pr vancomycin (Vancocin)	IV, 500 mg qid or 1 g bid; PO, 125–500 mg q6h

as effective as vancomycin against MRSA infections. Linezolid is administered intravenously or orally. Most clients can be converted from the IV to PO route in about 5 days. Linezolid is contraindicated in clients with hypersensitivity to the drug and in pregnancy, and it should be used with caution in clients who have hypertension. Cautious use is also necessary in clients taking monoamine oxidase (MAO) inhibitors or serotonin reuptake inhibitors because the drugs can interact, causing a hypertensive crisis. Linezolid can cause thrombocytopenia. The client should report significant side effects, including bleeding, diarrhea, headache, nausea, vomiting, rash, dizziness, and fever, to the healthcare provider immediately.

Vancomycin is usually reserved for severe infections from gram-positive organisms such as *S. aureus* and *S. pneumoniae*. It is often used after bacteria have become resistant to other, safer antibiotics. Vancomycin is the most effective drug for treating MRSA infections. Vancomycin is contraindicated in clients with known hypersensitivity to the drug and in clients with hearing loss. Due to ototoxicity, hearing must be evaluated frequently throughout the course of therapy. It should not be given to pregnant or lactating clients. Vancomycin can also cause nephrotoxicity leading to uremia.

Vancomycin is administered orally and IV, but not IM. A reaction that can occur with rapid IV administration is known as **red-man syndrome** and includes hypotension with flushing and a red rash on the face and upper body. The client should report significant side effects, including superinfections, generalized tingling after IV administration, chills, fever, skin rash, hives, hearing loss, and nausea, to the healthcare provider immediately.

In September 2003, the first in a new class of antibiotics, the cyclic lipopeptides, was approved. Daptomycin (Cubicin) is approved for the treatment of serious skin and skin structure infections such as major abscesses, post-surgical skin wound infections, and infected ulcers caused by *S. aureus, Streptococcus pyogenes, Streptococcus agalactiae,* and *E. faecalis*. The most common side effects are GI distress, injection site reactions, fever, headache, dizziness, insomnia, and rash.

See Nursing Process Focus: Clients Receiving Antibacterial Therapy for the nursing process applied to all antibacterials.

PROTOTYPE DRUG | Vancomycin (Vancocin)

Actions and Uses: Vancomycin is an antibiotic usually reserved for severe infections from gram-positive organisms such as *S. aureus* and *S. pneumoniae*. It is often used after bacteria have become resistant to other, safer antibiotics. It is bactericidal, inhibiting bacterial cell wall synthesis. Because vancomycin was not used frequently during the first 30 years following its discovery, the incidence of vancomycin-resistant organisms is less than with other antibiotics. Vancomycin is the most effective drug for treating MRSA infections, which have become a major problem in North America. However, vancomycin-resistant strains of *S. aureus* have begun to appear in recent years. Vancomycin is normally given intravenously, as it is not absorbed from the GI tract.

NCLEX Success Tips

Because vancomycin can affect the acoustic branch of the eighth cranial nerve, the client should report tinnitus. Vancomycin does not affect the vestibular branch of the acoustic nerve (which would cause vertigo and ataxia).

Caring for a client infected with vancomycin-resistant enterococci requires contact precautions. The nurse should wear a gown, gloves, a mask, and eye protection when entering the client's room. Because the gloves will be the most contaminated, the nurse should remove them first when exiting the room to prevent infection transmission.

Administration Alerts:

- Administer IV slowly at a rate of 10 mg/minute over not less than 60 minutes to avoid causing sudden hypotension.
- Vancomycin is pregnancy category B (oral), C (injection).

Adverse Effects and Interactions: Frequent, minor side effects include flushing, hypotension, and rash on the upper body, sometimes called the red-man syndrome. More serious adverse effects, including nephrotoxicity and ototoxicity, are possible

NURSING PROCESS FOCUS

Clients Receiving Antibacterial Therapy

Assessment	Potential Nursing Diagnoses/Identified Patterns
Prior to administration: • Obtain complete health history, including allergies, drug history, and possible drug interactions. • Obtain specimens for culture and sensitivity before initiating therapy. • Perform infection-focused physical examination, including vital signs, WBC count, and sedimentation rate.	• Alteration in nutrition and fluid intake • Need for knowledge regarding the disease process and transmission • Need for knowledge regarding drug therapy, management of side effects, and reporting of adverse effects • Need for knowledge regarding the importance of adherence to treatment for healing • Potential for injury related to side effects of drug therapy • Risk for superinfection

Planning: Client Goals and Expected Outcomes

The client will:

- Report reduction in symptoms related to the diagnosed infection and have negative results for laboratory and diagnostic tests for the presenting infection
- Demonstrate an understanding of the drug by accurately describing the drug's purpose, action, side effects, and precautions
- Immediately report significant side effects such as shortness of breath, swelling, fever, stomatitis, loose stools, vaginal discharge, or cough
- Complete the full course of antibiotic therapy and comply with follow-up care

Implementation

Interventions (Rationales)	Client Education/Discharge Planning
• Monitor vital signs and symptoms of infection to determine antibacterial effectiveness. (Another drug or different dosage may be required.) • Monitor for hypersensitivity reaction. (Immediate hypersensitivity reaction may occur within 2 to 30 minutes; accelerated occurs in 1 to 72 hours and delayed occurs after 72 hours.) • Monitor for severe diarrhea. (The condition may occur due to superinfection or the possible adverse effect of AAPMC.) • Administer drug around the clock (to maintain effective blood levels). • Monitor for superinfection, especially in elderly, debilitated, or immunosuppressed clients. (Increased risk for superinfections is due to elimination of normal flora.) • Monitor intake of OTC products such as antacids, calcium supplements, iron products, and laxatives containing magnesium. (These products interfere with absorption of many antibiotics.) • Monitor for photosensitivity. (Tetracyclines, fluoroquinolones, and sulfonamides can increase client's sensitivity to ultraviolet light and increase risk for sunburn.) • Determine the interactions of the prescribed antibiotics with various foods and beverages. • Monitor IV site for signs and symptoms of tissue irritation, severe pain, and extravasation. • Monitor for side effects specific to various antibiotic therapies. (See Nursing Considerations for each antibiotic classification in this chapter.) • Monitor renal function such as intake and output ratios and urine colour and consistency. Monitor lab work including serum creatinine and BUN. (Some antibiotics such as the aminoglycosides are nephrotoxic.) • Monitor for symptoms of ototoxicity. (Some antibiotics, such as the aminoglycosides and vancomycin, may cause vestibular or auditory nerve damage.) • Monitor client for compliance with antibiotic therapy.	• Instruct client to notify healthcare provider if symptoms persist or worsen • Instruct client to discontinue the medication and inform the healthcare provider if symptoms of hypersensitivity reaction, such as wheezing; shortness of breath; swelling of face, tongue, or hands; and itching or rash, develop Instruct client to: • Consult the healthcare provider before taking antidiarrheal drugs, which could cause retention of harmful bacteria • Consume cultured dairy products with live active cultures, such as kefir, yogurt, or buttermilk, to help restore and maintain normal intestinal flora Instruct client to: • Take medication on schedule • Complete the entire prescription, even if feeling better, to prevent development of resistant bacteria • Instruct client to report signs and symptoms of superinfection such as fever; black hairy tongue; stomatitis; loose, foul-smelling stools; vaginal discharge; or cough. • Advise client to consult with the healthcare provider before using OTC medications or herbal products Encourage client to: • Avoid direct exposure to sunlight during and after therapy • Wear protective clothing, sunglasses, and sunscreen when in the sun Instruct client regarding foods and beverages that should be avoided with specific antibiotic therapies: • Avoid acidic fruit juices with penicillins • Avoid alcohol intake with cephalosporins • Avoid dairy/calcium products with tetracyclines • Instruct client to report pain or other symptoms of discomfort immediately during intravenous infusion • Instruct client to report side effects specific to antibiotic therapy prescribed • Explain purpose of required laboratory tests and scheduled follow-up with the healthcare provider • Instruct client to increase fluid intake to 2000 to 3000 mL/day Instruct client to notify the healthcare provider of: • Changes in hearing, ringing in ears, or full feeling in the ears • Nausea and vomiting with motion, ataxia, nystagmus, or dizziness Instruct client in the importance of: • Completing the prescription as ordered • Follow-up care after antibiotic therapy is completed

Evaluation of Outcome Criteria

Evaluate the effectiveness of drug therapy by confirming that client goals and expected outcomes have been met (see "Planning").

See Tables 44.1 to 44.8 for lists of drugs to which these nursing actions apply.

with higher doses. Clients may experience acute allergic reactions, including anaphylaxis.

Vancomycin adds to the toxicity of aminoglycosides, amphotericin B, cisplatin, cyclosporine, polymyxin B, and other ototoxic and nephrotoxic medications. It interacts with cholestyramine and colestipol, causing a decrease in absorption of oral vancomycin. It may increase the risk for lactic acidosis when administered with metformin (Glucophage).

URINARY ANTISEPTICS

44.9 Urinary antiseptics are anti-infective drugs used exclusively for urinary tract infections.

As has been noted throughout this text, most medications are totally or partially excreted by the kidneys. The majority of drugs and their metabolites travel through the urinary system, producing little or no effect on the renal tubular cells or the other parts

◀ **Antibacterial Properties of Goldenseal**

Goldenseal (*Hydrastis canadensis*) was once a common plant found in woods in the eastern and midwestern United States. Native Americans used the root for a variety of medicinal applications, including wound healing, diuresis, and washes for inflamed eyes. In recent years, the plant has been harvested to near extinction. Goldenseal was reported to mask the appearance of drugs in the urine of clients who want to hide drug abuse. This claim has since been proven false.

The roots and leaves of goldenseal are dried and available as capsules, tablets, salves, and tinctures. One of the primary active ingredients in goldenseal is hydrastine, which is reported to have antibacterial and antifungal properties. When used topically or locally, it is purported to be of value in treating bacterial and fungal skin infections and oral conditions such as gingivitis and thrush. As an eyewash, it can soothe inflamed eyes. Considered safe for most people, it is contraindicated in pregnancy and hypertension.

of the kidney. For the small class of drugs known as the urinary antiseptics, however, the urinary system is their target tissue. Being able to reach the urinary tract in high concentrations is essential to their therapeutic success.

Urinary antiseptics are given by the PO route for their antibacterial action in the urinary tract. While they do not reach high enough levels in the blood to be effective for systemic infections, the kidney concentrates the drugs; therefore, their actions are specific to the urinary system. Urinary antiseptics reach therapeutic levels in the kidney tubules, and their anti-infective action continues as they travel to the urinary bladder.

The advantage of the urinary antiseptics is that they are able to treat local infections in the urinary tract without reaching high levels in the blood that might produce systemic toxicity. Although not considered first-line drugs for UTI, they serve important roles as secondary medications, especially in clients who present with infections resistant to TMP-SMZ or the fluoroquinolones.

PROTOTYPE DRUG | **Nitrofurantoin (Macrobid, Macrodantin)**

Actions and Uses: Nitrofurantoin is an older drug that is indicated for the treatment of uncomplicated acute cystitis, most commonly for the prophylaxis of recurrent UTI. Nitrofurantoin is active against *E. coli*, *Staphylococcus saprophyticus*, and many other strains of gram-positive and gram-negative aerobes. It is not effective against the *Pseudomonas*, *Proteus*, or *Serratia* species. It is not indicated for the treatment of pyelonephritis.

Nitrofurantoin is available in two formulations: a macrocrystalline form (Macrodantin) and a sustained-release macrocrystalline form (Macrobid). The macrocrystalline form is more slowly absorbed than the microcrystalline form and produces fewer GI-related adverse effects.

Development of resistance has not been a significant problem. The broad-based mechanism of action may explain the relative lack of acquired bacterial resistance to nitrofurantoin. Multiple mutations at diverse locations of the bacterial chromosome would be necessary for a bacterium to acquire such resistance. Cross-resistance with other antibiotics is very rare, if it occurs at all.

Nitrofurantoin acts by several unique mechanisms. When bacteria break down nitrofurantoin, the drug is converted to highly reactive intermediates. These intermediates attack bacterial ribosomal proteins. The drug inhibits bacterial protein synthesis, aerobic energy metabolism, DNA synthesis, RNA synthesis, and formation of the cell wall. Nitrofurantoin is bactericidal in the urine at therapeutic doses.

Pharmacokinetics: Nitrofurantoin is readily absorbed after PO administration. It is widely distributed to body fluids, crosses the placenta, and is secreted in breast milk. It is 60% bound to plasma protein. Onset of action is 30 minutes, with a half-life of 20 minutes. It is primarily metabolized by the liver and excreted by the kidney.

Administration Alerts:

- Because nitrofurantoin is excreted by the kidneys, significant renal impairment (creatinine clearance under 30 mL/minute or significant elevated serum creatinine) is a contraindication. Successful treatment depends on achieving high amounts of drug in the urine, which will not occur in clients with oliguria or anuria.

- Because of the possibility of hemolytic anemia due to immature erythrocyte enzyme systems, the drug is contraindicated in pregnant clients and in neonates younger than 1 month of age.

- This drug should be used with caution in clients with pre-existing pulmonary disease, and pulmonary function should be closely monitored throughout therapy. Although rare, reports have cited diffuse interstitial pneumonitis or pulmonary fibrosis as causes of death in clients who are receiving nitrofurantoin.

- Nitrofurantoin should be used with caution in clients with pre-existing hepatic disease. The drug should be discontinued immediately if changes in liver function tests are noted.

Adverse Effects and Interactions: Nitrofurantoin has the potential to produce many adverse effects. The most frequent include hypersensitivity reactions, anorexia, headache, rash, nausea, and vomiting. Acute and chronic pulmonary toxicity is a serious adverse effect and may include interstitial pneumonitis, persistent cough, and pulmonary fibrosis. Chronic pulmonary toxicity may not appear until months or years after therapy has been completed. Hepatotoxicity is rare, though potentially fatal, and may include cholestatic jaundice, hepatic necrosis, or hepatitis.

Nitrofurantoin should not be given with antacids that contain magnesium because absorption will be decreased. Concurrent administration with nalidixic acid, and possibly fluoroquinolones, may result in antagonism and a decreased drug effect.

TABLE 44.9 Antituberculosis Drugs

Drug	Route and Adult Dose
First-Line Agents	
ethambutol (Etibi)	PO, 15–25 mg/kg qd
Pr isoniazid	PO/IM, 5 mg/kg/day or 15 mg/kg 2–3 times weekly
	PO/IM, 5 mg/kg/day or 15 mg/kg 2–3 times weekly
pyrazinamide (Tebrazid)	PO, daily dosing based on weight (max 2 g/day)
rifampin (Rifadin, Rofact)	PO/IV, 10 mg/kg/day (max 600 mg/day)
rifater: combination of pyrazinamide with isoniazid and rifampin	PO, six tablets qd (for clients weighing 55 kg or more)
streptomycin	IM, 15–30 mg/kg/day or 1–2 g/day
Second-Line Agents	
amikacin (Amikin)	IV/IM, 5–7.5 mg/kg/dose q8h
ciprofloxacin (Cipro)	PO, 250–750 mg bid; IV, 400 mg q12h
ofloxacin	PO, 200–400 mg bid

TUBERCULOSIS

Tuberculosis is a highly contagious infection caused by *M. tuberculosis*. It is treated with multiple anti-infectives for a prolonged period. The antitubercular agents are listed in Table 44.9.

NCLEX Success Tips

Isoniazid (INH) and rifampin (Rifadin, Rofact) are hepatotoxic. The client should be warned to limit intake of alcohol during drug therapy. The medication should be taken on an empty stomach.

Antacids can inhibit the absorption of INH and should not be taken with the drug. If antacids are needed for gastrointestinal distress, they should be taken 1 hour before or 2 hours after the medication is administered. The client should not double the dose of the medication because of potential toxicity. The client taking the medication should avoid foods that are rich in tyramine—such as cheese, dairy products, alcohol (red wine and beer), bananas, raisins, and caffeine—or he or she may develop hypertension.

INH interferes with the effectiveness of hormonal contraceptives, and female clients of childbearing age should be counselled to use an alternative form of birth control while taking the medication.

All clients exposed to persons with tuberculosis should receive prophylactic isoniazid therapy in a daily dosage of 300 mg for 6 months to 1 year to avoid the deleterious effects of the latent mycobacterium. Taking the medication for less than 6 months may not provide adequate protection against tuberculosis. Daily oral doses of isoniazid and rifampin for 6 months to 2 years are appropriate for the client with active tuberculosis. Isolation for 2 to 4 weeks is warranted for a client with active tuberculosis.

Isoniazid competes for the available vitamin B6 in the body and leaves the client at risk for developing neuropathies related to vitamin deficiency. Supplemental vitamin B6 is routinely prescribed to address this issue.

Clients with a newly positive Mantoux skin test are aggressively treated with isoniazid for about 9 months. Repeat skin testing should not be performed as it will always be positive. Skin tests do not convert to negative once a positive response has been obtained.

Clients taking isoniazid may show signs of hepatic stress. The nurse should assess for signs of liver dysfunction. If jaundice is present, however, a client would potentially have pruritus; the early sign is sclera yellowing.

Pharmacotherapy of Tuberculosis

44.10 Multiple-drug therapy is needed in the treatment of tuberculosis since the complex microbes are slow growing and commonly develop drug resistance.

Tuberculosis is an infection caused by the organism *M. tuberculosis*. Although the microorganisms typically invade the lung, they may also enter other body systems, particularly bone. Mycobacteria activate cells of the immune response, which attempt to isolate the microorganisms by creating a wall around them. The slow-growing mycobacteria usually become dormant, existing inside cavities called **tubercles**. They may remain dormant during an entire lifetime, or they may become reactivated if the client's immune system becomes suppressed. When active, TB can be quite infectious, readily spread by contaminated sputum. With the immune suppression characteristic of acquired immune deficiency syndrome (AIDS), the incidence of TB has greatly increased; as many as 20% of all clients with AIDS develop active TB infections. Infection by a different species of mycobacterium, *M. leprae*, is responsible for a disease known as leprosy.

Drug therapy of TB differs from that of most other infections. Mycobacteria have a cell wall that is resistant to penetration by anti-infective drugs. For medications to reach the isolated microorganisms in the tubercles, therapy must continue for 6 to 12 months. Although the client may not be infectious this entire time and may have no symptoms, it is critical that therapy continue for the entire period. Some clients develop multidrug-resistant infections and require therapy for as long as 24 months.

A second difference in the pharmacotherapy of TB is that at least two, and sometimes four or more, antibiotics are administered concurrently. During the 6- to 24-month treatment period, different combinations of drugs may be used. Multiple-drug therapy is necessary because the mycobacteria grow slowly and resistance is common. Using multiple drugs in different combinations during the long treatment period lowers the potential for resistance and increases the success of the therapy. There are two broad categories of antitubercular agents. One class consists of first-line drugs, which are safer and generally the most effective. A second group of drugs, more toxic and less effective than the first-line agents, are used when resistance develops.

A third difference is that antituberculosis drugs are extensively used for *preventing* the disease in addition to treating it. Chemoprophylaxis is used for close contacts or family members of recently infected TB clients. Therapy usually begins immediately after a client receives a positive tuberculin test. Clients with immunosuppression, such as those with AIDS or those receiving immunosuppressant drugs, may receive preventive treatment with antituberculosis drugs. A short-term therapy of 2 months, consisting of a combination treatment with isoniazid and pyrazinamide (Tebrazid), is approved for TB prophylaxis in clients who are positive for human immunodeficiency virus (HIV).

A major concern with TB pharmacotherapy is ensuring that clients fully comply with the prescribed regimen. Nonadherence to pharmacotherapy is the most common cause of treatment failure in clients with TB. In high-risk clients, **directly observed therapy (DOT)** is necessary. DOT requires that a healthcare provider directly observe the client swallowing the pills, whether it is in the hospital, office, or home care setting. Nurses serve essential roles in providing education about this disorder to their clients and stressing the importance of adherence.

Nursing Considerations

The role of the nurse in antituberculosis therapy involves careful monitoring of the client's condition and providing education as it relates to the prescribed drug regimen. Before beginning therapy, assess the client for the presence or history of a positive tuberculin skin test, a positive sputum culture, or a close contact with a person recently infected with TB. These conditions are all indications for the use of antituberculosis drugs. Also assess the client for a history of alcohol abuse, AIDS, liver disease, or kidney disease because many antituberculosis drugs are contraindicated in those conditions. They are also contraindicated in clients who are receiving immunosuppressant drugs. A complete physical examination, including vital signs, should be performed.

Caution must be observed during pregnancy and lactation and in clients with renal dysfunction or a history of convulsive disorders. The drugs are used with caution in clients with chronic liver disease or alcoholism because of the risk for hepatic injury due to the production of toxic levels of drug metabolites. These drugs may cause asymptomatic hyperuricemia because they can inhibit the renal excretion of uric acid, which may lead to gouty arthritis. Ethambutol (Etibi) is contraindicated in clients with optic neuritis. Some antituberculosis drugs interact with oral contraceptives and decrease their effectiveness; therefore, female clients should use an alternative form of birth control while using these medications.

See Nursing Process Focus: Clients Receiving Antituberculosis Agents for specific teaching points.

PROTOTYPE DRUG | **Isoniazid**

Actions and Uses: Isoniazid has been a drug of choice for the treatment of *M. tuberculosis* for many years. It is bactericidal for actively growing organisms but bacteriostatic for dormant mycobacteria. It is selective for *M. tuberculosis*. Isoniazid is used alone for chemoprophylaxis or in combination with other antituberculosis drugs for treating active disease.

Pharmacokinetics: Isoniazid is well absorbed after PO or IM administration. It is widely distributed, crosses the blood-brain barrier and placenta, and enters breast milk. It is partly metabolized by the liver. About 50% is excreted unchanged in urine. Half-life is 1 to 4 hours.

NURSING PROCESS FOCUS

Clients Receiving Antituberculosis Agents

Assessment	Potential Nursing Diagnoses/Identified Patterns
Prior to administration: • Obtain complete health history, including allergies, drug history, and possible drug interactions. • Perform complete physical examination, including vital signs. • Assess for presence or history of the following: • Positive tuberculin skin test • Positive sputum culture or smear • Close contact with person recently infected with TB • HIV infection or AIDS • Immunosuppressant drug therapy • Alcohol abuse • Liver or kidney disease • Assess cognitive ability to comply with long-term therapy.	• Alteration in nutrition and fluid intake • Need for knowledge regarding drug therapy and adverse effects • Need for knowledge regarding the importance of adherence to treatment for healing and to protect the community • Potential for injury related to side effects of drug therapy • Risk for superinfection

Planning: Client Goals and Expected Outcomes

The client will:

• Report reduction in TB symptoms and have negative results for laboratory and diagnostic tests for TB infection
• Demonstrate an understanding of the drug by accurately describing the drug's purpose, action, side effects, and precautions
• Immediately report effects such as visual changes, difficulty voiding, changes in hearing, and symptoms of liver or kidney impairment
• Complete the full course of antitubercular therapy and comply with follow-up care

Implementation

Interventions (Rationales)	Client Education/Discharge Planning
• Monitor for hepatic side effects. (Antituberculosis agents, such as isoniazid and rifampin, cause hepatic impairment.) • Monitor for neurological side effects such as numbness and tingling of the extremities. (Antituberculosis agents, such as isoniazid, cause peripheral neuropathy and depletion of vitamin B_6.) • Collect sputum specimens as directed by thehealthcare provider. (This will determine the effectiveness of the antituberculosis agent.) • Monitor for dietary compliance when client is taking isoniazid. (Foods high in tyramine can interact with the drug and cause palpitations, flushing, and hypertension.) • Monitor for side effects specific to various antituberculosis drugs. • Establish infection control measures based on extent of disease condition and established protocol. • Establish therapeutic environment to ensure adequate rest, nutrition, hydration, and relaxation. (Symptoms of TB are manifested when the immune system is suppressed.) • Monitor client's ability and motivation to comply with therapeutic regimen. (Treatment must continue for the full length of therapy to eliminate all *M. tuberculosis* organisms.)	• Instruct client to report yellow eyes and skin, loss of appetite, dark urine, and unusual tiredness Instruct client to: • Report numbness and tingling of extremities • Take supplemental vitamin B_6 as ordered to reduce risk for side effects • Instruct client in technique needed to collect a quality sputum specimen • Advise clients taking isoniazid to avoid foods containing tyramine, such as aged cheese, smoked and pickled fish, beer and red wine, bananas, and chocolate Instruct client to report side effects specific to the antituberculosis therapy prescribed: • Blurred vision or changes in colour or vision field (ethambutol) • Difficulty in voiding (pyrazinamide) • Fever, yellowing of skin, weakness, dark urine (isoniazid, rifampin) • GI system disturbances (rifampin) • Changes in hearing (streptomycin) • Numbness and tingling of extremities (isoniazid) • Red discoloration of body fluids (rifampin) • Dark concentrated urine, weight gain, edema (streptomycin) • Instruct client in infectious control measures, such as frequent handwashing, covering the mouth when coughing or sneezing, and proper disposal of soiled tissues • Teach client to incorporate health-enhancing activities, such as adequate rest and sleep, intake of essential vitamins and nutrients, and intake of six to eight glasses of water per day Explain the importance of complying with the entire therapeutic plan, including: • Take all medications as directed by the healthcare provider • Do not discontinue medication until instructed • Wear a medical alert bracelet • Keep all appointments for follow-up care

Evaluation of Outcome Criteria

Evaluate the effectiveness of drug therapy by confirming that client goals and expected outcomes have been met (see "Planning").

See Table 44.9 for a list of drugs to which these nursing actions apply.

Administration Alerts:

• Give on an empty stomach, 1 hour after or 2 hours before meals.

• Give with meals if GI irritation occurs.

• For IM administration, administer deep into muscle and rotate sites.

• Isoniazid is pregnancy category C.

Adverse Effects and Interactions: The most common side effects of isoniazid are numbness of the hands and feet, rash, and fever. Although rare, liver toxicity is a serious adverse effect; therefore, be alert for signs of jaundice, fatigue, elevated hepatic enzymes, and loss of appetite. Liver enzyme tests are usually performed monthly during therapy to identify early hepatotoxicity.

Aluminum-containing antacids decrease the absorption of isoniazid. When disulfiram is taken with INH, lack of coordination or psychotic reactions may result. Drinking alcohol with INH increases the risk for hepatotoxicity.

DRUGS FOR LEPROSY

44.11 Leprosy is caused by a mycobacterium and is treated by a multidrug regimen.

Leprosy is a chronic infection caused by *M. leprae*. Leprosy has been known about for thousands of years, but the term *leper* has been used by different cultures to designate someone sinful or unclean, not necessarily someone with the disease we now call leprosy.

Although rare in Canada, it is estimated that 6 million people worldwide have leprosy. Clients with leprosy present with macular skin lesions that can become quite large. The organism invades peripheral nervous tissue, causing nerve thickening that results in loss of sensation or paresthesia. If left untreated, the infection causes extreme disfigurement and bone resorption, resulting in loss of digits. The disease is diagnosed through identification of the pathogen from a skin biopsy.

Leprosy may be infectious or non-infectious, depending on the stage of the disease and the progress of pharmacotherapy. Although the mode of transmission is not clear, *M. leprae* is likely spread by the respiratory route. The disease may have a very long incubation period extending from several months to years.

There are two presentations of leprosy, and pharmacotherapy differs for the different types. *Lepromatous* leprosy occurs in clients with defective cell-mediated immunity and is characterized by a slow, progressive development of nodular skin lesions and nerve involvement. Because the client has an impaired immune system, the mycobacteria may disseminate throughout the body and cause death. *Tuberculoid* leprosy is less progressive and may have long periods of remission followed by reactivation with more severe nerve involvement. These clients have an intact cell-mediated immune response; therefore, the disease is more benign and less often fatal.

Like TB, leprosy is treated with prolonged combination pharmacotherapy because monotherapy causes rapid development of resistant strains. Although improvement in skin lesions may occur within a few months, therapy must continue during the entire treatment period to eliminate all mycobacteria. A typical regimen includes the following:

- *Lepromatous leprosy.* Initial three-drug regimen that includes dapsone, clofazimine (Lamprene), and rifampin given for 2 to 5 years.
- *Tuberculoid leprosy.* Initial two-drug regimen with dapsone and rifampin for 6 to 12 months, followed by dapsone alone for 2 to 3 years.

Other drugs may be substituted when the client cannot tolerate the standard regimen. Ofloxacin, clarithromycin, and minocycline are antibacterials that have activity against *M. leprae* and may be used during the long course of leprosy pharmacotherapy.

During the first year of pharmacotherapy, skin lesions may actually worsen because of activation of the cell-mediated immune response. Skin edema may occur, and new lesions may appear on normal skin. Most of these reactions occur because immune cells are attacking antigens released by the mycobacteria. If this occurs, corticosteroids such as prednisone are added to the regimen to reduce the severe inflammation.

Clients with leprosy are examined monthly throughout the initial course of treatment and less frequently as therapy progresses. Follow-up may continue for 3 years or longer after the completion of pharmacotherapy. Close contacts of clients with leprosy normally do not receive chemoprophylaxis as do those of clients with TB, although follow-up examinations are conducted to ensure that they have not acquired the infection.

PROTOTYPE DRUG   **Dapsone**

Actions and Uses: Dapsone is a drug of choice for the treatment of *M. leprae* infections, usually in combination with other antileprosy drugs. It has several off-label uses that include the chemoprophylaxis of malaria in combination with pyrimethamine (Daraprim). In combination with trimethoprim, dapsone is used for the prophylaxis and treatment of *Pneumocystis jiroveci* pneumonia in clients with AIDS. It may take 3 to 6 months of dapsone therapy before symptoms begin to improve.

Pharmacokinetics: The mechanism of action of dapsone is incompletely understood but is thought to be the same as that of the sulfonamides: it inhibits folic acid metabolism. Route of administration is PO and it is readily absorbed and widely distributed. It crosses the placenta, is secreted into breast milk, and is up to 90% protein bound. Onset of action of dapsone is 4 to 8 hours, with a half-life of 20 to 30 hours. The primary site of metabolism is the liver, and it is excreted mainly by the kidney and in small amounts in feces.

Administration Alerts:

- Contraindications include hypersensitivity to dapsone or related drugs, such as sulfonamides.
- Because of its adverse effects on the hematological system, caution should be used in treating clients with pre-existing blood disorders.
- Frequent blood assessments are conducted during therapy to avoid serious adverse effects.
- Frequent liver enzyme testing should be conducted to monitor for hepatotoxicity, especially in clients with pre-existing liver impairment.

Adverse Effects and Interactions: The most frequent adverse effects of dapsone relate to the hematological system: dose-related hemolysis and methemoglobinemia with cyanosis. Aplastic anemia and agranulocytosis are rare, though potentially severe, adverse effects. Toxic hepatitis has been reported. The drug concentrates in the skin, causing dermatological reactions that include photosensitivity and toxic epidermal necrolysis.

Some clients who are receiving pyrimethamine and dapsone concurrently develop agranulocytosis during the second and third month of therapy; therefore, concurrent administration of these drugs must be carefully monitored. Increased dapsone levels have been reported in clients who are receiving trimethoprim, and clients receiving this combination may be at increased risk for dapsone toxicity. Rifampin may significantly reduce serum levels of dapsone. The H_2-receptor blockers such as ranitidine (Zantac) will decrease gastric pH and lower the effectiveness of dapsone.

CHAPTER
44

Understanding the Chapter

Key Concepts Summary

The numbered key concepts provide a succinct summary of the important points from the corresponding numbered section within the chapter. If any of these points are not clear, refer to the numbered section within the chapter for review.

44.1 Penicillins kill bacteria by disrupting the cell wall. Allergies occur most frequently with the penicillins.

44.2 The cephalosporins are similar in structure and function to the penicillins and are one of the most widely prescribed anti-infective classes. Cross-sensitivity may exist with the penicillins in some clients.

44.3 Tetracyclines have some of the broadest spectrums, but they are drugs of choice for relatively few diseases.

44.4 The macrolides are safe alternatives to penicillin for many diseases.

44.5 The aminoglycosides are narrow-spectrum drugs that have the potential to cause serious adverse effects such as ototoxicity, nephrotoxicity, and neuromuscular blockade.

44.6 The use of fluoroquinolones has expanded far beyond their initial role in treating urinary tract infections.

44.7 Once widely prescribed, resistance has limited the usefulness of sulfonamides to urinary tract infections and a few other specific infections.

44.8 A number of miscellaneous antibacterials have specific indications, distinct antibacterial mechanisms, and related nursing care.

44.9 Urinary antiseptics are anti-infective drugs used exclusively for urinary tract infections.

44.10 Multiple-drug therapy is needed in the treatment of tuberculosis since the complex microbes are slow growing and commonly develop drug resistance.

44.11 Leprosy is caused by a mycobacterium and is treated by a multidrug regimen.

Chapter 44 Scenario

Katie Dennison is an 83-year-old retired school teacher. She was recently seen by her healthcare provider for removal of a non-cancerous skin lesion. Now she suspects that the wound on her arm has become infected. She has attempted to report this condition to her healthcare provider. However, due to the holidays she has been unable to reach him. Ms. Dennison presents to a local urgent care centre for treatment.

The physical examination and diagnostic tests reveal the following findings. Vital signs are temperature, 38°C; pulse, 110 beats/minute; respiratory rate, 20 breaths/minute; and blood pressure, 108/68 mm Hg. The large dressing on her left arm is saturated with dried yellow-green exudate. She states that it is painful to move her left arm and that the pain has limited her range of motion in the affected extremity. She is pale and has "paper thin," fragile skin.

Ms. Dennison reports that she accidentally got the dressing wet while taking a shower. She did not change the dressing because she

was not told to do so by her healthcare provider when the skin lesion was removed. A series of laboratory tests were completed. A sterile dressing was applied to the wound. Ms. Dennison was given an injection of cefazolin (Ancef) and a prescription for antibiotics. She was also instructed to follow up with her healthcare provider within the next 2 to 3 days.

Critical Thinking Questions

1. What factors possibly contributed to the wound infection in this client?

2. What laboratory tests were probably obtained during this visit to the urgent care centre?

3. What information should the nurse provide to the client concerning the prescribed antibiotic?

4. Discuss the mechanism of action for cefazolin.

See Answers to Critical Thinking Questions in Appendix B.

NCLEX Practice Questions

1 Which instruction should the nurse give a 21-year-old female client being treated with ampicillin?

   a. Stop taking oral contraceptives because serious adverse effects could occur.

   b. Use oral contraceptives as prescribed because antibiotics do not react with birth control pills.

   c. The antibiotic may decrease the effectiveness of oral contraceptives.

   d. The antibiotic, when taken with oral contraceptives, causes toxicity.

2 The nurse is caring for a client who is receiving intravenous vancomycin (Vancocin). Which symptom, if present, may indicate that the client is experiencing drug-induced ototoxicity?

   a. Erythema of the earlobes and ear canal

   b. Inner ear pruritus after infusion is completed

   c. Tinnitus and dizziness when remaining still

   d. Ocular pain with purulent drainage

3 A client reports abnormal vaginal discharge after completing a prescription of cefotaxime (Claforan). For which condition is the client most likely exhibiting symptoms?

   a. Hypersensitivity reaction

   b. Superinfection (i.e., a yeast infection)

   c. Pseudomembranous colitis

   d. Antibiotic toxicity

4 A client who has been taking cefixime (Suprax) for the past week and a half returns to the provider with reports of "explosive diarrhea, very watery, sometimes with a lot of mucus" up to eight times in the last 2 days. The client reports significant weakness. For which condition is the client describing symptoms?

   a. Antibiotic-induced peptic ulcer disease

   b. Antibiotic-associated malabsorption

   c. GI-associated hypersensitivity

   d. *Clostridium difficile*–associated diarrhea

5 The nurse is teaching a client who recently was diagnosed with an upper respiratory infection and is prescribed ampicillin. The nurse will evaluate the session as being successful if the client states which of the following?

   a. "I should take this medication on an empty stomach with a full glass of water."

   b. "I can expect my tongue to become black and furry."

   c. "Once I stop coughing, I should stop taking this medication."

   d. "If I miss a dose, I should take two doses together to catch up."

See Answers to NCLEX Practice Questions in Appendix A.

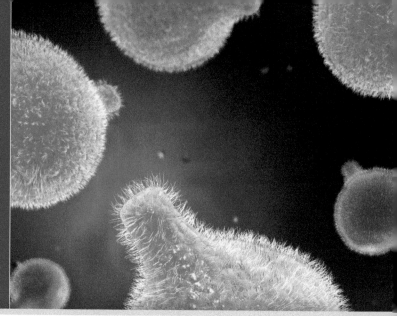

PROTOTYPE DRUGS

ANTIFUNGAL DRUGS
Agents for Systemic Infections
Pr *amphotericin B (Fungizone)*
Pr *fluconazole (Diflucan)*
Agents for Topical Infections
Pr *nystatin (Nyaderm)*

ANTIPROTOZOAN DRUGS
Antimalarial Agents
Non-Malarial Antiprotozoan Agents
Pr *metronidazole (Flagyl)*
Antiparasitic Agents

ANTHELMINTIC DRUGS
Pr *mebendazole (Vermox)*

Stocktrek Images, Inc./Alamy Stock Photo

CHAPTER
45
Pharmacotherapy of Fungal, Protozoan, and Helminthic Infections

LEARNING OUTCOMES

After reading this chapter, the student should be able to:

1. Compare and contrast the pharmacotherapy of superficial and systemic fungal infections.

2. Identify the types of clients at greatest risk for acquiring serious fungal infections.

3. Explain the therapeutic action of each class of drug used for fungal, protozoan, and helminthic infections in relation to the pathophysiology of the infection.

4. Discuss the role of the nurse regarding the non-pharmacological management of fungal infection, including identification of clients who are at greatest risk for acquiring serious fungal infections and client teaching.

5. Explain how an understanding of the *Plasmodium* life cycle is important to the effective pharmacotherapy of malaria.

6. Describe the nurse's role in the pharmacological management of clients who are receiving drugs for fungal, protozoan, malarial, and helminthic infections.

7. For each of the drug classes listed in Prototype Drugs, identify a representative drug and explain its mechanism of action, therapeutic effects, and important adverse effects.

8. Describe and explain, based on pharmacological principles, the rationale for nursing assessment, planning, and interventions for clients with fungal infection.

9. Use the nursing process to care for clients who are receiving drug therapy for fungal infection.

CHAPTER OUTLINE

▶ Characteristics of Fungi

▶ Classification of Mycoses

▶ Mechanism of Action of Antifungal Drugs

▶ Drugs for Systemic Antifungal Infections
  ▶ Pharmacotherapy of Systemic Fungal Diseases

▶ Azoles
  ▶ Pharmacotherapy with the Azole Antifungals

▶ Drugs for Superficial Fungal Infections
  ▶ Superficial Fungal Infections

▶ Protozoan Infections
  ▶ Pharmacotherapy of Malaria
  ▶ Pharmacotherapy of Non-Malarial Protozoan Infections

Fungi, protozoans, and multicellular parasites are more complex than bacteria. Because of structural and functional differences, most antibacterial drugs are ineffective against fungi. The past few decades have seen a dramatic rise in the incidence of fungal infections due to acquired immune deficiency syndrome (AIDS), aggressive cancer chemotherapy, the widespread use of indwelling intravenous (IV) catheters, and the use of broad-spectrum antibiotics. Although there are fewer drugs to treat fungal, protozoan, and helminthic diseases, the available drugs are usually effective.

Characteristics of Fungi

45.1 Fungi are more complex than bacteria and require special classes of drugs because they are unaffected by antibiotics.

Fungi are single-celled or multicellular organisms whose primary role on the planet is to serve as decomposers of dead plants and animals, returning the elements to the soil for recycling. Although 100 000 to 200 000 species exist in soil, air, and water, only about 300 are associated with disease in humans. A few species of fungi normally grow on skin and mucosal surfaces as part of the normal host flora.

Unlike bacteria, which grow rapidly to overwhelm hosts' defences, fungi grow slowly, and infections may progress for many months before symptoms develop. Fungi cause disease by replication; they do not secrete toxins like many bacterial species. With a few exceptions, fungal infections are not readily communicable to those who are in casual contact with the client.

The human body is remarkably resistant to infection by these organisms, and clients with a healthy immune system experience few serious fungal diseases. Clients who have a suppressed immune system, however, such as those infected with human immunodeficiency virus (HIV), may experience frequent fungal infections, some of which may require aggressive pharmacotherapy.

The species of pathogenic fungi that attack a host with a healthy immune system are somewhat distinct from those that infect clients who are immunocompromised. Clients with intact immune defences are afflicted with *community-acquired* infections such as sporotrichosis, blastomycosis, histoplasmosis, and coccidioidomycosis. *Opportunistic* fungal infections acquired in a nosocomial setting are more likely to be candidiasis, aspergillosis, cryptococcosis, and mucormycosis. Table 45.1 lists the most common fungi that cause disease in humans.

TABLE 45.1   Fungal Pathogens

Name of Fungus	Description of Disease
Systemic	
Aspergillus fumigatus, others	Aspergillosis: opportunistic; most commonly affects lung but can spread to other organs
Blastomyces dermatitidis	Blastomycosis: begins in the lungs and spreads to other organs
Candida albicans, others	Candidiasis: most common opportunistic fungal infection; may affect nearly any organ
Coccidioides immitis	Coccidioidomycosis: begins in the lungs and spreads to other organs
Cryptococcus neoformans	Cryptococcosis: opportunistic; begins in the lungs but is the most common cause of meningitis in AIDS clients
Histoplasma capsulatum	Histoplasmosis: begins in the lungs and spreads to other organs
Mucorales (various species)	Mucormycosis: opportunistic; affects blood vessels; causes sinus infections, stomach ulcers, and others
Pneumocystis carinii	Pneumocystis pneumonia: opportunistic; primarily causes pneumonia of the lung but can spread to other organs
Topical	
Candida albicans, others	Candidiasis: affects skin, nails, oral cavity (thrush), and vagina
Epidermophyton floccosum	Athlete's foot (tinea pedis), jock itch (tinea cruris), and other skin disorders
Microsporum audouinii, others	Ringworm of scalp (tinea capitis)
Sporothrix schenckii	Sporotrichosis: primarily affects skin and superficial lymph nodes
Trichophyton (various species)	Affects scalp, skin, and nails

Classification of Mycoses

45.2 Fungal infections are classified as either superficial—affecting hair, skin, nails, and mucous membranes—or systemic, affecting internal organs.

Fungal diseases are called **mycoses**. A simple and useful method of classifying fungal infections is to consider them as either superficial or systemic.

Superficial mycoses affect the scalp, skin, nails, and mucous membranes such as the oral cavity and vagina. Mycoses of this type are often treated with topical drugs, as the incidence of side effects is much lower using this route of administration. Superficial fungal infections are sometimes called **dermatophytic**.

Systemic mycoses are those that affect internal organs, typically the lungs, brain, and digestive organs. Although less common than superficial mycoses, systemic fungal infections affect multiple body systems and are sometimes fatal to clients with suppressed immune systems. Mycoses of this type often require aggressive oral or parenteral medications that produce more adverse effects than the topical agents.

Historically, the antifungal drugs used for superficial infections were clearly distinct from those prescribed for systemic infections. In recent years, this distinction has become blurred. Many of the newer antifungal agents may be used for either superficial or systemic infections. Furthermore, some superficial infections may be treated either systemically or topically.

Mechanism of Action of Antifungal Drugs

45.3 Antifungal medications act by disrupting aspects of growth or metabolism that are unique to these organisms.

Biologically, fungi are classified as eukaryotes; their cellular structure and metabolic pathways are more similar to those of humans than to bacteria. Antibiotics that are efficacious against bacteria are ineffective in treating mycoses. Therefore, an entirely different set of agents is needed.

One important difference between fungal cells and human cells is the steroid in their plasma membranes. Whereas cholesterol is essential for animal cell membranes, **ergosterol** is present in fungi. This difference allows antifungal agents such as amphotericin B (Fungizone) to be selective for fungal plasma membranes. The largest class of antifungals, the **azoles**, inhibits ergosterol synthesis, causing the fungal plasma membrane to become porous, or leaky.

Some antifungals act by mechanisms that take advantage of enzymatic differences between fungi and humans. For example, in fungi, flucytosine (Ancotil) is converted to the toxic antimetabolite 5-fluorouracil, which inhibits both DNA and RNA synthesis. Humans do not have the enzyme necessary for this conversion. Fluorouracil itself is a common antineoplastic drug (see Chapter 60).

DRUGS FOR SYSTEMIC ANTIFUNGAL INFECTIONS

Systemic or invasive fungal disease may require intensive pharmacotherapy for extended periods. Amphotericin B and fluconazole (Diflucan) are drugs of choice. Systemic antifungal drugs are shown in Table 45.2.

NCLEX Success Tip

Ketoconazole (Nizoral) suppresses adrenal steroid secretion and may cause acute hypoadrenalism. The adverse effect should reverse when the drug is discontinued. Ketoconazole does not destroy adrenal cells; it decreases adrenocorticotropic hormone (ACTH)-induced serum corticosteroid levels. Ketoconazole increases the duration of adrenal suppression when given with steroids.

TABLE 45.2 Drugs for Systemic Mycoses	
Drug	Route and Adult Dose
Pr amphotericin B (Fungizone)	IV, 0.3–1.5 mg/kg/day; therapy for 1–1.5 mg/kg over 4 to 6 hours every other day (qod) may be given once therapy is established
caspofungin acetate (Cancidas)	IV, loading dose 70 mg infused over 1 hour on day 1, followed by 50 mg infused over 1 hour four times a day (qid) for 30 days
Pr fluconazole (Diflucan)	Orally (PO)/IV: 150 mg once or a loading dose of 200–800 mg; maintenance of 200–800 mg every day (qd)
flucytosine (Ancotil)	PO, 50–150 mg/kg/day in divided doses every 6 hours (q6h)
itraconazole (Sporanox)	PO, 200 mg qd; may increase to 200 mg twice a day (bid) (max 400 mg/day)
ketoconazole (Nizoral)	PO, 200–400 mg qd
terbinafine (Apo-Terbinafine, Lamisil)	PO, 250 mg qd for 6–13 weeks
voriconazole (VFEND)	IV, 6 mg/kg every 12 hours (q12h) day 1, then 4 mg/kg q12h; may reduce to 3 mg/kg q12h if not tolerated

Pharmacotherapy of Systemic Fungal Diseases

45.4 Amphotericin B is a drug of choice for serious fungal infections of internal organs. Systemic mycoses affect the internal organs and may require prolonged and aggressive drug therapy.

Opportunistic fungal disease in clients with AIDS spurred the development of several new drugs for systemic fungal infections over the past 20 years. Others who may experience systemic mycoses include clients who are receiving prolonged therapy with corticosteroids, clients with extensive burns or indwelling vascular catheters, clients who are receiving antineoplastic agents, and clients who have received an organ transplant. Pharmacotherapy is often extended, lasting for several months. Systemic antifungal drugs have little or no antibacterial activity.

Amphotericin B has been the drug of choice for systemic fungal infections for many years; however, the newer azole drugs such as ketoconazole have replaced amphotericin B for the treatment of less severe systemic infections. Although rarely used as monotherapy, flucytosine is sometimes used in combination with amphotericin B in the pharmacotherapy of severe *Candida* infections. Flucytosine can cause immunosuppression and liver toxicity, and resistance has become a major problem.

Nursing Considerations

The role of the nurse in systemic antifungal therapy involves careful monitoring of the client's condition and providing education as it relates to the prescribed drug regimen. Prior to the initiation of therapy, the client's health history should be taken. This class of drug is contraindicated in clients with hypersensitivity and should be used cautiously in clients with renal impairment or severe bone marrow suppression. Obtain baseline culture and sensitivity tests prior to the beginning of therapy. Baseline and periodic laboratory tests including blood urea nitrogen (BUN), creatinine, complete blood count (CBC), electrolytes, and liver function tests should be obtained. Vital signs, especially pulse and blood pressure, should be obtained for baseline data, as clients with heart disease may develop fluid overload.

Amphotericin B causes some degree of kidney damage in 80% of the clients who take it; therefore, weight as well as intake and output should be monitored. Oliguria, changes in intake and output ratios, hematuria, and abnormal renal function tests should be reported to the physician immediately. Because amphotericin B can cause ototoxicity, assess for hearing loss, vertigo, unsteady gait, and tinnitus.

Electrolyte imbalance is a significant side effect due to excretion of the drug in the urine. Hypokalemia is common, so monitor for symptoms of low potassium levels, including dysrhythmias. Also evaluate all other medications taken by the client for compatibility with systemic antifungal medications. Concurrent therapy with medications that reduce liver or renal function is not recommended.

Client education as it relates to systemic antifungal medications should include goals, reasons for obtaining baseline data, and possible side effects. Instruct the client and caregivers to do the following:

- Complete the full course of treatment.
- Avoid drinking alcohol due to its effects on the liver.
- Use effective contraception measures to prevent pregnancy.
- Monitor urinary output and drink plenty of fluids.
- Use caution while performing hazardous activities.

See Nursing Process Focus: Clients Receiving Amphotericin B for specific points to include when teaching clients regarding this drug.

PROTOTYPE DRUG	Amphotericin B (Fungizone)

Actions and Uses: Amphotericin B has a wide spectrum of activity that includes most of the fungi pathogenic to humans; therefore, it is a drug of choice for most severe systemic mycoses. It may also be indicated as prophylactic antifungal therapy for clients with severe immunosuppression. It acts by binding to ergosterol in fungal cell membranes, causing them to become permeable (leaky). Treatment may continue for several months. Resistance to amphotericin B is not common.

To reduce toxicity, amphotericin B has been formulated with three lipid preparations: liposomal amphotericin B, amphotericin B lipid complex, and amphotericin B cholesteryl sulfate complex. The principal advantage of the lipid formulations is reduced nephrotoxicity and less infusion-related fever and chills. They are generally used only after therapy with other agents has failed, due to their expense.

Pharmacokinetics: Because amphotericin B is not absorbed from the GI tract, it is normally given by IV infusion. Topical preparations are available for superficial mycoses. Drug is distributed to most tissues and fluids except for cerebrospinal fluid (CSF). Half-life with regular dosing is about 2 weeks.

Administration Alerts:

- Infuse slowly. Cardiovascular collapse may result when medication is infused too rapidly.
- Administer premedication to help decrease the chance of infusion reactions.
- Withhold drug if BUN exceeds 40 mg/dL or serum creatinine rises above 3 mg/dL.
- Amphotericin B is pregnancy category B.

Adverse Effects and Interactions: Amphotericin B can cause a number of serious side effects. Many clients develop fever and chills, vomiting, and headache at the beginning of therapy, which subside as treatment continues. Phlebitis is common during IV therapy. Some degree of nephrotoxicity is observed in most clients, and kidney function tests are normally performed throughout the treatment period.

NURSING PROCESS FOCUS

Clients Receiving Amphotericin B (Fungizone)

Assessment	Potential Nursing Diagnoses/Identified Patterns
Prior to administration: • Obtain complete health history, including allergies, drug history, and possible drug interactions. • Obtain culture and sensitivity of suspected area of infection to determine need for therapy. • Obtain baseline vital signs, especially pulse and blood pressure. • Obtain renal function, including blood tests (CBC, chemistry panel, BUN, and creatinine).	• Risk for infection related to drug-induced leukopenia • Impaired skin integrity • Need for knowledge regarding drug therapy and adverse effects • Safety from injury related to side effects of drug therapy

Planning: Client Goals and Expected Outcomes

The client will:

- Report fewer symptoms of fungal infection
- Demonstrate an understanding of the drug's action by accurately describing drug side effects and precautions
- Immediately report effects such as fever, chills, fluid retention, dizziness, or decrease in urine output

Implementation

Interventions (Rationales)	Client Education/Discharge Planning
• Monitor vital signs, especially pulse and blood pressure, frequently during and after infusion. (Cardiovascular collapse may result when drug is infused too rapidly, which is caused by the drug binding to human cytoplasmic sterols.) • Monitor kidney function, including intake and output, urinalysis, and periodic blood work. (Amphotericin B is nephrotoxic. This medication is excreted in the urine and causes significant electrolyte loss from the kidneys.) • Monitor for gastrointestinal (GI) distress. • Monitor for fluid overload and electrolyte imbalance. (Clients with cardiac disease are at high risk.) • Monitor for signs/symptoms of toxicity and hypersensitivity. • Monitor IV site frequently for any signs of extravasation. (Medication is irritating to the vein. Use a central line if possible.)	• Advise client to report dizziness, shortness of breath, heart palpitations, or faintness immediately Instruct client to: • Keep all laboratory appointments for blood work (CBC, electrolytes every 2 weeks; BUN, creatinine weekly) • Keep an accurate record of intake and output • Drink at least 2.5 L of fluids daily • Report a decrease in urinary output, change in the appearance of urine, or weight gain or loss Instruct client to: • Take an antiemetic prior to drug therapy, if needed • Report GI distress such as anorexia, nausea, vomiting, extreme weight loss, and headache • Advise clients with any form of cardiac disease to report any palpitations, chest pain, swelling of extremities, and shortness of breath Instruct client to report the following: • IV: malaise; generalized pain; confusion; depression; hypotension tachycardia; respiratory failure; evidence of otoxicity such as hearing loss, tinnitus, vertigo, and unsteady gait • Topical: irritation, pruritus, dry skin, redness, burning, and itching • Advise client to report any pain at the IV site

Evaluation of Outcome Criteria

Evaluate the effectiveness of drug therapy by confirming that client goals and expected outcomes have been met (see "Planning").

Amphotericin B interacts with many drugs. For example, concurrent therapy with aminoglycosides, vancomycin (Vancocin), carboplatin, and furosemide (Lasix), which reduce renal function, is not recommended. Use with corticosteroids, skeletal muscle relaxants, and thiazole may potentiate hypokalemia. If hypokalemia is present, use with digitalis increases the risk for digitalis toxicity.

AZOLES

The azole drug class actually consists of two different chemical classes, the imidazoles and the triazoles. Azole antifungal drugs interfere with the biosynthesis of ergosterol, which is essential for fungal cell membranes. By depleting fungal cells of ergosterol, their growth is impaired. Several new azoles are in the final stages of clinical trials and should become available over the next few years.

Pharmacotherapy with the Azole Antifungals

45.5 The azole drugs have become widely used in the pharmacotherapy of both systemic and superficial mycoses due to their favourable safety profile.

Most azoles are given by the topical route, although fluconazole may be given orally or parenterally for systemic or superficial infections. Ketoconazole is only available orally, and it is the most hepatotoxic

of the azoles. Itraconazole (Sporanox) has begun to replace ketoconazole in the therapy of systemic mycoses because it has less hepatotoxicity and is given orally. It also has a broader spectrum of activity than the other systemic azoles. Clotrimazole (Canesten) is a drug of choice for fungal infections of the skin, vagina, and mouth.

The systemic azole drugs have a spectrum of activity similar to that of amphotericin B, are considerably less toxic, and have the major advantage that they can be administered orally. Topical formulations are available for superficial mycoses, although they may also be given by the oral route for these infections. Common side effects of the oral and parenteral azoles include nausea, vomiting, diarrhea, and rash.

Nursing Considerations

The role of the nurse in azole therapy involves careful monitoring of the client's condition and providing education as it relates to the prescribed drug regimen. Prior to the initiation of pharmacotherapy, the client's health history should be taken. These drugs are contraindicated in clients with hypersensitivity to azole antifungals and should be used with caution in clients with renal impairment. Laboratory tests, including BUN, creatinine, and liver function tests, should be obtained before therapy begins and throughout the course of treatment. Ketoconazole should not be given to clients with chronic alcoholism because this drug can be toxic to the liver.

Because the azoles can cause GI side effects, assess for nausea, vomiting, abdominal pain, and diarrhea. Monitor for signs and symptoms of hepatotoxicity, such as pruritus, jaundice, dark urine, and skin rash. Azoles may affect glycemic control in diabetic clients, so blood sugar should be monitored carefully in these clients.

Evaluate all other medications taken by the client for compatibility with antifungal drugs. Concurrent therapy with drugs that reduce liver or renal function is not recommended. Monitor for alcohol use, as it increases the risk for side effects such as nausea and vomiting and increases blood pressure.

Client education as it relates to azole drugs should include goals, reasons for obtaining baseline data, and possible side effects. Instruct the client and caregivers to do the following:

- Complete the full course of treatment.
- Report the use of any other prescription or over-the-counter (OTC) medications.
- Avoid drinking alcohol due to its effects on the liver.
- Use effective contraception measures to prevent pregnancy.
- Monitor urinary output and drink plenty of fluids.
- Use caution while performing hazardous activities.
- Advise diabetic clients to increase blood glucose monitoring and report hypoglycemia.

DRUGS FOR SUPERFICIAL FUNGAL INFECTIONS

Superficial fungal infections are generally not severe. If possible, superficial infections are treated with topical agents because they are safer than their systemic counterparts. Agents used to treat superficial mycoses are shown in Table 45.3.

NCLEX Success Tips

Griseofulvin is an antifungal agent that acts by binding to the keratin deposited in the skin, hair, and nails as they grow. This keratin is then resistant to the fungus. But as the keratin is normally shed, the fungus enters new, uninfected cells unless drug therapy continues.

Because griseofulvin is associated with photosensitivity reactions, the nurse should instruct the client to avoid intense sunlight. Griseofulvin is best absorbed when administered after a high-fat meal. Treatment with griseofulvin typically lasts for at least 1 month.

NCLEX Success Tip

Reducing gastric pH can decrease the absorption of ketoconazole and itraconazole (antifungal drugs).

PROTOTYPE DRUG | **Fluconazole (Diflucan)**

Actions and Uses: Like other azoles, fluconazole acts by inhibiting the synthesis of ergosterol. Fluconazole, however, offers several advantages over other systemic antifungals. It is rapidly and completely absorbed when given orally. Unlike itraconazole and ketoconazole, it is able to penetrate most body membranes to reach infections in the central nervous system (CNS), bone, eye, urinary tract, and respiratory tract.

A major disadvantage of fluconazole is its relatively narrow spectrum of activity. Although it is effective against *Candida albicans,* it may not be effective against other *Candida* species, which account for a significant percentage of opportunistic fungal infections.

TABLE 45.3 Drugs for Superficial Mycoses

Drug	Route and Adult Dose)
butoconazole (Gynazole)	Topical, one applicator intravaginally at bedtime (hs) for 3 days
ciclopirox (Loprox, Penlac)	Topical, apply bid for 4 weeks
clotrimazole (Canesten)	Topical, apply bid for 4 weeks; for vaginal mycoses, insert one applicator intravaginally hs for 7 days
econazole (Ecostatin)	Topical, apply bid for 4 weeks
Pr fluconazole (Diflucan)	PO/IV, 150 mg once or a loading dose of 200–800 mg; maintenance of 200–800 mg qd
griseofulvin	PO, 500 mg microsize or 330–375 mg ultra microsize qd
itraconazole (Sporanox)	PO, 200 mg qd; may increase to 200 mg bid (max 400 mg/day)
ketoconazole (Nizoral)	Topical, apply qd–bid to affected area; PO, 200 mg qd
miconazole (Micatin, Monistat)	Topical, apply bid for 2–4 weeks
naftifine (Naftin)	Topical, apply cream qd or gel bid for 4 weeks
Pr nystatin (Nyaderm)	PO, 500 000–1 000 000 units three times a day (tid)
terbinafine (Lamisil)	Topical, apply qd or bid for 7 weeks; PO, 250 mg qd
terconazole (Terazol)	Topical, insert one applicator intravaginally hs for 3–7 weeks
tolnaftate (Tinactin)	Topical, apply bid for 4–6 weeks
undecylenic acid	Topical, apply qd–bid

Pharmacokinetics: Fluconazole is well absorbed after oral administration. It is widely distributed into CSF, crosses the placenta, and enters breast milk. About 80% is excreted unchanged in urine and the rest is metabolized in the liver. Half-life is 30 hours in adults and 24 hours in children.

Administration Alerts:

- Do not mix IV fluconazole with other drugs.
- Fluconazole is pregnancy category C (single dose for vaginal candidiasis) and D (all other indications).

Adverse Effects and Interactions: Fluconazole causes few serious side effects. Nausea, vomiting, and diarrhea are reported at high doses. Because most of the drug is excreted by the kidneys, it should be used cautiously in clients with pre-existing kidney disease. Unlike ketoconazole, hepatotoxicity with fluconazole is rare.

Fluconazole interacts with several drugs. Use with warfarin may cause increased risk for bleeding. Hypoglycemic reaction may be seen with oral sulfonylureas. Fluconazole levels may be decreased with concurrent rifampin (Rifadin, Rofact) or cimetidine (Tagamet) use. The effects of fentanyl (Duragesic), alfentanil (Alfenta), and methadone (Metadol) may be prolonged with concurrent administration of fluconazole.

CONNECTIONS | Natural Therapies

◀ Remedies for Fungal Infections

Several natural products are reported to have antifungal properties:

- Grape seed extract: taken from the seeds of the grape *Vitis vinifera*; capsules are used orally for 3 to 6 months
- Garlic: in capsule or liquid extract form
- Probiotics: bacteria that compete with the fungi for resources; refrigerated supplements that contain *Lactobacillus acidophilus* and *Bifidobacterium bifidum* are the most potent
- Astragalus root: in capsule and tincture form
- Tea tree oil and thyme oil: used externally for fungal infections of the skin; these oils are powerful and should be diluted with another oil such as olive oil

Superficial Fungal Infections

45.6 Antifungal drugs to treat superficial mycoses may be given topically or orally. They are safe and effective in treating infections of the skin, nails, and mucous membranes.

Superficial fungal infections of the hair, scalp, nails, and mucous membranes of the mouth and vagina are rarely medical emergencies. Infections of the nails and skin, for example, may be ongoing for months or even years before a client seeks treatment. Unlike systemic fungal infections, superficial infections may occur in any client, not just those who have suppressed immune systems. About 75% of all female clients experience vulvovaginal candidiasis at least once in their lifetime.

Superficial antifungal drugs are much safer than their systemic counterparts because penetration into the deeper layers of the skin is generally poor and only small amounts are absorbed. Many are available as OTC creams, gels, and ointments. If the infection has grown into the deeper skin layers, oral antifungal drugs may be indicated. Extensive superficial mycoses are often treated with oral antifungal drugs along with the topical agents to be certain that the infection is eliminated.

Selection of a particular antifungal agent is based on the location of the infection and characteristics of the lesion. Griseofulvin is an inexpensive, older agent that is indicated for the oral therapy of mycoses of the hair, skin, and nails that have not responded to conventional topical preparations. Itraconazole and terbinafine (Lamisil) are oral preparations that have the advantage of accumulating in nail beds, allowing them to remain active many months after therapy is discontinued.

Although nystatin belongs to the same chemical class as amphotericin B, the **polyenes**, nystatin is available in a wider variety of formulations, including cream, ointment, powder, tablet, and lozenge. Too toxic for parenteral administration, it is primarily used topically for *Candida* infections of the vagina, skin, and mouth. When given topically, nystatin produces few adverse effects other than minor skin irritation. It may also be used orally to treat candidiasis of the intestine because it travels through the GI tract without being absorbed. When given orally, it may cause diarrhea, nausea, and vomiting.

Nursing Considerations

The role of the nurse in superficial antifungal therapy involves careful monitoring of the client's condition and providing education as it relates to the prescribed drug regimen. Prior to the initiation of therapy with antifungals, the client's health history should be obtained. Assess for signs of contact dermatitis; if this is present, the drug should be withheld and the physician notified.

There are few side effects to antifungals used for superficial mycoses. The medications may be "swished and swallowed" when used to treat oral candidiasis. Monitor for side effects such as nausea, vomiting, and diarrhea when the client is taking high doses. If GI side effects are especially disturbing, the client should be advised to spit out the medication rather than swallowing it. Some orders will be to "swish only" and then to spit out the medication. Monitor for signs of improvement in the mouth and on the tongue to evaluate the effectiveness of the medication.

Client education as it relates to superficial antifungal drugs should include goals, reasons for obtaining baseline data, and possible side effects. Instruct the client and caregivers to do the following:

- Complete the full course of treatment; some infections require pharmacotherapy for several months.
- If self-treating with OTC preparations, follow the directions carefully and notify the healthcare provider if symptoms do not resolve in 7 to 10 days.
- Abstain from sexual intercourse during treatment for vaginal infections.
- Teach clients with vaginal candidiasis the correct method for using vaginal suppositories, creams, and ointments.

See Nursing Process Focus: Clients Receiving Pharmacotherapy for Superficial Fungal Infections for specific points to include when teaching clients regarding this class of drugs.

PROTOTYPE DRUG | Nystatin (Nyaderm)

Actions and Uses: Nystatin binds to sterols in the fungal cell membrane, allowing leakage of intracellular contents as the membrane becomes weakened. Although it belongs to the same chemical class as amphotericin B, the polyenes, nystatin is available in a wider variety of formulations, including cream, ointment, powder, tablet, and lozenge. It is too toxic for parenteral administration and is primarily used topically for *Candida* infections of the vagina, skin, and mouth. It may also be used orally to treat candidiasis of the intestine because it travels through the GI tract without being absorbed.

NCLEX Success Tip

Nystatin oral solution is an antifungal medication used to treat fungal or yeast infections. Nystatin oral solution should be swished around the mouth after eating for the best contact with mucous membranes. Taking the drug before or with meals does not allow for optimal contact with mucous membranes.

Pharmacokinetics: Nystatin is poorly absorbed after oral administration. Distribution is unknown. It has a rapid onset and duration of about 2 hours when administered locally.

NURSING PROCESS FOCUS

Clients Receiving Pharmacotherapy for Superficial Fungal Infections

Assessment	Potential Nursing Diagnoses/Identified Patterns
Prior to administration: • Obtain complete health history, including allergies, drug history, and possible drug interactions. • Obtain culture and sensitivity of suspected area of infection to determine need for therapy. • Obtain baseline liver function tests.	• Risk for impaired skin integrity (rash) • Need for knowledge regarding drug therapy and adverse effects • Safety from injury related to side effects of drug therapy

Planning: Client Goals and Expected Outcomes

The client will:

• Report healing of fungal infection
• Demonstrate an understanding of the drug's action by accurately describing drug side effects and precautions
• Immediately report adverse effects such as hepatoxicity, GI distress, rash, or decreased urine output

Implementation

Interventions (Rationales)	Client Education/Discharge Planning
• Monitor for possible side effects or hypersensitivity. • Encourage adherence with instructions for taking oral antifungals (to increase medication effectiveness). • Monitor topical application. • Avoid occlusive dressings. (Dressings increase moisture in the infected area and encourage development of additional yeast infections.) • Monitor for contact dermatitis with topical formulations. (This is related to the preservatives found in many of the formulations.) • Encourage infection control practices (to prevent the spread of infection).	Instruct client to report: • Burning, stinging, dryness, itching, erythema, urticaria, angioedema, and local irritation for superficial drugs • Symptoms of hepatic toxicity—jaundice, dark urine, light-coloured stools, and pruritis • Nausea, vomiting, and diarrhea • Signs and symptoms of hypoglycemia or hyperglycemia Instruct client to: • Swish the oral suspension to coat all mucous membrane, then swallow medication • Spit out medication instead of swallowing if GI irritation occurs • Allow troche to dissolve completely, rather than chewing or swallowing; it may take 30 minutes for it to completely dissolve • Avoid food or drink for 30 minutes following administration • Remove dentures prior to using the oral suspension • Take ketoconazole with water, fruit juice, coffee, or tea to enhance dissolution and absorption • Instruct client to avoid wearing tight-fitting undergarments if using ointment in the vaginal or groin area • Instruct client to report any redness or skin rash Instruct client to: • Clean affected area daily • Apply medication with a glove • Wash hands properly before and after application • Change socks daily if rash is on feet

Evaluation of Outcome Criteria

Evaluate the effectiveness of drug therapy by confirming that client goals and expected outcomes have been met (see "Planning").

See Table 45.3, as well as the oral and topical systemic drugs listed in Table 45.2, for a list of drugs to which these nursing actions apply.

Administration Alerts:

• Apply with a swab to affected area in infants and children, as swishing is difficult or impossible.

• Nystatin is pregnancy category C.

Adverse Effects and Interactions: When given topically, nystatin produces few adverse effects other than minor skin irritation. There is a high incidence of contact dermatitis, which is related to the preservatives found in many of the formulations.

When given orally, it may cause diarrhea, nausea, and vomiting.

TABLE 45.4   Drugs for Malaria

Drug	Route and Adult Dose)
atovaquone (Mepron)	PO, 750 mg bid for 21 days
hydroxychloroquine (Plaquenil) (see Chapter 61, page 781, for the Prototype Drug box)	Prophylaxis: PO, 400 mg once weekly beginning 2 weeks before exposure; treatment: PO, 800 mg initially, followed by 400 mg at 6, 24, and 48 hours
mefloquine (Lariam)	Prophylaxis: PO, 250 mg weekly starting 1 week before arrival in endemic area, continuing weekly during travel and for 4 weeks after leaving endemic area; treatment: PO, 1250 mg (5 tablets) as a single dose
primaquine	PO, 15 mg qd for 2 weeks
atovaquone/proguanil (Malarone)	Prevention: 250 mg/100 mg qd; start 1–2 days prior to entering endemic area, continue throughout the stay and for 7 days after returning; treatment: PO, 1000 mg/400 mg as a single dose for 3 consecutive days
pyrimethamine (Daraprim)	PO, 25 mg once a week for 10 weeks
quinine	PO, 600 mg q8h for 3–7 days (use in combination with tetracycline, doxycline, or clindamycin)

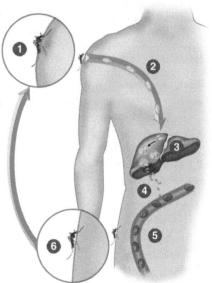

1. Infected mosquito bites person
2. Plasmodium travels to liver
3. Merozoites divide inside hepatocytes
4. Merozoites are released to bloodstream causing fever and chills
5. Merozoites enter red blood cells
6. Mosquito bites person and becomes infected to restart cycle

Figure 45.1   Life cycle of *Plasmodium.*

Superficial antifungals, such as nystatin, should not be used vaginally during pregnancy to treat infections caused by *Gardnerella vaginalis* or *Trichomonas* species. They should be used with caution in clients who are lactating.

PROTOZOAN INFECTIONS

Protozoans are single-celled animals. Although only a few of the more than 20 000 species cause disease in humans, they have a significant health impact in Africa, South America, and Asia. Travellers to these continents may acquire these infections overseas and bring them back to the United States and Canada. These parasites often thrive in conditions where sanitation and personal hygiene are poor and population density is high. In addition, protozoan infections often occur in clients who are immunocompromised, such as those in the advanced stages of AIDS. The most common protozoan disease in humans is malaria. Drugs for malarial infections are shown in Table 45.4.

NCLEX Success Tip

Difficulty seeing out of one eye in clients receiving hydroxychloroquine (Plaquenil) leads to the suspicion of possible retinal degeneration. The possibility of an irreversible retinal degeneration caused by deposits of hydroxychloroquine in the layers of the retina requires an ophthalmologic examination before therapy is begun and at 6-month intervals.

Pharmacotherapy of Malaria

45.7 Malaria is the most common protozoal disease and requires multidrug therapy due to the complicated life cycle of the parasite and to reduce resistance.

Drug therapy of protozoan infections is difficult due to the animals' complicated life cycles. When faced with adverse conditions, protozoans can form cysts that allow the animal to survive in harsh environments and infect other hosts. When cysts occur inside the host, the parasite is often resistant to pharmacotherapy. With few exceptions, antibiotics, antifungals, and antiviral drugs are ineffective against protozoans.

Malaria is caused by four species of the protozoan *Plasmodium.* Malaria is the second most common fatal infectious disease in the world, with 300 to 500 million cases occurring annually. Although an average of only 538 cases are treated per year in Canada, increased immigration and foreign travel have resulted in a gradual increase in cases.

Malaria begins with a bite from an infected female *Anopheles* mosquito. Once inside the human host, *Plasmodium* multiplies in the liver and transforms into progeny called **merozoites**. About 14 to 25 days after the initial infection, the merozoites are released into the blood. The merozoites infect red blood cells, which eventually rupture, releasing more merozoites and causing severe fever and chills. This is called the **erythrocytic stage** of the infection. *Plasmodium* can remain in body tissues for extended periods and cause relapses months, or even years, after the initial infection. The life cycle of *Plasmodium* is shown in Figure 45.1.

Pharmacotherapy of malaria attempts to interrupt the complex life cycle of *Plasmodium.* Although successful early in the course of the disease, therapy becomes increasingly difficult as the parasite enters different stages of its life cycle. Goals of antimalarial therapy include prevention of the disease, treatment of acute attacks, and prevention of relapses.

Prevention of malaria is the best therapeutic option because the disease is very difficult to treat after it has been acquired. Staying indoors from dusk to dawn when mosquitoes are biting most, wearing long-sleeved shirts and long pants, sleeping under a mosquito net, and using DEET-based insect repellents are recommended. Health Canada recommends that travellers to endemic areas receive prophylactic antimalarial drugs prior to and during their visit and for 1 to 4 weeks after leaving, depending on the specific drug. Because resistance has become a major problem in many regions of the world, in 2001 the World Health Organization

(WHO) recommended the use of artemisinin-based combination therapies in order to ensure high cure rates of *Plasmodium falciparum* malaria and to reduce the spread of drug resistance. In 2005, WHO called on all countries to develop combination drug therapies and begin the process of withdrawing monotherapies. Atovaquone/proguanil (Malarone) is a combination of two antimalarial drugs that is taken daily. It is used for treatment of malaria and prevention of chloroquine-resistant malaria. It is useful for those making short trips into areas with malaria risk.

During treatment of acute attacks, drugs are used to interrupt the erythrocytic stage and eliminate the merozoites from red blood cells. Treatment is most successful if it begins immediately after symptoms are recognized. Parenteral quinine is the drug of choice in Canada for the treatment of severe and complicated malaria. The Canadian Malaria Network was established to provide 24-hour access to this life-saving drug for persons with severe malaria. It also gathers surveillance data to improve the prevention, diagnosis, and management of malaria in Canada.

To prevent relapse, drugs are given to eliminate the latent forms of *Plasmodium* residing in the liver. Primaquine phosphate is one of the few drugs able to affect a total cure.

Nursing Considerations

The role of the nurse in antimalarial therapy involves careful monitoring of the client's condition and providing education as it relates to the prescribed drug regimen. Prior to the initiation of drug therapy, the client's health history should be taken. Those with hematological disorders and severe skin disorders such as psoriasis and those who are pregnant should not take antimalarial drugs. These drugs should be used cautiously in clients with preexisting cardiovascular disease and those who are lactating.

Initial laboratory work should include CBC, liver and renal function tests, and a test for glucose-6-phosphate dehydrogenase (G6PD) deficiency. Chloroquine (Aralen) may precipitate anemia in those with G6PD deficiency; furthermore, it concentrates in the erythrocytes and leukocytes and may cause bone marrow depression. A baseline electrocardiogram (ECG) should be taken because of potential cardiac complications associated with some antimalarial drugs. Other baseline information should include vital signs, especially temperature and blood pressure, and hearing and vision testing. All other medication taken by the client should be fully evaluated for compatibility with antimalarial medications, as drug-drug interactions are common.

During treatment, all vital signs should be closely monitored and periodic ECGs and CBCs should be obtained. Especially monitor for GI side effects such as vomiting, diarrhea, and abdominal pain; oral antimalarial drugs can be given with food to reduce GI distress. Assess for signs of allergic reaction, such as flushing, rashes, edema, and pruritus. Monitor for signs of toxicity, which include ringing in the ears with quinine and severe cardiac complications and/or CNS complications such as seizures and blurred vision.

Client education as it relates to antimalarial drugs should include goals, reasons for obtaining baseline data, and possible side effects. Instruct the client and caregivers to do the following:

- Complete the full course of treatment.
- Take with food to decrease GI upset.
- Change position slowly to decrease postural hypotension.
- Use effective contraception measures to prevent pregnancy.
- Abstain from alcohol.
- Do not perform hazardous tasks until the effects of the drug are known.
- Report significant side effects such as flushing, rashes, edema, itching, ringing in the ears, blurred vision, and seizures.

Pharmacotherapy of Non-Malarial Protozoan Infections

45.8 Treatment of non-malarial protozoan disease generally requires a different set of medications than those used for malaria. Other common protozoal diseases that may be indications for pharmacotherapy include amebiasis, toxoplasmosis, giardiasis, cryptosporidiosis, trichomoniasis, trypanosomiasis, and leishmaniasis.

Although infection by *Plasmodium* is the most significant protozoan disease worldwide, infections caused by other protozoans affect significant numbers of people in endemic areas. These infections include amebiasis, toxoplasmosis, giardiasis, cryptosporidiosis, trichomoniasis, trypanosomiasis, and leishmaniasis. Like *Plasmodium*, the non-malarial protozoan infections occur more frequently in areas where public sanitation is poor and population density is high. Several of these infections occur in severely immunocompromised clients. Each of the organisms has unique differences in its distribution pattern and physiology. Descriptions of common non-malarial protozoan infections are given in Table 45.5.

TABLE 45.5 Non-Malarial Protozoan Infections

Name of Protozoan	Description of Disease
Cryptosporidium (various species)	Cryptosporidiosis: primarily a disease of the intestines; often seen in immunocompromised clients
Entamoeba histolytica	Amebiasis: primarily a disease of the large intestine that may cause liver abscesses; rarely travels to other organs such as the brain, lungs, or kidney
Giardia lamblia	Giardiasis: primarily a disease of the intestines that may cause malabsorption, gas, and abdominal distention
Leishmania (various species)	Leishmaniasis: affects various body systems, including the skin, liver, spleen, or blood depending on the species
Pneumocystis carinii	Pneumocystosis: primarily causes pneumonia in immunocompromised clients
Toxoplasma gondii	Toxoplasmosis: causes a fatal encephalitis in immunocompromised clients
Trichomonas vaginalis	Trichomoniasis: causes inflammation of the vagina and urethra and is spread through sexual contact
Trypanosoma brucei	Trypanosomiasis: the African form, known as sleeping sickness, causes CNS depression in severe infections; the American form, known as Chagas disease, invades cardiac tissue

TABLE 45.6 Drugs for Non-Malarial Protozoan Infections

Drug	Route and Adult Dose
Pr metronidazole (Flagyl)	PO, 250–750 mg tid
pentamidine	IV, 4 mg/kg qd for 14–21 days; infuse over 60 minutes
tetracycline	PO, 250–500 mg q6h-q12h
doxycycline (Vibramycin)	IV/PO, 100–200 mg/day in 1 or 2 divided doses

One such protozoan infection, amebiasis, affects more than 50 million people and causes 100 000 deaths worldwide. Caused by the protozoan *Entamoeba histolytica,* amebiasis is common in Africa, Latin America, and Asia. Although primarily a disease of the large intestine, where it causes ulcers, *E. histolytica* can invade the liver and create abscesses. The primary symptom of amebiasis is amebic **dysentery**, a severe form of diarrhea. Drugs used to treat amebiasis include those that act directly on amoebas in the intestine and those that are administered for their systemic effects on the liver and other organs. Drugs for non-malarial protozoan infections are shown in Table 45.6.

Nursing Considerations

The role of the nurse in non-malarial antiprotozoan therapy involves careful monitoring of the client's condition and providing education as it relates to the prescribed drug regimen. Prior to the initiation of drug therapy, the client's health history should be taken. Antiprotozoan therapy is contraindicated in clients with blood dyscrasias and active organic disease of the CNS and during the first month of pregnancy. These drugs are contraindicated in alcoholics; the medication is not administered until more than 24 hours after the client's last drink of alcohol. It should be used cautiously in clients with peripheral neuropathy or pre-existing liver disease. These drugs should be used cautiously in clients who have a history of bone marrow depression because of the possibility of leukopenia. Safety and efficacy have not been established in children.

Initial laboratory work should include CBC and thyroid and liver function tests. Baseline vital signs should be obtained. Evaluate all other drugs taken by the client for compatibility with antiprotozoan drugs. Closely monitor vital signs and thyroid function during therapy because serum iodine may increase and cause thyroid enlargement with iodoquinol.

Monitor for GI distress; oral medications can be given with food to decrease unpleasant effects. Clients taking metronidazole (Flagyl) may complain of dryness of mouth and a metallic taste. Monitor for CNS toxicity such as seizures, paresthesia, nausea, and vomiting and for allergic responses such as urticaria and pruritus.

Client education as it relates to non-malarial antiprotozoan drug therapy should include goals, reasons for obtaining baseline data, and possible side effects. Instruct the client and caregivers to do the following:

- Complete the full course of treatment.
- Take with food to decrease GI upset.
- Use effective contraception measures to prevent pregnancy.
- Avoid using hepatotoxic drugs, including alcohol, which may cause a disulfiram (Antabuse)-like reaction.
- Recognize that urine may turn reddish-brown as an effect of the medication.
- Have any sexual partners treated concurrently to prevent reinfection.
- Immediately report seizures, numbness in limbs, nausea, vomiting, hives, or itching.

NURSING PROCESS FOCUS

Clients Receiving Metronidazole (Flagyl)

Assessment	Potential Nursing Diagnoses/Identified Patterns
Prior to administration: • Obtain complete health history, including allergies, drug and herbal history, and possible drug interactions. • Obtain results from serological studies, stool samples, or cultures of the suspected area of infection to determine the need for therapy. • Obtain baseline vital signs, especially pulse and blood pressure. • Obtain complete blood count.	• Nutritional adequacy • Risk for injury related to dizziness secondary to side effect of drug • Discomfort • Risk for dehydration and altered nutrition related to nausea and vomiting secondary to side effect of drug • Need for knowledge regarding drug therapy and adverse effects • Safety from injury related to side effects of drug therapy

Planning: Client Goals and Expected Outcomes

The client will:

- Report decreased signs and symptoms of amoebic or other infection
- Demonstrate an understanding of the drug's action by accurately describing drug side effects and precautions
- Immediately report effects such as seizures, numbness in limbs, nausea, vomiting, hives, or itching

Implementation

Interventions (Rationales)	Client Education/Discharge Planning
• Monitor CBC periodically. (The drug may cause leukopenia.) • Encourage treatment of sexual partner. (Asymptomatic trichomoniasis in the male is a frequent source of reinfection.) • Monitor use of alcohol. (Metronidazole interferes with the metabolism of alcohol and causes a disulfram-like reaction.) • Monitor CNS toxicity. (High doses may cause seizures and peripheral neuropathy possibly related to the medication's distribution into the CSF.) • Monitor for allergic reactions. • Monitor for GI distress. (This is the most common adverse effect.)	• Instruct client to notify the healthcare provider of fever or other signs of infection • Instruct client that simultaneous treatment of a sexual partner is necessary Instruct client to: • Abstain from alcohol, including any OTC medication that contains alcohol (liquid cough and cold products) • Report side effects such as cramping, vomiting, flushing, and headache, which may result with alcohol use • Instruct client to immediately report seizures, numbness of limbs, nausea, and vomiting • Instruct client to immediately report hives and itching, rash, flushing, fever, and/or joint pain Instruct client to: • Take medication with food to decrease GI distress • Recognize that medication may cause a metallic taste in the mouth

Evaluation of Outcome Criteria

Evaluate the effectiveness of drug therapy by confirming that client goals and expected outcomes have been met (see "Planning").

CONNECTIONS Special Considerations

◀ Parasitic Infections in Children

Many parasitic infections are common among children, with the national rates highest in children younger than 5 years of age. In public health laboratories, the most commonly diagnosed intestinal parasite is giardiasis. These cases are usually associated with water-related activities such as swimming and possibly the use of diapers.

Children adopted from Asian countries, Central and South America, and Eastern Europe also have a high rate of parasitic infection. Up to 35% of foreign-born adopted children are reported to be infected with *Giardia lamblia*. Environments in which these children have been living, particularly those from orphanages, often provide favourable conditions for infectious disease. The Centers for Disease Control and Prevention (CDC) recommends that internationally adopted children undergo examination of at least one stool sample, and three stool samples if GI symptoms are present. Unfortunately, evidence has shown that in communities where helminthic infections are common, poor nutritional status, anemia, and impaired growth and learning in children result.

PROTOTYPE DRUG **Metronidazole (Flagyl)**

Actions and Uses: Metronidazole is the prototype drug for most forms of amebiasis, being effective against both the intestinal and the hepatic stages of the disease. Resistant forms of *E. histolytica* have not yet emerged with metronidazole. The drug is unique among antiprotozoan drugs in that it also has antibiotic activity against anaerobic bacteria and thus is used to treat a number of respiratory, bone, skin, and CNS infections. Metronidazole

is a drug of choice for two other protozoan infections: giardiasis and trichomoniasis. It is used for *Helicobacter pylori* infections of the stomach. It is also used prophylactically in colorectal surgery. Topical forms of this agent are used to treat rosacea, a disease characterized by skin reddening and hyperplasia of the sebaceous glands, particularly around the nose and face.

NCLEX Success Tip

Metronidazole can cause a disulfiram-like reaction if it is taken with alcohol. Tachycardia, nausea, vomiting, and other serious interaction effects can occur. Metronidazole will cause a metallic taste in the mouth and make the urine a darker colour.

Pharmacokinetics: Metronidazole is about 80% absorbed after oral administration. It is widely distributed. It crosses the placenta and enters breast milk and the CSF. It is partially metabolized by the liver and partially excreted unchanged in urine and feces. Half-life is 6 to 12 hours.

Administration Alerts:
• Extended-release form must be swallowed whole.
• Metronidazole is contraindicated during the first trimester of pregnancy.
• Metronidazole is pregnancy category B.
• Abstain from using alcohol

Adverse Effects and Interactions: The most common side effects of metronidazole are anorexia, nausea, diarrhea, dizziness, and headache. Dryness of the mouth and an unpleasant metallic taste may be experienced. Although side effects are relatively common, most are not serious enough to cause discontinuation of therapy.

Metronidazole interacts with several drugs. For example, oral anticoagulants potentiate hypoprothrombinemia. In combination

TABLE 45.7 Drugs for Helminthic Infections

Drug	Route and Adult Dose
Pr mebendazole (Vermox)	PO, 100 mg for one dose or 100 mg bid for 3 days
praziquantel (Biltricide)	PO, 20–25 mg/kg/dose tid at 4–6 hour intervals for 1 day
pyrantel (Combantrin)	PO, 11 mg/kg for one dose (max 1 g)

with alcohol, metronidazole may elicit a disulfiram-like reaction. This would include other medications that may contain alcohol. The drug also may elevate lithium (Carbolith, Lithane) levels.

DRUGS FOR HELMINTHIC INFECTIONS

Helminths consist of various species of parasitic worms that have more complex anatomy, physiology, and life cycles than the protozoans. Diseases due to these pathogens affect more than 2 billion people worldwide and are quite common in areas that lack high standards of sanitation. Helminthic infections in Canada are neither common nor fatal, although drug therapy may be indicated. Drugs for helminthic infections are shown in Table 45.7.

Pharmacotherapy of Helminthic Infections

45.9 Helminths are parasitic worms that cause significant disease in certain regions of the world. The goals of pharmacotherapy are to kill the parasites locally and to disrupt their life cycle.

Helminths are classified as roundworms (nematodes), flukes (trematodes), or tapeworms (cestodes). The most common helminthic disease worldwide is caused by the roundworm *Ascaris lumbricoides*; however, infection by the pinworm *Enterobius vermicularis* is more common in North America. Drugs used to treat these infections are called anthelmintics.

Like protozoans, helminths have several stages in their life cycle, which includes immature and mature forms. Typically, the

CONNECTIONS | **Lifespan Considerations**

◀ **Prevention of Childhood Helminthic Infections**

Pinworms and roundworms (helminths) are more commonly seen in children because many of their hygiene and play habits contribute to transmission and reinfestation. Instruct parents and family members about ways to prevent exposure to and spread of helminths. Teach children correct handwashing techniques, emphasizing cleaning under the nails and washing before eating, after using the toilet, and after playing with pets. Discourage placing the fingers in the mouth, biting nails, and scratching the anal area. Children should wear shoes when playing outside. Avoid use of sandboxes that are accessed by dogs or cats; keep sandboxes covered when not in use. Clean all fruits and vegetables before eating. Keep diapers and undergarments clean and dry.

immature forms of helminths enter the body through the skin or digestive tract. Most attach to the human intestinal tract, although some form cysts in skeletal muscle or in organs such as the liver.

Pharmacotherapy is not indicated for all helminthic infections because the adult parasites often die without reinfecting the host. When the infestation is severe or complications occur, pharmacotherapy is initiated. Complications caused by extensive infections may include physical obstruction in the intestine, malabsorption, increased risk for secondary bacterial infections, and severe fatigue. Pharmacotherapy is aimed at eradicating the parasites locally in the intestine and systemically in the tissues and organs they have invaded. Some anthelmintics are effective against multiple organisms, whereas others are specific for a certain species.

Nursing Considerations

The role of the nurse in anthelmintic therapy involves careful monitoring of the client's condition and providing education as it relates to the prescribed drug regimen. Prior to the initiation of drug therapy, the client's health history should be taken. Anthelmintic therapy should be used cautiously in clients who are pregnant or lactating, have pre-existing liver disease, or are under the age of 2 years.

Initial laboratory tests should include a CBC and liver function studies. A stool specimen is obtained for verification and identification of the parasite and to determine the need for therapy. Other baseline information should include vital signs. Evaluate all other medications taken by the client for compatibility with anthelmintic drugs.

Closely monitor laboratory results and vital signs during therapy. Cases of leukopenia, thrombocytopenia, and agranulocytosis have been associated with the use of albendazole. Assessment of the client's health habits and living conditions should be done to locate and treat others who may be exposed and to identify means to prevent reinfection.

Monitor for GI symptoms such as abdominal pain and distention and diarrhea because these symptoms may occur as worms die. Such side effects are likely to occur more frequently in clients with Crohn's disease and ulcerative colitis because of the inflammatory process in the intestine. The nurse must monitor for CNS side effects such as drowsiness with thiabendazole (Mintezol). Allergic responses include urticaria and pruritus.

Client education as it relates to anthelmintic drug therapy should include goals, reasons for obtaining baseline data, and possible side effects. Instruct the client and caregivers to do the following:

- Complete the full course of treatment.
- Use effective contraception measures to prevent pregnancy during therapy.
- Avoid hazardous activities until the effects of the drug are known.
- Concurrently treat those who have close contact with the client in order to prevent reinfection.
- Report significant side effects such as itching and hives.

PROTOTYPE DRUG | **Mebendazole (Vermox)**

Actions and Uses: Mebendazole is used in the treatment of a wide range of helminthic infections, including those caused by roundworm (*Ascaris*) and pinworm (*Enterobiasis*) species. As a broad-spectrum drug, it is particularly valuable in mixed helminthic infections. It is effective against both the adult and the larval stages of these parasites.

Pharmacokinetics: Mebendazole is poorly absorbed after oral administration, which allows it to retain high concentrations in the intestine. For pinworm infections, a single dose is usually sufficient; other infections require 3 days of therapy. Half-life is 3 to 9 hours.

Administration Alerts:

- Drug is most effective when chewed and taken with a fatty meal.
- Mebendazole is pregnancy category C.

Adverse Effects and Interactions: Because so little of the drug is absorbed, mebendazole does not generally cause serious systemic side effects. As the worms die, some abdominal pain and distention and diarrhea may be experienced.

Carbamazepine (Tegretol) and phenytoin (Dilantin) can increase the metabolism of mebendazole.

NURSING PROCESS FOCUS

Clients Receiving Mebendazole (Vermox)

Assessment	Potential Nursing Diagnoses/Identified Patterns
Prior to administration: • Obtain complete health history, including allergies, drug history, and possible drug interactions. • Obtain a stool specimen for verification of parasite and need for therapy. • Obtain CBC. • Assess the client's living situation, including number of individuals in close contact with the client.	• Abdominal pain related to side effect of drug • Risk for dehydration related to diarrhea secondary to drug therapy • Need for knowledge regarding drug therapy and adverse effects

Planning: Client Goals and Expected Outcomes

The client will:

- Report decreased signs and symptoms of parasitic infection
- Demonstrate an understanding of the drug's action by accurately describing drug side effects and precautions
- Immediately report effects such as itching, hives, diarrhea, and fever

Implementation

Interventions (Rationales)	Client Education/Discharge Planning
• Monitor stools (to assess effectiveness of drug therapy). • Monitor for side effects. • Monitor CBC. (Thrombocytopenia, reversible neutropenia, and leukopenia may occur during therapy.) • Monitor for pregnancy. (Even one dose of this medication during the first trimester has been shown to cause fetal damage.) • Monitor self-administration of medication, including chewing tablets or crushing and mixing with fatty foods. (Drug is most effective when taken with fatty foods, which increase absorption.) • Evaluate health habits. (Lifestyle changes may be required to prevent the spread of infestation and prevent future infections.)	• Instruct client to bring stool sample to lab for testing • Instruct client to report transient abdominal pain, diarrhea, and fever • Instruct client to report any bleeding or signs of infection Instruct client to: • Use effective birth control during drug therapy • Notify the healthcare provider of any signs or suspicion of pregnancy • Instruct client that tablets can be chewed, swallowed, or crushed and mixed with food, especially fatty foods such as cheese or ice cream Instruct client: • That all family members should be treated at the same time to prevent reinfection • To wash all fruits and vegetables and to cook meat thoroughly • To carefully wash hands with soap and water before and after eating and toileting • To wash toilet seats with disinfectant • To keep nails clean and out of mouth • To wear tight underwear and change daily • To sleep alone and wash bedding • That it is extremely important to complete the entire course of drug therapy

Evaluation of Outcome Criteria

Evaluate the effectiveness of drug therapy by confirming that client goals and expected outcomes have been met (see "Planning").

CHAPTER
45

Understanding the Chapter

Key Concepts Summary

The numbered key concepts provide a succinct summary of the important points from the corresponding numbered section within the chapter. If any of these points are not clear, refer to the numbered section within the chapter for review.

45.1 Fungi are more complex than bacteria and require special classes of drugs because they are unaffected by antibiotics.

45.2 Fungal infections are classified as either superficial—affecting hair, skin, nails, and mucous membranes—or systemic, affecting internal organs.

45.3 Antifungal medications act by disrupting aspects of growth or metabolism that are unique to these organisms.

45.4 Amphotericin B is a drug of choice for serious fungal infections of internal organs. Systemic mycoses affect the internal organs and may require prolonged and aggressive drug therapy.

45.5 The azole drugs have become widely used in the pharmacotherapy of both systemic and superficial mycoses due to their favourable safety profile.

45.6 Antifungal drugs to treat superficial mycoses may be given topically or orally. They are safe and effective in treating infections of the skin, nails, and mucous membranes.

45.7 Malaria is the most common protozoal disease and requires multidrug therapy due to the complicated life cycle of the parasite and to reduce resistance.

45.8 Treatment of non-malarial protozoan disease generally requires a different set of medications than those used for malaria. Other common protozoal diseases that may be indications for pharmacotherapy include amebiasis, toxoplasmosis, giardiasis, cryptosporidiosis, trichomoniasis, trypanosomiasis, and leishmaniasis.

45.9 Helminths are parasitic worms that cause significant disease in certain regions of the world. The goals of pharmacotherapy are to kill the parasites locally and to disrupt their life cycle.

Chapter 45 Scenario

Sarah Williams is a 54-year-old female with lung cancer who recently finished her second round of chemotherapy. She comes to her appointment at the oncology clinic with concerns about white patches on her tongue and mouth. She states that her mouth is not sore but her throat burns when she swallows. This has made it very difficult for her to eat and drink.

A history and physical examination are completed. Sarah is 65 cm tall and weighs 52.7 kg. The healthcare provider evaluates Sarah for oropharyngeal candidiasis. Sarah was diagnosed with lung cancer several months earlier and is taking chemotherapy and corticosteroids. Upon initial assessment, her vital signs are normal, and she has no

complaints except her expressed concerns about her mouth and throat. She has worn dentures for about 5 years.

Critical Thinking Questions

1. What are the signs and symptoms that you, as the nurse, look for to determine if Sarah is experiencing oropharyngeal candidiasis?

2. Why do you think that Sarah is at risk for this type of infection?

3. What treatment do you anticipate Sarah will receive? What client teaching will she need regarding this treatment?

See Answers to Critical Thinking Questions in Appendix B.

NCLEX Practice Questions

1 A client is admitted to the intensive care unit for systemic fungal infections. Amphotericin B has been ordered and the nurse will administer this drug slowly IV. When administered too rapidly, amphotericin B may cause which significant adverse effects? Select all that apply.

a. Laryngeal spasms

b. Hypotension

c. Hypokalemia

d. Shock

e. Hypoglycemia

2 A client with AIDS has been given a prescription for oral fluconazole (Diflucan) to prevent *Candida* infection. Considering the client's primary diagnosis and the order for fluconazole, what essential teaching will the nurse provide?

a. Keep a food diary and request antinausea medication if eating becomes problematic.

b. Maintain regular low-impact exercise daily to avoid loss of muscle mass.

c. Wear a high-filtration mask if going out in public.

d. Avoid all fat-based soaps and allow the body to air-dry after bathing.

3 Nystatin suspension has been ordered for treatment of thrush (oropharyngeal *Candida*) in a 6-week-old infant. What instructions should the caregiver receive? Select all that apply.

a. Give the infant a small amount of water after feedings and before the drug to rinse the mouth.

b. Using an applicator or syringe, distribute the solution around the mouth and tongue, allowing the infant to swallow the remainder.

c. For a better taste, chill the suspension in the refrigerator before administering.

d. Give the suspension before feeding the infant to prevent adverse GI effects.

e. Add the suspension to a bottle of formula for easier administration.

4 The nurse is caring for a client with onychomycosis (nail fungus) who is receiving oral terbinafine (Lamisil) for treatment. The client questions the need for 3 months' worth of pills. What would the nurse's best response be?

a. "The healthcare provider will evaluate your nails monthly and stop treatment earlier if it's warranted."

b. "It is cheaper to buy more pills at one time than on a monthly schedule."

c. "The extensive prescription avoids the need for shorter term, potentially toxic doses."

d. "Nails grow slowly and the nail beds must receive an adequate length of treatment to eliminate the infection."

5 The nurse knows that pretreatment with corticosteroids, antihistamines, and antipyretics prior to the administration of amphotericin B is given for which effect?

a. To enhance the effectiveness of amphotericin B

b. To eliminate toxic by-products of amphotericin B

c. To reduce the severity of adverse effects associated with amphotericin B

d. To increase the half-life of amphotericin B

See Answers to NCLEX Practice Questions in Appendix A.

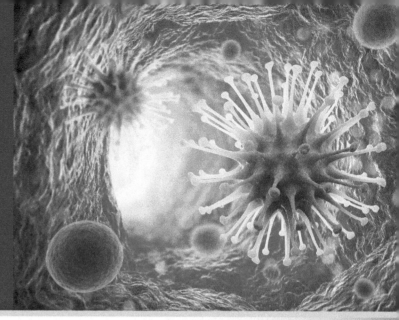

Andrzej Wojcicki/Science Photo Library/Brand X Pictures/Getty Images

PROTOTYPE DRUGS

AGENTS FOR HERPESVIRUSES	AGENTS FOR HEPATITIS
Pr *acyclovir (Zovirax)*	Interferons
AGENTS FOR INFLUENZA	Non-interferons
amantadine (Symmetrel)	

CHAPTER 46

Pharmacotherapy of Non-HIV Viral Infections

LEARNING OUTCOMES

After reading this chapter, the student should be able to:

1. Identify drug classes used for treating viral diseases.

2. Explain the five principal stages in the pathogenesis of a viral infection.

3. Explain general principles related to the pharmacotherapy of viral infections.

4. Describe the nurse's role in the pharmacological management of clients who are receiving medications for herpesviruses, influenza viruses, and hepatitis viruses.

5. Discuss the role of the nurse regarding the non-pharmacological management of viral diseases through client teaching.

6. For each of the drug classes listed in Prototype Drugs, identify a representative drug and explain its mechanism of action, therapeutic effects, and important adverse effects.

7. Describe and explain, based on pharmacological principles, the rationale for nursing assessment, planning, and interventions for clients who are receiving antiretroviral and antiviral drugs.

8. Use the nursing process to care for clients who are receiving antiretroviral and antiviral drugs.

CHAPTER OUTLINE

▸ Characteristics of Viruses

▸ Pharmacotherapy of Non-HIV Viral Infections

▸ Herpesviruses

  ▸ Pharmacotherapy of Herpesvirus Infections

▸ Influenza

  ▸ Pharmacotherapy of Influenza

▸ Hepatitis

  ▸ Pharmacotherapy of Hepatitis

Viruses are microscopic infectious agents capable of causing disease in humans and other organisms. After infecting an organism, viruses use host enzymes and cellular structures to replicate. Although the number of antiviral drugs has increased dramatically in recent years due to research on the epidemic of acquired immune deficiency syndrome (AIDS), antivirals remain the least effective of all anti-infective drug classes. This chapter examines the pharmacotherapy of non–human immunodeficiency virus (HIV) viral infections, including herpesviruses, influenza viruses, and hepatitis viruses. Drugs for HIV infection are discussed in Chapter 47.

Characteristics of Viruses

46.1 Viruses are non-living intracellular parasites that require host machinery to replicate.

Viruses are non-living agents that infect bacteria, plants, and animals. Viruses contain none of the cellular organelles necessary for self-survival that are present in living organisms. In fact, the structure of viruses is quite primitive compared to even the simplest cell. Surrounded by a protein coat, or **capsid**, a virus possesses only a few dozen genes, in the form of either ribonucleic acid (RNA) or deoxyribonucleic acid (DNA), that contain the information needed for viral replication. Some viruses also have a lipid envelope surrounding them. A mature infective particle is called a **virion**.

Although non-living and structurally simple, viruses are capable of remarkable feats. They infect their host by entering a target cell and then using the machinery inside that cell to replicate. Therefore, viruses are **intracellular parasites**—they must be inside a host cell to cause infection.

Despite their simple structures viruses are diverse, each having a distinct spectrum of infection. While some viruses are lethal, others can coexist with their host and produce no detectable symptoms. Only a handful of viruses cause significant disease in humans. Not all viral infections warrant pharmacotherapy. Viruses that may be treated with antiviral medications include herpes simplex, cytomegalovirus, Epstein-Barr, varicella zoster, respiratory syncytial virus, and hepatitis.

Despite their diversity, certain stages are common to most viral infections, as shown in Figure 46.1.

The first stage is attachment of the virus to its host cell. In this stage, the proteins on the surface of the virion fuse with protein receptors on the host cell. This attachment is very specific; the "attachment receptor" may be found only in a single species of plant, bacteria, or animal, or even on a single type of cell within an organism. This specificity is why most viruses infect only one species, although a few viruses can mutate and cross species, as is likely the case for HIV.

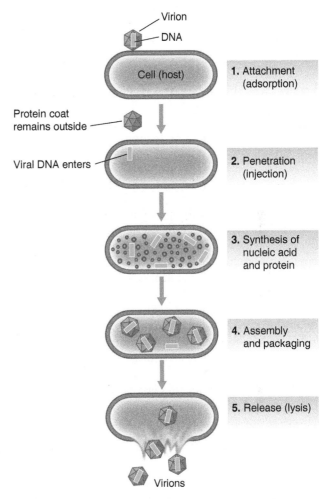

Figure 46.1 The five stages of viral infection.

From *Brock Biology of Microorganisms* (11th ed.), by M. Madigan and J. Martinko, 2006. Reprinted and Electronically reproduced by permission of Pearson Education, Inc., Upper Saddle River, NJ

The second stage of viral infection is penetration of the viral genes and enzymes into the host cell. With some viruses the entire virion enters the cell, whereas others simply "inject" their genes and enzymes into the host cell.

The third stage is synthesis of viral nucleic acid and proteins by the host cell. Immediately after penetration, a few viral proteins are constructed, which assist in duplication of the viral DNA or RNA. Following duplication of the viral genetic material, two possible events may occur. The virus may immediately begin replicating itself by making viral capsid proteins and viral enzymes and then assembling more virions. In some cases, however, the viral DNA enters the nucleus of the host cell, where it inserts into the chromosome and remains for a period of time ranging from weeks to years before it proceeds to the replication stage. Once the viral DNA integrates into the host chromosome, it is called a **provirus**.

Assembly is the fourth stage of viral infection. All viral components, structural proteins, enzymes, and nucleic acids are packaged and made ready for leaving the cell.

The final stage is the release of virions from the host cell. The number of virions may be so large that the cell bursts, releasing all infectious particles at one time, killing the cell. In other cases, the virions bud off of the host's plasma membrane in a slower, continuous process that does not result in death of the host cell.

Pharmacotherapy of Non-HIV Viral Infections

46.2 Pharmacotherapy can lessen the severity of non-HIV viral infections.

Viruses can produce significant effects on their host cells. Some viral infections, such as the common cold, cause acute symptoms but are self-limiting. While symptoms may be annoying, they resolve in 7 to 10 days and the virus causes no permanent effects if the client is otherwise healthy. For these viral infections, drug therapy is not warranted due to the expense and the possibility of producing adverse effects that may be worse than the symptoms of the viral infection itself.

Some viral infections are not self-limiting, and drug therapy can be used to prevent the infection or alleviate symptoms. For example, HIV is uniformly fatal if left untreated. Certain hepatitis viruses can result in permanent liver damage and increase a client's risk of hepatocellular carcinoma. Although not life threatening in most clients, herpesviruses can cause significant pain and, in the case of ocular herpes, permanent disability. Some viruses may even transform normal cells into tumour cells.

Antiviral therapy is targeted to a specific structure of the virus or an aspect of its replication cycle. For example, antiviral drugs are available that inhibit specific viral enzymes or change the shape of proteins that can prevent attachment to the host cell. Many of these drugs have become available only recently, due to research prompted by the AIDS epidemic.

Another approach to treating viral infections is to boost the immune system's response to viral antigens. Prevention of some viral infections can be accomplished through vaccines, which prepare body defences in advance of the infection. Treatment of acute disease may use immunomodulators such as interferons (IFNs) that enhance aspects of the immune response. These are of particular value in treating hepatitis.

Antiviral pharmacotherapy can be extremely challenging due to the rapid mutation rates of viruses, which can quickly render medications ineffective. Also complicating therapy is the intracellular nature of the virus, which makes it difficult for drugs to find their targets without giving excessively high doses that injure normal cells. Antiviral drugs have narrow spectrums of activity, usually limited to one specific virus. For most of the viral pathogens, pharmacological cures are not possible; therefore, antivirals remain the least effective of all anti-infective classes.

HERPESVIRUSES

Herpes simplex viruses (HSVs) are a family of DNA viruses that cause repeated, blister-like lesions on the skin, genitals, and other mucosal surfaces. Antiviral drugs can lower the frequency of acute herpes episodes and diminish the intensity of acute disease.

Pharmacotherapy of Herpesvirus Infections

46.3 Pharmacotherapy can lessen the severity of acute herpes simplex infections and prolong the latent period of the disease.

Herpesviruses are usually acquired through direct physical contact with an infected person. Herpesviruses can also be transmitted from infected mothers to their newborns, sometimes resulting in severe central nervous system (CNS) disease. The herpesvirus family includes the following:

- HSV type 1: primarily causes infections of the eye, mouth, and lips, although the incidence of genital infections is increasing
- HSV type 2: genital infections
- Cytomegalovirus (CMV): affects multiple body systems in immunosuppressed clients
- Varicella-zoster virus (VZV): shingles (zoster) and chickenpox (varicella)
- Epstein-Barr virus (EBV): mononucleosis and a form of cancer known as Burkitt's lymphoma

Pharmacotherapy of initial HSV type 1 and HSV type 2 infections is usually accomplished through oral antiviral therapy for 7 to 10 days (see Table 46.1 for a list of drugs for herpesviruses). Topical forms of several antivirals are available for local applications, though they are not as efficacious as the oral forms. In immunocompromised clients, intravenous (IV) acyclovir (Zovirax) may be indicated.

Following its initial entrance into the client, HSV may remain in a latent, asymptomatic, non-replicating state in ganglia for many years. Immunosuppression, physical challenges, or emotional stress can promote active replication of the virus and the

TABLE 46.1 Drugs for Herpesviruses	
Drug	**Route and Adult Dose**
Pr acyclovir (Zovirax)	HIV-infected patients: PO, 400 mg three times daily (tid) Herpes simplex virus and/or genital infection: PO, 200 mg five times daily while awake
docosanol (Abreva)	Topical, 10% cream applied to cold sore up to five times/day for 10 days
famciclovir (Famvir)	PO, 500 mg tid for 7 days
ganciclovir (Cytovene)	IV, 5 mg/kg infused over 1 hour twice a day (bid)
idoxuridine (Herplex)	Topical, one drop in each eye every hour (q1h) during the day and every 2 hours (q2h) at night
penciclovir (Denavir)	Topical, apply q2h while awake for 4 days
trifluridine (Viroptic)	Topical, one drop in each eye q2h during waking hours (max nine drops/day)
valacyclovir (Valtrex)	PO, 1 g tid for herpes zoster (shingles) PO, 2 g bid for 1 day for herpes labialis (cold sores)

reappearance of characteristic lesions. Although recurrent herpes lesions are usually mild and often require no drug treatment, clients who experience frequent recurrences may benefit from low doses of prophylactic antiviral therapy. It should be noted that the antiviral drugs used to treat herpesviruses do not cure clients; the virus remains with them for their lifetime.

Nursing Considerations

The following material provides a discussion of the nursing considerations for clients who are receiving antiviral medications not associated with HIV infection.

The role of the nurse in antiviral therapy involves careful monitoring of the client's condition and providing education as it relates to the prescribed drug regimen. Because many of these viral infections are systemic and not localized, perform a complete physical assessment prior to drug administration. Once a baseline assessment, including vital signs, weight, and laboratory studies (complete blood count [CBC], viral cultures, liver and kidney function) is completed, focus on the presenting symptoms of the viral infection. For clients with pre-existing renal or hepatic disease, the drugs should be used with extreme caution. Although many antiviral medications are listed as pregnancy category B or C, their judicious use is still warranted during pregnancy. Viral infections that can be treated with antiviral drugs include keratoconjunctivitis and infections that result from HSVs, CMV, EBV, VZV, and respiratory syncytial virus.

Depending on the specific antiviral drug, these agents can be administered intravenously, orally, topically, and through inhalation. Instruct the client in the proper administration techniques. In addition, it is important that the nurse emphasize adherence with antiviral therapy, such as taking the exact dose around the clock even if sleep is interrupted. Many antiviral drugs cause gastrointestinal (GI) distress and should be taken with food. Monitor the client for side effects throughout the course of the treatment and assist the client with managing antiviral-related problems. For example, because ganciclovir (Cytovene) may cause bone marrow suppression, clients should be monitored for anemia, thrombocytopenia, and neutropenia. Because many antiviral drugs are nephrotoxic and hepatotoxic, monitor the client for dysfunction of the kidneys and liver.

Client education as it relates to antiviral drugs should include goals, reasons for obtaining baseline data such as vital signs and tests for cardiac and renal disorders, and possible side effects. Teach the client modes of transmission and methods to prevent spreading the disease, and advise the client that these drugs do not prevent transmission of the virus to other individuals.

The following are other important points to include when teaching clients regarding antiviral agents:

- Report the following symptoms immediately: blood in urine, bruising, yellowing of the skin, fever, chills, confusion, nervousness, dizziness, nausea, and vomiting.
- Take the medication for the full course of therapy and continue taking it, even if symptoms improve, until the full prescription has been taken.
- Keep all appointments for follow-up care.
- Take necessary safety precautions while taking the drug because some antivirals may cause dizziness and drowsiness.

- Do not drive or perform hazardous activities until the effects of the drug are known.
- Consult the healthcare provider before taking any over-the-counter (OTC) medications or herbal supplements because of potentially toxic drug-drug interactions.
- Apply topical preparations with an applicator or a glove to prevent the spread of the virus to other areas.
- Do not apply any other types of cream, ointment, or lotion to the infected sites.

PROTOTYPE DRUG | **Acyclovir (Zovirax)**

Actions and Uses: Acyclovir was approved in 1982 as one of the first antiviral drugs. The activity of acyclovir is limited to the herpesviruses, for which it is a drug of choice. It is most effective against HSV type 1 and HSV type 2 and effective only at high doses against CMV and VZV. Acyclovir acts by inhibiting the viral enzyme thymidine kinase, thus preventing viral DNA synthesis. Acyclovir decreases the duration and severity of herpes episodes. When given for prophylaxis, it may decrease the frequency of herpes episodes, but it does not cure the client. It is available in topical form for direct treatment of active lesions, in oral form for prophylaxis, and in IV form for particularly severe episodes.

NCLEX Success Tips

A client with primary herpes genitalis should apply topical acyclovir ointment in sufficient quantities to cover the lesions every 3 hours, six times per day for 7 days.

Oral acyclovir may cause diarrhea, nausea, and vomiting.

Pharmacokinetics: Acyclovir is about 75% absorbed after oral administration. Distribution is wide. It crosses the placenta and enters breast milk. It enters the CNS. It is about 25% protein bound. A small amount is metabolized by the liver. More than 90% is excreted unchanged in urine. Its half-life is 2.5 to 4 hours. Because of its short half-life, acyclovir may be administered orally up to five times a day.

Administration Alerts:

- When given IV, the drug may cause painful inflammation of vessels at the site of infusion.
- Administer around the clock, even if sleep is interrupted.
- Administer with food.
- Acyclovir is pregnancy category B.

Adverse Effects and Interactions: There are few adverse effects of acyclovir when administered topically or orally. Because nephrotoxicity is possible when the medication is given IV, frequent laboratory tests may be performed to monitor kidney function. Resistance has developed to the drug, particularly in clients with HIV-AIDS.

Acyclovir interacts with several drugs. For example, probenecid (Benuryl) decreases acyclovir elimination, and zidovudine (AZT, Retrovir) may cause increased drowsiness and lethargy.

INFLUENZA

Influenza or flu is a viral infection characterized by acute symptoms that include sore throat, sneezing, coughing, fever, and chills. The infectious viral particles are easily spread via airborne droplets. In vulnerable and immunosuppressed clients, an influenza infection may be fatal. Influenza may be seasonal or pandemic. All of the influenza pandemics of the 20th century were avian in origin. In 1919, a worldwide outbreak of influenza killed approximately 20 million people. In China in 1997, the avian influenza virus A (H5N1 strain) was first transmitted from birds to humans. Since 2003, the virus has appeared in several different countries, causing deaths in humans. This is of global concern because sustained human-to-human transmission of the virus potentially may occur and result in a pandemic. Pandemics are caused by type A viruses. Seasonal influenza may be caused by type A or B viruses. The RNA-containing influenza viruses should not be confused with *Haemophilus influenzae*, which is a bacterium that causes respiratory disease.

Pharmacotherapy of Influenza

46.4 Drugs are available to prevent and to treat influenza infections. Vaccination is the best choice, as drugs are relatively ineffective once symptoms appear.

The best approach to influenza infection is prevention through annual vaccination. Those who benefit greatly from vaccinations include residents of long-term care facilities, those with chronic cardiopulmonary disease, pregnant women in their second or third trimester during the peak flu season, and healthy adults over age 50. Depending on the stage of the disease, HIV-positive clients usually benefit from vaccination. Adequate immunity is achieved about 2 weeks after vaccination and lasts for several months up to a year. Additional details on vaccines are presented in Chapter 41.

Antivirals may be used to prevent influenza or decrease the severity of symptoms. The drug amantadine has been available to prevent and treat influenza for many years. Chemoprophylaxis with amantadine (Symmetrel) is indicated for unvaccinated individuals after a confirmed outbreak of influenza type A. Therapy with these antivirals is sometimes started concurrently with vaccination; the antiviral offers protection during the period before therapeutic antibody titres are achieved from the vaccine. These drugs are generally prescribed for clients who are at greatest risk of the severe complications of influenza. Antivirals for influenza are listed in Table 46.2.

TABLE 46.2   Drugs for Treatment of Influenza

Drug	Route and Adult Dose
Influenza Prophylaxis	
amantadine (Symmetrel)	Orally (PO), 100 mg twice daily (bid)
Influenza Treatment: Neuraminidase Inhibitors	
oseltamivir (Tamiflu)	PO, 30 mg qd to 75 mg bid
zanamivir (Relenza)	Inhalation, two inhalations per day for 5 days

A new class of drug, the neuraminidase inhibitors, was introduced in 1999 to treat active influenza infections. Because seasonal as well as H5N1 viruses develop rapid resistance to amantadine, the neuraminidase inhibitors are often first-choice drugs if administered early in the disease. If given within 48 hours of the onset of symptoms, oseltamivir (Tamiflu) and zanamivir (Relenza) are reported to shorten the normal 7-day duration of influenza symptoms to 5 days. They may reduce complications of influenza such as bronchitis and pneumonia that could lead to death. Oseltamivir is given orally, whereas zanamivir is inhaled. Because these agents produce only modest effects on an active infection, prevention through vaccination remains the best alternative.

HEPATITIS

Hepatitis, or inflammation of the liver, may be caused by drugs, alcohol, autoimmune disorders, metabolic diseases, or infections. Viral hepatitis is a common infection caused by a number of different viruses. Although each virus has its own unique clinical features, they all invade hepatocytes, producing the same symptoms.

Hepatitis may be acute or chronic. Symptoms of acute hepatitis include fever, chills, fatigue, anorexia, nausea, and vomiting. Chronic hepatitis may result in prolonged fatigue, jaundice, liver cirrhosis, and ultimately hepatic failure. Neonates and immunocompromised clients are at higher risk for developing chronic hepatitis. Some clients who are infected with hepatitis viruses, especially children, are asymptomatic.

The three primary types of viral hepatitis are hepatitis A (HAV), hepatitis B (HBV), and hepatitis C (HCV). These are summarized in Table 46.3.

Pharmacotherapy of Hepatitis

46.5 Hepatitis A and B are best treated through immunization. Newer drugs for HBV and HBC have led to therapies for chronic hepatitis.

Hepatitis A virus (HAV), sometimes called infectious hepatitis, is caused by an RNA virus. It is spread by the oral-fecal route primarily in regions of the world that have poor sanitation. Hepatitis B virus (HBV), known as serum hepatitis, is caused by a DNA virus and is transmitted primarily through exposure to contaminated blood and body fluids. HBV has a much greater incidence of chronic hepatitis and a greater mortality rate than HAV. The hepatitis C, D, and E viruses are sometimes referred to as non A–non B viruses.

The best treatment for viral hepatitis is prevention through immunization, which is available for HAV and HBV. HAV vaccine is indicated for those who live in communities with high infection rates and for travellers to countries with high endemic

TABLE 46.3 Summary of Viral Hepatitis Types

Type	Transmission	People at Risk	Prevention	Treatment
Hepatitis A	Primarily through food or water contaminated by feces from an infected person. Rarely, it spreads through contact with infected blood	International travellers; people living in areas where hepatitis A outbreaks are common; people who live with or have sex with an infected person; and, during outbreaks, daycare children and employees, men who have sex with men, and injection drug users	Hepatitis A vaccine; also, avoiding tap water when traveling internationally, and practicing good hygiene and sanitation	Hepatitis A usually resolves on its own over several weeks
Hepatitis B	Through contact with infected blood, through sex with an infected person, and from mother to child during childbirth	People who have sex with an infected person, men who have sex with men, injection drug users, children of immigrants from disease-endemic areas, infants born to infected mothers, people who live with an infected person, health care workers, hemodialysis patients, people who received a transfusion of blood or blood products before July 1992 or clotting factors made before 1987, and international travellers	Hepatitis B vaccine	Chronic hepatitis B: drug treatment with alpha IFN, peginterferon (pegIFN), lamivudine, or adefovir dipivoxil Acute hepatitis B usually resolves on its own; severe cases can be treated with lamivudine
Hepatitis C	Primarily through contact with infected blood; less commonly, through sexual contact and childbirth	Injection drug users, people who have sex with an infected person, people who have multiple sex partners, healthcare workers, infants born to infected women, hemodialysis patients, and people who received a transfusion of blood or blood products before July 1992 or clotting factors made before 1987	There is no vaccine for hepatitis C; the only way to prevent the disease is to reduce the risk of exposure to the virus. This means avoiding behaviours like sharing drug needles or sharing personal items like toothbrushes, razors, and nail clippers with an infected person	Chronic hepatitis C: Drug treatment with pegIFN alone or combination treatment with pegIFN and the drug ribavirin or boceprevir Acute hepatitis C: Treatment is recommended if it does not resolve within 2 to 3 months
Hepatitis D	Through contact with infected blood; this disease occurs only in people who are already infected with hepatitis B	Anyone infected with hepatitis B; injection drug users who have hepatitis B have the highest risk. People who have hepatitis B are also at risk if they have sex with a person infected with hepatitis D or if they live with an infected person. Also at risk are people who received a transfusion of blood or blood products before July 1992 or clotting factors made before 1987	Immunization against hepatitis B for those not already infected; also, avoiding exposure to infected blood, contaminated needles, and an infected person's personal items	Chronic hepatitis D: Drug treatment with alpha IFN
Hepatitis E	Through food or water contaminated by feces from an infected person; uncommon in North America	International travellers, people living in areas where hepatitis E outbreaks are common, and people who live or have sex with an infected person	There is no vaccine for hepatitis E; the only way to prevent the disease is to reduce the risk of exposure to the virus. This means avoiding tap water when travelling internationally and practising good hygiene and sanitation	Hepatitis E usually resolves on its own over several weeks to months

HAV infection. Immunoglobulin, a concentrated solution of antibodies, is sometimes administered to close personal contacts of infected clients to prevent transmission of HAV. The immunoglobulins induce passive protection and provide prophylaxis for about 3 months.

Traditionally, HBV vaccine has been indicated for healthcare workers and others who are routinely exposed to blood and body fluids. Because this vaccination protocol failed to address hepatitis B in early childhood, universal vaccination of all children is now recommended. Post-exposure treatment of hepatitis B may include hepatitis B immunoglobulins and an antiviral agent such as interferon alfa-2a or lamivudine (3TC, Heptovir). Adefovir (Hepsera) is a recently approved therapy for chronic hepatitis B

infections. Following metabolism, adefovir is incorporated into the growing viral DNA strand, causing it to terminate prematurely.

Most clients recover completely from HAV and HBV infection without drug therapy, although complete recovery may take many months. The overall mortality rate is less than 1%. Neonates and immunocompromised clients are at higher risk for developing chronic hepatitis.

Transmitted primarily through exposure to infected blood or body fluid, hepatitis C virus (HCV) is more common than HBV. Up to 50% of all HIV-AIDS clients are co-infected with HCV. A large percentage of clients infected with HCV proceed to chronic hepatitis; HCV is the most common cause of liver transplants. A specific vaccine is not available for hepatitis C. Current pharmacotherapy for chronic HCV infection includes treatment with Rebetron, a combination agent consisting of interferon alfa-2b (Intron A) and ribavirin (Ibavyr). After 24 weeks of treatment with Rebetron, about 30% to 50% of clients will respond with increased liver function. If response is not attained, therapy may continue for as long as 12 to 18 months. Peginterferon alfa-2a (Pegasys) and peginterferon alfa-2b are recently approved therapies for chronic hepatitis C. **Pegylation** is a process that attaches polyethylene glycol to the interferon to extend its pharmacological activity. This permits the interferon to remain in the body longer and exert prolonged activity. Drugs for hepatitis are shown in Table 46.4.

NCLEX Success Tips

Interferon alfa-2b most commonly causes flu-like adverse effects, such as myalgia, arthralgia, headache, nausea, fever, and fatigue.

Clients are advised to administer the drug at bedtime and get adequate rest. The drug may also cause hematologic changes; therefore, laboratory tests such as a complete blood count and differential should be conducted monthly during drug therapy. Blood glucose laboratory values should be monitored for the development of hyperglycemia.

Pregnant clients should not take lamivudine.

TABLE 46.4 Drugs for Hepatitis

Drug	Route and Adult Dose
Interferons	
interferon alfa-2b (Intron A) (see Chapter 40, page 478 for the Prototype Drug box)	Intramuscular/subcutaneous (IM/SC), 2 million U/m^2 three times a week
peginterferon alfa-2a (Pegasys)	SC, 180 μg once a week for 48 weeks
Non-Interferons/Combinations	
adefovir dipivoxil (Hepsera)	PO, 10 mg every day (qd)
lamivudine (3TC, Heptovir)	PO, 150 mg bid
ribavirin/interferon alfa-2b (Ibavyr/Intron A)	Adults more than 75 kg: Rebeton PO, 3 × 200-mg capsules in the a.m. and 3 × 200-mg capsules in the p.m.; Intron A SC, 3 million IU three times a week

CHAPTER

46 Understanding the Chapter

Key Concepts Summary

The numbered key concepts provide a succinct summary of the important points from the corresponding numbered section within the chapter. If any of these points are not clear, refer to the numbered section within the chapter for review.

46.1 Viruses are non-living intracellular parasites that require host machinery to replicate.

46.2 Pharmacotherapy can lessen the severity of non-HIV viral infections.

46.3 Pharmacotherapy can lessen the severity of acute herpes simplex infections and prolong the latent period of the disease.

46.4 Drugs are available to prevent and to treat influenza infections. Vaccination is the best choice, as drugs are relatively ineffective once symptoms appear.

46.5 Hepatitis A and B are best treated through immunization. Newer drugs for HBV and HBC have led to therapies for chronic hepatitis.

Chapter 46 Scenario

Richard Palmer, a 19-year-old university student, has come to the health clinic. He states that he gets cold sores at least six to eight times per year. He informs the nurse that the cold sores usually start with lip pain or tingling, often followed by small, painful, fluid-filled blisters on a raised, red, painful area of his lip. The blisters usually last for 2 to 3 days, then form yellowish crusts that slough off to reveal pinkish skin.

With his final exams coming up, Richard admits to feeling stressed. He also works part time at a local restaurant to help meet the expenses of university. Like other students his age, Richard eats on the run and seldom sleeps more than 4 to 5 hours per night. His weekends are even more hectic, with the job, school, and social activities. Richard requests something to help rid him of the existing cold sore immediately.

Critical Thinking Questions

1. How would you explain the mode of transmission and onset of symptoms for herpes simplex viruses (HSVs) to Richard?

2. How would you respond when Richard asks, "Is there any medication I can take to prevent the cold sores from returning?"

3. Topical acyclovir is prescribed for this client. What client education would you provide?

See Answers to Critical Thinking Questions in Appendix B.

NCLEX Practice Questions

1 Acyclovir (Zovirax) has been ordered IV for a client with a herpes zoster infection to the upper torso and face. Which nursing intervention will help prevent a common adverse effect?

   a. Administering the drug slowly IV over an hour, and encouraging fluid intake throughout the day

   b. Keeping skin areas dry to prevent fungal overgrowth

   c. Administering antihistamines 1 hour before giving the infusion to prevent itching

   d. Assessing visual acuity periodically and providing for eye comfort (for example, with lubricating eye drops)

2 A client is receiving acyclovir (Zovirax) for genital herpes. Which statement by the client would indicate that client teaching for this condition has been successful?

   a. "Neither the topical nor the oral drug will prevent me from giving herpes to someone else."

   b. "I will clean the affected areas with soap and water every other day."

   c. "I should wear tight-fitting clothes over affected areas to prevent the spread of the infection."

   d. "I should start the antiviral therapy after the lesion forms a crust."

3 Which assessment data would be most important for the nurse to monitor frequently in a client receiving amantadine (Symmetrel)? Select all that apply.

   a. White blood cell and platelet counts

   b. Serum creatinine and urine output

   c. Mental status and level of consciousness

   d. Sodium and potassium levels

   e. Lung sounds and signs of peripheral edema

4 A client with chronic hepatitis B has been prescribed tenofovir (Viread). The nurse will teach the client to immediately report symptoms of which adverse and potentially life-threatening drug effect?

   a. Systemic yeast infection

   b. Lactic acidosis

   c. Heart failure

   d. Ventricular dysrhythmias

5 A client is receiving ribavirin (Ibavyr) for treatment of chronic hepatitis B. Which manifestation, if present in the client, would the nurse conclude is an adverse effect of this medication?

   a. Neurologic symptoms such as headaches and dizziness

   b. Respiratory symptoms such as dyspnea and congestion

   c. Skin disruptions such as acne and ulcerations

   d. Hematologic symptoms such as excessive fatigue or dizziness

See Answers to NCLEX Practice Questions in Appendix A.

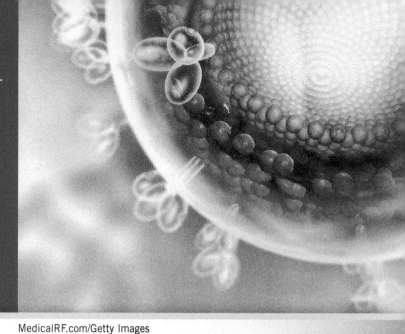

PROTOTYPE DRUGS

ANTIRETROVIRAL DRUGS

Nucleoside and Nucleotide Reverse Transcriptase Inhibitors
Pr *zidovudine (Retrovir, AZT)*

Non-Nucleoside Reverse Transcriptase Inhibitors
efavirenz (Sustiva)
Protease Inhibitors
lopinavir with ritonavir (Kaletra)

MedicalRF.com/Getty Images

CHAPTER 47

Pharmacotherapy of HIV-AIDS

LEARNING OUTCOMES

After reading this chapter, the student should be able to:

1. Describe the primary steps in the pathogenesis of HIV infection.
2. Explain the therapeutic goals for HIV-AIDS pharmacotherapy.
3. Identify reasons for treatment failure during HIV-AIDS pharmacotherapy.
4. Describe the advantages of highly active antiretroviral therapy in the pharmacotherapy of HIV infection.
5. Compare and contrast the classes of antiretroviral medications.
6. Explain the protocol and rationale for post-exposure prophylaxis following occupational exposure to HIV.
7. Explain recent advances in the pre-exposure prophylaxis of HIV infection.
8. Describe the antiretroviral protocols used to reduce the risk for perinatal transmission and for treating pediatric clients with HIV-AIDS.
9. Identify opportunistic infections commonly acquired by clients with AIDS and the drugs used to treat them.
10. Describe the nurse's role in the pharmacological management of clients who are receiving antiretroviral medications.
11. For each of the drug classes shown in Prototype Drugs, identify the prototype and representative drugs and explain the mechanism of drug action, therapeutic effects, and important adverse effects.
12. Apply the nursing process to care for clients who are receiving pharmacotherapy for HIV-AIDS.

CHAPTER OUTLINE

▶ HIV-AIDS

▶ General Principles of HIV Pharmacotherapy

▶ Classification of Drugs for HIV-AIDS

▶ Reverse Transcriptase Inhibitors

  ▶ Pharmacotherapy with Reverse Transcriptase Inhibitors

▶ Protease Inhibitors

  ▶ Pharmacotherapy with Protease Inhibitors

▶ Prophylaxis of HIV Infections

▶ Pharmacotherapy of Opportunistic Infections Associated with HIV-AIDS

HIV-AIDS

47.1 HIV attacks the T4 lymphocyte and uses reverse transcriptase to make viral DNA.

Acquired immune deficiency syndrome (AIDS) is characterized by profound immunosuppression that leads to opportunistic infections and malignancies not commonly found in clients with functioning immune defences. It results from infection with HIV. Antiretroviral drugs for **HIV-AIDS** slow the growth of human immunodeficiency virus (HIV) by several different mechanisms. Resistance to these drugs is a major clinical problem, and a pharmacological cure for HIV-AIDS is not yet achievable

AIDS is characterized by profound immunosuppression, leading to opportunistic infections (OIs) and malignancies not commonly acquired by people who have intact immune defences. The **human immunodeficiency virus (HIV)** was quickly identified as the causative agent for AIDS. HIV-AIDS has resulted in a tragic, worldwide epidemic that has caused the deaths of millions of people. The infection continues to be a major public health challenge.

The two primary types of HIV are HIV-1 and HIV-2. Because more than 99% of the global AIDS cases are caused by HIV-1, the discussion in this text will apply only to HIV-1. HIV uses the same stages of viral infection described in Chapter 46. There are, however, additional details that are important to understanding the pharmacotherapy of HIV infection.

Transmission

HIV infection occurs by exposure to contaminated body fluids, most commonly blood or semen, because these fluids have the highest concentration of the virus. Transmission may also occur through sexual activity or through contact of infected fluids with broken skin, mucous membranes, or needlesticks. Newborns of a mother infected with HIV may acquire the virus during birth or breastfeeding. Although in industrialized nations the majority of clients with HIV-AIDS are men who have sex with other men, heterosexual transmission is significant and is the predominant means of acquiring the infection in developing countries.

Replication Cycle

Like other viruses, HIV must infect a host cell to duplicate its genetic material and assemble more virus particles (virions). Knowledge of the replication cycle of HIV is critical to understanding the pharmacotherapy of HIV-AIDS (see Figure 47.1).

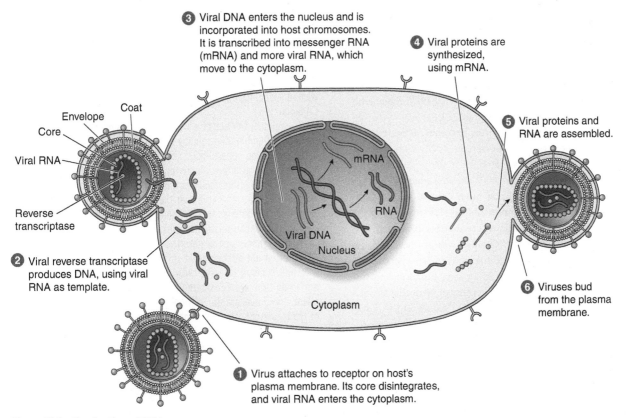

3 Viral DNA enters the nucleus and is incorporated into host chromosomes. It is transcribed into messenger RNA (mRNA) and more viral RNA, which move to the cytoplasm.

4 Viral proteins are synthesized, using mRNA.

5 Viral proteins and RNA are assembled.

6 Viruses bud from the plasma membrane.

2 Viral reverse transcriptase produces DNA, using viral RNA as template.

1 Virus attaches to receptor on host's plasma membrane. Its core disintegrates, and viral RNA enters the cytoplasm.

Coat
Envelope
Core
Viral RNA
Reverse transcriptase
mRNA
RNA
Viral DNA
Nucleus
Cytoplasm

Figure 47.1 Replication of HIV.

The first stage of HIV pathogenesis is the attachment of the virus to its preferred target: the **CD4 receptor** on the surface of T4 lymphocytes. (Note that the terms *CD4 cells*, *T4 cells*, and *T4 lymphocytes* are used interchangeably in this text.) During this initial stage, structural proteins on the surface of HIV fuse with the CD4 receptor. Because these receptors are also present on monocytes, macrophages, and dendritic cells, multiple cell types become infected. In addition to the CD4 receptor, coreceptors known as CCR5 and CXCR4 have been discovered that assist HIV in binding to the T4 lymphocyte.

The second stage of pathogenesis is the penetration of HIV into the T4 lymphocyte. The virus uncoats and the single-stranded ribonucleic acid (RNA) genetic material enters the host cell. HIV converts its RNA strands to double-stranded deoxyribonucleic acid (DNA), using the viral enzyme **reverse transcriptase**. Only a few viruses are able to construct DNA from RNA; no bacteria, plants, or animals are able to perform this unique metabolic function. All living organisms make RNA from DNA. Because of their "backward" or reverse DNA synthesis, these viruses are called *retroviruses* and drugs used to treat HIV infections are called **antiretrovirals**. Although unique to HIV, reverse transcriptase is an inefficient enzyme that makes many errors when converting the viral RNA to double-stranded DNA. The enzyme has no "proofreading" ability, which allows errors in the viral genetic code to accumulate. This produces a high mutation rate, making it difficult to develop effective vaccines.

The viral DNA eventually enters the nucleus of the T4 lymphocyte where it becomes incorporated into the host's chromosomes. This action is performed by HIV **integrase**, another enzyme unique to HIV. Once incorporated into human chromosomes, the HIV is called a provirus, and it remains for the lifetime of the cell. It is impossible to recognize the HIV provirus or remove it. Indeed, despite the fact that the T4 lymphocyte is infected with a deadly virus, the host's immune system is unable to effectively remove the defective cells.

This *latent phase* of the infection may last only a few weeks, or it may continue for decades. During this phase, clients are asymptomatic and do not realize that they are infected. It was once thought that the virus was truly "silent" during the latent phase, but research has demonstrated that continuous HIV replication and immune system damage are occurring.

At some point, the latent provirus becomes activated and produces large amounts of viral messenger RNA, with the first strands producing viral proteins that amplify the replication process. All structural components of HIV are subsequently synthesized, and the cell is ready to assemble more virions.

The individual structural components of HIV migrate to the plasma membrane of the host cell, where they are packaged, and eventually bud from the host cell. The new virions, however, are not yet infectious. As a final step, the viral enzyme **protease** cleaves some of the larger proteins to smaller, functional forms. Once budding occurs, the immune system recognizes that the cell is infected and kills the T4 lymphocyte. Unfortunately, it is too late; it is estimated that a client who is infected with HIV may produce as many as 10 billion new virions every day, and the immune system becomes overwhelmed by the infection.

Symptoms

Many people incorrectly assume that because the body cannot rid itself of HIV, the immune system does not recognize

invasion by the virus. Indeed, the immune system mounts an immediate, massive defence to the entry of HIV, producing an acute inflammatory response that rids the body of many of the infectious virions. It is estimated that 1 billion HIV virions are destroyed each day during this early stage. Clients experience sore throat, fever, rash, malaise, and weight loss that may last for several weeks. However, because clients often mistake these vague symptoms for the common cold or flu, they do not realize that HIV infection has occurred and rarely seek medical intervention. Symptoms during this initial phase are known as the **acute retroviral syndrome**. Although body defences may suppress the viral invasion, tragically they are unable to eliminate the virus.

Progression to AIDS is characterized by gradual destruction of the immune system, as measured by the steady decline in the number of CD4 lymphocytes. Unfortunately, the CD4 lymphocyte is the primary cell that coordinates the immune response for both the humoral and the cell-mediated branches of the immune system. When the CD4 cell count falls below a critical level, the client begins to experience opportunistic bacterial, fungal, and viral diseases and certain malignancies. Left untreated, the client eventually is unable to mount any immune defence, and death occurs.

CONNECTIONS | **Lifespan Considerations**

◀ HIV in Pregnant, Pediatric, and Geriatric Populations

Optimal care and maximal viral suppression during pregnancy may reduce the risk for HIV transmission to the fetus or infant from 25% to less than 1%. Combination antiretroviral therapy is the standard treatment in pregnancy, regardless of viral load and CD4 count. However, the safety of these drugs in pregnancy has yet to be established. Until the fetus is born and becomes an independent neonate, the woman's legal right to make a therapeutic decision has priority under Canadian law.

The younger the age at which a child acquires HIV, the poorer the prognosis. Combination therapy is also used with children. Because children develop opportunistic infections, including serious respiratory infections, at a much more rapid rate than do adults, prophylactic treatment against *Pneumocystis carinii* pneumonia may also be started early. Nurses can assist the caregivers of the child to learn to manage the intense medication regimen and to identify the early symptoms of opportunistic diseases.

The diagnosis of the geriatric client may be delayed because HIV is often not suspected in this population. The geriatric client who has become infected with HIV may be reluctant to disclose activities that are considered high-risk behaviours. The geriatric client may have greater difficulty handling the rigorous regimen of the treatment. The physiological changes associated with aging increase the possibility of drug toxicity in this population. The social factors must also be considered because these clients may be living alone or even be the primary caretaker of a disabled spouse. The ability of a client to be sexually active is not determined by age; therefore, it is very important to stress sexual activity precautions to prevent spread of HIV.

General Principles of HIV Pharmacotherapy

47.2 Antiretroviral drugs used in the treatment of HIV-AIDS do not cure the disease but do help many clients to live longer. Pharmacotherapy may be initiated in the acute (symptomatic) or chronic (asymptomatic) phase of HIV infection.

The widespread appearance of HIV infection in 1981 created enormous challenges for public health and an unprecedented need for the development of new antiviral drugs. HIV-AIDS is unlike any other infectious disease because it is sexually transmitted, is uniformly fatal, and demands a continuous supply of new drugs for client survival. The challenges of HIV-AIDS have resulted in the development of more than 18 new antiretroviral drugs, and many others are in various stages of clinical trials. Unfortunately, the initial hope of curing HIV-AIDS through antiretroviral therapy or vaccines has not been realized; none of these drugs produces a cure for this disease. HIV mutates extremely rapidly, and resistant strains develop so quickly that the creation of novel approaches to antiretroviral drug therapy must be an ongoing process.

While pharmacotherapy for HIV-AIDS has not produced a cure, it has resulted in a number of therapeutic successes. For example, many clients with HIV infection are able to live symptom-free lives for a much longer time due to medications. Furthermore, the transmission of the virus from an HIV-infected mother to her newborn has been reduced dramatically due to intensive drug therapy of the mother prior to delivery and of the baby immediately following birth. These two factors have resulted in a significant decline in the death rate due to HIV-AIDS. Unfortunately, this decline has not been observed in African countries, where antiviral drugs are not as readily available, largely due to their high cost.

The decision to begin treatment during the chronic phase has many negative consequences. Drugs for HIV-AIDS are expensive. These drugs produce a number of uncomfortable and potentially serious side effects. Therapy over many years promotes viral resistance: when the acute stage eventually develops, the drugs may no longer be effective. Two laboratory tests used to guide pharmacotherapy are measurement of the amount of HIV RNA in the plasma and the absolute CD4 lymphocyte count. In asymptomatic clients, initiation of therapy is based on laboratory criteria, primarily the **viral load** and secondly the CD4 lymphocyte count. A plasma viral load greater than 5000 to 10 000 HIV-1 RNA copies/mL, regardless of the CD4 count, is an indication for treatment. A CD4 count of less than 0.3×10^9/L is an indication for treatment regardless of the plasma viral load, to prevent further damage to the immune system. These tests are performed every 3 to 6 months to assess the degree of success of drug therapy.

The decision to begin therapy during the acute phase when symptoms are present is a much easier decision. The severe symptoms of AIDS can progress rapidly to death. Therefore, therapy is nearly always initiated during this phase.

The therapeutic goals for the pharmacotherapy of HIV-AIDS include the following:

- Evidence of reduction of HIV in the blood
- Increased lifespan
- Better quality of life
- Restoration and preservation of immunological function

Classification of Drugs for HIV-AIDS

47.3 Drugs from six drug classes are combined in the pharmacotherapy of HIV-AIDS. The nucleotide reverse transcriptase inhibitors and the fusion inhibitors have been recently developed.

Antiretroviral drugs block phases of the HIV replication cycle. The standard pharmacotherapy for HIV-AIDS includes aggressive treatment with as many as four drugs concurrently, a regimen called **highly active antiretroviral therapy (HAART)**. The goal of HAART is to reduce the plasma HIV RNA to its lowest possible level. It must be understood, however, that HIV is harboured in locations other than the blood, such as lymph nodes; therefore, elimination of the virus from the blood is not a cure. The simultaneous use of drugs from several classes also reduces the probability that the virus will become resistant to treatment. The antiretroviral drugs are shown in Table 47.1.

TABLE 47.1 Antiretroviral Drugs for HIV-AIDS

Drug	Route and Adult Dose
Non-Nucleoside Reverse Transcriptase Inhibitors	
delavirdine (Rescriptor)	Orally (PO), 400 mg three times a day (tid)
efavirenz (Sustiva)	PO, 600 mg every day (qd)
Pr nevirapine (Viramune)	PO, 200 mg qd for 14 days, then increase to twice a day (bid)
Nucleoside and Nucleotide Reverse Transcriptase Inhibitors	
abacavir (Ziagen)	PO, 300 mg bid
didanosine (Videx)	PO, 125–200 mg bid
emtricitabine (Emtriva)	PO, 200 mg once daily
lamivudine (3TC, Heptovir)	PO, 150 mg bid
stavudine (Zerit)	PO, 40 mg bid
tenofovir disoproxil fumarate (Viread)	PO, 300 mg once daily
Pr zidovudine (AZT, Retrovir)	PO, 300 mg bid; Intravenous (IV), 1 mg/kg/dose every 4 hours (q4h) around the clock (6 doses daily)
Protease Inhibitors	
atazanavir (Reyataz)	PO, 300–400 mg qd
indinavir (Crixivan)	PO, 800 mg q8h
nelfinavir (Viracept)	PO, 750 mg tid
ritonavir (Norvir)	PO, 50–600 mg bid
Pr saquinavir (Invirase)	PO, 500–1000 mg bid; always given in combination with ritonavir
Integrase Inhibitors	
enfuviride (Fuzeon)	Subcutaneous (SC), 90 mg bid
raltegravir (Isentress)	PO, 400 mg bid

NCLEX Success Tips

Didanosine (Videx): The nurse should withhold the medication and notify the physician immediately if the client develops manifestations of pancreatitis or hepatic failure, including nausea and vomiting, severe abdominal pain, elevated bilirubin, or elevated serum enzymes (e.g., amylase, aspartate transaminase [AST], alanine transaminase [ALT]).

Lamivudine (3TC, Heptovir): Fluid weight gain is of concern since the medication should be used with caution for clients with impaired renal function. Dosage adjustment may be needed for clients with renal insufficiency since the drug is excreted in the urine.

HIV-AIDS antiretroviral drugs are classified into the following six groups, based on their mechanism of activity:

- Nucleoside/nucleotide reverse transcriptase inhibitor (NRTI/NtRTI)
- Non-nucleoside reverse transcriptase inhibitor (NNRTI)
- Protease inhibitor
- Entry inhibitor (includes fusion inhibitors and CCR5 antagonists)
- Fusion inhibitor
- Integrase inhibitor

The last two classes include recently discovered agents that act by unique mechanisms. Tenofovir (Viread) is an NRTI that is structurally similar to adenosine monophosphate (AMP). After metabolism, tenofovir is incorporated into viral DNA in a manner similar to the NRTIs. Enfuvirtide blocks the fusion of the HIV virion to the CD4 receptor. Raltegravir (Isentress) blocks HIV integrase and prevents HIV from inserting its genes into uninfected DNA.

Pharmacokinetic variables become very important when treating clients with HIV-AIDS and can, in fact, contribute in a major way to the success or failure of pharmacotherapy. The bioavailability of some antiretrovirals is greatly affected by food in the stomach. The absorption of certain antiretrovirals (e.g., indinavir [Crixivan]) is decreased in the presence of food. Some antiretrovirals (e.g., lopinavir and ritonavir [Kaletra]) have a significantly increased absorption with high-fat meals, and others (e.g., nevirapine [Viramune]) are not affected by the presence of food.

In addition to changes in absorption, most antiretrovirals are metabolized by the liver. Several can significantly increase or decrease the hepatic metabolism of other drugs, resulting in large numbers of potential drug-drug interactions. These effects differ, even within the same drug class. For example, nevirapine induces the hepatic P450 enzyme system, thus decreasing the levels of other drugs. Delavirdine (Rescriptor), an antiretroviral in the same class, inhibits the P450 system, thus increasing the levels of other drugs. Predicting and avoiding complex drug interactions in clients with HIV requires truly skilled and dedicated nurses and other healthcare providers who are current on the most recent medical literature.

REVERSE TRANSCRIPTASE INHIBITORS

Drugs in the reverse transcriptase inhibitor class comprise agents that are structurally similar to nucleosides, the building blocks of DNA. This class includes non-nucleoside reverse transcriptase inhibitors, which bind directly to the viral enzyme reverse transcriptase and inhibit its function, and nucleotide reverse transcriptase inhibitors.

Pharmacotherapy with Reverse Transcriptase Inhibitors

47.4 The reverse transcriptase inhibitors block HIV replication at the level of the reverse transcriptase enzyme.

One of the early steps in HIV infection is the synthesis of viral DNA from the viral RNA inside the T4 lymphocyte. The enzyme that performs this step is reverse transcriptase. Because reverse transcriptase is a viral enzyme not found in animal cells, selective inhibition of viral replication is possible.

As viral DNA is synthesized, building blocks known as nucleosides are required. The NRTIs chemically resemble naturally occurring nucleosides. As reverse transcriptase uses these NRTIs to build the DNA, however, the viral DNA strand is prevented from lengthening. The prematurely terminated chain prevents the viral DNA from being inserted into the host chromosome.

As a class, the NRTIs are well tolerated, although nausea, vomiting, diarrhea, headache, and fatigue are common during the first few weeks of therapy. Some of the serious adverse effects of NRTIs are caused by **mitochondrial toxicity**. NRTIs inhibit a human enzyme called polymerase gamma, which is responsible for the replication of DNA in mitochondria. This small, obscure DNA molecule encodes subunits for mitochondrial enzymes in the respiratory chain, which generates adenosine triphosphate (ATP). All of the NRTIs have been associated with a low incidence of an unusual form of mitochondrial toxicity known as lactic acidosis/severe hepatomegaly with steatosis. This syndrome, which occurs more commonly in women and in those with pre-existing hepatic impairment, includes lipid deposits in the liver, elevated transaminase values, and possible hepatic failure. Symptoms are often vague and include nausea, right upper quadrant (RUQ) pain, and myalgia. The nurse must carefully monitor liver function tests and assess for hepatic disease, because some fatalities have resulted from this adverse effect.

Another manifestation of mitochondrial toxicity from NRTIs is **lipodystrophy**, a disorder in which fat is redistributed in specific areas in the body. Areas such as the face, arms, and legs tend to lose fat, while the abdomen, breasts, and base of the neck (buffalo hump) develop excess fat. The fat redistribution may be associated with hyperlipidemia and hyperglycemia.

A second mechanism for inhibiting reverse transcriptase is to affect the enzyme's function. Drugs in the NNRTI class act by binding near the active site of the enzyme, causing a structural change in the enzyme molecule. This causes a direct inhibition of enzyme function.

Although there are differences in their pharmacokinetic and toxicity profiles, no single NRTI or NNRTI offers a significant therapeutic advantage over any other. Choice of agent depends on client response and the experience of the healthcare provider. Because some of these drugs, such as zidovudine (AZT, Retrovir), have been used consistently for more than 15 years, the potential for resistance must be considered when selecting the specific agent. The NRTIs and NNRTIs are nearly always used in multidrug combinations in HAART.

NCLEX Success Tips

A mother who has human immunodeficiency virus (HIV) is strongly discouraged from breastfeeding because of the risk of transmitting the infection to the neonate. Newborns born to HIV-positive mothers are generally treated with the antiviral medication zidovudine for the first 6 weeks after birth.

Zidovudine interferes with replication of HIV and thereby slows progression of HIV infection to acquired immune deficiency syndrome (AIDS). There is no known cure for HIV infection. Today, clients are not treated with monotherapy but are usually on triple therapy due to a much-improved clinical response. Decreased viral loads with the drug combinations have improved the longevity and quality of life in clients with HIV-AIDS.

Because anemia is a major adverse effect of zidovudine, the nurse should monitor the client's red blood cell (RBC) count and assess for signs and symptoms of decreased cellular oxygenation. To be effective, zidovudine must be taken every 4 hours around the clock. Food does not affect absorption of this drug, so the client may take zidovudine either with food or on an empty stomach.

| PROTOTYPE DRUG | Zidovudine (AZT, Retrovir) |

Actions and Uses: Zidovudine was discovered in the 1960s, and its antiviral activity was demonstrated prior to the AIDS epidemic. Structurally, it resembles thymidine, one of the four nucleoside building blocks of DNA. As the reverse transcriptase enzyme begins to synthesize viral DNA, it mistakenly uses zidovudine as one of the nucleosides, thus creating a defective DNA strand. Because of its widespread use since the emergence of AIDS, resistant HIV strains are common. It is used in combination with other antiretrovirals for symptomatic and asymptomatic HIV-infected clients, for reducing transmission of HIV from pregnant woman to fetus, and for post-exposure prophylaxis in healthcare workers and others.

Pharmacokinetics: Zidovudine is well absorbed after oral administration. It is widely distributed, crosses the placenta, and enters the central nervous system (CNS). It is mostly metabolized by the liver. Less than 20% is excreted unchanged in urine. Its half-life is about 1 hour.

Administration Alerts:

- Administer on an empty stomach, with water only.
- Avoid administering with fruit juice.
- Zidovudine is pregnancy category C.

Adverse Effects and Interactions: Zidovudine can result in severe toxicity to blood cells at high doses; anemia and neutropenia are common and may limit therapy. Many clients experience anorexia, nausea, and diarrhea. Clients may report fatigue and generalized weakness.

Zidovudine interacts with many drugs. Acetaminophen (Tylenol) and ganciclovir (Cytovene) may worsen bone marrow suppression. The following drugs may increase the risk of zidovudine toxicity: atovaquone (Mepron), amphotericin B (Fungizone), acetylsalicylic acid (ASA [Aspirin]), doxorubicin (Adriamycin), fluconazole (Diflucan), methadone (Metadol), and valproic acid (Depakene, Epival). Other antiretroviral agents may cause lactic acidosis and severe hepatomegaly with steatosis.

Use with caution with herbal supplements, such as St. John's wort, which may cause a decrease in antiretroviral activity.

| PROTOTYPE DRUG | Nevirapine (Viramune) |

Actions and Uses: Nevirapine is an NNRTI that binds directly to reverse transcriptase, disrupting the enzyme's active site. This inhibition prevents viral DNA from being synthesized from HIV RNA. It is readily absorbed following an oral dose. Since resistance develops rapidly when used as monotherapy, nevirapine is nearly always used in combination with other antivirals in HAART.

Administration Alerts:

- Administer with food to minimize gastric distress.
- Nevirapine is pregnancy category B.

Pharmacokinetics: Nevirapine is well absorbed after oral administration. It crosses the placenta and enters breast milk. It enters the CNS. It is mostly metabolized by the liver. A small amount is excreted unchanged in urine. Its half-life is 25 to 30 hours.

Adverse Effects and Interactions: Nevirapine increases the levels of metabolic enzymes in the liver; therefore, it has the potential to interact with drugs metabolized by this organ. Therapy is sometimes contraindicated in clients with hepatic impairment. Gastrointestinal (GI)-related effects such as nausea, diarrhea, and abdominal pain are experienced by some clients. Skin rashes, fever, and fatigue are frequent side effects. Although rare, some clients acquire Stevens-Johnson syndrome, a sometimes fatal skin condition that affects mucous membranes and large areas of the body. Resistance can develop quite rapidly, which may extend to other NNRTIs.

Nevirapine interacts with several other drugs. For example, nevirapine may decrease plasma concentrations of protease inhibitors and oral contraceptives. It may also decrease methadone levels, inducing opiate withdrawal.

Use with caution with herbal supplements, such as St. John's wort, which may cause a decrease in antiretroviral activity.

PROTEASE INHIBITORS

Drugs in the protease inhibitor class block the viral enzyme protease, which is responsible for the final assembly of the HIV virions.

Pharmacotherapy with Protease Inhibitors

47.5 The protease inhibitors inhibit the final assembly of the HIV virion.

Near the end of its replication cycle, HIV has assembled all of the necessary molecular components for the creation of new virions. Using the metabolic machinery of the host cell, HIV RNA has been synthesized using the viral DNA that was incorporated into the host's genome. The structural and regulatory proteins of HIV have been synthesized using this viral RNA as a template.

As the newly formed virions bud from the host cell and are released into the surrounding extracellular fluid, one final step remains before the HIV is mature: a long polypeptide chain must

CONNECTIONS ◖ Special Considerations

◀ Cultural and Psychosocial Issues with Antiretroviral Drug Adherence

One key to success of antiretroviral therapy is client adherence to the prescribed medication plan. Drug adherence is difficult for most people once they feel well; clients may not feel sick while taking the medications and may be more prone to skip doses for various reasons. Many factors can enhance the probability that the client will adhere to treatment. For example, a multidisciplinary assessment can screen clients for depression, alcohol or drug abuse, or negative attitudes, and interventions can be initiated to minimize the impact on adherence. Cultural factors and personal beliefs may also influence adherence. Education at an appropriate level is essential so that the client can understand the disease process as well as the role the medications play in securing a positive outcome. Agencies such as the Canadian Aboriginal AIDS Network and Canadian AIDS Society provide resources for clients. Developing trust and open communication between the client and healthcare provider is essential to improve the chances of drug adherence and to reach common therapeutic goals.

be cleaved to produce the final HIV proteins. The enzyme that performs this step is HIV protease.

The protease inhibitors attach to the active site of the HIV protease enzyme and prevent the final maturation of the virions. When combined with other antiretroviral drug classes, the protease inhibitors are capable of lowering plasma HIV RNA to levels below the detectable range. The protease inhibitors are metabolized in the liver and have the potential to interact with many different drugs. In general, they are well tolerated, with GI complaints being the most common side effects. Various lipid abnormalities, or lipodystrophies, have been reported, including elevated cholesterol and triglyceride levels and abdominal obesity.

Of the six available protease inhibitors, all have equivalent efficacy and a similar range of adverse effects. Choice of protease inhibitor is generally based on clinical response and the experience of the healthcare provider. Cross-resistance among the various protease inhibitors has been reported.

Nursing Considerations

The following material provides a discussion of NRTIs, NNRTIs, and protease inhibitors. Because antiretrovirals are commonly prescribed for HIV infection, a Nursing Process Focus has been provided for them in this chapter.

Although NRTI, NNRTI, and protease inhibitors act by different mechanisms, the associated nursing care is similar. The role of the nurse involves careful monitoring of the client's condition and providing education as it relates to the prescribed drug regimen. The nurse is instrumental in providing client education, and psychosocial support will be crucial. Clients will experience tremendous emotional distress at various times during treatment. Denial and anger may be evident in the client's behaviour as he or she attempts to cope with the diagnosis.

Assess the client's understanding of the HIV disease process. Although drug therapies may slow the progression of the virus, they are not a cure. Prior to the administration of antiretroviral

drugs, assess for symptoms of HIV and for any opportunistic infections. Plasma HIV RNA (viral load) assays, CD4 counts, complete blood count (CBC), liver and renal profiles, and blood glucose levels should also be monitored. These diagnostic values will determine the effectiveness as well as the toxicity of the drugs used.

Verify the drug combination to determine potential side effects and precautions. All antiretroviral agents are contraindicated during pregnancy and lactation. The list of diseases and conditions that necessitate close observation is quite extensive for the antiretrovirals. Typically, agents classified as NTRI should be used cautiously in clients with pancreatitis, peripheral vascular disease, neuropathy, kidney disorders, liver disorders, cardiac disease, and alcohol abuse. NNTRI agents necessitate judicious use in clients with liver impairment and CNS diseases. Protease inhibitors are potentially problematic for clients who are suffering from sensitivity to sulfonamides, liver disorders, and renal insufficiency. It should be understood that in the acute stages of AIDS, treatment may proceed despite relative contraindications.

Some antiretroviral drugs vary in the way in which they should be taken. For example, clients who are taking an NRTI drug should be instructed to take the medication on an empty stomach. These drugs should always be taken with water only and never with fruit juice because acidic fruit juices interact with them. On the other hand, nevirapine and saquinavir (Invirase) should be taken with food to minimize gastric distress. With all antiretroviral drugs, it is critical that the client be instructed to consult with the healthcare provider before taking any over-the-counter (OTC) medication or herbal supplement to avoid drug interactions.

Many of the side effects of antiretrovirals can dramatically influence activities of daily living. Some of these drugs may cause dizziness or other troublesome CNS effects. When such side effects occur, the client may be instructed to take the medication just before sleep. The client should also be advised not to drive or perform hazardous activities until reaction to the medication is known. Specific side effects depend on the drugs used. The nurse must be vigilant in assessing for side effects and assisting clients to manage their therapeutic regimen.

Client education as it relates to antiretroviral drugs should include goals, reasons for obtaining baseline data such as vital signs and tests for cardiac and renal disorders, and possible side effects. Instruct the client to report adverse effects specific to the antiretroviral agent prescribed. For example, when teaching clients about NRTIs, instruct the client to report fever, skin rash, abdominal pain, nausea, vomiting, numbness, and burning of feet or hands. When teaching clients about NNRTIs, instruct the client to report fever, chills, rash, blistering of skin, reddening of skin, and muscle or joint pain to the healthcare provider. Clients who are taking protease inhibitors should report rash, abdominal pain, headache, insomnia, fever, constipation, cough, fainting, and visual changes.

The role of the nurse in teaching the client who is taking antiretroviral agents is critical and may enhance the quality of life of the individual. Because these clients are highly susceptible to infections, it is essential that the nurse describe the symptoms of infection, such as fever, chills, sore throat, and cough, and the importance of immediately seeking medical care should these signs develop. In addition, the client should be taught methods to minimize exposure to infection. Frequent handwashing, as well as avoiding crowds and people with colds, flu, and other infections, will greatly reduce the client's likelihood of becoming infected. The client should also be instructed to take additional measures to reduce microbial infections, such as increasing fluid intake, emptying the bladder frequently, and coughing and deep breathing several times per day to expel invading organisms.

Nurses should also incorporate health promotional teaching to the client receiving these drugs. Because clients on antiretroviral agents typically have impaired immune systems, instruct them to engage in activities that support immune function. These activities include adequate rest and sleep, consuming a diet that provides essential vitamins and minerals, and drinking six to eight glasses of water per day.

Another important factor in health teaching with these clients focuses on disease transmission. The client should be taught that antiretroviral agents may decrease the level of HIV infection in the blood but will not prevent the risk of transmission to other individuals. The nurse must discuss sensitive issues with the client, including abstinence, the use of barrier protection such as condoms during sexual activity, and the avoidance of sharing needles with other individuals. Open and honest dialogue will occur only if the nurse has developed a therapeutic rapport with the client based on trust and acceptance. Additional teaching points are discussed in Nursing Process Focus: Clients Receiving Antiretroviral Agents.

CONNECTIONS | Natural Therapies

◀ Complementary and Alternative Medicine for HIV

With no cure and the available drugs producing numerous adverse effects, it is not surprising that many clients infected with HIV turn to complementary and alternative medicine (CAM). It is estimated that as many as 70% of clients with HIV-AIDS use CAM during the course of their illness. Most clients use CAM in addition to antiretroviral therapy to control serious side effects, combat weight loss, and boost their immune system. Relieving stress and depression are also common reasons for seeking CAM. The most common herbal products reported by clients with HIV-AIDS are garlic, ginseng, echinacea, and aloe. Unfortunately, few controlled studies have examined the safety or efficacy of CAM in clients with HIV-AIDS.

Supportive education regarding the use of CAM should be provided. Although the use of these therapies should not be discouraged, clients must be strongly warned not to use CAM in place of conventional medical treatment. In addition, some herbs such as St. John's wort can increase the hepatic metabolism of antiretrovirals, resulting in an increased or decreased effect. Garlic co-administered with saquinavir has been shown to greatly reduce plasma levels of the antiretroviral. Urge the client to obtain CAM information from reliable sources and to always report the use of CAM therapies to the healthcare provider.

PROTOTYPE DRUG | Saquinavir (Invirase)

Actions and Uses: Saquinavir was the first protease inhibitor approved by the U.S. Food and Drug Administration (FDA) in 1995. By effectively inhibiting HIV protease, the final step in the assembly of an infectious HIV virion is prevented. The first formulation of saquinavir was a hard gelatin capsule that was poorly absorbed. The newer formulation is a soft gelatin capsule that gives a significantly higher absorption rate, particularly when taken with a high-fat, high-calorie meal. Because of its short half-life, it is usually taken every 8 hours.

Pharmacokinetics: Saquinavir undergoes rapid and extensive first-pass metabolism after oral administration. It is 98% bound to plasma proteins. A minor amount enters the CNS. It is mostly metabolized by the liver. Less than 1% is excreted unchanged in urine. Its half-life is 1 to 2 hours.

Administration Alerts:
- Administer with food to minimize gastric distress.
- Saquinavir is pregnancy category B.

NURSING PROCESS FOCUS

Clients Receiving Antiretroviral Agents

Assessment	Potential Nursing Diagnoses/Identified Patterns

Prior to administration:
• Obtain complete health history, including allergies, drug history, and possible drug interactions.
• Obtain complete physical examination.
• Assess for the presence or history of HIV infection.
• Obtain the following laboratory studies:
  • HIV RNA assay/CD4 count
  • CBC
  • Liver function
  • Renal function
  • Blood glucose
	• Need for knowledge regarding disease process, transmission, and drug therapy
	• Safety from injury related to side effects of drugs therapy
	• Risk for infection related to impaired immune system
	• Fear related to HIV diagnosis

Planning: Client Goals and Expected Outcomes

The client will:

- Exhibit a decrease in viral load and an increase in CD4 count
- Demonstrate knowledge of disease process, transmission, and treatment
- Demonstrate an understanding of the drug's action by accurately describing drug side effects and precautions
- Complete the full course of therapy and comply with follow-up care

Implementation

Interventions (Rationales)	Client Education/Discharge Planning
<ul><li>Monitor for symptoms of hypersensitivity reactions.</li><li>Monitor vital signs, especially temperature, and for symptoms of infection. Monitor white blood cell count. (Antiretroviral drugs such as delavirdine may cause neutropenia.)</li><li>Monitor client for signs of stomatitis. (Immunosuppression may result in the proliferation of oral bacteria.)</li><li>Monitor blood pressure. (Antiviral agents such as abacavir [Ziagen] may cause significant decrease in blood pressure.)</li><li>Monitor HIV RNA assay, CD4 count, liver function, kidney function, CBC, blood glucose, and serum amylase and triglyceride levels. (These will determine effectiveness and toxicity of drug.)</li><li>Determine potential drug-drug and drug-food interactions. (Antiretroviral medications have multiple drug-drug interactions and must be taken as prescribed.)</li><li>Monitor for symptoms of pancreatitis, including severe abdominal pain, nausea, vomiting, and abdominal distention. (Antiretroviral agents such as didanosine may cause pancreatitis.)</li><li>Monitor skin for rash; withhold medication and notify physician at first sign of rash. (Several antiretroviral drugs may cause Stevens-Johnson syndrome, which may be fatal.)</li><li>Establish therapeutic environment to ensure adequate rest, nutrition, hydration, and relaxation. (Support of the immune system is essential in clients with HIV to minimize opportunistic infections.)</li><li>Monitor blood glucose levels. (Antiretroviral drugs may cause hyperglycemia, especially in clients with type 1 diabetes.)</li><li>Monitor for neurological side effects such as numbness and tingling of the extremities. (Many NRTI agents cause peripheral neuropathy.)</li><li>Determine the effect of the prescribed antiretroviral agents on oral contraceptives. (Many agents reduce the effectiveness of oral contraceptives.)</li><li>Provide resources for medical and emotional support.</li><li>Assess client's knowledge level regarding use and effect of medication.</li></ul>	<ul><li>Instruct client to discontinue the medication and inform the healthcare provider if symptoms of hypersensitivity reaction develop, such as wheezing; shortness of breath; swelling of face, tongue, or hands; itching or rash</li></ul> Instruct client:<ul><li>To report symptoms of infection, such as fever, chills, sore throat, and cough</li><li>On methods to minimize exposure to infections such as frequent handwashing; avoiding crowds and people with colds, flu, and other infections; limiting exposure to children and animals; increasing fluid intake; emptying bladder frequently; and coughing and deep breathing several times per day</li><li>Advise client to be alert for mouth ulcers and to report their appearance</li></ul> Instruct client to:<ul><li>Rise slowly from lying or sitting position to minimize effects of postural hypotension</li><li>Report changes in blood pressure</li></ul> Instruct client:<ul><li>On the purpose of required laboratory tests and scheduled follow-ups with the healthcare provider</li><li>To monitor weight and presence of swelling</li><li>To keep all appointments for laboratory tests</li></ul> Instruct client:<ul><li>When to take the specific medication in relationship to food intake</li><li>About foods or beverages to avoid when taking medication; some antiretrovirals should not be taken with acidic fruit juice</li><li>To take medication exactly as directed; do not skip any doses</li><li>To consult with healthcare provider before taking any OTC medications or herbal supplements</li><li>Instruct client to report the following immediately: fever, severe abdominal pain, nausea/vomiting, and abdominal distention</li><li>Advise client to check skin frequently and notify the healthcare provider at first sign of any rash</li></ul> Teach client to incorporate the following health-enhancing activities:<ul><li>Adequate rest and sleep</li><li>Proper nutrition that provides essential vitamins and nutrients</li><li>Intake of six to eight glasses of water per day</li><li>Instruct client to report excessive thirst, hunger, and urination to the healthcare provider</li><li>Instruct diabetic clients to monitor blood glucose levels regularly</li></ul> Instruct client to:<ul><li>Report numbness and tingling of extremities</li><li>Use caution when in contact with heat and cold due to possible peripheral neuropathy</li><li>Instruct client to use an alternate form of birth control while taking antiretroviral medications</li><li>Advise client on community resources and support groups</li></ul> Advise client:<ul><li>That medication may decrease the level of HIV infection in the blood but will not prevent transmitting the disease</li><li>To use barrier protection during sexual activity</li><li>To avoid sharing needles</li><li>To not donate blood</li></ul>

Evaluate the effectiveness of drug therapy by confirming that client goals and expected outcomes have been met (see "Planning").

See Table 47.1 for a list of drugs to which these nursing actions apply.

Adverse Effects and Interactions: Saquinavir is well tolerated by most clients. The most frequently reported problems are GI related, such as nausea, vomiting, dyspepsia, and diarrhea. General fatigue and headache are possible. Though not common, reductions in platelets and erythrocytes have been reported. Resistance to saquinavir may develop with continued use and may include cross-resistance with other protease inhibitors.

Saquinavir interacts with several drugs, including rifampin (Rifadin, Rofact) and rifabutin (Mycobutin), which significantly decrease saquinavir levels. Phenobarbital (Phenobarb), phenytoin (Dilantin), and carbamazepine (Tegretol) may also reduce saquinavir levels. Conversely, ketoconazole (Nizoral) and ritonavir (Norvir) may increase levels.

Use with caution with herbal supplements, such as St. John's wort, which may cause a decrease in antiretroviral activity.

PROPHYLAXIS OF HIV INFECTIONS

Early in the history of the AIDS epidemic, scientists were optimistic that vaccines could be quickly developed that would prevent the spread of HIV infection. After all, scientists had totally eradicated the smallpox virus as a human threat and essentially controlled major viral infections such as measles and mumps. Such a vaccine could be given in childhood, offering lifetime protection against the fatal disease.

After decades of research, only a few HIV vaccines are currently in clinical trials, and none is expected to cause a major impact on the HIV epidemic. At best, the HIV vaccines produced thus far only boost the immune response; they are unable to prevent the infection. While this may help a client who is already infected with the virus to better control the disease, it does not prevent new infections. Why is this the case?

HIV has an extremely rapid replication rate, combined with a high "error" or mutation rate. While creating new viral DNA at a breakneck pace, reverse transcriptase frequently inserts an incorrect nucleotide. It is estimated that, given the size of the HIV genome at 10 000 base pairs, every possible mutation probably occurs at every nucleotide daily in an untreated client. These errors create huge numbers of genetic variants, or mutant strains, with new and different characteristics from the original. It is not unusual to find dozens of genetic variants of HIV replicating within the same client. Therefore, vaccine development, and indeed antiretroviral therapy, is trying to hit a "moving target" that is changing its genetic makeup literally every minute.

An additional challenge is to produce a vaccine-mediated immune response that will reach viruses lying latent inside T cells. HIV-infected cells reside in virtually every compartment in the

body and serve as reservoirs for the latent virus, protecting it from the immune response produced by the vaccine. How do scientists coax the immune system to recognize these infected cells and dispose of them? Perhaps a better question is: Can a vaccine be designed to prevent the entry of the virus into cells to begin with? And how can this vaccine be ethically tested, since no animals have the same immune system as humans to serve as an experimental model?

Vaccine research has not been a total failure. Scientists have learned an enormous amount about the immune system's response to HIV infection. This has promoted the development of new drugs and advanced our understanding of how to treat and control the infection. It is likely that a preventive vaccine will become available in the future, but not soon enough for the millions who are already infected.

Post-Exposure Prophylaxis of HIV Infection

Since the start of the AIDS epidemic, nurses and other healthcare workers caring for clients with HIV-AIDS have been concerned about acquiring the disease from these clients. Fortunately, if proper precautions are observed, the disease is rarely transmitted from client to healthcare worker. However, accidents have occurred in which the healthcare provider has acquired the infection by exposure to the blood or body fluids of clients infected with HIV. Although the risk is small, the question remains: Can HIV transmission be prevented following accidental occupational exposure to HIV? The answer is a qualified yes.

The success of post-exposure prophylaxis (PEP) for occupational HIV exposure is difficult to assess due to the lack of controlled studies and the small number of cases. Enough data have accumulated, however, to demonstrate that PEP is successful in certain circumstances. For prevention to be most successful, PEP should be started within 24 to 36 hours after exposure to a source person who is known to be HIV positive. Although the exact interval remains undefined, longer periods allow the infection to progress to stages where prophylaxis would not be successful. The healthcare worker should receive a baseline HIV viral load level as soon as possible after exposure.

If the HIV status of the source person is unknown, PEP is decided case by case, based on the type of exposure (percutaneous or mucous membrane) and the likelihood that the blood contained HIV. In some cases, PEP is initiated for a few days, until the source person can be tested. PEP should be initiated only if the exposure was sufficiently severe and the source fluid is known, or strongly suspected, to contain HIV. Using PEP outside established guidelines is both expensive and dangerous; the antiretrovirals used for PEP produce adverse effects in most recipients.

Low-risk PEP is initiated when the source person is asymptomatic for HIV or is known to have a low viral load (less than

1500 HIV RNA copies/mL). The basic PEP treatment includes one of the following regimens, conducted over a 4-week period:

- Zidovudine and lamivudine, *or*
- Zidovudine and emtricitabine (Emtriva), *or*
- Lamivudine and tenofovir, *or*
- Tenofovir and emtricitabine

If the accidental HIV exposure was severe and the source is a symptomatic HIV-infected person with a high viral load, a third drug may be added to the regimen. If available, the medical records of the source person should be consulted to determine the possibility of resistance to specific antiretrovirals. The enhanced PEP treatment includes one of the basic regimens listed previously, plus lopinavir-ritonavir.

Guidelines have also been established for the non-occupational post-exposure prophylaxis (nPEP) of HIV. These guidelines are largely based on animal studies and analysis of the existing data for occupational exposure. Because nPEP is expensive and may result in adverse drug effects, it is recommended only for specific non-occupational exposures. First, the person should have been exposed to the blood or body fluids of a person known to be infected with HIV. Second, the nature of the exposure must be such that there is a substantial risk for transmission. Third, the exposure must have occurred no later than 72 hours before antiretroviral therapy is initiated. The sooner nPEP is initiated, the more successful the outcome. The healthcare provider considers nPEP for exposures outside these guidelines on a case-by-case basis. Recommended therapy is a 28-day regimen with one of the following:

- Efavirenz (Sustiva) plus lamivudine, *or*
- Emtricitabine plus zidovudine or tenofovir, *or*
- Lopinavir/ritonavir plus lamivudine or emtricitabine, plus zidovudine

Reducing the Risk for Perinatal Transmission of HIV

Treatment regimens for HIV infection do not differ between men and women. Because some antiretrovirals have pharmacokinetic interactions with oral contraceptives, a second method of birth control is recommended.

Should pregnancy occur, the therapeutic outcomes focus on keeping the viral load low in the mother while aggressively protecting the transmission of HIV to the unborn child. Efavirenz has been shown to cause fetal malformations; therefore, its use is not recommended during pregnancy.

In 1994, clinical trials determined that perinatal transmission of HIV could be markedly reduced through pharmacotherapy. A reduction of approximately 70% in transmission from mother to infant was achieved using antepartum pharmacotherapy in the mother followed by aggressive treatment of the newborn child.

In pregnant women with HIV, antiretroviral therapy is recommended regardless of the viral level or CD4 count. Reducing the viral load in the mother has been shown to reduce the risk for HIV transmission to the fetus. Recommended protocols for the pregnant woman include two NRTIs (zidovudine and lamivudine) with either an NNRTI (nevirapine) or a protease inhibitor (lopinavir boosted with ritonavir). The specific regimen is adjusted based on resistance testing.

Regardless of the antepartum therapy, it is recommended that the woman receive a continuous infusion of zidovudine during labour. Zidovudine rapidly crosses the placenta. This may provide some protection for the fetus because most perinatal transmission of HIV occurs near to or during labour and delivery.

Therapy of neonates born to mothers infected with HIV should begin immediately after delivery, no later than 6 to 12 hours postpartum. HIV infection is established in infants by age 1 to 2 weeks, and beginning antiretroviral therapy more than 48 hours after birth has been shown to be ineffective in preventing the infection. It is recommended that zidovudine be given orally to the newborn for 6 weeks. In addition, three doses of nevirapine are given during the first week of life. As well, mothers must be advised not to breastfeed their infants, because this is a possible route of HIV transmission and many antiretrovirals are secreted in breast milk.

Although initial HIV antibody tests on the newborn may be positive, these antibodies may be due to maternal infection and not HIV infection in the child. Definitive diagnosis on infants younger than 18 months of age requires virological testing. If diagnostic testing reveals that the infant is not infected before the 6-week prophylactic treatment period is completed, zidovudine therapy is discontinued. On the other hand, if HIV diagnosis is confirmed during this period, the infant is switched to combination HAART therapy. In addition to antiretrovirals, all infants born to women with HIV infection should receive trimethoprim-sulfamethoxazole (TMP-SMZ [Bactrim, Septra]) to prevent *Pneumocystis jiroveci* pneumonia (PJP) at age 4 to 6 weeks.

Approximately 12 antiretrovirals are approved for pediatric indications. The other antiretrovirals are too toxic for pediatric use or not available in convenient formulations, or the doses remain to be established. Like adults, the specific regimen is chosen based on the experience of the prescriber and resistance patterns of the HIV strain. The possibility that the child may have inherited a strain already resistant to some of the antiretrovirals must be considered when developing the regimen.

PHARMACOTHERAPY OF OPPORTUNISTIC INFECTIONS ASSOCIATED WITH HIV-AIDS

47.7 Loss of immune function due to HIV often results in opportunistic infections that require anti-infective therapy.

In the early 1980s, all clients with AIDS acquired serious OIs from pathogenic bacteria, viruses, fungi, and protozoans. Profound loss of immune function allowed dormant pathogens to flourish and also lowered the defence barriers for infection by newly acquired organisms. Often, the presentation of an acute OI was the reason the client first sought medical attention for HIV disease. For example, in the early years of the epidemic, 70% to 80% of all clients with AIDS developed *Pneumocystis* pneumonia, which carried a mortality rate of up to 40% in these clients. Since the advent of HAART, *Pneumocystis* pneumonia is now rare.

OIs still occur in clients with HIV-AIDS; however, they are less common and mortality is diminished. This is because HAART increases the numbers of CD4 lymphocytes, allowing clients with HIV infection to maintain a higher level of immunological defence. In addition, the anti-infective pharmacotherapy of OIs has evolved due to a better understanding of these diseases. Clients with CD4 counts lower than 200 cells/mcL are placed on prophylactic antibiotics because the risk of an OI in these clients is very high. Most other clients with HIV-AIDS are monitored

carefully for signs of infectious disease and treated as symptoms indicate.

Drugs used for treating OIs have been presented in previous anti-infective chapters, and the student should refer to those chapters for specific drug information. A selected list of preferred drugs for selected OIs is provided in Table 47.2.

TABLE 47.2 Pharmacotherapy of Selected Opportunistic Infections in Patients with HIV-AIDS

Disease	Preferred Drug(s) for Prevention	Comments
Bacterial enteric infections	PO, fluoroquinolone (ciprofloxacin preferred) or TMP-SMZ	Most common pathogens are *Salmonella, Campylobacter,* and *Shigella*
Bacterial respiratory infections	Pneumococcal vaccine (PPV); inactivated influenza vaccine	Most common pathogens are *S. pneumoniae* and *H. influenzae*
Candidiasis (mucocutaneous)	PO, fluconazole	Topical azoles may be used for vulvovaginal or oropharyngeal disease
Cryptococcosis	No prevention recommended; treatment is with amphotericin B with flucytosine for 2 weeks, followed by fluconazole for 8 weeks	Lifelong prophylaxis with fluconazole is indicated in certain patients
Cryptosporidiosis	No specific anti-infective is indicated; clarithromycin or rifabutin may be effective	Therapy includes symptomatic treatment of diarrhea
Herpes simplex	PO, famciclovir or acyclovir for 7–14 days	IV therapy is indicated in severe infections
Histoplasmosis (disseminated)	PO, itraconazole daily	Lifelong prophylaxis with itraconazole is indicated in certain patients
Mycobacterial tuberculosis	PO, isoniazid plus pyridoxine for 9 months	Serious drug interactions can occur between rifamycin and the NNRTIs and protease inhibitors
Pneumocystis pneumonia (PJP)	PO, TMP-SMZ for 21 days	Lifelong prophylaxis is indicated in certain patients; pentamidine may be used for severe cases
Syphilis	IM, benzathine penicillin	If allergic to penicillin, penicillin desensitization is attempted or an alternate drug such as doxycycline is substituted
Toxoplasma gondii encephalitis	PO, TMP-SMZ	Clindamycin may be used instead of sulfadiazine

47 Understanding the Chapter

Key Concepts Summary

The numbered key concepts provide a succinct summary of the important points from the corresponding numbered section within the chapter. If any of these points are not clear, refer to the numbered section within the chapter for review.

47.1 HIV attacks the T4 lymphocyte and uses reverse transcriptase to make viral DNA.

47.2 Antiretroviral drugs used in the treatment of HIV-AIDS do not cure the disease but do help many clients to live longer. Pharmacotherapy may be initiated in the acute (symptomatic) or chronic (asymptomatic) phase of HIV infection.

47.3 Drugs from six drug classes are combined in the pharmacotherapy of HIV-AIDS. The nucleotide reverse

transcriptase inhibitors and the fusion inhibitors have been recently developed.

47.4 The reverse transcriptase inhibitors block HIV replication at the level of the reverse transcriptase enzyme.

47.5 The protease inhibitors inhibit the final assembly of the HIV virion.

47.6 Drugs are available to prevent and to treat influenza infections. Vaccination is the best choice, as drugs are relatively ineffective once symptoms appear.

47.7 Loss of immune function due to HIV often results in opportunistic infections that require anti-infective therapy.

Chapter 47 Scenario

Ryan Orre is a 37-year-old single male who has come to his healthcare provider because of the recent onset of a chronic sore throat and flu-like symptoms, including swollen lymph nodes in the neck and armpits, tiredness, fever, and night sweats. During this office visit, Ryan appears extremely anxious and troubled.

When questioned about his apparent nervousness, Ryan states, "You don't understand; I'm gay. But I've always been very careful and practise safe sex. What if I have AIDS? What will I do? I don't want to die." The healthcare provider acknowledges Ryan's fears and spends additional time allowing Ryan to express his concerns. The process of diagnosing HIV infection is discussed with the client and initiated.

Ryan's medical history reveals that he is allergic to penicillin, which results in rash and pruritus. Although Ryan does not currently take any prescribed medications, he recently started multivitamin and nutritional supplements due to a recent loss of weight. The client denies any current recreational drug use but admits that he occasionally used IV drugs during his university years. He has not used them in the past 8 years. No past history of medical or psychiatric illness exists. He has never had surgery.

Ryan does not use tobacco products. He reports drinking alcoholic beverages several times weekly but never to excess. Ryan explains that he has had several male sexual partners over the past 10 years but feels that he has been consistent in his use of condoms. He currently lives alone and works as a sales representative with a local computer firm. A series of laboratory diagnostic tests found the following abnormal results: white blood cell (WBC) count of 2950/mm^3 and CD4 count of 550/mm^3. Ryan is hospitalized with the preliminary diagnosis of sepsis and to rule out HIV infection. A test for HIV viral load is ordered.

Critical Thinking Questions

1. You are the nurse caring for Ryan in the hospital. On the evening he is hospitalized, Ryan asks if you think his provider will be prescribing antiretroviral therapy. Given this situation, how would you explain the factors that determine when antiretroviral therapy should be initiated?

2. Ryan's CD4 count is still within low-normal range but his HIV viral load comes back significantly increased, indicating HIV infection. After talking with the provider, Ryan asks you to explain again the difference between HIV infection and AIDS. How would you explain this?

3. Ryan's provider has decided to start him on antiretroviral therapy and Ryan will begin taking efavirenz (Sustiva), tenofovir (Viread), and emtricitabine (Emtriva). What will be the best method of teaching Ryan about these drugs? What other factors should be considered when talking with Ryan?

See Answers to Critical Thinking Questions in Appendix B.

NCLEX Practice Questions

1 Zidovudine (Retrovir, AZT) is prescribed for a client. Which statement by the client would indicate that further medication-related teaching is needed?

   a. "Antiretroviral therapy must be continued for the remainder of my life."

   b. "The human immunodeficiency virus vaccine creates only temporary immunity against the disease."

   c. "The medication schedule can be adjusted daily depending on my activities."

   d. "Many individuals infected with the human immunodeficiency virus are able to live symptom free due to the medication."

2 Emtricitabine (Emtriva) is included as part of a HAART regimen for a client newly diagnosed with HIV. While lower in toxicity than other NRTIs, a potentially fatal adverse effect known to occur is

   a. Ventricular cardiac dysrhythmias

   b. Pulmonary fibrosis

   c. Necrotic bowel syndrome

   d. Lactic acidosis

3 The nurse is aware that myelosuppression may be a problem for some clients receiving zidovudine (Retrovir). Which finding would indicate that this adverse effect was present?

   a. Increase in serum blood urea nitrogen levels

   b. Increase in white blood cell count

   c. Decrease in platelet count

   d. Decrease in blood pressure

4 The nurse is planning a teaching session with a client who will be receiving highly active antiretroviral therapy (HAART). Which of the following should be included in the teaching plan? Select all that apply.

   a. Avoid crowds and people with cold, flu, and other infections.

b. Notify the healthcare provider at the first sign of any rash.

c. The medications will reduce transmission of the disease.

d. The drugs will be stopped periodically to give the immune system a chance to respond.

e. Herbal supplements will not interfere with this therapy.

5 A client has been taking tenofovir (Viread) for the past 5 years as part of a HAART regimen. The client would like to include some alternative and complementary health activities to improve his overall health. Which activity may be contraindicated for this client?

a. Yoga and guided imagery

b. Massage therapy

c. Meditation and journalling

d. Weekly visits to a chiropractor

See Answers to NCLEX Practice Questions in Appendix A.

UNIT

11

Pharmacology of Alterations in the Cardiovascular System

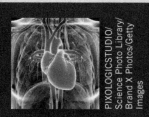

PIXOLOGICSTUDIO/
Science Photo Library/
Brand X Photos/Getty
Images

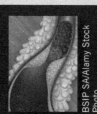

BSIP SA/Alamy Stock
Photo

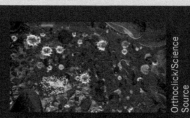

Orthoclick/Science
Source

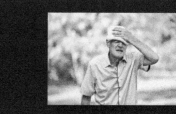

Robert Kneschke/
Shutterstock

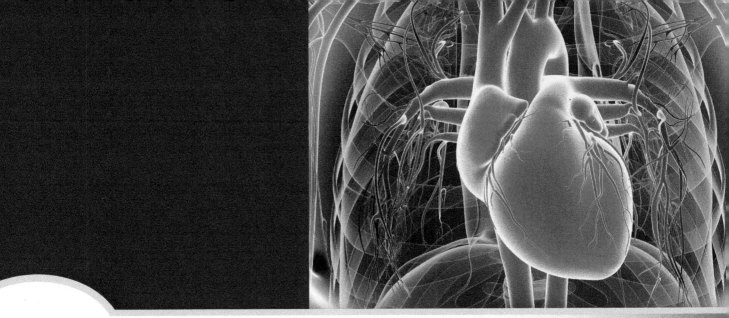

PIXOLOGICSTUDIO/Science Photo Library/Brand X Photos/Getty Images

CHAPTER 48

Brief Review of the Cardiovascular System

LEARNING OUTCOMES

After reading this chapter, the student should be able to:

1. Describe the major structures of the cardiovascular system.
2. Identify the components of blood and their functions.
3. Construct a flowchart that diagrams the primary steps of hemostasis.
4. Describe the structure of the heart and the function of the myocardium.
5. Describe the role of the coronary arteries in supplying the myocardium with oxygen.
6. Illustrate the flow of electrical impulses through the normal heart.
7. Explain the major factors that affect cardiac output.
8. Explain the effects of cardiac output, peripheral resistance, and blood volume on hemodynamics.
9. Discuss how the vasomotor centre, baroreceptors, chemoreceptors, and hormones regulate blood pressure.

CHAPTER OUTLINE

It is likely that the nurse will administer more cardiovascular drugs than any other class of medications. Why is this the case? First, healthcare providers have discovered the huge benefits of keeping blood pressure and blood lipid values within normal limits and how to prevent heart attacks and strokes. Second, the heart and vessels weaken over time and, as the average lifespan of the population increases, more pharmacotherapy will be needed to treat the chronic cardiovascular diseases of older adults.

A comprehensive knowledge of cardiovascular anatomy and physiology is essential to understanding cardiovascular pharmacology, which encompasses all chapters in this unit. The purpose of this chapter is to offer a brief review of the components of the structure and function of the cardiovascular system that are important to pharmacotherapy

Structure and Function of the Cardiovascular System

48.1 The cardiovascular system consists of the blood, heart, and blood vessels.

The three major components of the cardiovascular system are the blood, heart, and blood vessels, as shown in Figure 48.1. These three components work as an integrated whole to transport the essential oxygen, nutrients, and other substances that keep the body in homeostasis. Disruption of this flow for even brief periods can have serious, if not mortal, consequences. The functions of the cardiovascular system are diverse and include the following:

- Transport of nutrients and wastes
- Pumping of blood
- Regulation of blood pressure
- Regulation of acid-base balance
- Regulation of fluid balance
- Regulation of body temperature
- Protection against invasion by microbes

The cardiovascular system can function only with the cooperation of other body systems. For example, the role of the autonomic nervous system in controlling heart rate and blood vessel diameter is discussed in Chapter 12. The kidneys are intimately involved in assisting the cardiovascular system with fluid and acid-base balance, as discussed in Chapter 53. The respiratory system must bring oxygen to the blood and remove carbon dioxide from it.

Functions and Properties of Blood

48.2 Blood consists of formed elements and plasma.

Blood is a liquid connective tissue that consists of formed elements suspended in plasma. The solid, formed elements of the blood are the erythrocytes, leukocytes, and platelets. When combined, the formed elements comprise about 45% of the composition of blood.

The most numerous blood cells are erythrocytes, which comprise 99.9% of the formed elements. Carrying the iron-containing protein hemoglobin, the erythrocytes are responsible for transporting oxygen to the tissues and carbon dioxide from the tissues to the lungs. A single erythrocyte can carry as many as 1 billion molecules of oxygen. Erythrocyte homeostasis is controlled by **erythropoietin**, a hormone secreted by the kidney in response to low oxygen levels in the blood. Once secreted, erythropoietin stimulates the body's production of erythrocytes. Insufficient numbers of erythrocytes or structural defects such as sickle shapes lead to anemia, which is a common indication for pharmacotherapy (see Chapter 57).

Although small in number, white blood cells or leukocytes serve an essential role in the body's defence against infection. Unlike erythrocytes, which are all structurally identical, there are several types of leukocytes, each serving a different function. For example, neutrophils are the most common leukocyte and they respond to bacterial infections through phagocytosis of the microbes. The second most common leukocyte, the lymphocyte, is the key cell in the immune response that responds by secreting antibodies (B lymphocytes) or cytokines (T lymphocytes) that rid the body of the microbe. A review of body defences and the immune system is presented in Chapter 39.

The final formed elements of the blood are thrombocytes or platelets, which are actually fragments of larger cells called megakaryocytes. Platelets stick to the walls of damaged blood vessels

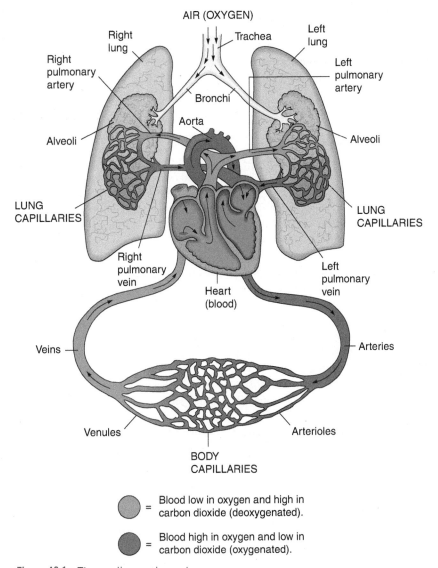

Figure 48.1 The cardiovascular system.

to begin the process of blood coagulation, which prevents excessive bleeding from sites of injury. Abnormally low numbers of platelets, or thrombocytopenia, can result in serious delays in blood clotting. Platelet homeostasis is controlled by the hormone **thrombopoietin**, which promotes the formation of additional platelets.

The production and maturation of blood cells, called **hemopoiesis** or hematopoiesis, occurs in red bone marrow. It is here that primitive stem cells of the blood become committed to forming erythrocytes, leukocytes, or platelets. This process occurs continuously throughout the lifespan and is subject to various homeostatic controls as well as certain drugs and physical agents. For example, ionizing radiation and a large number of drugs have the potential to adversely affect bone marrow and cause myelosuppression. Myelosuppression is a very serious adverse effect that reduces the number of erythrocytes, leukocytes, and thrombocytes (pancytopenia), leaving clients susceptible to anemia, infection, and bleeding. Many drugs used to treat cancer and those given to reduce the possibility of transplant rejection can produce profound myelosuppression as a dose-limiting adverse effect.

Plasma is the fluid portion of blood that consists of water, proteins, electrolytes, lipoproteins, carbohydrates, and other regulatory substances. The primary proteins in plasma are albumins (54%), globulins (38%), and fibrinogen (7%). Albumin is the primary regulator of blood osmotic pressure (also called oncotic pressure), which determines the movement of fluids among the vascular, interstitial, and cellular compartments or spaces. Globulins, also known as immunoglobulins or antibodies, are important in protecting the body from foreign agents such as bacteria or viruses. Fibrinogen is a critical protein in the coagulation of blood. The liver synthesizes more than 90% of the plasma proteins; therefore, clients with serious hepatic impairment will have deficiencies in coagulation and in maintaining body defences.

Serum is a term closely related to plasma. Serum contains all components of plasma, except that clotting factors such as fibrinogen have been removed. Serum is often used for blood typing and for determining blood levels of substances such as cholesterol, glucose, and hormones.

Fluid balance in the body is achieved by maintaining the proper amount of plasma in the blood. Too little water in plasma results in dehydration, whereas too much causes edema and hypertension (HTN). Various organs, including the kidneys, gastrointestinal (GI) tract, and skin, help to maintain normal fluid balance. The pharmacotherapy of fluid and electrolyte imbalances is an important topic in pharmacology and is discussed in Chapter 53.

Hemostasis

48.3 Hemostasis is a complex process involving multiple steps and a large number of enzymes and factors.

The process of **hemostasis** is complex, involving 13 different clotting factors that contribute to the stoppage of blood flow. Hemostasis occurs in a series of sequential steps, sometimes referred to as a cascade. Hemostasis is an essential mechanism that the body uses to prevent excessive bleeding after injury. Medications can be used to modify several of these steps, either to speed up or to delay the clotting process

Injury to a blood vessel triggers the clotting process. The vessel spasms, causing constriction, which slows blood flow to the injured area. Platelets have an affinity for the damaged vessel: they become sticky and adhere to each other and to the injured area. The clumping of platelets, or aggregation, is facilitated by adenosine diphosphate (ADP), the enzyme thrombin, and thromboxane A2. Platelet receptor sites and von Willebrand's factor make adhesion possible. The aggregated platelets disintegrate to initiate a platelet binding cascade. Blood flow is further slowed, thus allowing the process of **coagulation**, which is the formation of an insoluble clot, to occur.

When collagen is exposed at the site of vessel injury, the damaged cells initiate the coagulation cascade. Coagulation itself occurs when fibrin threads create a meshwork that fortifies the blood constituents so that clots can develop. During the cascade, various plasma proteins that are circulating in an inactive state are converted to their active forms. Two separate pathways, along with numerous biochemical processes, lead to coagulation. The **intrinsic pathway** is activated in response to injury and takes several minutes to complete. The **extrinsic pathway** is activated when blood leaks out of a vessel and enters tissue spaces. The extrinsic pathway is less complex and is completed within seconds. The two pathways share some common steps and the outcome is the same—the formation of the fibrin clot.

Near the end of the common pathway, a chemical called prothrombin activator (Active X) is formed. The prothrombin activator converts the clotting factor **prothrombin** to an enzyme called **thrombin**. Thrombin then converts **fibrinogen**, a plasma protein, to long strands of **fibrin**. The fibrin strands provide a framework to anchor the clot. Therefore, two of the factors essential to clotting, thrombin and fibrin, are formed only after injury to the vessels. The fibrin strands form an insoluble web over the injured area to stop blood loss. Normal blood clotting occurs in about 6 minutes.

It is important to note that several clotting factors, including thromboplastin and fibrinogen, are proteins made by the liver that are constantly circulating through the blood in an inactive form. Vitamin K, which is made by bacteria residing in the large intestine, is required for the liver to make four of the clotting factors.

Because of the crucial importance of the liver in creating these clotting factors, clients with serious hepatic impairment often have abnormal coagulation.

Cardiac Structure and Function

48.4 The heart is responsible for pumping blood throughout the circulatory system.

The heart is the hardest working organ in the body, pumping blood from before birth to the last minute of life. With the continuous workload, it is not surprising that this organ eventually weakens and that heart disease is the second leading cause of death in Canada. The heart is a frequent target for pharmacotherapy.

The heart may be thought of as a thick, specialized muscle. The muscular layer, called the **myocardium**, is the thickest of the heart layers and is responsible for the physical pumping action of the heart. The thickness of the myocardium is greatest in the left ventricle because this chamber performs the greatest amount of work. Cardiac muscle contains extensive branching networks of cellular structures that connect cardiac muscle cells to each other, allowing the entire myocardium to contract as a coordinated whole.

Should myocardial cells (myocytes) die, the body is unable to replace them because cardiac cells do not undergo mitosis. If a large area becomes deprived of oxygen and undergoes necrosis, the myocytes are replaced by fibrotic scar tissue and cardiac function becomes impaired. The different regions of the heart may not contract in a coordinated manner because conduction of the electrical potential may skip over areas of necrosis on the myocardium. This can result in heart failure or dysrhythmias, which are frequent indications for pharmacotherapy (see Chapters 54 and 55).

The heart has four chambers that receive blood prior to being pumped, as illustrated in Figure 48.2. These chambers differ in size, depending on their function. The left ventricle is the largest, because it must hold enough blood to pump to all body tissues. During heart failure, the size of the left ventricle and the thickness of the myocardial layer in this chamber can increase in size in clients, which is a condition known as left ventricular hypertrophy.

The Coronary Arteries

48.5 The coronary arteries bring essential nutrients to the myocardium.

Working continuously around the clock, the heart requires a bountiful supply of oxygen and other nutrients. These are provided by the right and left coronary arteries and their branches. The coronary arteries have the ability to rapidly adapt to the heart's needs for oxygen. For example, during exercise the heart rate and strength of contraction markedly increase, and healthy coronary arteries quickly dilate to provide oxygen to meet this increased workload on the myocardium.

The coronary arteries are subject to atherosclerosis, a buildup of fatty plaque, which narrows the lumen and restricts the blood supply that reaches myocytes. If allowed to progress, the narrowing results in chest pain, a condition known as angina pectoris. The first sign of angina is pain upon exercise or exertion, since this is

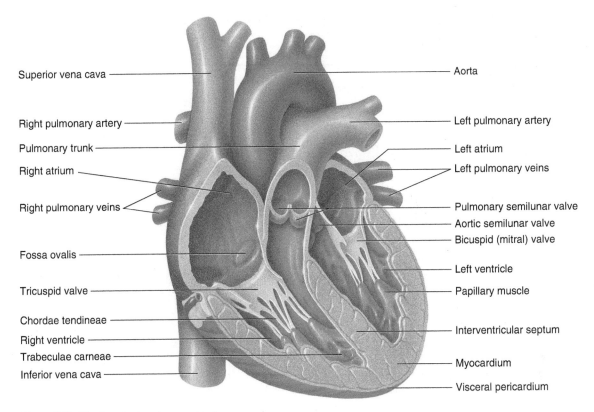

Superior vena cava

Right pulmonary artery

Pulmonary trunk

Right atrium

Right pulmonary veins

Fossa ovalis

Tricuspid valve

Chordae tendineae

Right ventricle

Trabeculae carneae

Inferior vena cava

Aorta

Left pulmonary artery

Left atrium

Left pulmonary veins

Pulmonary semilunar valve

Aortic semilunar valve

Bicuspid (mitral) valve

Left ventricle

Papillary muscle

Interventricular septum

Myocardium

Visceral pericardium

Figure 48.2 The heart: chambers and valves.

when the workload on the heart is increased. Continued narrowing increases the risk for a myocardial infarction.

The coronary arteries are important targets for pharmacotherapy. Chapter 49 explains how reducing lipid levels in the blood can decrease the risk of atherosclerosis of the coronary arteries (and other arteries). Chapter 50 discusses how drugs can be used to reduce angina pain and decrease the risk for mortality following a heart attack. Chapter 54 introduces drugs that reduce the cardiac workload in clients with heart failure so that the heart does not require as much oxygen from the coronary arteries.

The Cardiac Conduction System

48.6 The cardiac conduction system keeps the heart beating in a synchronized manner.

For the heart to function properly, the atria must contract simultaneously, sending their blood into the ventricles. Following atrial contraction, the right and left ventricles then must contract simultaneously. Lack of synchronization of the atria and ventricles or of the right and left sides of the heart may have profound consequences. Proper timing of chamber contractions is made possible by the cardiac conduction system, a branching network of specialized cardiac muscle cells that sends a synchronized, electrical signal across the myocardium. These electrical impulses, or action potentials, carry the signal for the cardiac muscle cells to contract and must be coordinated precisely for the chambers to beat in a synchronized manner. The cardiac conduction system is illustrated in Figure 48.3.

Control of the cardiac conduction system begins in a small area of tissue in the wall of the right atrium known as the sinoatrial (SA) node or cardiac pacemaker. Cells in the SA node have the property of **automaticity**, the ability to spontaneously generate action potentials without an outside signal from the nervous system. The SA node generates a new action potential approximately 75 times per minute under resting conditions. This is referred to as the normal **sinus rhythm**. The SA node is greatly influenced by the activity of the sympathetic and parasympathetic divisions of the autonomic nervous system.

Upon leaving the SA node, the action potential travels quickly across both atria and through internodal pathways to the atrioventricular (AV) node. Myocytes in the AV node also have the property of automaticity, although less so than those in the SA node. Should the SA node malfunction, the AV node has the ability to spontaneously generate action potentials and continue the heart's contraction at a rate of 40 to 60 beats per minute. Compared to other areas in the heart, impulse conduction through the AV node is slow. This allows the atria sufficient time to completely contract and empty their blood before the ventricles receive their signal to contract. If the ventricles should contract prematurely, the AV valves will close and the atria will be prevented from completely emptying their contents.

As the action potential leaves the AV node, it travels rapidly to the AV bundle or bundle of His. The pathway between the AV node and the bundle of His is the only electrical connection between the atria and the ventricles. The impulse is conducted down the right and left bundle branches to the Purkinje fibres, which rapidly carry the action potential to all regions of the ventricles almost simultaneously. Should the SA and AV nodes become

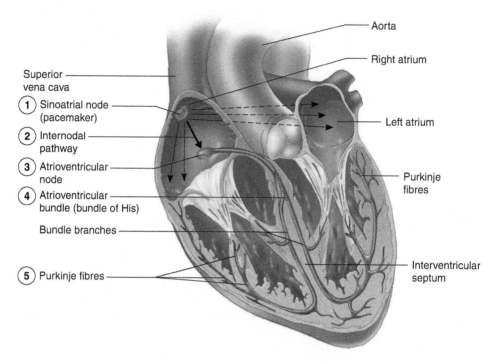

1. The sinoatrial (SA) node fires a stimulus across the walls of both left and right atria, causing them to contract.

2. The stimulus arrives at the atrioventricular (AV) node.

3. The stimulus is directed to follow the AV bundle (bundle of His).

4. The stimulus now travels through the apex of the heart through the bundle branches.

5. The Purkinje fibres distribute the stimulus across both ventricles, causing ventricular contraction.

Figure 48.3 The cardiac conduction system.

non-functional, cells in the AV bundle and Purkinje fibres can continue to generate myocardial contractions at a rate of about 30 beats per minute.

Although action potentials normally begin at the SA node and spread across the myocardium in a coordinated manner, other regions of the heart may also initiate beats. These **ectopic foci**, or *ectopic pacemakers*, may send waves of depolarization across the myocardium that compete with those from the normal conduction pathway. The timing and synchronization of atrial and ventricular contractions may be affected. Although healthy hearts occasionally experience an extra beat without incident, ectopic foci in diseased hearts have the potential to cause dysrhythmias, or disorders of cardiac rhythm. The events associated with the cardiac conduction system are recorded on an electrocardiogram (ECG).

It is important to understand that the underlying purpose of the cardiac conduction system is to keep the heart beating in a regular, synchronized manner so that cardiac output can be maintained. Dysrhythmias that profoundly affect cardiac output have the potential to produce serious, if not mortal, consequences. These types of dysrhythmias require pharmacological intervention, as discussed in Chapter 55.

Cardiac Output

48.7 Cardiac output is determined by stroke volume and heart rate.

To understand how medications act on the heart and to predict the consequences of pharmacotherapy, it is essential to have a comprehensive knowledge of normal cardiac physiology. This includes a thorough understanding of factors that determine the amount of blood pumped by the heart and the forces acting on the chambers.

The amount of blood pumped by each ventricle per minute is the **cardiac output (CO)**. The CO is essentially a measure of how effectively the heart is performing as a pump. The average CO is 5 L/minute. CO can be calculated by multiplying stroke volume by the heart rate.

CO = Stroke volume (mL/beat) × Heart rate (beats/minute)

Stroke volume is the amount of blood pumped by a ventricle in a single contraction. What types of factors might cause a ventricle to eject more blood during a contraction? To understand these factors, a simple comparison to a rubber band is useful. If you stretch a small rubber band 5 cm, it will snap back with a certain force. Stretching the band 10 cm will cause it to snap back with greater force. The force of the snap will continue to increase up to a certain limit, after which the rubber band has been stretched as far as possible and has reached maximum force (or it breaks!).

Cardiac muscle fibres are analogous to rubber bands. If you fill the chambers with more blood, the fibres will have more stretch and will "snap back" with greater force. This is known as Starling's law of the heart: the strength (force) of contraction, or **contractility**, is proportional to the muscle fibre length (stretch). The contractility determines the amount of blood ejected per beat, or the stroke volume. The degree to which the ventricles are filled with blood and the myocardial fibres are stretched just prior to contraction is called **preload**. Up to a physiological limit, drugs that increase preload and contractility will increase the CO. In addition to preload, the force of contraction can be increased by activation of beta$_1$-adrenergic receptors in the autonomic nervous system.

What causes the chambers to fill up with more blood, become stretched (more preload), and contract with greater force? Although several factors affect preload, the most important is **venous return**: the volume of blood returning to the heart from the veins. Giving a drug that constricts veins will increase venous return to the heart, as will simply increasing the total amount of blood in the vascular system (increased blood volume). Drugs or other mechanisms that constrict veins or increase blood volume will therefore increase stroke volume and CO. Conversely, drugs that dilate veins or reduce blood volume will lower CO.

Factors that increase cardiac contractility are called positive **inotropic drugs**. Examples of positive inotropic drugs include epinephrine (Adrenalin), norepinephrine (Levophed), thyroid hormone, and dopamine. Factors that decrease cardiac contractility are called negative inotropic drugs. Examples include quinidine (Quinate) and beta-adrenergic antagonists such as propranolol (Inderal).

A second primary factor that affects stroke volume is afterload. For the left ventricle to pump blood out of the heart, it must overcome a substantial "back pressure" in the aorta. **Afterload** is the systolic pressure in the aorta that must be overcome for blood to be ejected from the left ventricle. As afterload increases, the heart pumps less blood, and stroke volume (and thus CO) decreases. The most common cause of increased afterload is an increase in systemic blood pressure, or HTN. HTN creates an increased workload on the heart, which explains why clients with chronic HTN are more likely to experience heart failure. Antihypertensive drugs create less afterload, increase stroke volume, and result in less workload for the heart. Preload and afterload are illustrated in Figure 48.4.

Heart rate is the second primary factor that determines CO. Heart rate is generally controlled by the autonomic nervous system, which makes the minute-by-minute adjustments demanded by the circulatory system. Both sympathetic and parasympathetic fibres are found in the SA node, and heart rate is determined by which fibres are firing at a greater rate at any given moment. Circulating hormones such as epinephrine and thyroid hormone also affect heart rate. In theory, drugs that increase heart rate will increase CO, although compensatory mechanisms may prevent this effect. In addition, a very rapid heart rate may not give the chambers sufficient time to completely fill, thus reducing CO.

Hemodynamics and Blood Pressure

48.8 The primary factors responsible for blood pressure are cardiac output, peripheral resistance, and blood volume.

The homeostatic regulation of blood pressure is a key topic in pharmacology because HTN is so prevalent in the population.

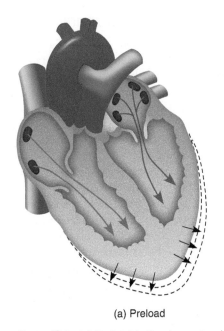

(a) Preload

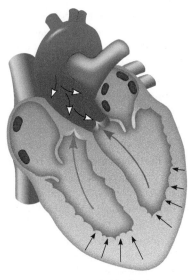

(b) Afterload

Figure 48.4 (a) Preload is the degree to which the ventricles are filled with blood and the myocardial fibres are stretched just prior to contraction. (b) Afterload is the systolic pressure in the aorta that must be overcome for blood to be ejected from the left ventricle.

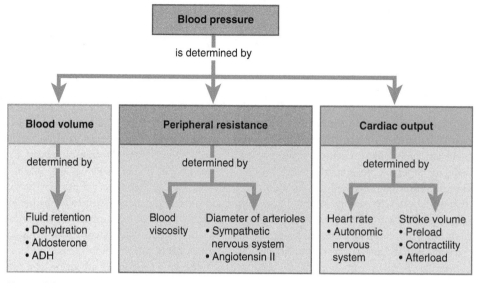

Figure 48.5   The primary factors affecting blood pressure.

Regulation of blood pressure is complex, with many diverse factors—both local and systemic—interacting to maintain adequate blood flow to the tissues. The three primary factors that regulate arterial blood pressure—CO, peripheral resistance, and blood volume—are shown in Figure 48.5. The following simple formula should be memorized (as well as understood) because it will help in predicting the actions and adverse effects of many classes of cardiovascular medications:

$$Blood\ pressure = CO \times Peripheral\ resistance$$

CO is determined by heart rate and stroke volume as discussed in section 48.7. From the preceding equation, it is easy to see that as CO increases, blood pressure also increases. This is important to pharmacology because medications that change the CO, stroke volume, or heart rate have the potential to influence a client's blood pressure.

As blood speeds through the vascular system, it exerts force against the walls of the vessels. Although the lining of the blood vessel is extremely smooth, friction reduces the velocity of the blood. Further friction is encountered as the stream of fast-moving blood narrows to enter smaller vessels, divides into two channels (arteries), or encounters fatty deposits on the vessel walls (plaque). Blood flow may exhibit turbulence, a chaotic, tumbling motion that greatly increases friction. The friction that blood encounters in the arteries is called **peripheral resistance**. Arteries have smooth muscle in their walls, which controls the total peripheral resistance. For example, if the smooth muscle constricts, the inside diameter or lumen of the arteries will become smaller and create more resistance and higher blood pressure. A large number of medications affect vascular smooth muscle. Some of these drugs cause vessels to constrict, thus raising blood pressure, whereas others relax smooth muscle, thereby opening the lumen and lowering blood pressure.

An additional factor responsible for blood pressure is the total amount of blood in the vascular system, or blood volume. Although the average person maintains a relatively constant blood volume of approximately 5 L, this can be changed by endogenous

regulatory factors, certain disease states, and pharmacotherapy. More fluid in the vascular system increases venous pressure and venous return to the heart, thus increasing CO and arterial blood pressure. Drugs are frequently used to adjust blood volume. For example, infusion of intravenous (IV) fluids quickly increases blood volume and raises blood pressure. This is used to advantage when treating hypotension due to shock. On the other hand, diuretics cause fluid loss through urination, thus decreasing blood volume and lowering blood pressure.

Neural Regulation of Blood Pressure

48.9 Neural regulation of blood pressure includes baroreceptor and chemoreceptor reflexes.

It is critical for the body to maintain a normal range of blood pressure and for it to be able to safely and rapidly change pressure as it proceeds through daily activities such as sleep and exercise. Hypotension can cause dizziness and lack of adequate urine formation, whereas extreme HTN can cause vessels to rupture and result in ischemia of critical organs. Figure 48.6 illustrates how the body maintains homeostasis during periods of blood pressure change.

The central and autonomic nervous systems are intimately involved in regulating blood pressure. On a minute-to-minute basis, blood pressure is regulated by a cluster of neurons in the medulla oblongata called the **vasomotor centre**. Sensory receptors in the aorta and the internal carotid artery provide the vasomotor centre with vital information on conditions in the vascular system. **Baroreceptors** have the ability to sense pressure within large vessels, whereas **chemoreceptors** recognize levels of oxygen, carbon dioxide, and the acidity or pH in the blood. The vasomotor centre reacts to information from baroreceptors and chemoreceptors by raising or lowering blood pressure accordingly. Nerve fibres travel from the vasomotor centre to the arteries, where the smooth muscle is directed to either constrict (raise blood pressure) or relax (lower blood pressure). As

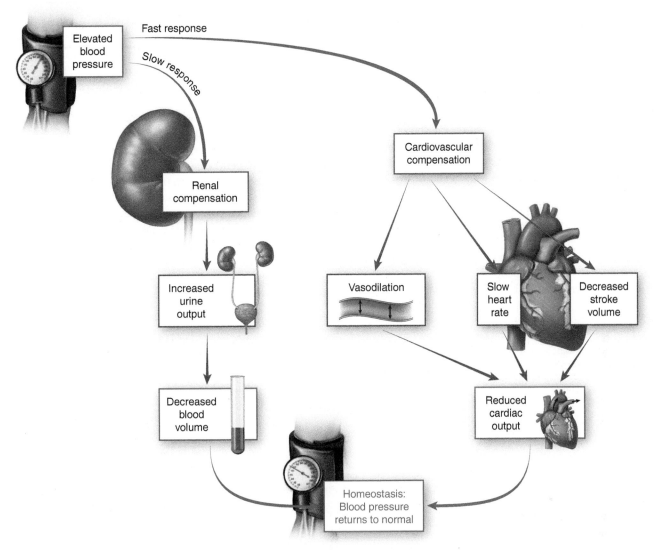

Figure 48.6 Cardiovascular and renal control of blood pressure.

discussed in Chapters 12 and 14, sympathetic outflow from the vasomotor centre stimulates alpha$_1$-adrenergic receptors on arterioles, causing vasoconstriction. Alpha$_2$-adrenergic agonists can also decrease blood pressure by their central effects on the vasomotor centre.

The baroreceptor reflex is an important mechanism used by the body for making rapid adjustments to blood pressure. If pressure in the vascular system increases, the baroreceptors in the aortic arch and carotid sinus trigger reflexes that constrict the arterioles and veins and accelerate the heart rate. Together, these actions return blood pressure to normal levels within seconds.

Drugs that raise or lower blood pressure can trigger the baroreceptor reflex. For example, antihypertensives administered by the IV route cause an immediate reduction in blood pressure that is recognized by the baroreceptors. The baroreceptors respond by attempting to return blood pressure back to the original level. The resulting accelerated heart rate, or **reflex tachycardia**, may cause the client to experience palpitations. The baroreceptors are not able to offer a continuous or sustained reduction in blood

pressure. Continued administration of an antihypertensive drug will "overcome" the reflex. In addition, with aging or certain disease states such as diabetes, the baroreceptor response may be diminished.

Another example of the baroreceptor reflex occurs when baroreceptors in the right atrium are triggered. These receptors recognize excess stretching of the right atrium, such as might occur when large amounts of IV fluids are administered. The **atrial reflex** causes the heart rate and CO to increase until the backlog of venous blood (or IV fluid) is distributed throughout the body.

The chemoreceptor reflex can also significantly affect blood pressure. Sensors in the carotid sinus and near the aortic arch recognize levels of oxygen and carbon dioxide and the acidity (pH) in the blood. Triggering these chemoreceptors activates the sympathetic nervous system and causes heart rate and CO to increase. The purpose of this reflex is to circulate blood faster so that the respiratory system can remove excess carbon dioxide (which returns pH to normal levels) and add more oxygen to the blood.

Hormonal Effects on Blood Pressure

48.10 Hormones may have profound effects on blood pressure.

Several hormones affect blood pressure, and certain classes of medications are given to either enhance or block the actions of these hormones. For example, injection of the catecholamine epinephrine or norepinephrine will immediately raise blood pressure, which is essential for clients who are experiencing shock.

Antidiuretic hormone (ADH) is a hormone released by the posterior pituitary gland when blood pressure falls or when the osmotic pressure of the blood increases. ADH, also known as vasopressin (Pressyn), is a potent peripheral vasoconstrictor that quickly increases blood pressure. The hormone also acts on the kidneys to conserve water and increase blood volume, thereby causing blood pressure to increase. The pharmacotherapy of ADH and related hormones is discussed in Chapter 51.

The **renin-angiotensin-aldosterone system (RAAS)** is particularly important in the drug therapy of HTN. As blood pressure falls, the enzyme renin is released by the kidneys. Through a two-step pathway, angiotensin II is formed, which subsequently increases CO and constricts arterioles to return blood pressure to original levels. Angiotensin II also promotes the release of aldosterone from the adrenal gland, which causes sodium and water retention. Drugs that block the RAAS are key drugs in the treatment of HTN and heart failure.

Atrial natriuretic peptide (ANP) is a hormone that is secreted by specialized cells in the right atrium when large increases in blood volume produce excessive stretch on the atrial wall. ANP has multiple effects, all of which attempt to return blood pressure to original levels. Sodium ion transport in the kidney is affected, resulting in enhanced sodium and water excretion. The release of ADH and aldosterone is suppressed by ANP. In addition, ANP reduces sympathetic outflow from the central nervous system, resulting in dilation of peripheral arteries. A summary of the various nervous and hormone factors influencing blood pressure is shown in Figure 48.7.

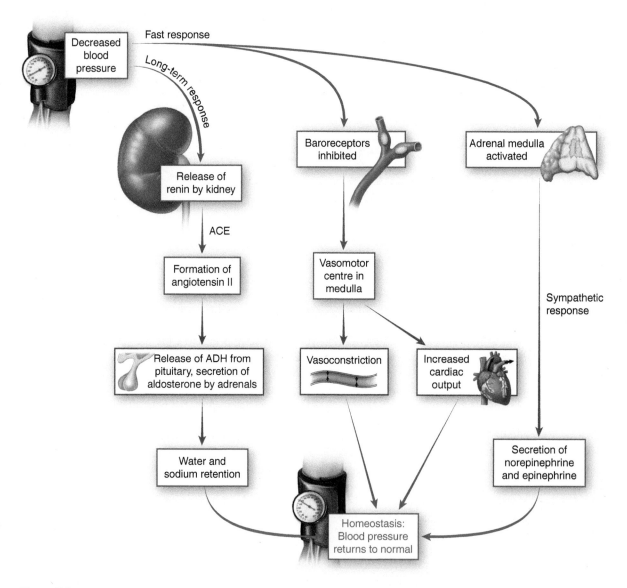

Figure 48.7 Endocrine and nervous control of blood pressure.

CHAPTER

48

Understanding the Chapter

Key Concepts Summary

The numbered key concepts provide a succinct summary of the important points from the corresponding numbered section within the chapter. If any of these points are not clear, refer to the numbered section within the chapter for review.

48.1   The cardiovascular system consists of the blood, heart, and blood vessels.

48.2   Blood consists of formed elements and plasma.

48.3   Hemostasis is a complex process involving multiple steps and a large number of enzymes and factors.

48.4   The heart is responsible for pumping blood throughout the circulatory system.

48.5   The coronary arteries bring essential nutrients to the myocardium.

48.6   The cardiac conduction system keeps the heart beating in a synchronized manner.

48.7   Cardiac output is determined by stroke volume and heart rate.

48.8   The primary factors responsible for blood pressure are cardiac output, peripheral resistance, and blood volume.

48.9   Neural regulation of blood pressure includes baroreceptor and chemoreceptor reflexes.

48.10   Hormones may have profound effects on blood pressure.

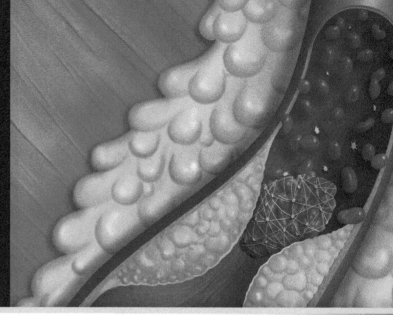

BSIP SA/Alamy Stock Photo

PROTOTYPE DRUGS

HMG-CoA REDUC-TASE INHIBITORS
Pr *atorvastatin*
(Lipitor)

BILE ACID RESINS
Pr *cholestyramine*
(Olestyr, Questran)

NICOTINIC ACID

FIBRIC ACID AGENTS
Pr *gemfibrozil (Lopid)*

CHAPTER 49

Pharmacotherapy of Lipid Disorders

LEARNING OUTCOMES

After reading this chapter, the student should be able to:

1. Summarize the link between high blood cholesterol, low-density lipoprotein (LDL) levels, and atherosclerosis

2. Identify drug classes used for treating lipid disorders.

3. Explain the therapeutic action of each class of drug used for lipid disorders in relation to the pathophysiology of the disorder requiring treatment.

4. Discuss the role of the nurse in teaching clients regarding control of cholesterol and LDL levels through non-pharmacological means.

5. Describe the nurse's role in the pharmacological management of clients who are receiving drugs for lipid disorders.

6. For each of the drug classes listed in Prototype Drugs, identify a representative drug and explain its mechanism of action, therapeutic effects, and important adverse effects.

7. Describe and explain, based on pharmacological principles, the rationale for nursing assessment, planning, and interventions for clients with lipid disorders.

8. Use the nursing process to care for clients who are receiving drug therapy for lipid disorders.

CHAPTER OUTLINE

▶ Types of Lipid

▶ Lipoproteins

▶ Achieving and Maintaining Desirable Lipid Levels

▶ Controlling Lipid Levels through Lifestyle Changes

▶ HMG-CoA Reductase Inhibitors (Statins)
  ▶ Pharmacotherapy with Statins

▶ Bile Acid Resins
  ▶ Bile Acid Resins for Reducing Cholesterol and LDL Levels

▶ Nicotinic Acid
  ▶ Pharmacotherapy with Nicotinic Acid

Research during the 1960s and 1970s brought about a nutritional revolution as new knowledge about lipids and their relationship to obesity and cardiovascular disease allowed people to make more intelligent lifestyle choices. Since then, advances in the diagnosis of lipid disorders have helped to identify those clients at greatest risk for cardiovascular disease and those most likely to benefit from pharmacological intervention. Research in pharmacology has led to safe and effective drugs for lowering lipid levels, thus decreasing the risk for cardiovascular-related diseases. As a result of this knowledge and advancement in pharmacology, the incidence of death due to most cardiovascular diseases has been declining, although cardiovascular disease remains the second leading cause of death in Canada.

Types of Lipid

49.1 Plasma lipids are organic compounds that are poorly soluble in water but miscible in organic solvents. They are the structural component in cells and are involved in metabolic and hormonal pathways.

The three types of lipid that are important to humans are illustrated in Figure 49.1. The most common are the **triglycerides**, which form a large family of different lipids all having three fatty acids attached to a chemical backbone of glycerol. Triglycerides are the major storage form of fat in the body and the only type of lipid that serves as an important energy source. They account for 90% of total lipids in the body.

The **phospholipids** are formed when a phosphorous group replaces one of the fatty acids in a triglyceride. These lipids are essential for building plasma membranes. The best-known phospholipids are **lecithins**, which are found in high concentration in egg yolks and soybeans. Lecithins were once promoted as a natural treatment for high cholesterol levels, but controlled studies have not shown lecithin to be of any benefit for this disorder. Likewise, lecithin has been proposed as a remedy for nervous system diseases such as Alzheimer's disease and bipolar disorder, but there is no definite evidence to support these claims.

The **steroids** are a diverse group of substances that have a common chemical structure called the **sterol nucleus**, or ring. **Cholesterol** is the most widely known of the steroids, and its role in promoting atherosclerosis has been clearly demonstrated.

Cholesterol is a natural and vital component of plasma membranes. Unlike the triglycerides that provide fuel for the body during times of energy need, cholesterol serves as the building block for a number of essential biochemicals, including vitamin D, bile acids, cortisol, estrogen, and testosterone. While clearly essential for life, the body needs only minute amounts of cholesterol. The liver is able to synthesize adequate amounts of cholesterol from other chemicals; it is not necessary to provide additional cholesterol in the diet. Dietary cholesterol is obtained solely from animal products; humans do not metabolize the sterols produced by plants. Health Canada recommends less than 300 mg of dietary cholesterol per day.

Lipoproteins

49.2 Lipids are carried through the blood as lipoproteins; VLDL and LDL are associated with an increased incidence of cardiovascular disease, whereas HDL exerts a protective effect.

Because lipid molecules are not soluble in plasma, they must be specially packaged for transport through the blood. To accomplish this, the body forms complexes called **lipoproteins** that consist of various amounts of cholesterol, triglycerides, and phospholipids, along with a protein carrier. The protein component is called an **apoprotein** (*apo*- means "separated from" or "derived from").

The three most common lipoproteins are classified according to their composition, size, and weight or density, which comes primarily from the amount of apoprotein present in the complex. Each type varies in lipid and apoprotein makeup and serves a different function in transporting lipids from sites of synthesis and absorption to sites of use. For example, **high-density lipoprotein (HDL)** contains the most apoprotein, up to 50% by weight. The highest amount of cholesterol is carried by **low-density lipoprotein (LDL)**. Figure 49.2 illustrates the three basic lipoproteins and their compositions.

To understand the pharmacotherapy of lipid disorders, it is important to learn the functions of the major lipoproteins and their roles in transporting cholesterol. LDL transports cholesterol from the liver to the tissues and organs, where it is used to build plasma membranes or to synthesize other steroids. Once in the tissues, it can also be stored for later use. However, storage of cholesterol in the lining of blood vessels is not desirable because it contributes

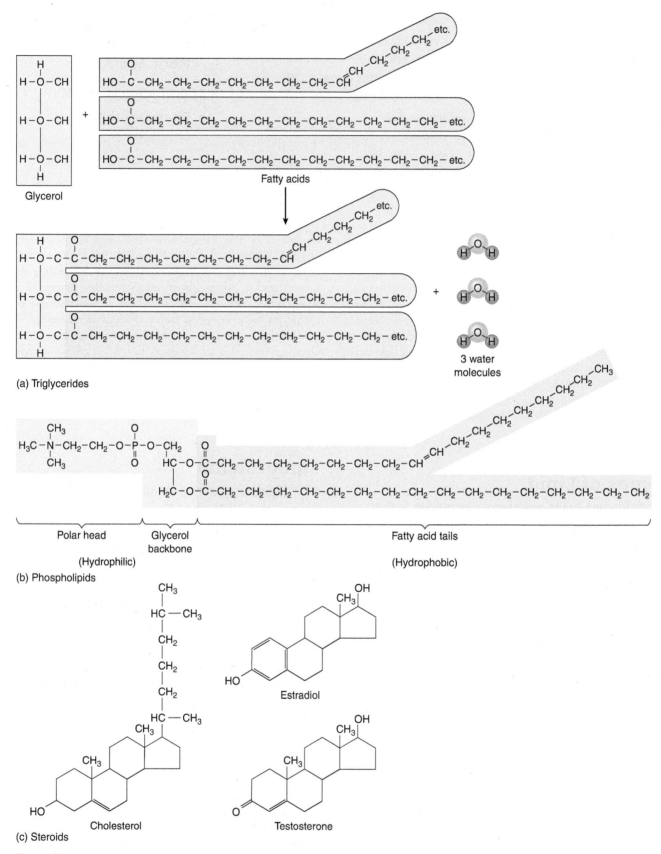

(a) Triglycerides

(b) Phospholipids

Polar head   Glycerol
              backbone

(Hydrophilic)

Fatty acid tails

(Hydrophobic)

Estradiol

Cholesterol

Testosterone

(c) Steroids

Figure 49.1   Chemical structure of the three types of lipid.

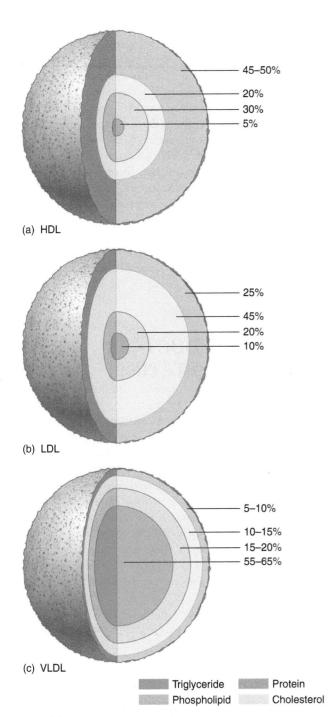

(a) HDL

45–50%
20%
30%
5%

(b) LDL

25%
45%
20%
10%

(c) VLDL

5–10%
10–15%
15–20%
55–65%

■ Triglyceride   ■ Protein
■ Phospholipid   ■ Cholesterol

Figure 49.2 Composition of the lipoproteins.

to plaque buildup and atherosclerosis. LDL is often called "bad" cholesterol because this lipoprotein contributes significantly to plaque deposits and coronary artery disease. Lowering LDL levels in the blood has been shown to decrease the incidence of coronary artery disease. **Very low–density lipoprotein (VLDL)** is the primary carrier of triglycerides in the blood. Through a series of steps, VLDL is reduced in size to become LDL.

HDL is manufactured in the liver and small intestine and assists in the transport of cholesterol away from the body tissues and back to the liver in a process called **reverse cholesterol transport**. The cholesterol component of HDL is then broken down

to unite with bile that is subsequently excreted in the feces. Excretion via bile is the only route the body uses to remove cholesterol. Because HDL transports cholesterol for destruction and removes it from the body, it is considered "good" cholesterol.

Hyperlipidemia, the general term meaning "high levels of lipids in the blood," is a major risk factor for cardiovascular disease. Elevated blood cholesterol, or **hypercholesterolemia**, is the type of hyperlipidemia that is most familiar to the general public. **Dyslipidemia** refers to abnormal (excess or deficient) levels of lipoproteins. The etiology may be inherited or acquired.

Achieving and Maintaining Desirable Lipid Levels

49.3 Blood lipid profiles are important diagnostic tools in guiding the therapy of dyslipidemia.

Achieving and maintaining optimal lipid levels are important for the prevention of cardiovascular disease. It is not adequate to simply measure total cholesterol in the blood. Because some cholesterol is being transported for destruction, a more accurate profile is obtained by measuring LDL cholesterol and the ratio of total cholesterol to HDL cholesterol in the blood. The goal in maintaining normal cholesterol levels is to maximize the HDL and minimize the LDL. The target LDL cholesterol level is less than 2.5 mmol/L. The target total cholesterol to HDL cholesterol ratio is less than 4.0. Triglyceride levels may also be assessed. The optimal serum triglyceride concentration is less than 1.7 mmol/L.

Scientists have further divided LDL into subclasses of lipoproteins. For example, one variety called lipoprotein (a) has been strongly associated with plaque formation and heart disease. It is likely that further research will discover other varieties, with the expectation that drugs will be designed to be more selective toward the "bad" lipoproteins.

CONNECTIONS Lifespan Considerations

◄ Pediatric Dyslipidemia

Most people consider dyslipidemia a condition that occurs with advancing age. Dyslipidemias, however, are also a concern for some pediatric clients. Children at risk include those with a family history of premature coronary artery disease or dyslipidemia and those who have hypertension or diabetes, or are obese. Lipid levels fluctuate in children, and they tend to be higher in girls. Nutritional intervention, regular physical activity, and risk factor management are warranted when the LDL cholesterol level reaches 2.85 to 3.34 mmol/L. More aggressive dietary therapy and pharmacotherapy may be warranted in pediatric clients with LDL cholesterol levels above 3.37 mmol/L. The long-term effects of lipid-lowering drugs in children have not been clearly established; therefore, drug therapy is not recommended for children under 10 years of age. Cholestyramine (Questran, Olestyr) and colestipol (Colestid) are the only approved drugs for hypercholesterolemia in children, although side effects sometimes result in poor adherence. Research into the use of niacin and low-dose statin pharmacotherapy in children is continuing.

Establishing treatment guidelines for dyslipidemia has been difficult, as the condition has no symptoms and the progression to cardiovascular disease may take decades. Based on years of research, the Canadian Working Group on Hypercholesterolemia and Other Dyslipidemias recently revised the recommended treatment guidelines for dyslipidemia. The new guidelines are based on accumulated evidence that reducing "borderline" high cholesterol levels can result in fewer heart attacks and fewer deaths. In addition, the guidelines recommend that high cholesterol levels be treated more aggressively in diabetic clients and other high-risk groups. These guidelines will likely lead to more widespread use of medications to treat dyslipidemia.

Controlling Lipid Levels through Lifestyle Changes

49.4 Before starting pharmacotherapy for hyperlipidemia, clients should seek to control the condition through lifestyle changes such as restriction of dietary saturated fats and cholesterol, increased exercise, and smoking cessation.

Lifestyle changes should always be included in any treatment plan for reducing blood lipid levels. Many clients with borderline laboratory values can control their dyslipidemia entirely through non-pharmacological means. It is important to note that all the lifestyle factors for reducing blood lipid levels also apply to cardiovascular disease in general. Because many clients taking lipid-lowering drugs also have underlying cardiovascular disease, these lifestyle changes are particularly important. The following are the most important lipid-reduction interventions:

- Monitor blood lipid levels regularly, as recommended by the healthcare provider.

- Maintain weight and waist circumference at an optimum level.

- Implement a medically supervised exercise plan.

- Reduce dietary saturated fat, trans fatty acids, and cholesterol to less than 7% of total calories, while increasing the proportion of monounsaturated and polyunsaturated fats.

- Increase soluble fibre in the diet, as found in oat bran, apples, beans, grapefruit, and broccoli.

- Limit alcohol use to no more than two standard drinks per day.

- Reduce or eliminate tobacco use.

Nutritionists recommend that the intake of dietary fat be less than 30% of the total caloric intake. Cholesterol intake should be reduced as much as possible and should not exceed 300 mg/day. It is interesting to note that restriction of dietary cholesterol alone will not result in a significant reduction in blood cholesterol levels. This is because the liver reacts to a low-cholesterol diet by making more cholesterol and by inhibiting its excretion when saturated fats are present. Therefore, the client must reduce saturated fat in the diet, as well as cholesterol, to control the amount made by the liver and to ultimately lower blood cholesterol levels.

The use of plant sterols and stanols is now approved in some countries to reduce blood cholesterol levels. These plant lipids have a similar structure to cholesterol and therefore compete with that substance for absorption in the digestive tract. When the body absorbs the plant sterols, cholesterol is excreted from the body. When less cholesterol is delivered to the liver, LDL uptake increases, thereby decreasing the serum LDL level. Plant sterols and stanols may be obtained from a variety of sources, including wheat, corn, rye, oats, and rice, as well as nuts and olive oil. In countries where they are approved, they may be found in some margarines, salad dressings, cereals, and fruit juices. The daily intake of plant sterols or stanols should not exceed 3 g. Health Canada advises that sterols may pose health risks for certain groups such as pregnant women, children, people who are predisposed to hemorrhagic strokes, and people who are taking cholesterol-lowering medication. Investigations are in progress to assess the safety of plant sterols and stanols.

HMG-CoA REDUCTASE INHIBITORS (STATINS)

The statin class of antihyperlipidemics interferes with a critical enzyme in the synthesis of cholesterol. Cholesterol is manufactured in the liver by a series of more than 25 metabolic steps, beginning with acetyl coenzyme A (acetyl CoA), a two-carbon unit that is produced from the breakdown of fatty acids. Of the many enzymes involved in this complex pathway, **HMG-CoA reductase** (3-hydroxy-3-methylglutaryl coenzyme A reductase) serves as the primary regulatory site for cholesterol biosynthesis. Under normal conditions, this enzyme is controlled through negative feedback: high levels of LDL cholesterol in the blood will shut down production of HMG-CoA reductase, thus turning off the cholesterol pathway. Figure 49.3 illustrates selected steps in cholesterol biosynthesis and the importance of HMG-CoA reductase.

The statins, which are also known as HMG-CoA reductase inhibitors, are listed in Table 49.1. They are first-line drugs in the treatment of lipid disorders.

NCLEX Success Tips

Simvastatin (Zocor): Liver function tests, including aspartate transaminase (AST), should be monitored before therapy, 6 to 12 weeks after initiation of therapy or after dose elevation, and then every 6 months. If AST levels increase to three times normal, therapy should be discontinued. Serum cholesterol and triglyceride levels should be evaluated before initiating therapy, after 4 to 6 weeks of therapy, and periodically thereafter.

If the serum cholesterol of a client taking simvastatin is within normal range, the medication is effective.

Simvastatin is used in combination with diet and exercise to decrease elevated total cholesterol. The client should take simvastatin in the evening, and the nurse should instruct the client that if a dose is missed, he or she should take it as soon as remembered but not at the same time as the next scheduled dose. The nurse should instruct the client to avoid grapefruit and grapefruit juice, which can increase the amount of the drug in the bloodstream.

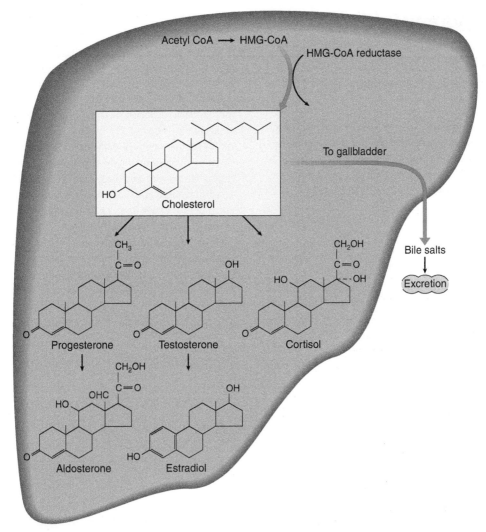

Figure 49.3 Cholesterol biosynthesis and excretion.

TABLE 49.1 Drugs for Dyslipidemia

Drug	Route and Adult Dose
HMG-CoA Reductase Inhibitors	
Pr atorvastatin (Lipitor)	Orally (PO), 10–80 mg every day (qd)
fluvastatin (Lescol)	PO, 20–80 mg qd
lovastatin (Mevacor)	PO, 20–80 mg qd–twice a day (bid)
pravastatin (Pravachol)	PO, 10–40 mg qd
rosuvastatin (Crestor)	PO, 5–40 mg qd
simvastatin (Zocor)	PO, 5–80 mg qd
Bile Acid–Binding Agents	
Pr cholestyramine (Olestyr, Questran)	PO, start with 4 g qd or bid; increase gradually over 1 month intervals; maintenance dose is 8-16 g/day divided in 2 doses
colestipol (Colestid)	PO, start with 5 g qd or bid; increase by 5 g/day at 1-2 month intervals; for clients with pre-existing constipation, start at 5 g qd for 5-7 days, then increase to 5 g bid; maintenance dose is 5-30 g qd or in divided doses
Fibric Acid Agents	
fenofibrate (Lipidil)	PO, 100–200 mg qd
Pr gemfibrozil (Lopid)	PO, 300–600 mg bid
Other Agents	
ezetimibe (Ezetrol)	PO, 10 mg/day
niacin (Niaspan)	Hyperlipidemia: PO, 1.5–3.0 g/day in divided doses (max 6 g/day)
orlistat (Xenical)	PO, 120 mg three times a day (tid) with meals

Pharmacotherapy with Statins

49.5 Statins, which inhibit HMG-CoA reductase, a critical enzyme in the biosynthesis of cholesterol, are drugs of first choice for reducing blood lipid levels.

In the late 1970s, compounds isolated from various species of fungi were found to inhibit cholesterol production in human cells in the laboratory. This class of drug, known as the statins, has since revolutionized the treatment of lipid disorders. Statins can produce a dramatic 20% to 40% reduction in LDL cholesterol levels. In addition to reducing the LDL cholesterol level in the blood, statins can also lower triglyceride and VLDL levels and raise the level of "good" HDL cholesterol.

The statins act by inhibiting HMG-CoA reductase, which results in less cholesterol biosynthesis. As the liver makes less cholesterol, it responds by making more LDL receptors on the surface of liver cells. The greater number of LDL receptors in liver cells results in increased removal of LDL from the blood. Blood levels of both LDL and cholesterol are reduced. The drop in lipid levels is not permanent, however, so clients need to remain on these drugs during the remainder of their lives or until their hyperlipidemia can be controlled through dietary or lifestyle changes. Statins have been shown to slow the progression of coronary artery disease and to reduce mortality from cardiovascular disease. The mechanisms of action of the statins and other drugs for dyslipidemia are illustrated in Figure 49.4.

All statins are given orally and are tolerated well by most clients. Because cholesterol biosynthesis in the liver is higher at night, statins with short half-lives, such as lovastatin (Mevacor), should be administered in the evening. The other statins, such as atorvastatin (Lipitor), have longer half-lives and are effective regardless of the time of day they are taken.

Much research is ongoing to determine other therapeutic effects of drugs in the statin class. For example, statins block the vasoconstrictive effect of the amyloid beta protein, a significant protein involved in Alzheimer's disease. Cholesterol and amyloid beta protein have similar effects on blood vessels, causing them to constrict. Preliminary research suggests that the statins may

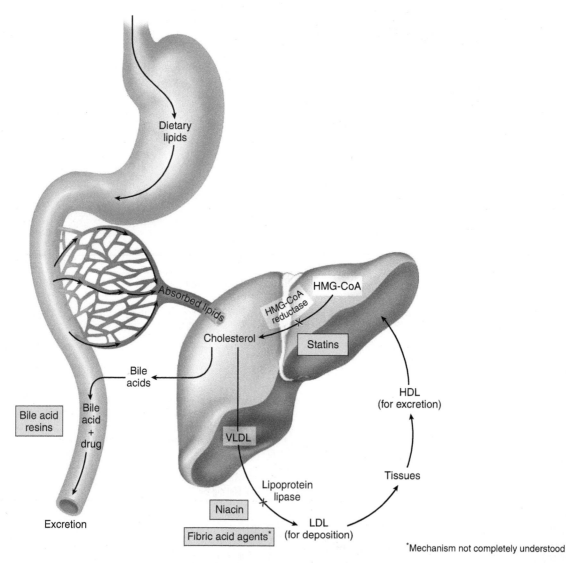

Figure 49.4 Mechanisms of action of lipid-lowering drugs.

protect against dementia by inhibiting the protein and thus slowing dementia caused by blood vessel constriction.

Severe myopathy and rhabdomyolysis are rare, although serious, adverse effects of the statins. **Rhabdomyolysis** is a breakdown of muscle fibres usually due to muscle trauma or ischemia. The mechanism by which statins cause this disorder is unknown. During rhabdomyolysis, the contents of muscle cells spill into the systemic circulation, causing potentially fatal acute renal failure. Macrolide antibiotics such as erythromycin (Eryc), azole antifungals, fibric acid drugs, and certain immunosuppressants should be avoided during statin therapy, because these interfere with statin metabolism and increase the risk for severe myopathy. Levels of creatine kinase (CK), an enzyme released during muscle injury, should be obtained if myopathy is suspected. If CK levels become elevated during therapy, the drug should be immediately discontinued. Statins may be discontinued if muscle weakness persists even without CK elevation. Nurses should urge all clients who develop unexplained muscle or joint pain during statin therapy to immediately report this to the prescriber.

Statins are pregnancy category X drugs because teratogenic effects have been reported in laboratory animals exposed to these drugs. Statins should not be used in clients who may become pregnant, are pregnant, or are breastfeeding.

NCLEX Success Tip

Myopathy/rhabdomyolysis is a potential side effect occurring with the use of statin medications.

Nursing Considerations

The role of the nurse in statin therapy involves careful monitoring of the client's condition and providing education as it relates to the prescribed drug regimen. Although statin drugs are effective in reducing blood lipid levels, there can be serious adverse effects in some clients. Statins are pregnancy category X and should not be used in clients who are pregnant or breastfeeding or who may become pregnant. Women taking statin drugs should use effective birth control and stop taking the medication if they suspect pregnancy.

Because liver dysfunction may occur with the use of statin drugs, the nurse should monitor liver function tests before and during therapy. Statin drugs should not be used in clients with active liver disease or unexplained elevations in liver function tests. This drug class should be used cautiously in clients who drink large quantities of alcohol, and alcohol use should be restricted or discontinued while on the medication. Because myopathy has been reported by some clients, the nurse should assess the client for muscle pain, tenderness, and weakness. Creatinine phosphokinase (CPK) levels should be obtained if myopathy is suspected and, if elevated, statin therapy should be discontinued. The drug may be discontinued if muscle weakness persists even without CPK elevation.

Nausea, vomiting, heartburn, dyspepsia, abdominal cramping, and diarrhea are common, though less serious, side effects. The statins can be taken with the evening meal to help alleviate gastrointestinal (GI) upset.

Client education as it relates to these drugs should include goals, reasons for obtaining baseline data such as vital signs and tests for cardiac and hepatic disorders, and possible side effects. The following are the important points the nurse should include when teaching clients regarding HMG-CoA reductase inhibitors:

- Keep all scheduled laboratory visits for liver function tests.
- Do not take other prescription drugs, over-the-counter (OTC) medications, herbal remedies, or vitamins or minerals without notifying the healthcare provider.
- Practise reliable contraception and notify the healthcare provider if pregnancy is planned or suspected.
- Immediately report unexplained muscle pain, tenderness, or weakness, especially if accompanied by malaise or fever.
- Immediately report unexplained numbness, tingling, weakness, or pain in the feet or hands.
- Take the drug with the evening meal to prevent GI disturbances.

NURSING PROCESS FOCUS

Clients Receiving HMG-CoA Reductase Inhibitor Therapy

Assessment	Potential Nursing Diagnoses/Identified Patterns
Prior to administration: • Obtain a complete health history, including allergies, drug history, and possible drug interactions. • Obtain baseline liver function tests, lipid studies, and a pregnancy test in women of childbearing age.	• Need for knowledge regarding drug therapy and lifestyle modifications • Nonadherence related to dietary and drug regimen • Chronic pain related to drug-induced myopathy

Planning: Client Goals and Expected Outcomes

The client will:

- Immediately report skeletal muscle pain, unexplained muscle soreness, or weakness
- Demonstrate adherence with appropriate lifestyle changes
- Demonstrate an understanding of the drug's action by accurately describing drug side effects and precautions

Implementation

Interventions (Rationales)	Client Education/Discharge Planning
• Monitor blood cholesterol and triglyceride levels at intervals during therapy (to determine effectiveness of therapy). • Monitor client adherence with dietary regimen. (Maintenance of controlled saturated fat in the diet is essential to effectiveness of medications.) • Monitor client for alcohol abuse. (Excessive alcohol intake may result in liver damage and interfere with drug effectiveness.) • Monitor CPK level. (Elevated CPK may be indicative of impending myopathy.) • Monitor liver function. (Liver dysfunction may occur with these drugs.) • Obtain client's smoking history. (Smoking increases risk for cardiovascular disease and may decrease HDL levels.)	• Advise client of the importance of keeping appointments for laboratory testing • Provide client with information needed to maintain a diet low in saturated fat and cholesterol • Instruct client to avoid or limit alcohol use • Instruct client to report symptoms of leg or muscle pain to the healthcare provider • Encourage smoking cessation if appropriate

Evaluation of Outcome Criteria

Evaluate the effectiveness of drug therapy by confirming that client goals and expected outcomes have been met (see "Planning").

See Table 49.1 for a list of drugs to which these nursing actions apply.

PROTOTYPE DRUG | **Atorvastatin (Lipitor)**

Actions and Uses: The primary indication for atorvastatin is hypercholesterolemia. The statins act by inhibiting HMG-CoA reductase. As the liver makes less cholesterol, it responds by making more LDL receptors on the surface of liver cells. The greater number of LDL receptors in liver cells results in increased removal of LDL from the blood. Blood levels of both LDL and cholesterol are reduced, although at least 2 weeks of therapy are required before these effects are realized.

Administration Alerts:

• Administer with food to decrease GI discomfort.

• Drug may be taken at any time of day.

• Atorvastatin is pregnancy category X.

Pharmacokinetics: Atorvastatin is rapidly absorbed. Bioavailability is 14% due to first-pass metabolism. It is excreted mostly in bile and feces. It has a half-life of 14 hours.

Adverse Effects and Interactions: Side effects of atorvastatin are rarely severe enough to cause discontinuation of therapy and include GI complaints such as intestinal cramping, diarrhea, and constipation. A small percentage of clients experience liver damage; therefore, hepatic function is monitored during the first few months of therapy.

Atorvastatin interacts with many other drugs. For example, it may increase digoxin (Lanoxin, Toloxin) levels by 20%, as well as increase levels of norethindrone (Micronor) and ethinyl estradiol (various oral contraceptives). Erythromycin may increase atorvastatin levels by 40%.

Grapefruit juice inhibits the metabolism of statins, allowing them to reach toxic levels. Since HMG-CoA reductase inhibitors also decrease the synthesis of coenzyme Q10 (CoQ10), clients may benefit from CoQ10 supplements.

BILE ACID RESINS

Bile acid resins bind bile acids, thus increasing the excretion of cholesterol. They are sometimes used in combination with the statins. These agents are listed in Table 49.1.

Bile Acid Resins for Reducing Cholesterol and LDL Levels

49.6 The bile acid resins bind bile acids (containing cholesterol) and accelerate their excretion. These agents can reduce cholesterol and LDL levels but are not drugs of choice due to their side effects.

Prior to the discovery of the statins, the primary means of lowering blood cholesterol was through use of bile acid–binding drugs called bile acid resins or sequestrants. These drugs bind bile acids, which contain a high concentration of cholesterol. Because of their large size, resins are not absorbed from the small intestine and the bound bile acids and cholesterol are eliminated in the feces. The liver responds to the loss of cholesterol by making more LDL receptors, which removes even more cholesterol from the blood in a mechanism similar to that of the statin drugs.

Although effective at producing a 20% drop in LDL cholesterol, the bile acid sequestrants tend to cause more frequent side effects than statins. Because of this, they are no longer considered first-line drugs for dyslipidemia.

The bile acid resins tend to cause more frequent adverse effects than statins. Because they are not absorbed into the systemic circulation, adverse effects are limited to the GI tract, causing symptoms such as abdominal pain, bloating, diarrhea, steatorrhea, and constipation. In addition to binding bile acids, these agents can bind drugs such as digoxin and warfarin (Coumadin) and increase the potential for drug-drug interactions. Bile acid resins also interfere with the absorption of vitamins and minerals, and nutritional deficiencies may occur with extended use. Other medications and vitamins should be taken at least 1 hour before or 4 hours after taking a bile acid resin to avoid drug interactions.

Bile acid resins may cause a transient increase in triglyceride levels. This effect is particularly prominent and often sustained in clients with pre-existing hypertriglyceridemia. Because of this, the bile acid resins are generally not prescribed for clients who have elevated triglycerides.

NCLEX Success Tips

Bile acid sequestrants can form insoluable complexes with other drugs, thereby severely limiting their absorption.

Bile acid sequestrants should be mixed with water, fruit juice, soup, or pulpy fruit to reduce esophageal irritation and impaction.

Nursing Considerations

The role of the nurse in bile acid resin therapy involves careful monitoring of the client's condition and providing education as it relates to the prescribed drug regimen. Because bile acid sequestrants act in the GI tract and are not absorbed, they have no systemic side effects. However, they can cause significant GI effects such as constipation, abdominal pain, bloating, nausea, vomiting, diarrhea, and steatorrhea. The nurse should assess bowel sounds and the presence of GI disturbance. Bile acid resins should be used cautiously in clients with GI disorders such as peptic ulcer disease, hemorrhoids, inflammatory bowel disease, or chronic constipation, as they may worsen or aggravate these conditions. These drugs are generally not used during pregnancy or lactation (pregnancy category C).

Bile acid resins decrease the absorption of vitamins and minerals; deficiencies may occur with extended use. Other medications should be taken more than 1 hour before or 4 hours after taking a bile acid sequestrant because of decreased absorption. Cholestyramine powder should be mixed with 60 to 180 mL of water, non-carbonated beverage, highly liquid soup, or pulpy fruit (applesauce, crushed pineapple) to prevent esophageal irritation. The nurse should place the contents of the packet on the surface of the fluid, allow it to stand (without stirring) for 2 minutes, occasionally twirling the glass, and then stir slowly (to prevent foaming) to form a suspension. The client should drink the medication immediately after stirring. The client should not inhale the powder, as it may irritate mucous membranes.

Constipation may occur with decreased bowel function. Nausea, vomiting, heartburn, dyspepsia, abdominal cramping, and diarrhea may also occur, so it is important to take this medication with lots of water. Clients with dysphagia or esophageal stricture could develop an obstruction while taking this medication.

Client education as it relates to bile acid resins should include goals; reasons for obtaining baseline data such as vital signs and cardiac, hepatic, and renal tests; and possible side effects. The following are important points the nurse should include when teaching clients regarding bile acid resins:

- Take the medication before meals.
- Take other medications 1 hour before or 4 hours after taking bile acid resins to avoid interference with absorption of other drugs.
- A high-bulk diet and adequate fluid intake will help to decrease constipation and bloating.

- Take vitamin supplements to replace folic acid, fat-soluble vitamins, and vitamin K.
- Do not take other prescription drugs, OTC medications, herbal remedies, or vitamins or minerals without notifying the healthcare provider.
- Report the following immediately: yellowing of skin or whites of eyes, severe constipation, flatulence, nausea, heartburn, straining with passing of stools, tarry stools, or abnormal bleeding.

PROTOTYPE DRUG	Cholestyramine (Olestyr, Questran)

Actions and Uses: Cholestyramine is a powder that is mixed with fluid before being taken once or twice daily. It lowers LDL cholesterol levels by increasing LDL receptors on hepatocytes. The resultant increase in LDL intake from plasma decreases circulating LDL levels.

Pharmacokinetics: Cholestyramine is not absorbed or metabolized once it enters the intestine, so it does not produce any systemic effects. It may take 30 days or longer to produce its maximum effect. It is excreted in the feces.

Administration Alerts:

- Mix the drug thoroughly with liquid and have the client drink it immediately to avoid potential irritation or obstruction in the GI tract.
- Other drugs should be taken more than 1 hour before or 4 hours after taking cholestyramine.
- Cholestyramine is pregnancy category C.

Adverse Effects and Interactions: Although cholestyramine rarely produces serious side effects, clients may experience constipation, bloating, gas, and nausea that sometimes limit its use. Cholestyramine needs to be taken with lots of water, and because it can bind to other drugs and interfere with their absorption, it should not be taken at the same time as other medications. Cholestyramine is sometimes combined with other cholesterol-lowering drugs such as the statins or nicotinic acid to produce additive effects.

NICOTINIC ACID

Nicotinic acid, or niacin (Niaspan), is a B complex vitamin that is occasionally used to lower lipid levels. It has a number of side effects that limit its use. The dose for nicotinic acid is given in Table 49.1.

Pharmacotherapy with Nicotinic Acid

49.7 Nicotinic acid, or niacin, can reduce LDL levels, but side effects limit its usefulness.

The ability of nicotinic acid to lower lipid levels is unrelated to its role as a vitamin since much higher doses are needed to produce its antilipidemic effects. For lowering cholesterol, the usual dose is 2 to 3 g/day. When taken as a vitamin, the dose is only 25 mg/day. The primary effect of nicotinic acid is to decrease VLDL levels; since LDL is synthesized from VLDL, the client experiences a reduction in LDL cholesterol levels. It also has the desirable effects of reducing triglycerides and increasing HDL levels. As with other lipid-lowering drugs, maximum therapeutic effect may take a month or longer to achieve.

Although effective at reducing LDL cholesterol by as much as 20%, nicotinic acid produces more side effects than the statins. Flushing and hot flashes occur in almost every client. In addition, a variety of uncomfortable intestinal effects such as nausea, excess gas, and diarrhea are commonly reported. More serious side effects such as hepatotoxicity and gout are possible. Niacin is not usually prescribed for clients with diabetes mellitus because severe hyperglycemia may result. Because of these adverse effects, nicotinic acid is most often used in lower doses in combination with a statin or bile acid sequestrant since the beneficial effects of these drugs are additive.

Because niacin is available without a prescription, clients should be instructed not to attempt self-medication with this drug. One form of niacin available OTC as a vitamin supplement called nicotinamide has no lipid-lowering effects. Clients should be informed that if nicotinic acid is to be used to lower cholesterol, it should be done under medical supervision.

NCLEX Success Tips

Niacin reduces low-density lipoprotein and triglyceride levels while increasing high-density lipoprotein better than any other drug.

Flushing is a side effect of niacin administration.

Nursing Considerations

The role of the nurse in nicotinic acid therapy involves careful monitoring of the client's condition and providing education as it relates to the prescribed drug regimen. Because there is a risk for liver toxicity, niacin therapy must be carefully monitored. This is particularly important with sustained-release versions, which have the highest risk for hepatotoxicity. The nurse should assess liver function prior to and during therapy. Clients with elevated liver enzymes, history of liver disease, or peptic ulcers should not take niacin to lower lipids, as this medication can worsen these conditions. In clients who are predisposed to gout, nicotinic acid may increase uric acid levels and precipitate acute gout.

Clients are most likely to discontinue nicotinic acid therapy due to the intense flushing and pruritus that occur 1 to 2 hours after taking the medication. This response may be caused by prostaglandin release; taking one acetylsalicylic acid (ASA [Aspirin]) tablet 30 minutes prior to the nicotinic acid dose will help to decrease this effect. The flushing effect decreases with time. Nicotinic acid may affect glycemic control in non–insulin-dependent diabetic clients. Diabetic clients should monitor their blood sugar levels more frequently until the effect of nicotinic acid is known. GI distress is a common side effect that may be decreased by taking the drug with food.

CONNECTIONS **Natural Therapies**

◀ **Coenzyme Q10 and Cardiovascular Disease**

Coenzyme Q10 (CoQ10) is a vitamin-like substance found in most animal cells. It is an essential component in the cell's mitochondria for producing energy in the form of adenosine triphosphate (ATP). Because the heart requires high levels of ATP, a sufficient level of CoQ10 is essential to that organ. Supplementation with CoQ10 is especially important to clients who are taking the HMG-CoA reductase inhibitors because these drugs significantly lower blood levels of CoQ10. CoQ10 and cholesterol share the same metabolic pathways. Inhibition of the enzyme HMG-CoA reductase concurrently decreases CoQ10 levels.

Foods richest in this substance are pork, sardines, beef heart, salmon, broccoli, spinach, and nuts. Older adults appear to have an increased need for CoQ10. Although CoQ10 can be synthesized by the body, many amino acids and other substances are required; therefore, clients with nutritional deficiencies may be in need of supplementation.

In 1978, a Nobel Prize was awarded for research proving the importance of CoQ10 in energy transfer, but it was not until the 1990s that the substance became the top-selling supplement in health food stores. CoQ10 has been purported to aid a wide range of conditions, including heart failure, hypertension, dysrhythmias, angina, diabetes, neurological disorders, cancer, and aging. A considerable body of research has begun to accumulate, particularly regarding the role of CoQ10 in heart disease. Some data have found below-normal levels of CoQ10 in clients with heart failure. Studies suggest that the frequency of pre-ventricular contractions may be reduced in some clients by supplementation with CoQ10. Although most studies have demonstrated positive results, CoQ10 has not been widely accepted in the conventional medical community.

Client education as it relates to nicotinic acid should include goals; reasons for obtaining baseline data such as vital signs and cardiac, hepatic, and renal tests; and possible side effects. The following are important points the nurse should include when teaching clients regarding nicotinic acid:

* Do not take megadoses of niacin due to the risk for serious toxic effects.
* Take niacin with cold water, as hot beverages increase flushing.
* Take with or after meals to prevent GI upset.
* Do not take other prescription drugs, OTC medications, herbal remedies, or vitamins or minerals without notifying the healthcare provider.
* Report the following immediately: flank, joint, or stomach pain; skin colour changes (advise the client to stay out of the sun if skin changes occur); and yellowing of the whites of the eyes.

FIBRIC ACID AGENTS

Fibric acid agents may be used to lower lipid levels. They are sometimes used in combination with the statins. The fibric acid agents are listed in Table 49.1.

Pharmacotherapy with Fibric Acid Agents

49.8 Fibric acid agents lower triglyceride levels but have little effect on LDL cholesterol levels. They are not drugs of choice due to their potential side effects.

Two fibric acid agents, fenofibrate (Lipidil) and gemfibrozil (Lopid), are sometimes prescribed for clients with excessive triglyceride (VLDL) levels. The mechanism of action of the fibric acid agents is largely unknown.

Nursing Considerations

The role of the nurse in fibric acid therapy involves careful monitoring of the client's condition and providing education as it relates to the prescribed drug regimen. Prior to administering fibric acid, the nurse should assess the client for abdominal pain, nausea, and vomiting, the most common adverse effects. Taking the medication with meals usually decreases GI distress. The nurse should obtain an accurate pharmacological history. The use of fibric acid agents with statin drugs increases the risk for myositis. If a client is taking warfarin, lower dosages will be needed because of competitive protein binding. More frequent monitoring of prothrombin time (PT) and international normalized ratio (INR) may be necessary until stabilization occurs. Fibric acid is generally not used in lactation or pregnancy (category C).

Client education as it relates to these drugs should include goals, reasons for obtaining baseline data such as vital signs and cardiac and renal tests, and possible side effects. The following are the important points the nurse should include when teaching clients about fibric acid agents:

- Keep appointments for medical follow-up and laboratory tests.
- Immediately report the following: unusual bruising or bleeding, right upper quadrant pain, changes in stool colour, or muscle cramping.

PROTOTYPE DRUG | **Gemfibrozil (Lopid)**

Actions and Uses: Effects of gemfibrozil include up to a 50% reduction in VLDL with an increase in HDL. The mechanism of action is unknown. It is less effective than the statins at lowering LDL, so it is not a drug of first choice for reducing LDL cholesterol levels. Gemfibrozil is taken orally at 300 to 600 mg bid.

Pharmacokinetics: Gemfibrozil is well absorbed, minimally metabolized by the liver, and eliminated mainly by the kidneys. It has a half-life of 1.5 hours.

Administrative Alert:
- Administer with meals to decrease GI distress.
- Gemfibrozil is pregnancy category C.

Adverse Effects and Interactions: Gemfibrozil produces few serious adverse effects, but it may increase the likelihood of gallstones and occasionally affect liver function. The most common side effects are GI related: diarrhea, nausea, and cramping.

Drug interactions with gemfibrozil include oral anticoagulants; concurrent use with gemfibrozil may potentiate anticoagulant effects. Lovastatin increases the risk for myopathy and rhabdomyolysis.

MISCELLANEOUS AGENTS

Newer strategies have been developed to treat dyslipidemias. The large number of people with elevated lipid values has encouraged the pharmaceutical industry to investigate new drugs for controlling LDL cholesterol and triglycerides. The search for new and improved antilipidemics has resulted in several new drugs for this condition.

Ezetimibe (Ezetrol)

Ezetimibe (Ezetrol) is the only drug in a class called the cholesterol absorption inhibitors. Cholesterol is absorbed from the intestinal lumen by cells in the jejunum of the small intestine. Ezetimibe blocks this absorption by as much as 50%, causing less cholesterol to enter the blood. Unlike the statins, the drug does not inhibit cholesterol biosynthesis in the liver or increase the excretion of bile acid.

When given as monotherapy, ezetimibe produces a modest reduction in LDL of about 20%. Adding a statin to the therapeutic regimen reduces LDL by an additional 15% to 20%. The drug produces a slight drop in serum triglycerides. Ezetimibe is available as a single tablet with a once-daily dosing regimen.

Nasopharyngitis, myalgia, upper respiratory tract infection, arthralgia, and diarrhea are the most common adverse effects of ezetimibe, although these rarely require discontinuation of therapy. Because bile acid sequestrants inhibit the absorption of ezetimibe, these drugs should not be taken together. In addition, ezetimibe and statins should not be given concurrently to clients with serious hepatic impairment or elevated serum transaminase levels. Ezetimibe is pregnancy category C.

Omega-3 Fatty Acids

Nutritionists have long reported the benefits of eating fish rich in omega-3 fatty acids such as tuna, salmon, and halibut. The two principal omega-3 fatty acids are eicosapentaenoic acid (EPA) and docosahexaenoic acid (DHA). Vegetarian sources of omega-3 fatty acids include flaxseed oil, soybeans, walnuts, and pumpkin seeds.

The role of omega-3 fatty acids in preventing cardiovascular disease is well established. When taken as dietary supplements, the omega-3 fatty acids are usually marketed as fish oil. Fish oil supplementation has been shown to decrease mortality due to myocardial infarction (MI) and stroke. A typical dose of omega-3 fatty acids in fish oil capsules is 180 mg of EPA and 120 mg of DHA.

Orlistat (Xenical) is a new class of antiobesity agent with a unique action. Orlistat is a reversible, long-acting inhibitor of GI lipases. These lipases are enzymes that are required for the systemic absorption of dietary triglycerides. By forming a bond with lipases in the stomach and small intestine, orlistat prevents absorption of about 30% of dietary fat, thus producing a weight loss effect.

Pharmacotherapy with Orlistat
49.9 Orlistat prevents absorption of triglycerides and may promote weight loss and help to lower LDL cholesterol.

In addition to contributing to weight loss, orlistat may reduce total cholesterol and LDL cholesterol in the blood. Orlistat is recommended as an adjunct to a weight loss program that includes exercise and a healthy diet. The dose is shown in Table 49.1.

Orlistat has negligible systemic absorption. About 97% of unabsorbed drug is excreted by fecal elimination, and less than 2% is excreted in urine. Because it is minimally absorbed, orlistat is a relatively safe antiobesity drug. Low-dose orlistat is being considered for OTC use. There is concern that OTC availability may lead to abuse by individuals with eating disorders. A multiple vitamin supplement is usually required, since orlistat reduces absorption of fat-soluble vitamins.

Side effects of orlistat include oily fecal spotting, oily stools, flatulence, fecal urgency, fecal incontinence, and abdominal pain. Side effects often diminish as the body adjusts. Use of orlistat is contraindicated in pregnant women (category X).

The role of the nurse in orlistat therapy includes client education. Clients should be advised to take orlistat during or immediately following a meal that contains fat. A fat-soluble vitamin supplement should be taken at least 2 hours before or after a dose of orlistat. Methods to reduce weight and LDL cholesterol through dietary modification and exercise should be emphasized.

CHAPTER 49

Understanding the Chapter

Key Concepts Summary

The numbered key concepts provide a succinct summary of the important points from the corresponding numbered section within the chapter. If any of these points are not clear, refer to the numbered section within the chapter for review.

49.1 Plasma lipids are organic compounds that are poorly soluble in water but miscible in organic solvents. They are the structural component in cells and are involved in metabolic and hormonal pathways.

49.2 Lipids are carried through the blood as lipoproteins; VLDL and LDL are associated with an increased incidence of cardiovascular disease, whereas HDL exerts a protective effect.

49.3 Blood lipid profiles are important diagnostic tools in guiding the therapy of dyslipidemia.

49.4 Before starting pharmacotherapy for hyperlipidemia, clients should seek to control the condition through lifestyle changes such as restriction of dietary saturated fats and cholesterol, increased exercise, and smoking cessation.

49.5 Statins, which inhibit HMG-CoA reductase, a critical enzyme in the biosynthesis of cholesterol, are drugs of first choice for reducing blood lipid levels.

49.6 The bile acid resins bind bile acids (containing cholesterol) and accelerate their excretion. These agents can reduce cholesterol and LDL levels but are not drugs of choice due to their side effects.

49.7 Nicotinic acid, or niacin, can reduce LDL levels, but side effects limit its usefulness.

49.8 Fibric acid agents lower triglyceride levels but have little effect on LDL cholesterol levels. They are not drugs of choice due to their potential side effects.

49.9 Orlistat prevents absorption of triglycerides and may promote weight loss and help to lower LDL cholesterol.

Chapter 49 Scenario

Belinda Cummings is a 39-year-old black female who feels fine. However, she recently had her cholesterol level checked at her church's health fair and was told that it exceeded the normal value. As directed, she made an appointment to see her healthcare provider for a checkup.

During the office visit, the nurse collects Belinda's social and health history. Belinda's vital signs are within normal limits, except that her blood pressure is elevated (142/90 mm Hg). She is also slightly overweight and has been on a low-carbohydrate diet for 1 week. Her favourite foods are potato chips and all dairy products, especially cheese. She admits to smoking less than a pack of cigarettes per day and occasionally drinks a glass of wine with dinner. Belinda is divorced and has one teenage son.

A series of laboratory tests is completed during the visit. Belinda's physical exam is normal, and there are no ECG abnormalities. The blood tests are unremarkable with the exception of the lipid profile.

	Client Value	Normal Range
Total cholesterol	6.5 mmol/L	Less than 5 mmol/L
Triglycerides	2.5 mmol/L	Less than 1.52 mmol/L
HDL cholesterol	1 mmol/L	Greater than 1.55 mmol/L
LDL cholesterol	4.7 mmol/L	3.5 mmol/L
Cholesterol-to-HDL ratio	6.6	Less than 4.5

The client is placed on a standard cholesterol-lowering diet and prescribed atorvastatin (Lipitor) 10 mg daily. Belinda is instructed to return to the office in 1 month for a follow-up visit.

Critical Thinking Questions

1. How would you respond to Belinda when she asks you, "Is high cholesterol due to heredity or from what I eat?"

2. What health teaching should you provide to the client about ways to reduce high blood lipid levels?

3. Create a list of potential adverse effects that this client should be taught to watch for related to the medication.

See Answers to Critical Thinking Questions in Appendix B.

NCLEX Practice Questions

1 The client taking atorvastatin (Lipitor) reports weakness and fatigue, pain in the shoulders, and aching joints. The nurse initially assesses the client for which condition?

  a. Rhabdomyolysis

  b. Renal failure

  c. Rheumatoid arthritis

  d. Hepatic insufficiency

2 A client is receiving cholestyramine (Questran) for elevated low-density lipoprotein levels. In the nurse's care plan, which adverse effect should the client be monitored for?

  a. Orange-coloured urine

  b. Abdominal pain

  c. Sore throat and fever

  d. Decreased capillary refill

3 The provider orders colestipol (Colestid) in combination with atorvastatin (Lipitor) for a client with elevated low-density lipoprotein levels. The nurse collaborates with the prescriber about which datum related to the client?

  a. Past history of peptic ulcer disease

  b. Recent myocardial infarction

  c. Laboratory value for serum sodium of 136 mEq/L

  d. Allergies to foods high in tyramine

4 Which assessment findings discovered by the nurse would be an expected adverse effect associated with niacin therapy? Select all that apply.

  a. Fever and chills

  b. Intense flushing and hot flashes

  c. Tingling of the fingers and toes

  d. Dry mucous membranes

  e. Hypoglycemia

5 The nurse is caring for a client receiving gemfibrozil (Lopid) for hyperlipidemia. The nurse would validate the order with the prescriber if the client reported a history of which of the following? Select all that apply.

  a. Gallbladder disease

  b. Angina

  c. Hypertension

  d. Diabetes

  e. Renal disease

See Answers to NCLEX Practice Questions in Appendix A.

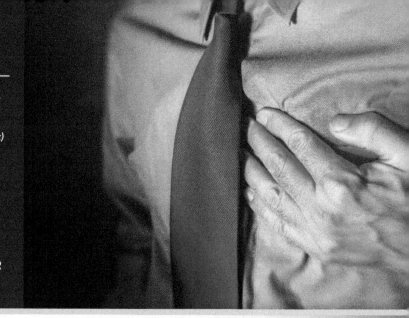

Igor Stevanovic/Alamy Stock Photo

CHAPTER 50

Pharmacotherapy of Angina Pectoris, Myocardial Infarction, and Cerebrovascular Accident

LEARNING OUTCOMES

After reading this chapter, the student should be able to:

1. Identify drug classes used for treating angina pectoris, myocardial infarction, and cerebrovascular accident.

2. Explain the therapeutic action of each class of drug used in the treatment of angina, myocardial infarction, and cerebrovascular accident in relation to the pathophysiology of these conditions.

3. Describe the nurse's role in the pharmacological management of clients who are receiving drugs used in the treatment of angina, myocardial infarction, and cerebrovascular accident.

4. For each of the drug classes listed in Prototype Drugs, identify a representative drug and explain its mechanism of action, therapeutic effects, and important adverse effects.

5. Describe and explain, based on pharmacological principles, the rationale for nursing assessment, planning, and interventions for clients with angina, myocardial infarction, and cerebrovascular accident.

6. Use the nursing process to care for clients who are receiving drug therapy for angina, myocardial infarction, and cerebrovascular accident.

CHAPTER OUTLINE

▶ Etiology of Coronary Artery Disease and Myocardial Ischemia

▶ Blood Supply to the Myocardium

▶ Pathogenesis of Angina Pectoris

▶ Non-Pharmacological Management of Angina

▶ Goals for the Pharmacotherapy of Angina

▶ Treating Angina with Organic Nitrates

▶ Treating Angina with Beta Blockers

▶ Treating Angina with Calcium Channel Blockers

▶ Diagnosis of Myocardial Infarction

The tissues and organs of the body are dependent on the arterial supply of oxygen and other vital nutrients to support life and health. Should the arterial blood supply become compromised, cardiovascular and cerebrovascular functioning may become impaired, resulting in angina pectoris, acute myocardial infarction, or cerebrovascular accident. Such conditions are associated with the development of atherosclerotic plaques or the aggregation of platelets on the intima of blood vessels, with resultant clot formation. Tissues and organs served by the arteries, distal to the site of involvement, become ischemic and suffer varying degrees of damage. This chapter focuses on the pharmacological and nursing interventions related to these conditions.

Etiology of Coronary Artery Disease and Myocardial Ischemia

50.1 Coronary artery disease includes both angina and myocardial infarction. It is caused by narrowing of the arterial lumen due to atherosclerotic plaque.

Coronary artery disease (CAD) is one of the leading causes of mortality. The primary characteristic defining CAD is narrowing or occlusion of the coronary arteries. The narrowing deprives heart cells of needed oxygen and nutrients, a condition known as **myocardial ischemia**. If it develops over a long period of time, the heart may compensate for its inadequate blood supply and the client may experience no symptoms. Indeed, coronary arteries may be occluded as much as 50% or more and cause no symptoms.

As CAD progresses, however, the heart does not receive enough oxygen to meet the metabolic demands of the myocardium. The oxygen deficiency signals the onset of anaerobic metabolism to generate the energy needed to maintain cardiac function. As a result, lactic acid accumulates. As with any muscle, the buildup of lactic acid produces pain and soreness. When lactic acid activates pericardial pain receptors, the body experiences the sensation of chest pain. Persistent myocardial ischemia may lead to heart attack.

The common etiology of CAD in adults is **atherosclerosis**, which is the presence of plaque within the walls of arteries. **Plaque** is a fatty, fibrous material that accumulates, thus producing varying degrees of intravascular narrowing—a situation that results in partial or total blockage of the blood vessel. In addition, the plaque impairs normal vessel elasticity. In CAD, the atherosclerotic coronary vessel is unable to dilate properly when the myocardium needs additional blood or oxygen. Plaque accumulation occurs gradually, possibly over periods of 40 to 50 years in some individuals, but actually begins to accrue early in life. As the material collects in the intima (inner layer) of a vessel, the cardiac muscle distal to the obstruction receives less oxygen, thus hindering its metabolic functions. The development of atherosclerosis is illustrated in Figure 50.1.

Blood Supply to the Myocardium

50.2 The myocardium requires a continuous supply of oxygen from the coronary arteries in order to function properly.

From the moment it begins to function in utero until death, the heart works to distribute oxygen and nutrients via its nonstop pumping action. Because the heart is a continually working muscle, it needs a steady supply of oxygen and nutrients. Any disturbance in blood flow to the vital organs or the myocardium itself—even for brief episodes—can result in life-threatening consequences.

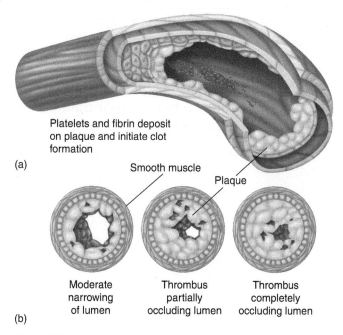

(a)

Platelets and fibrin deposit on plaque and initiate clot formation

Smooth muscle

Plaque

Moderate narrowing of lumen

Thrombus partially occluding lumen

Thrombus completely occluding lumen

(b)

Figure 50.1   Atherosclerosis in an artery.
Source: Pearson Education.

The myocardium receives its blood via two main arteries that arise within the right and left aortic sinuses at the base of the aorta, called the right and left coronary arteries. These arteries further divide into smaller branches that encircle the heart, bringing the myocardium a continuous supply of oxygen. The numerous smaller vessels serve as natural communication networks among the coronary arteries and are known as **anastomoses**. In the event that one of the vessels becomes restricted or blocked, blood flow to the myocardium may remain relatively uncompromised as a result of these channels functioning to bypass the block.

Pathogenesis of Angina Pectoris

50.3 Angina pectoris is chest pain, usually upon emotional or physical exertion. It is caused by the narrowing of a coronary artery, which results in lack of sufficient oxygen to the heart muscle.

Angina pectoris is acute chest pain caused by insufficient oxygen reaching a portion of the myocardium. About 2% of Canadians have angina pectoris, with more than 47 000 new cases each year. It is more prevalent in those over 55 years of age.

The classic presentation of angina pectoris is steady, intense pain, sometimes with a crushing or constricting sensation in the substernal region. Typically, the discomfort radiates to the left shoulder and proceeds down the left arm. It may also extend to the thoracic region of the back or move upward to the jaw. In some clients, the pain is experienced in the midepigastrium or abdominal area. Accompanying the discomfort is severe emotional distress—a feeling of panic with fear of impending death. There is usually pallor, dyspnea with cyanosis, diaphoresis, tachycardia, and elevated blood pressure.

Anginal pain is usually precipitated by physical exertion or emotional excitement—events associated with increased cardiorespiratory oxygen demand. Narrowed coronary arteries containing atherosclerotic deposits block the distribution of oxygen and nutrients to the stressed myocardium. Angina pectoris episodes are usually of short duration. With physical rest and stress reduction, the discomfort subsides within 10 to 15 minutes.

There are three basic types of angina. When anginal occurrences are fairly predictable as to frequency, intensity, and duration, the condition is described as classic or **stable angina**. The second type of angina, known as atypical or **variant angina** (Prinzmetal's angina), occurs when the decreased myocardial blood flow is caused by spasms of the coronary arteries. It often occurs at the same time each night, during rest or sleep. When episodes of angina arise more frequently, have added intensity, and occur during periods of rest, the condition is termed **unstable angina**. This condition requires more aggressive medical intervention and may be considered a medical emergency, as it is associated with an increased risk for myocardial infarction (MI).

Angina pain closely parallels the signs and symptoms of a heart attack. It is extremely important that the nurse know the characteristics that differentiate the two conditions because the pharmacological interventions related to angina differ considerably from those related to MI. Angina, while painful and distressing, rarely leads to a fatal outcome, and the chest pain is usually immediately relieved by nitroglycerin (Nitro-Dur, Minitran, Nitrostat, Trinipatch). MI, however, carries with it a high mortality rate if appropriate treatment is delayed. Pharmacological intervention must be initiated immediately and systematically maintained in the event of MI. Females may experience a heart attack as symptoms of fatigue and nausea rather than as distressing, crushing chest pain.

Any number of diverse situations—several unrelated to cardiac pathology—may cause chest pain. These include gallstones, peptic ulcer disease, pneumonia, musculoskeletal injuries, and certain cancers. The foremost objective for the healthcare provider when a person presents with chest pain is to quickly determine the cause of the pain so that proper, effective interventions can be delivered. This incorporates a detailed individual and family history, a complete physical examination, and laboratory and other diagnostic tests. All healthcare providers work collaboratively to quickly determine the cause of chest pain.

Non-Pharmacological Management of Angina

50.4 Angina management may include non-pharmacological therapies such as diet and lifestyle modifications, treatment of underlying disorders, angioplasty, or surgery.

A combination of variables, including dietary patterns and lifestyle circumstances, influences the development and progression of angina. The nurse is instrumental in assisting clients to control the rate of recurrence of anginal episodes. Such support includes the formulation of a comprehensive plan of care that incorporates psychosocial support and an individualized teaching plan. The client needs to understand the causes of angina, identify the conditions and situations that trigger it, and develop the motivation to modify behaviours associated with the condition.

In addition to drugs, treatment of angina includes therapies for conditions that worsen CAD, such as diabetes and hypertension. The practice of healthy lifestyle habits can prevent CAD in many individuals and slow the progression of the disease in those who have plaque buildup. The following factors have been shown to reduce the incidence of CAD:

- Limiting or abstaining from alcohol
- Eliminating foods that are high in cholesterol or saturated fat
- If blood lipids are high (hyperlipidemia), treating the condition
- Treating high blood pressure early
- Exercising regularly and maintaining optimum weight
- Maintaining blood glucose levels within the normal range
- Not using tobacco

When the coronary arteries are significantly obstructed, the two most common interventions are **percutaneous transluminal coronary angioplasty (PTCA)**, with stent insertion, and **coronary artery bypass graft (CABG)** surgery. PTCA is a procedure whereby the narrowed area of the artery is opened using either a balloon catheter or a laser. The basic concept is to place a catheter, with a small inflatable balloon on the end, within the narrowed section of the artery. Inflation of the balloon causes it to push outward against the narrowed wall of the artery. The stenosis is reduced until it no longer interferes with blood flow. Stenting is done in conjunction with a balloon angioplasty and/or atherectomy, a procedure in which plaque is removed from an artery. Angioplasty with stenting typically leaves less than 10% of the original blockage in the artery.

Coronary bypass surgery is reserved for severe cases of coronary blockage that cannot be dealt with by any other treatment modality. In CABG, a portion of a small blood vessel from the leg or chest is used to create a "bypass artery." One end of the graft is sewn to the aorta and the other end is sewn to the coronary artery beyond the narrowed area. Blood from the aorta then flows through the new grafted vessel to the heart muscle, "bypassing" the blockage in the coronary artery. The result is increased blood flow to the heart muscle, which reduces angina and the risk for heart attack.

CONNECTIONS | **Special Considerations**

◀ **The Influence of Gender and Ethnicity on Angina**

- Angina occurs more frequently in females than in males.
- Among racial-ethnic groups, the incidence of angina is highest among Aboriginal peoples and people of African descent.
- Females of African descent have a risk for angina that is twice that of their male counterparts.

Goals for the Pharmacotherapy of Angina

50.5 The pharmacological goals for the treatment of angina are to terminate acute attacks and prevent future episodes. This is usually achieved by reducing cardiac workload.

The pharmacological goals for a client with angina are twofold: to reduce the frequency of angina episodes and to terminate an incident of acute anginal pain once it is in progress. It is important to remember that interventions are directed toward symptomatic relief and management, as there is no drug treatment available to cure the underlying disorder. The primary means by which antianginal drugs accomplish these goals is to reduce the myocardial demand for oxygen. This can be accomplished by at least four different mechanisms:

1. Slowing the heart rate
2. Dilating veins so that the heart receives less blood (reduced preload)
3. Causing the heart to contract with less force (reduced contractility)
4. Dilating arterioles to lower blood pressure, thus giving the heart less resistance when ejecting blood from its chambers (reduced afterload)

The pharmacotherapy of angina uses three classes of drug: organic nitrates, beta-adrenergic blockers, and calcium channel blockers. For stable angina, the first line of pharmacotherapy is the rapid-acting organic nitrates that are administered during the anginal episode. If episodes become more frequent or severe, prophylactic treatment is initiated using oral or transdermal organic nitrates, beta-adrenergic blockers, or calcium channel blockers. Persistent angina sometimes requires drugs from two or more classes, such as a beta blocker combined with a long-acting nitrate or calcium channel blocker. Figure 50.2 illustrates the mechanisms of action of drugs used to prevent and treat angina.

Treating Angina with Organic Nitrates

50.6 The organic nitrates relieve angina by dilating veins and coronary arteries. They are drugs of choice for stable angina.

Since their medicinal properties were discovered in 1857, organic nitrates have remained the mainstay for the treatment of angina. The primary therapeutic action of the organic nitrates is their ability to relax both arterial and venous smooth muscle. With venous vasodilation, the amount of blood returning to the heart (preload) is reduced, and the chambers contain a smaller volume. With less blood for the ventricles to pump, cardiac output is reduced and the workload of the heart is decreased, thereby lowering myocardial oxygen demand. The therapeutic outcome is that chest pain

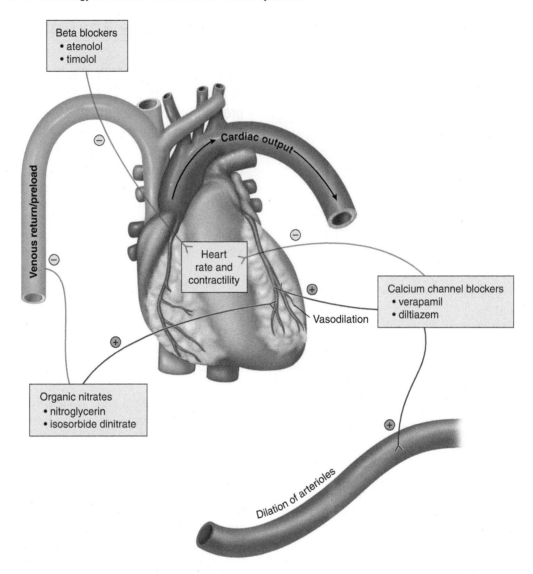

Figure 50.2   Mechanisms of action of drugs used to treat angina.

is alleviated and episodes of angina become less frequent. The organic nitrates are listed in Table 50.1.

NCLEX Success Tips

Nitroglycerin acts to decrease myocardial oxygen consumption. Vasodilation makes it easier for the heart to eject blood, resulting in decreased oxygen needs. Decreased oxygen demand reduces pain caused by the heart muscle not receiving sufficient oxygen.

Nitroglycerin in all dosage forms (sublingual, transdermal, or intravenous) should be shielded from light to prevent deterioration. The client should be instructed to keep the nitroglycerin in the dark container that is supplied by the pharmacy, and it should not be removed or placed in another container.

Clients should be instructed to use nitroglycerin at the first indication of chest pain and not to wait until pain becomes severe.

Nitroglycerin given for treatment of angina should be taken in 5-minute intervals for up to 3 doses. If the pain does not subside after 3 doses, 911 should be called to obtain an ambulance to take the client to the emergency department. The client should not drive or have a family member drive the client to the hospital.

Nitroglycerin tablets are not effective if chewed, swallowed, or placed between the cheek and gums.

Transdermal nitroglycerin can cause skin irritation. The client:

- should use the applicator paper to measure the amount of ointment to apply;

- should not rub or massage the ointment into the skin (the ointment should be allowed to absorb slowly);

- should rotate the patch application site daily to prevent sensitization and tolerance;

- should remove any remaining ointment with a tissue before applying a new dose;

- should avoid touching the medication-impregnated pad because touching it could cause drug absorption;

- should remove any remaining ointment with a tissue before applying a new dose; and

- should store pads away from temperature and humidity extremes, which may inactivate the drug.

Expected side effects of nitroglycerin include headache that should decrease over time, dizziness, and flushing. Acetaminophen (Tylenol) usually helps decrease nitroglycerin-induced headaches.

Hypotension and dizziness are also common adverse effects of nitroglycerin. To minimize these problems, the nurse should teach the client to take safety precautions, such as changing to an upright position slowly, climbing up and down stairs carefully, and lying down at the first sign of dizziness.

Blood pressure is the vital sign most likely to reflect an adverse effect of this drug. The nurse should check the client's blood pressure 1 hour after administering nitroglycerin ointment. A blood pressure decrease of 10 mm Hg is within the therapeutic range. If blood pressure falls more

TABLE 50.1   Drugs for Angina, Myocardial Infarction, and Cerebrovascular Accident

Drug	Route and Adult Dose
Organic Nitrates	
isosorbide dinitrate (Isordil, ISDN) (see Chapter 54, page 689, for the Prototype Drug box)	Orally (PO), start with 5-20 mg two to three times daily (bid-tid); maintenance dose is 5-80 mg bid-tid
isosorbide mononitrate (Imdur)	PO, 20–60 mg every day (qd)
Pr nitroglycerin (Nitro-Dur, Minitran, Nitrostat, Trinipatch)	Sublingual (SL), 1 tablet (0.3–0.6 mg) or 1 spray (0.4–0.8 mg) every 5 minutes (q5min) as needed (PRN); topical, 0.2-0.8 mg/hour; patch is applied for 12 hours then off for a period of 12 hours
Beta-Adrenergic Blockers	
Pr atenolol (Tenormin)	PO, 25–50 mg qd (max 100 mg/day)
Pr metoprolol (Lopressor)	PO, 50-200 mg bid (max 400 mg/day)
propranolol (Inderal) (see Chapter 55, page 704, for the Prototype Drug box)	PO, start with 40 mg bid; increase dosage every 3-7 days; usual dose is 120-240 mg in 2-3 divided doses (max 650 mg/day)
timolol (see Chapter 63, page 823, for the Prototype Drug box)	PO, start with 10 mg bid; increase gradually every 7 days; usual dosage is 20-40 mg/day in two divided doses (max 60 mg/day)
Calcium Channel Blockers	
amlodipine (Norvasc)	PO, 5–10 mg qd (max 10 mg/day)
Pr diltiazem (Cardizem, Tiazac)	PO, 30 mg qid (max 360 mg/day)
nifedipine (Adalat) (see Chapter 51, page 640, for the Prototype Drug box)	PO (immediate release), start with 10 mg tid; usual dose is 10-20 mg tid (max 180 mg/day); extended release, start with 30-60 mg qd (max 120 mg/day)
verapamil (Isoptin) (see Chapter 55, page 706, for the Prototype Drug box)	PO (immediate release), 80-160 mg tid; extended release, 120-240 mg qd
Glycoprotein IIb/IIIa Inhibitors	
abciximab (ReoPro)	Intravenous (IV), 0.25 mg/kg initial bolus over 5 minutes, then 10 μg/minute for 18-24 hours
eptifibatide (Integrilin)	IV, 180 μg/kg initial bolus over 1–2 minutes, then 2 μg/kg/minute for 24–72 hours
tirofiban (Aggrastat)	IV, loading dose, 25 μg/kg administered over 5 minutes or less; maintenance infusion is 0.15 μg/kg/minute continued for up to 18 hours

than 20 mm Hg below baseline, the nurse should remove the ointment and report the finding to the physician immediately.

Nitroglycerin causes vasodilation, which results in increased intra-ocular pressure. The vasodilatory effects of the medication can trigger an attack, causing pain and loss of vision.

Alcohol is prohibited because nitrates may enhance the effects of alcohol.

The client should report a change in the pattern of chest pain. It may indicate increasing severity of coronary artery disease. Pain occurring during stress or sexual activity would not be unexpected, and the client may be instructed to take nitroglycerin to prevent this pain.

To ensure the freshness of sublingual nitroglycerin, the client should replace tablets every 3 to 6 months, and store them in a tightly closed container in a cool, dark place. Many brands of sublingual nitroglycerin no longer produce a burning sensation.

Clients taking nitrate therapy, such as nitroglycerin, should avoid taking sildenafil (Viagra, which has an expected outcome of an erection that can last up to 4 hours) to prevent unsafe decreases in blood pressure.

Organic nitrates also have the ability to dilate coronary arteries, which was once thought to be their primary mechanism of action. It seems logical that dilating a partially occluded coronary vessel would allow more oxygen to get to the ischemic tissue. While this effect does indeed occur, it is no longer considered the primary mechanism of nitrate action in treating stable angina. However, this action is important in treating variant angina, in which the chest pain is caused by coronary artery spasm. The organic nitrates can relax these spasms and terminate the pain.

CONNECTIONS Special Considerations

◀ **Nitroglycerin Sublingual Tablets and Spray in Chest Pain**

Do the following if you are having chest pain (angina) and your healthcare provider has prescribed nitroglycerin:

1. Cease any activity and sit down. If driving, pull over safely and park the car—sometimes rest can help to relieve chest pain (angina), by reducing work demands on the heart. Take one nitroglycerin sublingual tablet or liquid spray. Wait 5 minutes.

2. If chest pain (angina) does not go away, take another nitroglycerin sublingual tablet or liquid spray and then call 911 or other emergency services for assistance, or go to a hospital emergency department. Do not attempt to drive yourself

3. If you still have chest pain (angina), you may take a third dose of nitroglycerin after 5 minutes.

4. Regardless of what happens, you should let your healthcare provider know that you had an episode of angina and continue to adhere to the recommended treatment.

Based on:

http://www.totalcardiology.ca/admin/sitefile/1/files/NitroProtocol-UpdatedJanuary2015(1).pdf.

http://www.webmd.com/heart-disease/tc/using-nitroglycerin-for-sudden-chest-pain-topic-overview?page=2 http://www.healthlinkbc.ca/healthtopics/content.asp?hwid=hw85228spec

http://www.health.harvard.edu/heart-health/take-nitroglycerin-to-ease-and-avoid-a-common-heart-disease-symptom

Organic nitrates are of two types: short acting and long acting. The short-acting nitrates, such as nitroglycerin, are taken sublingually to quickly terminate an acute angina attack in progress. Longer acting nitrates, such as isosorbide dinitrate (Isordil, ISDN), are taken orally or delivered through a transdermal patch to decrease the frequency and severity of angina episodes.

Tolerance is a common problem with prolonged use of the long-acting organic nitrates. The magnitude of the tolerance depends on the dosage and the frequency of drug administration. Clients are often instructed to remove the transdermal patch for 6 to 12 hours each day or to withhold the nighttime dose of the oral medications to delay the development of tolerance.

Most adverse effects of organic nitrates are extensions of their hypotensive action. Flushing of the face and headache are common effects, related to vasodilation. Orthostatic hypotension is a frequent adverse effect of this drug class, and clients should be advised to change positions gradually to prevent lightheadedness. Blood pressure should be carefully monitored, and the nurse should hold nitrates and remove topical forms if serious hypotension is discovered. Taking organic nitrates concurrently with alcohol may cause severe hypotension and even cardiovascular collapse.

An additional adverse effect that can be limiting in some clients is reflex tachycardia. When the organic nitrates dilate vessels and blood pressure falls, the baroreceptor reflex is triggered. Sympathetic stimulation of the heart increases heart rate and contractility, which are undesirable effects in a client with angina. This adverse effect is often transient and asymptomatic. Clients who report significant palpitations may be administered a beta blocker, which will prevent the reflex cardiac stimulation.

Long-acting organic nitrates such as isosorbide dinitrate are also useful in reducing the symptoms of heart failure (HF). Their role in the treatment of this disease is discussed in Chapter 54.

Nursing Considerations

The role of the nurse in nitrate therapy for angina involves careful monitoring of the client's condition and providing education as it relates to the prescribed drug regimen. Because the main action of nitrates is vasodilation, it is vital for the nurse to assess blood pressure prior to administration. IV nitrates have the greatest risk for causing severe hypotension. These drugs are contraindicated in aortic stenosis, pericardial tamponade, and constrictive pericarditis because the heart cannot increase cardiac output to maintain blood pressure as vasodilation occurs. In cases where increased vasodilation would be detrimental to the client (hypotension, shock, head injury with increased intracranial pressure), nitrates are contraindicated since they worsen the conditions. Nitrates should not be taken within 24 hours (before or after) of taking sildenafil (Viagra) or any of the phosphodiesterase-5 enzyme inhibitors, because life-threatening hypotension and cardiovascular collapse may occur. Sustained-release forms of these drugs should not be given to clients with glaucoma. Nitrates should be used with caution in clients who have severe liver or kidney disease or are in early MI.

Assessment should include the client's use of alcohol, as this agent can produce an additive vasodilation effect when taken concurrently with nitrates. Taking isosorbide dinitrate or isosorbide mononitrate (Imdur) with alcohol may cause severe hypotension and cardiovascular collapse.

With long-acting nitrates, monitor for orthostatic hypotension and advise clients to change positions gradually. With short-acting forms, ensure that clients are sitting or supine during administration and that blood pressure is taken after each dose. If hypotension occurs, withhold nitrates and remove transdermal forms until blood pressure has returned to normal. Frequent blood pressure measurements are done during therapy to monitor for hypotensive effects. Infusions of nitrates are frequently titrated to obtain pain relief for the client or a specific blood pressure level. Hold other forms of nitrates and remove transdermal forms during the infusion.

Client education as it relates to nitrates should include goals, reasons for obtaining baseline data such as vital signs and tests for cardiac and renal disorders, and possible side effects. The following are the important points to include when teaching clients regarding nitrates:

- Refrain from alcohol use; some clients experience flushing, weakness, and fainting.
- If using transdermal patches, rotate the application site and wash skin thoroughly after the patch is removed.
- If using a sublingual form, allow the tablet to dissolve under the tongue; do not chew or swallow the tablet.
- If chest pain is not relieved after two doses of nitroglycerin, 5 minutes apart, call emergency medical services (EMS).
- Contact the healthcare provider immediately if blurred vision, dry mouth, or severe headaches occur, which may be signs of overdose.
- Keep medication readily available in its original container, away from excess heat, light, and moisture. The prescription should be replaced every 6 months.

NURSING PROCESS FOCUS

Clients Receiving Nitroglycerin (Nitro-Dur, Minitran, Nitrostat, Trinipatch)

Assessment	Potential Nursing Diagnoses/Identified Patterns
Prior to administration: • Obtain complete health history, including allergies, drug history, and possible drug interactions. • Assess vital signs, electrocardiogram (ECG), frequency and severity of angina, and alcohol use. • Obtain history of cardiac disorders and lab tests, including cardiac enzymes, complete blood count (CBC), blood urea nitrogen (BUN), creatinine, and liver function tests. • Assess if client has taken sildenafil or any of the phosphodiesterase-5 enzyme inhibitors within the last 24 hours.	• Need for knowledge regarding drug therapy • Risk for injury (dizziness or fainting) related to hypotension from drug • Ineffective tissue perfusion related to hypotension from drug • Acute pain (headache) related to adverse effects of drug

---

Planning: Client Goals and Expected Outcomes

The client will:

- Experience relief or prevention of chest pain
- Report immediately any chest pain unrelieved by nitroglycerin
- Demonstrate an understanding of the drug's action by accurately describing drug side effects and precautions

---

Implementation

Interventions (Rationales)	Client Education/Discharge Planning
• Ask client to describe and rate pain prior to drug administration for description/documentation of anginal episode. • Obtain 12-lead ECG to differentiate between angina and infarction. (Pharmacotherapy depends on which disorder is presenting.) • Monitor blood pressure and pulse. Do not administer drug if client is hypotensive. (Drug will further reduce blood pressure.) • Monitor alcohol use. (Extremely low blood pressure may result, which could cause death.) • Monitor for headache in response to use of nitrates. • Monitor for use of sildenafil and phosphodiesterase-5 enzyme inhibitors concurrently with nitrates because cardiovascular disease is a major cause of erectile dysfunction in men. (Life-threatening hypotension may result with concurrent use of sildenafil.) • Monitor need for prophylactic nitrates.	Instruct client to: • Take one tablet every 5 minutes until pain is relieved during an acute angina attack • Call EMS if chest pain is not relieved after two doses • Place SL tablet or spray under tongue; do not inhale spray • Instruct client to sit or lie down before taking medication and to avoid abrupt changes in position. • Emphasize the importance of avoiding alcohol while taking nitroglycerin. Instruct client that: • Headache is a common side effect that usually decreases over time • Over-the-counter (OTC) medicines usually relieve the headache Instruct client to: • Not take sildenafil or a phosphodiesterase-5 enzyme inhibitors within 24 hours of taking nitrates • Wait at least 24 hours after taking sildenafil or any other phosphodiesterase-5 enzyme inhibitor to resume nitrate therapy • Advise client to take medication prior to a stressful event or physical activity to prevent angina.

Evaluation of Outcome Criteria

Evaluate the effectiveness of drug therapy by confirming that client goals and expected outcomes have been met (see "Planning").

PROTOTYPE DRUG | **Nitroglycerin (Nitro-Dur, Minitran, Nitrostat, Trinipatch)**

Actions and Uses: Nitroglycerin, the oldest and most widely used of the organic nitrates, can be delivered by a number of different routes: sublingual, oral (including extended-release forms), translingual, IV, transmucosal, transdermal, and topical. It may be taken while an acute anginal episode is in progress or just prior to physical activity. When given sublingually, it reaches peak plasma levels in approximately 4 minutes, thus terminating angina pain rapidly. Chest pain that does not respond to two or three doses of sublingual nitroglycerin may indicate MI.

Pharmacokinetics: Nitroglycerin is well absorbed. It is rapidly and almost completely metabolized by the liver and enzymes in the blood. It has a half-life of 1 to 3 minutes.

Administration Alerts:

- For IV administration, use glass IV bottle and special IV tubing because plastic absorbs nitrates significantly, thus reducing client dose.
- Cover IV bottle to reduce degradation of nitrates due to light exposure.
- Use gloves when applying nitroglycerin paste or ointment to prevent self-administration.
- Nitroglycerin is pregnancy category C.

Adverse Effects and Interactions: The side effects of nitroglycerin are usually cardiovascular in nature and are rarely life threatening. Because nitroglycerin can dilate cerebral vessels, headache is a common side effect and may be severe. Occasionally, the venodilation created by nitroglycerin causes reflex tachycardia. Some healthcare providers prescribe a beta-adrenergic blocker to diminish this undesirable heart rate increase. The side effects of nitroglycerin often diminish after a few doses.

Concurrent use with sildenafil or a phosphodiesterase 5-enzyme inhibitor may cause life-threatening hypotension and cardiovascular collapse. Nitrates should not be taken within 24 hours (before or after) of taking sildenafil.

Treating Angina with Beta Blockers

50.7 Beta-adrenergic blockers relieve angina by decreasing the oxygen demands on the heart. They are sometimes considered first-line drugs for chronic angina.

Because of their ability to reduce the workload of the heart by slowing heart rate (negative chronotropic effect) and reducing contractility (negative inotropic effect), beta blockers are used to decrease the frequency and severity of angina attacks caused by exertion. Unlike the nitrates, tolerance does not develop to the antianginal effects of beta blockers. They are first-line drugs in the pharmacotherapy of chronic stable angina. Clients should be advised against abruptly stopping beta blocker therapy, as this may result in a sudden increase in cardiac workload and worsen angina. The beta blockers used for angina are listed in Table 50.1. The beta blockers are widely used in medicine, and additional details may be found in Chapter 14.

Beta-adrenergic blockers offer several advantages over the organic nitrates. Tolerance does not develop to the antianginal effects of the beta blockers during prolonged therapy. They possess antidysrhythmic properties, which help to prevent cardiac conduction abnormalities that are common complications of clients with ischemic heart disease. Beta blockers are ideal for clients who have both hypertension and CAD due to their antihypertensive action. They have also been shown to reduce the incidence of MI. Because of these cardioprotective actions, beta blockers are considered drugs of choice for the prophylaxis of chronic angina.

Beta-adrenergic antagonists are well tolerated by most clients. In some clients, fatigue, lethargy, and depression are reasons for discontinuation of beta blocker therapy. At high doses, drugs in this class can cause shortness of breath and respiratory distress due to bronchoconstriction, and they should be used cautiously in clients with asthma or chronic obstructive pulmonary disease (COPD). Because beta blockers slow the heart rate and myocardial conduction velocity, they are contraindicated in clients with bradycardia and greater than first-degree heart block. Heart rate should be closely monitored so that it does not fall below 50 to 60 beats/minute at rest or 100 beats/minute during exercise. Beta blockers are also contraindicated in cardiogenic shock and overt cardiac failure.

Clients with diabetes who are prescribed beta blockers should be aware that the actions of beta blockers can obscure the initial symptoms of hypoglycemia (palpitations, diaphoresis, and nervousness). Because of this, blood glucose levels should be monitored more frequently, and insulin doses may need to be adjusted accordingly.

Nursing Considerations

The role of the nurse in beta blocker therapy for angina involves careful monitoring of the client's condition and providing education as it relates to the prescribed drug regimen. Before administering beta blockers, assess the client's apical pulse, especially if the client is also taking digoxin (Lanoxin, Toloxin), since both drugs slow atrioventricular (AV) conduction. Because beta blockers lower blood pressure, vital signs should be monitored. Monitor the client for shortness of breath and respiratory distress. Side effects occur more often with higher doses of beta blockers.

Because beta blockers slow heart rate and conduction velocity, they are contraindicated in bradycardia, second- and third-degree heart block, and cardiogenic shock. Beta blockers should be used with caution in clients with asthma, COPD, or impaired renal function. Diabetic clients should be aware that initial symptoms of hypoglycemia, such as palpitations, diaphoresis, and nervousness, may not be evident with beta blockade. Blood glucose levels should be monitored frequently in clients with diabetes mellitus because insulin doses may need to be decreased when using beta blockers.

Beta blockers should not be abruptly discontinued because with long-term use the heart adapts to the catecholamines blocked by these drugs. When they are withdrawn abruptly, adrenergic receptors are stimulated, causing excitation. This may exacerbate angina and precipitate tachycardia or even an MI in clients with cardiovascular disease. One side effect of beta blockers is fatigue during exercise because these drugs prevent the heart rate from increasing with activity.

Client education as it relates to beta blockers should include goals, reasons for obtaining baseline data such as vital signs and tests for cardiac and renal disorders, and possible side effects. The following are important teaching points to include regarding beta blockers:

- Change positions slowly; report dizziness or lightheadedness.
- Do not take OTC medications or herbal products without discussing them with the healthcare provider.
- Do not discontinue medication abruptly.
- If pulse falls below 50 beats/minute, notify the healthcare provider. This rate may be 60 beats/minute in some agencies.
- Alternate periods of activity with periods of rest in order to avoid fatigue.
- See also Nursing Process Focus: Clients Receiving Adrenergic Therapy in Chapter 14, page 150, for the complete nursing process applied to caring for clients who are receiving beta-adrenergic agonists.

NCLEX Success Tips

Sudden discontinuation of a beta-adrenergic antagonist is dangerous because it may exacerbate symptoms. The medication should not be discontinued without a prescription.

There is a direct interaction between the effects of insulin and those of beta blockers. The nurse must be aware that there is a potential for increased hypoglycemic effects of insulin when a beta blocker is added to the client's medication regimen. The client's blood sugar should be monitored.

Erectile dysfunction is a potential adverse effect of beta blockers.

As a long-acting, selective beta$_1$-adrenergic blocker, atenolol decreases cardiac output and systolic and diastolic blood pressure; however, like other beta-adrenergic blockers, it increases peripheral vascular resistance at rest and with exercise. Atenolol (Tenormin) may cause bradycardia.

PROTOTYPE DRUG | **Atenolol (Tenormin)**

Actions and Uses: Atenolol selectively blocks beta$_1$-adrenergic receptors in the heart. Its effectiveness in angina is attributed to its ability to slow heart rate and reduce contractility, both of which lower myocardial oxygen demand. It is also used in the treatment of hypertension and in the prevention of MI. Because of its 6- to 9-hour half-life, it may be taken once a day.

Administration Alerts:

- During IV administration, monitor ECG continuously; blood pressure and pulse should be assessed before, during, and after dose is administered.
- Assess pulse and blood pressure before oral administration. Hold drug if pulse is below 50 beats/minute (60 beats/minute in some agencies) or if client is hypotensive.
- Initial doses of atenolol may precipitate bronchospasm in susceptible clients.
- Atenolol is pregnancy category D.

Pharmacokinetics: Bioavailability of oral atenolol is 50% to 60%. Unabsorbed drug is excreted in the feces and the remainder is excreted by the kidneys.

Adverse Effects and Interactions: Being a cardioselective beta$_1$-adrenergic blocker, atenolol has few adverse effects on the lung. Like other beta blockers, therapy generally begins with low doses, which are gradually increased until the therapeutic effect is achieved. The most common side effects of atenolol include fatigue, weakness, and hypotension. Anticholinergics may cause decreased absorption from the gastrointestinal (GI) tract.

Concurrent use with calcium channel blockers may cause excessive cardiac suppression. Concurrent use with digitalis may cause slowed AV conduction, leading to heart block. Clients should avoid concurrent use of this drug with nicotine or caffeine due to their vasoconstricting effects.

In case of beta blocker overdose, glucagon IV may be administered to reduce cardiac depression and increase myocardial contractibility, heart rate, and AV node conduction.

NCLEX Success Tips

The effect of a beta blocker is a decrease in heart rate, contractility, and afterload, which leads to a decrease in blood pressure. The client at first may have an increase in fatigue when starting the beta blocker.

Aspirin and other nonsteroidal antiinflammatory drugs (NSAIDs) counteract the blood pressure–reducing effects of beta blockers by reducing the effects of prostaglandins.

Metoprolol (Lopressor) is indicated in the treatment of hemodynamically stable clients with an acute MI to reduce cardiovascular mortality. Cardiogenic shock causes severe hemodynamic instability, and a beta blocker will further depress myocardial contractility. The metoprolol should be discontinued. The decrease in cardiac output will impair perfusion to the kidneys.

Metoprolol masks the common signs of hypoglycemia, such as palpitations, tachycardia, and tremor. Therefore, glucose levels would be monitored closely in diabetic clients.

When used to treat an MI, metoprolol is contraindicated in clients with heart rates less than 45 beats/minute and any degree of heart block, so the nurse would monitor the client for bradycardia and heart block.

Metoprolol masks common signs and symptoms of shock, such as decreased blood pressure, so blood pressure would also be monitored closely.

Although metoprolol would not be mixed with other drugs, studies have shown that it is compatible when mixed with morphine sulfate or when administered with alteplase infusion at a Y-site connection. The nurse would give the drug undiluted by direct injection. Metoprolol should be taken with food at same time each day; it should not be chewed or crushed. The physician should be notified if the client's pulse falls below 50 beats/minute for several days.

Use of any OTC decongestants, asthma and cold remedies, and herbal preparations must be avoided. Fainting spells may occur due to exercise or stress, and the dosage of the drug may need to be reduced or discontinued.

Metoprolol may cause increased PR interval and bradycardia.

PROTOTYPE DRUG	Metoprolol (Lopressor)

Actions and Uses: Metoprolol is a selective beta$_1$ antagonist available in tablet, sustained-release tablet, and IV forms. At high doses it may also affect beta$_2$ receptors in bronchial smooth muscle. When given IV, it quickly acts to reduce myocardial oxygen demand. Following an acute MI, metoprolol is infused slowly until a target heart rate is reached, usually between 60 and 90 beats/minute. Upon hospital discharge, clients can be switched to oral forms of the drug. Metoprolol is also approved for angina, hypertension, and MI.

Administration Alerts:

- During IV administration, monitor ECG, blood pressure, and pulse frequently.
- Assess pulse and blood pressure before oral administration. Hold drug if pulse is below 50 beats/minute (60 beats/minute in some agencies) or if client is hypotensive.
- Do not crush or chew sustained-release tablets.
- Metoprolol is pregnancy category C.

Pharmacokinetics: Metoprolol is well absorbed, widely distributed, and mostly metabolized by the liver. It has a half-life of 3 to 7 hours.

Adverse Effects and Interactions: Because it is selective for blocking beta$_1$ receptors in the heart, metoprolol has few adverse effects on other autonomic targets and thus is preferred over non-selective beta blockers, such as propranolol (Inderal), for clients with lung disorders. Side effects are generally minor and relate to its autonomic activity, such as slowing of the heart rate and hypotension. Because of its multiple effects on the heart, clients with HF should be carefully monitored. This agent is contraindicated in cardiogenic shock, sinus bradycardia, and heart block greater than first degree. Concurrent use with digoxin may result in bradycardia. Oral contraceptives may increase metoprolol's effects.

Treating Angina with Calcium Channel Blockers

50.8 Calcium channel blockers relieve angina by dilating the coronary vessels and reducing the workload of the heart. They are drugs of first choice for treating variant angina.

Blockade of calcium channels has a number of effects on the heart, most of which are similar to those of beta blockers. Like beta blockers, the value of calcium channel blockers (CCBs) is presented for several other conditions, including hypertension (Chapter 51) and dysrhythmias (Chapter 55). The first approved use of CCBs was for the treatment of angina. The CCBs used for angina are listed in Table 50.1.

CCBs have several cardiovascular actions that benefit the client with angina. Dihydropyridine CCBs such as amlodipine (Norvasc) and nifedipine (Adalat) relax arteriolar smooth muscle, thus lowering blood pressure. This reduction in afterload decreases myocardial oxygen demand. Non-dihydropyridine CCBs such as verapamil (Isoptin) and diltiazem (Cardizem, Tiazac) also relax arteriolar smooth muscle, but in addition they slow conduction velocity through the heart, decreasing heart rate and further reducing cardiac workload. An additional effect of the CCBs is their ability to dilate the coronary arteries, bringing more oxygen to the myocardium. Because they are able to relieve the acute vasospasm of variant angina, CCBs are considered drugs of choice for clients with vasospastic angina. For stable angina, CCBs may be used as monotherapy in clients who are unable to tolerate beta blockers. In clients with persistent symptoms, dihydropyridine CCBs may be combined with beta blockers. Non-dihydropyridine CCBs are not generally used with beta blockers or in heart block because of their effects on conduction.

Nursing Considerations

The role of the nurse in CCB therapy for angina involves careful monitoring of the client's condition and providing education as it relates to the prescribed drug regimen. Because of the effects on blood pressure and heart rate, vital signs should be assessed before administering these medications. Take blood pressure in both arms while the client is lying, sitting, and standing in order to monitor for orthostatic hypotension. Because CCBs, especially when administered IV, can affect myocardial conduction, they are not used in clients with sick sinus syndrome or third-degree AV block without the presence of a pacemaker. The ECG should be assessed prior to initiating therapy for any indication of conduction disturbances.

Some CCBs reduce myocardial contractility and can worsen HF. Monitor the client for signs and symptoms of worsening HF such as peripheral edema, shortness of breath, and lung congestion. Also monitor the client's weight for a sudden increase, which indicates fluid retention. Bowel function should be assessed, as some CCBs cause constipation. Extended-release tablets or capsules should not be crushed or split because this can result in a large dose being released and cause serious hypotension.

Client education as it relates to CCBs should include goals, reasons for obtaining baseline data such as vital signs and tests for cardiac and renal disorders, and possible side effects. The following are important points to include when teaching clients regarding CCBs:

- Take blood pressure and pulse before self-administering the medication. Withhold drug if either pulse or blood pressure is below established parameters and notify the healthcare provider.
- Keep a record of frequency and severity of each angina attack.
- Change positions slowly and be cautious when performing hazardous activities until effects of the drug are known.
- Notify the healthcare provider of any symptoms of HF such as shortness of breath, weight gain, and slow heartbeat.
- Do not crush or break extended-release capsules or tablets.
- Avoid grapefruit juice, as it can cause CCBs to rise to toxic levels.

NCLEX Success Tips

Diltiazem is a calcium channel blocker that blocks the influx of calcium into the cell during phase 0 of the cardiac action potential. This action causes the sinoatrial node and AV node to slow their response times, which results in slowed AV conduction, decreased ventricular depolarization, and arrhythmias. The primary use of diltiazem is to promote vasodilation and prevent spasms of the arteries. As a result of the vasodilation, blood, oxygen, and nutrients can reach the muscle and tissues. Calcium channel blockers are first-line drug therapy for the treatment of vasospasms with Raynaud's phenomenon when other therapies are ineffective.

The chief complications of diltiazem are hypotension, atrioventricular blocks, heart failure, and elevated liver enzyme levels.

| PROTOTYPE DRUG | Diltiazem (Cardizem, Tiazac) |

Actions and Uses: Like other calcium channel blockers, diltiazem inhibits the transport of calcium into myocardial cells. It has the ability to relax both coronary and peripheral blood vessels. It is useful in the treatment of atrial dysrhythmias and hypertension as well as angina. When given as extended-release capsules, it can be administered once daily.

Administration Alerts:

- During IV administration, the client must be continuously monitored and cardioversion equipment must be available.
- Extended-release tablets and capsules should not be crushed or split.
- Diltiazem is pregnancy category C.

Pharmacokinetics: Diltiazem is well absorbed. It is 70% to 80% protein bound. It is metabolized by the liver. It has a half-life of 3.5 to 9 hours.

Adverse Effects and Interactions: Side effects of diltiazem are generally not serious and are related to vasodilation: headache, dizziness, and edema of the ankles and feet. Although diltiazem produces few adverse effects on the heart or vessels, it should be used with caution in clients who are taking other cardiovascular drugs, particularly digoxin or beta-adrenergic blockers. The combined effects of these drugs may cause partial or complete heart block, HF, or dysrhythmias.

This drug may increase digoxin and quinidine (Quinate) levels when taken concurrently.

Use with caution with herbal supplements, such as dong quai and ginger, as these products interfere with blood clotting. Calcium chloride can be administered by slow IV push to reverse hypotension or heart block *if* induced by CCBs.

Diagnosis of Myocardial Infarction

50.9 The early diagnosis of myocardial infarction increases chances of survival. Early pharmacotherapy may include thrombolytics, ASA, beta blockers, and antidysrhythmics.

Heart attack, also known as **myocardial infarction (MI)**, is responsible for a substantial number of deaths each year. Some clients die before reaching a medical facility for treatment, and many others die within 1 to 2 days following the initial MI. Clearly, MI is a serious and frightening disease and one responsible for a large percentage of sudden deaths.

The primary cause of MI is advanced coronary artery disease. Plaque buildup can severely narrow one or more branches of the coronary arteries. Pieces of plaque can break off and lodge in a small vessel serving a portion of the myocardium. Deprived of its oxygen supply, this area of myocardium becomes ischemic and the tissue can die unless its blood supply is quickly restored. Figure 50.3 illustrates the pathogenesis and treatment of MI.

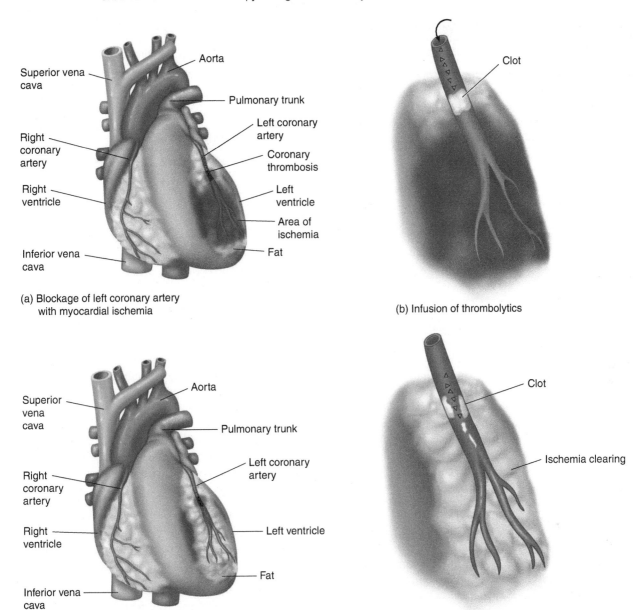

(a) Blockage of left coronary artery with myocardial ischemia

(b) Infusion of thrombolytics

(c) Blood supply restarted to myocardium

(d) Thrombus dissolving

Figure 50.3 Blockage and reperfusion following myocardial infarction: (a) blockage of left coronary artery with resultant myocardial ischemia; (b) infusion of thrombolytics; (c) blood supply returning to the myocardium; (d) thrombus dissolving and ischemia clearing. *Source:* Figures (a) and (c), Pearson Education.

Goals for the pharmacological treatment of acute MI are as follows:

- Restore blood supply (perfusion) to the damaged myocardium as quickly as possible through the use of thrombolytics.
- Reduce myocardial oxygen demand with organic nitrates and beta blockers, to prevent further MIs.
- Control or prevent associated dysrhythmias with beta blockers or other antidysrhythmics.
- Reduce post-MI mortality with acetylsalicylic acid (ASA [Aspirin]) and angiotensin-converting enzyme (ACE) inhibitors.
- Control MI pain and associated anxiety with narcotic analgesics.

Laboratory test results are used to aid in diagnosis and to monitor progress after an MI. Table 50.2 describes important laboratory values.

Treating Myocardial Infarction with Thrombolytics

50.10 If given within hours after the onset of MI, thrombolytic agents can dissolve clots and restore perfusion to affected regions of the myocardium.

In the treatment of MI, the goal of thrombolytic therapy is to dissolve clots obstructing the coronary arteries and restore circulation to the myocardium. Quick restoration of cardiac circulation has been found to reduce mortality caused by acute MI. Thrombolytics are most effective when administered from 20 minutes to 12 hours after the onset of MI symptoms. If administered after 24 hours, the drugs are mostly ineffective. After the clot is successfully dissolved, anticoagulant therapy is initiated to prevent the

TABLE 50.2   Changes in Blood Test Values with Acute MI

Blood Test	Initial Elevation after MI	Peak Elevation after MI	Duration of Elevation	Normal Range
Cholesterol			4 weeks, during stress response	5.2 mmol/L
Creatine kinase (CK)	3–8 hours	12–24 hours	2–4 days	Males: 12–80 U/L Females: 10–70 U/L
Creatinine phosphokinase (CPK)	4–8 hours	18–24 hours	2–3 days	0%–3% of CK
Erythrocyte sedimentation rate (ESR)	First week		Several weeks	
Glucose			Duration of stress response	Fasting: 3.3–5.8 mmol/L
Lactase dehydrogenase (LDH)	8–72 hours	3–6 days	8–14 days	95–195 U/L
Myoglobin	1–3 hours	4–6 hours	1–2 days	0–57 µg/mL
Troponin I	2–4 hours	24–36 hours	7–10 days	3.1 µg/L
Troponin T	2–4 hours	24–36 hours	10–14 days	0.01–0.1 µg/L
White blood cell (WBC) count	Few hours		3–7 days	$4–10 \times 10^9$/L

formation of additional clots. Dosages and descriptions of the various thrombolytics are provided in Chapter 56.

Thrombolytics have a narrow margin of safety between dissolving "normal" and "abnormal" clots. It must be understood that once infused in the blood, the drugs travel to all vessels and may cause adverse effects anywhere in the body. The primary risk associated with thrombolytics is excessive bleeding from interference with the normal clotting process. Vital signs must be monitored continuously, and any signs of bleeding generally call for discontinuation of therapy. Because these drugs are rapidly destroyed in the blood, discontinuation of the drug normally results in the rapid termination of adverse effects.

Thrombolytic therapy is contraindicated for many conditions, including recent trauma or surgery, internal bleeding (other than menses), active peptic ulcer, postpartum (within 10 days), history of intracranial hemorrhage, suspected ischemic stroke within the past 3 months, bleeding disorders, severe liver disease, or thrombocytopenia. Caution should be used when administering thrombolytics to clients who are taking anticoagulants or antiplatelet drugs.

Nursing Considerations

The role of the nurse in thrombolytic therapy for MI involves careful monitoring of the client's condition and providing education as it relates to the prescribed drug regimen. Assess for conditions that would be contraindicated, including recent trauma or surgery/biopsy, GI bleeding, postpartum (within 10 days), cerebral hemorrhage, bleeding disorders, and thrombocytopenia, because thrombolytics would place the client at risk for increased bleeding. In septic thrombophlebitis, a favourable clot is in place that would be dissolved by thrombolytics, resulting in client injury, so the drugs are contraindicated in this condition. These drugs should be used with caution in any condition where bleeding could be a significant hazard, such as severe renal or liver disease.

IV lines, arterial lines, and Foley catheters should be established prior to beginning thrombolytic therapy to decrease the chance of bleeding from those sites. Monitor vital signs and changes in laboratory values, including hemoglobin, hematocrit (Hct), platelets, and coagulation studies, that are indicative of bleeding. Because cerebral hemorrhage is a major concern, changes in level of consciousness should be carefully monitored and neurological status assessed. Monitor for dysrhythmias that may occur as cardiac tissue is reperfused after MI. Monitor laboratory work such as CBC during and after therapy for indications of blood loss due to internal bleeding. The client has an increased risk for bleeding for 2 to 4 days post-therapy.

Client education as it relates to thrombolytics should include goals, reasons for obtaining baseline data such as vital signs and tests for cardiac and renal disorders, and possible side effects. The following are the important points to include when teaching clients about thrombolytics:

- Keep movement of IV sites to a minimum to prevent bleeding.
- Minimize physical activity during the infusion.
- Report immediately any bleeding from gums, rectum, or vagina during and for at least 4 days following completion of the infusion.

See also Nursing Process Focus: Clients Receiving Thrombolytic Therapy in Chapter 56, page 721, for the complete nursing process applied to caring for clients who are receiving thrombolytics.

PROTOTYPE DRUG   Reteplase (Retavase)

Actions and Uses: Reteplase acts as a catalyst in the cleavage of plasminogen to plasmin, a substance responsible for degrading the fibrin matrix of a clot. Reteplase is one of the newer thrombolytics. Like other drugs in this class, reteplase should be given as soon as possible after the onset of MI symptoms. It usually acts within 20 minutes, and restoration of circulation to the ischemic site may be faster than with other thrombolytics. After the clot has been dissolved, heparin therapy is often started to prevent additional clots from forming.

Pharmacokinetics: Reteplase is rapidly metabolized by the liver and is excreted by the kidneys. It has a half-life of 13 to 16 minutes.

Administration Alerts:

- Drug must be reconstituted just prior to use with diluent provided by the manufacturer; swirl to mix—do not shake.
- Do not give any other drug simultaneously through the same IV line.

- Drug must be administered within 6 hours of onset of MI symptoms and within 3 hours of thrombotic cerebrovascular accident in order to be effective.
- Reteplase is pregnancy category C.

Adverse Effects and Interactions: Reteplase is contraindicated in clients with active bleeding. The healthcare provider must be vigilant in recognizing and responding to abnormal bleeding during therapy.

Drug interactions with anticoagulants and platelet aggregation inhibitors will produce an additive effect and increase the risk for bleeding.

Treating Myocardial Infarction with Antiplatelets and Anticoagulants

50.11 Glycoprotein IIb/IIIa inhibitors are antiplatelet agents for the treatment of myocardial ischemia.

Unless contraindicated, 160 to 325 mg of ASA is given as soon as an MI is suspected. ASA use in the weeks following an acute MI dramatically reduces mortality, probably because of its antiplatelet action. The low doses used in maintenance therapy (75 to 150 mg/day) rarely cause GI bleeding.

Clopidogrel (Plavix) and ticlopidine (Ticlid) are antiplatelet agents that block adenosine diphosphate. They may be used for the prevention of thrombotic stroke and MI. Because these drugs are considerably more expensive than ASA, they are usually considered for clients allergic to ASA or who are at risk for GI bleeding from ASA.

Glycoprotein IIb/IIIa inhibitors are antiplatelet agents with a mechanism of action different from that of ASA. **Glycoprotein IIb/IIIa** is a receptor found on the surface of platelets. Glycoprotein IIb/IIIa inhibitors occupy this receptor and inhibit clot formation. These agents are sometimes used for unstable angina or MI or for clients who are undergoing PTCA. Clopidogrel, the most common drug in this class, is infused during PTCA and for 12 hours following the procedure.

Heparin is an anticoagulant that is often initiated following an MI to prevent additional thrombi from forming. Heparin therapy is usually continued for about 3 days, after which clients are switched to warfarin (Coumadin). An alternative is to administer a low-molecular-weight heparin, such as dalteparin (Fragmin). Refer to Chapter 56 for a comparison of anticoagulants and their dosages.

Treating Myocardial Infarction with Beta Blockers

50.12 When given within 24 hours after the onset of myocardial infarction, beta-adrenergic blockers can improve survival.

The use of the beta-adrenergic blockers in the treatment of cardiovascular disease has been discussed in a number of chapters in this textbook. This section will focus on their use in the treatment of MI. The beta blockers used for MI are listed in Table 50.1.

Beta blockers have the ability to slow heart rate, decrease contractility, and reduce blood pressure. These three factors reduce myocardial oxygen demand, which is beneficial for clients who have experienced a recent MI. In addition, beta blockers slow impulse conduction through the heart, which tends to suppress dysrhythmias, which are serious and sometimes fatal complications following an MI. Beta blockers have been shown to reduce mortality when given within 8 hours of MI onset.

Nursing Considerations

See Nursing Considerations for beta blockers in Section 50.7.

Drugs for Symptoms and Complications of Acute Myocardial Infarction

50.13 A number of additional drugs are used to treat the symptoms and complications of acute MI. These include analgesics, anticoagulants (including ASA), and ACE inhibitors.

Several additional drugs have proven useful in treating the client who presents with an acute MI. Unless contraindicated, 180 to 325 mg of ASA is given as soon as an MI is suspected. ASA use in the weeks following an acute MI reduces mortality dramatically. Additional actions of ASA may be found in Chapters 23 and 42.

Two ACE inhibitors, captopril (Capoten) and lisinopril (Prinivi, Zestrill), also have been determined to improve survival following acute MI. These drugs are most effective when therapy is started within 1 to 2 days following the onset of symptoms. Oral doses are normally begun after thrombolytic therapy is completed and the client's condition has stabilized. Additional indications for ACE inhibitors may be found in Chapters 51 and 54.

Pain control is essential following acute MI to ensure client comfort and reduce stress. Narcotic analgesics such as morphine sulfate (Kadian, M-Eslon, MS Contin, MS-IR, Statex) or fentanyl (Duragesic) are sometimes given to ease extreme pain associated with acute MI and to sedate the anxious client. The pharmacology of the analgesics is presented in Chapter 23.

Pathogenesis of Cerebrovascular Accident

50.14 Cerebrovascular accident, also known as stroke and brain attack, is a major cause of death and disability. CVAs may be caused by a clot or by rupture of a cerebral vessel.

Cerebrovascular accident (CVA), also called **stroke** or **brain attack**, is a major cause of permanent disability. It is the third leading cause of death in North America, following heart disease and cancer. The majority of CVAs are **thrombotic strokes**, which are caused by a thrombus (clot) in a blood vessel serving the brain. Tissues distal to the clot lose their oxygen supply, and neural tissue will die unless circulation is quickly restored. A smaller percentage of CVAs, about 20%, are caused by rupture of a cerebral vessel with associated bleeding into neural tissue, known as a **hemorrhagic stroke**. Symptoms are the same for the two types of stroke. Mortality from CVA is very high: more than 30% of clients die within the first year following the CVA. Most of the risk factors associated with CVA are the same as for other cardiovascular disease, such as hypertension and coronary artery disease.

The signs and symptoms of a CVA depend on a number of factors, the most important of which are the location of the obstruction and how much brain tissue is affected. A stroke affecting one side of the brain will result in neurological deficits on the opposite side of the body. For example, if the stroke occurs in the right side of the brain, the left side of the body will be affected. The five warning signs of stroke are:

1. Paralysis or weakness on one side of the body
2. Vision problems
3. Dizziness
4. Speech or language problems
5. Headache

Pharmacotherapy of Thrombotic CVA

50.15 Aggressive treatment of thrombotic CVA with thrombolytics, to restore perfusion, and anticoagulants, to prevent additional clots from forming, can increase survival.

Drug therapy for thrombotic CVA focuses on two main goals: prevention of CVA through the use of anticoagulants and antihypertensive agents, and restoration of blood supply to the affected neurons as quickly as possible after a CVA through the use of thrombolytics.

Sustained, chronic hypertension is closely associated with CVA. Antihypertensive drugs such as the beta-adrenergic blockers, calcium channel blockers, diuretics, and ACE inhibitors can help to control blood pressure and reduce the probability of CVA. Diet and lifestyle factors that reduce blood pressure should be implemented concurrently with antihypertensive pharmacotherapy.

ASA, through its anticoagulant properties, reduces the incidence of stroke. When given in very low doses, ASA discourages the formation of clots by inhibiting platelets. Clients are often placed on a daily regimen of low-dose ASA therapy following a transient ischemic attack or following their first CVA. Many healthcare providers recommend low-dose ASA therapy as a prophylactic measure for the prevention of MI and CVA. Ticlopidine, or the use of clopidogrel, which is more commonly seen in clinical practice, is an antiplatelet drug that may be used to provide anticoagulation in clients who cannot tolerate ASA. Other anticoagulants, such as warfarin, may be given to prevent CVA in high-risk individuals, such as those with prosthetic heart valves. More detailed information on anticoagulants can be found in Chapter 56.

The single most important breakthrough in the pharmacotherapy of CVA was the development of the thrombolytic drugs called "clot busters." Prior to the advent of these drugs, the treatment of CVA was largely a passive, wait-and-see strategy. Care was directed at habilitation or rehabilitation after the fact. Stroke is now aggressively treated with thrombolytics as soon as the client arrives at the hospital. Such agents are most effective if administered within 3 hours of the attack. The use of aggressive thrombolytic therapy can completely restore brain function in a significant number of stroke victims. As a result, CVA is now considered a condition that mandates immediate treatment. The condition is often referred to by its newer title, brain attack, which reflects the need for urgent treatment.

CONNECTIONS | **Special Considerations**

◀ **Cultural, Gender, and Age Considerations in Stroke**

- Overall, the incidence and prevalence of stroke are about equal for men and women.
- At all ages, however, more women than men die from stroke.
- Risk for stroke is greater in people who have a family history of stroke.
- Aboriginal peoples and those of African or South Asian descent have a higher risk for disability and death from stroke than the general population, in part because they have a greater incidence of hypertension, diabetes, and related complications.

CONNECTIONS | **Natural Therapies**

◀ **Ginseng**

Ginseng is one of the oldest known herbal remedies, with at least six species being reported to have medicinal properties. *Panax ginseng* is distributed throughout China, Korea, and Siberia, whereas *Panax quinquefolius* is native to Canada and the United States. The plant's popularity has led to its extinction from certain regions, and much of the available ginseng is now grown commercially.

Standardization of ginseng focuses on a group of chemicals called ginsenosides, although there are many other chemicals in the root, which is the harvested portion of the plant. The *German Commission E Monographs* (a therapeutic guide to herbal medicine) recommend a dose of 20 to 30 mg ginsenosides. This is sometimes reported as a percent, with 5% being the recommended standard amount of ginsenosides.

There are differences in chemical composition among the various species of ginseng: American ginseng is not considered equivalent to Siberian ginseng. Ginseng is reported to be a calcium channel antagonist. By increasing the conversion of L-arginine to nitric oxide, ginseng improves blood flow to the heart in times of low oxygen supply, such as with myocardial ischemia. The Chinese have found that nitric oxide is a potent antioxidant that combats free radical injury to the heart muscle. The nurse should caution clients who take ginseng because herb–drug interactions are possible with warfarin and loop diuretics.

CHAPTER 50

Understanding the Chapter

Key Concepts Summary

The numbered key concepts provide a succinct summary of the important points from the corresponding numbered section within the chapter. If any of these points are not clear, refer to the numbered section within the chapter for review.

50.1 Coronary artery disease includes both angina and myocardial infarction. It is caused by narrowing of the arterial lumen due to atherosclerotic plaque.

50.2 The myocardium requires a continuous supply of oxygen from the coronary arteries in order to function properly.

50.3 Angina pectoris is chest pain, usually upon emotional or physical exertion. It is caused by the narrowing of a coronary artery, which results in lack of sufficient oxygen to the heart muscle.

50.4 Angina management may include non-pharmacological therapies such as diet and lifestyle modifications, treatment of underlying disorders, angioplasty, or surgery.

50.5 The pharmacological goals for the treatment of angina are to terminate acute attacks and prevent future episodes. This is usually achieved by reducing cardiac workload.

50.6 The organic nitrates relieve angina by dilating veins and coronary arteries. They are drugs of choice for stable angina.

50.7 Beta-adrenergic blockers relieve angina by decreasing the oxygen demands on the heart. They are sometimes considered first-line drugs for chronic angina.

50.8 Calcium channel blockers relieve angina by dilating the coronary vessels and reducing the workload of the heart. They are drugs of first choice for treating variant angina.

50.9 The early diagnosis of myocardial infarction increases chances of survival. Early pharmacotherapy may include thrombolytics, ASA, beta blockers, and antidysrhythmics.

50.10 If given within hours after the onset of MI, thrombolytic agents can dissolve clots and restore perfusion to affected regions of the myocardium.

50.11 Glycoprotein IIb/IIIa inhibitors are antiplatelet agents for the treatment of myocardial ischemia.

50.12 When given within 24 hours after the onset of myocardial infarction, beta-adrenergic blockers can improve survival.

50.13 A number of additional drugs are used to treat the symptoms and complications of acute MI. These include analgesics, anticoagulants (including ASA), and ACE inhibitors.

50.14 Cerebrovascular accident, also known as stroke and brain attack, is a major cause of death and disability. CVAs may be caused by a clot or by rupture of a cerebral vessel.

50.15 Aggressive treatment of thrombotic CVA with thrombolytics, to restore perfusion, and anticoagulants, to prevent additional clots from forming, can increase survival.

Chapter 50 Scenario

Early one morning, 60-year-old Michael Graff began to feel severe anterior crushing chest pain that lasted for 35 minutes. He experienced dizziness, cold sweats, and nausea. Although he considered driving to the local emergency department, his family insisted on calling an ambulance for emergency transport to the hospital.

Michael, a general contractor, is a 2-pack-per-day smoker and consumes alcohol (beer) two to three times per week. He has a family history of coronary artery disease, diabetes mellitus, and hyperlipidemia. It has been at least 10 years since his last physical examination.

Upon arrival at the emergency department, he presented with symptoms of anxiety, moderate chest pain, and cold extremities. Auscultation of the thorax revealed tachycardia and clear lung fields. Blood pressure was slightly above normal at 156/90 mm Hg. He had no neck venous distention. His white blood cell count was 7600/mm^3, hematocrit 43.8%, platelets 256 000/mm^3, creatine phosphokinase (CPK)

87 international units/L, and troponin-I <4.1 µg/L. An ECG showed ST-segment elevation.

Once stabilized, Michael is transported to the coronary care unit with the admission diagnosis of unstable angina and to rule out MI. In the coronary care unit, he receives IV nitroglycerin 50 mg in D_5W 25 mL. The nurse begins the infusion at 10 µg/minute and titrates the rate based on his report of chest pain every 5 to 10 minutes (5–10 µg/minute).

Critical Thinking Questions

1. Michael and his family ask you to explain what is occurring with his heart. How would you describe the pathophysiology of Michael's condition to them?

2. Discuss the reason Michael is receiving nitroglycerin.
3. What adverse effects should the nurse monitor with clients who are receiving IV nitroglycerin?
4. How do nitroglycerin infusions differ from other IV infusions?

See Answers to Critical Thinking Questions in Appendix B.

NCLEX Practice Questions

1 Nitroglycerin topical ointment is being initiated for a client with angina. Which health teaching would be most appropriate for that client?

a. Keep the medication in the refrigerator.
b. Only take this medication when chest pain is severe.
c. Remove the old paste before applying the next dose.
d. Apply the ointment on the chest wall only.

2 A client with chest pain is receiving sublingual nitroglycerin. The nurse's care plan will include monitoring the client for which adverse effect?

a. Photosensitivity
b. Elevated blood pressure
c. Vomiting and diarrhea
d. Decreased blood pressure

3 A client states, "I always put my nitroglycerin patch in the same place so that I won't forget to take it off." The nurse's response will be based on which of the following physiological concepts?

a. Clients are more likely to remember to apply the patch if it is applied to the same site daily.
b. Repeated use of the same application site will enhance medication absorption.

c. Rebound phenomenon is likely to occur when the same site is used more than once.
d. Skin irritation due to the nitroglycerin patch can occur if the same site is used repeatedly.

4 The client asks how atenolol (Tenormin) helps angina. The nurse's response is based on which concept? This medication

a. Slows the heart rate and reduces contractility
b. Increases the heart rate and diminishes contractility
c. Blocks sodium channels and elevates depolarization
d. Decreases blood pressure and blocks the $alpha_2$ receptors

5 Which of the following assessment findings, if discovered in a client receiving verapamil (Isoptin) for angina, would cause the nurse to withhold the medication? Select all that apply.

a. Bradycardia: heart rate 40 beats/minute
b. Tachycardia: heart rate 126 beats/minute
c. Hypotension: blood pressure 76/46 mm Hg
d. Tinnitus with hearing loss
e. Hypertension: blood pressure 156/92 mm Hg

See Answers to NCLEX Practice Questions in Appendix A.

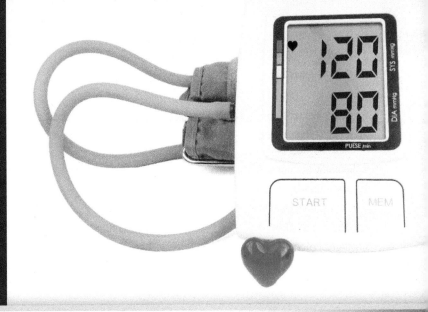

hasan eroglu/Shutterstock

CHAPTER

51

Pharmacotherapy of Hypertension

LEARNING OUTCOMES

After reading this chapter, the student should be able to:

1. Summarize the long-term consequences of untreated hypertension.
2. Identify drug classes used for treating hypertension.
3. Describe general principles guiding the pharmacotherapy of hypertension.
4. Explain the therapeutic action of each class of antihypertensive drug in relation to the pathophysiology of hypertension.
5. Discuss the role of the nurse regarding the non-pharmacological control of hypertension through client teaching.
6. Describe the nurse's role in the pharmacological management of clients who are receiving drugs for hypertension.
7. For each of the drug classes listed in Prototype Drugs, identify a representative drug and explain its mechanism of action, therapeutic effects, and important adverse effects.
8. Describe and explain, based on pharmacological principles, the rationale for nursing assessment, planning, and interventions for clients with hypertension.
9. Use the nursing process to care for clients who are receiving drug therapy for hypertension.

CHAPTER OUTLINE

▸ Risk Factors for Hypertension

▸ Factors Responsible for Blood Pressure

▸ Normal Regulation of Blood Pressure

▸ Indications and Guidelines for Hypertension Therapy

▸ Non-Pharmacological Therapy of Hypertension

▸ Risk Factors and Selection of Antihypertensive Drugs

▸ Diuretics

  ▸ Treating Hypertension with Diuretics

▸ Calcium Channel Blockers

  ▸ Treating Hypertension with Calcium Channel Blockers

Cardiovascular disease, which includes all conditions that affect the heart and blood vessels, is the most common cause of death in Canada. **Hypertension (HTN)**, or high blood pressure, is the most common of the cardiovascular diseases. About one in five Canadians has HTN, yet more than 40% do not know they have it. Although mild HTN can often be controlled with lifestyle modifications, moderate to severe HTN requires pharmacotherapy. Because nurses encounter numerous clients with this disease, having an understanding of the underlying principles of antihypertensive therapy is critical. Nurses play a vital role in teaching the client safe principles of pharmacotherapy as it relates to HTN.

Risk Factors for Hypertension

51.1 High blood pressure is classified as essential (primary) or secondary. Uncontrolled hypertension can lead to chronic and debilitating disorders such as stroke, heart attack, and heart failure.

Hypertension that has no identifiable cause is called primary, idiopathic, or essential. This classification accounts for 90% of all cases. Secondary hypertension, which accounts for only 10% of all cases, is caused by identifiable factors such as excessive secretion of epinephrine by the adrenal glands or by narrowing of the renal arteries.

Because chronic HTN may produce no identifiable symptoms for as long as 10 to 20 years, many people are not aware of their condition. Convincing clients to control their diets, buy costly medications, and take drugs on a regular basis when they are feeling healthy is an important yet challenging task for the nurse. In addition, many clients do not take HTN medications because of their undesirable side effects. However, failure to control this condition can result in serious consequences. Prolonged or improperly controlled HTN can damage small blood vessels, leading to accelerated narrowing of the arteries that can result in angina, myocardial infarction (MI), and peripheral vascular disease. One of the most serious consequences of chronic HTN is that the heart must work harder to pump blood to the various organs and

tissues. This excessive cardiac workload can cause the heart to fail and the lungs to fill with fluid, a condition known as heart failure (HF). Drug therapy of HF is discussed in Chapter 54.

Damage to the vessels that supply blood and oxygen to the brain can result in transient ischemic attacks and cerebral vascular accidents or strokes. Renal damage and retinal damage are also common sequelae of sustained HTN.

The death rate from cardiovascular-related diseases has dropped significantly over the past 20 years due, in large part, to the recognition and treatment of HTN, as well as the acceptance of healthier lifestyle habits. Early treatment is essential, as the long-term cardiovascular damage caused by HTN may be irreversible if the disease is allowed to progress unchecked.

Factors Responsible for Blood Pressure

51.2 The three primary factors controlling blood pressure are cardiac output, peripheral resistance, and blood volume.

Although many factors can influence blood pressure, the three factors truly responsible for creating the pressure are cardiac output, peripheral resistance, and blood volume. These are shown in Figure 51.1.

The volume of blood pumped per minute is called the **cardiac output**. The higher the cardiac output, the higher the blood pressure. Cardiac output is determined by heart rate and **stroke volume**, which is the amount of blood pumped by a ventricle in one contraction. This is important to pharmacology because drugs that change the cardiac output, stroke volume, or heart rate have the potential to influence a client's blood pressure.

As blood flows at high speeds through the vascular system, it exerts force against the walls of the vessels. Although the inner layer of the blood vessel lining, known as the **endothelium**, is extremely smooth, this friction reduces the velocity of the blood. This turbulence-induced friction in the arteries is called **peripheral resistance**. Arteries have smooth muscle in their walls that,

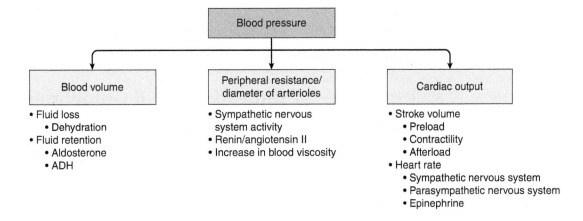

Figure 51.1 Primary factors affecting blood pressure.

when constricted, will cause the inside diameter (lumen) to become smaller, thus creating more resistance and higher pressure. A large number of drugs affect vascular smooth muscle, causing vessels to constrict and raising blood pressure. Other drugs cause the smooth muscle to relax, thereby opening the lumen and lowering blood pressure. Chapter 14 presents the role of the autonomic nervous system in controlling peripheral resistance.

The third factor responsible for blood pressure is the total amount of blood in the vascular system, or blood volume. While the average person maintains a relatively constant blood volume of approximately 5 L, this can change due to many regulatory factors and certain disease states. More blood in the vascular system will exert additional pressure on the walls of the arteries and raise blood pressure. For example, high-sodium diets may cause water to be retained by the body, thus increasing blood volume and raising blood pressure. On the other hand, substances known as **diuretics** can cause fluid loss through urination, thus decreasing blood volume and lowering blood pressure. Loss of blood volume during hemorrhage or shock also lowers blood pressure (see Chapter 58).

Normal Regulation of Blood Pressure

51.3 Many factors help to regulate blood pressure, including the vasomotor centre, baroreceptors and chemoreceptors in the aorta and internal carotid arteries, and the renin-angiotensin-aldosterone system.

It is critical for the body to maintain a normal range of blood pressure and to have the ability to safely and rapidly change pressure as it proceeds through daily activities such as sleep and exercise. Low blood pressure can cause dizziness and lack of adequate urine formation, whereas excessively high pressure can cause vessels to rupture. How the body maintains homeostasis of blood pressure during periods of change is shown in Figure 51.2.

Blood pressure is regulated on a minute-to-minute basis by a cluster of neurons in the medulla oblongata called the

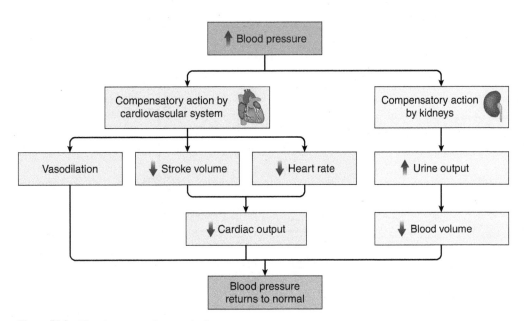

Figure 51.2 Blood pressure homeostasis.

vasomotor centre. Nerves travel from the vasomotor centre to the arteries, where the smooth muscle is instructed to either constrict (raise blood pressure) or relax (lower blood pressure). Potent vasoconstrictors, such as angiotensin II and endothelin, and potent vasodilators, such as nitric oxide and vasodilator prostaglandins, that are released in the vascular endothelium exert local effects on blood pressure.

Receptors in the aorta and the internal carotid artery act as sensors to provide the vasomotor centre with vital information on conditions in the vascular system. **Baroreceptors** have the ability to sense pressure within large vessels, and **chemoreceptors** recognize pH and levels of oxygen and carbon dioxide in the blood. The vasomotor centre reacts to information from baroreceptors and chemoreceptors by raising or lowering blood pressure accordingly.

Emotions can also have a profound effect on blood pressure. Anger and stress can cause blood pressure to rise, whereas mental depression and lethargy may cause it to fall. Strong emotions, if present for a prolonged period, may become important contributors to chronic HTN.

A number of hormones and other endogenous agents affect blood pressure on a daily basis. When given as medications, some of these agents may have a profound effect on blood pressure. For example, injection of epinephrine (Adrenalin) or norepinephrine (Levophed) will immediately raise blood pressure. **Antidiuretic hormone (ADH)** is a potent vasoconstrictor that can also increase blood pressure by raising blood volume. The **renin-angiotensin-aldosterone system (RAAS)** is particularly important in the

pharmacotherapy of HTN and is discussed later in this chapter. A summary of the various nervous and hormonal factors that influence blood pressure is shown in Figure 51.3.

Indications and Guidelines for Hypertension Therapy

51.4 Hypertension has been recently redefined as a sustained blood pressure of 140/90 mm Hg after multiple measurements made over several clinic visits. A person with sustained blood pressure of 120–139/80–89 mm Hg is said to be prehypertensive and is at increased risk for developing hypertension.

When the ventricles of the heart contract and eject blood, the pressure created in the arteries is called **systolic blood pressure**. When the ventricles relax and the heart is not ejecting blood, pressure in the arteries will fall, and this is called **diastolic blood pressure**. For many years, blood pressure measuring 120/80 mm Hg had been considered optimal. However, the risk for cardiovascular disease (CVD) beginning at 115/75 mm Hg *doubles* with each increment of 20/10 mm Hg. Individuals with prehypertension are at increased risk for progression to HTN; those in the 130–139/80–89 mm Hg blood pressure range are at twice the risk for developing HTN as those with lower values. Individuals with

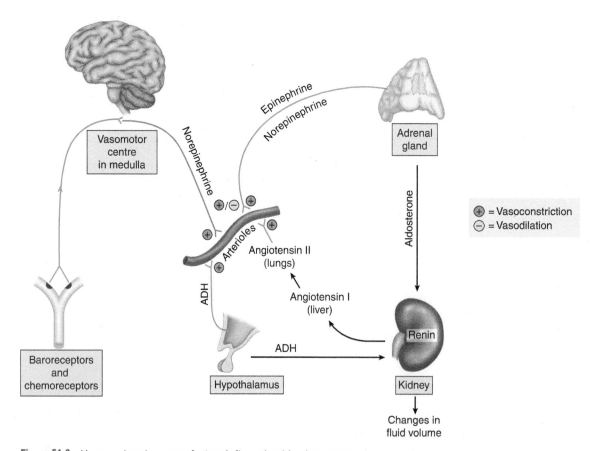

Figure 51.3 Hormonal and nervous factors influencing blood pressure.

systolic blood pressure of 120 to 139 mm Hg or diastolic blood pressure of 80 to 89 mm Hg may be considered *prehypertensive*. These clients should be strongly encouraged by the nurse to adopt health-promoting lifestyle modifications to prevent CVD.

The diagnosis of chronic HTN is rarely made on a single blood pressure measurement. A client who has a sustained systolic pressure of 140 to 159 mm Hg or diastolic pressure of 90 to 99 mm Hg, after multiple measurements made over several clinic visits, is said to have stage 1 hypertension. In low-risk clients with stage 1 hypertension, lifestyle modification can be the sole therapy. The *Canadian Hypertension Education Program Recommendations* (Hypertension Canada, 2016) state that pharmacotherapy for HTN is indicated in clients with any of the following:

- Other cardiovascular risk factors, if blood pressure remains equal to or above 140/90 mm Hg with lifestyle modification
- Target organ damage (e.g., proteinuria), if blood pressure is equal to or above 140/90 mm Hg
- Known atherosclerotic disease (e.g., previous stroke), even if blood pressure is normal
- Diabetes or chronic kidney disease (CKD), if blood pressure is equal to or above 130/80 mm Hg

Lifestyle modification is the cornerstone of HTN prevention and management. In clients who do not have conditions that may require special treatment, the first-line drugs are thiazide diuretics, angiotensin-converting enzyme (ACE) inhibitors, angiotensin II receptor blockers (ARBs), and calcium channel blockers. An example of dual combination therapy is the combination of a thiazide diuretic with an ACE inhibitor or ARB for an additive hypotensive effect. Treatment recommendations from the Canadian Hypertension Education Program (Hypertension Canada, 2016) are summarized in Figure 51.4. The nurse should

check http://guidelines.hypertension.ca/prevention-treatment/ for the recommendations that are revised annually.

Research-based guidelines have been developed to aid the healthcare provider in providing optimum treatment for clients with HTN. When most people use the word *hypertension*, they are referring to systemic HTN, that which is measured routinely by a conventional blood pressure cuff on the upper arm over the brachial artery. Systemic HTN is a general measurement of arterial blood pressure in the body. Localized HTN may also occur. For example, clients with cirrhosis of the liver often develop portal HTN, which occurs in the portal vein and its branches serving the liver. Pulmonary HTN occurs in the pulmonary artery and its branches and is most often observed in clients with left-sided heart failure. These localized types of HTN respond to many of the same antihypertensive drugs used for systemic HTN.

To develop guidelines for treatment, many attempts have been made to define HTN and to determine when medical intervention is beneficial in reducing mortality due to cardiovascular disease.

Late in 2013, the Eighth Joint National Committee (JNC-8) significantly revised the HTN guidelines, based on newer research (James et al., 2014). The JNC-8 committee kept the same definition of hypertension as was used by JNC-7: 140/90 mm Hg. The primary difference is that research has shown that not all people with a blood pressure higher than 140/90 mm Hg need pharmacotherapy. For example, clients over age 60 years who do not have CKD or diabetes do not need pharmacotherapy until the 150/90 mm Hg threshold. Furthermore, the classes of medications recommended as first-line therapy have changed: beta-adrenergic blockers are no longer considered first-line drugs.

In the past decade, research has determined that there are racial differences in response to antihypertensive medications. To account for these differences, the JNC-8 guidelines make a distinction between drugs used for black and non-black clients.

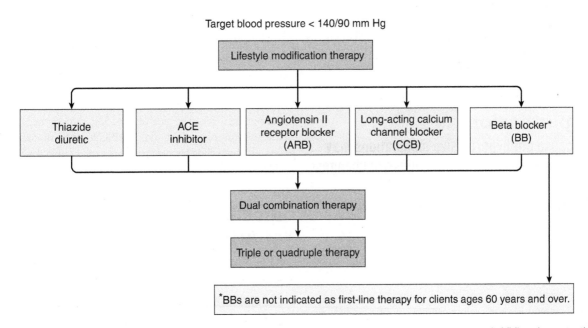

Figure 51.4 Guidelines for the management of hypertension.
Based on http://guidelines.hypertension.ca/prevention-treatment/

TABLE 51.1 Recommendations for Treating Hypertension

| Group | Blood Pressure Goal | First-Line Drugs (Alone or in Combination) | |
		Non-black	Black
Age 60 or greater without DM or CKD	Less than 150/90 mm Hg	Thiazide diuretic, ACEI, ARB, or CCB	Thiazide diuretic or CCB
Age 59 or lower without DM or CKD	Less than 140/90 mm Hg	Thiazide diuretic, ACEI, ARB, or CCB	Thiazide diuretic or CCB
All ages with DM present (no CKD)	Less than 130/80 mm Hg	Thiazide diuretic, ACEI, ARB, or CCB	Thiazide diuretic or CCB
All ages with CKD present (with or without DM)	Less than 130/80 mm Hg	ACEI or ARB	ACEI or ARB

DM = diabetes mellitus; CKD = chronic kidney disease; ACEI = angiotensin-converting enzyme inhibitor; ARB = angiotensin receptor blocker; CCB = calcium channel blocker

TABLE 51.2 Drug Classes for Hypertension

Type	Class
First-line drugs	Diuretics
	Angiotensin-converting enzyme (ACE) inhibitors
	Angiotensin receptor blockers (ARBs)
	Calcium channel blockers (CCBs)
Second-line drugs	Alpha$_2$-adrenergic agonists
	Alpha$_1$- adrenergic blockers
	Beta-adrenergic blockers
	Centrally acting alpha and beta blockers
	Direct-acting vasodilators
	Direct renin inhibitors
	Peripherally acting adrenergic neuron blockers

Non-black clients without CKD should be treated with thiazide diuretics, calcium channel blockers (CCBs), ACE inhibitors, or ARBs. Black clients without CKD are more effectively treated with thiazide diuretics either alone or in combination with CCBs. For clients with CKD, the therapy for black and non-black clients is the same. See Tables 51.1 and 51.2 for recommendations for treating HTN and drug classes for HTN.

Non-Pharmacological Therapy of Hypertension

51.5 Because antihypertensive medications may have uncomfortable side effects, lifestyle changes such as proper diet and exercise should be implemented prior to and during pharmacotherapy to allow lower drug doses.

When a client is first diagnosed with HTN, a comprehensive medical history is necessary to determine whether the disease can be controlled by non-pharmacological means. In many cases, modifying certain health-related lifestyle habits, such as increasing physical activity, lowering salt consumption, eating a balanced diet, minimizing the consumption of alcohol, avoiding smoking, and maintaining a healthy body weight, may eliminate the need for pharmacotherapy. Even if pharmacotherapy is required to manage the HTN, it is important that the client continue positive

CONNECTIONS **Special Considerations**

◀ **Lifestyle Recommendations for the Management of Hypertension**

1. Healthy diet in accordance with the DASH diet: high in fresh fruits and vegetables and low-fat dairy products; low in saturated fat and salt
2. Regular physical activity: 30 to 60 minutes of moderate cardio-respiratory activity (such as walking, jogging, cycling, or swimming) four to seven times per week
3. Limited alcohol intake: no more than 2 standard drinks per day (less than 14 per week for men and less than 9 per week for women)
4. Healthy weight: maintain an ideal body weight (body mass index [BMI] of 18.5 to 24.9 kg/m^2; waist circumference <102 cm for men and <88 cm for women)
5. Restricted salt intake: less than 100 mg/day for individuals who are considered salt-sensitive (such as those over age 45 years, of African descent, or with impaired renal function or diabetes)
6. Smoke-free environment
7. Stress management

Based on 2016 Canadian Hypertension Education Program Recommendations. http://guidelines.hypertension.ca/prevention-treatment/health-behaviour-management/

lifestyle changes so that dosages can be minimized, thus lowering the potential for drug side effects. The nurse is key in educating clients about controlling their HTN. Non-pharmacological methods for controlling hypertension are presented in the Special Considerations box.

Risk Factors and Selection of Antihypertensive Drugs

51.6 Pharmacotherapy of HTN often begins with low doses of a single medication. If ineffective, a second agent from a different class may be added to the regimen.

The goal of antihypertensive therapy is to reduce blood pressure in order to avoid serious, long-term consequences of HTN. Keeping blood pressure within acceptable limits reduces the risk for

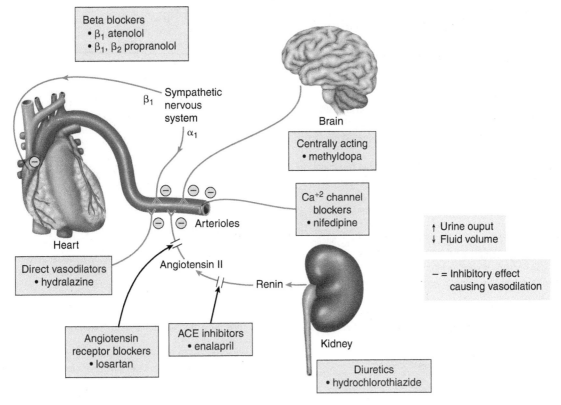

Figure 51.5 Mechanism of action of antihypertensive drugs.

hypertension-related diseases such as stroke and heart failure. Several strategies that are used to achieve this goal are summarized in Figure 51.5.

The pharmacological management of HTN is individualized with regard to the client's risk factors, concurrent medical conditions, and degree of blood pressure elevation. Once the appropriate drug has been chosen, a low dose is prescribed. Depending on the expected response time of the drug, the client will be re-evaluated, and the dosage may be adjusted. A second drug from a different class may be added if the client has not responded to the initial medication.

It is common practice for healthcare providers to prescribe two antihypertensives concurrently to manage resistant HTN.

The advantage of using two drugs is that lower doses may be used, resulting in fewer side effects and better client adherence. Unfortunately, adherence decreases when clients need to take more than one drug or need to take them more often. In an effort to minimize nonadherence, drug manufacturers sometimes combine two drugs into a single pill or capsule. These combination drugs are quite common in the treatment of HTN. It is important for the client to receive education on all drugs in combination formulas. Selected combination drugs are listed in Table 51.3. Strategies that may be used to promote adherence with antihypertensive therapy are summarized in the Special Considerations box.

TABLE 51.3   Combination Drugs Commonly Used to Treat Hypertension

Trade Name	Thiazide Diuretic	Adrenergic Agent	Potassium-Sparing Diuretic	ACE Inhibitor or Angiotensin II Receptor Blocker	Other
Aldactazide	hydrochlorothiazide		spironolactone		
Moduret	hydrochlorothiazide		amiloride		
Hyzaar HCT	hydrochlorothiazide			losartan	
Lopressor HCT	hydrochlorothiazide	metoprolol			
Lotensin HCT	hydrochlorothiazide			benazepril	
Dyazide	hydrochlorothiazide		triamterene		
Tarka				trandolapril	verapamil
Vaseretic	hydrochlorothiazide			enalapril	
Zestoretic	hydrochlorothiazide			lisinopril	

CONNECTIONS   Special Considerations

◀ Strategies to Promote Adherence with HTN Pharmacotherapy

- Teach clients to take their pills on a regular schedule that is associated with a routine daily activity such as brushing the teeth.
- Help clients to get more involved in their treatment, for example, by measuring their own blood pressure.
- Teach clients and their families about the disease and treatment regimens, verbally and in writing (audio recordings are often helpful).
- Assess adherence to pharmacological and non-pharmacological therapy.
- Simplify medication regimens (e.g., by using long-acting, once-daily, or fixed-dose combination tablets).
- Use unit-of-use packaging such as blister packs.
- Follow up with telephone contact, particularly during the first 3 months of therapy.
- Collaborate with other healthcare providers to promote adherence with pharmacological and lifestyle modification prescriptions.

Based on 2016 Canadian Hypertension Education Program.
http://guidelines.hypertension.ca/prevention-treatment/adherence/

The types of drugs used to treat chronic HTN generally fall into five primary classes, as follows:

1. Diuretics
2. Calcium channel blockers
3. Agents affecting the renin-angiotensin-aldosterone system
4. Adrenergic agents
5. Direct-acting vasodilators

DIURETICS

Diuretics act by increasing the volume of urine production. They are widely used in the treatment of HTN and HF. These agents are shown in Table 51.4.

NCLEX Success Tips

Spironolactone (Aldactone) is a potassium-sparing diuretic; therefore, clients should be monitored closely for hyperkalemia.

Daily weight measurement is the most accurate indicator of fluid status; a loss of 1 kg (2.2 lb) indicates a loss of 1 L (34 oz.) of fluid. Because spironolactone is a diuretic, weight loss is the best indicator of its effectiveness. Acidosis is also an adverse reaction to spironolactone.

Spironolactone is a potassium-sparing diuretic often used to counteract potassium loss caused by other diuretics. If foods or fluids are ingested that are high in potassium, hyperkalemia may result and lead to cardiac arrhythmias.

Spironolactone can cause menstrual irregularities and decreased libido. Men may experience gynecomastia and impotence.

Diarrhea, hyponatremia, and hyperkalemia are also adverse effects of spirolactone.

Diuretics, in general, reduce total blood volume and circulatory congestion.

To minimize the effects of orthostatic hypotension, the nurse should instruct the client on diuretics to rise slowly, such as by sitting for several minutes before standing.

It is recommended that diuretics are given early in the day, as the client will void frequently during the daytime hours and will not need to void frequently during the night. Therefore, the client's sleep will not be disturbed.

Furosemide (Lasix) is a potassium-wasting diuretic. The nurse must monitor the serum potassium level and assess for signs of low potassium.

The therapeutic effect of furosemide is to mobilize excess fluid that can be manifested by a decrease in peripheral edema and a decrease in fluid in the lungs; the client's crackles should decrease.

After an intravenous injection of furosemide, diuresis normally begins in about 5 minutes and reaches its peak within about 30 minutes. Medication effects last 2 to 4 hours. When furosemide is given intramuscularly or orally, drug action begins more slowly and lasts longer than when it is given intravenously.

Furosemide can cause pancreatitis. Furosemide is nephrotoxic, so parents of children taking the medication should be taught to inform the healthcare provider if the child has no urine output in 8 hours.

Furosemide can cause ringing in the ears, or tinnitus, as a sign of ototoxicity. The nurse should stop furosemide and notify the physician. If the drug is stopped soon enough, permanent hearing loss can be avoided, and the tinnitus should subside. The nurse should note the observation in the medical record.

Reducing dietary sodium intake in clients receiving loop diuretic will help increase the effectiveness of diuretic medication and may allow smaller doses to be ordered.

TABLE 51.4   Diuretics for Hypertension

Drug	Route and Adult Dose
Potassium-Sparing Type	
amiloride (Midamor)	Orally (PO), 5–10 mg qd (max 20 mg/day)
spironolactone (Aldactone) (see Chapter 52, page 660, for the Prototype Drug box)	PO, 25–100 mg in one to two divided doses (max 200 mg/day)
triamterene	PO, 100–300 mg/day in one to two divided doses (max 300 mg/day)
Thiazide and Thiazide-Like Agents	
chlorothiazide (Diuril) (see Chapter 52, page 658, for the Prototype Drug box)	PO, 500-2000 mg/day in one to two divided doses (max 2 g/day)
chlorthalidone	PO, 50–100 mg every day (qd) (max 100 mg/day)
Pr hydrochlorothiazide (HCTZ, Urozide)	PO, 25–100 mg in one to two divided doses (max 100 mg/day)
indapamide (Lozide)	PO, 1.25–5.0 mg qd (max 5 mg/day)
metolazone (Zaroxolyn)	PO, 5–20 mg qd
Loop (High-Ceiling) Type	
bumetanide (Burinex)	PO, 0.5–2.0 mg qd or twice a day (bid) (max 10 mg/day)
	IM/IV, 0.5-1 mg/dose, may repeat in 2-3 hours if diuretic response is not achieved for up to 2 doses (max 10 mg/day)
furosemide (Lasix) (see Chapter 54, page 692, for the Prototype Drug box)	PO, 20–80 mg given in increments of 6-24 hours (max 600 mg/day)
	IM/IV, 20-40 mg/dose; can be given as frequent as every 6 hours (q6h) if needed

Compliance is very important with diuretics. In order to effectively monitor therapy, the nurse would encourage the client to take the medication exactly as prescribed. Salt substitutes are not recommended because they contain potassium instead of sodium and may cause serious cardiovascular effects.

Treating Hypertension with Diuretics

51.7 Diuretics are often the first-line medications for HTN because they have few side effects and can control minor to moderate hypertension.

Diuretics were the first class of drug used to treat HTN in the 1950s. Despite many advances in pharmacotherapy, diuretics are still considered first-line drugs for this disease because they produce few adverse effects and are very effective at controlling mild to moderate HTN. Although sometimes used alone, they are frequently prescribed with other antihypertensive drugs to enhance their effectiveness. Diuretics are also used to treat heart failure (Chapter 54) and kidney disorders (Chapter 52).

Although many different diuretics are available for hypertension, all produce a similar result: the reduction of blood volume through the urinary excretion of water and electrolytes. **Electrolytes** are ions such as sodium (Na^+), calcium (Ca^{+2}), chloride (Cl^-), and potassium (K^+). The mechanism by which diuretics reduce blood volume (specifically where and how the kidney is affected) differs among the various classes of diuretic. Details of the mechanisms of action of the diuretic classes are discussed in Chapter 53.

When a drug changes urine composition or output, electrolyte depletion is possible; the specific electrolyte lost is dependent on the mechanism of action of the particular drug. Potassium loss (hypokalemia) is of particular concern for loop and thiazide diuretics. Others such as triamterene have less tendency to cause potassium depletion and, for this reason, are called potassium-sparing diuretics. Taking potassium supplements with potassium-sparing diuretics may result in dangerously high potassium levels in the blood (hyperkalemia), leading to cardiac conduction abnormalities.

Nursing Considerations

The role of the nurse in diuretic therapy for HTN involves careful monitoring of the client's condition and providing education as it relates to the prescribed drug regimen. Diuretics decrease circulating blood volume, causing the potential development of dehydration and hypovolemia. **Orthostatic hypotension** (postural hypotension) may occur because of the reduced blood volume. The client may experience dizziness and faintness after rising too quickly from a sitting or lying position.

Because diuretics act by altering the physiological balance of fluid and electrolytes in the body, careful monitoring of laboratory values and body weight is essential. The client should be weighed daily and changes should be reported. The nurse must measure fluid intake and output and assess insensible losses that may occur

due to exercise or illness, such as high fever. The ankles and lower legs should be examined for signs of pitting edema, which signifies fluid retention. Auscultate breath and heart sounds when taking vital signs; rales or rhonchi may indicate pulmonary edema, and "crackles" and murmurs may indicate impending heart failure. Electrolyte levels, particularly sodium and potassium, should be monitored carefully during diuretic therapy. Diuretics can reduce the renal excretion of lithium, causing this drug to build up to toxic levels. Most diuretics are contraindicated in clients who are unable to produce urine (anuria).

Because diuretics cause frequent urination, assess the client's ability to safely go to the bathroom, or secure a urinal or bedside commode as needed. Diuretics should be administered early in the day so that sleep is not interrupted by frequent urination.

Photosensitivity is also a side effect of many diuretics. Photosensitization occurs when a drug, absorbed into the bloodstream, enters the skin. Sunlight, also absorbed by the skin, chemically changes the drug, and the new compound triggers a reaction in the body.

Potassium-Sparing Diuretics Potassium-sparing diuretics should not be used in clients with renal insufficiency or hyperkalemia since potassium levels may rise to life-threatening levels. Potassium-sparing diuretics are not normally used for pregnant or lactating women, as they are pregnancy category C (triamterene, spironolactone). Uric acid levels may increase, and clients with a history of gout or kidney stones may not tolerate these diuretics. Complete blood counts (CBCs) should be obtained periodically throughout therapy, as agranulocytosis and other hematological disorders may occur. Because white blood cell levels may be too low to combat infections, clients should report fever, rash, and sore throat. Spironolactone can cause gynecomastia (breast enlargement) and androgenic effects such as testicular atrophy or accelerated hair growth (hirsutism) in females. Clients should avoid excess potassium in their diet and salts that contain potassium (e.g., KCl).

Thiazide and Thiazide-Like Diuretics Because thiazide and thiazide-like diuretics alter blood chemistry, including fluid and electrolyte balance, laboratory values (K^+, Cl^-, Na^+, Ca^{+2}, Mg^{+2}, CBC, blood urea nitrogen [BUN], creatinine, cholesterol, and serum lipids) should be closely monitored. These drugs may cause excess potassium excretion; therefore, clients should increase potassium in their diet. Potassium supplements may be necessary. These diuretics can cause hyperglycemia and decrease the effectiveness of oral antidiabetic drugs. Because uric acid levels may increase, clients should be monitored for signs and symptoms of gout.

Because thiazides may increase blood lipids, these agents should be used cautiously in clients with existing hyperlipidemia. Cautious use is advised during pregnancy (category B) and lactation, as these diuretics cross the placenta and are secreted into breast milk. Thiazides may exacerbate systemic lupus erythematosus (SLE) and therefore are contraindicated in this condition. Elderly clients are at increased risk for electrolyte imbalances due to physiological changes in the kidneys related to aging. Losses of potassium and magnesium caused by thiazide diuretics increase the risk for digoxin (Lanoxin, Toloxin) toxicity.

Loop (High-Ceiling) Diuretics The efficacious loop, or high-ceiling, group of diuretics is more likely to cause severe potassium loss, hypovolemia, and hypotension compared to other diuretic classes. The client's blood pressure should be monitored frequently, especially with intravenous (IV) administration. Loop diuretics are ototoxic—an effect more likely to occur in clients with renal insufficiency or when high doses are administered. Hearing loss usually reverses when the drug is discontinued. Loop diuretics may also increase glucose and uric acid levels; therefore, these laboratory values should be monitored during therapy.

See Nursing Process Focus: Clients Receiving Diuretic Therapy for specific teaching points.

NCLEX Success Tips

Treatment of Ménière's disease may include diuretics, such as hydrochlorothiazide (Urozide, HCTZ), which may reduce potassium levels. The nurse should instruct the client to increase his or her intake of bananas, tomatoes, and oranges because these foods are high in potassium.

Hydrochlorothiazide causes increased urination and decreased swelling (if there is edema) and weight loss. It is important to check and record weight two to three times per week at the same time of day with similar amount of clothing.

Hydrochlorothiazide is a diuretic that is prescribed for lower blood pressure and may cause dizziness and faintness when the client stands up suddenly. This can be prevented or decreased by changing positions slowly.

NURSING PROCESS FOCUS

Clients Receiving Diuretic Therapy

Assessment	Potential Nursing Diagnoses/Identified Patterns
Prior to administration: • Obtain complete health history, including allergies, drug history, and possible drug interactions. • Obtain vital signs; assess in context of client's baseline values. • Obtain baseline weight. • Auscultate chest sounds for rales or rhonchi indicative of pulmonary edema. • Assess lower limbs for edema; note character and level (e.g., "++ pitting"). • Obtain blood and urine specimens for laboratory analysis.	• Need for knowledge regarding drug therapy • Risk for fluid and electrolyte imbalance • Increased urinary elimination related to diuretic use • Fatigue

Planning: Client Goals and Expected Outcomes

The client will:

• Exhibit a reduction in systolic and diastolic blood pressure
• Demonstrate an understanding of the drug's action by accurately describing drug side effects and precautions
• Maintain normal serum electrolyte levels during drug therapy

Implementation

Interventions (Rationales)	Client Education/Discharge Planning
• Monitor laboratory values. (Diuretic therapy affects the results of laboratory tests.) • Monitor vital signs, especially blood pressure. (Diuretics reduce circulating blood volume, resulting in lowered blood pressure.) • Observe for changes in level of consciousness, dizziness, fatigue, postural hypotension. (These are caused by reduction in circulating blood volume.) • Monitor for fluid overload and signs of HF. (Increased blood volume causes increased cardiac workload and pulmonary edema.) • Measure intake and output and daily body weight. • Monitor nutritional status. (Electrolyte imbalances may be counteracted by dietary measures.) • Observe for signs of hyperglycemia. Use drug with caution in diabetics. • Monitor liver and kidney function. (Drugs are metabolized by the liver and excreted by the kidneys.) • Observe for hypersensitivity reaction. • Observe for signs of infection. • Monitor hearing and vision. (Loop diuretics such as furosemide are ototoxic. Thiazide diuretics increase serum digitalis levels, which may produce visual changes.)	Instruct client to: • Inform laboratory personnel of diuretic therapy when providing blood or urine samples • Carry a wallet card or wear medical identification jewellery to indicate diuretic therapy Instruct client to: • Monitor vital signs, particularly blood pressure, as specified by the nurse, ensuring proper use of home equipment • Withhold medication for severe hypotensive readings as specified by the nurse (e.g., "hold for levels below 88/50") Instruct client to: • Report dizziness or lightheadedness • Rise slowly from prolonged periods of sitting or lying down • Obtain blood pressure readings in sitting, standing, and supine positions to monitor fluctuations in blood pressure Instruct client: • To immediately report any severe shortness of breath, frothy sputum, profound fatigue, and edema in extremities

- Monitor for alcohol and caffeine use. (Alcohol potentiates the hypotensive action of some thiazide diuretics. Caffeine is a mild diuretic that could increase diuresis.)
- Ensure client safety. Monitor ambulation until effects of drug are known. (Postural hypotension can be caused by drug.)
- Monitor reactivity to light exposure. (Drug causes photosensitivity.)

- To measure and monitor fluid intake and output and to weigh self daily
- To consume enough *plain* water to remain adequately, but not overly, hydrated
- To avoid excessive heat, which contributes to excessive sweating and fluid loss
- That increased urine output and decreased weight indicate that the drug is working

For clients who are taking potassium-wasting diuretics, instruct them to:

- Eat foods high in potassium, such as bananas, apricots, kidney beans, sweet potatoes, and peanut butter

For clients who are taking potassium-sparing diuretics, instruct them to:

- Avoid foods high in potassium
- Consult with the nurse before using vitamin/mineral supplements or electrolyte-fortified sports drinks
- Instruct client to report signs and symptoms of diabetes mellitus to the healthcare provider

Instruct client to:

- Immediately report symptoms of metabolic imbalances: nausea and vomiting, profound weakness, lethargy, muscle cramps, depression or disorientation, hallucinations, heart spasms, palpitations, numbness or tingling in limbs, extreme thirst, changes in urine output
- Adhere to laboratory testing regimen as ordered by the healthcare provider
- Instruct client to immediately report difficulty breathing, throat tightness, hives or rash, muscle cramps, or tremors
- Instruct client or caregiver to report any flu-like symptoms: shortness of breath, fever, sore throat, malaise, joint pain, or profound fatigue

Instruct client to:

- Report changes in hearing such as ringing or buzzing in the ears or becoming "hard of hearing"
- Report dimness of sight, seeing halos, or "yellow vision"
- Instruct client to restrict consumption of alcohol and caffeine

Instruct client to:

- Obtain help before getting out of bed or attempting to walk alone
- Avoid sudden changes of position to prevent dizziness caused by postural hypotension
- Avoid driving and other activities requiring mental alertness or physical coordination until effects of the drug are known

Instruct client to:

- Limit exposure to the sun
- Wear dark glasses and light-coloured, loose-fitting clothes when outdoors

---

Evaluation of Outcome Criteria

Evaluate the effectiveness of drug therapy by confirming that client goals and expected outcomes have been met (see "Planning").

See Table 51.4 for a list of drugs to which these nursing actions apply.

| PROTOTYPE DRUG | Hydrochlorothiazide (HCTZ, Urozide) |

Actions and Uses: Hydrochlorothiazide is the most widely prescribed diuretic for HTN, belonging to a large class known as the thiazides. Like many diuretics, it produces few adverse effects and is effective at producing a 10 to 20 mm Hg reduction in blood pressure.

However, clients with severe HTN may require the addition of a second drug from a different class to control their blood pressure.

HCTZ acts on the kidney tubule to decrease the reabsorption of sodium. Normally, more than 99% of the sodium entering the kidney is reabsorbed by the body so that very little leaves via the urine. When HCTZ blocks this reabsorption, more sodium is sent into the urine. When sodium moves across the tubule, water flows with it; as a result, blood volume decreases and blood pressure falls. The volume of urine produced is directly proportional to the amount of sodium reabsorption blocked by the diuretic.

Administration Alerts:

* Administer the drug early in the day to prevent nocturia.
* Hydrochlorothiazide is pregnancy category B.

Pharmacokinetics: HCTZ is rapidly absorbed, widely distributed, and excreted mainly unchanged by the kidneys. It has a half-life of 6 to 15 hours.

Adverse Effects and Interactions: The most common side effects of HCTZ involve potential electrolyte imbalances; potassium is lost along with the sodium. Because hypokalemia may cause conduction abnormalities in the heart, clients must closely monitor their dietary potassium and are usually asked to increase their potassium intake as a precaution.

HCTZ potentiates the action of other antihypertensives and increases responsiveness to skeletal muscle relaxants. Thiazides may reduce the effectiveness of anticoagulants, sulfonylureas, antigout drugs, and antidiabetic drugs, including insulin. Cholestyramine (Questran, Olestyr), colestipol (Colestid), and nonsteroidal anti-inflammatory drugs (NSAIDs) reduce the effectiveness of HCTZ.

Central nervous system (CNS) depressants such as alcohol, barbiturates, and opioids may exacerbate the orthostatic hypotension caused by HCTZ. Steroids or amphotericin B (Fungizone) increase potassium loss when given with HCTZ, leading to hypokalemia.

HCTZ increases the risk for serum toxicity of the following drugs: digitalis, lithium (Carbolith, Lithane), allopurinol (Zyloprim), diazoxide (Proglycem), anesthetics, and antineoplastics. HCTZ alters vitamin D metabolism and causes calcium conservation; use of calcium supplements may cause hypercalcemia.

Use with caution with herbal supplements, such as ginkgo, which may produce a paradoxical increase in blood pressure.

CALCIUM CHANNEL BLOCKERS

Calcium channel blockers exert a number of beneficial effects on the heart and blood vessels by blocking calcium ion channels. They are widely used in the treatment of hypertension and other cardiovascular diseases. These agents are shown in Table 51.5.

TABLE 51.5 Calcium Channel Blockers for Hypertension

Drug	Route and Adult Dose
Selective: For Blood Vessels	
amlodipine (Norvasc)	PO, 5–10 mg qd (max 10 mg/day)
felodipine (Plendil)	PO, 5–10 mg qd (max 10 mg/day)
Pr nifedipine (Adalat)	PO, 10–20 mg three times a day (tid) (max 180 mg/day)
Non-Selective: For Blood Vessels and Heart	
diltiazem (Cardizem, Tiazac) (see Chapter 50, page 620, for the Prototype Drug box)	PO, 60–120 mg sustained release bid; 120-360 mg/day extended release
verapamil (Isoptin) (see Chapter 55, page 706, for the Prototype Drug box)	PO, 80–160 mg tid (max 360 mg/day)

Treating Hypertension with Calcium Channel Blockers

51.8 Calcium channel blockers block calcium ions from entering cells and cause smooth muscle in arterioles to relax, thus reducing blood pressure. CCBs have emerged as major drugs in the treatment of hypertension.

Calcium channel blockers (CCBs) comprise a group of drugs used to treat a number of cardiovascular diseases, including angina pectoris, dysrhythmias, and HTN. After CCBs were first approved for the treatment of angina in the early 1980s, it was quickly noted that a "side effect" was the lowering of blood pressure in hypertensive clients. CCBs have since become a widely prescribed class of drug for hypertension.

Contraction of muscle is regulated by the amount of calcium ion inside the cell. When calcium enters the cell through channels in the plasma membrane, muscular contraction is initiated. CCBs block these channels and inhibit calcium from entering the cell, limiting muscular contraction. At low doses, CCBs cause the smooth muscle in arterioles to relax, lowering peripheral resistance and decreasing blood pressure. Some CCBs such as nifedipine (Adalat) are selective for calcium channels in arterioles, while others such as verapamil (Isoptin) affect channels in both arterioles and the myocardium. CCBs vary in their potency and by the frequency and types of side effects they produce. Uses of CCBs in the treatment of angina and dysrhythmias are discussed in Chapters 50 and 55, respectively.

Nursing Considerations

The role of the nurse in CCB therapy for HTN involves careful monitoring of the client's condition and providing education as it relates to the prescribed drug regimen. CCBs affect the coronary arteries and myocardial conductivity and contractility. Electrocardiogram (ECG), heart rate, and blood pressure should be assessed prior to therapy; vital signs should be monitored regularly thereafter. CCBs reduce myocardial contractility and can increase the risk for, and worsen, heart failure. CCBs are contraindicated in clients with certain types of heart conditions, such as sick sinus syndrome or third-degree atrioventricular (AV) block without the presence of a pacemaker. Due to their potent vasodilating effects, CCBs can cause reflex tachycardia, a condition that occurs when the heart rate increases due to the rapid fall in blood pressure created by the drug. CCBs are pregnancy category C.

Tachycardia and hypotension are most pronounced with IV administration of CCBs. Grapefruit juice increases absorption of these drugs from the gastrointestinal (GI) tract, causing greater than expected effects from the dose. Grapefruit juice taken with a sustained-release CCB could result in rapid toxic overdose, which is a medical emergency.

Teaching strategies regarding calcium channel blockers should include goals; reasons for obtaining baseline data such as vital signs, tests for cardiac and renal disorders (including ECG), and laboratory values; and possible side effects. See Nursing Process Focus: Clients Receiving Calcium Channel Blocker Therapy for specific teaching points.

NURSING PROCESS FOCUS

Clients Receiving Calcium Channel Blocker Therapy

Assessment	Potential Nursing Diagnoses/Identified Patterns
Prior to administration: • Obtain complete health history, including data on recent cardiac events, allergies, drug history, and possible drug interactions. • Obtain ECG and vital signs; assess in context of client's baseline values. • Assess neurological status and level of consciousness. • Auscultate chest sounds for rales or rhonchi indicative of pulmonary edema. • Assess lower limbs for edema; note character and level.	• Need for knowledge regarding drug therapy • Decreased cardiac output • Altered tissue perfusion

Planning: Client Goals and Expected Outcomes

The client will:

• Exhibit a reduction in systolic and diastolic blood pressure
• Demonstrate an understanding of the drug's action by accurately describing drug side effects and precautions.

Implementation

Interventions (Rationales)	Client Education/Discharge Planning
• Monitor vital signs. • Observe for changes in level of consciousness, dizziness, fatigue, postural hypotension (caused by vasodilation). • Observe for paradoxical increase in chest pain or angina symptoms (related to severe hypotension). • Obtain blood pressure readings in sitting, standing, and supine positions to monitor fluctuations in blood pressure. • Monitor for signs of heart failure. (CCBs can decrease myocardial contractility, increasing the risk for heart failure.) • Monitor for fluid accumulation. • Measure intake and output and daily body weight. (Edema is a side effect of some CCBs.) • Observe for hypersensitivity reaction. • Monitor liver and kidney function. (CCBs are metabolized in the liver and excreted by the kidneys.) • Observe for constipation. Client may need an increase in dietary fibre, or laxatives. • Ensure client safety. • Monitor ambulation until response to drug is known (due to postural hypotension caused by drug).	Instruct client to: • Monitor vital signs, particularly blood pressure, as specified by the nurse, ensuring proper use of home equipment • Withhold medication for severe hypotensive readings as specified by the nurse (e.g., "hold for levels below 88/50") • Immediately report palpitations or rapid heartbeat Instruct client to: • Report dizziness or lightheadedness • Report chest pain or other angina-like symptoms • Rise slowly from prolonged periods of sitting or lying • Instruct client to immediately report any severe shortness of breath, frothy sputum, profound fatigue, and swelling. These may be signs of heart failure or fluid accumulation in the lungs Instruct client to: • Avoid excessive heat, which contributes to excessive sweating and fluid loss • Measure and monitor fluid intake and output and to weigh self daily • Consume enough *plain* water to remain adequately, but not overly, hydrated • Instruct client to immediately report difficulty breathing, throat tightness, hives or rash, muscle cramps, or tremors Instruct client to: • Report signs of liver toxicity: nausea, vomiting, anorexia, bleeding, severe upper or abdominal pain, heartburn, jaundice, or a change in the colour or character of stools • Report signs of renal toxicity: fever; flank pain; changes in urine output, colour, or character (e.g., cloudy, with sediment) • Adhere to laboratory testing regimens as ordered by the healthcare provider Advise client to: • Maintain adequate fluid and fibre intake to facilitate stool passage • Use a bulk laxative or stool softener, as recommended by the healthcare provider • Instruct client to avoid driving and other activities requiring mental alertness or physical coordination until effects of the drug are known

Evaluation of Outcome Criteria

Evaluate the effectiveness of drug therapy by confirming that client goals and expected outcomes have been met (see "Planning").

See Table 51.5 for a list of drugs to which these nursing actions apply.

NCLEX Success Tip

Headache is a common side effect of nifedipine but is not an indicator to stop taking the drug.

| PROTOTYPE DRUG | Nifedipine (Adalat) |

Actions and Uses: Nifedipine is a CCB generally prescribed for HTN and variant or vasospastic angina. It is occasionally used to treat Raynaud's phenomenon and hypertrophic cardiomyopathy. Nifedipine acts by selectively blocking calcium channels in myocardial and vascular smooth muscle, including that in the coronary arteries. This results in less oxygen use by the heart, an increase in cardiac output, and a fall in blood pressure. Nifedipine is as effective as diuretics and beta-adrenergic blockers at reducing blood pressure.

Administration Alerts:

* Do not administer immediate-release formulations of nifedipine if an impending MI is suspected or within 2 weeks following a confirmed MI.

* Administer nifedipine capsules or tablets whole. If capsules or extended-release tablets are chewed, divided, or crushed, the entire dose will be delivered at once.

* Nifedipine is pregnancy category C.

Pharmacokinetics: Nifedipine is well absorbed, but bioavailability is reduced due to first-pass metabolism. It is 92% to 98% protein bound and is mostly metabolized by the liver. It has a half-life of 2 to 5 hours.

Adverse Effects and Interactions: Side effects of nifedipine are generally minor and related to vasodilation, such as headache, dizziness, and flushing. Fast-acting forms of nifedipine can cause reflex tachycardia. To avoid rebound hypotension, discontinuation of the drug should occur gradually. In rare cases, nifedipine may cause a paradoxical increase in anginal chest pain possibly related to hypotension or HF.

Nifedipine may increase serum levels of digitalis, cimetidine (Tagamet), and ranitidine. Nifedipine may potentiate the effects of warfarin (Coumadin), resulting in increased international normalized ratio (INR). Potentiation may also occur with fentanyl (Duragesic) anesthesia, resulting in severe hypotension and increased fluid volume requirements. Grapefruit juice may cause enhanced absorption of nifedipine. Nifedipine may reduce serum levels of quinidine.

Alcohol potentiates the vasodilating action of nifedipine and could lead to syncope caused by a severe drop in blood pressure. Nicotine causes vasoconstriction, counteracting the desired effect of nifedipine.

Use with caution with melatonin, which may increase blood pressure and heart rate.

DRUGS AFFECTING THE RENIN-ANGIOTENSIN-ALDOSTERONE SYSTEM

Drugs that affect the renin-angiotensin-aldosterone pathway decrease blood pressure and increase urine volume. They are widely used

TABLE 51.6 ACE Inhibitors and Angiotensin II Receptor Blockers for Hypertension

Drug	Route and Adult Dose
ACE Inhibitors	
benazepril (Lotensin)	PO, 10–40 mg in one to two divided doses (max 40 mg/day)
captopril (Capoten)	PO, 6.25–25 mg tid (max 450 mg/day)
Pr enalapril (Vasotec)	PO, 5–40 mg in one to two divided doses (max 40 mg/day)
fosinopril (Monopril)	PO, 5–40 mg qd (max 40 mg/day)
lisinopril (Prinivil, Zestril) (see Chapter 54, page 687, for the Prototype Drug box)	PO, 2.5–40 mg qd (max 80 mg/day)
quinapril (Accupril)	PO, 10–20 mg qd (max 80 mg/day)
ramipril (Altace)	PO, 2.5–20 mg qd (max 20 mg/day)
trandolapril (Mavik)	PO, 1–4 mg qd (max 8 mg/day)
Angiotensin II Receptor Blockers	
candesartan (Atacand)	PO, start at 16 mg qd (range 8–32 mg divided once or twice daily)
eprosartan (Teveten)	PO, 400–800 mg/day in one to two divided doses (max 800 mg/day)
irbesartan (Avapro)	PO, 150–300 mg qd (max 300 mg/day)
losartan (Cozaar)	PO, 25–100 qd (max 100 mg/day)
telmisartan (Micardis)	PO, 40 mg qd, may increase to 80 mg/day
valsartan (Diovan)	PO, 80–320 mg qd (max 320 mg/day)

in the treatment of HTN, HF, and MI. These agents are listed in Table 51.6.

Pharmacotherapy with ACE Inhibitors and Angiotensin II Receptor Blockers

51.9 Drugs blocking the renin-angiotensin-aldosterone system prevent the intense vasoconstriction caused by angiotensin II. These drugs also decrease blood volume, which enhances their antihypertensive effect.

The renin-angiotensin-aldosterone system is a key homeostatic mechanism that controls blood pressure and fluid balance. This mechanism is illustrated in Figure 51.6. Renin is an enzyme secreted by specialized cells in the kidney when blood pressure falls or when there is a decrease in sodium flowing through the kidney tubules. Once in the blood, renin converts the inactive liver protein angiotensinogen to angiotensin I. When passing through the lungs, angiotensin I is converted to **angiotensin II**, one of the most potent natural vasoconstrictors known. The enzyme responsible for the final step in this system is **angiotensin-converting enzyme (ACE)**. The intense vasoconstriction of arterioles caused by angiotensin II raises blood pressure by increasing peripheral resistance.

Angiotensin II also stimulates the secretion of two hormones that markedly affect blood pressure: aldosterone and ADH.

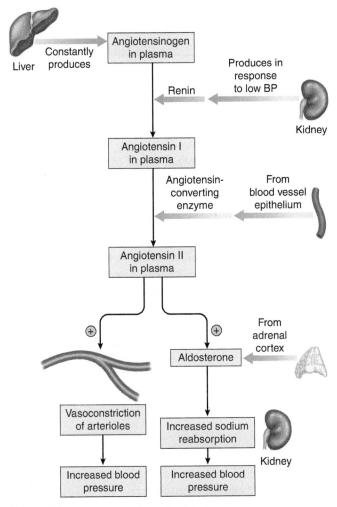

Figure 51.6 The renin-angiotensin-aldosterone pathway.

Aldosterone, a hormone from the adrenal cortex, increases sodium reabsorption in the kidney. The enhanced sodium reabsorption helps the body to retain water, thus increasing blood volume and raising blood pressure. ADH, a hormone from the posterior pituitary, enhances the conservation of water by the kidneys. This raises blood pressure by increasing blood volume. Pharmacotherapy with ADH is discussed in Chapter 27.

First detected in the venom of pit vipers in the 1960s, ACE inhibitors have been approved as drugs for hypertension since the 1980s. Since then, drugs in this class have become key agents in the treatment of HTN. ACE inhibitors block the effects of angiotensin II, decreasing blood pressure through two mechanisms: lowering peripheral resistance and decreasing blood volume. Some ACE inhibitors have also been approved for the treatment of myocardial infarction and heart failure, as discussed in Chapters 50 and 54, respectively.

Side effects of ACE inhibitors are usually minor and include persistent cough and postural hypotension, particularly following the first few doses of the drug. The most serious adverse effect is the development of angioedema, an acute hypersensitivity reaction featuring non-inflammatory swelling of the skin, mucous membranes, and other organs. Angioedema may be life-threatening; laryngeal swelling can lead to asphyxia and death. The development of angioedema usually occurs within days of taking an

ACE inhibitor; however, it can occur as a delayed reaction months or even years into therapy.

A second method of altering the renin-angiotensin-aldosterone pathway is by blocking the action of angiotensin II *after* it is formed. The **angiotensin II receptor blockers (ARBs)** block receptors for angiotensin II in arteriolar smooth muscle and in the adrenal gland, thus causing blood pressure to fall. Their effects of arteriolar dilation and increased sodium excretion by the kidneys are similar to those of the ACE inhibitors. ARBs differ in how they are distributed and eliminated from the body. Some ARBs need to be converted to an active form in the body before they can lower blood pressure. Drugs in this class are often combined with drugs from other classes for the management of HTN.

The most common side effects of ARBs are cough, elevated potassium levels, low blood pressure, dizziness, headache, drowsiness, diarrhea, abnormal taste sensation (metallic or salty taste), and rash. Since ARBs may increase blood levels of potassium, the use of potassium supplements, salt substitutes that contain potassium, or other drugs that increase potassium may result in excessive blood potassium levels. ARBs may also increase the blood concentration of lithium. Compared to ACE inhibitors, cough occurs less often with ARBs. ARBs may cause birth defects if used during pregnancy.

New drugs that use different methods of altering the renin-angiotensin-aldosterone system are in clinical trials and show promise for the pharmacotherapy of HTN. Aldosterone receptor blockers prevent aldosterone from reaching its receptors in the kidneys, resulting in less sodium reabsorption and a fall in blood pressure. Vasopeptidase inhibitors have dual inhibition of both ACE and the enzyme neutral endopeptidase (NEP). Inhibiting NEP leads to a buildup of natriuretic peptides, which causes both vasodilation and diuresis.

Nursing Considerations

The role of the nurse in ACE inhibitor therapy for HTN involves careful monitoring of the client's condition and providing education as it relates to the prescribed drug regimen. ACE inhibitors act on the vasodilator bradykinin, causing a chronic, dry or "tickling," non-productive cough. Because cough is a significant symptom, it should always be investigated. For example, dry cough may result from vasovagal stimulation related to angina or impending MI. Severe paroxysms of dry cough may indicate laryngeal swelling and the onset of life-threatening angioedema. Suspected angioedema requires immediate discontinuance of ACE inhibitor therapy. Due to the risk for angioedema, resuscitative equipment and oxygen apparatus should remain accessible during initiation of ACE

CONNECTIONS | **Special Considerations**

◀ Ethnicity and ACE Inhibitor Action

ACE inhibitors can have unique idiosyncratic effects on individuals of particular racial and/or ethnic groups. In particular, African-Canadian clients experience reduced efficacy and a higher incidence of angioedema. Inform clients of African descent of the variations in drug effectiveness and increased risk for angioedema.

inhibitor therapy, especially during IV administration. Intravenous administration may initiate an immediate, profound hypotensive response and possible loss of consciousness.

Contraindications to ACE inhibitors include hypersensitivity and any history of angioedema (idiopathic, familial, or drug induced). They should not be given to clients with heart failure who are presently taking a potassium-sparing diuretic. ACE inhibitors increase the risk for stroke, angina, peripheral artery disease (PAD), and GI bleeding. ACE inhibitors are also contraindicated in pregnancy (category D), in lactation, and in clients with renal insufficiency.

See Nursing Process Focus: Clients Receiving ACE Inhibitor Therapy for specific teaching points.

| PROTOTYPE DRUG | **Enalapril (Vasotec)** |

Actions and Uses: Enalapril is one of the most frequently prescribed ACE inhibitors for HTN. Unlike captopril (Capoten)—the first ACE inhibitor to be marketed—enalapril has a prolonged half-life, which permits administration once or twice daily. Enalapril acts by reducing angiotensin II and aldosterone levels to produce a significant reduction in blood pressure with few side effects. Enalapril may be used by itself or in combination with other antihypertensives to minimize side effects.

Administration Alerts:

- Enalapril may produce a first-dose phenomenon resulting in profound hypotension, which may lead to syncope.
- Enalapril is pregnancy category D.

Pharmacokinetics: Enalapril is converted by the liver to its active metabolite, enalaprilat. All ACE inhibitors cross the placenta. Enalapril and enalaprilat have a half-life of 11 hours and are excreted by the kidneys.

Adverse Effects and Interactions: ACE inhibitors such as enalapril can cause potassium and creatine levels in the blood to increase. They cause fewer cardiac side effects than beta-adrenergic blockers. Enalapril may cause orthostatic hypotension when moving quickly from a supine to an upright position. A rapid fall in blood pressure may occur following the first dose. Other side effects include headache and dizziness.

ACE inhibitors can cause life-threatening angioedema, neutropenia, and agranulocytosis. Renin-releasing antihypertensives potentiate the action of enalapril and can cause profound hypotension.

Thiazide diuretics increase potassium loss; potassium-sparing diuretics increase serum potassium and may be prescribed with thiazide diuretics to decrease risk for hypokalemia. Enalapril may induce lithium toxicity by reducing renal clearance of lithium. NSAIDs may reduce the effectiveness of ACE inhibition.

NURSING PROCESS FOCUS

Clients Receiving ACE Inhibitor Therapy

Assessment	Potential Nursing Diagnoses/Identified Patterns
Prior to administration: - Obtain complete health history, including data on recent cardiac events and any incidence of angioedema, allergies, drug history, and possible drug interactions. - Obtain ECG and vital signs; assess in context of client's baseline values. - Assess neurological status and level of consciousness. - Obtain blood and urine specimens for laboratory analysis.	- Need for knowledge regarding drug therapy - Risk for injury related to orthostatic hypotension - Ineffective tissue perfusion - Risk for hyperkalemia

Planning: Client Goals and Expected Outcomes
The client will: - Exhibit a reduction in systolic and diastolic blood pressure - Maintain normal serum electrolyte levels during drug therapy - Demonstrate an understanding of the drug's action by accurately describing drug side effects and precautions

Implementation

Interventions (Rationales)	Client Education/Discharge Planning
- Monitor for first-dose phenomenon of profound hypotension. - Observe for hypersensitivity reaction, particularly angioedema. (Angioedema may arise at any time during ACE inhibitor therapy but is generally expected shortly after initiation of therapy.) - Monitor for the presence of blood dyscrasia. - Observe for signs of infection: fever, sore throat, malaise, joint pain, ecchymoses, profound fatigue, shortness of breath, or pallor. (Bruising is a sign of bleeding, which can indicate the presence of a serious blood disorder.)	- Warn the client about the first-dose phenomenon; reassure that this effect diminishes with continued therapy Instruct client: - That changes in consciousness may occur due to rapid reduction in blood pressure; immediately report a feeling of faintness - That the drug takes effect in approximately 1 hour and peaks in 3 to 4 hours; rest in the supine position beginning 1 hour after administration and for 3 to 4 hours after the first dose - To always arise slowly, avoiding sudden posture changes

- Monitor for changes in level of consciousness, dizziness, drowsiness, or lightheadedness. (Signs of decreased blood flow to the brain are due to the drug's vasodilating hypotensive action. Sudden syncopal collapse is possible.)
- Monitor for persistent dry cough. (This may be triggered by bradykinin's proinflammatory action.)
- Monitor changes in cough pattern. (This may indicate another disease process.)
- Monitor for dehydration or fluid overload. (Dehydration causes low circulating blood volume and will exacerbate hypotension. Severe dehydration may trigger syncope and collapse. Pitting edema indicates fluid retention and can be a sign of HF; it may also indicate reduced drug efficacy.)
- Monitor for hyperkalemia (may occur due to reduced aldosterone levels).
- Monitor for liver and kidney function. (ACE inhibitors are metabolized by the liver and excreted by the kidneys.)
- Ensure client safety (due to postural hypotension caused by drug).
- Monitor ambulation until response to the drug is known.

Instruct client:

- To immediately report difficulty breathing, throat tightness, muscle cramps, hives or rash, and tremors. These symptoms can occur with the first dose or much later as a delayed reaction
- That angioedema can be life-threatening and to call emergency medical services if severe dyspnea or hoarseness is accompanied by swelling of the face or mouth

Instruct client to:

- Immediately report any flu-like symptoms
- Observe for bruising; signs of bleeding from the nose, mouth, or GI tract ("coffee grounds" vomit or tarry stools); menstrual flooding; or bright red rectal bleeding

Instruct client to:

- Report dizziness or fainting that persists beyond the first dose, as well as unusual sensations (e.g., numbness and tingling) or other changes in the face or limbs
- Contact the healthcare provider, before the next scheduled dose of the drug, if fainting occurs

Instruct client to:

- Expect persistent dry cough
- Report any change in the character or frequency of cough. Any cough accompanied by shortness of breath, fever, or chest pain should be reported *immediately* because it may indicate MI
- Sleep with head elevated if cough becomes troublesome when in supine position
- Use non-medicated, sugar-free lozenges or hard candies to relieve cough

Instruct client to:

- Observe for signs of dehydration such as oliguria, dry lips and mucous membranes, or poor skin turgor
- Report any bodily swelling that leaves sunken marks on the skin when pressed
- Measure and monitor fluid intake and output and weigh self daily
- Monitor increased need for fluid caused by vomiting, diarrhea, or excessive sweating
- Avoid excessive heat, which contributes to sweating and fluid loss
- Consume adequate amounts of *plain* water

Instruct client to:

- Immediately report signs of hyperkalemia: nausea, irregular heartbeat, profound fatigue or muscle weakness, and slow or faint pulse
- Avoid consuming electrolyte-fortified snacks or sports drinks that may contain potassium
- Avoid using salt substitute (KCl) to flavour foods
- Consult the healthcare provider before taking any nutritional supplements containing potassium

Instruct client to:

- Report signs of liver toxicity: nausea; vomiting; anorexia; diarrhea; rash; jaundice; abdominal pain, tenderness, or distention; or change in the colour or character of stools
- Discontinue drug immediately and contact the healthcare provider if jaundice occurs
- Adhere to laboratory testing regimen as ordered by the healthcare provider

Instruct client to:

- Obtain help prior to getting out of bed or attempting to walk alone
- Avoid driving or other activities that require mental alertness or physical coordination until effects of the drug are known

---

Evaluation of Outcome Criteria

Evaluate the effectiveness of drug therapy by confirming that client goals and expected outcomes have been met (see "Planning").

See Table 51.6 under "ACE Inhibitors" for a list of drugs to which these nursing actions apply.

ADRENERGIC AGENTS

The adrenergic receptor has been a site of pharmacological action in the treatment of HTN since the first such drugs were developed in the 1950s. Blockade of adrenergic receptors results in a number of beneficial effects on the heart and blood vessels, and these autonomic drugs are used for a wide variety of cardiovascular disorders. Table 51.7 lists the adrenergic agents used for hypertension.

NCLEX Success Tips

Clonidine (Catapres), a central-acting adrenergic antagonist, is used as adjunctive therapy in opioid withdrawal. It reduces sympathetic outflow from the central nervous system. It is mainly used for the treatment of blood pressure. Dry mouth, impotence, and sleep disturbances are possible adverse effects.

Pheochromocytoma causes excessive production of epinephrine and norepinephrine, natural catecholamines that raise the blood pressure. Phentolamine (OraVerse, Rogitine), an alpha-adrenergic given by IV bolus or drip, antagonizes the body's response to circulating epinephrine and norepinephrine, reducing blood pressure quickly and effectively. Although methyldopa is an antihypertensive agent available in parenteral form, it is not effective in treating hypertensive emergencies.

The combination of antipsychotics with beta blockers may lead to an increase in the effect of both medications, therefore caution should be taken before combining these drugs.

Pharmacotherapy with Adrenergic Agents

51.10 Antihypertensive autonomic agents are available to block alpha$_1$, beta$_1$, and/or beta$_2$ receptors, or stimulate alpha$_2$ receptors in the brainstem (centrally acting).

As discussed in Chapter 12, the autonomic nervous system controls involuntary functions of the body such as heart rate, pupil size, and smooth muscle contraction, including that in the arterial walls. Stimulation of the sympathetic division causes fight-or-flight responses such as faster heart rate, an increase in blood pressure, and bronchodilation. Peripheral blood vessels are innervated only by sympathetic nerves.

Antihypertensive drugs have been developed that affect the sympathetic division through a number of distinct mechanisms, although they all have in common the effect of lowering blood pressure. These mechanisms include the following:

- Blockade of alpha$_1$ receptors in the arterioles
- Selective blockade of beta$_1$ receptors in the heart
- Non-selective blockade of both beta$_1$ and beta$_2$ receptors
- Non-selective blockade of both alpha and beta receptors

TABLE 51.7 Adrenergic Agents for Hypertension

Drug	Route and Adult Dose
Beta Blockers	
atenolol (Tenormin): beta$_1$ (see Chapter 50, page 618, for the Prototype Drug box)	PO, 25–50 mg qd (max 100 mg/day)
bisoprolol: beta$_1$	PO, 2.5–10 mg qd (max 20 mg/day)
metoprolol (Lopressor): beta$_1$ (see Chapter 50, page 619, for the Prototype Drug box)	PO, 50–200 mg qd–bid (max 450 mg/day)
propranolol (Inderal): beta$_1$ and beta$_2$ (see Chapter 55, page 704, for the Prototype Drug box)	PO, immediate release, 120-240 mg/day in two to three divided doses (max 640 mg/day); extended release, 120-160 mg qd (max 640 mg/day)
timolol: beta$_1$ and beta$_2$ (see Chapter 63, page 823, for the Prototype Drug box)	PO, 20-40 mg in two divided doses (max 60 mg/day)
Alpha$_1$ Blockers	
Pr doxazosin (Cardura)	PO, 1–2 mg at bedtime (hs), (max 16 mg/day)
prazosin (Minipress) (see Chapter 14, page 152, for the Prototype Drug box)	PO, 0.5 mg bid-tid (max 20 mg/day)
terazosin (Hytrin)	PO, 1 mg hs, usual dosage range is 1-2 mg/day (max 20 mg/day)
Alpha$_2$-Adrenergic Agonists	
clonidine (Catapres)	PO, start with 0.1 mg bid; usual dose is 0.1-0.2 mg bid (max 2.4 mg/day)
methyldopa	PO, 250 mg bid or tid (max 3 g/day)
Alpha$_1$ and Beta Blockers (Centrally Acting)	
labetalol (Trandate)	PO, 100 mg bid, may increase to 200–400 mg bid (max 1200–2400 mg/day)

- Stimulation of alpha$_2$ receptors in the brainstem (centrally acting)
- Blockade of peripheral adrenergic neurons

The earliest drugs for HTN were non-selective agents, blocking nerve transmission at the ganglion or blocking both alpha and beta receptors. Although these non-selective agents revolutionized the treatment of HTN, they produced significant side effects. They are rarely used today because the selective agents are more efficacious and better tolerated by clients.

The side effects of adrenergic blockers are generally predictable extensions of the fight-or-flight response. The alpha$_1$-adrenergic blockers tend to cause orthostatic hypotension when moving quickly from a supine to an upright position. Dizziness, nausea, bradycardia, and dry mouth are also common. Less common, though sometimes a major cause for nonadherence, is their adverse effect on male sexual function. These agents can cause decreased libido and erectile dysfunction (impotence). Non-selective beta blockers will slow the heart rate and cause bronchoconstriction. They should be used with caution in clients with asthma or HF. Some beta blockers are associated with clinical depression.

Some adrenergic agents cause blood pressure reduction by acting on alpha$_2$ receptors in the CNS. Methyldopa is converted to a "false" neurotransmitter in the brainstem, thus causing a shortage of the "real" neurotransmitter and inhibition of the sympathetic nervous system. Clonidine, an alpha$_2$ agonist, affects alpha-adrenergic receptors in the cardiovascular control centres in the brainstem. The centrally acting agents have a tendency to produce sedation and may cause depression. They are not considered first-line drugs in the pharmacotherapy of HTN.

Nursing Considerations

The role of the nurse in adrenergic agent therapy for HTN involves careful monitoring of the client's condition and providing education as it relates to the prescribed drug regimen. Because of their widespread therapeutic applications, discussions of adrenergic antagonists appear in many chapters in this text. Prototype drugs include atenolol (Tenormin), metoprolol (Lopressor), carvedilol (Coreg), propranolol (Inderal), and timolol.

Alpha$_1$ Antagonists Alpha$_1$ antagonists are indicated for HTN. These drugs are also used to treat benign prostatic hyperplasia (BPH) and urinary obstruction because they relax smooth muscle in the prostate and bladder neck, thus reducing urethral resistance. The client may experience hypotension with the first few doses of these medications, and orthostatic hypotension may persist throughout treatment. The first-dose phenomenon, especially syncope, can occur. Therefore, it remains important to assess blood pressure prior to and routinely during therapy in order to maintain client safety. Assess for common side effects such as weakness, dizziness, headache, and GI complaints such as nausea and vomiting. Older adults are especially prone to the hypotensive and hypothermic effects related to vasodilation caused by these drugs. Drugs in this group are pregnancy category C (terazosin [Hytrin], prazosin [Minipress]). See Nursing Process Focus: Clients Receiving Adrenergic Antagonist Therapy in Chapter 14 for more information.

Alpha$_2$ Agonists Alpha$_2$ agonists are centrally acting and have multiple side effects. These drugs are usually reserved to treat HTN uncontrolled by other drugs. Assess for the presence of common adverse effects such as orthostatic hypotension, sedation, decreased libido, impotence, sodium/water retention, and dry mouth. Alpha$_2$ agonists are pregnancy category B/C; these drugs are distributed into breast milk.

Beta Blockers Adrenergic antagonists may be cardioselective (beta$_1$) or non-specific (beta$_1$ and beta$_2$) receptor blockers. Cardioselective beta blockers decrease heart rate and affect myocardial conduction and contractility. Reduction in myocardial contractility reduces myocardial oxygen demand. Non-specific beta blockers produce the same effects but also act on the respiratory system and the blood vessels, producing vasoconstriction and bronchoconstriction. Be alert for signs of respiratory distress, including shortness of breath and wheezing, in clients on non-specific beta-blocking drugs. These side effects tend to occur at high doses and with older drugs. Beta blockers have several other important therapeutic applications. By decreasing the cardiac workload, beta blockers can ease the symptoms of angina pectoris (Chapter 50). By slowing conduction through the myocardium, beta blockers are able to treat certain types of dysrhythmia (Chapter 55). Other therapeutic uses include the treatment of heart failure (Chapter 54), myocardial infarction (Chapter 50), and migraines (Chapter 23).

Because all beta blockers affect myocardial contractility, monitor heart rate, rhythm, and sounds as well as the ECG. Beta blockers can produce bradycardia and heart block. Reduction in heart rate can also contribute to fatigue and activity intolerance. Beta blockers cause the heart rate to become less responsive to exertion. Clients should be advised to monitor their pulse and blood pressure daily. Because beta blockers inhibit the sympathetic response to low blood glucose, diabetic clients should be warned that symptoms of hypoglycemia (diaphoresis, nervousness, and palpitation) may be less observable while on beta-blocker therapy.

See Nursing Process Focus: Clients Receiving Beta-Adrenergic Antagonist Therapy for more information.

NURSING PROCESS FOCUS

Clients Receiving Beta-Adrenergic Antagonist Therapy

Assessment	Potential Nursing Diagnoses/Identified Patterns
Prior to administration: • Obtain complete health history, including allergies, drug history, and possible drug interactions. • Assess vital signs, urinary output, and cardiac output (initially and throughout therapy). • Assess for presence of respiratory disease, including asthma and chronic obstructive pulmonary disease.	• Need for knowledge regarding drug therapy • Decreased cardiac output • Risk for injury related to orthostatic hypotension • Sexual dysfunction • Nonadherence with therapeutic regimen

---

Planning: Client Goals and Expected Outcomes

The client will:

- Exhibit a reduction in systolic and diastolic blood pressure
- Report a decrease in cardiac symptoms such as chest pain and dyspnea on exertion
- Demonstrate an understanding of the drug's action by accurately describing drug side effects and precautions

---

Implementation

Interventions (Rationales)	Client Education/Discharge Planning
<ul><li>Monitor vital signs and pulse; observe for signs of bradycardia, heart failure, and pulmonary edema. (Beta blockers affect heart rate.)</li><li>Monitor for orthostatic hypotension when assisting client up from a supine position.</li><li>Observe for additional side effects such as fatigue and weakness.</li><li>In diabetic clients, monitor for hypoglycemia. (Beta-adrenergic blockers may prevent clients from experiencing common signs of low blood glucose levels.)</li><li>Observe for side effects such as drowsiness.</li><li>Measure intake and output; measure daily weight.</li></ul>	<ul><li>Instruct client to monitor vital signs, particularly blood pressure, as specified by the nurse, ensuring proper use of home equipment</li></ul>Instruct client to:<ul><li>Withhold medication for severe hypotensive readings as specified by the nurse (e.g., "hold for levels below 88/50")</li><li>Always arise slowly, avoiding sudden posture changes</li><li>Instruct client to report side effects such as slow pulse, difficulty breathing, dizziness, confusion, fatigue, weakness, and impotence</li><li>Instruct the diabetic client to check blood glucose levels and be more alert for and report signs of hypoglycemia</li><li>Instruct client to avoid driving and other activities requiring mental alertness or physical coordination until effects of the drug are known</li></ul>Instruct client to:<ul><li>Measure and monitor fluid intake and output and to weigh self daily</li><li>Consume enough *plain* water to remain adequately, but not overly, hydrated</li></ul>

Evaluation of Outcome Criteria

Evaluate the effectiveness of drug therapy by confirming that client goals and expected outcomes have been met (see "Planning").

See Table 51.7 under "Beta Blockers" for a list of drugs to which these nursing actions apply.

PROTOTYPE DRUG | **Doxazosin (Cardura)**

Actions and Uses: Doxazosin is a selective alpha$_1$-adrenergic blocker available only in oral form. Because it is selective for alpha$_1$ receptors in vascular smooth muscle, it has few adverse effects on other autonomic organs and is preferred over nonselective beta blockers. Doxazosin dilates arteries and veins and is capable of causing a rapid, profound fall in blood pressure. Clients who have difficulty urinating due to an enlarged prostate (e.g., BPH) sometimes receive this drug to relieve symptoms of dysuria.

Administration Alerts:

- Doxazosin may produce a first-dose phenomenon resulting in profound hypotension, which may lead to syncope.
- The first-dose phenomenon can recur when medication is resumed after a period of withdrawal and with dosage increases.
- Doxazosin is pregnancy category C.

Pharmacokinetics: Doxazosin is well absorbed and is 98% protein bound. It is extensively metabolized by the liver. It has a half-life of 22 hours.

Adverse Effects and Interactions: Upon starting doxazosin therapy, some clients experience orthostatic hypotension, although tolerance normally develops to this side effect after a few doses. Dizziness and headache are also common side effects, although they are rarely severe enough to cause discontinuation of therapy.

Oral cimetidine may cause a mild increase (10%) in the half-life of doxazosin. This increase is not considered to be clinically significant.

DIRECT VASODILATORS

Drugs that directly affect arteriolar smooth muscle are highly effective at lowering blood pressure but produce too many side effects to be drugs of first choice. These agents are shown in Table 51.8.

TABLE 51.8	Direct-Acting Vasodilators for Hypertension
Drug	**Route and Adult Dose**
Pr hydralazine (Apresoline)	PO, 10–50 mg qid (max 300 mg/day)
minoxidil (Loniten)	PO, 5–40 mg/day in a single or divided doses (max 100 mg/day)
nitroprusside (Nipride)	IV, start with 0.3-0.5 µg/kg/minute; increase every few minutes to achieve desired effect; average range is 1.5-10 µg/kg/minute (max 10 µg/kg/minute)

Treating Hypertension with Direct Vasodilators

51.11 A few medications lower blood pressure by acting directly to relax arteriolar smooth muscle, but these are not widely used due to their numerous side effects.

All antihypertensive classes discussed thus far lower blood pressure through indirect means by affecting enzymes (ACE inhibitors), autonomic nerves (alpha and beta blockers), or fluid volume (diuretics). It would seem that a more efficient way to reduce blood pressure would be to cause a direct relaxation of arteriolar smooth muscle; unfortunately, the direct vasodilator drugs have the potential to produce serious adverse effects. All direct vasodilators can produce **reflex tachycardia** as a compensatory response to the sudden decrease in blood pressure. Hydralazine (Apresoline) can induce a lupus-like syndrome. Pericardial effusions have been reported with minoxidil use. Because safer drugs are available, oral direct vasodilators are rarely prescribed.

One direct-acting vasodilator, nitroprusside (Nipride), is specifically used for those clients who have aggressive, life-threatening hypertension that must be quickly controlled. Nitroprusside, with a half-life of only 2 minutes, has the capability of lowering blood pressure almost instantaneously upon IV administration. It is essential to continuously monitor clients receiving this drug in order to avoid hypotension because of overtreatment. In conditions such as malnutrition or surgery or high rates of infusion, nitroprusside may lead to depletion of sulphur stores and accumulation of cyanide and its toxic metabolites.

Nursing Considerations

Direct vasodilators are primarily used in emergency situations when it is necessary to reduce blood pressure quickly. In the critical care or emergency department setting, the client will likely undergo continuous monitoring of vital signs, ECG, and pulse oximetry. The nurse may also be expected to auscultate blood pressures every 5 to 15 minutes during the drug infusion. Closely observe monitoring equipment to assess heart rate and ECG for reflex tachycardia.

Contraindications include hypersensitivity, coronary artery disease, rheumatic mitral valve disease, cerebrovascular disease, renal insufficiency, and systemic lupus erythematosus. Direct vasodilators can cause priapism, a sustained, painful penile erection unrelieved by orgasm. Clients may feel embarrassed by priapism and

CONNECTIONS | Natural Therapies

◀ Hawthorn for Hypertension

A number of botanicals have been reported to possess antihypertensive activity, including hawthorn, which is sometimes called mayflower. Hawthorn (*Crataegus laevigata*) is a thorny shrub or small tree that is widespread in North America, Europe, and Asia. In some cultures, the shrub is surrounded in magic and religious rites and is thought to ward off evil spirits. The ship *Mayflower* was named after this shrub.

Leaves, flowers, and berries of the plant are dried or extracted in liquid form. Active ingredients are flavonoids and procyanidins. Hawthorn has been purported to lower blood pressure after 4 weeks or longer of therapy, although the effect has been small. The mechanism of action may be inhibition of ACE or reduction of cardiac workload. Clients who are taking cardiac glycosides should avoid hawthorn because it has the ability to decrease cardiac output. Clients should be advised not to rely on any botanical for the treatment of hypertension without frequent measurements of blood pressure to be certain therapy is effective.

be reluctant to report this side effect. They should be warned that priapism constitutes a medical emergency; if not treated promptly, permanent impotence may result.

There are specific considerations for the various types of direct vasodilators. For minoxidil (Loniten) therapy, monitor blood pressure and pulse in both arms while the client is lying, sitting, and standing to assess for orthostatic hypotension. The client should be informed that these agents may cause elongation, thickening, and increased pigmentation of body hair. This is normal and will stop when the drug is discontinued.

Intravenous nitroprusside is a chemically unstable solution. The only diluent compatible with nitroprusside is 5% dextrose in water (D_5W). This drug should never be mixed with any other drugs or diluents. Once dissolved in the vial, nitroprusside solution should be further diluted (in a 250 mL to 1 L bag of D_5W) to prevent phlebitis. Reconstituted nitroprusside solution is brown and considered stable for up to 24 hours, but the drug is exceptionally light sensitive. Once reconstituted, wrap the IV bag and tubing in an opaque substance (e.g., aluminum foil); labelling should appear on the wrap as well as on the bag itself. The drug solution should be checked periodically and the drug discarded if the colour of the solution changes.

See Nursing Process Focus: Clients Receiving Direct Vasodilator Therapy for specific teaching points.

PROTOTYPE DRUG | Hydralazine (Apresoline)

Actions and Uses: Hydralazine was one of the first oral antihypertensive drugs marketed in North America. It acts through direct vasodilation of vascular smooth muscle. Although it produces an effective reduction in blood pressure, drugs in other antihypertensive classes have largely replaced hydralazine. The drug is available in both oral and parenteral formulations.

NURSING PROCESS FOCUS

Clients Receiving Direct Vasodilator Therapy

Assessment	Potential Nursing Diagnoses/Identified Patterns
Prior to administration: • Obtain complete health history, including allergies, drug history, and possible drug interactions. • Obtain ECG and vital signs; assess in context of client's baseline values. • Auscultate heart and chest sounds. • Assess neurological status and level of consciousness. • Obtain blood and urine specimens for laboratory analysis.	• Need for knowledge regarding drug therapy • Risk for fluid and electrolyte imbalance • Ineffective tissue perfusion • Excess fluid volume • Risk for injury related to orthostatic hypotension • Risk for impaired skin integrity (e.g., IV vasodilators)

Planning: Client Goals and Expected Outcomes

The client will:

• Exhibit a reduction in systolic and diastolic blood pressure
• Demonstrate an understanding of the drug's action by accurately describing drug side effects and precautions

Implementation

Intervention (Rationales)	Client Education/Discharge Planning
• Observe for signs and symptoms of lupus. • Monitor client vital signs every 5 to 15 minutes and titrate infusion based on prescribed parameters. (These drugs cause rapid hypotension.) • Use with caution with impaired cardiac/cerebral circulation. (The hypotension produced by vasodilators may further compromise individuals who already suffer from ischemia.) • Monitor for dizziness. (This is a sign of hypotension that occurs because the brain is not getting enough blood flow.) • Evaluate need for lifestyle modifications. • Discontinue medication gradually. (Abrupt withdrawal of drug may cause rebound hypertension and anxiety.)	• Instruct client to report classic "butterfly rash" over the nose and cheeks, muscle aches, and fatigue when taking hydralazine • Instruct client to report any burning or stinging pain, swelling, warmth, redness, or tenderness at the IV insertion site, which may signal phlebitis Instruct client to: • Report angina-like symptoms: chest, arm, back and/or neck pain, palpitations • Report faintness; dizziness; drowsiness; any sensation of cold, numbness, or tingling; pale or dusky look to the hands and feet • Report headache or signs of stroke: facial drooping, visual changes, limb weakness, or paralysis • Monitor vitals signs (especially blood pressure) daily or as often as advised by the nurse Instruct client to: • Avoid driving and other activities requiring mental alertness or physical coordination until effects of the drug are known • Always arise slowly, avoiding sudden posture changes • Instruct client to comply with additional interventions for HTN such as weight reduction, modification of sodium intake, smoking cessation, exercise, and stress management • Instruct client to not suddenly stop taking the drug

Evaluation of Outcome Criteria

Evaluate the effectiveness of drug therapy by confirming that client goals and expected outcomes have been met (see "Planning").

See Table 51.8 for a list of drugs to which these nursing applications apply.

Administration Alerts:

• Abrupt withdrawal of the drug may cause rebound hypertension and anxiety.

• Hydralazine is pregnancy category C.

Pharmacokinetics: Hydralazine is rapidly absorbed, widely distributed, and mostly metabolized by the GI mucosa and liver. It has a half-life of 2 to 8 hours.

Adverse Effects and Interactions: Hydralazine may produce serious side effects, including severe reflex tachycardia.

Clients taking hydralazine sometimes receive a beta-adrenergic blocker to counteract this effect on the heart. The drug may produce a lupus-like syndrome with extended use. Sodium and fluid retention is a potentially serious adverse effect. Because of these side effects, the use of hydralazine is mostly limited to clients whose HTN cannot be controlled with other, safer medications.

Monoamine oxidase (MAO) inhibitors may potentiate hypotensive action. Other antihypertensive drugs given concomitantly can cause profound hypotension. NSAIDs may decrease the antihypertensive response.

CHAPTER
51

Understanding the Chapter

Key Concepts Summary

The numbered key concepts provide a succinct summary of the important points from the corresponding numbered section within the chapter. If any of these points are not clear, refer to the numbered section within the chapter for review.

51.1 High blood pressure is classified as essential (primary) or secondary. Uncontrolled hypertension can lead to chronic and debilitating disorders such as stroke, heart attack, and heart failure.

51.2 The three primary factors controlling blood pressure are cardiac output, peripheral resistance, and blood volume.

51.3 Many factors help to regulate blood pressure, including the vasomotor centre, baroreceptors and chemoreceptors in the aorta and internal carotid arteries, and the renin-angiotensin-aldosterone system.

51.4 Hypertension has been recently redefined as a sustained blood pressure of 140/90 mm Hg after multiple measurements made over several clinic visits. A person with sustained blood pressure of 120–139/80–89 mm Hg is said to be prehypertensive and is at increased risk for developing hypertension.

51.5 Because antihypertensive medications may have uncomfortable side effects, lifestyle changes such as proper diet and exercise should be implemented prior to and during pharmacotherapy to allow lower drug doses.

51.6 Pharmacotherapy of HTN often begins with low doses of a single medication. If ineffective, a second agent from a different class may be added to the regimen.

51.7 Diuretics are often the first-line medications for HTN because they have few side effects and can control minor to moderate hypertension.

51.8 Calcium channel blockers block calcium ions from entering cells and cause smooth muscle in arterioles to relax, thus reducing blood pressure. CCBs have emerged as major drugs in the treatment of hypertension.

51.9 Drugs blocking the renin-angiotensin-aldosterone system prevent the intense vasoconstriction caused by angiotensin II. These drugs also decrease blood volume, which enhances their antihypertensive effect.

51.10 Antihypertensive autonomic agents are available to block $alpha_1$, $beta_1$, and/or $beta_2$ receptors, or stimulate $alpha_2$ receptors in the brainstem (centrally acting).

51.11 A few medications lower blood pressure by acting directly to relax arteriolar smooth muscle, but these are not widely used due to their numerous side effects.

Chapter 51 Scenario

Elmer Foley is a 72-year-old Caucasian male with a 10-month history of uncontrolled HTN. Initially, Elmer was prescribed the thiazide diuretic HCTZ (Urozide). However, after 1 week of therapy his blood pressure has remained at 168/102 mm Hg. Next, Elmer's healthcare provider added an ACE inhibitor, captopril (Capoten), to the regimen. Still, Elmer's blood pressure remained above normal limits. Then the healthcare provider discontinued the captopril and started Elmer on hydralazine (Apresoline). With this visit, his blood pressure is 146/90 mm Hg.

When Elmer was first told he had HTN, he began many of the suggested lifestyle changes encouraged by his healthcare provider. He has lost a total of 15 kg (33 lb) since starting his diet 10 months ago. Elmer started walking daily for exercise and can now walk up to 1 mile without fatigue. He avoids all salty foods and diligently checks food labels for fat and salt content. Elmer occasionally drinks a glass of wine, although never more than 1 to 2 glasses per month. Although it was difficult for Elmer to stop smoking totally, he proudly claims that he has been smokeless for 8 months.

Critical Thinking Questions

1. How would you respond to Elmer's question, "What else can I do?" Is there anything else he can do to reduce his blood pressure?

2. Elmer wants to know why the previous therapies were unsuccessful. What would you say as his nurse?

3. As the nurse, how can you support Elmer before he leaves the clinic?

See Answers to Critical Thinking Questions in Appendix B.

NCLEX Practice Questions

1 Methyldopa is being initiated for a client with hypertension. Which health teaching would be most appropriate for this drug?

a. Avoid hot baths and showers and prolonged standing in one position.

b. This drug may discolour the urine a pinkish brown.

c. This drug may cause bloating and weight gain.

d. The tablet should be taken only with food or milk.

2 A client is receiving hydralazine (Apresoline) for elevated blood pressure levels. The nurse's care plan will include monitor the client for which adverse effect?

a. Atelectasis

b. Crystalluria

c. Photosensitivity

d. Orthostatic hypotension

3 The nurse determines that her client understands an important principle in self-administration of hydralazine (Apresoline) when the client makes which statement?

a. "I should not drive until my response to the drug therapy is determined."

b. "I can stop taking this medication once I begin to feel better."

c. "If I experience dizziness, I should take only half the dose."

d. "I should avoid air travel while taking this medication."

4 A client with hypertensive crisis is started on nitroprusside (Nipride) therapy. During the course of this treatment, the nurse will perform which priority intervention?

a. Monitoring for the presence or absence of bowel sounds

b. Obtaining urine samples for specific gravity measurements and glucose levels

c. Observing skin pressure points for turgor and integrity

d. Titrating intravenous infusion rate according to the blood pressure response

5 A 65-year-old Caucasian client has been newly diagnosed with hypertension, with an average blood pressure of 164/92 mm Hg. Which of the following drug groups will potentially be ordered initially? Select all that apply.

a. Beta blockers

b. Calcium channel blockers

c. Thiazide diuretics

d. Angiotensin-converting enzyme (ACE) inhibitors or angiotensin II receptor blockers (ARBs)

e. Direct-acting vasodilators

See Answers to NCLEX Practice Questions in Appendix A.

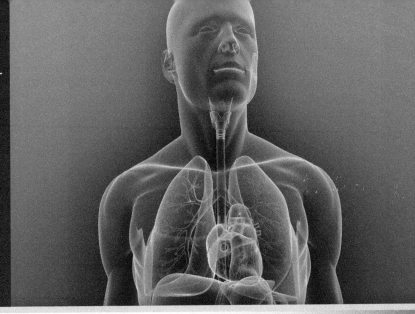

Sebastian Kaulitzki/Shutterstock

CHAPTER 52

Diuretic Therapy and Pharmacotherapy of Renal Failure

LEARNING OUTCOMES

After reading this chapter, the student should be able to:

1. Explain the role of the urinary system in maintaining fluid and electrolyte homeostasis.
2. Identify drug classes used for treating renal disorders and fluid excesses.
3. Explain the therapeutic action of each class of diuretic in relation to underlying pathophysiology.
4. Compare and contrast the loop, thiazide, and potassium-sparing diuretics in terms of action and indications for their use.
5. Discuss the role of the nurse regarding non-pharmacological care and client teaching.
6. Describe the nurse's role in the pharmacological management of clients who are receiving diuretics and other therapies for renal disorders.
7. Describe the adjustments in pharmacotherapy that must be considered in clients with renal failure.
8. For each of the drug classes listed in Prototype Drugs, identify a representative drug and explain its mechanism of action, therapeutic effects, and important adverse effects.
9. Describe and explain, based on pharmacological principles, the rationale for nursing assessment, planning, and interventions for clients who are receiving diuretics.
10. Use the nursing process to care for clients who are receiving therapy for fluid excess and renal disorders.

CHAPTER OUTLINE

▸ Brief Review of Renal Physiology

▸ Changes in Renal Filtrate Composition as a Result of Reabsorption and Secretion

▸ Renal Failure
  ▸ Pharmacotherapy of Renal Failure

▸ Diuretics
  ▸ Mechanism of Action of Diuretics
  ▸ Pharmacotherapy with Loop (High-Ceiling) Diuretics
  ▸ Pharmacotherapy with Thiazide and Thiazide-Like Diuretics
  ▸ Pharmacotherapy with Potassium-Sparing Diuretics
  ▸ Miscellaneous Diuretics for Specific Indications

The kidneys serve an amazing role in maintaining proper homeostasis. By filtering a volume equivalent to all of the body's extracellular fluid every 100 minutes, the kidneys are able to make immediate adjustments to fluid volume, electrolyte composition, and acid-base balance. When the kidney fails to adjust to changing internal conditions of the body, consequences of this become very serious and pharmacotherapy is often used to correct these imbalances. The purpose of this chapter is to examine agents that influence kidney function by increasing urine output or that treat clients with renal dysfunction. Chapter 53 covers agents that more specifically affect fluid, electrolyte, and acid-base imbalances.

Brief Review of Renal Physiology

52.1 The kidneys regulate fluid volume, electrolytes, and acid-base balance.

The urinary system consists of two kidneys, two ureters, one urinary bladder, and a urethra. Each kidney contains more than 1 million **nephrons**, the functional units of the kidney. As blood enters a nephron, it is filtered through a semipermeable membrane known as **Bowman's capsule**. Water and other small molecules readily pass through Bowman's capsule and enter the first section of the nephron, the **proximal tubule**. Once in the nephron, the fluid is called **filtrate**. After leaving the proximal tubule, the filtrate travels through the **loop of Henle** and, subsequently, the **distal tubule**. Nephrons empty their filtrate into common collecting ducts, which empty into larger collecting structures inside the kidney. Fluid that leaves the collecting ducts and enters subsequent portions of the kidney is called urine. Parts of the nephron are illustrated in Figure 52.1.

When most people think of the kidney, what comes to mind readily is excretion. Although this is certainly true, the kidneys have many other homeostatic functions. They are the primary organs that regulate fluid and electrolytes. They secrete renin (an enzyme that helps to regulate blood pressure), erythropoietin (a hormone that stimulates red blood cell production), and calcitrol (the active form of vitamin D). About 25% of the total cardiac output passes

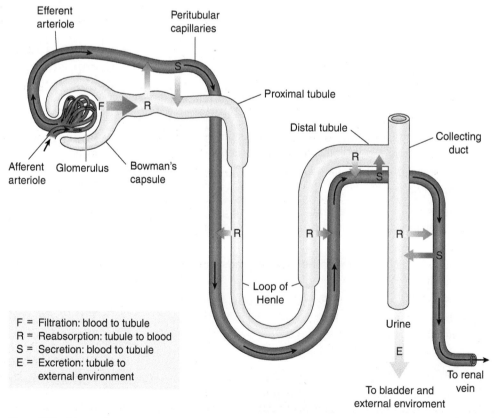

F = Filtration: blood to tubule
R = Reabsorption: tubule to blood
S = Secretion: blood to tubule
E = Excretion: tubule to external environment

Figure 52.1 The nephron.

through the kidneys each minute, and the nephrons perform the role of filtration, reabsorption, and secretion at the glomerulus, loop of Henle, proximal and distal tubules, and collecting tubules.

During filtration, substances that are too large to pass through the pores of Bowman's capsule, such as plasma proteins and the formed elements of the blood (erythrocytes, leucocytes and platelets), continue to circulate in the blood, which account for the oncotic pressure. The appearance of these substancess in urine is a sign of kidney pathology, as seen in glomerulonephritis. Water and other small molecules in plasma readily pass through the glomerular pores and enter the next section of the nephron.

The initial filtrate inside the nephron enters the proximal tubule, then the loop of Henle, and then the distal tubule. The composition of this filtrate continuously changes as it travels through the tubules, until it leaves the collecting ducts as urine. Approximately 1 mL of urine is produced each minute under normal circumstances.

Many drugs are small enough to pass through the glomerulus and enter the filtrate for excretion. If the drug is bound to a plasma protein, the resulting drug-protein complex becomes too large to be filtered and will continue circulating in the blood, thus prolonging the duration of action of such drugs. Plasma proteins such as albumin are too large to pass through the filter and will not be present in the urine of a healthy individual. The appearance of excess plasma proteins in urine (proteinuria or albuminuria) is a sign of kidney pathology. A common example is inflammation of the glomerulus (glomerulonephritis), when as a result of the inflammation the pores become larger and allow larger substances such as proteins to filter into the urine.

Changes in Renal Filtrate Composition as a Result of Reabsorption and Secretion

52.2 As filtrate travels through the nephron, its composition changes dramatically as a result of the processes of reabsorption and secretion.

When filtrate passes through Bowman's capsule, its composition is the same as plasma minus large proteins, such as albumin, that are too large to pass through the filter. As the filtrate travels through the nephron, its composition changes dramatically. Some substances in the filtrate pass across the walls of the nephron to re-enter the blood, a process known as **reabsorption**. Water is the most important molecule reabsorbed in the tubule. For every 178 L of water that enter the filtrate each day, 172 L are reabsorbed, leaving only 1.5 L to be excreted in the urine. Glucose, amino acids, and essential ions such as sodium, chloride, calcium, and bicarbonate are also reabsorbed.

Certain ions and molecules that are too large to pass through Bowman's capsule may still enter the urine by crossing from the blood to the filtrate by a process known as **secretion**. Potassium, phosphate, hydrogen, ammonium ions, and many organic acids enter the filtrate through this mechanism.

Reabsorption and secretion are critical to the pharmacokinetics of many drugs. Some drugs are reabsorbed, whereas others are secreted into the filtrate. For example, approximately 90% of a dose of penicillin G enters the urine through secretion. The

processes of reabsorption and secretion are shown in Figure 52.1. Hormones can markedly affect the degree of reabsorption in the renal tubule. Aldosterone, for example, exerts a major effect on the tubule by stimulating sodium reabsorption in the distal portions of the nephron. Under the influence of aldosterone, potassium excretion is increased because this ion is "exchanged" for sodium ions, which are reabsorbed. Antidiuretic hormone (ADH) also affects kidney function, increasing water reabsorption by making the collecting ducts become more permeable to water. The formation of urine is indeed a dynamic process that undergoes continuous modification as the filtrate travels down the tubule. Many drugs have the ability to either enhance or block the effects of hormones on tubular processes.

RENAL FAILURE

Renal failure is a decrease in kidney function that results in an inability to maintain electrolyte and fluid balance and excrete nitrogenous waste products. Renal failure may be acute or chronic and may result from disorders of other body systems or be intrinsic to the kidney itself. The primary treatment goal is to maintain blood flow through the kidney and adequate urine output. Renal failure may significantly affect the success of pharmacotherapy.

Pharmacotherapy of Renal Failure

52.3 The dosage levels for most medications must be adjusted in clients with renal failure. Diuretics may be used to maintain urine output while the cause of the hypoperfusion is treated.

Before pharmacotherapy may be considered in a client with renal failure, an accurate diagnosis of the kidney impairment is necessary. The basic diagnostic test is a **urinalysis**, which examines urine for the presence of blood cells, proteins, pH, specific gravity, ketones, glucose, and microorganisms. Although it is easy to perform, the urinalysis is nonspecific and does not identify the etiology of the kidney disease. Many diseases can cause abnormal urinalysis values. Serum creatinine and blood urea nitrogen (BUN) are additional laboratory measures used to detect kidney diseases. To provide a more definitive diagnosis, diagnostic imaging such as computed tomography, sonography, or magnetic resonance imaging may be necessary. Renal biopsy may be performed to obtain a more specific diagnosis. The best marker for estimating kidney function is the **glomerular filtration rate (GFR)**, which is the volume of water filtered through the Bowman's capsules per minute. The GFR can be used to predict the onset and progression of kidney failure, and it indicates the ability of the kidneys to excrete drugs from the body. With normal values ranging from 90 to 120 mL/minute, a progressive decline in GFR indicates a reduction in the number of functioning nephrons. As nephrons "die," however, the remaining healthy ones have the ability to compensate by increasing their filtration capacity. Because of this, clients with significant kidney damage may be asymptomatic until 50% or more of the nephrons have become non-functional and the GFR has fallen to less than half its normal value.

Renal failure is classified as acute or chronic. Acute renal failure requires immediate treatment because retention of nitrogenous waste products such as urea and creatinine in the body, known as **azotemia**, can result in death if untreated. The most common cause of acute renal failure is renal hypoperfusion—lack of sufficient blood flowing through the kidneys. Hypoperfusion can lead to permanent damage to kidney cells. To correct this type of renal failure, the cause of the hypoperfusion must be quickly identified and corrected. Potential causes include heart failure, dysrhythmias, hemorrhage, and dehydration. Pharmacotherapy with nephrotoxic drugs can also lead to either acute or chronic renal failure. It is good practice for the nurse to remember common nephrotoxic drugs so that kidney function may be continuously monitored during therapy with these drugs.

Chronic renal failure occurs over a period of months or years. More than half of the cases of chronic renal failure occur in clients with long-standing hypertension or diabetes mellitus. Due to its long development and nonspecific symptoms, chronic renal failure may go undiagnosed for many years, until the impairment becomes irreversible. In end-stage renal disease, dialysis and kidney transplantation become treatment alternatives.

Pharmacotherapy of renal failure attempts to treat the cause of the dysfunction. Diuretics are given to increase urine output as long as renal function is possible, and cardiovascular drugs are commonly administered to treat underlying hypertension or heart failure. Dietary management is often necessary to prevent worsening of renal impairment. Depending on the stage of the disease, dietary management may include protein restriction and reduction of sodium, potassium, phosphorus, and magnesium. A summary of the pharmacological agents used to treat kidney failure is given in Table 52.1.

The nurse serves a key role in recognizing and responding to renal failure. Once a diagnosis is established, all nephrotoxic medications should be either discontinued or used with extreme caution. Common nephrotoxic drugs include nonsteroidal anti-inflammatory drugs (NSAIDs), aminoglycoside antibiotics, amphotericin B (Fungizone), many antineoplastic agents, and angiotensin-converting enzyme (ACE) inhibitors in volume-depleted clients. Because the kidneys excrete most drugs, medications will require a significant dosage reduction in clients who have moderate to severe renal

failure. The importance of this cannot be overemphasized: administering the "average" dose to a client who is in severe renal failure can have fatal consequences.

DIURETICS

Diuretics are drugs that adjust the volume and/or composition of body fluids. They are of particular value in the treatment of renal failure, hypertension, and heart failure (by removing edema fluid).

Mechanism of Action of Diuretics

52.4 Diuretics are drugs that increase urine output, usually by blocking sodium reabsorption.

A **diuretic** is a drug that increases urine output. Mobilizing excess fluid in the body for the purpose of excretion is particularly desirable in the following conditions:

- Hypertension
- Heart failure

TABLE 52.1 Pharmacological Management of Renal Failure

Complication	Pathogenesis	Treatment
Anemia	Hypoperfusion of kidneys results in less erythropoietin synthesis	erythropoietin (epoetin alfa, Procrit, Epogen)
Hyperkalemia	Kidneys are unable to adequately excrete potassium	Dietary restriction of potassium; polystyrene sulfate (Kayexalate) with sorbitol
Hyperphosphatemia	Kidneys are unable to adequately excrete phosphate	Dietary restriction of phosphate; phosphate binders such as calcium carbonate (Os-Cal 500, others), calcium acetate (PhosLo), or sevelamer HCl (Renagel)
Hypervolemia	Hypoperfusion of kidneys leads to water retention	Dietary restriction of sodium; loop diuretics in acute conditions, thiazide diuretics in mild conditions
Hypocalcemia	Hyperphosphatemia leads to loss of calcium	Usually corrected by reversing the hyperphosphatemia but additional calcium supplements may be necessary
Metabolic acidosis	Kidneys are unable to adequately excrete metabolic acids	sodium bicarbonate or sodium citrate

- Kidney failure
- Liver failure or cirrhosis
- Pulmonary edema

Most diuretics act by blocking sodium (Na^+) reabsorption in the nephron, thus sending more Na^+ to the urine. Chloride ion (Cl^-) follows sodium. Because water molecules also tend to travel with sodium ions, blocking the reabsorption of Na^+ will increase the volume of urination, known as diuresis. Some drugs, such as furosemide (Lasix), act by preventing the reabsorption of sodium in the loop of Henle. Because of the abundance of sodium in the filtrate within the loop of Henle, furosemide is capable of producing large increases in urine output. Other drugs, such as the thiazides, act on the distal tubule. Because most Na^+ has already been reabsorbed from the filtrate by the time it reaches the distal tubule, the thiazides produce less diuresis than furosemide. The sites in the nephron at which the various diuretics act are shown in Figure 52.2.

The amount of diuresis produced by a diuretic is directly related to the amount of sodium reabsorption that is blocked: those that block the most sodium are the most effective at increasing urine output. Diuretics also affect the renal excretion of ions such as magnesium, potassium, phosphate, calcium, and bicarbonate. It is important to remember that imbalances in virtually any electrolyte may occur during diuretic therapy.

Diuretics are classified into five major groups, based on differences in their chemical nature and mechanism of action.

- *Loop or high-ceiling.* These drugs prevent the reabsorption of Na^+ in the loop of Henle; therefore, they are called loop diuretics. Because there is an abundance of Na^+ in the filtrate within the loop of Henle, drugs in this class are capable of producing large increases in urine output.
- *Thiazides.* The largest diuretic class, the thiazides act by blocking Na^+ in the distal tubule. Because most Na^+ has already been reabsorbed from the filtrate by the time it reaches this part of the nephron, the thiazides produce less diuresis than loop diuretics.
- *Potassium-sparing.* The third major class is named potassium-sparing diuretics, because these drugs have minimal effect on potassium ion (K^+) excretion. These drugs produce a mild diuresis.

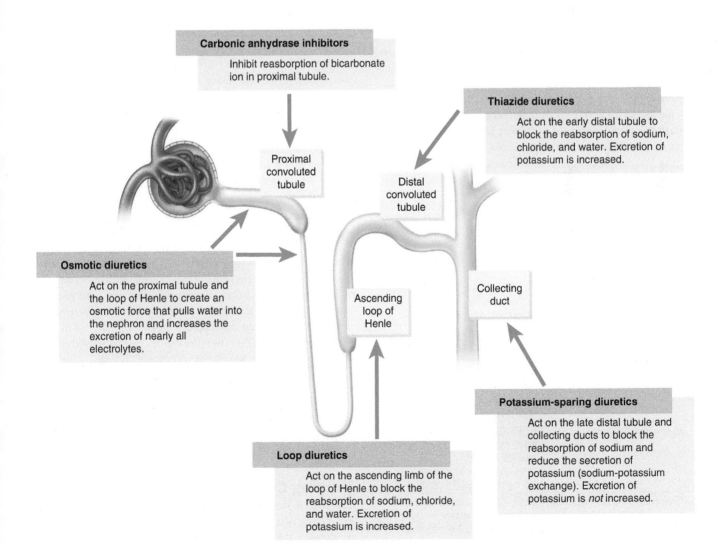

Figure 52.2 Sites of action of the diuretics.

- *Osmotic.* These drugs are relatively inert drugs that change the osmolality of filtrate, causing water to remain in the nephron for excretion. These drugs are very effective but are rarely prescribed because they can produce potentially serious adverse effects.
- *Carbonic anhydrase inhibitors.* These drugs block the enzyme in the nephron responsible for bicarbonate reabsorption. They produce a weak diuresis and are rarely used.

It is common practice to combine two or more drugs in the pharmacotherapy of hypertension and fluid retention disorders. The primary rationales for combination therapy are that the incidence of side effects is decreased and the pharmacological effect may be enhanced. For client convenience, some of these drugs are combined in single-tablet formulations. Examples of single-tablet diuretic combinations include the following:

- Aldactazide: hydrochlorothiazide and spironolactone
- Dyazide, Maxzide: hydrochlorothiazide and triamterene

Pharmacotherapy with Loop (High-Ceiling) Diuretics

52.5 The most efficacious diuretics are the loop (high-ceiling) agents that block the reabsorption of sodium in the loop of Henle.

The most effective diuretics are called loop (high-ceiling) diuretics. Drugs in this class act by blocking the reabsorption of sodium and chloride in the loop of Henle. When given intravenously (IV), they have the ability to cause large amounts of fluid to be excreted by the kidney in a very short time. Loop diuretics are used to reduce the edema associated with heart failure, hepatic cirrhosis, or chronic renal failure. The loop diuretics are listed in Table 52.2.

NCLEX Success Tip

Loop diuretics block sodium reabsorption in the ascending loop of Henle, which promotes water diuresis. They also dilate renal blood vessels. Although loop diuretics block potassium reabsorption, this is not usually a therapeutic action.

TABLE 52.2   Loop Diuretics

Drug	Route and Adult Dose
bumetanide (Burinex)	Orally (PO), 0.5–2 mg once (qd) or twice (bid) per day; may repeat at 4- to 5-hour intervals if needed (max 10 mg/day) IV/intramuscular (IM), 0.5–1 mg over 1–2 minutes, repeated every 2 to 2 hours (q2–3h) as needed (PRN) (max 10 mg/day)
ethacrynic acid (Edecrin)	PO, 50–200 mg/day in 1–2 divided doses; may increase by 25–50 mg PRN (max 400 mg/day) IV, 0.5–1 mg/kg or 50 mg up to 100 mg, may repeat if necessary
furosemide (Lasix) (see Chapter 54, page 692, for the Prototype Drug box)	PO, 20–80 mg in 1 or more divided doses (max 600 mg/day) IV/IM, 20–40 mg in 1 or more divided doses (max 600 mg/day)
torsemide (Demadex)	PO/IV, 10–20 mg/day (max 200 mg/day)

NCLEX Success Tip

Loop (high-ceiling) diuretics can lead to severe hypokalemia, which sometimes needs to be corrected to prevent alterations in cardiac rhythm by IV potassium chloride. When administering IV potassium chloride, the administration should not exceed 10 mEq/hour (10 mmol/L) or a concentration of 40 mEq/L (40 mmol/L) via a peripheral line.

Furosemide is the most commonly prescribed loop diuretic. A Prototype Drug box for furosemide is provided in Chapter 54 (page 692). Unlike the thiazide diuretics, furosemide is able to increase urine output even when blood flow to the kidneys is diminished, which makes it of particular value in clients with renal failure. All loop diuretics are available for either oral or parenteral administration and are extensively bound to plasma proteins. They have relatively short half-lives, and extended-release preparations are not available. Furosemide and torsemide (Demadex) are also approved for hypertension, although their short half-lives make them less suitable for this indication than thiazide diuretics.

NCLEX Success Tip

When administering furosemide, the nurse must keep in mind that as water and sodium are lost in the urine, blood pressure decreases, blood volume decreases, and urine output increases.

Torsemide has a longer half-life than furosemide, which offers the advantage of once-a-day dosing. Bumetanide (Burinex) is 40 times more potent than furosemide but has a shorter duration of action.

NCLEX Success Tip

The nurse should teach clients taking potassium-wasting diuretics to include dietary sources of potassium or to take a potassium supplement. Bananas, dried fruit, and oranges are examples of food high in potassium.

The rapid excretion of large amounts of water has the potential to produce serious adverse effects such as dehydration and electrolyte imbalances. Signs of dehydration include thirst, dry mouth, weight loss, and headache. Hypotension, dizziness, and fainting can result from the fluid loss. Excess potassium loss may result in dysrhythmias; potassium supplements may be indicated to prevent **hypokalemia**. Potassium loss is of particular concern to clients who are also taking digoxin (Lanoxin, Toloxin). Although rare, ototoxicity is possible and other ototoxic drugs such as the aminoglycoside antibiotics should be avoided during loop diuretic therapy. Because of the potential for serious side effects, the loop diuretics are normally reserved for clients with moderate to severe fluid retention or when other diuretics have failed to achieve therapeutic goals.

Nursing Considerations

The role of the nurse in loop diuretic therapy involves careful monitoring of the client's condition and providing education as it relates to the prescribed drug regimen. Prior to initiation of therapy, obtain baseline values for weight, blood pressure (sitting and supine), pulse, respiration, and electrolytes. Any sites of edema, and its extent, should be recorded. Measure the abdominal girth of clients with fluid in the abdomen (ascites). Loop diuretics should be used with caution in clients with cardiovascular disease, renal impairment, diabetes mellitus, or a history of gout. They should also be used with caution in clients who are pregnant or who are concurrently taking digoxin, lithium (Carbolith, Lithane), ototoxic drugs, NSAIDs, or other antihypertensives.

NCLEX Success Tips

The main reason to give a diuretic to a client with heart failure is to promote sodium and water excretion through the kidneys. As a result, the excessive body water that tends to accumulate in a client with heart failure is reduced, leading to weight loss. Monitoring the client's weight daily helps evaluate the effectiveness of diuretic therapy. The nurse should instruct the client to weigh himself or herself daily and to keep a record of the findings.

It is essential to check the client's serum potassium level when administering digoxin. Digoxin increases contractility of the heart and increases renal perfusion, resulting in a diuretic effect with increased loss of potassium and sodium. Hypokalemia increases the risk of digoxin toxicity.

Blood pressure and pulse rate should be monitored regularly. If a substantial drop in blood pressure occurs, the medication should be withheld and the blood pressure reported to the physician. Intake and output should be monitored, including weighing the client daily and evaluating for decreased edema. Potassium levels should be monitored closely, as loop diuretics cause potassium depletion. Closely observe elderly clients for weakness, hypotension, and confusion. Monitor laboratory results for electrolyte imbalance, elevated BUN, hyperglycemia, and anemia, which can be side effects of diuretics. Monitor vital signs and intake and output carefully to establish effectiveness of the medication. Rapid and excessive diuresis can result in dehydration, hypovolemia, and circulatory collapse.

Client education as it relates to loop diuretics should include goals, reasons for obtaining baseline data such as vital signs and tests for renal disorders, and possible side effects. The following are important points to include when teaching clients regarding loop diuretics:

- Weigh self daily, preferably in the morning before eating.
- Maintain a weight record.
- Monitor blood pressure and report substantial pressure drops.
- Make position changes slowly because diuretics in combination with other drugs can cause dizziness.
- Report any hearing loss or ringing in the ears.
- Monitor blood glucose diligently (for diabetic clients).
- Report tenderness or swelling in joints, which may indicate gout.

NCLEX Success Tip

Complete blood count (CBC) should be monitored in clients receiving furosemide because furosemide can cause agranulocytosis, anemia, leukopenia, and thrombocytopenia.

◄ Diuretic Therapy in Older Adult Clients

Diuretic therapy is commonly used to treat older adults with chronic diseases such as heart failure. The target goal for diuretic therapy is removal of excess fluid to reduce the cardiac workload. This can be a problem for older adults for several reasons. Diuretics can cause frequent urination, which can be inconvenient and increase the likelihood of incontinence in an elderly person. With the threat of this embarrassment, the older adult may opt for less participation in activities, resulting in social isolation. Depression may result. In addition to these risks, diuretics can cause electrolyte imbalances, making older adults susceptible to faintness, dizziness, and falls. Again, fear of these adverse effects can promote isolation. Nurses must assess for these concerns and work with older adults to help them maintain both diuretic therapy and the quality of their lives.

See Nursing Process Focus: Clients Receiving Diuretic Therapy at the end of the chapter for the complete nursing process applied to caring for clients who are receiving diuretic therapy.

Pharmacotherapy with Thiazide and Thiazide-Like Diuretics

52.6 The thiazides act by blocking sodium reabsorption in the distal tubule of the nephron, and they are the most widely prescribed class of diuretics.

The thiazides comprise the largest, most commonly prescribed class of diuretics. These drugs act on the distal tubule to block Na^+ reabsorption and increase potassium and water excretion. Their primary use is for the treatment of mild to moderate hypertension; however, they are also indicated for edema due to mild to moderate heart failure, liver failure, or renal failure. They are less efficacious than the loop diuretics because more than 90% of the Na^+ has already been reabsorbed by the time the filtrate reaches the distal tubule, and therefore they are not effective in clients with severe renal failure. The thiazide diuretics are listed in Table 52.3.

TABLE 52.3 Thiazide and Thiazide-Like Diuretics	
Drug	**Route and Adult Dose**
Short Acting	
Pr chlorothiazide (Diuril)	PO/IV, 500-1000 mg/day in 1–2 divided doses
hydrochlorothiazide (HCTZ, Urozide) (see Chapter 51, page 637, for the Prototype Drug box)	PO, 25–100 mg/day in 1–2 divided doses
Intermediate Acting	
metolazone (Zaroxolyn)	PO, 5–20 mg qd
Long Acting	
chlorthalidone	PO, 50–100 mg qd
indapamide (Lozide)	PO, 2.5–5 mg qd
methyclothiazide	PO, 2.5–10 mg qd

Thiazides are available only by the PO route with the exception of chlorothiazide (Diuril), which may be administered parenterally. All of the thiazide diuretics have equivalent effectiveness and safety profiles. They differ, however, in their potency and duration of action. For example, metolazone (Zaroxolyn) is 10 times more potent than hydrochlorothiazide (Urozide). At therapeutic doses, all thiazides produce the same level of diuresis.

Four drugs—chlorthalidone, indapamide (Lozide), metolazone, and quinethazone—are not true thiazides, but they are included with this drug class because they have similar actions and side effects.

Other than lack of ototoxicity, the side effects of the thiazides are identical to those of the loop diuretics, although their frequency is less. Diabetic clients should be made aware that thiazide diuretics sometimes raise blood glucose levels.

Nursing Considerations

The role of the nurse in thiazide diuretic therapy involves careful monitoring of the client's condition and providing education as it relates to the prescribed drug regimen. Prior to administering diuretics, assess for hypotension and withhold the medication if low blood pressure is present. Assess for hypersensitivity to thiazides or sulfonamides, anuria, and hypokalemia because thiazides are contraindicated in clients with these conditions. They should be used with caution in clients who are allergic to sulfa, are diabetic, or have impaired renal or hepatic function. Baseline laboratory tests such as CBC, electrolytes, BUN, creatinine, uric acid, and blood glucose should be obtained. All diuretics, including thiazide diuretics, reduce circulating blood volume, which may cause orthostatic hypotension and changes in serum electrolyte levels. Examine the skin and mucous membranes for turgor and moisture because diuretics are notorious for causing dehydration. Monitor vital signs, especially blood pressure, when caring for clients who are taking thiazides. Nursing Process Focus: Clients Receiving Diuretic Therapy at the end of the chapter provides a guide to the care of all individuals who are receiving diuretic therapy.

Because the effectiveness of diuretic therapy is measured in weight loss and fluid output, the client should be weighed at the same time of day, wearing the same type of clothing. A weight gain of more than 1 kg should be reported, as it may indicate fluid retention. The nurse must carefully monitor intake and output to determine hydration status and effectiveness of the medication. Conditions such as diarrhea, vomiting, or profuse sweating will increase fluid loss and put the client at greater risk for dehydration.

Assess for signs and symptoms of dehydration and excessive loss of sodium, potassium, and chloride ions. Concurrent therapy with digoxin requires careful monitoring to avoid excessive potassium loss. Like loop diuretics, the thiazides cause potassium depletion, so clients should be monitored for signs of hypokalemia. Dietary intake of high-sodium foods may negate the effects of thiazide diuretics in reducing blood pressure or relieving excessive fluid volume.

Some thiazide diuretics may cause hyperglycemia and glycosuria in diabetic clients. Blood glucose levels should be monitored closely and dosage adjustments of hypoglycemic drugs may be indicated. Also, some clients with gout may experience hyperuricemia secondary to the thiazide's interference with uric acid excretion. Monitor uric acid levels and assess for symptoms of gout such as pain, swelling, and redness in the joints.

Client education as it relates to thiazides should include goals, reasons for obtaining baseline data such as vital signs and laboratory work, and possible side effects. The following are important points to include when teaching clients regarding thiazide diuretics:

- Monitor blood pressure on a regular basis; withhold medication and report a blood pressure below specific written parameters.
- Weigh self every morning before breakfast, wearing the same weight of clothing.
- Consume foods that are high in potassium content, such as oranges, peaches, bananas, dried apricots, potatoes, tomatoes, and broccoli.
- Avoid foods that are high in sodium content, such as canned foods, "fast" foods, and frozen dinners.
- Protect skin from exposure to direct sunlight because these medications can cause photosensitivity.
- Take thiazide diuretics in the morning, when possible, to prevent the need to get up through the night to urinate.
- Keep a symptom log during the initial phase of therapy to assist the healthcare provider in tailoring dosage as needed.
- Use additional health promotional activities, in addition to diuretics, to help reduce blood pressure, such as smoking cessation, exercise, weight control, stress management, and moderate consumption of alcohol, if any.

See Nursing Process Focus: Clients Receiving Diuretic Therapy at the end of the chapter for the complete nursing process applied to caring for clients who are receiving diuretic therapy.

NCLEX Success Tips

Hydrochlorothiazide is a thiazide diuretic used in the management of mild to moderate hypertension and in the treatment of edema associated with heart failure, renal dysfunction, cirrhosis, corticosteroid therapy, and estrogen therapy.

Hydrochlorothiazide increases the excretion of sodium and water by inhibiting sodium reabsorption in the distal tubule of the kidneys. It promotes the excretion of chloride, potassium, magnesium, and bicarbonate. Side effects include drowsiness, lethargy, and muscle weakness.

PROTOTYPE DRUG	Chlorothiazide (Diuril)

Actions and Uses: The most common indication for chlorothiazide is mild to moderate hypertension. It may be combined with other antihypertensives in the multidrug therapy of severe hypertension. It is also prescribed to treat fluid retention due to heart failure, liver disease, and corticosteroid or estrogen therapy.

Administration Alerts:

- Give oral doses in the morning to avoid interrupted sleep due to nocturia.
- Give IV at a rate of 0.5 g over 5 minutes when administering intermittently.
- When administering IV, take special care to avoid extravasation, as this drug is highly irritating to tissues.
- Chlorothiazide is pregnancy category C.

Pharmacokinetics: Chlorothiazide is well absorbed after oral administration. When given orally, it may take as long as 4 weeks to obtain the optimum therapeutic effect. When given IV, results are seen in 15 to 30 minutes. It is widely distributed, crosses the placenta, and enters breast milk. It is excreted mainly unchanged in urine. Its half-life is 1.5 hours.

Adverse Effects and Interactions: Excess loss of water and electrolytes can occur during chlorothiazide pharmacotherapy. Symptoms include thirst, weakness, lethargy, muscle cramping, hypotension, and tachycardia. Due to the potentially serious consequences of hypokalemia, clients taking digoxin concurrently should be monitored carefully. The intake of potassium-rich foods should be increased, and potassium supplements may be indicated.

Chlorothiazide interacts with several drugs. For example, when administered with amphotericin B or corticosteroids, hypokalemic effects are increased. Antidiabetic medications such as sulfonylureas and insulin may be less effective when taken with chlorothiazide. Cholestyramine (Questran, Olestyr) and colestipol (Colestid) decrease absorption of chlorothiazide. Concurrent administration with digoxin may cause digitoxin toxicity due to increased potassium and magnesium loss. Alcohol potentiates the hypotensive action of some thiazide diuretics, and caffeine may increase diuresis.

Use with caution with herbal supplements, such as licorice, which, in large amounts, will create an additive effect of hypokalemia. Aloe may increase potassium loss.

Pharmacotherapy with Potassium-Sparing Diuretics

52.7 Though less efficacious than the loop diuretics, potassium-sparing diuretics are used in combination with other agents and help to prevent hypokalemia.

Hypokalemia is one of the most serious adverse effects of the thiazide and loop diuretics. The therapeutic advantage of the potassium-sparing diuretics is that mild diuresis can be obtained without affecting blood potassium levels. The potassium-sparing diuretics are listed in Table 52.4.

There are two distinct subclasses of potassium-sparing diuretics: sodium ion channel inhibitors and aldosterone antagonists.

Sodium Ion Channel Inhibitors

In the distal tubule, Na^+ is reabsorbed from the filtrate through sodium ion channels. As the sodium ion in the filtrate travels across the renal tubule cell and returns to the bloodstream, potassium ion moves in the opposite direction. In other words, as sodium ion is reabsorbed, potassium ion is secreted.

TABLE 52.4   Potassium-Sparing Diuretics

Drug	Route and Adult Dose
amiloride (Midamor)	PO, 5 mg qd (max 20 mg/day)
Pr spironolactone (Aldactone)	PO, 25–200 mg/day in 1–2 divided doses
triamterene	PO, 100–300 mg/day in 1–2 divided doses (max 300 mg/day)

Triamterene and amiloride (Midamor) block the Na^+ channel, causing sodium to stay in the filtrate. Because water always follows sodium ions, additional water remains in the filtrate and ultimately leaves in the urine. When the sodium ion channel is blocked, another important action occurs: potassium ion is not secreted to the filtrate. The body, therefore, does not lose potassium, as is the case with the thiazide and loop diuretics. Because most of the sodium ion has already been removed before the filtrate reaches the distal tubule, these potassium-sparing diuretics produce only a mild diuresis. Drugs in this class are rarely prescribed alone, but they may be used in combination with thiazide or loop diuretics to minimize loss of potassium ions in the pharmacotherapy of hypertension or edema.

Aldosterone Antagonists

Aldosterone is the primary mineralocorticoid hormone secreted by the adrenal gland. The physiological targets, or membrane receptors (MRs), for aldosterone are located in the distal tubule and collecting ducts of the nephron. Once bound to its receptors, the MR-aldosterone complex causes the renal tubule cells to synthesize more Na^+ channels, thereby allowing for more reabsorption of Na^+ from the filtrate. Simply stated, aldosterone increases sodium reabsorption.

Spironolactone (Aldactone) and eplerenone (Inspra) prevent the formation of the MR-aldosterone complex and are called aldosterone antagonists. By blocking the actions of aldosterone, these drugs enhance the excretion of sodium and the retention of potassium. Like the sodium ion channel inhibitors, spironolactone and eplerenone produce only a weak diuresis, and they are normally combined with drugs from other classes when treating hypertension or edema. Spironolactone has also been found to significantly reduce mortality in clients with heart failure and, because of this important beneficial effect, its use has increased. The aldosterone antagonists are also used to treat hyperaldosteronism, a rare disorder in which a tumour of the adrenal gland secretes large amounts of aldosterone.

NCLEX Success Tip

Spironolactone is a potassium-sparing diuretic; therefore, clients should be monitored closely for hyperkalemia. When taking this drug, clients must be careful to avoid foods high in potassium to avoid elevating serum potassium levels. There is no need for the client to restrict sodium intake as the drug promotes sodium excretion.

Normally, sodium and potassium are exchanged in the distal tubule: Na^+ is reabsorbed into the body, and K^+ is secreted into the tubule. Potassium-sparing diuretics block this exchange, causing sodium to stay in the tubule and ultimately leave through the urine. When sodium is blocked, the body retains more K^+. Because most of the sodium has already been removed before the filtrate reaches the distal tubule, potassium-sparing diuretics produce only mild diuresis. Their primary use is in combination with thiazide or loop diuretics, to minimize potassium loss.

Unlike the loop and thiazide diuretics, clients who are taking potassium-sparing diuretics should not take potassium supplements or be advised to add potassium-rich foods to their diet. Intake of excess potassium when taking these medications may lead to hyperkalemia. Signs and symptoms of hyperkalemia include muscle weakness, ventricular tachycardia, or fibrillation. Other minor adverse effects of the drugs include headache, dizziness, nausea, and vomiting. Spironolactone binds to progesterone and androgen receptors, resulting in a small incidence of gynecomastia, menstrual abnormalities, and impotence. Gynecomastia, abnormal enlargement of the breasts in males, appears to be related to dosage level and duration of therapy; it may persist after the drug is discontinued. The incidence of adverse reproductive system effects is lower with eplerenone.

Nursing Considerations

The role of the nurse in potassium-sparing diuretic therapy involves careful monitoring of the client's condition and providing education as it relates to the prescribed drug regimen. The nurse must constantly monitor the client for signs of hyperkalemia, such as irritability, anxiety, abdominal cramping, and irregularities in pulse, because these diuretics prevent potassium from being excreted. Also assess for anuria, acute renal insufficiency, and impaired kidney function because potassium-sparing diuretics are contraindicated in these conditions. They should be used with caution in clients who have a BUN of 40 mg/dL or greater and in clients with liver disease. As with thiazide diuretics, monitor blood pressure before administering these drugs, as they cause a reduction in circulating blood volume and decreased blood pressure. Electrolyte levels, especially potassium and sodium, and renal function tests should be obtained before initiating therapy and frequently during early therapy. Also assess for signs of hypersensitivity reaction, such as fever, sore throat, malaise, joint pain, ecchymoses, profound fatigue, shortness of breath, and pallor.

Some potassium-sparing diuretics cause dizziness when first prescribed, so the nurse must be careful to ensure client safety when the client is changing position and ambulating. The client should be instructed to continue taking the medication even though he or she may be feeling well.

Clients who are taking potassium-sparing diuretics may experience decreased libido. Additional hormonal side effects that may occur with these diuretics include hirsutism, irregular menses, amenorrhea, and postmenopausal bleeding in females and gynecomastia and impotence in males. Report these side effects to the healthcare provider immediately, and provide emotional support.

Follow-up care is critical with clients who are taking potassium-sparing diuretics. The client should have weekly blood pressure monitoring and electrocardiogram (ECG) tests as directed by the healthcare provider, especially if therapy is prolonged.

Client education as it relates to potassium-sparing diuretics should include goals, reasons for obtaining baseline data such as vital signs and laboratory tests for electrolytes, and possible side effects. The following are important points to include when teaching clients regarding potassium-sparing diuretics:

- Report signs of hyperkalemia immediately, including irritability, anxiety, abdominal cramping, and irregular heartbeat.
- Avoid using salt substitutes that are potassium based.
- Avoid eating excess amounts of foods that are high in potassium, such as oranges, peaches, potatoes, tomatoes, broccoli, bananas, and dried apricots.

- Avoid performing tasks that require mental alertness until effects of the medication are known.
- Do not abruptly discontinue taking the diuretic unless recommended by the healthcare provider.
- Take the medication exactly as ordered and keep all appointments for follow-up care.
- Keep a symptom log during the initial phase of therapy to assist the healthcare provider in tailoring dosage as needed.
- Use additional health promotional activities to help reduce blood pressure, such as smoking cessation, exercise, weight control, stress management, and moderate consumption of alcohol, if any.

See Nursing Process Focus: Clients Receiving Diuretic Therapy for the complete nursing process applied to caring for clients who are receiving diuretic therapy.

| PROTOTYPE DRUG | Spironolactone (Aldactone) |

Actions and Uses: Spironolactone acts by blocking sodium reabsorption in the distal tubule. It accomplishes this by inhibiting aldosterone, the hormone secreted by the adrenal cortex that is responsible for increasing the renal reabsorption of sodium in exchange for potassium, thus causing water retention. When blocked by spironolactone, sodium and water excretion is increased and the body retains more potassium. The other two potassium-sparing diuretics do not exert an antialdosterone effect, but instead act by directly inhibiting the sodium-potassium exchange mechanism in the renal tubule.

Pharmacokinetics: Spironolactone is well absorbed after oral administration. It is widely distributed, crosses the placenta, and enters breast milk. It is mostly metabolized by the liver to canrenone, its active diuretic compound. Its half-life is 13 to 24 hours.

Administration Alerts:

- Give with food to increase absorption of drug.
- Do not give potassium supplements.
- Spironolactone is pregnancy category C.

Adverse Effects and Interactions: Spironolactone does such an efficient job of retaining potassium that hyperkalemia may develop. The probability of hyperkalemia is increased if the client takes potassium supplements or is concurrently taking ACE inhibitors. Signs and symptoms of hyperkalemia include muscle weakness, ventricular tachycardia, and fibrillation. When serum potassium levels are monitored carefully and maintained within normal values, side effects of spironolactone are uncommon.

Spironolactone interacts with several drugs. For example, when combined with ammonium chloride, acidosis may occur. Acetylsalicylic acid (ASA [Aspirin]) and other salicylates may decrease the diuretic effect of the medication. Concurrent use of spironolactone and digoxin may decrease the effects of digoxin. When taken with potassium supplements, ACE inhibitors, and angiotensin II receptor blockers, hyperkalemia may result.

Miscellaneous Diuretics for Specific Indications

52.8 Several less commonly prescribed classes, such as the osmotic diuretics and the carbonic anhydrase inhibitors, have specific indications in reducing intraocular fluid pressure (acetazolamide) or reversing severe renal hypoperfusion (mannitol).

Carbonic Anhydrase Inhibitors

A few diuretics, shown in Table 52.5, cannot be classified as loop, thiazide, or potassium-sparing agents. These diuretics have limited and specific indications. Three of these drugs inhibit **carbonic anhydrase**, an enzyme that affects acid-base balance by its ability to form carbonic acid from water and carbon dioxide. For example, acetazolamide is a carbonic anhydrase inhibitor used to decrease intraocular fluid pressure in clients with open-angle glaucoma (see Chapter 63). Unrelated to its diuretic effect, acetazolamide also has applications as an anticonvulsant and in treating motion sickness.

Although once used as diuretics, the carbonic anhydrase inhibitors are now rarely prescribed for that purpose because they produce only a weak, short-lived diuresis and can contribute to metabolic acidosis. Carbonic anhydrase inhibitors that are given by the oral route include acetazolamide (Diamox) and methazolamide (Neptazane). Acetazolamide, also used to decrease intraocular fluid pressure, has several other indications. Two drugs in this class, dorzolamide (Trusopt) and brinzolamide (Azopt), are

administered topically to the eye for open-angle glaucoma. The antiglaucoma drugs in this class are discussed in Chapter 63.

Osmotic Diuretics

The osmotic diuretics, listed in Table 52.5, are a small class of drugs that are reserved for very specific indications. Unlike the thiazides and loop diuretics that block transport proteins, osmotic diuretics are mostly inert and act by raising the osmolality, which is a measure of the amount of dissolved particles, or solutes, in a solution. This in turn increases the **osmotic pressure**, which creates a force that moves substances between compartments. Osmotic diuretics cause water to shift compartments by creating a difference in osmotic pressure across a membrane or between two body compartments.

When given IV, osmotic diuretics are filtered at the glomerulus and readily enter the renal filtrate. Once in the tubule, they remain unchanged. As normal sodium and water reabsorption progresses in the proximal tubule, the diuretic remains behind, and its concentration in the tubule begins to increase. The osmolality of the filtrate increases due to the presence of the osmotic diuretic in the tubule. This osmotic force draws water into the filtrate, resulting in increased diuresis.

A second action of osmotic diuretics is their ability to raise the osmolality of the plasma. This creates an osmotic force that moves water from the intracellular and extravascular spaces to the plasma. The increased volume of water in the plasma is filtered by the kidney, resulting in enhanced diuresis. This action is used to advantage in the treatment of two conditions where fluid has accumulated in extravascular spaces. For example, following a traumatic head injury, fluid accumulates in the brain, causing dangerously high intracranial pressure. Osmotic diuretics create an osmotic force that promotes the fluid to leave the brain and enter the blood, thus reducing cerebral edema. A second example is high intraocular pressure caused by excess fluid accumulation in the eye (glaucoma). Osmotic diuretics can cause the fluid to leave the eye and enter the blood, thus relieving the high intraocular pressure.

NCLEX Success Tip

Mannitol (Osmitrol) is an osmotic diuretic that works by increasing osmotic pressure and drawing fluid into the vascular space. Monitoring hourly urine output is a priority nursing assessment when administering this medication. Electrolyte levels should also be monitored, most specifically sodium, chloride, and potassium.

TABLE 52.5 Miscellaneous Diuretics

Drug	Route and Adult Dose
Carbonic Anhydrase Inhibitors	
acetazolamide (Diamox)	PO/IV, 250–375 mg qd
Osmotic Type	
mannitol (Osmitrol)	For intracranial pressure (ICP), cerebral edema reduction (off label dosing): IV, 0.25–1 g/kg/dose; may repeat q6h-q8h. For intraocular pressure (IOP) reduction: IV, 1.5–2 g/kg administered over 30–60 minutes 1–1.5 hours before surgery

NURSING PROCESS FOCUS

Clients Receiving Diuretic Therapy

Assessment	Potential Nursing Diagnoses/Identified Patterns
Prior to administration: • Obtain complete health history (mental and physical), including data on recent surgeries or trauma. • Obtain vital signs; assess in context of client's baseline values. • Obtain client's medication history, including nicotine and alcohol consumption to determine possible drug allergies and/or interactions. • Obtain blood and urine specimens for laboratory analysis.	• Risk for fluid and electrolyte imbalance • Risk for deficient fluid volume related to excess diuresis • Need for knowledge regarding drug therapy and adverse effects • Safety from injury related to side effects of drug therapy • Fatigue • Decreased cardiac output • Risk for falls related to dizziness and hypotension • Risk for urge urinary incontinence

---

Planning: Client Goals and Expected Outcomes (Examples)

The client will:

- Exhibit normal fluid balance and maintain electrolyte levels within normal limits during drug therapy
- Demonstrate an understanding of the drug's action by accurately describing drug side effects and precautions
- Immediately report effects such as symptoms of hyperkalemia or hypokalemia and hypersensitivity

---

Implementation

Interventions (Rationales)	Client Education/Discharge Planning
- Monitor laboratory values. (Diuretics can cause electrolyte imbalances.) - Monitor vital signs, especially blood pressure. (Diuretics reduce blood volume, resulting in lowered blood pressure.) - Observe for changes in level of consciousness (LOC), dizziness, fatigue, and postural hypotension. (Reduction in blood volume due to diuretic therapy may produce changes in LOC or syncope.) - Monitor for fluid overload by measuring intake, output, and daily weight. (Intake, output, and daily body weight are indications of the effectiveness of diuretic therapy.) - Monitor potassium intake. (Potassium is vital to maintaining proper electrolyte balance and can become depleted with thiazide or loop diuretics.) - Observe for signs of hypersensitivity reaction. - Monitor hearing and vision. (Loop diuretics are ototoxic. Thiazide diuretics increase serum digitalis levels; elevated levels produce visual changes.) - Monitor reactivity to light exposure. (Some diuretics cause photosensitivity.)	- Instruct client to inform laboratory personnel of diuretic therapy when providing blood or urine samples Instruct client to: - Monitor blood pressure as specified by the healthcare provider, and ensure proper use of home equipment - Withhold medication for severe hypotensive readings as specified by the healthcare provider (e.g., "hold for levels below 88/50") Instruct client to: - Immediately report any change in LOC, especially feeling faint - Avoid abrupt changes in posture; rise slowly from prolonged periods of sitting or lying down - Obtain blood pressure readings in sitting, standing, and supine positions Instruct client to: - Immediately report any severe shortness of breath, frothy sputum, profound fatigue and edema in extremities, potential signs of heart failure, or pulmonary edema - Accurately measure intake, output, and body weight and report weight gain of 1 kg or more within 2 days or a decrease in output - Avoid excessive heat, which contributes to fluid loss through perspiration - Consume adequate amounts of *plain water* For clients receiving loop or thiazide diuretics, encourage foods high in potassium For clients receiving potassium-sparing diuretics: - Instruct client to avoid foods high in potassium - Consult with healthcare provider before using vitamin/mineral supplements or electrolyte-fortified sports drinks Instruct client or caregiver to report: - Difficulty breathing, throat tightness, hives or rash, and bleeding - Flu-like symptoms: shortness of breath, fever, sore throat, malaise, joint pain, profound fatigue - Instruct client to report any changes in hearing or vision such as ringing or buzzing in the ears, becoming "hard of hearing," experiencing dimness of sight, seeing halos, or having "yellow vision" Instruct client to: - Limit exposure to the sun or wear sunscreen - Wear dark glasses and light-coloured, loose-fitting clothes when outdoors

---

Evaluation of Outcome Criteria

Evaluate the effectiveness of drug therapy by confirming that client goals and expected outcomes have been met (see "Planning").

See Tables 52.2 to 52.5 for lists of drugs to which these nursing actions apply.

Osmotic diuretics are rarely the drugs of first choice due to their potential toxicity. Mannitol is given by the IV route under controlled conditions during which the client can be closely monitored. Although as diuretics they are useful in increasing urine output, these drugs are contraindicated in clients with severe renal impairment. The rapid movement of water from the extravascular spaces to the blood can result in severe dehydration in the tissues and cause a serious fluid overload in clients with severe heart failure. Electrolyte imbalances, especially hyponatremia, may occur with these agents.

The osmotic diuretics also have very specific applications. For example, mannitol is used to maintain urine flow in clients with acute renal failure or during prolonged surgery. Since this agent is not reabsorbed in the tubule, it is able to maintain the flow of filtrate even in cases of severe renal hypoperfusion. Mannitol can also be used to lower intraocular pressure in certain types of glaucoma. It is a highly potent diuretic that is given only by the IV route. Unlike other diuretics that draw excess fluid away from tissue spaces, mannitol can worsen edema and thus must be used with caution in clients with pre-existing heart failure or pulmonary edema.

CHAPTER 52 Understanding the Chapter

Key Concepts Summary

The numbered key concepts provide a succinct summary of the important points from the corresponding numbered section within the chapter. If any of these points are not clear, refer to the numbered section within the chapter for review.

52.1 The kidneys regulate fluid volume, electrolytes, and acid-base balance.

52.2 As filtrate travels through the nephron, its composition changes dramatically as a result of the processes of reabsorption and secretion.

52.3 The dosage levels for most medications must be adjusted in clients with renal failure. Diuretics may be used to maintain urine output while the cause of the hypoperfusion is treated.

52.4 Diuretics are drugs that increase urine output, usually by blocking sodium reabsorption.

52.5 The most efficacious diuretics are the loop (high-ceiling) agents that block the reabsorption of sodium in the loop of Henle.

52.6 The thiazides act by blocking sodium reabsorption in the distal tubule of the nephron, and they are the most widely prescribed class of diuretics.

52.7 Though less efficacious than the loop diuretics, potassium-sparing diuretics are used in combination with other agents and help to prevent hypokalemia.

52.8 Several less commonly prescribed classes, such as the osmotic diuretics and the carbonic anhydrase inhibitors, have specific indications in reducing intraocular fluid pressure (acetazolamide) or reversing severe renal hypoperfusion (mannitol).

Chapter 52 Scenario

Katherine Crosland, a 79-year-old widow, has lived alone for the past 5 years. Although her son and daughters all reside in distant locations, they check on her at least weekly by telephone. Katherine is fairly independent; however, she does not drive and is dependent on a neighbour to get her groceries and medications.

Three years ago, Katherine was hospitalized for a myocardial infarction (MI), which resulted in heart failure. She is adherent with her medications, which include digoxin (Lanoxin) 0.125 mg daily, furosemide (Lasix) 20 mg/day, and potassium supplements (K-Dur) 20 mEq daily.

Recently Katherine's neighbour went on an extended, out-of-town trip. Katherine was certain that she had enough of her medicine to last through that time. However, before the neighbour returned, Katherine discovered that she had miscalculated her potassium supplement and only had enough for 10 days. Katherine figured that because the potassium was only a "supplement," she would be able to wait until her neighbour returned to get the medication refilled.

Today, she presents to the clinic with generalized weakness and fatigue. She has lost 3.6 kg (8 lb) since her last clinic visit 6 weeks ago. Her blood pressure is 104/62 mm Hg, her heart rate is 98 beats/

minute, she has a slightly irregular respiratory rate of 20 breaths/minute, and her body temperature is 36.2°C. The blood specimen collected for diagnostic studies showed several outstanding findings, such as a serum sodium level of 150 mEq/L and potassium level of 3.2 mEq/L. Katherine is diagnosed with dehydration and hypokalemia induced by diuretic therapy.

Critical Thinking Questions

1. Discuss fluid and electrolyte imbalances related to the following diuretic therapies:
   a. Loop diuretics
   b. Thiazide diuretics

c. Potassium-sparing diuretics
d. Osmotic diuretics

2. What relationship exists between this client's diuretic therapy, digoxin therapy, and hypokalemia?

3. What client education should the nurse provide about diuretic therapy?

See Answers to Critical Thinking Questions in Appendix B.

NCLEX Practice Questions

1 The nurse is teaching a group of clients with cardiac conditions who are taking diuretic therapy. The nurse explains that individuals prescribed furosemide (Lasix) should

   a. Avoid consuming large amounts of cabbage, cauliflower, and kale.

   b. Rise slowly from sitting or lying positions.

   c. Count their pulse for 1 full minute before taking the medication.

   d. Restrict fluid intake to no more than 1000 mL in a 24-hour period.

2 While preparing a client for discharge, which of the following statements should the nurse include in the instructions regarding the client's new prescription of hydrochlorothiazide (Urozide)?

   a. "There are no limitations on your salt and fluid intake."

   b. "Ingest vitamin K–rich foods, such as green leafy vegetables and broccoli, every day."

   c. "Report muscle cramps or weakness to the healthcare provider."

   d. "Antihypertensive drugs taken concurrently may produce sleepiness."

3 Clients prescribed spironolactone (Aldactone) are often at risk for electrolyte imbalance. The nurse assesses for this adverse effect because this drug may cause the body to

   a. Retain potassium

   b. Release magnesium

   c. Excrete potassium

   d. Bind calcium

4 Which nursing measures should be a nursing priority for a client first beginning mannitol (Osmitrol)?

   a. Keeping the urinal or bedpan available for clients with limited mobility

   b. Assessing for hypokalemia and encouraging the intake of foods high in potassium

   c. Monitoring intake and output ratio and weighing the client daily

   d. Monitoring blood pressure and assessing for level of consciousness

5 The nurse is monitoring a client receiving acetazolamide (Diamox). Which acid-base imbalance is a potential risk for this client?

   a. Metabolic acidosis

   b. Metabolic alkalosis

   c. Respiratory acidosis

   d. Respiratory alkalosis

See Answers to NCLEX Practice Questions in Appendix A.

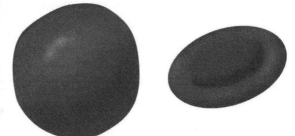
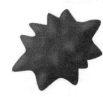

PROTOTYPE DRUGS

FLUID REPLACE-MENT AGENTS	ACID-BASE AGENTS
Colloids	Pr *sodium bicarbonate*
Pr *dextran 40*	Pr *ammonium chloride*
Crystalloids	
ELECTROLYTES	
Pr *sodium chloride*	
Pr *potassium chloride (K-Dur, Slow-K, Micro-K)*	

Monica Schroeder/Science Source

Pharmacotherapy of Fluid and Electrolyte Imbalances and Acid-Base Disorders

LEARNING OUTCOMES

After reading this chapter, the student should be able to:

1. Explain how changes in the osmolality or tonicity of a fluid can cause water to move to a different compartment.

2. Compare and contrast colloids and crystalloids used in intravenous (IV) therapy.

3. Explain the importance of electrolyte balance in the body.

4. Discuss causes of sodium imbalance and the medications used to treat this condition.

5. Discuss causes of potassium imbalance and the medications used to treat this condition.

6. Discuss common causes of alkalosis and acidosis and the medications used to treat these disorders.

7. Describe the nurse's role in the pharmacological management of clients who are receiving drugs for fluid, electrolyte, and acid-base disorders.

8. For each of the drug classes listed in Prototype Drugs, identify a representative drug and explain its mechanism of action, therapeutic effects, and important adverse effects.

9. Describe and explain, based on pharmacological principles, the rationale for nursing assessment, planning, and interventions for clients with fluid, electrolyte, and acid-base disorders.

10. Use the nursing process to care for clients who are receiving drug therapy for fluid, electrolyte, and acid-base disorders.

CHAPTER OUTLINE

▶ Fluid Balance
  ▶ Body Fluid Compartments
  ▶ Osmolality, Tonicity, and the Movement of Body Fluids
  ▶ Regulation of Fluid Intake and Output

▶ Fluid Replacement Agents
  ▶ Intravenous Therapy with Crystalloids and Colloids
  ▶ Transfusions of Blood Products

▶ Electrolytes
  ▶ Normal Functions of Electrolytes
  ▶ Pharmacotherapy of Sodium Imbalances
  ▶ Pharmacotherapy of Potassium Imbalances
  ▶ Magnesium Imbalances

The maintenance of normal fluid volume, electrolyte composition, and acid-base balance is essential to life. Conditions such as hemorrhage and dehydration must be quickly treated; otherwise fluids and electrolytes will be rapidly depleted. Disorders of acid-base balance may be acute, as in diabetic ketoacidosis, or they may proceed more slowly, over a period of months. Fortunately, safe and effective drugs are available to quickly reverse most symptoms of fluid volume, electrolyte, and acid-base imbalance.

FLUID BALANCE

Body fluids travel between compartments, which are separated by semipermeable membranes. Control of water balance in the various compartments is essential to homeostasis. Fluid imbalances are frequent indications for pharmacotherapy.

Body Fluid Compartments

53.1 There is a continuous exchange of fluids across membranes separating the intracellular and extracellular fluid compartments. Large molecules and those that are ionized are less able to cross membranes.

The bulk of body fluid consists of water, which serves as the universal solvent in which most of the body's nutrients, electrolytes, and minerals are dissolved. Water alone is responsible for about 60% of the total body weight.

In a simple model, water in the body can be located in one of two places, or compartments. The **intracellular fluid (ICF) compartment**, which contains water that is *inside* cells, accounts for about two-thirds of the total body water. The remaining one-third of body fluid resides *outside* cells in the **extracellular fluid (ECF) compartment**. The ECF compartment is further divided into two parts: fluid in the *plasma* and fluid in the *interstitial spaces* between cells. The relationship between these fluid compartments is illustrated in Figure 53.1.

A continuous exchange and mixing of fluids occurs between the compartments, which are separated by membranes. The plasma membranes of the cells separate the ICF from the ECF. The capillary membranes separate plasma from the interstitial fluid. Although water travels freely among the compartments, the

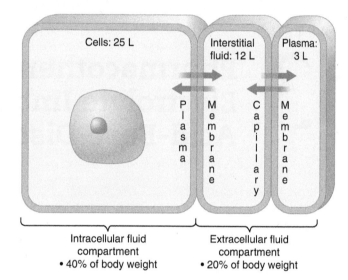

Figure 53.1   Major fluid compartments in the body.

movement of large molecules and those with electrical charges is governed by processes of diffusion and active transport. Movement of ions and drugs across membranes is a primary concern of pharmacokinetics (see Chapter 3).

Osmolality, Tonicity, and the Movement of Body Fluids

53.2 Changes in the osmolality of body fluids can cause water to move to different compartments.

Osmolality and *tonicity* are two related terms central to understanding fluid balance in the body. Large changes in the osmolality or tonicity of a body fluid can cause significant shifts in water balance between compartments. The nurse will often administer intravenous (IV) fluids to compensate for these changes.

The **osmolality** of a fluid is determined by the number of dissolved particles, or solutes, in 1 kg (1 L) of water. In most body fluids, three solutes determine the osmolality: sodium, glucose, and urea. Sodium is the greatest contributor to osmolality due to its abundance in most body fluids. The normal osmolality of body fluids ranges from 275 to 295 milliosmoles per kilogram (mOsm/kg).

The term *tonicity* is sometimes used interchangeably with osmolality, although they are somewhat different. Whereas osmolality is a laboratory value that can be precisely measured, **tonicity** is a general term used to describe the *relative* concentration of IV fluids. Tonicity is the ability of a solution to cause a change in water movement across a membrane due to osmotic forces. The tonicity of the plasma is used as the reference point when administering IV solutions: normal plasma is considered isotonic. Solutions that are isotonic have the same concentration of solutes (same osmolality) as the blood. Hypertonic solutions have a greater concentration of solutes than plasma, whereas hypotonic solutions have a lesser concentration of solutes than plasma.

Through **osmosis**, water moves from areas of low solute concentration (low osmolality) to areas of high solute concentration (high osmolality). If a hypertonic (hyperosmolar) IV solution is administered, the plasma gains more solutes than the interstitial fluid. Water will move, by osmosis, from the interstitial fluid to the plasma. Water will move in the opposite direction, from plasma to interstitial fluid, if a hypotonic solution is administered. Isotonic solutions will produce no net fluid shift. These movements are illustrated in Figure 53.2.

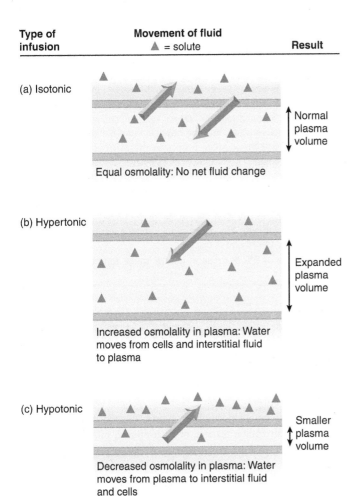

Type of infusion	Movement of fluid ▲ = solute	Result

(a) Isotonic

Equal osmolality: No net fluid change

↕ Normal plasma volume

(b) Hypertonic

Increased osmolality in plasma: Water moves from cells and interstitial fluid to plasma

↕ Expanded plasma volume

(c) Hypotonic

Decreased osmolality in plasma: Water moves from plasma to interstitial fluid and cells

↕ Smaller plasma volume

Figure 53.2 Movement of fluids and solution tonicity.

Regulation of Fluid Intake and Output

53.3 Water balance is achieved through complex mechanisms that regulate fluid intake and output. The greatest contributor to osmolality is sodium, although glucose and urea also contribute.

The average adult has a water intake of approximately 2500 mL/day from food and beverages. Water output is achieved through the kidneys, lungs, skin, feces, and sweat. To maintain water balance, water intake must equal water output. Gains or losses of water can be estimated by changes in total body weight.

The most important physiological regulator of fluid intake is the thirst mechanism. The sensation of thirst occurs when osmoreceptors in the hypothalamus sense a hypertonic ECF. As saliva secretion diminishes and the mouth dries, the individual is driven to ingest liquid. As the ingested water is absorbed, the osmolality of the ECF falls and the thirst centre in the hypothalamus is no longer stimulated.

The kidneys are the primary regulators of fluid output. Through the renin-angiotensin-aldosterone mechanism (see Chapter 51), the hormone aldosterone is secreted by the adrenal cortex. Aldosterone causes the kidneys to retain sodium and water, thus increasing the osmolality of the ECF. A second hormone, antidiuretic hormone (ADH), is released during periods of high plasma osmolality. ADH acts directly on the distal tubules of the kidney to increase water reabsorption.

Failure to properly balance intake with output can result in fluid volume disorders that are indications for pharmacological intervention. Fluid deficit disorders can cause dehydration or shock, which are treated by administering oral or IV fluids. Fluid excess disorders are treated with diuretics (see Chapter 52). When treating fluid volume disorders, the ultimate goal is to diagnose and correct the *cause* of the disorder, while administering supporting fluids and medications to stabilize the client.

FLUID REPLACEMENT AGENTS

Loss of fluids from the body can result in dehydration and shock. Fluid replacement solutions are used to maintain blood volume and support blood pressure.

Intravenous Therapy with Crystalloids and Colloids

53.4 Intravenous fluid therapy using crystalloids and colloids is used to replace lost fluids. Colloids such as dextran have the ability to rapidly expand plasma volume.

When fluid output exceeds fluid intake, volume deficits may result. Shock, dehydration, or electrolyte loss may occur; large deficits are fatal unless treated. The following are some common reasons for fluid loss:

- Loss of gastrointestinal (GI) fluids due to vomiting, diarrhea, chronic laxative use, or GI suctioning

- Excessive sweating during hot weather, athletic activity, or prolonged fever
- Severe burns
- Trauma resulting in significant blood loss
- Excessive renal fluid loss due to diuretic therapy or uncontrolled diabetic ketoacidosis
- Surgical procedures

The immediate goal in treating a volume deficit disorder is to replace the missing fluid. In non-acute circumstances, this may be achieved by administering fluids via the oral route or through a nasogastric tube. In acute situations, IV fluid therapy is indicated. Regardless of the route, careful attention must be paid to restoring normal levels of electrolytes as well as fluid volume.

Intravenous replacement fluids are of two basic types: colloids and crystalloids. **Colloids** are proteins or other large molecules that remain in the blood for a long time because they are too large to cross the capillary membrane. While circulating, they draw water molecules from the cells and tissues into the plasma through their ability to increase plasma osmolality and osmotic pressure. These agents are sometimes called plasma volume expanders. They are particularly important in treating hypovolemic shock due to burns, hemorrhage, or surgery. Several of these products contain dextran, a synthetic polysaccharide. Dextran infusions can double the plasma volume within a few minutes, although its effects last only about 12 hours. Plasma protein fraction contains 83% albumin and 17% plasma globulins. Plasma protein fraction and albumin are also indicated in clients with hypoproteinemia. Select colloid solutions are given in Table 53.1.

Crystalloids are IV solutions that contain electrolytes and other agents that are used to replace lost fluids and to promote urine output. Unlike colloids, crystalloid solutions are capable of quickly diffusing across membranes, leaving the plasma and entering the interstitial fluid and ICF. Isotonic, hypotonic, and hypertonic solutions are available. Some crystalloids contain dextrose, a form of glucose, commonly in concentrations of 2.5%, 5%, or 10%. Dextrose is added to provide nutritional value: 1 L of 5% dextrose supplies 170 calories. In addition, water is formed during the metabolism of dextrose, adding to the rehydration of the client.

Infusion of crystalloids will increase total fluid volume in the body, but the compartment that is most expanded depends on the solute (sodium) concentration. Infusion of hypertonic crystalloids will draw water from the cells and tissues and expand plasma volume. Hypotonic crystalloids will cause water to move out of the plasma to the tissues and cells; therefore, these solutions are not

TABLE 53.1 Select Colloid IV Solutions (Plasma Volume Expanders)

Solution	Tonicity
5% albumin	isotonic
dextran 40 in normal saline	isotonic
dextran 40 in 5% dextrose in water (D₅W)	isotonic
dextran 70 in normal saline	isotonic
hetastarch 6% in normal saline	isotonic
plasma protein fraction	isotonic

TABLE 53.2 Select Crystalloid IV Solutions

Solution	Tonicity
normal saline (0.9% NaCl)	isotonic
hypertonic saline (3% NaCl)	hypertonic
hypotonic saline (0.45% NaCl)	hypotonic
lactated Ringer's	isotonic
Plasma-Lyte 148	isotonic
Plasma-Lyte 56	hypotonic
Dextrose Solutions	
5% dextrose in water (D₅W)	hypotonic/isotonic*
5% dextrose in normal saline	hypertonic
5% dextrose in 0.2% saline	isotonic
5% dextrose in lactated Ringer's	hypertonic
5% dextrose in Plasma-Lyte 56	hypertonic

*Because dextrose is metabolized quickly, the solution is sometimes considered hypotonic.

considered efficient plasma volume expanders. Select crystalloid solutions are given in Table 53.2.

NCLEX Success Tips

Normal saline (0.9%) solution is the only IV solution that is compatible with any blood products.

Lactated Ringer's and dextrose solutions are incompatible with blood products.

When dextrose is abruptly discontinued, the nurse should assess the client for symptoms of hypoglycemia because rebound hypoglycaemia can occur.

When a transfusion reaction occurs, the transfusion should be immediately stopped, normal saline solution should be infused to maintain venous access, and the physician and blood bank should be notified immediately.

The ideal solution in the case of an extensive burn is lactated Ringer's solution because it replaces lost sodium and corrects metabolic acidosis.

Infiltration is manifested by slowing of the infusion and swelling, pain, hardness, pallor, and coolness of the skin at the site. If these signs happen, the IV line should be discontinued and restarted at another infusion site. The nurse should apply a warm soak to the site but only after the IV line is discontinued.

Each litre of 5% dextrose in normal saline solution contains 170 calories.

Transfusions of Blood Products

53.5 Transfusions of blood products are used to treat serious conditions that cannot be managed effectively by other means.

Blood products include whole blood, packed red blood cells (RBCs), fresh frozen plasma, cryoprecipitate, immune globulins, and platelet infusions. A single unit of whole blood can be separated into its specific constituents (erythrocytes, leukocytes, platelets, plasma proteins, fresh frozen plasma, and globulins), which can be used to treat multiple clients. Indications for the various blood products are shown in Table 53.3.

TABLE 53.3 Indications for Blood Products

Product	Description	Indication(s)
Whole blood	Contains all blood components	Rapid, massive blood loss when safer agents are not available
Packed RBCs	One unit of packed RBCs increases hemoglobin by about 1 g/dL and hematocrit by about 3% Washed RBCs are nearly free of plasma, WBCs, and platelets and are reserved for patients who have severe reactions to plasma components	Product of choice to increase serum hemoglobin level
Fresh frozen plasma (FFP)	An unconcentrated source of all clotting factors, without platelets	Correction of bleeding secondary to factor deficiencies for which specific factor replacements are unavailable, multifactor deficiency states, and rapid warfarin reversal FFP should not be used for simple volume expansion
Cryoprecipitate	A concentrate prepared from FFP Each concentrate contains about 80 units each of Factor VIII and von Willebrand factor and about 250 mg of fibrinogen It also contains fibronectin and Factor XIII	Originally used for hemophilia and von Willebrand's disease, it is currently used as a source of fibrinogen in acute disseminated intravascular coagulation with bleeding, treatment of uremic bleeding, cardiothoracic surgery, and obstetric emergencies such as abruptio placentae
Immune globulins	Antibody preparations used to provide an immediate boost to the immune system	Rho [D] immune globulin (RhoGAM) prevents development of maternal Rh antibodies that can result from fetomaternal hemorrhage Other immune globulins are available for postexposure prophylaxis for patients exposed to certain infectious diseases, including cytomegalovirus, hepatitis A and B, measles, rabies, respiratory syncytial virus, rubella, tetanus, smallpox, and varicella
Platelets	One platelet concentrate increases the platelet count by about 10 000/mcL	Used to prevent bleeding in asymptomatic severe thrombocytopenia, for bleeding patients with less severe thrombocytopenia, for bleeding patients with platelet dysfunction due to antiplatelet drugs but with normal platelet count, for patients receiving a massive transfusion that causes dilutional thrombocytopenia, and before invasive surgery

Blood products may be administered to restore deficient numbers of blood cells or proteins or to increase fluid volume, depending on the clinical situation. Whole blood is indicated for the treatment of acute, massive blood loss (depletion of more than 30% of the total volume) when there is a need to replace plasma volume as well as supply erythrocytes to increase the blood's oxygen-carrying capacity.

The administration of whole blood has been largely replaced by the use of blood components. Whole blood is rarely administered for several reasons. If the client needs only one specific component in blood, there is no need to expose the client to unnecessary components that could potentially trigger an adverse effect. The supply of blood products depends on human donors and requires careful crossmatching to ensure compatibility between the donor and the recipient.

The most common complications of whole blood transfusion include febrile non-hemolytic and chill-rigour reactions. The client experiences symptoms of an allergic reaction that include back pain and low-grade fever and chills. Dizziness, urticaria, and headache may occur during or immediately after the transfusion. Symptoms are generally mild and treated with acetaminophen (Tylenol) and diphenhydramine (Benadryl) as needed.

The most serious adverse effect from administration of whole blood is an acute hemolytic transfusion reaction. This occurs when the client receiving the transfusion develops antibodies against donor RBC antigens. ABO blood type incompatibility is the most common cause of this rare, though sometimes fatal, disorder. Another uncommon, though serious, adverse effect from whole blood is transfusion-related acute lung injury. This injury occurs when the client receives donor antibodies that attack normal granulocytes in the lung. Acute respiratory symptoms develop and may be fatal.

Whole blood, despite being carefully screened, also has the potential to transmit serious infections such as hepatitis, cytomegalovirus, malaria, or human immunodeficiency virus. In addition, platelet concentrates are stored at room temperature, which may promote the growth of bacteria in the sample. Although disease transmission from donor to recipient is possible, the risk is very low.

NCLEX Success Tips

Before administering any blood product, the nurse should validate the client information and the blood product with another nurse to prevent administration of the wrong blood transfusion.

Blood transfusion should be initiated slowly for the first 10 to 15 minutes, during which the nurse should stay with the client and monitor the client's vital signs frequently for any indication of hemolytic reaction. The nurse should use at least a 19G catheter to prevent hemolysis of red blood cells. If there is no evidence of a reaction, the nurse can adjust the rate of infusion to ensure that the blood product is infused over 2 to 4 hours.

If a blood transfusion reaction does occur, it is imperative to keep an established IV line so that medication can be administered to prevent or treat cardiovascular collapse in case of anaphylaxis.

Warming to room temperature is not necessary because refrigerating blood until infusion prevents bacterial growth.

Nursing Considerations

The role of the nurse in fluid replacement therapy involves careful monitoring of the client's condition and providing education as it relates to the prescribed drug regimen. Prior to administration of colloids (plasma volume expanders), obtain a complete health history, drug history, and a physical examination. Laboratory tests, including complete blood count (CBC), serum electrolytes, blood urea nitrogen (BUN), and creatinine, should be obtained. Evaluate the client's fluid balance before initiating therapy. Administration of colloid solutions to dehydrated clients can lead to renal failure.

Colloidal solutions are contraindicated in clients with renal failure, hypervolemic conditions, severe heart failure, or thrombocytopenia, and in those with clotting abnormalities. They should be used with caution in clients with active hemorrhage, severe dehydration, chronic liver disease, or impaired renal function. Carefully monitor vital signs and observe the client for the first 30 minutes of the infusion for hypersensitivity reactions. The nurse should stop the infusion at the first sign of hypersensitivity.

Some colloidal solutions decrease platelet adhesion and lead to decreased coagulation. Plasma expanders will lower hematocrit and hemoglobin levels because of increased intravascular volume. Immediately report a hematocrit below 30% to the physician.

The primary nursing responsibility when caring for the client who is receiving plasma volume expanders is monitoring fluid volume status. The client should be closely monitored for both fluid volume deficit and fluid volume excess. Vital signs and hemodynamic status should be monitored frequently during the infusion, until the client's condition stabilizes. The client's neurological status and urinary output should also be closely assessed, as these two systems are critically dependent on proper fluid balance. The infusion of the solutions can create a multitude of problems for the critically ill client.

These medications are most often used to treat shock, so the client may not be alert. However, caregivers may need emotional support from the nurse, including updates about the client's condition and psychosocial support.

Client education as it relates to colloidal solutions should include goals, reasons for obtaining baseline data such as vital signs and lab tests, and possible side effects. The following are important points to include when teaching clients and families about colloidal solutions:

- Immediately report any signs of bleeding, such as easy bruising, blood in the urine, or dark, tarry stools.
- Immediately report flushing, shortness of breath, or itching, which could indicate hypersensitivity to the medication.
- Immediately report shortness of breath, cough, chest congestion, or heart palpitations, which could indicate circulatory overload.

PROTOTYPE DRUG | Dextran 40

Actions and Uses: Dextran 40 is a polysaccharide that is too large to pass through capillary walls. It is identical to dextran 70, except that dextran 40 has a lower molecular weight. Dextran 40 acts by raising the osmotic pressure of the blood, thereby causing fluid to move from the tissues to the vascular spaces. Cardiovascular responses include increased blood pressure, increased cardiac output, and improved venous return to the heart. Indications include fluid replacement for clients who are experiencing hypovolemic shock due to hemorrhage, surgery, or severe burns. When given for acute shock, it is infused as rapidly as possible until blood volume is restored.

Dextran 40 also reduces platelet adhesiveness and improves blood flow through its ability to reduce blood viscosity. These properties have led to its use in preventing deep vein thromboses and pulmonary emboli.

Pharmacokinetics: Given as an IV infusion, it has the capability of expanding plasma volume within minutes after administration. Dextran 40 is excreted rapidly by the kidneys.

Administration Alerts:

- Emergency administration may be given at a rate of 1.2 to 2.4 g/minute.
- Non-emergency administration should be infused no faster than 240 mg/minute.
- Once opened, discard unused portion because dextran contains no preservatives.
- Dextran 40 is pregnancy category C.

Adverse Effects: Vital signs should be monitored continuously to avoid hypertension caused by the plasma volume expansion. Signs of fluid overload such as tachycardia, peripheral edema, distended neck veins, dyspnea, or cough should be reported immediately. Because of its extensive renal excretion, dextran 40 is contraindicated in clients with renal failure. Due to its ability to quickly draw water from tissues, it is also contraindicated in clients with severe dehydration. A small percentage of clients are allergic to dextran 40, with urticaria being the most common sign.

There are no clinically significant interactions.

NURSING PROCESS FOCUS

Clients Receiving Fluid Replacement Therapy

Assessment	Potential Nursing Diagnoses/Identified Patterns
Prior to administration: - Obtain complete health history, including allergies, drug history, and possible drug interactions. - Obtain complete physical examination. - Assess for the presence of fluid volume deficit. - Obtain the following laboratory studies: CBC, serum electrolytes, renal function (BUN and serum creatinine).	- Risk for infection at IV site - Risk for fluid imbalance - Need for knowledge regarding drug therapy and adverse effects - Safety from injury related to side effects of drug therapy

---

Planning: Client Goals and Expected Outcomes

The client will:

- Exhibit signs of normal fluid volume such as stable blood pressure and adequate urinary output
- Demonstrate an understanding of the drug by accurately describing the drug's purpose, action, side effects, and precautions
- Immediately report effects such as itching, shortness of breath, flushing, cough, and heart palpitations

---

Implementation

Interventions (Rationales)	Client Education/Discharge Planning
<ul><li>Monitor hemodynamic status every 15 to 60 minutes, including blood pressure, urinary output, and invasive pressure monitoring devices. (Plasma volume expanders cause rapid movement of water into the circulatory system.)</li><li>Monitor for hypersensitivity reactions such as urticaria, pruritus, dyspnea, flushing, and anaphylaxis.</li><li>Monitor for signs of circulatory overload such as dyspnea, cyanosis, cough, crackles, wheezes, and neck vein distention. (Medication may cause fluid overload quickly.)</li><li>Monitor for changes in CBC results. (Plasma volume expanders can inhibit coagulation and lower hematocrit and hemoglobin levels. Report reduction of hematocrit below 30%.)</li></ul>	Instruct client about:<ul><li>Why vital signs and other assessments are being monitored frequently</li><li>Expected outcomes of plasma volume expansion therapy</li><li>Instruct client to report itching, shortness of breath, or flushing as symptoms occur</li><li>Instruct client to report shortness of breath, cough, or heart palpitation as soon as such symptoms occur</li><li>Instruct client of the need for frequent laboratory studies</li></ul>

Evaluation of Outcome Criteria

Evaluate the effectiveness of drug therapy by confirming that client goals and expected outcomes have been met (see "Planning").

See Table 53.1 for a list of drugs to which these nursing actions apply.

TABLE 53.4 Electrolytes Important to Human Physiology

Compound	Formula	Cation	Anion
calcium chloride	$CaCl_2$	Ca^{+2}	Cl^-
disodium phosphate	Na_2HPO_4	Na^+	HPO_4^{-2}
Pr potassium chloride	KCl	K^+	Cl^-
sodium bicarbonate	$NaHCO_3$	Na^+	HCO_3^-
Pr sodium chloride	$NaCl$	Na^+	Cl^-
sodium sulfate	Na_2SO_4	Na^+	SO_4^{-2}

ELECTROLYTES

Electrolytes are small, charged molecules that are essential to homeostasis. Too little or too much of an electrolyte may result in serious disease and must be quickly corrected. Table 53.4 lists inorganic substances and their electrolytes that are important to human physiology.

Normal Functions of Electrolytes

53.6 Electrolytes are charged substances that are essential to nerve conduction, membrane permeability, water balance, and other critical body functions.

Chapter 37 discusses the role of minerals in health and wellness. In certain body fluids, some of these minerals become ions and possess a charge. Small, inorganic molecules that possess a positive or negative charge are called **electrolytes**. Positively charged

electrolytes are called **cations**; those with a negative charge are called **anions**.

Inorganic compounds are held together by ionic bonds. When placed in aqueous solution, these bonds break and the compound undergoes dissociation, or ionization. The resulting ions have charges and are able to conduct electricity, hence the name *electrolyte*. Electrolyte levels are measured in milliequivalents per litre (mEq/L).

Electrolytes are essential to many body functions, including nerve conduction, membrane permeability, muscle contraction, water balance, and bone growth and remodelling. Levels of electrolytes in body fluids must be maintained within narrow ranges. As electrolytes are lost due to normal excretory functions, they must be compensated by adequate intake, otherwise electrolyte imbalances can result. The major electrolyte imbalance states are shown in Table 53.5. Calcium, phosphorous, and magnesium imbalances are discussed in Chapter 37; the role of calcium in bone homeostasis is presented in Chapter 61.

Pharmacotherapy of Sodium Imbalances

53.7 Sodium is essential to maintain osmolality, water balance, and acid-base balance. Hypernatremia may be corrected with hypotonic IV fluids or diuretics, and hyponatremia is corrected with infusions of sodium chloride.

Sodium is the major electrolyte in extracellular fluid. Due to sodium's central roles in neuromuscular function, acid-base balance,

TABLE 53.5   Electrolyte Imbalances

Ion	Condition	Abnormal Serum Value (mEq/L)	Supportive Treatment*
Calcium	Hypercalcemia	>11	Hypotonic fluid or calcitonin
	Hypocalcemia	<4	Calcium supplements or vitamin D
Chloride	Hyperchloremia	>112	Hypotonic fluid
	Hypochloremia	<95	Hypertonic salt solution
Magnesium	Hypermagnesemia	>4	Hypotonic fluid
	Hypomagnesemia	<0.8	Magnesium supplements
Phosphate	Hyperphosphatemia	>6	Dietary phosphate restriction
	Hypophosphatemia	<1	Phosphate supplements
Potassium	Hyperkalemia	>5	Hypotonic fluid, buffers, or dietary potassium restriction
	Hypokalemia	<3.5	Potassium supplements
Sodium	Hypernatremia	>145	Hypotonic fluid or dietary sodium restriction
	Hyponatremia	<135	Hypertonic salt solution or sodium supplement

*For all electrolyte imbalances, the primary therapeutic goal is to identify and correct the cause of the imbalance.

and overall fluid distribution, sodium imbalances can have serious consequences. Although definite sodium monitors or sensors have yet to be discovered in the body, the regulation of sodium balance is well understood.

Sodium balance and water balance are intimately connected. As sodium levels increase in a body fluid, solute particles accumulate and the osmolality increases. Water will move toward this area of relatively high osmolality. In simplest terms, water travels toward or with sodium. The physiological consequences of this relationship cannot be overstated: as water content of the plasma increases, so does blood volume and blood pressure. Therefore, sodium movement provides an important link between water retention, blood volume, and blood pressure.

In healthy individuals, sodium intake is equal to sodium output, which is under the regulation of the kidneys. High levels of aldosterone secreted by the adrenal cortex promote sodium and water retention by the kidneys. Inhibition of aldosterone promotes sodium and water excretion. When a client ingests high amounts of sodium, aldosterone secretion decreases and more sodium enters the urine. This relationship is illustrated in Figure 53.3.

Sodium excess, or **hypernatremia**, is a serum sodium level greater than 145 mEq/L. The most common cause of hypernatremia is kidney disease resulting in decreased sodium excretion. Hypernatremia may also be caused by excessive intake of sodium, either through dietary consumption or by overtreatment with IV fluids containing sodium chloride or sodium bicarbonate. Another cause of hypernatremia is high net water loss, such as that occurring from inadequate water intake, watery diarrhea, fever, or burns. In addition, high doses of glucocorticoids or estrogens promote sodium retention.

A high serum sodium level increases the osmolality of the plasma and draws fluid from interstitial spaces and cells, thus causing cellular dehydration. Manifestations of hypernatremia include thirst, fatigue, weakness, muscle twitching, convulsions, weight

gain, and dyspnea. For minor hypernatremia, a low-salt diet may be effective in returning serum sodium to normal levels. In clients with acute hypernatremia, however, treatment goals are to rapidly return the osmolality of the plasma to normal and to excrete the excess sodium. If the client is hypovolemic, the administration of hypotonic fluids such as D_5W or 0.45% NaCl will increase plasma volume and at the same time reduce plasma osmolality. For the client who is hypervolemic, diuretics may be used to remove sodium from the body.

Sodium deficiency, or **hyponatremia**, is a serum sodium level less than 135 mEq/L. Hyponatremia may occur through excessive dilution of the plasma or by increased sodium loss due to disorders of the skin, GI tract, or kidneys. Excessive ADH secretion or administration of hypotonic IV solutions can increase plasma volume and lead to hyponatremia. Significant loss of sodium by the skin may occur in burn clients and in those with excessive sweating or prolonged fever. Gastrointestinal losses occur from vomiting, diarrhea, or GI suctioning, and renal sodium loss may occur with diuretic use and in certain advanced kidney disorders. Early symptoms of hyponatremia include nausea, vomiting, anorexia, and abdominal cramping. Later signs include altered neurological function such as confusion, lethargy, convulsions, and muscle twitching or tremors. Tachycardia, hypotension, and dry skin and mucous membranes may also occur. Hyponatremia is usually treated with solutions of sodium chloride.

Nursing Considerations

The role of the nurse in sodium replacement therapy involves careful monitoring of the client's condition and providing education as it relates to the prescribed drug regimen. Because sodium and body water are so closely related, the nurse's primary role when caring for clients with sodium imbalances is monitoring fluid balance. Hyponatremia is seldom caused from inadequate

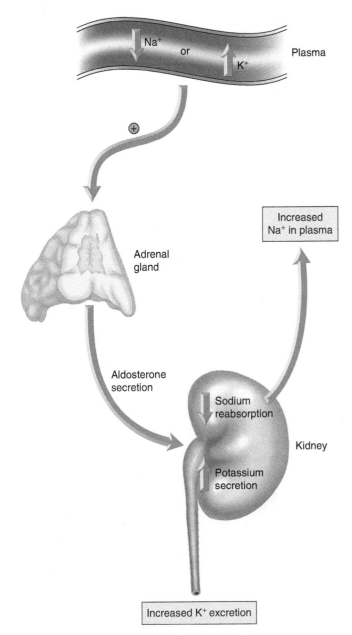

Figure 53.3 Renal regulation of sodium and potassium balance.

dietary intake; however, in rare instances, this may occur in individuals who are following sodium-restricted diets or receiving diuretic therapy. In most cases, infusion of 0.45% or 0.9% sodium solutions are used to restore extracellular fluid balance.

Prior to and during administration of sodium solutions, assess sodium and electrolyte balance. When assessing for hyponatremia, observe for signs of nausea, vomiting, muscle cramps, tachycardia, dry mucous membranes, and headache. The nurse must also be alert for signs indicating hypernatremia, such as weakness, restlessness, irritability, seizures, coma, hypertension, tachycardia, fluid accumulation, pulmonary edema, and respiratory arrest.

Serum sodium levels, urine specific gravity, and serum and urine osmolarity should be monitored closely when administering hypertonic solutions. The client should be taught to report any symptoms that may relate to fluid overload during infusion

of hypertonic saline solutions. The symptoms of this condition include shortness of breath, palpitation, headache, and restlessness.

Side effects of sodium chloride when given as an electrolyte replacement are rare. Some clients have self-induced hypernatremia by taking salt tablets, believing that they will replace sodium lost due to sweating. Those who sweat profusely due to working outdoors or exercising can avoid heat-related problems if they consume adequate amounts of water or balanced electrolyte solutions contained in sports drinks. The client should consume salt tablets only when instructed to do so by the healthcare provider.

Client education as it relates to sodium replacement should include goals, reasons for obtaining baseline data such as vital signs and tests for cardiac and renal function, and possible side effects. The following are the important points to include when teaching clients regarding sodium replacements:

- Avoid taking sodium chloride (salt) tablets to replace sodium lost through perspiration.

- Drink adequate amounts of water or balanced sports drinks to replenish lost fluids and electrolytes.

- Immediately report symptoms of low sodium such as nausea, vomiting, muscle cramps, rapid heart rate, and headache.

- Immediately report symptoms of high sodium such as weakness, restlessness, irritability, seizures, hypertension, and fluid retention.

PROTOTYPE DRUG | **Sodium Chloride**

Actions and Uses: Sodium chloride (NaCl) is administered during periods of hyponatremia when serum levels fall below 130 mEq/L. Sodium chloride is available in several concentrations to treat different levels of hyponatremia. Normal saline consists of 0.9% NaCl and is used to treat mild hyponatremia. When serum sodium falls below 115 mEq/L, a 3% NaCl solution may be infused. Other concentrations include 0.45% and 0.22%, and both hypotonic and isotonic solutions are available. The decision about which NaCl concentration to administer is driven by the severity of the sodium deficiency. Infusions of high concentrations of NaCl are contraindicated in clients with heart failure or impaired renal function.

Pharmacokinetics: Sodium chloride is well absorbed after oral administration. It is widely distributed. It is excreted by the kidneys.

Administration Alert:

- Sodium chloride is pregnancy category C.

Adverse Effects: Clients who are receiving NaCl infusions must be monitored frequently to avoid symptoms of hypernatremia. Symptoms of excessive sodium include lethargy, confusion, muscle tremor or rigidity, hypotension, and restlessness. Because some of these symptoms are also common to hyponatremia, the healthcare provider must rely on periodic laboratory assessments to be certain that sodium values lie within the normal range. When infusing 3% NaCl solutions, continuously check for signs of pulmonary edema.

There are no clinically significant drug interactions.

Pharmacotherapy of Potassium Imbalances

53.8 Potassium is essential for proper nervous and muscle function as well as for maintaining acid-base balance. Hyperkalemia may be treated with glucose and insulin or by administration of polystyrene sulfonate.

Potassium is the most abundant intracellular cation and serves important roles in regulating intracellular osmolality and in maintaining acid-base balance. Potassium levels must be carefully balanced between adequate dietary intake and renal excretion. Like sodium, potassium excretion is influenced by the effect of aldosterone on the kidney. In fact, the renal excretion of sodium and potassium ions is closely linked—for every sodium ion that is reabsorbed, one potassium ion is secreted into the renal tubules. Serum potassium levels must be maintained within narrow limits; excess or deficiency states can be serious or fatal.

Hyperkalemia is a serum potassium level greater than 5 mEq/L, which may be caused by high consumption of potassium-rich foods or dietary supplements, particularly when clients are taking potassium-sparing diuretics such as spironolactone (Aldactone; see Chapter 52). Excess potassium may also accumulate when renal excretion is diminished due to kidney pathology. The most serious consequences of hyperkalemia are related to cardiac function: dysrhythmias and heart block are possible. Other symptoms are muscle twitching, fatigue, paresthesias, dyspnea, cramping, and diarrhea.

In mild cases of hyperkalemia, potassium levels may be returned to normal by restricting major dietary sources of potassium such as bananas, dried fruits, peanut butter, broccoli, and green leafy vegetables. If the client is taking a potassium-sparing diuretic, the dose must be lowered or an alternate drug may be considered. In severe cases, serum potassium levels may be temporarily lowered by administering glucose and insulin, which cause potassium to leave the extracellular fluid and enter cells. Calcium gluconate or calcium chloride may be administered on an emergency basis to counteract potential potassium toxicity on the heart. Sodium bicarbonate is sometimes infused to correct any acidosis that may be concurrent with the hyperkalemia. Elimination of excess potassium may be enhanced by giving polystyrene sulfonate orally or rectally. This agent, which exchanges sodium ion for potassium ion in the intestine, is given concurrently with a laxative such as sorbitol to promote rapid evacuation of the potassium.

Hypokalemia occurs when the serum potassium level falls below 3.5 mEq/L. Hypokalemia is a relatively common adverse effect resulting from high doses of loop diuretics such as furosemide (Lasix). In addition, strenuous muscular activity and severe vomiting or diarrhea can result in significant potassium loss. Because the body does not have large stores of potassium, adequate daily intake is necessary. Neurons and muscle fibres are most sensitive to potassium loss, and muscle weakness, lethargy, anorexia, dysrhythmias, and cardiac arrest are possible consequences. Mild hypokalemia is treated by increasing the dietary intake of potassium-rich foods, whereas more severe deficiencies require higher doses of oral or parenteral potassium supplements.

NCLEX Success Tips

Potassium chloride is never given by IV push because it could cause cardiac arrest. Administration guidelines require no more than 10 mEq (10 mmol/L) of potassium chloride be infused per hour on a general medical-surgical unit. An infusion device or pump is required for safe administration.

Cardiac monitoring and electrocardiogram should be provided while client is receiving potassium because of the risk for dysrhythmias.

Potassium-sparing diuretics may lead to hyperkalemia because they affect the kidney's ability to excrete excess potassium.

Metabolic alkalosis can cause potassium to shift into the cells, thus decreasing the client's serum potassium levels.

Potassium chloride is readily excreted in the urine. Before hanging IV fluids with potassium chloride, the nurse should ascertain whether the client can void; if not, potassium chloride may build up in the serum and cause hyperkalemia.

Nursing Considerations

The role of the nurse in potassium replacement therapy involves careful monitoring of the client's condition and providing education as it relates to the prescribed drug regimen. Potassium imbalances are probably the most common electrolyte disturbance that clients experience. Quick recognition of potassium imbalance will prevent life-threatening complications such as dysrhythmias, heart blocks, and cardiac arrest.

Potassium supplements are contraindicated in conditions that predispose the client to hyperkalemia, such as severe renal impairment and use of potassium-sparing diuretics. Potassium supplements are also contraindicated in acute dehydration, in heat cramps, and in clients with digitalis intoxication with atrioventricular (AV) node disturbance. They should be used with caution in clients with kidney disease, cardiac disease, and systemic acidosis.

Oral potassium administration is used for the prevention and treatment of mild deficiency. Oral forms, especially tablets and capsules, which can produce high local concentrations of potassium, are irritating to the GI tract and may cause peptic ulcers. This is less likely with the use of tablets and capsules that contain microencapsulated particles. To minimize GI irritation, instruct the client to administer oral forms with meals. Prior to oral or IV administration of potassium chloride, serum potassium levels should be measured. Check for the most recent potassium level before administering any form of potassium. Too much potassium can be just as dangerous for the client as too little. In either case, the consequences can be fatal.

Intravenous potassium administration is used for clients with severe deficiency or for those who cannot tolerate oral forms. Monitor serum potassium levels throughout treatment to reduce the risk of hyperkalemia. Assess renal function prior to and during treatment; if renal failure develops, the infusion should be stopped immediately. Monitor for electrocardiogram (ECG) changes, which can be an early indication of developing hyperkalemia. Clients who experience potassium imbalances must be taught to avoid the underlying problems, comply with the medication regimen, and use dietary interventions to correct and maintain normal electrolyte balance.

Client education as it relates to potassium replacement should include goals, reasons for obtaining baseline data such as vital signs and tests for cardiac and renal function, and possible side effects. The following are important points to include when teaching clients regarding potassium replacements:

- Report symptoms of hypokalemia such as weakness, fatigue, lethargy, or anorexia.
- Report symptoms of hyperkalemia such as nausea, abdominal cramping, oliguria, weakness, changes in heart rate, and numbness or tingling of arms or legs.
- Report decreased urinary output since this can lead to hyperkalemia.
- Keep all laboratory appointments to assess serum potassium level.
- If taking a potassium supplement, avoid potassium-rich foods and salt substitutes that are potassium based.
- Take potassium supplements with food to decrease GI distress.

| PROTOTYPE DRUG | Potassium Chloride (K-Dur, Slow-K, Micro-K) |

Actions and Uses: Potassium chloride (KCl) is the drug of choice for treating or preventing hypokalemia. It is also used to treat mild forms of alkalosis. Oral formulations include tablets, powders, and liquids, usually heavily flavoured due to the unpleasant taste of the drug. Because the drug can cause peptic ulcers, the supplement should be diluted with plenty of water. When given IV, potassium preparations must be administered slowly since bolus injections can overload the heart and cause cardiac arrest. Because pharmacotherapy with loop or thiazide diuretics is the most common cause of potassium loss, clients who are taking these diuretics are usually instructed to take oral potassium supplements to prevent hypokalemia.

Pharmacokinetics: Potassium chloride is well absorbed after oral administration. It is widely distributed. It is excreted by the kidneys.

Administration Alerts:

- Always give oral medication while the client is upright in order to avoid esophagitis.
- Tablets should not be crushed or chewed.
- Dilute liquid forms before giving through a nasogastric tube.
- Never administer IV push or in concentrated amounts.
- Be extremely careful to avoid extravasation and infiltration.
- Potassium chloride is pregnancy category C.

Adverse Effects and Interactions: Nausea and vomiting are common because potassium chloride irritates the GI mucosa. The drug may be taken with meals or antacids to lessen gastric distress. The most serious side effects of potassium chloride are related to the possible accumulation of potassium. Hyperkalemia may occur if the client takes potassium supplements concurrently with potassium-sparing diuretics. Kidney function should be assessed periodically. Since the kidneys perform more than 90% of the body's potassium excretion, reduced renal function can

rapidly lead to hyperkalemia, particularly in clients who are taking potassium supplements.

Potassium supplements interact with potassium-sparing diuretics and angiotensin-converting enzyme (ACE) inhibitors to increase the risk for hyperkalemia.

Magnesium Imbalances
53.9 Magnesium imbalances significantly affect cardiovascular and neuromuscular function.

Magnesium imbalances significantly affect cardiovascular and neuromuscular function.

Magnesium is the second most abundant intracellular cation and, like potassium, it is essential for proper neuromuscular function. Magnesium also serves a metabolic role in activating certain enzymes in the breakdown of carbohydrates and proteins; it is a cofactor in more than 300 biochemical reactions. Clients with disorders of magnesium homeostasis generally present with cardiovascular and neuromuscular symptoms. Because the majority of magnesium is found in bone, serum magnesium levels are not accurate indicators of total body magnesium.

Magnesium levels are primarily controlled by the kidney. The ion is freely filtered and reabsorbed in the loop of Henle, and loop diuretics such as furosemide can cause significant magnesium loss. Renal impairment is a major cause of magnesium imbalances. Magnesium is absorbed by the small intestine, and small amounts are secreted in intestinal fluid.

Hypomagnesemia
Because it produces few symptoms until serum levels fall below 1 mEq/L, hypomagnesemia is sometimes called the most common undiagnosed electrolyte abnormality. Although the overall incidence for magnesium deficiency is 6% to 12%, the majority of critically ill clients present with this condition. Renal causes of hypomagnesemia include kidney failure and therapy with loop diuretics. Gastrointestinal causes include malabsorption disorders and loss of significant amounts of body fluids due to diarrhea, chronic laxative abuse, or nasogastric suctioning. Hypomagnesemia may also present in alcoholics and in those who are receiving prolonged parenteral feeding with magnesium-free solutions. Clients may experience general weakness, dysrhythmias, hypertension, loss of deep tendon reflexes, and respiratory depression—signs and symptoms that are sometimes mistaken for hypokalemia. Additional signs include muscle twitches, tetany, or seizures.

Magnesium supplements are available by both oral and parenteral routes. Oral formulations are used for minor hypomagnesemia. Because intramuscular (IM) preparations produce significant pain at the injection site, severe cases of hypomagnesemia are normally treated using the IV route. Pharmacotherapy with magnesium sulfate can quickly reverse symptoms of hypomagnesemia. Magnesium sulfate is a central nervous system (CNS) depressant and is sometimes given to prevent or terminate seizures associated with eclampsia.

Hypermagnesemia

Advanced renal failure is the only major cause of hypermagnesemia, although overtreatment with magnesium supplements may also lead to excessive serum magnesium levels. Clinical signs include CNS depression, respiratory depression, hypotension, dysrhythmias, bradycardia, complete heart block, and coma. Infusions of calcium salts will immediately reverse the neuromuscular and cardiovascular signs. If the magnesium elevation is minor, treatment with furosemide to increase urinary excretion may be sufficient to reverse the hypermagnesemia

ACID-BASE BALANCE

Unless quickly corrected, acidosis and alkalosis can have serious and even fatal consequences. Acidic and basic agents may be given to rapidly correct pH imbalances in body fluids.

CONNECTIONS | Special Considerations

◀ Laxatives and Fluid-Electrolyte Balance

With aging, peristalsis slows, food intake diminishes, and physical activity declines; these factors can change bowel movement regularity. Many older adults believe that they must have a bowel movement every day, and so they take daily laxatives. Chronic use of laxatives may result in fluid depletion and hyperkalemia. Stimulant laxatives, in particular, are the most frequently prescribed class of laxatives, and these agents alter electrolyte transport in the intestinal mucosa. Older adults are especially susceptible to fluid and electrolyte depletion with chronic laxative use. Teach the client to drink plenty of fluids when taking a laxative and that overuse of laxatives can result in adverse side effects, so they should be used only as directed. Recommend that older clients increase exercise (as tolerated) and add insoluble fibre to the diet to maintain elimination regularity.

Buffers and the Maintenance of Body pH

53.10 The body uses buffers to maintain overall pH within narrow limits.

The degree of acidity or alkalinity of a solution is measured by its **pH**. A pH of 7.0 is defined as neutral; above 7.0 is basic or alkaline, and below 7.0 is acidic. To maintain homeostasis, the pH of plasma and most body fluids must be kept within the narrow range of 7.35 to 7.45. Nearly all proteins and enzymes in the body function optimally within this narrow range of pH. A few enzymes, most notably those in the digestive tract, require pH values outside the 7.35 to 7.45 range to function properly. The correction of acid-base imbalance is illustrated in Figure 53.4.

The body generates significant amounts of acid during normal metabolic processes. Without sophisticated means of neutralizing these metabolic acids, the overall pH of body fluids would quickly fall below the normal range. **Buffers** are chemicals that help to maintain normal body pH by neutralizing strong acids and bases. The two primary buffers that the body uses to keep pH within normal limits are bicarbonate ions and phosphate ions.

The body uses two mechanisms to remove acid. The carbon dioxide (CO_2) produced during body metabolism is efficiently removed by the lungs during exhalation. The kidneys remove excess acid in the form of hydrogen ion (H^+) by excreting it in the urine. If retained in the body, CO_2 and/or H^+ would lower body pH. Therefore, the lung and the kidneys collaborate in the removal of acids to maintain normal acid-base balance.

Pharmacotherapy of Acidosis

53.11 Pharmacotherapy of acidosis, a plasma pH below 7.35, includes the administration of sodium bicarbonate.

Acidosis occurs when the pH of the plasma falls below 7.35, which is confirmed by measuring arterial pH, partial pressure of

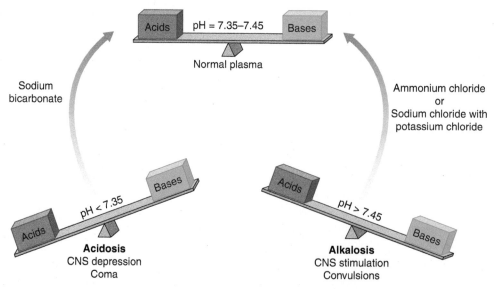

Figure 53.4 Acid-base imbalances.

TABLE 53.6 Causes of Alkalosis and Acidosis

Acidosis	Alkalosis
Respiratory Origins	**Respiratory Origin**
• Hypoventilation or shallow breathing	• Hyperventilation due to asthma, anxiety, or high altitude
• Airway constriction	
• Damage to respiratory centre in medulla	
Metabolic Origins	**Metabolic Origins**
• Severe diarrhea	• Constipation for prolonged periods
• Kidney failure	• Ingestion of excess sodium bicarbonate
• Diabetes mellitus	• Diuretics that cause potassium depletion
• Excess alcohol ingestion	• Severe vomiting
• Starvation	

carbon dioxide (PCO_2), and plasma bicarbonate levels. Diagnosis must differentiate between respiratory etiology and metabolic (renal) etiology. Occasionally, the cause has mixed respiratory and metabolic components. The most profound symptoms of acidosis affect the CNS and include lethargy, confusion, and CNS depression leading to coma. A deep, rapid respiration rate indicates an attempt by the lungs to rid the body of excess acid. Common causes of acidosis are shown in Table 53.6.

Nursing Considerations

The role of the nurse in drug therapy of acidosis involves careful monitoring of the client's condition and providing education as it relates to the prescribed drug regimen. The focus of nursing care is directed toward correction and maintenance of acid-base status. Assess the arterial blood gas analysis, which reports pH, carbon dioxide levels (PCO_2), bicarbonate levels (HCO_3^-), and oxygenation status (PO_2 and O_2 saturation). Also assess the client for symptoms associated with acidosis, such as sleepiness, coma, disorientation, dizziness, headache, seizures, and hypoventilation. The nurse will further assess the client for causative factors that could produce acidosis, such as diabetes mellitus, shock, diarrhea, and vomiting. Acidosis is frequently corrected when the underlying disease condition is successfully managed.

The client who is receiving sodium bicarbonate is prone to alkalosis, especially if an excessive amount has been administered. Monitor the client for symptoms of alkalosis such as irritability, confusion, cyanosis, slow respirations, irregular pulse, and muscle twitching. These symptoms would warrant withholding the medication and notifying the healthcare provider.

There are several contraindications and precautions related to the administration of sodium bicarbonate. Clients who have lost chloride due to vomiting or continuous GI suctioning and clients who are receiving diuretic therapy that may cause hypochloremia should not be given sodium bicarbonate. Clients who have hypocalcemia should not receive sodium bicarbonate because it may produce alkalosis. Due to the sodium content of this drug, it

should be used judiciously in clients with cardiac disease and renal impairment.

Sodium bicarbonate may also be used to alkalinize the urine. This process is useful in the treatment of overdoses of certain acidic medications such as acetylsalicylic acid (ASA [Aspirin]) and phenobarbital (Phenobarb). When IV sodium bicarbonate is given, it causes the urine to become more alkaline. Less acid is reabsorbed in the renal tubules, so more acid and acidic medicine is excreted. This process is known as ion trapping. Closely monitor the client's acid-base status and report symptoms of imbalance to the healthcare provider. Provide care directed toward supporting critical body functions such as cardiovascular, respiratory, and neurological status that may be impaired secondary to the drug overdose.

Sodium bicarbonate (baking soda) is used as a home remedy to neutralize gastric acid in order to relieve heartburn or sour stomach. Although occasional use is acceptable, be aware that clients may misinterpret cardiac symptoms as heartburn and may overuse sodium bicarbonate, leading to systemic alkalosis.

Client education as it relates to sodium bicarbonate should include goals, reasons for obtaining baseline data such as vital signs and electrolyte levels, and possible side effects. The following are important points to include when teaching clients regarding sodium bicarbonate:

- Contact a healthcare provider immediately if gastric discomfort continues or is accompanied by chest pain, dyspnea, or diaphoresis.

- Use non–sodium bicarbonate over-the-counter antacids to prevent the problem of excess sodium or bicarbonate being absorbed into systemic circulation.

- Do not use any antacid, including sodium bicarbonate, for longer than 2 weeks without consulting the healthcare provider.

NCLEX Success Tips

Metabolic alkalosis increases plasma pH because of accumulated base bicarbonate or decreased hydrogen ion concentrations. A client's regular use of baking soda (sodium bicarbonate) may place him or her at risk for this condition.

Metabolic acidosis decreases plasma pH because of increased organic acids (acids other than carbonic acid) or decreased bicarbonate.

Respiratory acidosis is caused by excess carbonic acid.

Respiratory alkalosis results from a carbonic acid deficit that occurs when rapid breathing releases more CO_2 than necessary with expired air.

Metabolic acidosis occurs in clients with end-stage renal disease because the kidneys can't excrete increased loads of acid. Decreased acid secretion results from the inability of the kidney tubules to excrete ammonia (NH_3^-) and to reabsorb sodium bicarbonate (HCO_3^-). There is also decreased excretion of phosphates and other organic acids.

Hyperkalemia is a life-threatening common complication of acute renal failure that needs immediate action to reverse it. Administering glucose and regular insulin, with sodium bicarbonate if necessary, can prevent cardiac arrest by moving potassium into the cells and reducing serum potassium levels.

PROTOTYPE DRUG   **Sodium Bicarbonate**

Actions and Uses: Sodium bicarbonate is the drug of choice for correcting acidosis. After dissociation, the bicarbonate ion acts by directly raising the pH of body fluids. Sodium bicarbonate may be given orally, if acidosis is mild, or IV in cases of acute disease. Although sodium bicarbonate neutralizes gastric acid, it is rarely used to treat peptic ulcers due to its tendency to cause uncomfortable gastric distention. After absorption, sodium bicarbonate makes the urine more alkaline, which aids in the renal excretion of acidic drugs such as barbiturates and salicylates.

Pharmacokinetics: Sodium bicarbonate is readily absorbed. It is widely distributed in extracellular fluid. It is excreted in urine. The half-life is unknown.

Administration Alerts:

- Do not add oral preparation to calcium-containing solutions.
- Sodium bicarbonate is pregnancy category C.

Adverse Effects and Interactions: Most of the side effects of sodium bicarbonate therapy are the result of metabolic alkalosis caused by too much bicarbonate ion. Symptoms may include confusion, irritability, slow respiration rate, and vomiting. Simply discontinuing the sodium bicarbonate infusion often reverses these symptoms; however, potassium chloride or ammonium chloride may be administered to reverse the alkalosis. During sodium bicarbonate infusions, serum electrolytes should be carefully monitored, as sodium levels may give rise to hypernatremia and fluid retention. In addition, high levels of bicarbonate ion passing through the kidney tubules increase potassium secretion, and hypokalemia is possible.

Sodium bicarbonate interacts with several drugs. For example, it may decrease absorption of ketoconazole (Nizoral) and may decrease elimination of dextroamphetamine (Dexedrine), ephedrine, pseudoephedrine (Sudafed), and quinidine (Quinate). Sodium bicarbonate may increase elimination of lithium (Carbolith, Lithane), salicylates, and tetracyclines.

Pharmacotherapy of Alkalosis

53.12 Pharmacotherapy of alkalosis, a plasma pH above 7.45, includes the administration of ammonium chloride, or sodium chloride with potassium chloride.

At plasma pH values above 7.45, **alkalosis** develops. Like acidosis, alkalosis may have both respiratory and metabolic causes, as shown in Table 53.6. Also like acidosis, the CNS is greatly affected. Symptoms of CNS stimulation include nervousness, hyperactive reflexes, and convulsions. Slow, shallow breathing indicates that the body is attempting to retain acid and lower internal pH. In mild cases, alkalosis may be corrected by administering sodium chloride combined with potassium chloride. This combination increases the renal excretion of bicarbonate ion, which indirectly increases the acidity of the blood. More severe alkalosis may be treated with infusions of ammonium chloride.

Nursing Considerations

The role of the nurse in drug therapy with ammonium chloride involves careful monitoring of the client's condition and providing education as it relates to the prescribed drug regimen. The major treatment for both metabolic alkalosis and respiratory alkalosis is to first attempt to correct the underlying disease condition creating

---

CONNECTIONS   Natural Therapies

◀ **Sea Vegetables for Acidosis**

Sea vegetables, or seaweeds, are a form of marine algae that grows in the upper levels of the ocean, where sunlight can penetrate. Examples of these edible seaweeds include kelp, arame, and nori, which are used a great deal in Japanese cooking. Sea vegetables are found in coastal locations throughout the world. Kelp (*Laminaria*) is found in the cold waters of the North Atlantic and Pacific oceans.

Sea vegetables contain a multitude of vitamins, as well as protein. However, their most notable nutritional aspect is their mineral content. Plants from the sea contain more minerals than most other food sources, including calcium, magnesium, phosphorus, iron, potassium, and all essential trace elements. Because they are so rich in minerals, seaweeds act as alkalizers of the blood, helping to rid the body of acidic conditions (acidosis). Kelp is a particularly rich source of iron.

---

the imbalance. The administration of ammonium chloride is only used in clinical practice when the alkalosis is so severe that the pH must be restored quickly to prevent life-threatening consequences. This drug is contraindicated in the presence of liver disease since its acidifying action depends on proper liver functioning to convert ammonium ions to urea.

During the IV infusion of ammonium chloride, the nurse must continually assess for metabolic acidosis and ammonium toxicity. Symptoms of toxic levels of ammonium include pallor, sweating, irregular breathing, retching, bradycardia, twitching, and convulsions. If the client exhibits any of these symptoms, the nurse should immediately stop the infusion and contact the healthcare provider.

The nurse must also closely monitor the client's renal status during the administration of ammonium chloride because the excretion of this drug depends on normal kidney function. Monitor intake and output ratio, body weight, electrolyte status, and renal function studies for any sign of renal impairment.

When ammonium chloride is administered IV, closely monitor the IV infusion site because this drug is extremely irritating to veins and may cause severe inflammation. The drug must be infused slowly, no more than 5 mL/minute, to prevent ammonia toxicity.

Like sodium bicarbonate, ammonium chloride is used as an ionic trapping agent in the treatment of drug overdoses. Ammonium chloride acidifies urine, which increases the excretion of alkaline substances such as amphetamines, phencyclidine (PCP/angel dust), and other basic substances. Overdoses of alkaline substances can greatly compromise the cardiovascular, respiratory, and neurological status, and the nursing role in these situations will be directed toward monitoring the client's acid-base status and supporting critical body functions.

Client education as it relates to ammonium chloride should include goals, reasons for obtaining baseline data such as vital signs and renal status, and possible side effects. The following are the important points to include when teaching clients and families regarding ammonium chloride:

- Report pain at the IV site.
- If medication is taken orally, report anorexia, nausea, vomiting, and thirst.

- If medication is given parenterally, report rash, headache, bradycardia, drowsiness, confusion, depression, and excitement alternating with coma.

- Take ammonium chloride tablets for no longer than 6 days.

- Report severe GI upset, fever, chills, and changes in urine or stool colour.

- Take medication after meals or use enteric-coated tablets to decrease GI upset; swallow tablets whole.

| **PROTOTYPE DRUG** | **Ammonium Chloride** |

Actions and Uses: Severe alkalosis may be reversed by the administration of acidic agents such as ammonium chloride. During the hepatic conversion of ammonium chloride to urea, Cl^- and H^+ are formed, and the pH of body fluids decreases. Ammonium chloride acidifies the urine, which is beneficial in treating certain urinary tract infections. Historically, it has been used as a diuretic, though safer and more efficacious agents have made its use for this indication obsolete. By acidifying the urine, ammonium chloride promotes the excretion of alkaline drugs such as amphetamines. When given for acidosis, the IM or IV route is preferred.

Pharmacokinetics: Ammonium chloride is administered PO or IV. Ammonium chloride is rapidly absorbed. It is mostly metabolized in the liver. Excretion is by the kidneys.

Administration Alerts:
- IV solution should be infused slowly (no faster than 5 mL/ minute) to prevent ammonia toxicity.
- Ammonium chloride is pregnancy category C.

Adverse Effects and Interactions: Ammonium chloride is generally infused slowly to minimize the potential for producing acidosis. Observe for signs of CNS depression characteristic of acidosis. Ammonium chloride may interact with several drugs; for example, it may cause crystalluria when taken with aminosalicylic acid. Ammonium chloride increases excretion of amphetamines, flecainide (Tambocor), mexiletine (Mexitil), methadone (Metadol), ephedrine, and pseudoephedrine and decreases urinary excretion of sulfonylureas and salicylates.

CHAPTER

53 Understanding the Chapter

Key Concepts Summary

The numbered key concepts provide a succinct summary of the important points from the corresponding numbered section within the chapter. If any of these points are not clear, refer to the numbered section within the chapter for review.

53.1 There is a continuous exchange of fluids across membranes separating the intracellular and extracellular fluid compartments. Large molecules and those that are ionized are less able to cross membranes.

53.2 Changes in the osmolality of body fluids can cause water to move to different compartments.

53.3 Water balance is achieved through complex mechanisms that regulate fluid intake and output. The greatest contributor to osmolality is sodium, although glucose and urea also contribute.

53.4 Intravenous fluid therapy using crystalloids and colloids is used to replace lost fluids. Colloids such as dextran have the ability to rapidly expand plasma volume.

53.5 Transfusions of blood products are used to treat serious conditions that cannot be managed effectively by other means.

53.6 Electrolytes are charged substances that are essential to nerve conduction, membrane permeability, water balance, and other critical body functions.

53.7 Sodium is essential to maintain osmolality, water balance, and acid-base balance. Hypernatremia may be corrected with hypotonic IV fluids or diuretics, and hyponatremia is corrected with infusions of sodium chloride.

53.8 Potassium is essential for proper nervous and muscle function as well as for maintaining acid-base balance. Hyperkalemia may be treated with glucose and insulin or by administration of polystyrene sulfonate.

53.9 Magnesium imbalances significantly affect cardiovascular and neuromuscular function.

53.10 The body uses buffers to maintain overall pH within narrow limits.

53.11 Pharmacotherapy of acidosis, a plasma pH below 7.35, includes the administration of sodium bicarbonate.

53.12 Pharmacotherapy of alkalosis, a plasma pH above 7.45, includes the administration of ammonium chloride, or sodium chloride with potassium chloride.

Chapter 53 Scenario

Peggy Hover is 26 years old and has been admitted to the short-stay surgical unit for an elective laparoscopic cholecystectomy. She has been in good health except for repeated bouts of gallbladder attacks, and it is anticipated that she will be able to go home this afternoon after the surgery is completed.

As the nurse admitting Peggy, you have orders to start a D_5W infusion prior to surgery, to run at 15 mL/hour. You have started the IV in her right hand. Peggy asks you why she needs it, especially since she will be returning home that afternoon.

Critical Thinking Questions

1. Why do you think an IV was ordered for Peggy, and what will you explain to her?

2. What are the two main categories of IV solutions? Which category was ordered for Peggy?

3. D_5W (5% dextrose in water) is a common solution. What precautions should be taken with this fluid type?

See Answers to Critical Thinking Questions in Appendix B.

NCLEX Practice Questions

1 A client with a disorder causing metabolic acidosis is being treated with intravenous sodium bicarbonate. The nurse monitors for therapeutic effectiveness by noting which laboratory values?

   a. Serum pH

   b. Red blood cell count

   c. Liver function test

   d. Blood urea nitrogen

2 The nurse is teaching a client about a liquid potassium chloride supplement. Which statement by the client would indicate that further teaching is necessary?

   a. "I should avoid salt substitutes unless they're approved by my healthcare provider."

   b. "Liquid preparations should not be diluted with other fluids."

   c. "I should report signs of potassium deficit, such as weakness and fatigue."

   d. "Persistent vomiting will result in significant losses of potassium."

3 The client will be receiving 5% dextrose in water (D_5W) intravenous infusion. Which statement about this therapy is correct?

   a. D_5W can cause hypoglycemia in a client who has diabetes.

   b. D_5W may be used to dilute mixed intravenous drugs.

   c. D_5W is considered a colloid solution.

   d. D_5W has a sufficient number of calories to supply metabolic needs.

4 The healthcare provider orders intravenous magnesium sulfate for a pregnant client with preeclampsia. The nurse should consult with the prescriber about how the drug therapy may be affected by which client assessment?

   a. Pupil constriction to direct light

   b. Chest congestion and coughing

   c. Elevated blood pressure

   d. Decreased patellar deep tendon reflexes

5 Which of the following nursing actions should be included in the care plan for a client receiving normal serum albumin? Select all that apply.

   a. Documenting past history of blood transfusion reactions

   b. Restricting dietary intake of food high in potassium

   c. Monitoring blood pressure and pulse rate

   d. Measuring urinary output hourly

   e. Observing for signs related to potassium deficit

See Answers to NCLEX Practice Questions in Appendix A.

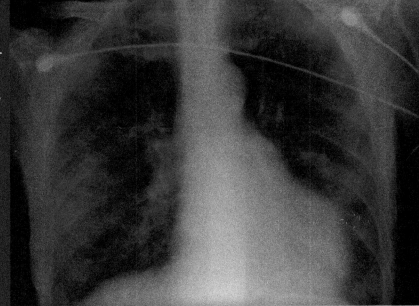

PROTOTYPE DRUGS

ANGIOTENSIN-CONVERTING ENZYME INHIBITORS
Pr *lisinopril (Prinivil, Zestril)*

ANGIOTENSIN II RECEPTOR BLOCKERS

BETA-ADRENERGIC BLOCKERS
Pr *carvedilol (Coreg)*

VASODILATORS
Pr *isosorbide dinitrate (Isordil, ISDN)*

CARDIAC GLYCOSIDES
Pr *digoxin (Lanoxin, Toloxin)*

DIURETICS
Loop (high ceiling)
Pr *furosemide (Lasix)*
Thiazide and thiazide-like
Potassium-sparing

PHOSPHODIESTERASE INHIBITORS
Pr *milrinone*

Cultura RM/Alamy Stock Photo

Pharmacotherapy of Heart Failure

LEARNING OUTCOMES

After reading this chapter, the student should be able to:

1. Identify the major diseases associated with heart failure.
2. Relate how the symptoms associated with heart failure may be caused by a weakened heart muscle and diminished cardiac output.
3. Identify drug classes used for treating heart failure.
4. Explain the therapeutic action of each class of drug used for heart failure in relation to the pathophysiology of heart failure.
5. Describe the nurse's role in the pharmacological management of clients who are receiving drugs for heart failure.
6. For each of the drug classes listed in Prototype Drugs, identify a representative drug and explain its mechanism of action, therapeutic effects, and important adverse effects.
7. Describe and explain, based on pharmacological principles, the rationale for nursing assessment, planning, interventions, and teaching for clients with heart failure.
8. Use the nursing process to care for clients who are receiving drug therapy for heart failure.

CHAPTER OUTLINE

Heart failure is one of the most common and fatal of the cardiovascular diseases, and its incidence is expected to increase as the population ages. Despite the dramatic decline in mortality for most cardiovascular diseases that has occurred over the past 2 decades, the death rate for heart failure has only recently begun to decrease. Although improved treatment of myocardial infarction and hypertension has led to declines in mortality due to heart failure, approximately one in five clients still dies within 1 year of diagnosis of heart failure, and 50% die within 5 years. Historically, this condition was called congestive heart failure; however, because heart failure can be diagnosed without evidence of volume overload or congestion, it is now called heart failure.

The Etiology of Heart Failure

54.1 The central cause of HF is weakened heart muscle. Diminished contractility reduces cardiac output.

Heart failure (HF) is the inability of the ventricles to pump enough blood to meet the body's metabolic demands. HF can be caused by any disorder that decreases the ability of the heart to receive or eject blood. These disorders include:

- Mitral stenosis
- Myocardial infarction (MI)
- Chronic hypertension
- Coronary artery disease (CAD)
- Diabetes mellitus

The ability to prevent major causes of morbidity and mortality through control of healthy lifestyle choices is a common theme in cardiovascular pharmacology. Controlling lipid levels, implementing a regular exercise program, maintaining optimum body weight, and keeping blood pressure within recommended limits reduce the incidences of CAD and MI. Maintaining blood glucose within the normal range reduces the consequences of uncontrolled diabetes. Thus, for many clients, HF is a preventable condition; controlling associated diseases will greatly reduce the risk of development and progression of HF.

Since there is no cure for HF, the treatment goals are to prevent, treat, or remove the underlying causes whenever possible and to treat its symptoms, so that the client's quality of life can be improved. Advances in understanding the pathophysiology of HF during the past 2 decades have led to a change in pharmacotherapeutic goals. No longer is therapy of HF focused on end stages of the disorder. Pharmacotherapy is now targeted at prevention and slowing the progression of HF. This change in emphasis has led to significant improvements in survival and quality of life in clients with HF.

Cardiovascular Changes in Heart Failure

54.2 The three primary characteristics of heart function are force of contraction, heart rate, and speed of impulse conduction.

Although a number of diseases can lead to HF, the end result is the same: the heart is unable to pump the volume of blood required to meet the body's metabolic needs. To understand how medications act on the weakened myocardium, it is essential to understand the underlying cardiac physiology.

The right side of the heart receives blood from the venous system and pumps it to the lungs, where the blood receives oxygen and loses its carbon dioxide. The blood returns to the left side of the heart, which pumps it to the rest of the body via the aorta. The amount of blood received by the right side should exactly equal that sent out by the left side. If this does not happen, HF may occur. The amount of blood pumped by each ventricle per minute is the **cardiac output**. The relationship between cardiac output and blood pressure is explained in Chapter 51.

Although many variables affect cardiac output, the two most important factors are preload and afterload. Just before the chambers of the heart contract (systole), they are filled to their maximum capacity with blood. The degree to which the myocardial fibres are stretched just prior to contraction is called **preload**. The more these fibres are stretched, the more forcefully they will contract, a principle called the **Frank-Starling law**. This is somewhat similar to a rubber band—the more it is stretched, the more forcefully it will snap back. The strength of contraction of the heart is called **contractility**. Drugs that increase preload and contractility help to increase cardiac output. Drugs such as norepinephrine (Levophed), epinephrine (Adrenalin), and thyroid hormone that increase contractility are called positive inotropic agents. Drugs such as beta-adrenergic blockers and quinidine (Quinate) decrease contractility and are called negative inotropic agents.

The second important factor affecting cardiac output is afterload. **Afterload** is the pressure in the aorta that must be overcome for blood to be ejected from the left ventricle. Hypertension increases afterload and workload of the heart. Drugs that treat hypertension are explained in Chapter 51.

In HF, the myocardium becomes weakened, and the heart cannot eject all the blood it receives. This weakening may occur on the left side, the right side, or both sides of the heart. If it occurs on the left side, excess blood accumulates in the left ventricle. The wall of the left ventricle may become thicker (hypertrophies) in an attempt to compensate for the extra blood retained in the chamber. Since the left ventricle has limits to its ability to compensate for the increased preload, blood "backs up" into the lungs, resulting in the classic symptoms of cough and shortness of breath. Left heart failure is sometimes called congestive heart failure (CHF). The pathophysiology of HF is shown in Figure 54.1.

Although left heart failure is more common, the right side of the heart can also weaken, either simultaneously with the left side or independently. In right heart failure, the blood backs up into the peripheral veins, resulting in **peripheral edema** and engorgement of organs such as the liver. The symptoms of HF are listed in Figure 54.2.

PHARMACOTHERAPY OF HEART FAILURE

Drugs can relieve the symptoms of heart failure by a number of different mechanisms, including slowing the heart rate, increasing contractility, and reducing workload. These mechanisms are illustrated in Figure 54.3.

The 2007 Canadian Cardiovascular Society Consensus Conference recommendations for the management of HF are outlined in

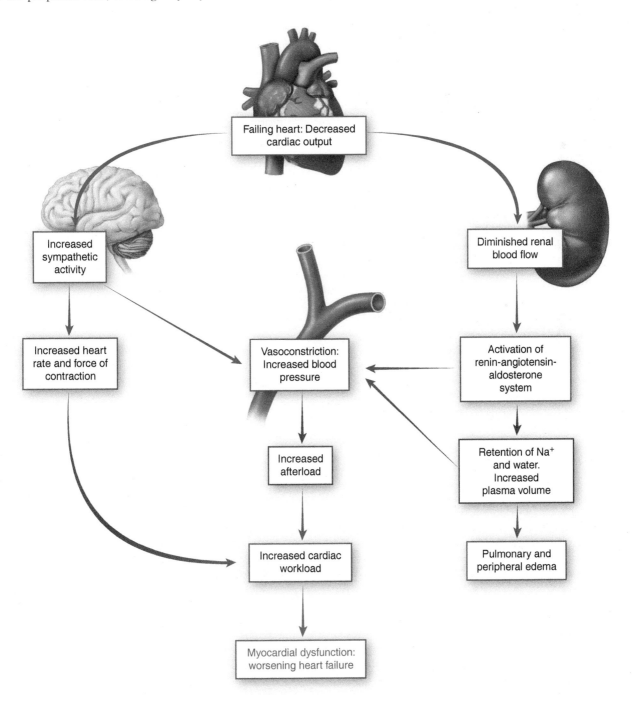

Figure 54.1 Pathophysiology of heart failure.

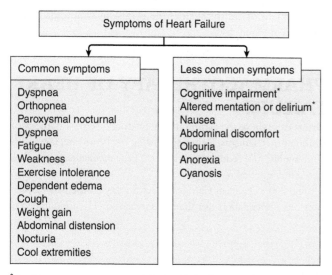

Figure 54.2 as a flowchart:

Symptoms of Heart Failure

Common symptoms
- Dyspnea
- Orthopnea
- Paroxysmal nocturnal Dyspnea
- Fatigue
- Weakness
- Exercise intolerance
- Dependent edema
- Cough
- Weight gain
- Abdominal distension
- Nocturia
- Cool extremities

Less common symptoms
- Cognitive impairment*
- Altered mentation or delirium*
- Nausea
- Abdominal discomfort
- Oliguria
- Anorexia
- Cyanosis

*May be a more common presentation in elderly clients.

Figure 54.2 Symptoms of heart failure.

Source: Based on JMO Arnold, P Liu, C Demers, et al. Canadian Cardiovascular Society consensus conference recommendations on heart failure 2006: Diagnosis and management. *Can J Cardiol* 2006;22(1):23-45.

Figure 54.4. Non-pharmacological recommendations include client education about HF, lifestyle modifications to reduce risk factors and symptoms, and control of salt intake. Pharmacological recommendations include that all HF clients with a left ventricle that ejects less than 40% of received blood should be treated with both an angiotensin-converting enzyme (ACE) inhibitor and a beta blocker, unless a specific contraindication exists. Usually, ACE inhibitor therapy is initiated before the beta blocker is added. Angiotensin receptor blockers (ARBs) may be used when symptoms persist despite optimal treatment with ACE inhibitors and beta blockers or when these agents cannot be used. Diuretics should be used for most clients with HF who have peripheral edema or pulmonary congestion. Once acute congestion is cleared, the lowest dose that maintains stable signs and symptoms should be used. Digoxin (Lanoxin, Toloxin) may be used to relieve symptoms and reduce hospitalizations in clients in sinus rhythm who have persistent moderate to severe symptoms despite optimized therapy with other HF drugs. Also, clients with HF should be immunized against influenza (annually) and pneumococcal pneumonia (if not done in the last 6 years) to reduce the risk for respiratory infections that may seriously aggravate HF.

Pharmacotherapy of HF focuses on three primary goals:

1. Reduction of preload
2. Reduction of systemic vascular resistance (afterload reduction)

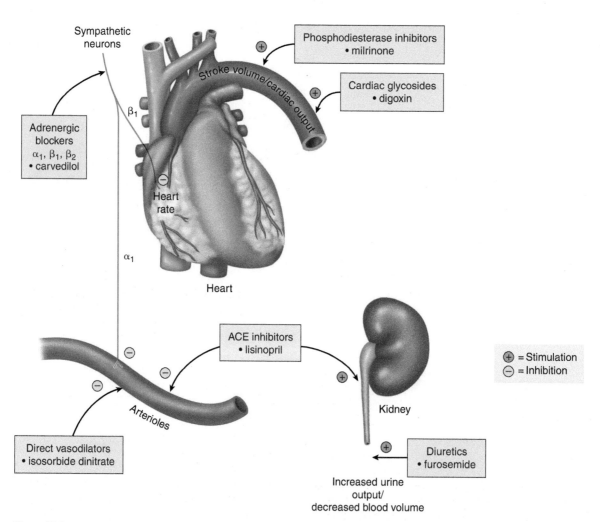

Figure 54.3 Mechanisms of action of drugs used for heart failure.

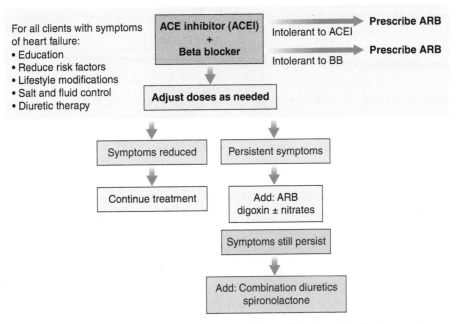

Figure 54.4 Treatment of heart failure: recommendations of the Canadian Cardiovascular Society Consensus Conference.

Source: Based on JMO Arnold, P Liu, C Demers, et al. Canadian Cardiovascular Society consensus conference recommendations on heart failure 2006: Diagnosis and management. *Can J Cardiol* 2006;22(1):23-45.

3. Inhibition of both the renin-angiotensin-aldosterone system (RAAS) and the vasoconstrictor mechanisms of the sympathetic nervous system.

The first two goals provide symptomatic relief but do not reverse the progression of the disease. In addition to reducing symptoms, inhibition of the RAAS and vasoconstriction by the sympathetic nervous system also result in a significant reduction in morbidity and mortality from HF.

ACE INHIBITORS AND ANGIOTENSIN RECEPTOR BLOCKERS

Drugs that affect the renin-angiotensin-aldosterone system reduce the afterload on the heart and lower blood pressure. They are often drugs of choice in the treatment of HF. The ACE inhibitors and ARBs used for HF are listed in Table 54.1.

NCLEX Success Tips

Nonsteroidal anti-inflammatory drugs (NSAIDs) decrease the antihypertensive effect of ACE inhibitors and put the client at risk for developing acute renal failure. Lab tests used to evaluate the function of the kidneys are blood urea nitrogen (BUN), creatinine, and creatinine clearance.

Captopril (Capoten) is an ACE inhibitor, and hyperkalemia is a side effect. The BUN and creatinine should be viewed prior to administration because renal insufficiency is another potential side effect of an ACE inhibitor.

White blood cell count should be monitored in clients who are receiving captopril before the initiation of the drug and every 2 weeks for the first 3 months. The client should notify the physician if they develop a fever, sore throat, leukopenia, or tachycardia.

When ACE inhibitors are used with potassium-sparing diuretics, potassium supplements, or salt substitutes, hyperkalemia can occur.

Angioedema is an indication that the ACE inhibitor should be discontinued.

ACE inhibitors act by preventing the conversion of angiotensin I to angiotensin II. Angiotensin II is a potent vasoconstrictor and also contributes to aldosterone secretion. Thus, ACE inhibitors decreases blood pressure through systemic vasodilation.

ACE inhibitors can cause a characteristic dry, nonproductive cough that reverses when therapy is stopped.

Facial swelling or difficulty breathing would be reported immediately in clients who are receiving ACE inhibitors because they may be signs of angioedema, which would require discontinuation of the drug.

The nurse should teach the client taking ACE inhibitors to change positions slowly to minimize the risk of orthostatic hypotension. The nurse would tell the client to report light-headedness.

Pharmacotherapy with ACE Inhibitors and ARBs

54.3 ACE inhibitors improve HF by reducing peripheral edema and increasing cardiac output. They are first-line drugs for the treatment of HF.

ACE inhibitors were approved for the treatment of hypertension in the 1980s. Since then, research has shown that they can prevent the occurrence of HF in clients at risk and slow the progression of HF. Because of their relative safety and efficacy, they have replaced digoxin as drugs of choice for the treatment of HF. Unless specifically contraindicated, ACE inhibitors should be given to all clients with HF and many clients at high risk for HF.

The primary action of the ACE inhibitors is to lower blood pressure by their action on the renin-angiotensin-aldosterone system. ACE inhibitors inhibit aldosterone excretion, enhancing the excretion of sodium and water and decreasing blood volume. The resultant

TABLE 54.1   Drugs for Heart Failure

Drug	Route and Adult Dose
ACE Inhibitors	
captopril (Capoten)	Orally (PO), start with 6.25 mg three times a day (tid); target is 50 mg tid (max 450 mg/day)
enalapril (Vasotec) (see Chapter 51, page 642, for the Prototype Drug box)	PO, start with 2.5 mg twice a day (bid); usual range is 5–40 mg in two divided doses (max 40 mg/day)
fosinopril (Monopril)	PO, 5–40 mg every day (qd) (max 40 mg/day)
Pr lisinopril (Prinivil, Zestril)	PO, start with 2.5–5 mg/day; usual dosage is 5–40 mg/day (max 80 mg/day)
quinapril (Accupril)	PO, start with 5 mg bid; target range is 20–40 mg in two divided doses (max 40 mg/day)
ramipril (Altace)	PO, 2.5–5.0 mg bid (max 10/day)
Angiotensin II Receptor Blockers	
candesartan (Atacand)	PO, start with 4 mg qd; usual dosage is 4–32 mg qd
eprosartan (Teveten)	PO, 600–800 mg/day in one to two divided doses
irbesartan (Avapro)	PO, 150–300 mg qd (max 300 mg/day)
losartan (Cozaar)	PO, 25–100 mg/day in one to two divided doses (max 100 mg/day)
valsartan (Diovan)	PO, start with 40 mg bid; target dose is 160 mg bid (max 320 mg/day)
Beta-Adrenergic Blockers	
Pr carvedilol (Coreg)	PO, 3.125–6.25 mg bid (max 100 mg/day)
metoprolol: beta$_1$ (Lopressor, Lopressor SR)	PO, 12.5–200 mg/day
Vasodilators	
hydralazine (Apresoline) (see Chapter 51, page 648, for the Prototype Drug box)	PO, 10–50 mg four times a day (qid) (max 300 mg/day)
Pr isosorbide dinitrate (Isordil, ISDN)	PO, start with 20-30 mg tid-qid (max 120 mg/day)
Diuretics	
Loop (High Ceiling)	
bumetanide (Burinex)	PO, 0.5–2 mg qd–bid (max 10 mg/day); IM/IV, 0.5–1 mg/dose, may repeat in 2–3 hours up to two doses (max 10 mg/day)
Pr furosemide (Lasix)	PO, 20–80 mg in one or more divided doses (max 600 mg/day); IM/IV, start with 20–40 mg/dose, can administer another 20 mg/day and administer 1–2 hours after previous dose (max 200 mg/day)
Thiazide and Thiazide-Like	
hydrochlorothiazide (HCTZ, Urozide) (see Chapter 51, page 637, for the Prototype Drug box)	PO, 25–100 mg/day in one to two divided doses (max 200 mg/day)
Potassium-Sparing	
spironolactone (Aldactone) (see Chapter 52, page 660, for the Prototype Drug box)	PO, start with 12.5–25 mg/day (max 50 mg/day)
triamterene	PO, 100–300 mg/day in one or two divided doses (max 300 mg/day)
Cardiac Glycosides	
Pr digoxin (Lanoxin, Toloxin)	PO, 0.125–0.25 mg qd
Phosphodiesterase Inhibitors	
Pr milrinone	Intravenous (IV), 50 µg/kg over 10 minutes; then 0.375–0.75 µg/kg/minute

reduction in arterial blood pressure reduces the afterload of the heart, thus increasing cardiac output. An additional effect of the ACE inhibitors is dilation of the veins returning blood to the heart. This action, which is probably not directly related to their inhibition of angiotensin, decreases preload and reduces peripheral edema. The combined reductions in preload, afterload, and blood volume substantially decrease the workload of the heart and allow it to work more efficiently for the HF client. Several ACE inhibitors have been shown to reduce mortality following acute myocardial infarction when therapy is started soon after the onset of symptoms (Chapter 50).

Another mechanism for decreasing the effects of angiotensin is the use of ARBs. The actions of the ARBs are similar to those of the ACE inhibitors, as would be expected since both classes inhibit angiotensin. In clients with HF, ARBs show equivalent efficacy to the ACE inhibitors. Their use in the treatment of HF is usually reserved for clients who are unable to tolerate the side effects of ACE inhibitors or who have persistent HF symptoms despite optimal treatment

with ACE inhibitors and beta blockers. More information on ACE inhibitors and ARBs can be found in Chapter 51.

Nursing Considerations

The role of the nurse in ACE inhibitor or ARB therapy for HF involves careful monitoring of the client's condition and providing education as it relates to the prescribed drug regimen. Prior to beginning therapy, a thorough health history should be taken. These drugs are contraindicated in pregnancy and lactation and in clients with a history of angioedema. A complete blood count should be obtained before starting therapy and repeated every month for the first 3 to 6 months of treatment, then at periodic intervals for 1 year. ACE inhibitors should be withheld if the neutrophil count drops below 1000/mm^3 because they may cause neutropenia. An increase in serum creatinine of up to 30% is not unexpected when ACE inhibitor or ARB therapy is initiated. Diuretics should be discontinued before the nurse initially administers ACE inhibitors, to prevent severe hypotension. Because ACE inhibitors can cause severe hypotension with initial doses, monitor the client closely for several hours afterwards. If severe hypotension does occur, place the client in a supine position and notify the healthcare provider. A lower dose is indicated for elderly clients and those with renal insufficiency. Use with caution in clients with impaired kidney function, hyperkalemia, and autoimmune diseases, especially systemic lupus erythematosus.

Client education as it relates to ACE inhibitors or ARBs used to treat HF should include goals, reasons for obtaining baseline data such as vital signs and tests for cardiac and renal function, and possible side effects. The following are the important points to include when teaching clients regarding ACE inhibitors or ARBs:

- Check with the healthcare provider before taking additional prescription medications or over-the-counter (OTC) drugs.
- It may take weeks or months for maximum therapeutic response to be reached.
- Follow prescribed dietary modifications, including sodium and potassium restrictions, to prevent side effects of hyponatremia and hyperkalemia.
- Do not take salt or potassium supplements unless ordered by the healthcare provider.
- Avoid driving until the effect of the drug is known.

Refer to Nursing Process Focus: Clients Receiving ACE Inhibitor Therapy in Chapter 51 for additional information.

CONNECTIONS Special Considerations

◀ Points to Consider in Educating Clients with HF

- Regular physical activity is recommended for all clients with stable symptoms and impaired left ventricular systolic function.
- Before starting a physical activity program, all clients should have a graded exercise stress test to assess functional capacity, ischemia, and optimal heart rate.
- Erect and supine blood pressure should be assessed.
- All clients with symptomatic HF should not add salt to their diet, and clients with advanced HF should reduce salt to less than 2 g/day.
- Fluid intake beyond normal needs to prevent thirst is *not* recommended.
- Daily morning weight should be monitored in HF clients with fluid retention or congestion not easily controlled with diuretics and in clients with significant renal dysfunction or hyponatremia.
- Restriction of daily fluid intake to 1.5 to 2 L/day should be considered for clients with fluid retention or congestion not easily controlled with diuretics and in clients with severe renal dysfunction or hyponatremia.
- Clients with HF should be immunized against influenza (annually) and pneumococcal pneumonia (if not done in the last 6 years) to reduce the risk for respiratory infections that may seriously aggravate HF.
- Clients should be aware of which symptoms to report immediately to the healthcare provider.

Based on Canadian Cardiovascular Society Consensus Conference recommendations on heart failure (Arnold et al., 2006).http://www.ncbi.nlm.nih.gov/pmc/articles/PMC2538984/

PROTOTYPE DRUG Lisinopril (Prinivil, Zestril)

Actions and Uses: Due to its value in the treatment of both HF and hypertension, lisinopril has become one of the most commonly prescribed drugs. Like other ACE inhibitors, doses of lisinopril may require 2 to 3 weeks of adjustment to reach maximum efficacy, and several months of therapy may be needed for a client's cardiac function to return to normal. Because of their synergistic hypotensive action, combined therapy with lisinopril and diuretics should be carefully monitored.

Pharmacokinetics: Absorption of lisinopril is about 25% but varies. It is excreted unchanged by the kidneys. It has a half-life of 12 hours.

Administration Alerts:
- Measure blood pressure just prior to administering lisinopril to be certain that effects are lasting for 24 hours and to determine if the client's blood pressure is within acceptable range.
- Lisinopril is pregnancy category D.

Adverse Effects and Interactions: Although lisinopril causes few side effects, hyperkalemia may occur during therapy; therefore, electrolyte levels are usually monitored periodically. Other side effects include cough, taste disturbances, headache, dizziness, chest pain, nausea, vomiting, diarrhea, and hypotension.

Lisinopril interacts with indomethacin (Indocin) and other NSAIDs, causing decreased antihypertensive activity. When taken concurrently with potassium-sparing diuretics, hyperkalemia may result. Lisinopril may increase lithium levels and toxicity.

BETA-ADRENERGIC BLOCKERS (ANTAGONISTS)

Only two beta blockers are approved for the treatment of HF: carvedilol and metoprolol extended-release form. The doses of these agents are shown in Table 54.1. They reduce the cardiac workload by decreasing afterload.

Pharmacotherapy with Beta-Adrenergic Blockers

54.4 Beta-adrenergic blockers play a role in the treatment of HF by slowing the heart rate and decreasing blood pressure. They are used in combination with ACE inhibitors as first-line drugs for HF.

Beta-adrenergic blockers improve the symptoms of HF by reducing cardiac workload. The negative inotropic effect (decreased heart contractility) of beta blockers is in contrast to the positive inotropic effect (increased heart contractility) of cardiac glycosides and some other drugs that may be used to treat HF.

Clients with HF have excessive activation of the sympathetic nervous system, which weakens the heart and leads to progression of the disease. Beta blockers block the cardiac actions of the sympathetic nervous system, thus slowing the heart rate and reducing blood pressure. The decreased afterload that results reduces cardiac workload; after several months of therapy, heart size, shape, and function return to normal in some clients. Extensive clinical research has demonstrated that the proper use of beta blockers can dramatically reduce HF-associated hospitalizations and deaths.

To benefit clients with HF, however, beta blockers must be administered in a very specific manner. Initial doses must be one-tenth to one-twentieth of the target dose. Doses are doubled every 2 weeks until the optimum dose is reached. If therapy is begun with too high a dose or the dose is increased too rapidly, beta blockers can worsen HF. Beta blockers are rarely used as monotherapy for HF. The 2007 Canadian Cardiovascular Society Consensus Conference recommends that they be used in combination with ACE inhibitors as first-line therapy for HF.

The basic pharmacology of the beta blockers is presented in Chapter 14. Other uses of beta blockers are discussed elsewhere in this text: hypertension in Chapter 51, dysrhythmias in Chapter 55, and angina and myocardial infarction in Chapter 50.

Nursing Considerations

The role of the nurse in beta blocker therapy involves careful monitoring of the client's condition and providing education as it relates to the prescribed drug regimen. Beta blockers are contraindicated in clients with decompensated HF, chronic obstructive pulmonary disease, bradycardia, or heart block. Beta blockers are also contraindicated in pregnant or lactating clients. These medications should be used with caution in clients with diabetes, peripheral vascular disease, and hepatic impairment. Caution is needed with elderly clients, who may need a reduced dose.

The nurse should monitor for worsening signs and symptoms of HF and for signs of hepatic toxicity. Liver function tests should be assessed periodically. Notify the healthcare provider if signs or symptoms of liver impairment become apparent.

Client education as it relates to beta blockers should include goals, reasons for obtaining baseline data such as liver function tests, and possible side effects. The following are the important points to include when teaching clients regarding beta blockers:

- Monitor blood pressure and pulse. Notify the healthcare provider if pulse is less than 50 to 60 beats/minute.
- Report immediately signs and symptoms of worsening HF, such as shortness of breath, edema of feet and ankles, and chest pain.
- Do not stop taking the drug abruptly without consulting with the healthcare provider.
- Diabetic clients should monitor serum glucose carefully because these drugs may cause changes in blood sugar levels.
- Report significant side effects such as fainting, difficulty breathing, weight gain, and slow, irregular heart rate.

See Nursing Process Focus: Clients Receiving Adrenergic Antagonist Therapy in Chapter 14 for additional information.

PROTOTYPE DRUG	Carvedilol (Coreg)

Actions and Uses: Carvedilol is the first beta blocker approved for the treatment of HF. It has been found to reduce symptoms, slow the progression of the disease, and increase exercise tolerance when combined with other HF drugs such as the ACE inhibitors. Unlike many drugs in this class, carvedilol blocks beta$_1$- and beta$_2$- as well as alpha$_1$-adrenergic receptors. The primary therapeutic effects relevant to HF are a reduction in heart rate and a drop in blood pressure. The lower blood pressure decreases afterload and reduces the workload of the heart.

Administration Alerts:
- To minimize the risk of orthostatic hypotension, give the drug with food to slow absorption.
- Carvedilol is pregnancy category C.

Pharmacokinetics: The bioavailability of carvedilol is 25% to 35% due to first-pass metabolism. It is 98% protein bound and is excreted mostly in bile and feces. Its half-life is 7 to 10 hours.

Adverse Effects and Interactions: The ability of carvedilol to decrease the heart rate combined with its ability to reduce contractility has the potential to worsen HF; therefore, dosage must be carefully monitored. Because of the potential for adverse cardiac effects, beta blockers such as carvedilol are not considered first-line drugs alone in the treatment of HF.

Carvedilol interacts with many drugs. For example, levels of carvedilol are significantly increased when taken concurrently with rifampin. Monoamine oxidase inhibitors, clonidine (Catapres), and reserpine can cause hypotension or bradycardia when given with carvedilol. When given with digoxin, carvedilol may increase digoxin levels. It may also enhance the hypoglycemic effects of insulin and oral hypoglycemic agents.

VASODILATORS

Through their hypotensive effects, vasodilators play a minor role in the pharmacotherapy of HF. They are also used for hypertension and angina pectoris. Doses for the vasodilators are given in Table 54.1.

Pharmacotherapy with Direct Vasodilators

54.5 Vasodilators can help to reduce symptoms of HF by reducing preload and decreasing the oxygen demand of the heart.

The two drugs in this class, hydralazine (Apresoline) and isosorbide dinitrate (Isordil, ISDN), act directly to relax blood vessels and lower blood pressure. Hydralazine acts on arterioles, while isosorbide dinitrate acts on veins. Because the two drugs act synergistically, isosorbide dinitrate is usually combined with hydralazine in the treatment of HF. Because of the high incidence of side effects, they are generally reserved for clients who cannot tolerate ACE inhibitors.

Nursing Considerations

The role of the nurse in the care of clients receiving drug therapy with hydralazine for the treatment of hypertension is discussed in Chapter 51 (see Nursing Considerations and Nursing Process Focus: Clients Receiving Direct Vasodilator Therapy). The use of isosorbide dinitrate for therapy of angina pectoris is presented in Chapter 50 (see Nursing Considerations).

NCLEX Success Tip

Adverse effects of isosorbide are lightheadedness, dizziness, and orthostatic hypotension. Clients should be instructed to change positions slowly to prevent these adverse effects and to avoid fainting.

PROTOTYPE DRUG	Isosorbide Dinitrate (Isordil, ISDN)

Actions and Uses: Isosorbide dinitrate acts directly and selectively on veins to cause venodilation. This reduces venous return (preload), thus decreasing cardiac workload. The resultant improvement in cardiac output reduces pulmonary congestion and peripheral edema and improves exercise tolerance. Isosorbide dinitrate also dilates the coronary arteries to bring more oxygen to the myocardium. Isosorbide dinitrate belongs to a class of drugs called organic nitrates that are widely used in the treatment of angina.

Pharmacokinetics: Isosorbide dinitrate is well absorbed and mostly metabolized by the liver. Its half-life is 50 minutes.

Administration Alerts:

* Do not confuse this drug with isosorbide (Ismotic), which is an oral osmotic diuretic.

* If administered sublingually, advise the client not to eat, drink, talk, or smoke while the tablet is dissolving.

* Isosorbide dinitrate is pregnancy category C.

Adverse Effects and Interactions: Common side effects of isosorbide dinitrate include headache and reflex tachycardia. Orthostatic hypotension may cause dizziness and falling, particularly in older adults. Use is contraindicated if the client is also taking sildenafil (Viagra) because serious hypotension may result.

CARDIAC GLYCOSIDES

The cardiac glycosides were once used as arrow poisons by African tribes and as medicines by the ancient Egyptians and Romans. The value of the cardiac glycosides in treating heart disorders has been known for more than 2000 years. The chemical classification draws its name from three sugars, or glycosides, which are attached to a steroid nucleus. Information on doses of the cardiac glycosides is provided in Table 54.1.

Pharmacotherapy with Cardiac Glycosides

54.6 Cardiac glycosides increase the force of myocardial contraction and are the traditional drugs of choice for HF. Due to a low safety margin, their use has declined.

Extracted from the flowering plants *Digitalis purpurea* (purple foxglove) and *Digitalis lanata* (woolly foxglove), drugs in this class are also called digitalis glycosides. Cardiac glycosides were once the mainstay of HF treatment. Currently, they are reserved for use in clients whose symptoms persist despite first-line therapy

with other drugs. The cardiac glycosides cause the heart to beat more forcefully and more slowly, improving cardiac output. The two primary cardiac glycosides—digoxin and digitoxin—are quite similar in efficacy; the primary difference is that the latter has a more prolonged half-life.

NCLEX Success Tips

Digoxin inhibits the action of the sodium-potassium pump and slows the electrical impulses through the atrioventricular node.

Because digoxin may reduce the heart rate and heart failure may cause a pulse deficit, the nurse should measure the client's apical pulse before administering the drug to prevent further slowing of the heart rate.

Digoxin is metabolized in the liver, and the kidneys eliminate any remaining digoxin as unchanged drug. Therefore, a client with renal failure will require a decreased digoxin dosage. Digoxin is not eliminated by the lungs, feces, or skin.

Hypokalaemia increases the risk for digoxin toxicity and potential dysrhythmias. Abdominal pain, anorexia, nausea, and vomiting are common symptoms of digoxin toxicity. Flickering flashes of light, coloured or halo vision, photophobia, blurring, diplopia, and scotomata and seeing yellow spots are also symptoms of digoxin toxicity. Digoxin toxicity can cause many types of cardiac dysrhythmias, such as atrial fibrillation or bradycardia, due to the increased intracellular calcium release and decreased atrioventricular (AV) conduction time slowing the heart rate.

The earliest clinical signs of digoxin toxicity are anorexia, nausea, and vomiting.

The margin of safety between a therapeutic dose and a toxic dose of digitalis is quite narrow, and severe adverse effects may result from unmonitored treatment. Digitalization refers to a procedure in which the dose of cardiac glycoside is gradually increased until tissues become saturated with the drug and the symptoms of HF diminish. If the client is critically ill, digitalization can be accomplished rapidly with IV doses in a controlled clinical environment where side adverse effects are carefully monitored. For

---

CONNECTIONS	**Natural Therapies**

◀ Hawthorn for Heart Failure

Hawthorn (sometimes spelled hawthorne) is a bush found throughout the United States, Canada, Europe, and Asia. This plant is readily available and may be used to treat symptoms of HF. Research supports its use in HF. In a meta-analysis of randomized clinical trials, it was concluded that there is a significant benefit from hawthorn extract as an adjunctive treatment for chronic HF (Pittler et al., 2003). Its cardiovascular effects are believed to be due to its antioxidant flavonoid components, which increase the integrity of the blood vessel walls, improve coronary blood flow, and increase oxygen use (Chang et al., 2005; Jie et al., 2013; Mary et al., 2010).

Reported adverse effects include nausea, vomiting, and dizziness. Because hawthorn is effective at reducing blood pressure, this vital sign must be monitored. Clients who are concurrently taking an antihypertensive medication should especially be aware of this side effect.

Concurrent use with digoxin may be a concern. However, one interaction study showed that at dosages of 0.25 mg of digoxin per day and 450 mg of hawthorn twice daily, hawthorn did not significantly alter the pharmacokinetic parameters of digoxin (Tankanow et al., 2003).

outpatients, digitalization with digoxin may occur over a period of 7 days, using oral dosing. In either case, the goal is to determine the proper dose of drug that may be administered without undue adverse effects.

Nursing Considerations

The role of the nurse in cardiac glycoside therapy involves careful monitoring of the client's condition and providing education as it relates to the prescribed drug regimen. Prior to beginning therapy with cardiac glycosides, the client should be evaluated for ventricular dysrhythmias not caused by HF and for any history of hypersensitivity to cardiac glycosides. Renal function should be assessed because the drug is excreted by the kidneys. Administer these drugs with caution in elderly clients; those with acute myocardial infarction, incomplete heart block, and renal insufficiency; and in pregnant or lactating clients.

Side effects that the nurse must monitor for when caring for clients who are taking these drugs include fatigue, drowsiness, dizziness, visual disturbances, anorexia, nausea, and vomiting. Advise clients to carry or wear identification describing their medical diagnosis and drug regimen. Instruct clients to eat potassium-rich foods, as hypokalemia may predispose the client to digoxin toxicity. Antacids and antidiarrheal medications should not be taken within 2 hours of cardiac glycoside administration because they decrease the absorption of digoxin.

It is common for dysrhythmias to occur when high doses of digoxin are administered. The nurse should be prepared to administer digoxin immune Fab (Digibind) in the case of life-threatening dysrhythmia. This drug binds and subsequently removes digoxin from the body and prevents toxic effects of overdose.

See Nursing Process Focus: Clients Receiving Cardiac Glycoside Therapy for specific teaching points.

NURSING PROCESS FOCUS

Clients Receiving Cardiac Glycoside Therapy

Assessment	Potential Nursing Diagnoses/Identified Patterns
Prior to administration: • Obtain complete health history, including allergies, drug history, and possible drug interactions. • Assess vital signs, urinary output, and cardiac output, initially and throughout therapy. • Determine the reason the medication is being administered.	• Need for knowledge regarding drug therapy and lifestyle modifications • Need for knowledge related to dietary and drug regimen • Risk for fluid excess and electrolyte imbalance • Ineffective tissue perfusion related to decreased cardiac output • Risk for injury related to decreased cardiac function • Risk for falls related to drug side effects

Planning: Client Goals and Expected Outcomes

The client will:

• Report decreased symptoms of cardiac decompensation related to fluid overload
• Exhibit evidence of improved organ perfusion, including kidney, heart, and brain
• Demonstrate an understanding of the drug's action by accurately describing drug side effects and precautions
• Immediately report side effects such as nausea, vomiting, diarrhea, heart rate below 50, and vision changes

Implementation

Interventions (Rationales)	Client Education/Discharge Planning
• Monitor electrocardiogram (ECG) for rate and rhythm changes during initial digitalization therapy. (Drug has a strong positive inotropic effect.) • Observe for side effects such as nausea, vomiting, diarrhea, anorexia, shortness of breath, vision changes, and leg muscle cramps. • Weigh client daily. • Administer precise ordered dose at same time each day. (Overdose may cause serious toxicity.) • Monitor serum drug level (to determine therapeutic concentration and toxicity). • Report serum drug levels greater than 1.8 ng/mL to the healthcare provider. • Monitor levels of potassium, magnesium, calcium, BUN, and creatinine. (Hypokalemia predisposes the client to digoxin toxicity.) • Monitor for signs and symptoms of digoxin toxicity.	Instruct client to: • Count pulse for 1 full minute and record pulse with every dose • Contact healthcare provider if pulse rate is less than 50 or greater than 100 (or as determined by local agency policies; some providers specify reporting pulse less than 60 and withholding the drug) • Instruct client to report side effects immediately to prevent toxicity • Instruct client to report weight gain of 1 kg or more per day Instruct client to: • Take as directed; do not double dose • Not discontinue drug without advice of the healthcare provider • Instruct client to report to laboratory as scheduled by the healthcare provider for ongoing drug level determinations • Instruct client to consume foods high in potassium such as bananas, apricots, kidney beans, sweet potatoes, and peanut butter • Instruct client to immediately report visual changes, mental depression, palpitations, weakness, loss of appetite, vomiting, and diarrhea

---

Evaluation of Outcome Criteria

Evaluate the effectiveness of drug therapy by confirming that client goals and expected outcomes have been met (see "Planning").

See Table 54.1 (under "Cardiac Glycosides") for a list of drugs to which these nursing actions apply.

PROTOTYPE DRUG	Digoxin (Lanoxin, Toloxin)

Actions and Uses: The primary benefit of digoxin is its ability to increase the contractility of myocardial contraction—a positive inotropic action. Digoxin accomplishes this by inhibiting Na$^+$/K$^+$-ATPase, the critical enzyme responsible for pumping sodium ion out of the myocardial cell in exchange for potassium ion. As sodium accumulates, calcium ions are released from their storage areas in the cell. The release of calcium ion produces a more forceful contraction of the myocardial fibres.

By increasing myocardial contractility, digoxin directly increases cardiac output, thus alleviating symptoms of HF and improving exercise tolerance. The improved cardiac output results in increased urine production and a desirable reduction in blood volume, relieving the distressing symptoms of pulmonary congestion and peripheral edema.

In addition to its positive inotropic effect, digoxin also affects impulse conduction in the heart. Digoxin has the ability to suppress the sinoatrial (SA) node and slow electrical conduction through the AV node. Because of these actions, digoxin is sometimes used to treat dysrhythmias, as discussed in Chapter 55.

Pharmacokinetics: Digoxin taken orally has 60% to 80% bioavailability and peaks in 2 to 8 hours. It is widely distributed and excreted almost completely unchanged by the kidneys. It has a half-life of 36 to 48 hours.

Administration Alerts:
- Take the client's apical pulse for 1 full minute, noting rate, rhythm, and quality before administering. If pulse is below 60 beats/minute, the drug is usually withheld and the healthcare provider is notified.
- Check for recent serum digoxin level results before administering. If the level is higher than 1.8, withhold dose and notify the healthcare provider.
- Digoxin is pregnancy category C.

Adverse Effects and Interactions: The most dangerous adverse effect of digoxin is its ability to create dysrhythmias, particularly in clients who have low potassium levels in the blood (hypokalemia). Because diuretics can cause hypokalemia and may also be used to treat HF, concurrent use of digoxin and diuretics must be carefully monitored. Other adverse effects of digoxin therapy include nausea, vomiting, anorexia, fatigue, and visual disturbances such as seeing haloes, a yellow/green tinge, or blurring. Periodic serum drug levels should be obtained to determine if the digoxin level is within the therapeutic range, so the dosage may be adjusted based on the laboratory results. Because a small increase in digoxin levels can produce serious adverse effects, the nurse must constantly be on the alert for drug-drug interactions and for changes in renal function.

Digoxin interacts with a number of drugs. Antacids and cholesterol-lowering drugs can decrease absorption of digoxin. If calcium is administered IV together with digoxin, it can increase the risk for dysrhythmias. When the client is also receiving quinidine, verapamil (Isoptin), or flecainide (Tambocor), digoxin levels will be significantly increased, and the digoxin dose should be decreased by 50%.

Use with caution with herbal supplements, such as ginseng, which may increase the risk of digoxin toxicity. Ma huang and ephedra may induce dysrhythmias. Clients on cardiac glycosides should be strongly advised not to take any other prescription or OTC medication or herbal product without notifying the healthcare provider.

DIURETICS

Diuretics increase urine flow, thereby reducing blood volume and cardiac workload. They are widely used in the treatment of cardiovascular disease. Select diuretics are shown in Table 54.1.

Pharmacotherapy with Diuretics
54.7 Diuretics relieve symptoms of HF by reducing fluid volume and decreasing blood pressure.

Diuretics are common drugs for the treatment of clients with HF because they produce few adverse effects and are effective at reducing blood volume, edema, and pulmonary congestion. As diuretics reduce fluid volume and lower blood pressure, the workload of the heart is reduced and cardiac output increases. Diuretics are rarely used alone but are prescribed in combination with ACE inhibitors or other HF drugs.

The mechanism by which diuretics reduce blood volume, specifically where and how the nephron is affected, differs among the various drugs. Differences in mechanisms among the classes of diuretics are discussed in Chapter 52. The role of the thiazide diuretics in the treatment of hypertension is discussed in Chapter 51.

Nursing Considerations
The role of the nurse in diuretic therapy for HF involves careful monitoring of the client's condition and providing education as it relates to the prescribed drug regimen. Prior to initiation of diuretic therapy, the client should be questioned about past history of kidney disease. Diuretics are contraindicated in pregnancy and lactation and in clients with renal dysfunction, fluid and electrolyte depletion, and hepatic coma. Diuretics should be used cautiously in clients with hepatic cirrhosis or nephritic syndrome and in infants and older adults.

Potassium levels should be monitored closely since non–potassium-sparing diuretics cause hypokalemia with diuresis. Closely observe older clients for weakness, hypotension, and confusion. Monitor for electrolyte imbalance, elevated BUN, hyperglycemia, and anemia, which can all be side effects of diuretics. Monitor vital signs and carefully monitor intake and output to establish effectiveness of the medication. Rapid and excessive diuresis can result in dehydration, hypovolemia, and circulatory collapse.

Client education as it relates to diuretics should include goals, reasons for obtaining baseline data such as vital signs and tests for renal function, and possible side effects. The following are important points to include when teaching clients about diuretics:

- Monitor total sodium intake daily. The recommended daily intake should be no more than 4000 mg/day.
- Report weight loss of more than 1 kg a week.
- Report fatigue and muscle cramping.
- Change positions slowly because diuretics in combination with other drugs can cause dizziness.

See Nursing Process Focus: Clients Receiving Diuretic Therapy in Chapter 52 for additional information.

NCLEX Success Tips

Loop diuretics can cause the excretion of potassium, sodium, and magnesium.

Furosemide (Lasix) is a potassium-wasting diuretic. The nurse must monitor the serum potassium level and assess for signs of low potassium. Cardiac complications can result from the loss of potassium.

Diuretics, such as furosemide, are commonly used to treat acute heart failure. Most diuretics increase the renal excretion of potassium. The nurse should check the client's potassium level before administering diuretics and obtain an order to replace potassium if the level is low.

Furosemide may cause ototoxicity. The nurse should tell the client to immediately report any hearing loss, dizziness, or tinnitus to prevent permanent ear damage.

PROTOTYPE DRUG	Furosemide (Lasix)

Actions and Uses: Furosemide is often used in the treatment of acute HF because it has the ability to remove large amounts of edematous fluid from the client in a short period of time. When given IV, diuresis begins within 5 minutes. Clients often experience quick relief from their distressing symptoms. Furosemide acts by preventing the reabsorption of sodium and chloride, primarily in the loop of Henle region of the nephron. Compared to other diuretics, furosemide is particularly beneficial when cardiac output and renal flow are severely diminished.

Pharmacokinetics: Furosemide given orally is 47% to 64% bioavailable and 91% to 97% protein bound. It is partly metabolized by the liver and is excreted by the kidneys. It has a half-life of 0.5 to 2 hours.

Administration Alerts:

- Check the client's serum potassium levels before administering drug. If potassium levels are falling or are below normal, notify the physician before administering.
- Furosemide is pregnancy category C.

Adverse Effects and Interactions: Side effects of furosemide, like those of most diuretics, involve potential electrolyte imbalances, the most important of which is hypokalemia. Because hypokalemia may cause dysrhythmias in clients who are taking cardiac glycosides, combination therapy with furosemide and digoxin must be carefully monitored. Because furosemide is so efficacious,

fluid loss must be carefully monitored to avoid possible dehydration and hypotension.

When furosemide is given with corticosteroids and amphotericin B (Fungizone), it can potentiate hypokalemia. When given with lithium (Carbolith, Lithane), elimination of lithium is decreased, causing higher risk for toxicity. When given with sulfonylureas and insulin, furosemide may diminish their hypoglycemic effects.

PHOSPHODIESTERASE INHIBITORS

Phosphodiesterase inhibitors became available in the 1980s. They have a short half-life and are used for the short-term control of acute HF. The dose of milrinone, the prototype drug, is shown in Table 54.1.

Pharmacotherapy with Phosphodiesterase Inhibitors

54.8 Phosphodiesterase inhibitors increase the force of contraction and cause vasodilation. They are highly toxic and reserved for acute situations.

Phosphodiesterase inhibitors block the enzyme **phosphodiesterase** in cardiac and smooth muscle. Blocking phosphodiesterase has the effect of increasing the amount of calcium available for myocardial contraction. The inhibition results in two main actions that benefit clients with HF: a positive inotropic response and vasodilation. Cardiac output is increased due to the increase in contractility and the decrease in left ventricular afterload. Due to their toxicity, phosphodiesterase inhibitors are normally reserved for clients who have not responded to ACE inhibitors or cardiac glycosides, and they are generally used for only 2 to 3 days.

Nursing Considerations

The role of the nurse in drug therapy with phosphodiesterase inhibitors involves careful monitoring of the client's condition and providing education as it relates to the prescribed drug regimen. Prior to administration of phosphodiesterase inhibitors, assess potassium levels. If hypokalemia is present, it should be corrected before administering these drugs. Evaluate the client for history of renal impairment and dysrhythmias. Baseline vital signs, especially blood pressure, should be obtained because these drugs can cause hypotension. During IV administration, the client should be continuously monitored for ventricular dysrhythmias such as ectopic beats, supraventricular dysrhythmias, preventricular contractions (PVCs), ventricular tachycardia, and ventricular fibrillation. If ordered for elderly, pregnant, or pediatric clients, the healthcare provider should be consulted, as safety has not been established in these populations or conditions.

Client education as it relates to phosphodiesterase inhibitors should include goals, reasons for obtaining baseline data such as vital signs and tests for cardiac and renal function, and possible side effects. The following are the important points to include when teaching clients about phosphodiesterase inhibitors:

- Report the following immediately: irregular, fast heartbeat; pain or swelling at the infusion site; and fever of 38.3°C or higher.
- Report immediately any increase in chest pain that might indicate angina.

Special Considerations

◀ Psychosocial Issues and Adherence in Clients with HF

Clients with depression and lack of social support who have HF have been shown to be less compliant with their drug therapy regimen. When clients can no longer maintain what they consider an acceptable lifestyle, they may become depressed. Clients are less likely to adhere to lifestyle modifications when depressed. Their choices may place their health and safety at risk. Reduced sexual desire and performance problems are frequently related to side effects of drug therapy and may reduce adherence to drug therapy. Clients may weigh the side effects against the drug's benefits and determine that the risks outweigh the benefits. Assess these issues in all clients with HF. Clients may be referred to cardiac rehabilitation programs, which have been shown to increase adherence.

PROTOTYPE DRUG	Milrinone

Actions and Uses: Milrinone is primarily used for the short-term support of advanced HF. It is only given intravenously. Peak effects occur in 2 minutes. Immediate effects of milrinone include an increased force of myocardial contraction and an increase in cardiac output.

Pharmacokinetics: Its half-life is 2.3 hours.

Administration Alerts:
* When administering this medication IV, a microdrip set and an infusion pump should be used.
* Milrinone is pregnancy category C.

Adverse Effects and Interactions: The most serious side effect of milrinone is ventricular dysrhythmia, which may occur in at least 1 of every 10 clients taking the drug. The client's ECG is usually monitored continuously during infusion of the drug. Milrinone interacts with disopyramide (Rhythmodan), causing excessive hypotension.

In 2001, nesiritide (Natrecor) was approved for treatment of HF. Nesiritide is a small peptide hormone produced through recombinant DNA technology that is structurally identical to endogenous human B-type natriuretic peptide (hBNP).

When HF occurs, the ventricles begin to secrete hBNP in response to the increased stretch of the ventricular walls. This results in diuresis and renal excretion of sodium and decreased preload. In therapeutic doses, exogenous hBNP also causes vasodilation and afterload. By reducing preload and afterload, hBNP reduces cardiac workload.

CHAPTER

54 Understanding the Chapter

Key Concepts Summary

The numbered key concepts provide a succinct summary of the important points from the corresponding numbered section within the chapter. If any of these points are not clear, refer to the numbered section within the chapter for review.

54.1 The central cause of HF is weakened heart muscle. Diminished contractility reduces cardiac output.

54.2 The three primary characteristics of heart function are force of contraction, heart rate, and speed of impulse conduction.

54.3 ACE inhibitors improve HF by reducing peripheral edema and increasing cardiac output. They are first-line drugs for the treatment of HF.

54.4 Beta-adrenergic blockers play a role in the treatment of HF by slowing the heart rate and decreasing blood pressure. They are used in combination with ACE inhibitors as first-line drugs for HF.

54.5 Vasodilators can help to reduce symptoms of HF by reducing preload and decreasing the oxygen demand of the heart.

54.6 Cardiac glycosides increase the force of myocardial contraction and are the traditional drugs of choice for HF. Due to a low safety margin, their use has declined.

54.7 Diuretics relieve symptoms of HF by reducing fluid volume and decreasing blood pressure.

54.8 Phosphodiesterase inhibitors increase the force of contraction and cause vasodilation. They are highly toxic and reserved for acute situations.

Chapter 54 Scenario

Jim Mabry, 77 years old, currently takes the following medications daily: digoxin (Lanoxin) 0.125 mg; furosemide (Lasix) 20 mg; and potassium supplementation (K-Dur) 20 mEq. As his nurse, you will be discussing Jim's medication regimen and his next healthcare provider office visit after discharge from the hospital.

Critical Thinking Questions

1. Discuss the relationship among the three medications.

2. Jim will have a digoxin serum level collected during the healthcare provider office visit. What does he need to know about this procedure?

3. Jim asked you to compile a list of foods that are rich in potassium. Prepare this list.

See Answers to Critical Thinking Questions in Appendix B.

NCLEX Practice Questions

1 A client newly diagnosed with heart failure following an acute myocardial infarction has a prescription for enalapril (Vasotec). This drug class is frequently used in early heart failure because of which clinical improvement?

  a. It strengthens the force of myocardial contraction to improve cardiac output.

  b. It decreases peripheral resistance, increasing cardiac output.

  c. It slows the heart rate, improving filling time and increasing cardiac output.

  d. It has diuretic effects, decreasing peripheral edema and pulmonary congestion.

2 In providing a client with heart failure information prior to discharge, the nurse will discuss digoxin (Lanoxin) therapy. Which point would the nurse include in teaching the client?

  a. Take the drug in the morning before rising.

  b. Monitor the pulse daily prior to taking the drug.

  c. Discontinue the drug if the pulse rate is 70 beats per minute.

  d. Eat a diet high in bran fibre and calcium.

3 A client is receiving hydralazine with isosorbide for heart failure. The nurse should monitor this client for

  a. Confusion and agitation

  b. Bleeding

  c. Tingling or cramping in the legs

  d. Dizziness and rapid heart rate

4 A client will begin taking carvedilol (Coreg) for heart failure. Before teaching the client about this drug, the nurse will discuss with the healthcare provider which recommended routine for beta-adrenergic blockers in heart failure?

  a. Significantly lower dosages are used first, then gradually increased to a target dose.

  b. A loading dose that is higher than the subsequent daily dose must be given.

  c. The beta-adrenergic blocker dosage must be lowered if the client is also on ACE inhibitors.

  d. Beta-adrenergic blockers are almost never used in HF, and the order must be confirmed.

5 When planning client education, the nurse knows that client adherence to beta-adrenergic blocker therapy in heart failure may be difficult to achieve, despite the usefulness of these drugs. Which of the following points will the nurse need to address in the teaching plan? Select all that apply.

  a. The dosage must be gradually adjusted over time to a beneficial dose.

  b. The client may not notice significant improvement during early therapy.

  c. The drug therapy may require changes to many other medications the client is taking.

  d. The drug has significant benefits in reducing mortality from heart failure.

  e. The drug will require extensive lifestyle changes.

See Answers to NCLEX Practice Questions in Appendix A.

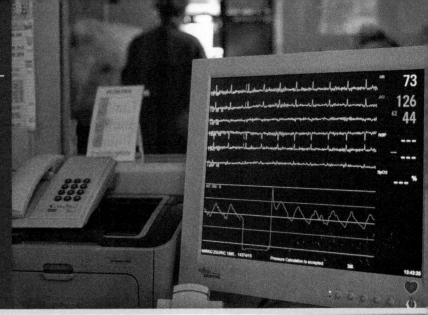

PROTOTYPE DRUGS

SODIUM CHANNEL BLOCKERS
Pr procainamide (Procan)

BETA-ADRENERGIC BLOCKERS
Pr propranolol (Inderal)

POTASSIUM CHANNEL BLOCKERS
Pr amiodarone (Cordarone)

CALCIUM CHANNEL BLOCKERS
Pr verapamil (Isoptin)

MISCELLANEOUS DRUGS

Ivan Batinic / Alamy Stock Photo

CHAPTER
55

Pharmacotherapy of Dysrhythmias

LEARNING OUTCOMES

After reading this chapter, the student should be able to:

1. Explain how rhythm abnormalities can affect cardiac function.

2. Identify drug classes used for treating dysrhythmias.

3. Explain the therapeutic action of each class of antidysrhythmic drug in relation to the pathophysiology of dysrhythmias.

4. Discuss the role of the nurse regarding non-pharmacological therapies for the treatment of dysrhythmias.

5. Describe the nurse's role in the pharmacological management of clients with dysrhythmias.

6. For each of the drug classes listed in Prototype Drugs, identify a representative drug and explain its mechanism of action, therapeutic effects, and important adverse effects.

7. Describe and explain, based on pharmacological principles, the rationale for nursing assessment, planning, and interventions for clients with dysrhythmias.

8. Use the nursing process to care for clients who are receiving drug therapy for dysrhythmias.

CHAPTER OUTLINE

▶ Frequency of Dysrhythmias in the Population

▶ Classification of Dysrhythmias

▶ Conduction Pathways in the Myocardium

▶ The Electrocardiograph

▶ Sodium, Potassium, and the Myocardial Action Potential

▶ Non-Pharmacological Therapy of Dysrhythmias

▶ Classification of Dysrhythmias and Antidysrhythmic Drugs

▶ Sodium Channel Blockers (Class I)

 ▶ Treating Dysrhythmias with Sodium Channel Blockers

▶ Beta-Adrenergic Blockers (Class II)

 ▶ Treating Dysrhythmias with Beta-Adrenergic Blockers

Dysrhythmias, sometimes called arrhythmias, encompass a number of different disorders that range from harmless to life-threatening. **Dysrhythmias** are abnormalities of electrical conduction that may result in disturbances in heart rate or cardiac rhythm. Diagnosis is often difficult because clients usually must be connected to an electrocardiograph (ECG) and be experiencing symptoms in order to determine the exact type of rhythm disorder. Proper diagnosis and optimum pharmacological treatment can significantly affect the frequency of dysrhythmias and their consequences.

Frequency of Dysrhythmias in the Population

55.1 The frequency of dysrhythmias in the population is difficult to predict because many clients experience no symptoms. Persistent or severe dysrhythmias may be lethal.

While some dysrhythmias produce no symptoms and have negligible effects on cardiac function, others are life-threatening and require immediate treatment. Typical symptoms include dizziness, weakness, decreased exercise tolerance, shortness of breath, and fainting. Many clients report palpitations or a sensation that their heart has skipped a beat. Persistent dysrhythmias are associated with increased risk for stroke and heart failure (HF). Severe dysrhythmias may result in sudden death. Since asymptomatic clients may not seek medical attention, it is difficult to estimate the frequency of the disease, although it is likely that dysrhythmias are quite common in the population.

Classification of Dysrhythmias

55.2 Dysrhythmias are classified by location (atrial or ventricular) or type of rhythm abnormality produced (flutter, fibrillation, block).

Dysrhythmias are classified by a number of different methods. The simplest method is to name dysrhythmias according to the

CONNECTIONS | Lifespan Considerations

◀ Dysrhythmias

- A large majority of sudden cardiac deaths is thought to be caused by ventricular dysrhythmias.
- Atrial dysrhythmias occur more commonly in men than in women.
- The incidence of atrial dysrhythmias increases with age. They affect:
  - Less than 0.5% of those aged 25 to 35.
  - 1.5% of those under age 60.
  - 9% of those over age 75.
- About 15% of strokes occur in clients with atrial dysrhythmias.
- Sudden cardiac death occurs three to four times more frequently in black individuals.
- Atrial fibrillation affects 0.6% of the Canadian population.

Based on Statistics Canada, Humphries et al., 2004. Humphries, K., Jackevicius, C., Gong, Y., Svensen, L., Cox, J., Tu, J., Laupacis, A. (2004). Population rates of hospitalization for atrial fibrillation/flutter in Canada. *Canadian Journal of Cardiology*, 20(9), 869–876. Elsevier BV Publishing c/o ScienceDirect Publishing

type of rhythm abnormality produced and its *location*. Dysrhythmias that originate in the atria are sometimes referred to as **supraventricular**. Those that originate in the ventricles are generally more serious, as they more often interfere with the normal function of the heart. **Atrial fibrillation**, a complete disorganization of rhythm, is thought to be the most common type of dysrhythmia. A summary of common dysrhythmias with a brief description of each is given in Table 55.1. Although obtaining a correct diagnosis of the type of dysrhythmia is sometimes difficult, it is essential for effective treatment.

While the actual cause of most dysrhythmias is elusive, dysrhythmias are associated with certain conditions, primarily heart disease and myocardial infarction. The following are diseases and conditions associated with dysrhythmias:

- Hypertension
- Cardiac valve disease such as mitral stenosis
- Coronary artery disease

TABLE 55.1 Types of Dysrhythmia

Dysrhythmia	Description
Premature atrial contractions or premature ventricular contractions (PVCs)	An extra beat often originating from a source other than the sinoatrial (SA) node; not normally serious unless it occurs at high frequency
Atrial or ventricular tachycardia	Rapid heart beat greater than 150 beats/minute (bpm); ventricular is more serious than atrial
Atrial or ventricular flutter and/or fibrillation	Very rapid, uncoordinated beats; atrial may require treatment but is not usually fatal; ventricular requires immediate treatment
Sinus bradycardia	Slow heartbeat, less than 50 bpm; may require a pacemaker
Heart block	Area of non-conduction in the myocardium; may be partial or complete; classified as first, second, or third degree

TABLE 55.2 Selected Prodysrhythmic Drugs

Class of Medication	Example Drugs
Antidysrhythmic drugs	amiodarone, disopyramide, dofetilide, flecainide, ibutilide, procainamide, propafenone, quinidine, sotalol
Autonomic drugs	atenolol, clonidine, methyldopa, nadolol, propranolol
Calcium channel blockers	diltiazem, nifedipine, verapamil
Cardiac glycosides	digoxin
Miscellaneous drugs	amitriptyline, chloroquine, cimetidine, haloperidol, lithium carbonate, phenothiazines

- Low potassium levels in the blood
- Myocardial infarction
- Stroke
- Diabetes mellitus
- Congestive heart failure

In addition to the preceding list, a number of medications have been found to cause new dysrhythmias or worsen existing ones. Caution must be used when administering prodysrhythmic drugs to clients with pre-existing cardiac impairment or who may have any of the above conditions. Table 55.2 lists selected drugs known to have prodysrhythmic properties.

Conduction Pathways in the Myocardium

55.3 The electrical conduction pathway from the SA node, to the AV node, to the bundle branches and Purkinje fibres keeps the heart beating in a synchronized manner. Some myocardial cells in these regions have the property of automaticity.

Although there are many types of dysrhythmia, all have in common a defect in the generation or conduction of electrical impulses across the myocardium. These electrical impulses, or **action potentials**, carry the signal for the cardiac muscle cells to contract and must be coordinated precisely for the chambers to beat in a synchronized manner. For the heart to function properly, the atria must contract simultaneously, sending their blood into the ventricles. Following atrial contraction, the right and left ventricles must contract simultaneously. Lack of synchronization of the atria and ventricles or of the right and left sides of the heart may have profound consequences. The total time for the electrical impulse to travel across the heart is about 0.22 seconds. The normal conduction pathway in the heart is illustrated in Figure 55.1.

Normal control of this synchronization begins in a small area of tissue in the wall of the right atrium known as the **sinoatrial (SA) node**. The SA node, or pacemaker, of the heart has a property called **automaticity**, which is the ability to spontaneously generate an action potential without direction from the nervous system. The SA node generates a new action potential approximately 75 times per minute under resting conditions. This is referred to as the normal **sinus rhythm**.

Upon leaving the SA node, the action potential travels quickly across both atria and then to the **atrioventricular (AV) node**. The AV node also has the property of automaticity, although less so than the SA node. Should the SA node malfunction, the AV node has the ability to spontaneously generate action potentials and continue the heart's contraction at a rate of 40 to 60 bpm. Compared to other areas in the heart, impulse conduction through the AV node is slow. This allows the atrial contraction to completely empty blood into the ventricles, thereby optimizing cardiac output.

As the action potential leaves the AV node, it travels rapidly to the **atrioventricular bundle**, or bundle of His. The impulse is

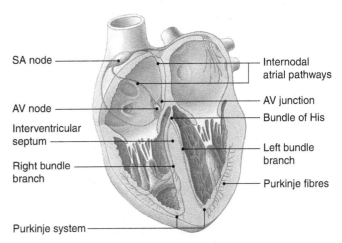

Figure 55.1 Normal conduction pathway in the heart.
Pearson Education.

then conducted down the right and left **bundle branches** to the **Purkinje fibres**, which carry the action potential to all regions of the ventricles almost simultaneously. Should the SA and AV nodes become non-functional, cells in the AV bundle and Purkinje fibres can continue to generate myocardial contractions at a rate of about 30 bpm.

Although action potentials normally begin in the SA node and spread across the myocardium in a coordinated manner, other regions of the heart may begin to initiate beats. These areas, known as **ectopic foci** or **ectopic pacemakers**, may begin to send impulses across the myocardium that compete with those from the normal conduction pathway, thereby affecting the normal flow of impulses. Ectopic foci have the potential to cause many of the types of dysrhythmias noted in Table 55.1.

It is important to understand that the underlying purpose of this conduction system is to keep the heart beating in a regular, synchronized manner so that cardiac output can be maintained. Some dysrhythmias occur sporadically, elicit no symptoms, and do not affect cardiac output. Others, however, profoundly affect cardiac output, result in client symptoms, and have the potential to produce serious if not fatal consequences. It is these types of dysrhythmias that require pharmacological treatment.

The Electrocardiograph

55.4 The electrophysiological events in the heart can be measured with an electrocardiograph.

The wave of electrical activity across the myocardium can be measured using the electrocardiograph. The graphic recording from this device is an **electrocardiogram (ECG)**, and it is useful in diagnosing many types of heart conditions, including dysrhythmias. An ECG may also be referred to as an EKG.

Three distinct waves are produced on a normal ECG: the P wave, the QRS complex, and the T wave. Changes to the wave patterns or their timing can reveal certain pathologies. For example, an exaggerated R wave suggests enlargement of the ventricles, and a flat T wave indicates ischemia to the myocardium. A normal ECG and its relationship to impulse conduction in the heart are shown in Figure 55.2.

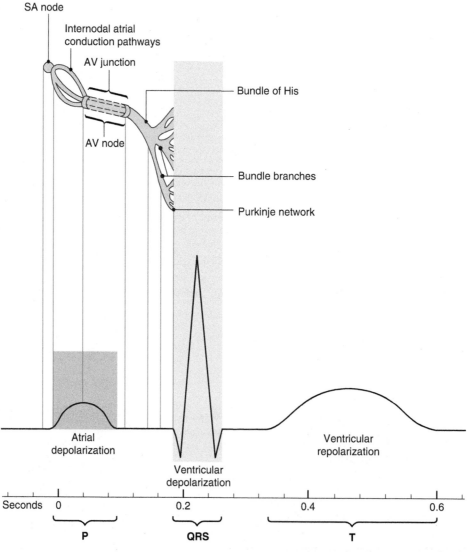

Figure 55.2 Relationship of the electrocardiogram to electrical conduction in the heart.
Pearson Education.

Sodium, Potassium, and the Myocardial Action Potential

55.5 Changes in sodium and potassium levels generate the action potential in myocardial cells. Depolarization occurs when sodium (and calcium) rushes in; repolarization occurs when potassium is removed.

Dysrhythmias are alterations in the normal generation or conduction of electrical impulses, or action potentials, across the myocardium. Because antidysrhythmic drugs act by correcting or modifying impulse conduction, a firm grasp of cardiac electrical properties is essential to understanding drug mechanisms. Before proceeding, the student should review the normal pathway of impulse conduction in the heart.

An action potential illustrating the steps in electrical conduction is shown in Figure 55.3. The changes in ions, or fluxes, that occur during an action potential may be grouped into five phases.

Phase 4: It is easiest to begin with phase 4 because this is the period during which the myocyte is "resting" and the action potential has not yet occurred. Note in Figure 55.3, however, that during phase 4 the membrane potential is slowly increasing toward a potential that will trigger an action potential: the **threshold potential**. Sodium is slowly "leaking" into the cell during this period, causing the change in potential, which gives certain regions such as the SA node the property of automaticity, the ability to depolarize spontaneously, without input from the nervous system.

Phase 0: An action potential begins when the threshold potential is reached and gated **sodium ion channels** located in the plasma membrane become activated and open. Sodium ions rush into the cell, producing a rapid **depolarization**, or loss of membrane potential. Because they open and close rapidly, these sodium channels are sometimes referred to as "fast" channels. During this period, Ca^{2+} also enters the cell through

calcium ion channels, although the influx is slower than that of sodium. In myocytes located in the SA and AV nodes, it is the influx of Ca^{2+}, rather than Na^+, that generates the rapid depolarization of the membrane.

Phase 1: During depolarization, the inside of the plasma membrane temporarily reverses its charge, becoming positive. This is a brief, transient phase.

Phase 2: During phase 2, a plateau is reached in which depolarization is maintained. The entry of Ca^{2+} into the cells signals the release of additional calcium ions that had been held in storage inside the sarcoplasmic reticula. This large and sudden increase in intracellular Ca^{2+} is responsible for the contraction of cardiac muscle. Gated **potassium ion channels** open, causing an efflux of K^+ from the cells. The plateau is maintained for as long as the positive calcium ions entering the myocytes are balanced by the positive potassium ions leaving the cell. Action potentials in skeletal muscle lack this plateau phase.

Phase 3: During phase 3, the calcium channels close and additional potassium channels open, thus causing a net loss of positive ions from the cell. This **repolarization** returns the negative resting membrane potential to the cell.

The synchronized pumping action of the heart requires alternating periods of contraction and relaxation. There is a brief period of time following depolarization and most of repolarization during which the cell cannot initiate a subsequent action potential. This **refractory period** ensures that the myocardial cell finishes contracting before a second action potential begins.

Although learning about the different ions involved in an action potential may seem complicated, they are very important to cardiac pharmacology. Blocking potassium, sodium, or calcium ion channels is a pharmacological strategy used to terminate or prevent dysrhythmias. In addition, the therapeutic effect of some antidysrhythmic drugs is due to their prolongation of the refractory period. It is not possible to understand drug mechanisms

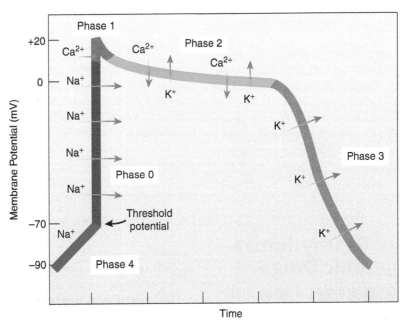

Figure 55.3 Phases of the myocardial action potential. Ion movements during each phase are shown.

without adequate knowledge of the normal electrical conduction properties of the heart. In general, most cardiac drugs:

* Increase impulse formation (or automaticity)
* Increase conduction velocity
* Increase both impulse formation and conduction velocity

OR

* Decrease impulse formation or automaticity
* Decrease conduction velocity
* Decrease both impulse formation or automaticity and conduction

Non-Pharmacological Therapy of Dysrhythmias

55.6 Non-pharmacological therapy of dysrhythmias, including cardioversion, ablation, and implantable cardioverter defibrillators, are often the treatments of choice.

The therapeutic goals of antidysrhythmic pharmacotherapy are to terminate existing dysrhythmias and to prevent abnormal rhythms to reduce the risk of sudden death, stroke, and other complications resulting from the disorder. Because of their potential to cause serious side effects, antidysrhythmic drugs are normally reserved for those clients who are experiencing overt symptoms or for those whose condition cannot be controlled by other means. There is little or no benefit to the client in treating asymptomatic dysrhythmias with medication. Healthcare providers use several non-pharmacological strategies to eliminate dysrhythmias.

The more serious types of dysrhythmia are corrected through electrical shock of the heart, with treatments such as elective **cardioversion** and **defibrillation**. The electrical shock momentarily stops all electrical impulses in the heart, both normal and abnormal. Under ideal conditions, the temporary cessation of electrical activity will allow the SA node to automatically return conduction to a normal sinus rhythm.

Other types of non-pharmacological treatment include identification and destruction of the myocardial cells responsible for the abnormal conduction through a surgical procedure called catheter ablation. Cardiac pacemakers are sometimes inserted to correct the types of dysrhythmia that cause the heart to beat too slowly. Implantable cardioverter defibrillators (ICDs) are placed in clients to restore normal rhythm by either pacing the heart or giving it an electric shock when dysrhythmias occur. In addition, the ICD is capable of storing information regarding the heart rhythm for the healthcare provider to evaluate.

Classification of Dysrhythmias and Antidysrhythmic Drugs

55.7 Antidysrhythmic drugs are classified by their mechanism of action into classes I through IV.

There are many types of dysrhythmias and they are classified by a number of different methods. The two broad categories of

rhythm abnormalities are those that affect impulse formation and those that affect impulse conduction. Although a correct diagnosis of the type of dysrhythmia is sometimes difficult, it is essential for effective treatment.

Bradydysrhythmias are disorders characterized by a heart rate of less than 60 bpm. Bradydysrhythmias are very common in older adults because the number of cells in the SA node declines progressively such that by age 75 about 90% of the cells are non-functional. Similar age-related changes occur in the AV node, where normal cells progressively die and are replaced by fibrotic tissue. Bradydysrhythmias are the major indication for pacemaker implantation. Common bradydysrhythmias include the following:

* *Sinus bradycardia.* The most common slow heart rhythm. Sinus bradycardia generally does not require treatment unless the client is experiencing syncope or dizziness due to lack of sufficient blood flow to the brain, or if the heart rate fails to increase during periods of exertion.

* *Sinoatrial node dysfunction (sick sinus syndrome).* The SA node fails to generate or transmit sufficient electrical impulses. Clients with this condition may experience severe bradycardia (less than 40 bpm resting), failure of the heart rate to increase with exercise, or significant sinus "pauses." Severe episodes of bradycardia may alternate with periods of abnormally rapid heart rates.

* *Atrioventricular conduction block.* The AV node fails to conduct impulses to the rest of the myocardium. AV blocks are classified by degree. In first-degree AV block, the AV node conducts the impulse slowly, and conduction is delayed. In second-degree AV block, some, but not all, impulses are prevented (blocked) from leaving the AV node. Second-degree AV block results in non-conducted P waves. A third-degree AV block results in total stoppage of impulses through the AV node. None of the impulses originating in the atria can make their way through the block into the ventricles. Second- and third-degree blocks require pharmacotherapy or the insertion of a temporary or permanent pacemaker. Some AV blocks are temporary in origin and can be due to cardiac drug toxicity. Any drug that slows AV conduction can cause a temporary form of AV block.

Tachydysrhythmias are disorders exhibiting a heart rate greater than 100 bpm. The incidence of tachydysrhythmias increases in older adults and in clients with pre-existing cardiovascular disease. The simplest method for categorizing tachydysrhythmias is according to the type of rhythm abnormality produced and its location. Dysrhythmias that originate in the atria are sometimes referred to as supraventricular. Those that originate in the ventricles are generally more serious because they are more likely to interfere with the normal function of the heart.

* *Atrial tachycardia.* May be caused by a rapidly firing SA node or by an ectopic focus in the atria that suppresses the SA node and establishes a rapid heart rate, often between 160 and 200 bpm. When these episodes alternate with periods of normal rhythm, it is called paroxysmal atrial tachycardia (PAT), or **paroxysmal supraventricular tachycardia (PSVT)**.

* *Atrial flutter.* A rapid, regular heartbeat in which the atria may beat 250 to 350 times per minute. During atrial flutter, the job of the AV node is to selectively block some of the impulses

coming from the atria, so the ventricular rate (pulse) is 125 to 175 bpm (usually two, three, or four atrial beats for each ventricular beat).

- *Atrial fibrillation.* A complete disorganization of rhythm, this is the most common type of dysrhythmia. It is caused by multiple sites of impulse formation in the atria, all firing in a chaotic fashion. The atrial rate can range from 300 to 600 bpm, causing an irregular ventricular rate ranging from 50 to 200 bpm. The rapid atrial rate causes a loss of organized atrial contraction and results in quivering (fibrillation). This lack of contraction causes blood to lie dormant in parts of the atria and may give rise to clots. Because of the potential for clot formation, atrial fibrillation is a leading risk factor for stroke.

- *Ventricular tachycardia.* Usually recognized by regular, rapid, wide beats with a ventricular rate of 100 to 200 bpm. Clients with sustained or symptomatic ventricular tachycardia must be treated immediately because this condition is associated with a high risk for sudden death. **Torsades de pointes** is a specific type of ventricular tachycardia that is characterized by rates between 200 and 250 bpm and "twisting of the points" of the QRS complex on the ECG.

- *Ventricular fibrillation.* A complete disorganization of rhythm in which the ventricles pump little or no blood, quickly starving the tissues of oxygen. Ventricular fibrillation is now considered cardiac arrest.

Antidysrhythmic drugs act by altering electrophysiological properties of the heart. They do this in two basic ways: blocking ion flow through ion channels or altering autonomic activity.

Antidysrhythmic drugs are grouped according to the stage in which they affect the action potential. These drugs fall into four primary classes, referred to as I, II, III, and IV, and a fifth group that includes miscellaneous drugs not acting by one of the other four mechanisms. The phases of the action potential at which antidysrhythmic drugs act are shown in Figure 55.4. Categories of antidysrhythmics include the following:

1. Sodium channel blockers (class I)
2. Beta-adrenergic blockers (class II)

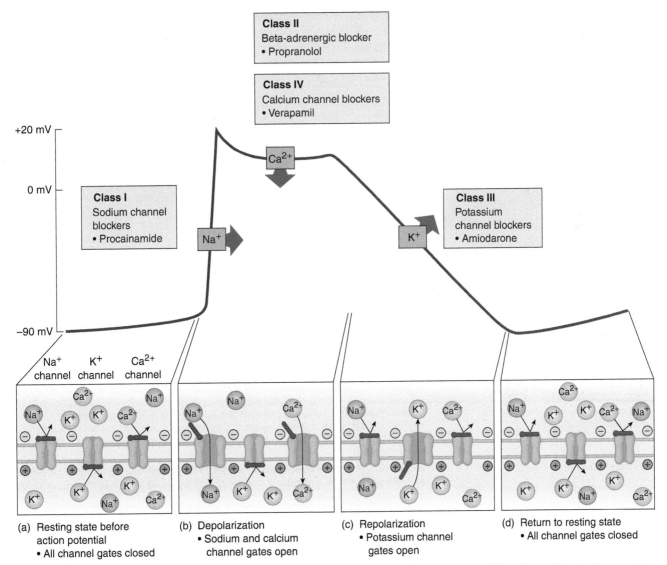

Figure 55.4 Ion channels in myocardial cells: (a) resting state before action potential (all channel gates closed); (b) depolarization (sodium and calcium channel gates open); (c) repolarization (potassium channel gates open); (d) return to resting state (all channel gates closed).

3. Potassium channel blockers (class III)

4. Calcium channel blockers (class IV)

5. Miscellaneous antidysrhythmic drugs

Drugs that affect cardiac electrophysiology have a narrow margin between a therapeutic effect and a toxic effect. They have the ability not only to correct dysrhythmias, but also to worsen or even create new dysrhythmias. The nurse must carefully monitor clients who are taking antidysrhythmic drugs. Often, the client is hospitalized during the initial stages of therapy so that the optimum dose can be accurately determined.

SODIUM CHANNEL BLOCKERS (CLASS I)

The first medical uses of the sodium channel blockers were recorded in the 18th century. This is the largest class of antidysrhythmics, and many are still widely prescribed. The sodium channel blockers are shown in Table 55.3.

NCLEX Success Tips

Procainamide (Procan) can lead to increased QRS complexes and QT intervals. If the QRS duration increases by more than 50%, the

TABLE 55.3 Antidysrhythmic Drugs

Drug	Route and Adult Dose
Class IA: Sodium Channel Blockers	
disopyramide (Rythmodan)	Orally (PO), 100–200 mg four times a day (qid) (max 800 mg/day)
Pr procainamide (Procan)	Intramuscular (IM), 50 mg/kg/day divided every 3 to 6 hours (q3h–q6h) or 0.5–1 g q4h–q8h Intravenous (IV), loading dose 500–600 mg administered as a slow infusion over 25–30 minutes or 100 mg/dose at a rate not to exceed 50 mg/minute repeated every 5 minutes as needed (PRN) to a total dose of 1000 mg PO, 50 mg/kg/24 hours given in divided doses q6h
quinidine gluconate	PO, 324–648 mg q8h–q12h (max 3–4 g/day)
quinidine polygalacturonate	PO, 275–825 mg every 3 to 4 hours (q3–4h) for four or more doses until dysrhythmia terminates, then 137.5–275 mg twice a day (bid) or tid
quinidine sulfate	PO, 200–400 mg q6h–q12h (max 3–4 g/day)
Class IB: Sodium Channel Blockers	
lidocaine (Xylocaine) (see Chapter 24, page 279, for the Prototype Drug box)	IV, start with 1–1.5 mg/kg; if refractory ventricular fibrillation or pulseless ventricular tachycardia, repeat 0.5–0.75 mg/kg bolus every 5–10 minutes (max cumulative dose 3 mg/kg); follow with continuous infusion (1–4 mg/minute) after return of perfusion
mexiletine	PO, 200–300 mg tid (max 1200 mg/day)
Class IC: Sodium Channel Blockers	
flecainide (Tambocor)	PO, 50–100 mg bid; increase by 50 mg bid every 4 days (max 400 mg/day)
propafenone (Rythmol)	PO, 150–300 mg tid (max 900 mg/day)
Class II: Beta Blockers	
acebutolol (Rhotral, Sectral)	PO, 200–600 mg bid (max 1200 mg/day)
esmolol (Brevibloc)	IV, 50 µg/kg/minute maintenance dose (max 200 µg/kg/minute)
Pr propranolol (Inderal)	PO, 10–30 mg tid or qid (max 320 mg/day); IV, 1–3 mg/dose slowly, repeat every 2 to 5 minutes up to a total of 5 mg, once response is achieved or max dose is administered additional doses should not be given for at least 4 hours; alternate dosing, 0.5–1 mg over 1 minute, may repeat if necessary up to max of 0.1 mg/kg
Class III: Potassium Channel Blockers	
Pr amiodarone (Cordarone)	PO, 800–1600 mg/day in 1–2 divided doses for 1–3 weeks; when adequate arrhythmia control is achieved decrease to 600–800 mg/day in 1–2 doses; usual maintenance dose is 400–600 mg/day
sotalol (Rylosol)	PO, 80 mg bid (max 320 mg/day)
Class IV: Calcium Channel Blockers	
diltiazem (Cardizem, Tiazac) (see Chapter 50, page 620, for the Prototype Drug box)	IV, inital bolus dose 0.25 mg/kg over 2 minutest (average adult dose is 20 mg); repeat bolus may be given after 15 minutes if the response is inadequate, 0.35 mg/kg over 2 minutes (average adult dose is 25 mg); continuous infusions, start with rate of 10 mg/hour (infusions > 24 hours or infusion rates > 15mg/hour are not recommended)
Pr verapamil (Isoptin)	PO, 240–480 mg/day in 3–4 divided doses; IV, 0.075–0.15 mg/kg (usual dose is 5–10 mg) administered as a bolus over 2 minutes; if no response, may give an additional 10 mg after 15–30 minutes; continuous infusion, start with 5 mg/hour
Miscellaneous Antidysrhythmics	
adenosine (Adenocard)	IV (rapid, over 1–2 seconds via peripheral line), start with 6 mg; if not effective within 1–2 minutes, 12 mg may be given; may repeat 12 mg bolus if needed (max single dose 12 mg)
digoxin (Lanoxin, Toloxin) (see Chapter 54, page 691, for the Prototype Drug box)	PO, 0.125–0.25 mg qd
ibutilide (Corvert)	IV, 1 mg infused over 10 minutes

nurse should stop the medication and notify the physician. The drug is contraindicated in complete heart block and systemic lupus erythematosus and must be used with caution in heart failure and myasthenia gravis, as those conditions may be worsened by the medication.

Metoprolol (Lopressor) may cause increased PR interval and bradycardia.

Propafenone (Rythmol) and verapamil (Isoptin) may cause bradycardia and atrioventricular blocks.

Treating Dysrhythmias with Sodium Channel Blockers

55.8 Sodium channel blockers are the largest group of antidysrhythmics and act by slowing the rate of impulse conduction across the heart.

Sodium channel blockers, the class I drugs, are divided into three subgroups, IA, IB, and IC, based on subtle differences in their mechanism of action. Since progression of the action potential is dependent on the opening of sodium ion channels, a blockade of these channels will prevent depolarization. The spread of the action potential across the myocardium will slow, and areas of ectopic pacemaker activity will be suppressed.

Nursing Considerations

The role of the nurse in sodium channel blocker therapy is included in Nursing Process Focus: Clients Receiving Antidysrhythmic Therapies at the end of this chapter. Additional nursing considerations will vary depending on the drug used.

Because class I antidysrhythmics have profound effects on the heart, a complete health history and physical examination, including baseline ECG, vital signs, hepatic and urinary function tests, and electrolyte values, should be obtained before initiating therapy. Assess for HF, hypotension, myasthenia gravis, and renal or hepatic impairment, as these are contraindicated in class I antidysrhythmic therapy. A thorough drug history should be obtained because these agents interact with a large number of other drugs, including cardiac glycosides, cimetidine (Tagamet), anticonvulsants, nifedipine (Adalat), and warfarin (Coumadin).

During pharmacotherapy, monitor the client for changes in the ECG such as an increase in PR and QT intervals and widening of the QRS complex. Blood pressure should be monitored frequently, as some agents can cause hypotension. Some drugs in this class can cause arterial embolism. This adverse effect is related to the formation of small blood clots in the atrium that occur while the client is being treated for atrial fibrillation. For this reason, current research and 2007 Canadian Consensus Conference guidelines for HF and associated atrial fibrillation support the use of anticoagulant (e.g., warfarin) therapy to prevent stroke in clients with atrial fibrillation. Nurses should monitor the client for changes in level of consciousness and respiratory status and report these to the physician immediately.

Monitor drug plasma levels during therapy. Also, the client should be monitored for diarrhea, which occurs in approximately one-third of clients on quinidine (Quinate). This adverse effect is due to the fact that quinidine is chemically related to quinine in structure and action. Because diarrhea may be intense, implement appropriate interventions related to the diarrhea to maintain fluid and electrolyte balance.

Client education as it relates to sodium channel blockers should include goals, reasons for obtaining baseline data such as vital signs and tests for cardiac and renal function, and possible side effects. Include the following points when teaching clients regarding sodium channel blockers:

* Do not skip doses of the medication, even if feeling well. Do not take two doses at a time if the first dose is missed.
* Avoid the use of alcohol, caffeine, and tobacco.
* Comply with monitoring of laboratory tests as ordered.
* Report the following symptoms immediately: shortness of breath, signs of bleeding, excessive bruising, fever, nausea, persistent headache, changes to vision or hearing, diarrhea, or dizziness.

PROTOTYPE DRUG	Procainamide (Procan)

Actions and Uses: Procainamide blocks sodium ion channels in myocardial cells, thus reducing automaticity and slowing conduction of the action potential across the myocardium. This slight delay in conduction velocity prolongs the refractory period and can suppress dysrhythmias. Procainamide is referred to as a broad-spectrum drug because it has the ability to correct many different types of atrial and ventricular dysrhythmia. Procainamide is available in capsule, extended-release tablet, IV, and intramuscular (IM) formulations. The therapeutic serum drug level is 4 to 8 μg/mL.

Pharmacokinetics: Procainamide is well absorbed and is 15% to 20% protein bound. It is mostly metabolized by the liver and excreted by the kidneys. It has a half-life of 3 hours.

Administration Alerts:
* The supine position should be used during IV administration because severe hypotension may occur.
* Do not break or crush extended-release tablets.
* Procainamide is pregnancy category C.

Adverse Effects and Interactions: Nausea, anorexia, diarrhea, hypotension, abdominal pain, and headache are common adverse effects. Like all antidysrhythmic drugs, procainamide has the ability to produce new dysrhythmias or worsen existing ones. A lupus-like syndrome may occur in 30% to 50% of clients who take the drug over a year. High doses may produce central nervous system (CNS) effects such as confusion or psychosis. Hypotension due to overdosage may be treated with vasopressors. Procainamide is contraindicated in clients with complete AV block, severe HF, blood dyscrasias, and myasthenia gravis.

BETA-ADRENERGIC BLOCKERS (CLASS II)

Beta-adrenergic blockers are widely used for cardiovascular disorders. Their ability to slow the heart rate and conduction velocity can suppress several types of dysrhythmia. The beta blockers are shown in Table 55.3.

Treating Dysrhythmias with Beta-Adrenergic Blockers

55.9 Beta-adrenergic blockers act by reducing automaticity and by slowing conduction velocity across the myocardium.

Beta blockers are used to treat a large number of cardiovascular diseases, including hypertension, MI, HF, and dysrhythmias. Because of potentially serious side effects, however, only a few beta blockers are approved to treat dysrhythmias. Beta blockers slow the heart rate (negative chronotropic effect) and decrease conduction velocity through the AV node. Myocardial automaticity is reduced, and many types of dysrhythmias are stabilized. The main value of beta blockers as antidysrhythmic agents is to treat atrial dysrhythmias associated with heart failure. Abrupt discontinuation of beta blockers can lead to dysrhythmias and hypertension. The basic pharmacology of beta-adrenergic blockers is explained in Chapter 14.

Nursing Considerations

The role of the nurse caring for clients who are receiving beta-adrenergic antagonists for dysrhythmias is included in Nursing Process Focus: Clients Receiving Antidysrhythmic Therapies at the end of this chapter. For additional nursing considerations, refer to Nursing Process Focus: Clients Receiving Adrenergic Antagonist Therapy in Chapter 14.

All drugs in this class are contraindicated in clients with heart block, severe bradycardia, AV block, and asthma. The action of beta blockers is to decrease the contractions of the myocardium and to lessen the speed of conduction through the AV node. This action predisposes clients with certain existing heart problems to experience a significant decrease in heart rate that may not be well tolerated. The most common adverse reaction to these drugs is hypotension.

Monitor elderly clients for cognitive dysfunction and depression, as well as for hallucinations and psychosis, which are more likely with higher doses. These reactions appear to be related to the lipid solubility of this medication and its ability to cross the blood-brain barrier. Monitor for hypoglycemia. There is an increased incidence of hypoglycemia in clients with type 1 diabetes mellitus because beta blockers may inhibit glycogenolysis.

Client education as it relates to beta-adrenergic blockers should include goals, reasons for obtaining baseline data such as vital signs and tests for cardiac and renal function, and possible side effects. Provide the following information when teaching clients about beta-adrenergic blockers:

- Take pulse prior to drug administration. Report pulse rate less than 50 to the healthcare provider.
- Slowly rise from a sitting or lying position to avoid dizziness.
- Report the following symptoms immediately: shortness of breath, feeling of skipping a heartbeat, painful or difficult urination, frequent nighttime urination, weight gain of 1 kg or more, dizziness, insomnia, drowsiness, or confusion.

NCLEX Success Tips

In addition to lowering blood pressure by blocking sympathetic nervous system stimulation, propranolol's (Inderal) therapeutic effect is to lower the heart rate. The nurse should teach the client about how to take his or her own pulse and instruct the client to call his or her healthcare provider if heart rate drops below 55 bpm.

One of the actions of propranolol, a drug used in the treatment of migraine headaches, is to inhibit arterial vasodilation. The nurse should assess the client's blood pressure to evaluate overall circulatory response to the medication.

The client who is taking propranolol should also be assessed for bradycardia and other arrhythmias.

The client needs to be instructed not to discontinue medication because sudden withdrawal of propranolol hydrochloride may cause rebound hypertension and tachycardia.

PROTOTYPE DRUG | **Propranolol (Inderal)**

Actions and Uses: Propranolol is a non-selective beta-adrenergic blocker, affecting beta$_1$ receptors in the heart and beta$_2$ receptors in pulmonary and vascular smooth muscle. Propranolol reduces heart rate, slows conduction velocity, and lowers blood pressure. Propranolol is most effective against tachycardia caused by excessive sympathetic stimulation. It is approved to treat a wide variety of diseases, including hypertension, angina, and migraine headaches, and to prevent myocardial infarction.

Administration Alerts:
- Abrupt discontinuation may cause myocardial infarction, severe hypertension, and ventricular dysrhythmias because of a potential rebound effect.
- If pulse is less than 50 bpm (or as per agency policy), withhold the dose and notify the physician.
- Propranolol is pregnancy category C.

Pharmacokinetics: Propranolol undergoes extensive first-pass metabolism and is 93% protein bound. It is almost completely metabolized by the liver. Its onset of action is 1 to 2 hours, and the half-life is 3 to 6 hours.

Adverse Effects and Interactions: Common side effects of propranolol include fatigue, hypotension, and bradycardia. Because of its ability to slow the heart rate, clients with other cardiac disorders such as HF must be carefully monitored. Side effects such as diminished libido and impotence may result in nonadherence in male clients.

Propranolol interacts with many other drugs, including phenothiazines, which have additive hypotensive effects. Propranolol should not be given within 2 weeks of a monamine oxidase (MAO) inhibitor. Beta-adrenergic agonists such as salbutamol (Ventolin) antagonize the actions of propranolol.

Intravenous glucagon reverses the cardiac depression caused by beta blocker overdose by increasing myocardial contractibility, heart rate, and improving AV node conduction.

POTASSIUM CHANNEL BLOCKERS (CLASS III)

Although a small drug class, the potassium channel blockers have important applications to the treatment of dysrhythmias. These drugs prolong the refractory period, which stabilizes certain types of dysrhythmia. The potassium channel blockers are listed in Table 55.3.

Treating Dysrhythmias with Potassium Channel Blockers

55.10 Potassium channel blockers act by prolonging the refractory period of the heart.

The drugs in class III exert their actions by blocking potassium ion channels in myocardial cells. After the action potential has passed and the myocardial cell is in a depolarized state, repolarization depends on removal of potassium from the cell. The class III medications delay repolarization of the myocardial cells and lengthen the refractory period, which tends to stabilize dysrhythmias. In addition to blocking potassium channels, sotalol is also a beta-adrenergic blocker. Drugs in this class generally are not first-line therapy due to potentially serious side effects.

Nursing Considerations

The role of the nurse caring for clients who are receiving potassium channel blockers for dysrhythmias is included in Nursing Process Focus: Clients Receiving Antidysrhythmic Therapies at the end of this chapter. Additional nursing considerations will vary depending on the specific drug. Be aware of the specific mechanism of action, side effects, administration requirements, and client teaching for each drug prescribed. These drugs are not recommended for use during pregnancy (category C) or lactation.

Client education as it relates to potassium channel blockers should include goals, reasons for obtaining baseline data such as vital signs and tests for liver and renal function, and possible side effects. Provide the following information when teaching clients about potassium channel blockers:

- Have regular eye exams, due to possible vision changes.
- Avoid prolonged sun exposure and use sunscreen.
- Take medication with meals or a small snack.
- Report the following symptoms immediately: shortness of breath, feeling that the heart has skipped a beat, cough, vision changes, yellow eyes and skin (jaundice), right upper abdominal pain, or dizziness.

NCLEX Success Tips

Amiodarone (Cordarone) is used for the treatment of premature ventricular contractions, ventricular tachycardia with a pulse, atrial fibrillation, and atrial flutter. It also increases the ventricular fibrillation threshold.

Amiodarone is contraindicated in sinus node dysfunction, heart block, and severe bradycardia and pulseless dysrhythmia. Adverse effects of amiodarone includ thyroid disorders, bradycardia, hypotension, SA node dysfunction, QT prolongation, blue-grey colouring of the skin (face, arms, neck), and constipation. The nurse must monitor pulmonary function in clients taking amiodarone because the drug may also cause pulmonary fibrosis.

The nurse must monitor blood glucose levels closely in clients with type 2 diabetes who are taking beta-adrenergic blockers such as carvedilol because beta-adrenergic blockers may mask the signs of hypoglycemia.

Amiodarone is metabolized in the liver and excreted in the bile and feces. As such, it may cause liver toxicity so the nurse should monitor the client's liver enzymes.

PROTOTYPE DRUG | **Amiodarone (Cordarone)**

Actions and Uses: Amiodarone is structurally similar to thyroid hormone. It is approved for the treatment of resistant ventricular tachycardia that may prove life-threatening, and it has become a drug of choice for the treatment of atrial dysrhythmias in clients with heart failure. In addition to blocking potassium ion channels, some of this drug's actions on the heart relate to its blockade of sodium ion channels.

Pharmacokinetics: Amiodarone is 96% protein bound, accumulates in body tissues, and is metabolized by the liver. Its onset of action may take several weeks when taken orally. The therapeutic serum level of amiodarone is 0.5 to 2.5 µg/mL. Its effects can last 4 to 8 weeks after the drug is discontinued since it has a long half-life that may exceed 100 days.

Administration Alerts:
- Hypokalemia and hypomagnesemia should be corrected prior to initiating therapy.
- Amiodarone is pregnancy category D.

Adverse Effects and Interactions: The most serious adverse effect of amiodarone occurs in the lung; the drug causes a pneumonia-like syndrome. The drug also causes blurred vision, rashes, photosensitivity, nausea, vomiting, anorexia, fatigue, dizziness, and hypotension. Amiodarone is stored in certain tissues; therefore, adverse effects may be slow to resolve. As with other antidysrhythmics, clients must be closely monitored to avoid serious toxicity.

Amiodarone interacts with many other drugs and herbals. For example, it increases digoxin (Lanoxin, Toloxin) levels in the blood and enhances the actions of anticoagulants. Use with beta-adrenergic blockers may potentiate sinus bradycardia, sinus arrest, or AV block. Amiodarone may increase phenytoin (Dilantin) levels twofold to threefold. Use with echinacea may cause an increase in hepatotoxicity. Aloe may cause an increased effect of amiodarone. Grapefruit juice may decrease metabolism and worsen hypotension.

CALCIUM CHANNEL BLOCKERS (CLASS IV)

Like the beta blockers, the calcium channel blockers are widely prescribed for various cardiovascular disorders. By slowing conduction velocity, they are able to stabilize certain dysrhythmias. The antidysrhythmic calcium channel blockers are listed in Table 55.3.

Treating Dysrhythmias with Calcium Channel Blockers

55.11 Calcium channel blockers act by reducing automaticity and by slowing myocardial conduction velocity. Their actions and effects are similar to the beta blockers.

Although about 10 calcium channel blockers (CCBs) are available to treat cardiovascular disease, only a limited number have been approved for dysrhythmias. A few CCBs such as diltiazem (Cardizem, Tiazac) and verapamil (Isoptin) block calcium ion channels in the heart; the remaining CCBs are specific to calcium channels in vascular smooth muscle. The basic pharmacology of this drug class is presented in Chapter 50.

Blockade of calcium ion channels has a number of effects on the heart, most of which are similar to those of beta-adrenergic blockers. Effects include reduced automaticity in the SA node and slowed impulse conduction through the AV node. This prolongs the refractory period and stabilizes many types of dysrhythmia. CCBs are only effective against supraventricular dysrhythmias.

Nursing Considerations

The role of the nurse caring for clients who are receiving CCBs for dysrhythmias is included in Nursing Process Focus: Clients Receiving Antidysrhythmic Therapies at the end of this chapter. For additional nursing considerations, refer to Nursing Process Focus: Clients Receiving Calcium Channel Blocker Therapy in Chapter 51.

CCB therapy should never be initiated in clients with sick sinus syndrome, heart block, severe hypotension, cardiogenic shock, or severe HF. The desired action of this drug class is to decrease oxygen demand, reduce cardiac workload, and increase oxygen to the myocardium. These therapeutic actions may cause clients with existing heart abnormalities to experience adverse effects on the heart. These drugs may produce lethal ventricular dysrhythmias. Calcium chloride may be administered by slow IV push to reverse hypotension or heart block *if* induced by CCBs.

Because CCBs cause vasodilation of peripheral arterioles and decrease total peripheral vascular resistance, some clients, especially older adults, may not be able to tolerate the rapid decrease in blood pressure and are at increased risk for falls. Older clients should be informed about the importance of changing positions slowly and using hand rails and other safety devices as required. Because constipation is a common side effect of these drugs, the nurse also should instruct the client to eat foods that are high in fibre. These drugs are not recommended for use during pregnancy (category C) or lactation.

Client education as it relates to CCBs used to treat dysrhythmias should include goals, reasons for obtaining baseline data such as vital signs, and possible side effects. Provide the following information when teaching clients about CCBs:

- Report any feelings that the heart has skipped a beat.
- Take blood pressure frequently and report changes: either low blood pressure or elevated blood pressure.
- Take pulse frequently and notify the healthcare provider if it falls below 60 bpm.
- Observe for swelling (edema).
- Report any shortness of breath.

PROTOTYPE DRUG	Verapamil (Isoptin)

Actions and Uses: Verapamil, a CCB, acts by inhibiting the flow of Ca^{+2} into both myocardial cells and vascular smooth muscle cells. In the heart, this action slows conduction velocity and stabilizes dysrhythmias. In the vessels, calcium ion channel inhibition lowers blood pressure, which reduces cardiac workload. Verapamil also dilates the coronary arteries, an action that is important when the drug is used to treat angina (see Chapter 50).

Pharmacokinetics: Verapamil is readily absorbed, but its bioavailability is less than 25% due to rapid metabolism by the liver. It is 90% protein bound. When taken PO, its onset of action is 1 to 2 hours. Its therapeutic serum level is 0.08 to 0.3 µg/mL. Its half-life is 4.5 to 12 hours.

Administration Alerts:

- Capsule contents should not be dissolved or chewed.
- For IV administration, inspect drug preparation to make sure solution is clear and colourless.
- Verapamil is pregnancy category C.

Adverse Effects and Interactions: Side effects are generally minor and may include headache, constipation, and hypotension. Because verapamil can cause bradycardia, clients with HF should be carefully monitored. Clients should notify their healthcare provider if their heart rate falls below 50 bpm or if systolic blood pressure falls below 90 mm Hg. Like many other antidysrhythmics, verapamil has the ability to elevate blood levels of digoxin. Since both digoxin and verapamil have the effect of slowing conduction through the AV node, their concurrent use must be carefully monitored.

Grapefruit juice may decrease metabolism of CCBs and increase their serum concentration, thus worsening hypotension. Use with caution with herbal supplements, such as hawthorn, which may have additive hypotensive effects.

TREATING DYSRHYTHMIAS WITH DIGOXIN AND MISCELLANEOUS DRUGS

55.12 Digoxin, adenosine, and ibutilide are used for specific dysrhythmias but do not act by blocking ion channels.

Several other drugs are occasionally used to treat specific dysrhythmias but do not act by the mechanisms previously described. These miscellaneous agents are listed in Table 55.3. Although digoxin is primarily used to treat heart failure, it is also prescribed for certain types of atrial dysrhythmia because of its ability to decrease automaticity of the SA node and slow conduction through the AV node. Because excessive levels of digoxin can produce serious dysrhythmias, and interactions with other medications are common, clients must be carefully monitored during therapy. Additional information on the mechanism of action and the adverse effects of digoxin may be found in Chapter 54.

Adenosine (Adenocard) and ibutilide (Corvert) are two additional drugs used for specific dysrhythmias. Adenosine is a naturally occurring nucleoside. When given as a 1- to 2-second bolus IV injection, adenosine terminates serious atrial tachycardia by slowing conduction through the AV node and decreasing automaticity of the SA node. Although dyspnea is common, side effects are generally self-limiting because of its 10-second half-life.

Ibutilide is also used as a short-acting IV intervention, infused over 10 minutes to terminate atrial flutter and fibrillation by prolonging the duration of the cardiac action potential. The infusion is stopped as soon as the dysrhythmia is terminated.

CONNECTIONS Natural Therapies

◀ Magnesium for Dysrhythmias

Magnesium has been shown to be effective in the treatment of certain cardiac dysrhythmias in those clients who are magnesium deficient. Magnesium deficiency is associated with a number of dysrhythmias, including atrial fibrillation, premature atrial and ventricular beats, ventricular tachycardia, and ventricular fibrillation. The mechanism of magnesium's antidysrhythmic action is not fully understood, but it may be related to its role in maintaining intracellular potassium. It may also be related to its role as a natural calcium channel blocker. Magnesium may be administered intravenously or in liquid or capsule form. Foods that are rich in magnesium include unpolished grains, nuts, and green vegetables.

NURSING PROCESS FOCUS

Clients Receiving Antidysrhythmic Therapies

Assessment	Potential Nursing Diagnoses/Identified Patterns
Prior to administration: • Obtain complete health history, including allergies, drug history, and possible drug interactions. • Assess to determine if cardiac alteration is producing a symptomatic effect on cardiac output, including vital signs, level of consciousness, urinary output, skin temperature, and peripheral pulses. • Obtain baseline ECG to compare throughout therapy.	• Need for knowledge regarding drug therapy and adverse effects • Safety from injury related to decreased cardiac output and cardiac conduction abnormalities

Planning: Client Goals and Expected Outcomes

The client will:

• Exhibit improved cardiac output as evidenced by stabilization of heart rate, heart rhythm, sensorium, urinary output, and vital signs
• State expected outcomes of drug therapy
• Demonstrate an understanding of the drug's action by accurately describing drug side effects and precautions

Implementation

Interventions (Rationales)	Client Education/Discharge Planning
• Monitor cardiac rate and rhythm continuously if administering drug IV. (IV route is used when rapid therapeutic effects are needed. Constant monitoring is needed to detect any potential serious dysrhythmias.) • Monitor IV site. Administer all parenteral medication via infusion pump. • Investigate possible causes of the dysrhythmia such as electrolyte imbalances, hypoxia, pain, anxiety, caffeine ingestion, and tobacco use. • Observe for side effects specific to the antidysrhythmic used. • Monitor for proper use of medication.	• Explain the need for continuous ECG monitoring when administering the medication intravenously • Instruct client to report any burning or stinging pain, swelling, warmth, redness, or tenderness at the IV insertion site Instruct client to: • Maintain a diet low in sodium and fat, with sufficient potassium • Report illness such as flu, vomiting, diarrhea, and dehydration to the healthcare provider to avoid adverse effects • Restrict use of caffeine and tobacco products Instruct client to: • Report adverse effects specific to prescribed antidysrhythmic • Report palpitations, chest pain, dyspnea, unusual fatigue, weakness, and visual disturbances Instruct client to: • Never discontinue the drug abruptly • Take the drug exactly as prescribed, even if feeling well • Take pulse prior to taking the drug (instruct client regarding the normal range and rhythm of pulse; instruct to consult the healthcare provider regarding "reportable" pulse)

Evaluation of Outcome Criteria

Evaluate the effectiveness of drug therapy by confirming that client goals and expected outcomes have been met (see "Planning").

See Table 55.3 for a list of drugs (classes I to IV) to which these nursing actions apply.

CHAPTER

55 Understanding the Chapter

Key Concepts Summary

The numbered key concepts provide a succinct summary of the important points from the corresponding numbered section within the chapter. If any of these points are not clear, refer to the numbered section within the chapter for review.

55.1 The frequency of dysrhythmias in the population is difficult to predict because many clients experience no symptoms. Persistent or severe dysrhythmias may be lethal.

55.2 Dysrhythmias are classified by location (atrial or ventricular) or type of rhythm abnormality produced (flutter, fibrillation, block).

55.3 The electrical conduction pathway from the SA node, to the AV node, to the bundle branches and Purkinje fibres keeps the heart beating in a synchronized manner. Some myocardial cells in these regions have the property of automaticity.

55.4 The electrophysiological events in the heart can be measured with an electrocardiograph.

55.5 Changes in sodium and potassium levels generate the action potential in myocardial cells. Depolarization occurs when sodium (and calcium) rushes in; repolarization occurs when potassium is removed.

55.6 Non-pharmacological therapy of dysrhythmias, including cardioversion, ablation, and implantable cardioverter defibrillators, are often the treatments of choice.

55.7 Antidysrhythmic drugs are classified by their mechanism of action into classes I through IV.

55.8 Sodium channel blockers are the largest group of antidysrhythmics and act by slowing the rate of impulse conduction across the heart.

55.9 Beta-adrenergic blockers act by reducing automaticity and by slowing conduction velocity across the myocardium.

55.10 Potassium channel blockers act by prolonging the refractory period of the heart.

55.11 Calcium channel blockers act by reducing automaticity and by slowing myocardial conduction velocity. Their actions and effects are similar to the beta blockers.

55.12 Digoxin, adenosine, and ibutilide are used for specific dysrhythmias but do not act by blocking ion channels.

Chapter 55 Scenario

The day had been busy as Jada prepared for her daughter's upcoming wedding. There were so many arrangements to be made, and Jada felt overwhelmed. During the day she experienced heaviness in her chest, but she attributed it to the stress of the wedding and perhaps a touch of bronchitis. Nonetheless, she knew that there was no time to stop and rest; there was too much to do.

Later that afternoon, she realized that she had to take it easy. Then she experienced that strange sensation once again. As she sat in a chair,

Jada suddenly felt dizzy, with extreme weakness and difficulty breathing. Her family members report that she became pale and unexpectedly collapsed. Emergency personnel were called to the scene, and Jada was taken to the nearest hospital.

In the emergency department, Jada's physical examination revealed the following findings: weak, middle-aged Asian female; vital signs: blood pressure 102/68 mm Hg, heart rate 116 beats/minute, respiratory rate 18 breaths/minute, afebrile; weight 53 kg (116 lb). She has clear bilateral breath sounds and active bowel sounds heard in all four quadrants. Her ECG reveals atrial fibrillation with a ventricular rate of 116 beats/minute. She is admitted to the coronary care unit for further testing and observation.

Critical Thinking Questions

1. Jada's ECG shows atrial fibrillation. Trace the electrical conduction system through the heart. What part of the ECG complex would be most affected with this client's medical diagnosis?

2. While in the coronary care unit, Jada will receive amiodarone (Cordarone) IV infusion. She wants to know how long she will need to receive the IV medication and how it works. How would you respond to this client's questions?

3. Jada is being discharged on amiodarone 400 mg twice daily. What instructions should this client receive?

4. List any drug-food interaction concerns you should discuss with Jada.

See Answers to Critical Thinking Questions in Appendix B.

NCLEX Practice Questions

1 A healthcare provider has ordered procainamide for each of four clients. The nurse should question the order for a client with which condition?

   a. Ventricular tachycardia

   b. Paroxysmal atrial tachycardia

   c. Atrial fibrillation

   d. Severe heart failure

2 A client is receiving intravenous lidocaine for ventricular dysrhythmias. Which nursing intervention is appropriate for this therapy?

   a. Monitoring the client for decreased platelet levels.

   b. Placing the client in a supine position during administration.

   c. Monitoring for paresthesias, drowsiness, or confusion.

   d. Encouraging coughing and deep breathing to remove secretions.

3 A client with a rapid atrial dysrhythmia is being treated with verapamil (Isoptin). The nurse will monitor for therapeutic effectiveness by noting which of the following in the client?

   a. Change in the blood pressure

   b. Increase in the serum potassium level

   c. Changes in the cardiac rhythm

   d. Reduction in the urine output

4 The client is prescribed propranolol (Inderal) for the treatment of atrial dysrhythmias associated with heart failure. The nurse knows this drug is used cautiously in clients with heart failure because of which effect?

   a. It causes sodium retention, worsening congestion.

   b. Its adverse effects include hypertension and worsening heart failure.

   c. It is a negative inotropic drug and will decrease myocardial contractility and cardiac output.

   d. It may cause bronchoconstriction.

5 A client is being discharged with a diagnosis of dysrhythmias. The nurse is teaching the client about amiodarone (Cordarone). What client teaching about this medication is needed?

   a. Avoid crowds while taking this medication.

   b. Avoid birth control pills and use an alternate form of birth control.

   c. Wear protective clothing and adequate sunscreen.

   d. Use an electric razor to shave.

See Answers to NCLEX Practice Questions in Appendix A.

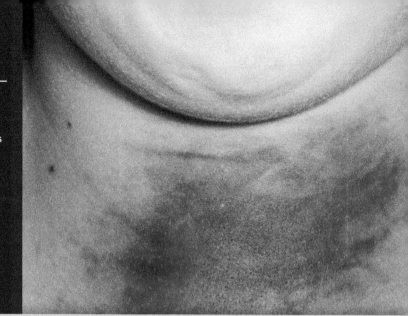

PROTOTYPE DRUGS

ANTICOAGULANTS
Parenteral
Anticoagulants
Pr *heparin*

Oral Anticoagulants
Pr *warfarin*
(Coumadin)

ANTIPLATELET AGENTS
ADP Receptor
Blockers

Pr *clopidogrel*
(Plavix)
Glycoprotein IIb/IIIa
Receptor Blockers

THROMBOLYTICS
Pr *alteplase*
(Activase)

ANTIFIBRINOLYTICS
Pr *aminocaproic
acid* (Amicar)

CHAPTER 56

Pharmacotherapy of Coagulation Disorders

LEARNING OUTCOMES

After reading this chapter, the student should be able to:

1. Identify drug classes used for treating coagulation disorders.

2. Explain the therapeutic action of each class of drug used in relation to the pathophysiology of coagulation (thromboembolic) disorders.

3. Explain how laboratory testing of coagulation parameters is used to monitor anticoagulant pharmacotherapy.

4. Describe the nurse's role in the pharmacological management of clients with coagulation disorders.

5. For each of the drug classes listed in Prototype Drugs, identify a representative drug and explain its mechanism of action, therapeutic effects, and important adverse effects.

6. Describe and explain, based on pharmacological principles, the rationale for nursing assessment, planning, and interventions for clients with coagulation disorders.

7. Use the nursing process to care for clients who are receiving drug therapy for coagulation disorders.

CHAPTER OUTLINE

▶ The Process of Hemostasis

▶ Removal of Blood Clots

▶ Diseases of Hemostasis

▶ Mechanisms of Coagulation Modification

▶ Anticoagulants

  ▶ Pharmacotherapy with Parenteral and Oral Anticoagulants

▶ Antiplatelet Agents

  ▶ Inhibition of Platelet Function

▶ Thrombolytics

  ▶ Pharmacotherapy with Thrombolytics

▶ Antifibrinolytics

  ▶ Pharmacotherapy with Antifibrinolytics

The process of hemostasis, or the stopping of blood flow, is an essential mechanism protecting the body from both external and internal injury. Without efficient hemostasis, bleeding from wounds or internal injuries would lead to shock and perhaps death. Too much clotting, however, can be just as dangerous. The physiological processes of hemostasis must maintain a delicate balance between fluidity and coagulation.

A number of diseases and conditions, including myocardial infarction (MI), cerebrovascular accident (CVA), venous thrombus, valvular heart disease, and indwelling catheters, can affect hemostasis. Because these disorders are so prevalent, nurses will have frequent occasions to administer and monitor coagulation-modifying drugs. Drugs may be used to enhance coagulation, inhibit coagulation, or dissolve existing clots to restore blood flow.

The Process of Hemostasis

56.1 Hemostasis is a complex process involving multiple steps and a large number of enzymes and factors. The final product is a fibrin clot that stops blood loss.

The process of hemostasis is complex, involving a number of substances called **clotting factors**. **Hemostasis** occurs in a series of sequential steps, sometimes referred to as a cascade. Drugs can be used to modify several of these steps.

When a blood vessel is injured, a series of events initiate the clotting process. The vessel spasms cause constriction, which limits blood flow to the injured area. Platelets have an affinity for the damaged vessel. They become sticky, adhering to each other and to the injured area. Aggregation is facilitated by adenosine diphosphate (ADP), the enzyme thrombin, and thromboxane A_2, while adhesion is made possible by platelet receptor sites and von Willebrand's factor. As the bound platelets break down, they release substances that attract more platelets to the area. Blood flow is further slowed, thus allowing the process of **coagulation**, which is the formation of an insoluble clot. The basic steps of hemostasis are shown in Figure 56.1.

When collagen is exposed at the site of vascular injury and platelets adhere to the damaged cells, a series of complex reactions called the **coagulation cascade** is initiated. Coagulation occurs when fibrin threads form to create a meshwork that fortifies the blood constituents so that they develop the clot. During the cascade, various plasma proteins that are circulating in an inactive state are converted to their active forms. Two separate pathways, along with numerous biochemical processes, lead to coagulation. The intrinsic pathway is activated in response to injury. The extrinsic pathway is activated when blood leaks out of a vessel and enters tissue spaces. There are common steps between the two pathways and the outcome is the same—the formation of the fibrin clot. The steps in each coagulation cascade are shown in Figure 56.2.

Near the end of the common pathway, a chemical called **prothrombin activator**, or prothrombinase, is formed. Prothrombin activator converts the clotting factor **prothrombin** to an enzyme called **thrombin**. Thrombin then converts **fibrinogen**, a plasma protein, to long strands of **fibrin**. The fibrin strands provide a framework for the structure of the clot. Therefore, two of the factors essential to clotting, thrombin and fibrin, are only formed after injury to the vessel. The fibrin strands form an insoluble web over the injured area to stop blood loss. Normal blood clotting occurs in approximately 6 minutes.

It is important to note that several clotting factors, including thromboplastin and fibrinogen, are proteins made by the liver that are constantly circulating through the blood in an inactive form. Vitamin K, which is made by bacteria residing in the large intestine, is required for the liver to make four of the clotting factors. Because of the crucial importance of the liver in creating these clotting factors, clients with serious liver disorders often have abnormal coagulation.

Removal of Blood Clots

56.2 Fibrinolysis, or removal of a blood clot, is an enzymatic process initiated by the release of tPA. Plasmin digests the fibrin strands, thus restoring circulation to the injured area.

Hemostasis has been achieved once a blood clot is formed, protecting the body from excessive hemorrhage. The clot, however, stops most or all of the blood flow to the affected area; circulation must eventually be restored so that the tissue can resume normal

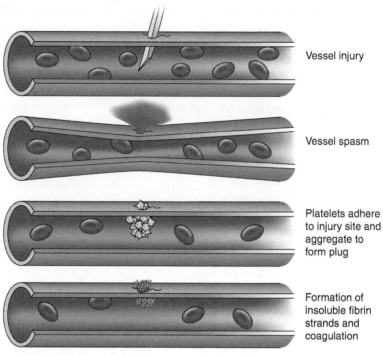

Figure 56.1 Basic steps of hemostasis.

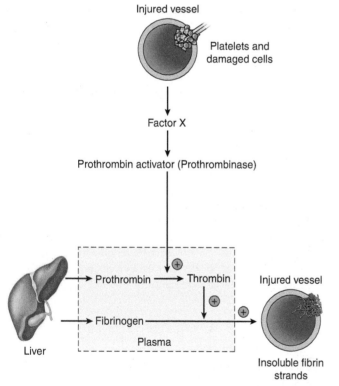

Figure 56.2 Major steps in the coagulation cascade: common pathway.

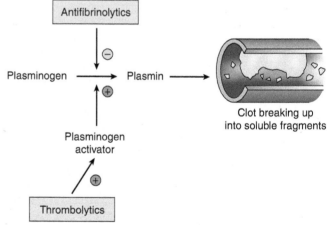

Figure 56.3 Primary steps of fibrinolysis.

tissue plasminogen activator (tPA), which converts the inactive protein **plasminogen** in the fibrin clot to its active enzymatic form called **plasmin**. Plasmin then digests the fibrin strands to remove the clot. The body normally regulates fibrinolysis such that unwanted fibrin clots are removed but fibrin present in wounds is left to maintain hemostasis. The steps of fibrinolysis are shown in Figure 56.3.

Diseases of Hemostasis

56.3 Diseases of hemostasis include thromboembolic disorders caused by thrombi and emboli and bleeding disorders such as hemophilia and von Willebrand's disease.

To diagnose bleeding disorders, a thorough health history and physical examination is necessary. Laboratory tests that measure

activities. The process of clot removal is called **fibrinolysis**. It is initiated within 24 to 48 hours of clot formation and continues until the clot is dissolved.

Fibrinolysis also involves several cascading steps. When the fibrin clot is formed, nearby blood vessel cells secrete the enzyme coagulation must be obtained. These usually include a whole blood clotting time, **prothrombin time (PT)**, thrombin time, **activated partial thromboplastin time (aPTT)**, liver function tests, and in some instances a bleeding time. Platelet count is also of interest in assessing bleeding disorders. Additional tests may be indicated based on the results of these laboratory analyses.

Thromboembolic disorders occur when undesirable clots are formed. Once a stationary clot, called a **thrombus**, forms in a vessel, it often grows larger as more fibrin is added. Arterial thrombi are particularly problematic, as they deprive an area of blood flow. Cessation of blood flow results in an infarction and tissue death will result. This is the case in MIs and many CVAs.

Pieces of a thrombus may break off and travel in the bloodstream to affect other vessels. A travelling clot is called an **embolus**. Thrombi in the venous system usually form in the veins of the legs in susceptible clients, a condition called **deep vein thrombosis (DVT)**. Thrombi can also form in the atria during atrial fibrillation. A thrombus in the right atrium can dislodge and travel to the lung, causing a pulmonary embolism. A thrombus in the left atrium can dislodge and cause a CVA or an arterial infarction elsewhere in the body. Arterial thrombi and emboli can also result from procedures involving arterial punctures, such as angiography. Thromboembolic disorders are the most common indications for pharmacotherapy with anticoagulants.

When thrombosis occurs in the legs it is called DVT. Because blood flow is slowest in the deep veins of the lower limbs, these vessels are the most common sites for venous thromboembolism (VTE). Conditions associated with venous stasis and DVT include the following:

- *Extended immobility*. During major illness or following surgery, clients may be supine or otherwise immobile for extended periods of time. Because the movement of blood through the deep veins is entirely dependent on the squeezing action from skeletal muscular contraction, blood in the deep veins of these clients has difficulty returning to the heart.

- *Major trauma*. Trauma often causes serious bleeding that activates pro-coagulation factors. In addition, stasis will likely occur surrounding the injured area, promoting the development of DVT. Trauma involving the lower extremities places the client at high risk for DVT.

- *Major surgery*. Surgery of the lower extremities, especially knee and hip replacements, are common causes of DVT for the same reasons as trauma; bleeding activates pro-coagulation factors and stasis occurs around the surgical site.

- *Hypercoagulability states*. Malignancy, lupus, and pregnancy are examples of conditions associated with an increased risk for coagulation and DVT. Certain genetic disorders also produce hypercoagulability, the most common being a genetic deficiency of protein C, a natural anticoagulant.

- *Drug therapy*. High amounts of estrogen, prescribed as replacement therapy or as a component of oral contraceptives, have been associated with DVT in numerous studies. Selective estrogen receptor modulators, such as raloxifene (Evista), are also associated with a higher risk for DVT.

The second primary thromboembolic disorder is **pulmonary embolism**, which occurs when a venous clot dislodges, migrates

to the pulmonary vessels, and blocks arterial circulation to the lungs. Pulmonary emboli are the most serious consequence of VTE because death may occur within minutes after the onset of symptoms. The factors associated with an increased risk for pulmonary embolism are the same as those for clients with DVT: prolonged immobility, major trauma, lower extremity surgery, hypercoagulability states, and estrogen therapy. Prevention of pulmonary embolism is a primary goal for all clients with VTE and a major indication for pharmacotherapy.

Clients with DVT are sometimes asymptomatic, or report nonspecific symptoms such as pain, swelling, or warmth of the legs. The disorder may be present for years, causing progressive damage to venous valves, thus worsening blood flow in the region and increasing the risk for an acute episode. However, a pulmonary embolism produces a sudden onset of cough, chest pain, tachypnea, dyspnea, tachycardia, and hemoptysis. Symptoms of pulmonary embolism resemble an MI, and rapid diagnosis and treatment are essential.

Arterial thromboembolism may deprive an area of blood flow and is a medical emergency because tissue hypoxia and cellular death will result soon after blood stoppage. The most serious arterial thromboembolism disorders are MI and stroke.

Arterial thrombi and emboli commonly result from procedures involving arterial punctures such as angiography and stent placement. They may also originate from the heart. Emboli are common complications of mitral valve disease, prosthetic heart valves, and atrial dysrhythmias. Emboli originating from the left side of the heart may lodge in any organ in the body.

CONNECTIONS **Special Considerations**

◀ Secondary Causes of Thrombocytopenia

Diseases
Acquired immune deficiency syndrome (AIDS)
Alcoholism
Anemia (aplastic, folic acid, vitamin B_{12})
Disseminated intravascular coagulation (DIC)
Infectious mononucleosis
Leukemia
Viral infections

Drugs
Acetylsalicylic acid (ASA [Aspirin])
Cimetidine (Tagamet)
Digitalis
Furosemide (Lasix)
Heparin
Ibuprofen (Advil, Motrin)
Indomethacin (Indocin)
Morphine sulfate (Kadian, M-Eslon, MS Contin, MS-IR, Statex)
Naproxen (Aleve, Naprosyn)
Quinidine (Quinate)
Sulfonamides
Thiazide diuretics

Therapeutic Regimens
Chemotherapy
Radiation therapy

Bleeding disorders are characterized by abnormal clot formation. The most common bleeding disorder is a deficiency of platelets known as **thrombocytopenia**, which results from any condition that suppresses bone marrow function. Certain drugs, such as immunosuppressants and most anticancer agents, can cause this condition.

Hemophilias are bleeding disorders caused by genetic deficiencies in certain clotting factors. They are typified by prolonged coagulation times that result in persistent bleeding that can be acute. The classic form, hemophilia A, is caused by a lack of clotting factor VIII and accounts for approximately 80% of all cases. Hemophilia B, or Christmas disease, is caused by a deficiency of factor IX and makes up about 20% of cases. Hemophilia is treated with the administration of the absent clotting factor and, in acute situations, transfusions of fresh frozen plasma. Of the other inherited bleeding disorders, **von Willebrand's disease (vWD)** is the most common. This disorder results in a decrease in the quantity or quality of von Willebrand factor (vWF), which has a role in platelet aggregation. This type of bleeding disorder is treated with factor VIII concentrate as well as desmopressin (DDAVP, Nocdurna), which promotes the release of stored vWF. For the most severely affected clients, plasma products containing vWF may be required.

Mechanisms of Coagulation Modification

56.4 The normal coagulation process can be modified by a number of different mechanisms, including inhibiting clotting factors, dissolving fibrin, and influencing platelet function.

Drugs can modify hemostasis by four basic mechanisms, as summarized in Table 56.1. The most commonly prescribed coagulation modifiers are the **anticoagulants**, which are used to prevent the formation of clots. To accomplish clot prevention, drugs can either inhibit specific clotting factors in the coagulation cascade or diminish the clotting action of platelets. Regardless of the mechanism, all anticoagulant drugs will increase the normal time the body takes to form clots.

Once an abnormal clot has formed in a blood vessel, it may be critical to quickly remove it to restore normal function. This is particularly important for vessels that serve the heart, lungs, and brain. A specific class of drug, the **thrombolytics**, has been developed to dissolve such life-threatening clots.

Occasionally, it is necessary to actually promote the formation of clots. These drugs, called **antifibrinolytics**, inhibit the normal removal of fibrin, thus keeping the clot in place for a longer

period of time. Antifibrinolytics are primarily used to speed clot formation in order to limit bleeding from a surgical site.

Since hemostasis involves a delicate balance of factors favouring clotting versus those inhibiting clotting, pharmacotherapy with coagulation modifiers is individualized to each client. Clients who are receiving coagulation-modifying drugs require regular physical and laboratory assessments.

ANTICOAGULANTS

Anticoagulants are drugs used to prolong bleeding time in order to prevent blood clots from forming. They are widely used in the treatment of thromboembolic disease.

Pharmacotherapy with Parenteral and Oral Anticoagulants

56.5 Anticoagulants prevent clot formation. The primary drugs in this category are heparin (parenteral) and warfarin (oral).

Anticoagulants lengthen clotting time and prevent thrombi from forming or growing larger by inhibiting certain clotting factors. Thromboembolic disease can be life-threatening; therefore, therapy is often begun by administering anticoagulants intravenously or subcutaneously to achieve a rapid onset of action. The most commonly prescribed parenteral anticoagulant is heparin. As the disease stabilizes, the client is switched to an oral anticoagulant, with careful monitoring of appropriate laboratory coagulation studies. Warfarin (Coumadin) is the most commonly prescribed oral anticoagulant.

Anticoagulants act by a number of different mechanisms, as illustrated in Figure 56.4. These drugs are often referred to as blood thinners, which is actually not the case, because they do not change the viscosity of the blood. Instead, anticoagulants exert a negative charge on the surface of the platelets, so that the clumping action or aggregation of these cells is inhibited. Heparin acts by enhancing the inhibitory actions of **antithrombin III**. Warfarin acts by inhibiting the hepatic synthesis of coagulation factors II, VII, IX, and X. Table 56.2 lists the primary anticoagulants.

In recent years, the heparin molecule has been shortened and modified to create a new class of drug called **low-molecular-weight heparins (LMWHs)**. The mechanism of action of these agents is similar to that of heparin, except that their inhibition is more specific to active factor X (see Figure 56.2). LMWHs possess the same degree of anticoagulant activity as heparin but have several advantages. LMWHs are less likely to cause thrombocytopenia. The duration of action of LMWHs is two to four times longer,

TABLE 56.1 Mechanisms of Coagulation Modification

Type of Modification	Mechanism	Drug Classification
Prevention of clot formation	Inhibition of specific clotting factors	Anticoagulant
Prevention of clot formation	Inhibition of platelet actions	Anticoagulant/antiplatelet
Removal of an existing clot	Dissolving of the clot	Thrombolytic
Promotion of clot formation	Inhibition of the destruction of fibrin	Antifibrinolytic

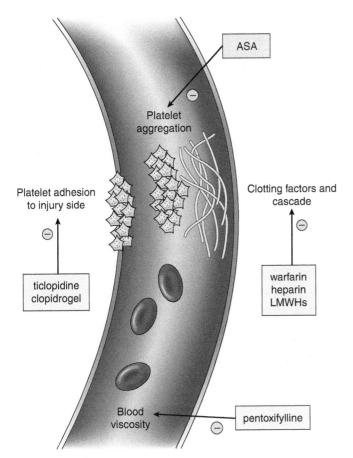

Figure 56.4 Mechanisms of action of anticoagulants.

and they produce a more stable response than heparin; therefore, fewer follow-up laboratory tests are needed, and the client or family members can be trained to give the necessary SC injections at home. LMWHs have become the drugs of choice for a number of clotting disorders, including the prevention of DVT following surgery.

Other parenteral anticoagulants include the direct thrombin inhibitors argatroban (Novastan) and bivalirudin (Angiomax). Thrombin inhibitors bind to both clot-bound and circulating thrombin,

preventing the formation of fibrin clots. The therapeutic aPTT value for these drugs is usually one and a half to three times the control value. Bivalirudin is administered in combination with acetylsalicylic acid (ASA [Aspirin]) to prevent thrombi in clients who are undergoing angioplasty. Argatroban is indicated for prevention or treatment of thrombocytopenia induced by heparin therapy. There is no specific antidote for these agents. Blood transfusion may be required if excessive bleeding occurs.

Although parenteral anticoagulants have the advantage of an almost immediate onset of action, drugs given by this route require close medical supervision because adverse effects such as bleeding can rapidly ensue. When the client's condition allows, oral anticoagulants are used due to their convenience and greater safety.

Warfarin has been available as an anticoagulant for more than 50 years and is the most frequently used drug in this class. In acute situations, clients begin anticoagulation therapy with heparin and are switched to warfarin when their condition stabilizes. When transitioning, the two drugs must be administered concurrently for 2 to 3 days. This is because heparin has a brief half-life (90 minutes), and aPTT returns to normal within 2 to 3 hours following discontinuation of heparin. Warfarin, on the other hand, takes 1 to 3 days of therapy to achieve optimum anticoagulation. Therefore, concomitant pharmacotherapy is necessary to ensure continuous anticoagulation. During this transition, there is increased risk for bleeding, due to the additive anticoagulant action of the two drugs.

Unlike heparin, which is monitored with aPTT values, PT is the standard laboratory test used to monitor the effectiveness of warfarin. The normal PT range is 12 to 15 seconds. During therapeutic anticoagulation, PT should increase to 1.5 to 2 times the client's baseline. Because laboratory testing methods for PT vary, however, PT time is also reported as an international normalized ratio (INR) value; INR values averaging 2.5 are considered therapeutic for most indications. PT is measured daily until the desired level of therapeutic anticoagulation is achieved. Then, the frequency of laboratory testing is decreased to weekly or monthly as the client's condition stabilizes. Home monitoring devices are available to provide convenient and reliable INR values, which can guide the clients to adjust their own medication amounts. Self-monitoring

TABLE 56.2	Anticoagulants
Drug	**Route and Adult Dose**
Pr heparin	Intravenous (IV), infusion: 5000–40 000 units/day; subcutaneous (SC), 15 000–20 000 units twice a day (bid)
pentoxifylline (Trental)*	Orally (PO), 400 mg three times a day (tid)
Pr warfarin (Coumadin)	PO, 1–10 mg/day
Low-Molecular-Weight Heparins (LMWHs)	
dalteparin (Fragmin)	SC, 2500–5000 units/day for up to 14 days
danaparoid (Orgaran)	SC, 750 units bid for up to 14 days
enoxaparin (Lovenox)	SC, 40 mg once a day (qd) or 30 mg every 12 hours (q12h)
tinzaparin (Innohep)	SC, 175 units/kg every day for at least 6 days
Direct Thrombin Inhibitors	
argatroban (Novastan)	IV, 2 µg/kg/minute (max 10 µg/kg/minute)
bivalirudin (Angiomax)	IV, start with 0.75 mg/kg bolus immediately prior to procedure, followed by 1.75 mg/kg/hour for the duration of the procedure; after the procedure, may continue the infusion at 1.75 mg/kg/hour for up to 4 hours if needed

Sometimes classified as a hemorrheological drug.

has its limitations, however. The devices are expensive and the client or their caregiver must be capable of understanding how to properly adjust the dosage.

Several newer drugs have emerged as significant alternatives to warfarin for stroke prevention; rivaroxaban (Xarelto), apixaban (Eliquis), and dabigatran (Pradaxa) are examples. The three newer alternatives do not require INR monitoring and they do not exhibit extensive drug interactions compared to warfarin. Perhaps more important is that the three alternatives appear to be more effective than warfarin at preventing strokes. The alternatives are more expensive than warfarin and they have a much shorter half-life; therefore, missing a single dose may increase stroke risk.

The primary advantage of a direct thrombin inhibitor is that it is given at a fixed dose with no titrating or coagulation monitoring. Compared to available anticoagulants, it has low potential for food and drug interactions.

Nursing Considerations

The role of the nurse in anticoagulant therapy involves careful monitoring of the client's condition and providing education as it relates to the prescribed drug regimen. The most serious side effect of anticoagulants is bleeding. Assess the client for signs of bleeding, including bruising, nosebleeds, excessive menstrual flow, "coffee grounds" emesis, tarry stools, tea-coloured urine, bright red bleeding from the rectum, dizziness, fatigue, or pale, pasty-looking skin. The risk for bleeding is dose dependent—the higher the dose, the higher the risk.

Hypotension accompanied by declining complete blood count (CBC) values (red blood cells [RBCs], platelets, hemoglobin [Hgb], and hematocrit [Hct]) may signal internal bleeding. Lumbar pain and unilateral abdominal wall bulges or swelling could indicate retroperitoneal hemorrhage. Guaiac tests can be performed on stool to identify occult blood. Use of heparin during breastfeeding can trigger bleeding from the nipples and should be avoided. Use of warfarin during pregnancy is contraindicated, as it can cause hemorrhage or other abnormalities in the fetus.

Monitoring of laboratory values during anticoagulant therapy is essential to client safety. For heparin, aPTT is measured, with normal values ranging from 25 to 40 seconds. For therapeutic anticoagulation, the aPTT should be one to two times the client's baseline. During continuous IV heparin therapy, the aPTT is measured daily and 6 to 8 hours after any changes in dosage.

PT is a laboratory test used to monitor the effectiveness of warfarin. The normal PT range is 12 to 15 seconds. During therapeutic anticoagulation, PT should increase to one to two times the client's baseline. Because laboratory testing methods for PT vary, PT is also reported as an INR value; INR values of 2.0 to 3.5 are considered therapeutic. PT is measured daily until the therapeutic dose is determined, and then the frequency of testing is decreased to weekly or monthly as therapy progresses.

When transitioning from IV heparin to PO warfarin, the two drugs must be administered simultaneously for 2 to 3 days. Heparin has a brief half-life (90 minutes) and warfarin has a long one (1 to 3 days). The aPTT returns to normal within 2 to 3 hours following discontinuation of heparin, so concomitant pharmacotherapy is necessary to ensure continuous therapeutic anticoagulation. During this transition, there is increased risk for bleeding due to the potentiated action of the combined drugs.

LMWHs are given subcutaneously, with dosage calculations based on the client's weight rather than laboratory values. Follow the manufacturer's recommendations for sites of injection. There is an increased risk for bleeding if injected into muscle. For example, enoxaparin is given in the subcutaneous tissue of the anterolateral or posterolateral abdominal wall (the "love handles"). To administer safely, gently grasp a skinfold between the thumb and forefinger, insert a 1-cm (3/8-inch) needle fully at a 90-degree angle, and hold the skin fold throughout the injection. For exceptionally lean clients, a longer needle is used and is carefully inserted at a 45-degree angle to avoid inadvertent intramuscular (IM) injection of the medication. To prevent tissue injury and bruising, an injection site should never be massaged.

Client education should include goals, reasons for obtaining baseline data such as vital signs and blood tests, and possible side effects. The following are important points to include when teaching clients about heparin and warfarin:

- Immediately report burning, stinging, tightness, tenderness, warmth, or other pain at heparin injection or IV insertion sites; these signs may signal drug infiltration into sensitive tissues.

- Notify the nurse of excessive bruising or evidence of swelling at a heparin injection site.

- Take warfarin at the same time each day.

- Moderate daily intake of vitamin K–rich foods when taking warfarin.

- Avoid strenuous and hazardous activities that could result in bleeding injury.

General teaching strategies for anticoagulants can be found in Nursing Process Focus: Clients Receiving Anticoagulant Therapy.

NURSING PROCESS FOCUS

Clients Receiving Anticoagulant Therapy

Assessment	Potential Nursing Diagnoses/Identified Patterns
Prior to administration: • Obtain complete health history, including recent surgeries or trauma, allergies, drug history, and possible drug interactions. • Obtain vital signs; assess in context of client's baseline values.	• Adequate knowledge regarding drug therapy and adverse effects • Safety from injury (bleeding, bruising) related to adverse effects of anticoagulant therapy • Safety from physical injury such as falls • Effective tissue perfusion • Tissue integrity • Safety from infection

---

Planning: Client Goals and Expected Outcomes

The client will:

- Experience a decrease in blood coagulability as evidenced by laboratory values and signs of effective blood circulation
- Experience a safe environment with no evidence of physical injury
- Demonstrate an understanding of the drug's action by accurately describing drug side effects and precautions

---

Implementation

Interventions (Rationales)	Client Education/Discharge Planning
• Monitor for adverse clotting reactions. (Heparin can cause thrombus formation with thrombocytopenia, or "white clot syndrome." Warfarin may cause cholesterol microemboli, which result in gangrene, localized vasculitis, or "purple toes syndrome.") • Observe for signs of skin necrosis such as blue or purple mottling of the feet that blanches with pressure or fades when the legs are elevated. (Clients on anticoagulant therapy remain at risk for developing emboli, resulting in CVA or pulmonary embolism.) • Use with caution in clients with gastrointestinal (GI), renal, and/or liver disease; alcoholism; diabetes; hypertension; or hyperlipidemia, and in the elderly and premenopausal women. (Clients with coronary artery disease [CAD] risk factors are at increased risk for developing cholesterol microemboli.) • Monitor for signs of bleeding: flu-like symptoms, excessive bruising, pallor, epistaxis, hemoptysis, hematemesis, menorrhagia, hematuria, melena, frank rectal bleeding, or excessive bleeding from wounds or in the mouth. (Bleeding is a sign of anticoagulant overdose.) • Monitor vital signs. (Increase in heart rate accompanied by low blood pressure or subnormal temperature may signal bleeding.) • Monitor laboratory values (aPTT, PT) for therapeutic values. (Because heparin is metabolized by the liver and may cause significant elevations of serum glutamic oxaloacetic transaminase [serum aspartate aminotransferase] and serum glutamic pyruvic transaminase [serum alanine transferase], also assess these enzyme values.) • Monitor CBC, especially in premenopausal women.	Instruct client to: • Immediately report sudden dyspnea, chest pain, temperature or colour change in the hands, arms, legs, and feet (gangrene may occur between day 3 and 8 of warfarin therapy; purple toes syndrome usually occurs within weeks 3 to 10 or later) • Feel pedal pulses daily to check circulation • Protect feet from injury by wearing loose-fitting socks; avoid going barefoot • Instruct elderly clients, menstruating women, and those with peptic ulcer disease, alcoholism, or kidney or liver disease that they have an increased risk for bleeding • Diabetics and clients with high blood pressure or cholesterol are at risk for developing microscopic clots despite anticoagulant therapy Advise client to: • Immediately report flu-like symptoms (dizziness, chills, weakness, pale skin); blood coming from a cough, the nose, mouth, or rectum; menstrual "flooding"; "coffee grounds" vomit; tarry stools; excessive bruising; bleeding from wounds that cannot be stopped within 10 minutes; all physical injuries • Avoid all contact sports and amusement park rides that cause intense or violent bumping or jostling • Use a soft toothbrush and an electric shaver • Keep a "pad count" during menstrual periods to estimate blood loss • Instruct client to immediately report palpitations, fatigue, or feeling faint, which may signal low blood pressure related to bleeding Instruct client to: • Always inform laboratory personnel of heparin therapy when providing samples • Carry a wallet card or wear medical identification (ID) jewellery indicating heparin therapy

---

Evaluation of Outcome Criteria

Evaluate the effectiveness of drug therapy by confirming that client goals and expected outcomes have been met (see "Planning").

See Table 56.2 for a list of drugs to which these nursing actions apply.

NCLEX Success Tips

Heparin dosage is usually determined by the physician based on the client's PT. Monitoring of the client's PT is done when the client is receiving warfarin sodium. Administering aspirin when the client is on heparin is contraindicated.

Green leafy vegetables are high in vitamin K and therefore are not recommended for clients receiving warfarin sodium.

Teach the client to use a soft toothbrush while brushing his or her teeth as heparin therapy can cause the gums to bleed.

Use of aspirin and other nonsteroidal anti-inflammatory medications (NSAIDs) should be avoided in clients who are on heparin because of the increased risk for possible hemorrhage.

Protamine sulfate is the antidote for heparin therapy. Vitamin K is the antidote for warfarin excess.

Alcohol can inhibit the metabolism of oral anticoagulants and should be avoided.

PROTOTYPE DRUG | **Heparin**

Actions and Uses: Heparin is a natural substance found in the liver and the lining of blood vessels. Its normal function is to prolong coagulation time, thereby preventing excessive clotting within blood vessels. As a result, it prevents the enlargement of existing clots and the formation of new ones. The binding of heparin to antithrombin III inactivates several clotting factors and inhibits thrombin activity.

Administration Alerts:

- Heparin is poorly absorbed by the GI mucosa because of rapid metabolism by the hepatic enzyme heparinase. Therefore, it must be given either by the SC route or through IV bolus injection or continuous infusion.

- When administering heparin SC, never draw back the syringe plunger once the needle has entered the skin, and never massage the site after injection. Doing either can contribute to bleeding or tissue damage.
- IM administration is contraindicated due to bleeding risk.
- Heparin is pregnancy category C.

Pharmacokinetics: The onset of action for IV heparin is immediate, whereas SC heparin may take up to 1 hour for maximum therapeutic effect. It does not cross the placenta or enter breast milk. It is metabolized by the liver and reticuloendothelial system (lymph nodes, spleen). Half-life is 1.5 hours.

Adverse Effects and Interactions: Abnormal bleeding is not uncommon with heparin therapy. Should aPTT become prolonged or toxicity be observed, discontinuation of the drug will result in loss of anticoagulant activity within hours. If serious hemorrhage occurs, a specific antagonist, protamine sulfate, may be administered to neutralize the anticoagulant activity of heparin. Protamine sulfate has an onset of action of 5 minutes and is also an antagonist to the LMWHs.

Oral anticoagulants, including warfarin, potentiate the action of heparin. Drugs that inhibit platelet aggregation, such as ASA, indomethacin (Indocin), and ibuprofen (Advil, Motrin), may induce bleeding. Nicotine, digitalis, tetracyclines, and antihistamines may inhibit anticoagulation.

Use with caution with herbal supplements, such as arnica, which contains a coumarin component and may increase the anticoagulant effect.

NCLEX Success Tips

PROTOTYPE DRUG | **Warfarin (Coumadin)**

Actions and Uses: Unlike heparin, the anticoagulant activity of warfarin can take several days to reach its maximum effect. This explains why heparin and warfarin therapy are overlapped. Warfarin inhibits the action of vitamin K. Without adequate vitamin K, the synthesis of clotting factors II, VII, IX, and X is diminished. Because these clotting factors are normally circulating in the blood, it takes several days for their plasma levels to fall and for the anticoagulant effect of warfarin to appear. Another reason for the slow onset is that 99% of the warfarin is bound to plasma proteins and is thus unavailable to produce its effect.

Pharmacokinetics: The onset of action is 24 to 72 hours with full therapeutic effect achieved within 5 to 7 days. Warfarin crosses the placenta but does not enter breast milk. Protein binding is 99%. It is metabolized by the liver. Half-life is 42 hours.

Administration Alerts:

- Should life-threatening bleeding occur during therapy, the anticoagulant effects of warfarin can be reduced in 6 hours

through the IM or SC administration of its antagonist, vitamin K_1.

- Warfarin is pregnancy category X unless the client has a mechanical heart valve, in which case it is category D.

Adverse Effects and Interactions: The most serious adverse effect of warfarin is abnormal bleeding. Upon discontinuation of therapy, the anticoagulant activity of warfarin may persist for up to 10 days.

Extensive protein binding is responsible for numerous drug-drug interactions, some of which include NSAIDs, diuretics, selective serotonin reuptake inhibitors (SSRIs) and other antidepressants, steroids, antibiotics, vaccines, and vitamins (e.g., vitamin K). Concurrent use with NSAIDs may increase bleeding risk.

Use with caution with herbal supplements, such as arnica, feverfew, garlic, and ginger, which may increase the risk of bleeding.

ANTIPLATELET AGENTS

Antiplatelet drugs cause an anticoagulant effect by interfering with various aspects of platelet function—primarily platelet aggregation. Unlike the anticoagulants, which are used primarily to prevent thrombosis in veins, antiplatelet agents are used to prevent clot formation in arteries. The antiplatelet agents are listed in Table 56.3.

NCLEX Success Tips

TABLE 56.3 Antiplatelet Agents

Drug	Route and Adult Dose
acetylsalicylic acid (ASA [Aspirin]) (see Chapter 23, page 266, for the Prototype Drug box) dipyridamole (Persantine)	PO, 81–325 mg/day PO, 75–100 mg qid
ADP Receptor Blockers	
Pr clopidogrel (Plavix) ticlopidine (Ticlid)	PO, 75 mg qd PO, 250 mg bid
Glycoprotein IIb/IIIa Receptor Blockers	
abciximab (ReoPro) eptifibatide (Integrilin) tirofiban (Aggrastat)	PCI: IV, 0.25 mg/kg bolus administered 10–60 minutes prior to start of PCI followed by an infusion of 0.125 µg/kg/minute (max 10 µg/min) for 12 hours UA/NSTEMI: IV, 0.25 mg/kg bolus followed by an 18–24 hour infusion of 10 µg/minute concluding 1 hour after PCI IV, 180 µg/kg initial bolus over 1–2 minutes, then 2 µg/kg/minute for 24–72 hours IV, loading dose, 25 µg/kg administered over 5 minutes or less; maintenance infusion 0.15 µg/kg/minute continued for up to 18 hours

Inhibition of Platelet Function

56.6 Several drugs prolong bleeding time by interfering with the aggregation of platelets. Antiplatelet agents include ASA, ADP blockers, and glycoprotein IIb/IIIa receptor blockers.

Platelets are a central component of the hemostasis process, and too few platelets or diminished platelet function can profoundly increase bleeding time. The antiplatelet drugs are classified as such due to their inhibition of platelet function:

* ASA
* ADP receptor blockers
* Glycoprotein IIb/IIIa receptor blockers
* Drugs for intermittent claudication

ASA deserves special mention as an antiplatelet agent. Because it is available over the counter (OTC), clients may not consider ASA a potent medication; however, its anticoagulant activity is well documented. ASA acts by binding irreversibly to the enzyme cyclooxygenase in platelets. This binding inhibits the formation of thromboxane A_2, a powerful inducer of platelet aggregation. The anticoagulant effect of a single dose of ASA may persist for as long as a week. Concurrent use of ASA with other coagulation modifiers should be avoided unless medically approved. The primary uses of ASA are described in relation to several conditions in this textbook: pain relief in Chapter 23, prevention of strokes and MI in Chapter 50, and reduction of inflammation in Chapter 42.

The ADP receptor blockers comprise a small group of drugs that irreversibly alter receptors for ADP on the plasma membrane of platelets. ADP is unable to bind to the altered receptors and thus the platelets are unable to receive the chemical signals required for them to aggregate. Both ticlopidine and clopidogrel are given orally to prevent thrombi formation in clients who have experienced a recent thromboembolic event such as a stroke or MI. Ticlopidine can cause life-threatening neutropenia and agranulocytosis. Clopidogrel is much safer, having side effects comparable to those of ASA.

Glycoprotein IIb/IIIa inhibitors are relatively new additions to the treatment of thromboembolic disease. **Glycoprotein IIb/IIIa** is an enzyme necessary for platelet aggregation. Inhibition of this enzyme has the effect of preventing thrombus formation in clients who have

experienced a recent MI, stroke, or PTCA. Although these drugs are the most efficacious antiplatelet agents, they are very expensive. Another major disadvantage is that they can be given only by the IV route.

Intermittent claudication (IC) is a condition caused by insufficient blood flow to skeletal muscles in the lower limbs. Ischemia of skeletal muscles causes severe pain on walking, particularly in the calf muscles. Although some of the therapies for myocardial ischemia are beneficial in treating IC, two drugs are used *only* for this disorder. Pentoxifylline (Trental) has antiplatelet action and acts on RBCs to reduce their viscosity and increase their flexibility, thus allowing them to enter vessels that are partially occluded and reduce hypoxia and pain in the muscle. Cilostazol (Pletal) inhibits platelet aggregation and promotes vasodilation, which brings additional blood to ischemic muscles. Both drugs are given orally and show only modest improvement in IC symptoms. Exercise and therapeutic lifestyle changes are necessary for maximum benefit.

Nursing Considerations

The role of the nurse in antiplatelet therapy involves careful monitoring of the client's condition and providing education as it relates to the prescribed drug regimen. Drugs that affect platelet aggregation increase the risk for bleeding when the client sustains trauma or undergoes medical procedures or surgery. These drugs are sometimes given in addition to anticoagulants, which further increases bleeding risk. Injection or venipuncture wounds will require prolonged direct pressure to control bleeding. Observe for ecchymoses and monitor bleeding time following venipunctures. Bleeding that lasts more than 10 minutes may require special medical or nursing interventions, such as suturing or "sand-bagging" a large venipuncture site.

ASA may cause gastritis or GI bleeding due to inhibition of prostaglandins in the GI tract (prostaglandins increase bicarbonate and mucous layer production). ASA and ticlopidine may cause nausea and GI upset. Nursing interventions for ASA therapy can be found in Nursing Process Focus: Clients Receiving NSAID Therapy in Chapter 23.

Client education as it relates to antiplatelet agents should include goals; reasons for obtaining baseline data such as vital signs, diagnostic procedures, and laboratory tests; and possible side effects. The following are important points to include when teaching clients regarding antiplatelet agents:

* Avoid strenuous and hazardous activities that could result in bleeding injury.

- Do not take OTC products containing ASA, due to increased risk for bleeding, unless otherwise directed by the healthcare provider.
- If taking antiplatelet agents concurrently with anticoagulants, be aware that the risk for bleeding is greater.
- Report spontaneous nosebleeds, bleeding gums, excessive bruising, and other signs of bleeding to the healthcare provider.

PROTOTYPE DRUG | **Clopidogrel (Plavix)**

Actions and Uses: Clopidogrel prolongs bleeding time by inhibiting platelet aggregation. It is used to prevent thrombi formation in clients at risk for stroke or MI and to prevent postoperative DVT. Because the drug is expensive but has anticoagulant activity similar to ASA, it is usually prescribed for clients who are unable to tolerate ASA. It is given orally.

Pharmacokinetics: The onset of action is less than 24 hours. The active metabolite of clopidogrel, rather than the parent compound, is responsible for the antiplatelet action. Clopidogrel is a prodrug. The active metabolite is 94% protein bound and, once metabolized, it is excreted in urine and feces. Half-life of the active metabolite is 8 hours.

Administration Alerts:
- Do not crush or split tablets.
- Discontinue drug 1 week before surgery.
- Clopidogrel is pregnancy category B.

Adverse Effects and Interactions: Side effects are similar to ASA and include headache, dizziness, rash, pruritus, and cough. Upon discontinuation of therapy, the anticoagulant activity may persist for up to 5 days. Overdose with risk for hemorrhage may be treated with platelet infusions.

Numerous drug-drug and drug-herbal interactions may occur. Increased risk for bleeding may occur with concurrent use of NSAIDs, other anticoagulants, and natural products such as arnica, chamomile, clove, feverfew, ginger, ginkgo, garlic, ginseng, and others.

THROMBOLYTICS

Thrombolytics promote fibrinolysis, or clot destruction, by converting plasminogen to plasmin. The enzyme plasmin digests fibrin and breaks down fibrinogen, prothrombin, and other plasma proteins and clotting factors. Unlike the anticoagulants, thrombolytics actually bring about dissolution (lysis) of the insoluble fibrin within intravascular emboli and thrombi. Their therapeutic effect is proportional to the time frame in which they are administered—they are more effective when given as soon as possible after clot formation occurs, preferably within 4 hours.

NCLEX Success Tip

Garlic has anticoagulant properties and can potentially cause bleeding if enough has been taken too close to surgery. If the client reports garlic intake, the nurse should obtain more quantifiable details about the amounts and frequency of garlic intake. Garlic and ginger increase the bleeding time and must be avoided when a client is on anticoagulant therapy.

CONNECTIONS | **Natural Therapies**

◀ Garlic for Cardiovascular Health

Garlic (*Allium sativum*) is one of the best-studied herbs. Purported indications for garlic include arteriosclerosis, common cold, cough/bronchitis, high cholesterol, hypertension, and tendency to infection. It has been proven to be of value in only a few of these disorders.

Several different substances, known as alliaceous oils, have been isolated from garlic and shown to have pharmacological activity. Dosage forms include eating prepared garlic oil or the fresh bulbs from the plant.

Garlic has been shown to decrease the aggregation or "stickiness" of platelets, thus producing an anticoagulant effect. Platelet aggregation on roughened walls of arteries damaged by atherosclerosis commonly initiates the formation of blood clots that lead to heart attacks and strokes. Claims that garlic can reduce heart disease and the incidence of stroke may be related to this action. Clients who are taking anticoagulant medications should limit their intake of garlic to avoid bleeding complications.

Pharmacotherapy with Thrombolytics

56.7 Thrombolytics are used to dissolve existing intravascular clots in clients with MI and CVA.

It is often mistakenly believed that the purpose of anticoagulants such as heparin or warfarin is to dissolve pre-existing clots, but this is not the case. A totally different class of drugs is needed for this purpose. The thrombolytics, shown in Table 56.4, are administered quite differently than the anticoagulants and produce their effects by different mechanisms. Thrombolytics are prescribed for disorders in which an intravascular clot has already formed, such as acute myocardial infarction, pulmonary embolism, acute ischemic cerebrovascular accident, and deep vein thrombosis.

NCLEX Success Tips

Hematocrit, hemoglobin level, and platelet count are baseline laboratory data that must be checked before a client is started on tissue plasminogent activator or alteplase recombinant.

The thrombolytic agent alteplase (Activase) is given intravenously to break down (lyse) the clot blocking the coronary or cerebral artery. The drug is most effective when administered within the first 6 hours after onset of MI to salvage the client's myocardium and 3 to 4.5 hours after the onset of a nonhemorrhagic stroke.

Physicians initiate IV heparin therapy after administration of a thrombolytic agent and this is usually continued for 5 to 7 days.

The nurse needs to assess the client's neurological status while administering thrombolytic agent tPA. Altered sensorium or neurological changes may indicate intracranial bleeding for the client who has received tissue plasminogen activator or alteplase.

The nurse should carefully check for bleeding every 15 minutes during the first hour of therapy, every 15 to 30 minutes during the next 9 hours, and at least every 4 hours during the duration of therapy. Bleeding may occur from sites of invasive procedures or from body orifices. Arterial punctures are avoided due to the invasiveness of the procedure and the potential for excessive bleeding.

TABLE 56.4 Thrombolytics

Drug	Route and Adult Dose
Pr alteplase (Activase)	Acute ischemic stroke: recommended total dose: 0.9 mg/kg (max 90 mg); for clients less than 100 kg, load with 0.09 mg/kg (10% of 0.9 mg/kg dose) as an IV bolus over 1 minute, followed by 0.81 mg/kg (90% of 0.9 mg/kg dose) as a continuous infusion over 60 minutes STEMI: For clients over 67 kg, total dose is 100 mg over 1.5 hours administered as 15 mg IV bolus over 1 to 2 minutes followed by infusions of 50 mg over 30 minutes, then 35 mg over 1 hour (max 100 mg); for clients less than 67 kg, infuse 15 mg IV bolus over 1 to 2 minutes followed by infusions of 0.75 mg/kg (not to exceed 50 mg) over 30 minutes, then 0.5 mg/kg (not to exceed 35 mg) over 1 hour (max 100 mg)
reteplase (Retavase) (see Chapter 50, page 622, for the Prototype Drug box)	IV, 10 units over 2 minutes; repeat dose in 30 minutes
urokinase (Abbokinase)	IV, 4400–6000 units administered over several minutes to 12 hours

Some of the contraindications for tPA or alteplase recombinant therapy are current active internal bleeding, 3 hours or longer since the onset of symptoms of a stroke, and severe hypertension and a recent stroke (within 2 months). Age greater than 65 years is not a contraindication for the therapy.

If withdrawing blood for arterial blood gases (ABGs) is necessary, the nurse should use the radial artery to obtain blood gas samples because it is easier to maintain firm pressure there than on the femoral artery.

IM injections are contraindicated during thrombolytic therapy. The nurse should prevent physical manipulation of the client, which can cause bruising.

Thrombolytics are nonspecific; that is, they will dissolve whatever clots they encounter. Because clotting is a natural and desirable process to prevent excessive bleeding, thrombolytics have a narrow margin of safety between dissolving "abnormal" and "normal" clots. Vital signs must be monitored continuously and any signs of bleeding may call for discontinuation of therapy. Because these drugs are rapidly destroyed in the bloodstream, discontinuation normally results in immediate termination of thrombolytic activity. After the clot is successfully dissolved with the thrombolytic, anticoagulant therapy is generally initiated to prevent the reformation of clots.

Since the discovery of streptokinase, the first thrombolytic, there have been a number of ensuing generations of thrombolytics. The newer drugs such as tenecteplase (TNKase), or TNK tPA, are more fibrin specific and are reported to have fewer side effects than streptokinase. Tissue plasminogen activator, marketed as alteplase, has replaced urokinase as the drug of choice in clearing thrombosed central IV lines. Urokinase was removed from the market due to the possibility of viral contamination, because it is obtained from pooled human donors.

Nursing Considerations

The role of the nurse in thrombolytic therapy involves careful monitoring of the client's condition and providing education as it relates to the prescribed drug regimen. Thrombolytics are generally administered in the critical care or emergency department setting. Identify conditions that exclude the client from receiving thrombolytics, such as recent trauma, surgery, biopsy, arterial emboli, cerebral embolism, hemorrhage, thrombocytopenia, septic thrombophlebitis, or childbirth (within 10 days). Baseline coagulation tests (aPTT, bleeding time, PT, and/or INR) should be obtained prior to therapy. Baseline Hct, Hgb, and platelet counts should be obtained so that they may be compared to later values to assess for bleeding. Cerebral hemorrhage is a major concern; therefore, assess for changes in level of consciousness and check neurological status. When given for MI, observe for dysrhythmias that may occur as cardiac tissue perfusion is re-established. IM injections are contraindicated during thrombolytic therapy due to the risk for bleeding.

See Nursing Process Focus: Clients Receiving Thrombolytic Therapy for specific teaching points.

These drugs are often given in acute situations when time for client teaching may be limited and the client may be unable to focus on information due to the stress of the situation. This information can be discussed further when the client is ready.

NURSING PROCESS FOCUS

Clients Receiving Thrombolytic Therapy

Assessment	Potential Nursing Diagnoses/Identified Patterns
Prior to administration: • Obtain complete health history, including recent surgeries or trauma, allergies, drug history, and possible drug interactions. • Obtain vital signs; assess in the context of the client's baseline values. • Assess lab values: aPTT, PT, Hgb, Hct, platelet count.	• Adequate knowledge regarding drug therapy and adverse effects • Safety from injury (bleeding) related to adverse effects of thrombolytic therapy • Effective tissue perfusion with decrease in size of thrombus

Planning: Client Goals and Expected Outcomes

The client will:

• Experience dissolving of pre-existing blood clot(s) as evidenced by laboratory values ordered by the healthcare provider
• Demonstrate an understanding of the drug's action by accurately describing drug side effects and precautions

Implementation

Interventions (Rationales)	Client Education/Discharge Planning
• If necessary, start IV lines, arterial line, and Foley catheter prior to beginning therapy. (This decreases the risk for bleeding from those sites.) • Monitor vital signs every 15 minutes during first hour of infusion, then every 30 minutes during remainder of infusion. • Client should be moved as little as possible during the infusion. (This is done to prevent internal injury.) • If given for thrombotic CVA, monitor neurological status frequently. • Monitor cardiac response while medication is infusing. (Dysrhythmias may occur with reperfusion of myocardium.) • Monitor blood tests (Hct, Hgb, platelet counts) during and after therapy for indications of blood loss due to internal bleeding. (Client has increased risk for bleeding for 2 to 4 days post-infusion.)	• Instruct client about procedures and why they are necessary prior to beginning thrombolytic therapy Advise client: • Of the need for frequent taking of vital signs • That activity will be limited during infusion, and a pressure dressing may be needed to prevent any active bleeding • Advise client about assessments and why they are necessary • Advise client that cardiac rhythm will be monitored during therapy • Instruct client of increased risk for bleeding and need for activity restriction and frequent monitoring during this time

Evaluation of Outcome Criteria

Evaluate the effectiveness of drug therapy by confirming that client goals and expected outcomes have been met (see "Planning").

See Table 56.4 for a list of drugs to which these nursing actions apply.

PROTOTYPE DRUG	Alteplase (Activase)

Actions and Uses: Produced through recombinant DNA technology, alteplase is identical to the enzyme human tPA. Like other thrombolytics, the primary action of alteplase is to convert plasminogen to plasmin, which then dissolves fibrin clots. To achieve maximum effect, therapy should begin immediately after the onset of symptoms. Alteplase does not exhibit the allergic reactions seen with streptokinase. An unlabelled use is for restoration of patency of IV catheters.

Pharmacokinetics: The onset of action for IV alteplase is 5 to 10 minutes. It is rapidly metabolized by the liver. Initial half-life is 5 minutes.

Administration Alerts:

• Drug must be given within 6 hours of the onset of symptoms of MI and within 3 hours of thrombotic CVA for maximum effectiveness.

• Avoid IM injections, IV punctures, and arterial punctures during infusion to decrease the risk for bleeding.

• Alteplase is pregnancy category C.

Adverse Effects and Interactions: Thrombolytics such as alteplase are contraindicated in clients with active bleeding or with a history of recent trauma. Trauma may include, but is not limited to, physical injury, surgery, biopsies, or childbirth (within the 10-day postpartum period). The nurse must carefully monitor the client for signs of bleeding every 15 minutes for the first hour of therapy and every 30 minutes thereafter. Signs of bleeding such as spontaneous ecchymoses, hematomas, or epistaxis should be reported to the healthcare provider immediately.

Use with caution with herbal supplements, such as ginkgo, which may cause an increased thrombolytic effect.

ANTIFIBRINOLYTICS

Antifibrinolytics have an action opposite to that of anticoagulants: to shorten bleeding time. They are used to prevent excessive bleeding following surgery.

Pharmacotherapy with Antifibrinolytics

56.8 Antifibrinolytics are used to promote the formation of clots in clients with excessive bleeding from surgical sites.

The final class of coagulation modifiers, the antifibrinolytics, is a small group of drugs used to prevent and treat excessive bleeding from surgical sites. All of the antifibrinolytics have very specific indications for use and none are commonly prescribed. Although their mechanisms differ, all drugs in this class prevent fibrin from dissolving, thus enhancing the stability of the clot. Because of their ability to slow blood flow, they are sometimes classified as hemostatic agents.

Desmopressin differs from the others in being a hormone similar to vasopressin, a hormone naturally present in the body that promotes the renal conservation of water. Unlike the other antifibrinolytics, it has uses beyond hemostasis that include the control of excessive or nocturnal urination (enuresis). The antifibrinolytics are listed in Table 56.5.

Nursing Considerations

The role of the nurse in antifibrinolytic therapy involves careful monitoring of the client's condition and providing education as it relates to the prescribed drug regimen. Assess for clotting. Changes in peripheral pulses, paresthesias, positive Homans' sign, and prominence of superficial veins indicate clotting occurring in peripheral arterial or venous vasculature. Chest pain and shortness of breath may indicate pulmonary thrombus or embolus. Use is

TABLE 56.5 Antifibrinolytics

Drug	Route and Adult Dose
Pr aminocaproic acid (Amicar)	PO/IV, loading dose of 4–5 g during first hour, followed by 1 g/hour for 8 hours (or 1.25 g/hour using oral solution) or until bleeding is controlled (max 30 g/day)
aprotinin (Trasylol)	IV, 15 000 units as a test dose, then give 500 000 units during surgery
tranexamic acid (Cyklokapron)	PO, 1000–1500 mg q6h–q12h

contraindicated in clients with disseminated intravascular clotting and severe renal impairment.

Antifibrinolytics are administered intravenously. Monitor injection sites frequently for thrombophlebitis and extravasation. Antifibrinolytics may affect the muscles, causing wasting and weakness. Identify and report the presence of myopathy and myoglobinuria, manifesting as reddish-brown urine.

Client education as it relates to antifibrinolytic agents should include goals; reasons for obtaining baseline data such as vital signs, diagnostic procedures, and laboratory tests; and possible side effects. The following are important points to include when teaching clients regarding antifibrinolytic agents:

- Report renewed bleeding episodes.
- Avoid the use of ASA and OTC medications containing ASA.
- Report the following immediately: excessive bleeding following a medical or dental procedure, altered colour vision, decreased amounts of urine, and pain, numbness, or tingling in the extremities.

PROTOTYPE DRUG **Aminocaproic Acid (Amicar)**

Actions and Uses: Aminocaproic acid acts by inactivating plasminogen, the precursor of the enzyme plasmin that digests the fibrin clot. Aminocaproic acid is prescribed in situations where there is excessive bleeding due to clots being dissolved prematurely. During acute hemorrhages, it can be given IV to reduce bleeding in 1 to 2 hours. It is most commonly prescribed following surgery to reduce postoperative bleeding. The therapeutic serum level is 100 to 400 µg/mL.

Pharmacokinetics: The onset and duration of action and half-life for oral aminocaproic acid are unknown. It is widely distributed and excreted mostly unchanged by the kidneys.

Administration Alerts:

- This drug may cause hypotension and bradycardia when given IV. Assess vital signs frequently and place the client on cardiac monitor to assess for dysrhythmias.
- Aminocaproic acid is pregnancy category C.

Adverse Effects and Interactions: Since aminocaproic acid tends to stabilize clots, it should be used cautiously in clients with a history of thromboembolic disease. Side effects are generally mild.

Drug interactions include hypercoagulation with concurrent use of estrogens and oral contraceptives.

CHAPTER
56 Understanding the Chapter

Key Concepts Summary

The numbered key concepts provide a succinct summary of the important points from the corresponding numbered section within the chapter. If any of these points are not clear, refer to the numbered section within the chapter for review.

56.1 Hemostasis is a complex process involving multiple steps and a large number of enzymes and factors. The final product is a fibrin clot that stops blood loss.

56.2 Fibrinolysis, or removal of a blood clot, is an enzymatic process initiated by the release of tPA. Plasmin digests the fibrin strands, thus restoring circulation to the injured area.

56.3 Diseases of hemostasis include thromboembolic disorders caused by thrombi and emboli and bleeding disorders such as hemophilia and von Willebrand's disease.

56.4 The normal coagulation process can be modified by a number of different mechanisms, including inhibiting

clotting factors, dissolving fibrin, and influencing platelet function.

56.5 Anticoagulants prevent clot formation. The primary drugs in this category are heparin (parenteral) and warfarin (oral).

56.6 Several drugs prolong bleeding time by interfering with the aggregation of platelets. Antiplatelet agents include ASA, ADP blockers, and glycoprotein IIb/IIIa receptor blockers.

56.7 Thrombolytics are used to dissolve existing intravascular clots in clients with MI and CVA.

56.8 Antifibrinolytics are used to promote the formation of clots in clients with excessive bleeding from surgical sites.

Chapter 56 Scenario

You are attending an annual family reunion and begin talking to your favourite uncle, Lewis, about his recent hospitalization. Lewis Kinard, a 55-year-old man, was recently discharged from the hospital following an episode of atrial fibrillation. He returned home with instructions to take warfarin (Coumadin) 10 mg daily. He has many questions for you, his favourite relative.

Critical Thinking Questions

1. Why would someone with atrial fibrillation be prescribed Coumadin?

2. What special precautions should Lewis take while on this drug?

3. Are there any foods that he should avoid or limit in his diet?

4. What laboratory testing will be done to determine this drug's effectiveness?

See Answers to Critical Thinking Questions in Appendix B.

NCLEX Practice Questions

1 A client with deep venous thrombosis is being treated with a heparin infusion. The nurse will monitor for therapeutic effectiveness by noting which of the following?

  a. Activated partial thromboplastin time (aPTT)

  b. Prothrombin time (PT)

  c. Platelet counts

  d. International normalized ratio (INR)

2 Which of the following should the nurse include in the teaching plan for a client receiving subcutaneous heparin? Select all that apply.

  a. Inject medication into the deep, fatty layer of the abdomen.

  b. When brushing your teeth, use a soft toothbrush.

  c. Hold direct pressure on any puncture sites for 15 minutes.

  d. Use dental floss daily after brushing.

  e. Take a daily aspirin tablet, 325 mg, to prevent inflammation at the injection site.

3 A client who is taking warfarin (Coumadin) states, "I wake up every morning with arthritis pain and I always take aspirin or ibuprofen." The nurse's response would be based on which physiological concepts?

  a. Aspirin and ibuprofen (Motrin) will counteract the therapeutic effects of many anticoagulants.

  b. Anticoagulants will reduce the half-life of drugs such as aspirin and ibuprofen.

  c. Many substances, such as aspirin and ibuprofen, will increase the risk of bleeding.

  d. The combination of aspirin products with anticoagulants will worsen arthritis pain.

4 A client who is taking clopidogrel (Plavix) to prevent another stroke asks the nurse how the medication works. The nurse's response should be based on an understanding that Plavix

  a. Inhibits platelet aggregation to prevent clot formation.

  b. Activates antithrombin III and subsequently inhibits thrombin.

  c. Inhibits enzymes involved in the formation of vitamin K.

  d. Converts plasminogen to plasmin to dissolve fibrin clots.

5 A client will be receiving dabigatran (Pradaxa). Which of the following is true about this drug therapy? Select all that apply.

  a. Ginger, garlic, and green tea may increase the risk of bleeding.

  b. Vitamin B_{12} is used to augment this drug's response.

  c. Pradaxa is used for DVT.

  d. Activated partial thromboplastin time may be monitored to determine its effectiveness.

  e. This drug is contraindicated for clients with gastritis.

See Answers to NCLEX Practice Questions in Appendix A.

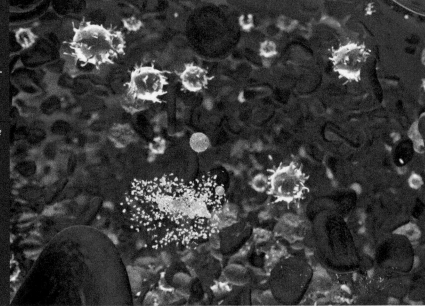

Orthoclick/Science Source

PROTOTYPE DRUGS

HEMATOPOIETIC GROWTH FACTORS	ANTIANEMIC AGENTS
Erythropoietin	Pr cyanocobala-
Pr *epoetin alfa*	min: vitamin B$_{12}$
(Epogen, Eprex)	Iron Salts
Colony-Stimulating	Pr *ferrous sulfate*
Factors	*(Fer-In-Sol)*
Pr *filgrastim*	
(Neupogen,	
Grastofil)	
Platelet Enhancers	

CHAPTER

57 Pharmacotherapy of Hematopoietic Disorders

LEARNING OUTCOMES

After reading this chapter, the student should be able to:

1. Identify drug classes used for treating hematopoietic disorders.
2. Explain the therapeutic action of each class of drug used for anemias and hematopoietic disorders in relation to the pathophysiology of the disorder.
3. Explain why hematopoietic agents are often administered to clients following chemotherapy or organ transplant.
4. Explain the role of intrinsic factor in the absorption of vitamin B$_{12}$.
5. Describe the metabolism, storage, and transfer of iron in the body.
6. Describe the nurse's role in the pharmacological management of clients who are receiving drugs for hematopoietic disorders.
7. For each of the drug classes listed in Prototype Drugs, identify a representative drug and explain its mechanism of action, therapeutic effects, and important adverse effects.
8. Describe and explain, based on pharmacological principles, the rationale for nursing assessment, planning, and interventions for clients with hematopoietic disorders.
9. Use the nursing process to care for clients who are receiving drug therapy for hematopoietic disorders.

CHAPTER OUTLINE

▶ Hematopoiesis

▶ Hematopoietic Growth Factors

  ▶ Pharmacotherapy with Erythropoietin

  ▶ Pharmacotherapy with Colony-Stimulating Factors

  ▶ Pharmacotherapy with Platelet Enhancers

▶ Anemias

  ▶ Classification of Anemias

▶ Antianemic Agents

  ▶ Pharmacotherapy with Vitamin B$_{12}$ and Folic Acid

▶ Iron

  ▶ Pharmacotherapy with Iron

The blood serves all other cells in the body and is the only fluid tissue. Because of its diverse functions, diseases that affect blood constituents have widespread effects on the body. Correspondingly, drugs for treating blood disorders will affect cells in many different tissues.

Hematopoiesis

57.1 Hematopoiesis is the process of erythrocyte production that begins with primitive stem cells in the bone marrow. Homeostatic control of erythropoiesis is through hematopoietic growth factors.

Blood is a highly dynamic tissue; more than 200 billion new blood cells are formed every day. The process of blood cell formation is called **hematopoiesis** or hemopoiesis. Hematopoiesis occurs primarily in red bone marrow and requires B vitamins, vitamin C, copper, iron, and other nutrients.

Hematopoiesis is responsive to the demands of the body. For example, the production of white blood cells (WBCs) can increase to 10 times the normal number in response to infection. The number of red blood cells (RBCs) can also increase as much as 5 times in response to anemia or hypoxia. Homeostatic control of hematopoiesis is influenced by a number of hormones and growth factors, which allow for points of pharmacological intervention. The process of hematopoiesis is illustrated in Figure 57.1.

The process of hematopoiesis begins with a hematopoietic **stem cell**, which is capable of maturing into any type of blood cell. The specific path taken by the stem cell, whether it becomes an erythrocyte, leukocyte, or platelet, depends on the internal needs of the body. Regulation of hematopoiesis occurs through messages from certain hormones, such as erythropoietin; chemicals secreted by leukocytes, known as colony-stimulating factors; and other circulating substances. Through recombinant DNA technology, some of these growth agents are now available in sufficient quantity to be used as medications.

The pharmacological management of hematopoietic disorders often involves simply replacing a deficient substance that is essential to hematopoiesis. In some cases, the drug is identical, or very closely resembles, the deficient endogenous factor. For example, the drug epoetin alfa (Epogen, Eprex) is identical to the natural hormone erythropoietin and stimulates the production of RBCs in the same manner. Administration of antianemic medications such as ferrous sulfate or vitamin B_{12} supplies essential factors that may be deficient.

Some of the hematopoietic drugs have become important adjunct medications in the pharmacotherapy of malignancies.

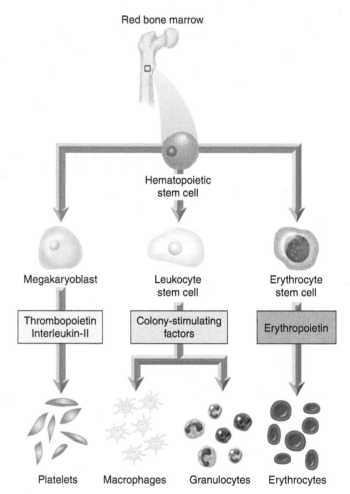

Figure 57.1 Hematopoiesis.

Antineoplastic drugs often are toxic to bone marrow and cause neutropenia, a reduced number of WBCs. Neutropenia is a primary cause of client morbidity and mortality in the treatment of cancer. Hematopoietic drugs can be used to boost the WBC counts in these clients.

Natural hormones that regulate some aspect of blood formation are called hematopoietic growth factors.

HEMATOPOIETIC GROWTH FACTORS

Natural hormones that promote some aspect of blood formation are called hematopoietic growth factors. Several growth factors, listed in Table 57.1, are used pharmacologically to stimulate erythrocyte, leukocyte, or platelet production.

TABLE 57.1 Hematopoietic Growth Factors

Drug	Route and Adult Dose
Pr epoetin alfa (Epogen, Eprex): erythropoietin	Individualize dosing and use the lowest dose necessary to reduce the risk for RBC transfusions; consider initiating treatment when hemoglobin is < 10 g/dL Subcutaneous/intravenous (SC/IV), start with 50–100 units/kg three times a week
darbepoetin alfa (Aranesp)	Consider initiating treatment when hemoglobin is < 10g/dL; use only if rate of hemoglobin decline would likely result in RBC transfusion and desire is to reduce risk SC/IV, start with 0.45 µg/kg once per week or 0.75 µg/kg once every 2 weeks
Colony-Stimulating Factors	
Pr filgrastim (Neupogen, Grastofil): G-CSF	SC/IV, 5 µg/kg/day; doses may be increased by 5 µg/kg (for each chemotherapy cycle) according to the duration and severity of the neutropenia; continue for up to 14 days until the absolute neutrophil count (ANC) reaches 10 000/mm³ IV infusion, 10 µg/kg/day (administer more than 24 hours after chemotherapy and more than 24 hours after bone marrow infusion); adjust the dose according to the duration and severity of neutropenia
sargramostim (Leukine): GM-CSF	IV, 250 µg/m²/day infused over 2 hours for 21 days, begin 2–4 hours after bone marrow transfusion and not less than 24 hours after last dose of chemotherapy or 12 hours after last radiation therapy
Platelet Enhancers	
oprelvekin (Neumega)	SC, 50 µg/kg once daily starting 6–24 hours after completing chemotherapy

NCLEX Success Tips

Chronic renal failure decreases the production of erythropoietin by the kidneys and leads to a subnormal hemoglobin (Hgb) level. An effective pharmacological treatment for this is epoetin alfa, a recombinant erythropoietin. Because the client's anemia is caused by a deficiency of erythropoietin and not a deficiency of iron, administering ferrous sulfate would be ineffective.

The hematocrit, not the hemoglobin level, is used for monitoring the effectiveness of erythropoietin therapy. Erythropoietin is given to decrease the need for blood transfusions by stimulating RBC production.

Erythropoietin must be given through a single IV line without other medications to avoid adverse interactions. When initiating IV erythropoietin therapy, the nurse should monitor the hematocrit level so that it rises no more than four points in any 2-week period. In addition, the initial doses of erythropoietin are adjusted according to the client's changes in blood pressure. The nurse should teach the client to avoid driving and performing hazardous activity during the initial treatment due to possible dizziness and headaches secondary to the adverse effect of hypertension.

The vial of erythropoietin should not be shaken because it may be biologically inactive. The solution should not be used if it is discoloured. Any remaining erythropoietin should be discarded because the vial does not contain preservatives.

Chemotherapy causes myelosuppression with a decrease in RBCs, WBCs, and platelets. An absolute neutrophil count (ANC) of 500 to 1000/mm³ (0.5 to 1 × 10⁹/L) indicates a moderate risk of infection; less than 500/mm³ (0.5 × 10⁹/L) indicates severe neutropenia and a high risk for infection. Precautions to protect the client from life-threatening infections may be instituted when ANC is less than 1000/mm³ (1 × 10⁹/L). Granulocyte colony-stimulating factors or granulocyte macrophage colony-stimulating factors are useful for treating neutropenia.

Oprelvekin (Neumega) is used for thrombocytopenia, which would be assessed as bruising and fatigue.

Pharmacotherapy with Erythropoietin

57.2 Erythropoietin is a hormone that stimulates the production of red blood cells and is used, as epoetin alfa, to treat specific anemias.

The process of RBC formation, or erythropoiesis, is primarily regulated by the hormone **erythropoietin**. Secreted by the kidney, erythropoietin travels to the bone marrow, where it interacts with receptors on hematopoietic stem cells to increase erythrocyte production. The primary signal for the increased secretion of erythropoietin is a reduction in oxygen reaching the kidney. Serum levels of erythropoietin may increase as much as 1000-fold in response to severe hypoxia. Hemorrhage, chronic obstructive pulmonary disease, anemia, or high altitude may cause this hypoxia. Human erythropoietin is marketed as epoetin alfa.

Darbepoetin alfa (Aranesp) is closely related to erythropoietin (epoetin alfa). It has the same pharmacological action, efficacy, and safety profile as these other agents; however, it has an extended duration of action that allows it to be administered once weekly. Darbepoetin alfa is only approved for the treatment of anemia associated with chronic renal failure.

Nursing Considerations

The role of the nurse in hematopoietic growth factor therapy involves careful monitoring of the client's condition and providing education as it relates to the prescribed drug regimen. Since its development, epoetin alfa has significantly improved the quality of life of clients with cancer, acquired immune deficiency syndrome (AIDS), and chronic renal failure. Although this drug does not cure the primary disease condition, it helps to reduce the anemia that dramatically affects the client's ability to perform daily activities. Assess for food or drug allergies because epoetin alfa is contraindicated in individuals who are hypersensitive to many protein-based products. Also assess for a history of uncontrolled hypertension, as the drug can raise blood pressure to dangerous levels. Baseline laboratory tests, especially a complete blood count (CBC), and vital signs should be obtained. Hct and Hgb levels provide a reference for evaluating the drug's effectiveness. Epoetin alfa should be used with caution in pregnant and lactating clients (pregnancy category C). Premature infants are especially sensitive to benzyl alcohol, which may be used as a preservative in multidose vials; they must be given the preservative-free formulation to prevent "fetal gasping" syndrome.

Because this drug increases the risk for thromboembolic disease, the client should be monitored for early signs of stroke or heart attack. Clients on dialysis are at higher risk for transient ischemic attack (TIA), stroke, and myocardial infarction (MI) and may need increased doses of heparin while receiving epoetin alfa. Monitor for side effects such as nausea and vomiting, constipation, injection site reaction, and headache.

See Nursing Process Focus: Clients Receiving Epoetin Alfa (Epogen, Eprex) for specific teaching points.

NURSING PROCESS FOCUS

Clients Receiving Epoetin Alfa (Epogen, Eprex)

Assessment	Potential Nursing Diagnoses/Identified Patterns
Prior to administration: • Obtain complete health history, including allergies, drug history, and possible drug reactions. • Assess reason for drug administration, such as presence or history of anemia secondary to chronic renal failure, malignancy, chemotherapy, autologous blood donation, and treatment with zidovudine in clients infected with human immunodeficiency virus (HIV). • Assess vital signs, especially blood pressure. • Assess CBC, specifically Hct and Hgb levels, to establish baseline values. • Assess activity tolerance and dietary patterns.	• Adequate knowledge regarding drug therapy and adverse effects • Safety from physical injury such as falls related to anemia symptoms (weakness, dizziness, syncope) • Effective tissue perfusion • Reduced physical activity related to RBC deficiency

Planning: Client Goals and Expected Outcomes

The client will:

• Exhibit an increase in Hct level and improvement in anemia-related symptoms
• Immediately report effects such as severe headache, chest pain, confusion, numbness, or loss of movement in an extremity
• Demonstrate an understanding of drug therapy by accurately describing the drug's intended effects, side effects, and precautions

Implementation

Interventions (Rationales)	Client Education/Discharge Planning
• Monitor vital signs, especially blood pressure. (The rate of hypertension is directly related to the rate of rise of the hematocrit. Clients who have existing hypertension are at higher risk for stroke and seizures. Hypertension is also much more likely in clients with chronic renal failure.) • Monitor for side effects, especially symptoms of neurological or cardiovascular events. • Monitor client's ability to self-administer medication. • Monitor laboratory values such as Hct and Hgb to evaluate effectiveness of treatment. (Increases in Hct and Hgb values indicate increased RBC production.) • Monitor client for signs of seizure activity. (Seizures can result from a rapid rise in Hct—especially during first 90 days of treatment.) • Monitor client for signs of thrombus, such as swelling, warmth, and pain in an extremity. (As Hct rises, there is an increased chance of thrombus formation, particularly for clients with chronic renal failure.) • Monitor dietary intake. Ensure adequate intake of all essential nutrients. (Response to this medication is minimal if blood levels of iron, folic acid, and vitamin B_{12} are deficient.)	Instruct client: • On the importance of periodic blood pressure monitoring and in the proper use of home blood pressure monitoring equipment • On "reportable" blood pressure ranges ("Call healthcare provider when blood pressure is greater than... ") • Instruct client to report side effects such as nausea, vomiting, constipation, redness or pain at injection site, confusion, numbness, chest pain, and difficulty breathing Instruct client: • In the technique for SC injection if client is to self-administer the medication • In proper disposal of needles and syringes Instruct client: • Of the need for initial and continuing laboratory blood monitoring • To keep all laboratory appointments • Of latest Hct value so that physical activities may be adjusted accordingly • Instruct client to not drive or perform hazardous activities until the effects of the drug are known Instruct client: • To report any increase in size, pain, and/or warmth in an extremity • On signs and symptoms of blood clots • Not to rub or massage calves and to report leg discomfort Instruct client to: • Maintain adequate dietary intake of essential vitamins and nutrients • Continue to follow necessary dietary restrictions if receiving renal dialysis

Evaluation of Outcome Criteria

Evaluate the effectiveness of drug therapy by confirming that client goals and expected outcomes have been met (see "Planning").

<table>
<tr><td>PROTOTYPE DRUG</td><td>Epoetin Alfa (Epogen, Eprex)</td></tr>
</table>

Actions and Uses: Epoetin alfa is made through recombinant DNA technology and is functionally identical to human erythropoietin. Because of its ability to stimulate erythropoiesis, epoetin alfa is effective in treating specific disorders caused by a deficiency in RBC formation. Clients with chronic renal failure often cannot secrete enough endogenous erythropoietin and thus will benefit from epoetin administration. Epoetin is sometimes given to clients who are undergoing cancer chemotherapy, to counteract the anemia caused by antineoplastic agents. It is occasionally prescribed for clients prior to blood transfusions or surgery and to treat anemia in HIV-infected clients.

Pharmacokinetics: Epoetin alfa is administered SC or IV. It is usually administered three times per week until a therapeutic response is achieved. Dose is adjusted according to Hct (target is 30% to 36%). Distribution, metabolism, and excretion are unknown. Half-life is 4 to 13 hours.

Administration Alerts:

- The SC route is generally preferred over IV since lower doses are needed and absorption is slower.
- Premature infants are especially sensitive to benzyl alcohol, which may be used as a preservative in multidose vials; therefore, they must be given the preservative-free formulation to prevent "fetal gasping" syndrome.
- Do not shake vial because this may deactivate the drug. Visibly inspect solution for particulate matter.
- Epoetin alfa is pregnancy category C.

Adverse Effects and Interactions: The most common adverse effect of epoetin alfa is hypertension, which may occur in as many as 30% of clients receiving the drug. Blood pressure should be monitored during therapy, and an antihypertensive drug may be indicated. The risk for thromboembolic events is increased. Clients who are on dialysis may require increased doses of heparin. TIAs, heart attacks, and strokes have occurred in clients with chronic renal failure who are on dialysis and also being treated with epoetin alfa. The effectiveness of epoetin alfa will be greatly reduced in clients with iron deficiency or other vitamin depleted states since erythropoiesis cannot be enhanced without these vital nutrients. There are no clinically significant drug interactions with epoetin alfa.

Pharmacotherapy with Colony-Stimulating Factors

57.3 Colony-stimulating factors (CSFs) are growth factors that stimulate the production of leukocytes and are used following chemotherapy or organ transplants.

Control of WBC production, or leukopoiesis, is more complicated than erythropoiesis due to the many different types of leukocytes

in the blood. The two basic categories of growth factors are interleukins and **colony-stimulating factors (CSFs)**. Because the primary action of the interleukins is to modulate the immune system rather than enhance leukopoiesis, they are presented in Chapter 40. One interleukin stimulates the production of platelets and is discussed in Section 57.4.

The leukopoietic growth factors are active at very low concentrations. It is believed that each stem cell stimulated by these growth factors is capable of producing as many as 1000 mature leukocytes. The growth factors not only increase the production of leukocytes, but also activate existing WBCs. Examples of enhanced functions include increased migration of leukocytes to antigens, increased antibody toxicity, and increased phagocytosis.

CSFs are named according to the types of blood cells they stimulate. For example, granulocyte colony-stimulating factor (G-CSF) increases the production of neutrophils, the most common type of granulocyte. Granulocyte-macrophage colony-stimulating factor (GM-CSF) stimulates both neutrophil and macrophage production. Made through recombinant DNA technology, the two CSFs available as medications are filgrastim (Neupogen, Grastofil) and sargramostim (Leukine). Filgrastim is primarily used for chronic neutropenia or neutropenia secondary to chemotherapy. Sargramostim is used specifically to treat non-Hodgkin's lymphoma, acute lymphoblastic leukemia, and clients with Hodgkin's disease who are having autologous bone marrow transplantation.

Nursing Considerations

The role of the nurse in CSF therapy involves careful monitoring of the client's condition and providing education as it relates to the prescribed drug regimen. Prior to administration of filgrastim, assess for hypersensitivity to certain foreign proteins, specifically those in *Escherichia coli*. Due to its structural components, the drug is contraindicated in clients with this type of hypersensitivity. Obtain a health history, especially checking for myeloid cancers such as leukemia because filgrastim may stimulate proliferation of these malignant cells. This drug should not be administered simultaneously with chemotherapy. A baseline CBC with differential and platelet count should be obtained for baseline data to evaluate drug effectiveness. Usage of filgrastim may cause dysrhythmias and tachycardia; therefore, a thorough initial and ongoing cardiac assessment should be performed throughout the treatment regimen.

Assess for both hypertension and skeletal pain, which are adverse effects of filgrastim therapy. The electrocardiogram (ECG) readings should be monitored for abnormal ST segment depression, which is also a side effect of the drug. See Nursing Process Focus: Clients Receiving Filgrastim for further details on this drug.

A CBC should be obtained prior to administration of sargramostim because this drug is contraindicated when excessive leukemic myeloid blasts are present in blood or bone marrow. Obtain a health history, specifically for any known hypersensitivity to GM-CSF or yeast products. Sargramostim should be used cautiously in clients with cardiac disease such as dysrhythmias or heart failure (HF) because this agent may cause supraventricular dysrhythmias. This is usually a temporary side effect that disappears when the drug is discontinued. It should also be used with caution in clients with kidney and liver impairment.

It is often difficult to assess the adverse effects of CSF medications because the symptoms may also be attributed to the chemotherapy or the disease itself. A serious side effect of sargramostim is respiratory distress that occurs during the IV infusion, which develops because granulocytes become trapped in the pulmonary circulation. If this occurs, it is recommended that the nurse decrease the infusion rate. Occasionally, clients will develop a syndrome that occurs the first time the drug is administered. The client develops difficulty breathing, tachycardia, low blood pressure, and lightheadedness. This also appears to be related to the trapping of granulocytes in the pulmonary circulation. If these symptoms occur during the first infusion, restart the infusion at half the rate after all symptoms have resolved.

Client education as it relates to CSFs should include goals, reasons for obtaining baseline data such as vital signs, and possible side effects. Include the following general points when teaching clients regarding CSFs:

- Wash hands frequently and avoid people with infections such as colds and flu.
- Immediately report symptoms such as chest pain or palpitations, respiratory difficulty, nausea, vomiting, fever, chills, and malaise.
- Keep all physician and laboratory appointments.

See Nursing Process Focus: Clients Receiving Filgrastim for specific teaching points.

| PROTOTYPE DRUG | Filgrastim (Neupogen, Grastofil) |

Actions and Uses: Filgrastim is human G-CSF produced through recombinant DNA technology. Its two primary actions are to increase neutrophil production in the bone marrow and to enhance the phagocytic and cytotoxic functions of existing neutrophils. This is particularly important for clients with neutropenia, which is a reduction in circulating neutrophils that often results in severe bacterial and fungal infections. Administration of filgrastim will shorten the length of neutropenia in cancer clients whose bone marrow has been suppressed by antineoplastic agents or in clients following organ transplants. It may also be used in clients with AIDS-related immunosuppression.

Pharmacokinetics: Filgrastim is administered daily as a single SC injection or continuously as a slow SC or IV infusion. Dose is adjusted according to absolute neutrophil count (target is sustained count of $1000/mm^3$). Distribution, metabolism, and excretion are unknown. Half-life is 3.5 hours.

Administration Alerts:
- Do not administer within 24 hours before or after chemotherapy with cytotoxic agents, as this will greatly decrease the effectiveness of filgrastim.
- Filgrastim is pregnancy category C.

Adverse Effects and Interactions: Bone pain is a common side effect of high-dose filgrastim therapy. A small percentage of clients may develop an allergic reaction. Frequent laboratory tests are conducted to ensure that excessive numbers of neutrophils, or leukocytosis, does not occur. Because the antineoplastic drugs and CSFs produce opposite effects, filgrastim is not administered until at least 24 hours after a chemotherapy session.

NURSING PROCESS FOCUS

Clients Receiving Filgrastim (Neupogen, Grastofil)

Assessment	Potential Nursing Diagnoses/Identified Patterns
Prior to administration: • Obtain complete health history, including allergies, drug history, and possible drug reactions. • Assess reason for drug administration, such as presence or history of severe bacterial or fungal infections, chemotherapy-induced neutropenia, or AIDS-related immunosuppression. • Assess vital signs. • Assess CBC, specifically WBC with differential, to establish baseline values.	• Adequate knowledge regarding drug therapy and adverse effects • Safety from injury related to side effects of drug therapy • Risk for infection related to impaired immune defence (low WBCs)

Planning: Client Goals and Expected Outcomes

The client will:

- Exhibit an increase in leukocyte levels and experience a decrease in the incidence of infection
- Demonstrate an understanding of drug therapy by accurately describing drug's intended effects, side effects, and precautions
- Immediately report significant adverse effects from the medication such as nausea, vomiting, fever, chills, malaise, and skeletal pain, and allergic-type responses such as rash, urticaria, wheezing, and dyspnea

Implementation	
Interventions (Rationales)	**Client Education/Discharge Planning**
• Monitor vital signs. (MI and dysrhythmias have occurred in a small number of clients because the drug has been known to cause abnormal ST segment depression.) • Monitor for signs and symptoms of infection. • Limit the client's exposure to pathogenic microorganisms. (Clients are more susceptible to infection until WBC response is achieved.) • Monitor CBC with differential until WBC count is at an acceptable level. • Monitor hepatic status during pharmacotherapy. (Filgrastim may cause an elevation in liver enzymes.) • Assess for bone pain. (Drug works by stimulating bone marrow cells.) • Monitor for significant side effects and allergic-type reactions. (Client may be hypersensitive to *E. coli*.) • Monitor client's ability to self-administer medication.	• Instruct client to report any chest pain or palpitations Instruct the client to: • Wash hands frequently • Avoid crowds and people with colds, flu, and infections • Cook all foods completely and thoroughly • Clean surfaces touched by raw foods • Avoid fresh fruits, vegetables, and plants until WBC level is within normal limits • Limit exposure to children and animals • Increase fluid intake and empty bladder frequently • Cough and deep breathe several times per day • Inform clients of WBC status during the course of the treatment so they may take necessary precautions to avoid infection Instruct client: • Of the need for initial and continuing laboratory blood monitoring • To keep all laboratory appointments • Instruct client to report any pain not relieved by over-the-counter (OTC) analgesics Instruct client to immediately report: • Side effects such as nausea, vomiting, fever, chills, and malaise • Symptoms of allergic reaction such as rash, urticaria, wheezing, and dyspnea Instruct client about: • Self-injection technique • Proper disposal of needles and syringes
Evaluation of Outcome Criteria	
Evaluate the effectiveness of drug therapy by confirming that client goals and expected outcomes have been met (see "Planning").	

Pharmacotherapy with Platelet Enhancers

57.4 Platelet enhancers stimulate the activity of megakaryocytes and thrombopoietin and increase the production of platelets.

The production of platelets, or thrombocytopoiesis, begins when megakaryocytes in the bone marrow start shedding membrane-bound packets. These packets enter the bloodstream and become platelets. A single megakaryocyte can produce thousands of platelets.

Megakaryocyte activity is controlled by the hormone **thrombopoietin**, which is produced by the kidneys. Thrombopoietin may be used to increase platelets. Because it is a new drug, clients who are taking thrombopoietin require careful monitoring for adverse effects.

Oprelvekin is a drug produced through recombinant DNA technology that stimulates the production of megakaryocytes and thrombopoietin. Although it differs slightly from endogenous interleukin 11, the two are considered functionally equivalent.

Oprelvekin is used to stimulate the production of platelets in clients who are at risk for thrombocytopenia caused by cancer chemotherapy. The onset of action is 5 to 9 days, and platelet counts will remain elevated for about 7 days after the last dose. Oprelvekin is only given by the SC route.

Nursing Considerations

The role of the nurse in platelet enhancer therapy involves careful monitoring of the client's condition and providing education as it relates to the prescribed drug regimen. Oprelvekin should not be given to clients with hypersensitivity to this drug. It is used with caution in clients with cardiac disease, especially HF, dysrhythmias, and left ventricular dysfunction, since fluid retention is a common side effect.

As with the CSFs, oprelvekin should not be used within 24 hours of chemotherapy because the cytotoxic effects of the antineoplastic agents decrease the effectiveness of the drug. Adverse effects are related to fluid retention and may be severe, including pleural effusion and papilledema. Clients should be advised to report edema to the nurse and to avoid activities that could cause bleeding until the platelet count has returned to normal.

Oprelvekin should be withheld for 12 hours before or after radiation therapy because the breakdown of cells after radiation will decrease the effectiveness of the medication. Monitor clients with a history of edema, as this drug aggravates fluid retention and may cause pleural effusion or congestive heart failure.

See Nursing Process Focus: Clients Receiving Filgrastim for additional teaching points.

ANEMIAS

Anemia is a condition in which RBCs have a diminished capacity to carry oxygen. Although there are many different causes of anemia, they fall into one of the following categories:

- Blood loss due to hemorrhage
- Excessive erythrocyte destruction
- Diminished erythrocyte synthesis due to a deficiency in a substance needed for erythropoiesis

Classification of Anemias

57.5 Anemias are disorders in which blood has a reduced capacity to carry oxygen, due to hemorrhage, excessive erythrocyte destruction, or insufficient erythrocyte synthesis.

Classification of anemia is generally based on a description of erythrocyte size and colour. Size is described as normal (normocytic), small (microcytic), or large (macrocytic). Colour is based on the amount of hemoglobin present and is described as normal red (normochromic) or light red (hypochromic). This classification is shown in Table 57.2.

Each type of anemia has specific characteristics, but all have common signs and symptoms. The client often exhibits pallor, which is a paleness of the skin and mucous membranes due to hemoglobin deficiency. Decreased exercise tolerance, fatigue, and lethargy occur because of insufficient oxygen reaching the muscles. Dizziness and fainting are common because the brain is not receiving enough oxygen to function properly. The cardiovascular system attempts to compensate for the oxygen depletion by increasing respiration rate and heart rate. Long-standing or severe disease can result in HF.

ANTIANEMIC AGENTS

Several vitamins and minerals are given to enhance the oxygen-carrying capacity of blood in clients with certain anemias. The two most common agents are cyanocobalamin, a purified form of vitamin B_{12}, and ferrous sulfate (Fer-In-Sol), an iron supplement. These agents are listed in Table 57.3.

Pharmacotherapy with Vitamin B_{12} and Folic Acid

57.6 Deficiencies in either vitamin B_{12} or folic acid can lead to pernicious anemia. Treatment with cyanocobalamin or folate can reverse these anemias in many clients.

Vitamin B_{12} and folic acid are dietary nutrients essential for rapidly dividing cells. Because erythropoiesis is occurring at a continuously high rate throughout the lifespan, deficiencies in these nutrients often manifest as anemias.

Vitamin B_{12} is an essential component of two coenzymes that are required for normal cell growth and replication. Vitamin B_{12} is not synthesized by either plants or animals; only bacteria serve this function. Because only miniscule amounts of vitamin B_{12} are required (3 μg/day), deficiency of this vitamin is usually not due to insufficient dietary intake. Instead, the most common cause of vitamin B_{12} deficiency is lack of **intrinsic factor**, a protein secreted

TABLE 57.3 Antianemic Agents

Drug	Route and Adult Dose
Pr cyanocobalamin: vitamin B_{12}	Orally (PO), 1000 μg/day; intramuscular (IM)/deep SC, 100–1000 μg monthly (or if treating active anemia may give 100 μg/day for 6–7 days; if client improves, administer same dose on alternate days for 7 doses, then every 3–4 days for 2–3 weeks, then maintenance of 100-1000 μg/month)
folic acid	PO/IM/SC/IV, 0.4–1.0 mg/day
Iron Salts	
ferrous fumarate (Palafer, Eurofer) ferrous gluconate **Pr** ferrous sulfate (Fer-In-Sol)	(Dosing is the same for all three types of iron; the difference between the three types is the amount of elemental iron in each product) PO, 100–200 mg/day in 2-3 divided doses; to avoid GI upset, start with a single daily dose and increase by 1 tablet/day each week or as tolerated until desired daily dose is achieved

TABLE 57.2 Classification of Anemia

Morphology	Description	Examples
Normocytic-normochromic	Loss of normal erythroblasts or mature erythrocytes	Aplastic anemia
		Hemorrhagic anemia
		Sickle cell anemia
		Hemolytic anemia
Macrocytic-normochromic	Large, abnormally shaped erythrocytes with normal hemoglobin	Pernicious anemia Folate deficiency anemia
Microcytic-hypochromic	Small, abnormally shaped erythrocytes with diminished haemoglobin	Iron-deficiency anemia Thalassemia

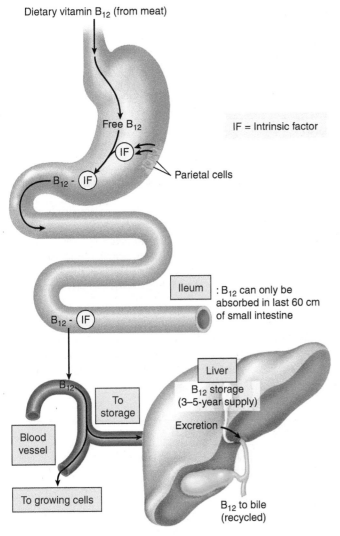

Dietary vitamin B₁₂ (from meat)

Free B₁₂

IF = Intrinsic factor

B₁₂ - IF

Parietal cells

Ileum : B₁₂ can only be absorbed in last 60 cm of small intestine

B₁₂ - IF

Liver
B₁₂ storage (3–5-year supply)

B₁₂

To storage

Excretion

Blood vessel

To growing cells

B₁₂ to bile (recycled)

Figure 57.2 Metabolism of vitamin B₁₂.

by stomach cells. Intrinsic factor is required for vitamin B₁₂ to be absorbed from the intestine. Figure 57.2 illustrates the metabolism of vitamin B₁₂. Inflammatory diseases of the stomach or surgical removal of the stomach may result in deficiency of intrinsic factor. Inflammatory diseases of the small intestine that affect food and nutrient absorption may also cause vitamin B₁₂ deficiency.

The most profound consequence of B₁₂ deficiency is a condition called **pernicious**, or **megaloblastic**, **anemia** that affects both the hematological and the nervous systems. The stem cells produce abnormally large erythrocytes that do not fully mature. RBCs are most affected, though lack of maturation of all blood cell types may occur in severe disease. Nervous system symptoms may include memory loss, confusion, unsteadiness, tingling or numbness in the limbs, delusions, mood disturbances, and even hallucinations in severe deficiencies. Permanent nervous system damage may result if the disease remains untreated.

Folic acid, or **folate**, is another vitamin essential for normal DNA and RNA synthesis. Like B₁₂ deficiency, insufficient folic acid can manifest itself as anemia. In fact, the metabolism of vitamin B₁₂ and folic acid is intricately linked: a B₁₂ deficiency will create a lack of activated folic acid.

Unlike vitamin B₁₂, folic acid does not require intrinsic factor for intestinal absorption, and the most common cause of folate deficiency is insufficient dietary intake. This is most commonly observed in chronic alcoholism, although other absorption diseases of the small intestine can result in folate anemia. Hematopoietic signs of folate deficiency are the same as those for B₁₂ deficiency; however, no neurological signs are present. Folate deficiency during pregnancy has been linked to neural birth defects such as spina bifida; therefore, advise pregnant clients and those planning to become pregnant to take adequate amounts of this vitamin. Treatment is often accomplished by increasing the dietary intake of folic acid through fresh green vegetables and wheat products. In cases when adequate dietary intake cannot be achieved, therapy with folate sodium or folic acid is warranted. Folic acid is discussed further in Chapter 61.

Nursing Considerations

The role of the nurse in antianemic therapy involves careful monitoring of the client's condition and providing education as it relates to the prescribed drug regimen. Although most vitamin B₁₂ deficiencies are caused by a lack of intrinsic factor, investigate the possibility of inadequate dietary intake of the vitamin, particularly in vegans. Prior to administration, assess for other causes of anemia, including gastrointestinal (GI) dysfunction, GI surgery, tapeworm infestation, and gluten enteropathy.

Prior to and at regular intervals during treatment, a CBC is needed to evaluate the effectiveness of vitamin B₁₂ therapy. This drug is not an effective treatment for iron-deficiency anemias.

Potassium levels should be monitored during pharmacotherapy because hypokalemia is a possible side effect of this drug. Assess clients for additional side effects such as itching, rash, or flushing. Clients who are taking this drug may develop pulmonary edema and HF, so cardiovascular status must be monitored.

See Nursing Process Focus: Clients Receiving Cyanocobalamin: Vitamin B₁₂ for specific teaching points.

NURSING PROCESS FOCUS

Clients Receiving Cyanocobalamin: Vitamin B₁₂

Assessment	Potential Nursing Diagnoses/Identified Patterns
Prior to administration: • Obtain complete health history, including allergies, drug history, and possible drug reactions. • Assess vital signs. • Assess for other causes of anemia.	• Adequate knowledge regarding drug therapy and adverse effects • Safety from physical injury such as falls related to anemia symptoms (weakness, dizziness, syncope) • Effective tissue perfusion related to effective drug therapy

---

Planning: Client Goals and Expected Outcomes

The client will:

- Report a decrease in symptoms of vitamin B_{12} deficiency
- Immediately report significant side effects such as dyspnea, palpitations, fatigue, muscle weakness, and dysrhythmias
- Demonstrate an understanding of drug therapy by accurately describing the drug's intended effects, side effects, and precautions

---

Implementation

Interventions (Rationales)	Client Education/Discharge Planning
• Monitor vital signs. (Altered potassium levels and overexertion may produce cardiovascular complications, especially irregular rhythm.) • Monitor potassium levels during first 48 hours of therapy. (Conversion to normal RBC production increases the need for potassium.) • Monitor respiratory pattern. (Pulmonary edema may occur early in therapy related to a possible sensitivity to the drug. Reactions may take up to 8 days to occur.) • Monitor serum vitamin B_{12}, RBC, and Hgb levels to determine effectiveness of drug. (Initial doses of B_{12} stimulate rapid RBC regeneration, and level should return to near normal within 2 weeks.) • Assist client to plan activities and allow for periods of rest to conserve energy. • Encourage client to maintain adequate dietary intake of essential nutrients and vitamins. • Monitor for side effects such as palpitations, fatigue, muscle weakness, and dysrhythmias.	• Instruct client to monitor pulse rate and report irregularities and changes in rhythm • Instruct client on the need for initial and continuing laboratory blood monitoring, and to keep all laboratory appointments • Instruct client to immediately report any respiratory difficulty • Advise client that treatment for pernicious anemia (usually IM injection) must be continued throughout life to prevent neurological damage • Instruct client to rest when he or she begins to feel tired and to avoid strenuous activities Instruct client: • That dietary control, by itself, is not possible in treating pernicious anemia • To consume adequate dietary intake of essential nutrients and vitamins • Teach client to immediately report side effects to the healthcare provider

---

Evaluation of Outcome Criteria

Evaluate the effectiveness of drug therapy by confirming that client goals and expected outcomes have been met (see "Planning").

NCLEX Success Tip

A low folic acid level in the presence of a normal vitamin B_{12} level is indicative of a primary folic acid deficiency anemia. Factors that affect the absorption of folic acid are drugs such as methotrexate, oral contraceptives, antiseizure drugs, and alcohol.

PROTOTYPE DRUG | **Cyanocobalamin: Vitamin B_{12}**

Actions and Uses: Cyanocobalamin is a purified form of vitamin B_{12} that is administered in deficiency states. Treatment of vitamin B_{12} deficiency is most often by weekly, biweekly, or monthly IM or SC injections. Although oral B_{12} supplements are available, they are only effective in clients who have sufficient intrinsic factor and normal absorption in the small intestine. Parenteral administration rapidly reverses most signs and symptoms of B_{12} deficiency. If the disease has been prolonged, symptoms may take longer to resolve, and some neurological damage may be permanent. In most cases, treatment must often be maintained for the remainder of the client's life.

Pharmacokinetics: Cyanocobalamin is well absorbed after SC, IV, or intranasal administration. Calcium and intrinsic factor are necessary for PO absorption. It is stored in the liver, crosses the placenta, and enters breast milk. Excess drug is excreted unchanged in the urine. Half-life is 6 days.

Administration Alerts:

- If PO preparations are mixed with fruit juices, administer quickly because ascorbic acid affects the stability of vitamin B_{12}.
- Cyanocobalamin is pregnancy category C when used parenterally.

Adverse Effects and Interactions: Side effects from cyanocobalamin are uncommon. Hypokalemia is possible, so serum potassium levels are monitored periodically. A small percentage of clients who receive B_{12} exhibit rashes, itching, or other signs of allergy. Anaphylaxis is possible, though rare.

Drug interactions with cyanocobalamin include a decrease in absorption when given concurrently with alcohol, aminosalicylic acid (ASA [Aspirin]), neomycin, and colchicine. Chloramphenicol (Chloromycetin) may interfere with therapeutic response to cyanocobalamin.

IRON

Iron is a mineral essential to the function of several biological molecules, the most significant of which is hemoglobin. Of all iron in the body, 60% to 80% is associated with the hemoglobin in erythrocytes. Iron is also essential for a number of mitochondrial enzymes involved in metabolism and energy production in the cell. Because free iron is toxic, the body binds the mineral to the protein complexes **ferritin**, **hemosiderin**, and **transferrin**.

Ferritin and hemosiderin maintain iron stores *inside* cells, whereas transferrin *transports* iron to sites in the body where it is needed.

Pharmacotherapy with Iron

57.7 Iron deficiency is the most common cause of nutritional anemia and can be successfully treated with iron supplements.

The most common cause of nutritional anemia is iron deficiency. A primary cause of iron-deficiency anemia is blood loss, such as may occur from peptic ulcer disease. Certain individuals, including those who are pregnant, experiencing heavy menstruation, or undergoing intensive athletic training, have an increased demand for iron. These conditions may require more than the recommended daily intake of iron. The most significant effect of iron deficiency is a reduction in erythropoiesis, resulting in symptoms of anemia.

CONNECTIONS | **Lifespan Considerations**

◀ **Iron Deficiency in Children**

Iron deficiency and iron-deficiency anemia have been identified as significant problems among children 1 to 2 years of age. Inadequate iron intake and storage is the main reason for this condition. Extremely low levels of iron can cause permanent mental and psychomotor impairment; therefore, prevention is of utmost importance. Primary prevention of iron deficiency can be accomplished by daily supplementation of 10 mg of elemental iron with iron-fortified vitamins, iron drops, or an iron-fortified nutritional drink. Accidental overdose due to ingestion of products that contain iron is one of the leading causes of fatal poisoning in children. It is extremely important that iron be kept out of the reach of children. If overdosing occurs, caregivers should call the healthcare provider or poison control centre.

After erythrocytes die, nearly all of the iron in their hemoglobin is incorporated into transferrin and recycled for later use. Because of this efficient recycling, only about 1 mg of iron is excreted from the body per day, making daily dietary iron requirements in most individuals quite small. However, the amount of iron lost by some women during menstruation may be significant enough to produce anemic symptoms. Ferrous sulfate, ferrous gluconate, and ferrous fumarate are the most commonly used oral iron preparations.

Nursing Considerations

The role of the nurse in iron therapy involves careful monitoring of the client's condition and providing education as it relates to the prescribed drug regimen. All iron preparations have essentially the same nursing considerations. Before initiating therapy with these medicines, obtain vital signs and a CBC, including Hgb and Hct levels, to establish baseline values. Obtain a health history, assessing for peptic ulcer, regional enteritis, ulcerative colitis, and cirrhosis of the liver because these drugs are contraindicated in such disorders.

Iron dextran (Dexiron) can be given as an IM injection or as an IV infusion and is often used for clients who cannot tolerate oral iron preparations. Prior to administering an infusion, the client must receive a test dose to determine possible allergic reaction, which may cause respiratory arrest and circulatory collapse. Vital signs must be monitored during this initial infusion.

Possible GI reactions such as nausea, vomiting, constipation, and diarrhea are common with the oral iron preparations. Inform the client that these effects will diminish over time and that iron will turn stools a harmless dark green or black colour. Taking oral iron with food reduces GI distress but also greatly reduces absorption. Common adverse reactions of iron dextran are headache and muscle and joint pain; these are more severe when the drug is given IV and are lessened when given IM. Iron dextran appears to increase bone density in the joints, which is the probable cause of the muscle and joint pain.

See Nursing Process Focus: Clients Receiving Iron Products for specific teaching points.

NURSING PROCESS FOCUS

Clients Receiving Iron Products

Assessment	Potential Nursing Diagnoses/Identified Patterns
Prior to administration: • Obtain complete health history, including allergies, drug history, and possible drug reactions. • Assess reason for drug administration, such as presence or history of anemia or prophylaxis during infancy, childhood, or pregnancy. • Assess CBC, specifically Hct and Hgb levels, to establish baseline values. • Assess vital signs.	• Adequate knowledge regarding drug therapy and adverse effects • Safety from physical injury such as falls related to anemia symptoms (weakness, dizziness, syncope) • Adequate tissue oxygenation (may be impaired related to low RBC count) • Balanced intake of iron and other nutrients

Planning: Client Goals and Expected Outcomes

The client will:

• Exhibit an increase in Hct level and improvement in anemia-related symptoms
• Demonstrate an understanding of drug therapy by accurately describing the drug's intended effects, side effects, and precautions
• Immediately report significant side effects such as GI distress

Implementation

Intervention (Rationales)	Client Education/Discharge Planning
• Monitor vital signs, especially pulse. (Increased pulse is an indicator of decreased oxygen content in the blood.) • Monitor CBC to evaluate effectiveness of treatment. (Increases in Hct and Hgb values indicate increased RBC production.) • Monitor changes in stool. (Drug may cause constipation, changes in stool colour, and false positives when stool is tested for occult blood.) • Plan activities and allow for periods of rest to help client conserve energy. (Diminished iron levels result in decreased formation of Hgb, leading to weakness.) • Administer medication on an empty stomach (if tolerated) at least 1 hour before bedtime. (This maximizes absorption; taking drug closer to bedtime may increase the chance of GI distress.) • Administer liquid iron preparations through a straw or place on the back of the tongue (to avoid staining the teeth). • Monitor dietary intake to ensure adequate intake of foods high in iron. • Monitor for potential of child access to medication. (Iron poisoning can be fatal to young children.)	• Instruct client to monitor pulse rate and report irregularities and changes in rhythm Instruct client: • On the need for initial and continuing laboratory blood monitoring • To keep all laboratory appointments Instruct client: • That stool colour may change (usually a dark brown or black colour) and this is not a cause for alarm • On measures to relieve constipation, such as including fruits and fruit juices in diet and increasing fluid intake and exercise Instruct client to: • Rest when feeling tired and not to overexert • Plan activities to avoid fatigue Instruct client: • Not to crush or chew sustained-release preparations • That medication may cause GI upset • To take medication with food if GI upset becomes a problem • To take medication at least 1 hour before bedtime Instruct client to: • Dilute liquid medication before using and to use a straw to take medication • Rinse the mouth after swallowing to decrease the chance of staining the teeth • Instruct client to increase intake of iron-rich foods such as liver, egg yolks, brewer's yeast, wheat germ, and muscle meats • Advise parents to store iron-containing vitamins out of reach of children and in childproof containers

Evaluation of Outcome Criteria

Evaluate the effectiveness of drug therapy by confirming that client goals and expected outcomes have been met (see "Planning").

NCLEX Success Tips

Iron supplements should be administered orally between meals because gastric acidity and the absence of food promote iron absorption (food containing calcium will decrease iron absorption). Iron supplements are preferably administered on an empty stomach if tolerated by the client. However, the client should take iron supplements with vitamin C (in citrus juice) to improve absorption—the citrus juice may also improve the taste as well. The client should take iron supplements and an antacid at least 2 hours apart because antacids bind with iron in the GI tract, decreasing the rate or extent of iron absorption.

Staining of the teeth is a common side effect when iron supplements are taken in liquid form. Drinking from a straw helps to minimize this effect. Constipation is also a common side effect of iron supplements. The client is encouraged to drink plenty of fluids.

Contraindications for the use of iron supplements include primary hemochromatosis, infectious kidney disease in the acute phase, peptic ulcer, regional enteritis, ulcerative colitis, and known hypersensitivity to iron.

Iron dextran requires cautious use in pregnant or breastfeeding clients and in those with severely impaired liver function, significant allergies, or asthma.

PROTOTYPE DRUG **Ferrous Sulfate (Fer-In-Sol)**

Actions and Uses: Ferrous sulfate is an iron supplement containing about 30% elemental iron. It is available in a wide variety of dosage forms to prevent or rapidly reverse symptoms of iron-deficiency anemia. Other forms of iron include ferrous fumarate (Palafer, Eurofer), which contains 33% elemental iron, and ferrous gluconate, which contains 12% elemental iron. The doses of these various preparations are based on their iron content.

Laboratory evaluation of Hgb or Hct values is conducted regularly, as excess iron is toxic. Although a positive therapeutic response may be achieved in 48 hours, therapy may continue for several months.

Pharmacokinetics: Up to 60% of ferrous sulfate taken PO is absorbed. It crosses the placenta and enters breast milk. It is about 90% protein bound. Ferrous sulfate may be retained in the body for many months because it is mostly recycled, with only small amounts being excreted.

Administration Alerts:

- When administering IV, be careful to prevent infiltration, as iron is highly irritating to tissues.
- Use the Z-track method (deep muscle) when giving IM injection.
- Do not crush tablet or empty contents of capsule when administering.
- Do not give tablets or capsules within 1 hour of bedtime.
- Ferrous sulfate is pregnancy category A.

Adverse Effects and Interactions: The most common side effect of ferrous sulfate is GI upset. Taking the drug with food will diminish GI upset but can decrease the absorption of iron by as much as 70%. In addition, antacids should not be taken with ferrous sulfate because they also reduce absorption of the mineral. Ideally, iron preparations should be administered 1 hour before or 2 hours after a meal. Clients should be advised that iron preparations may darken stools, but this is a harmless side effect. Constipation is also a common side effect. Excessive doses of iron are very toxic, so advise clients to take their medication exactly as directed.

Drug interactions with ferrous sulfate include reduced absorption when given concurrently with antacids. Iron decreases the absorption of tetracyclines, thyroid hormone, levodopa-carbidopa (Sinemet), and methyldopa. It is advisable to take iron supplements *at least* 1 hour before or after other medications.

CHAPTER 57 Understanding the Chapter

Key Concepts Summary

The numbered key concepts provide a succinct summary of the important points from the corresponding numbered section within the chapter. If any of these points are not clear, refer to the numbered section within the chapter for review.

57.1 Hematopoiesis is the process of erythrocyte production that begins with primitive stem cells in the bone marrow. Homeostatic control of erythropoiesis is through hematopoietic growth factors.

57.2 Erythropoietin is a hormone that stimulates the production of red blood cells and is used, as epoetin alfa, to treat specific anemias.

57.3 Colony-stimulating factors (CSFs) are growth factors that stimulate the production of leukocytes and are used following chemotherapy or organ transplants.

57.4 Platelet enhancers stimulate the activity of megakaryocytes and thrombopoietin and increase the production of platelets.

57.5 Anemias are disorders in which blood has a reduced capacity to carry oxygen, due to hemorrhage, excessive erythrocyte destruction, or insufficient erythrocyte synthesis.

57.6 Deficiencies in either vitamin B_{12} or folic acid can lead to pernicious anemia. Treatment with cyanocobalamin or folate can reverse these anemias in many clients.

57.7 Iron deficiency is the most common cause of nutritional anemia and can be successfully treated with iron supplements.

Chapter 57 Scenario

A real people-person who never met a stranger. That is how family and friends have always described Carl Guenther. His positive and outgoing personality is well known in the community. When Carl was informed about his prostate cancer, he handled the diagnosis well and with his usual optimism. He was confident that the chemotherapy would be successful. His mantra for years had been "Live every day as if it were your last." However, the treatment for the cancer had adverse effects that he did not expect and his enthusiasm diminished.

Carl is a 72-year-old retired sales representative for a chain of department stores. His entire career centred on interacting with all kinds of people. When he retired, his outgoing nature was an asset for the many community agencies at which he volunteered. He was active in the local Lions Club, his church's outreach ministry, and at the children's hospital. He had even considered working as a greeter at his neighbourhood department store.

As he went through chemotherapy, the associated nausea and vomiting were well managed with antiemetic agents. His physical appearance did not change much since Carl had minimal hair loss due to the chemotherapy. Now he faces an exceedingly low WBC count and has been advised to avoid potential sources of infection, including people. By far, this is the worst adverse effect of the chemotherapy for Carl. He feels socially isolated and depressed. Is this the end, he wonders? Am I to die lonely?

Critical Thinking Questions

1. The healthcare provider orders filgrastim (Neupogen) 10 μg/kg daily for 4 days. Carl asks you, his nurse, "How does this drug work?" What is your response?

2. List interventions that should be followed during this period of chemotherapy-induced neutropenia to protect Carl from infection.

3. What adverse effects would you monitor in clients receiving Neupogen?

See Answers to Critical Thinking Questions in Appendix B.

NCLEX Practice Questions

1 Which statement would the nurse include in the care plan for a client receiving epoetin alfa?

a. Avoid fresh fruit and vegetables, or partially cooked meats.

b. Encourage frequent rest periods to minimize fatigue.

c. Limit exposure to direct sunlight and use sunscreen when outdoors.

d. Protect tissues and mucous membranes from traumatic injury.

2 A client is being treated with filgrastim (Neupogen). Which of the following would the nurse monitor to determine the effectiveness of this drug?

a. Red blood cell counts

b. Platelet counts

c. White blood cell counts

d. Reticulocyte count and mean cell volume (MCV)

3 The nurse is teaching a client about oprelvekin (Neumega). Which statement by the client would indicate that additional health teaching is needed?

a. "This drug stimulates the production of platelets."

b. "I should weigh myself and watch for fluid retention."

c. "I will report vision changes to my healthcare provider."

d. "I will add more iron-rich foods to my diet."

4 A client who regularly consumes significant amounts of alcohol and has been prescribed cyanocobalamin states, "I don't understand why my healthcare provider has prescribed B_{12} injections." The nurse's response will be based on which physiological concept?

a. Clients who regularly consume large amounts of alcohol are often deficient in this nutrient.

b. Alcohol facilitates folate metabolism in the liver, which destroys vitamin B_{12}.

c. Clients who regularly consume large amounts of alcohol are at high risk for neutropenia, a condition that develops from vitamin B_{12} loss.

d. Liver cirrhosis caused by large amounts of alcohol ingestion diminishes natural physiological deposits of B_{12}.

5 The nurse is teaching a client about ferrous sulfate (Fer-In-Sol). Which statement should be included in the teaching plan? Select all that apply.

a. This drug should be taken on an empty stomach at least 1 hour before or 2 hours after a meal.

b. Getting liquid iron on teeth should be avoided because the drug can cause brown stains.

c. Iron preparation may darken stools and cause constipation.

d. Vitamin E is added to many oral iron supplements because it enhances iron absorption.

e. This drug can be taken with caffeinated beverages.

See Answers to NCLEX Practice Questions in Appendix A.

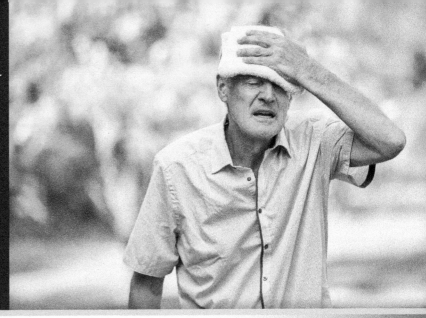

Robert Kneschke/Shutterstock

PROTOTYPE DRUGS

FLUID REPLACEMENT AGENTS
Blood and Blood
    Products
Crystalloid Solutions
Colloid Solutions
    Pr *normal human
        serum albumin
        (Albuminar,
        Alburex, Plasbumin)*

VASOCONSTRICTORS
    Pr *norepinephrine
        (Levophed)*
CARDIOTONIC AGENTS
    Pr *dopamine*

CHAPTER

58

Pharmacotherapy of Shock

LEARNING OUTCOMES

After reading this chapter, the student should be able to:

1. Relate the symptoms of the different types of shock to their physiological causes.

2. Explain the initial treatment for a client who is in shock.

3. Identify drug classes used for treating shock.

4. Explain the therapeutic action of each class of drug used for shock in relation to the pathophysiology of shock.

5. Compare and contrast the use of colloids and crystalloids in fluid replacement therapy.

6. Describe the nurse's role in the pharmacological management of clients receiving drugs for shock.

7. For each of the drug classes listed in Prototype Drugs, identify a representative drug and explain its mechanism of action, therapeutic effects, and important adverse effects.

8. Describe and explain, based on pharmacological principles, the rationale for nursing assessment, planning, and interventions for clients being treated for shock.

9. Use the nursing process to care for clients receiving drug therapy for shock.

CHAPTER OUTLINE

▶ Characteristics of Shock

▶ Causes of Shock

▶ Fluid Replacement Agents

   ▶ Treatment Priorities for Shock

   ▶ Treating Shock with Crystalloids and Colloids

▶ Vasoconstrictors

   ▶ Treating Shock with Vasoconstrictors

▶ Cardiotonic Agents

   ▶ Treating Shock with Cardiotonic Agents

KEY TERMS

albumin, 744	crystalloids, 743	oncotic pressure, 743
anaphylactic shock, 741	hypovolemic shock, 741	septic shock, 741
cardiogenic shock, 741	inotropic agents, 746	shock, 740
colloids, 743	neurogenic shock, 741	

Shock is a condition in which vital tissues are not receiving enough blood to function properly. Without adequate oxygen and other nutrients, cells cannot carry out normal metabolic processes. Shock is considered a medical emergency; failure to reverse the causes and symptoms of shock may lead to irreversible organ damage and death. This chapter examines how drugs are used to aid in the treatment of different types of shock.

Characteristics of Shock

58.1 Shock is a clinical syndrome characterized by the inability of the cardiovascular system to pump enough blood to meet the metabolic needs of the tissues.

Shock is a collection of signs and symptoms, many of which are nonspecific, that occur when vital tissues are not receiving enough blood to function. Although symptoms vary somewhat among the different kinds of shock, some similarities exist. The client appears pale and may claim to feel sick or weak without reporting specific complaints. Behavioural changes are often some of the earliest symptoms and may include restlessness, anxiety, confusion, depression, and apathy. Lack of sufficient blood flow to the brain may result in fainting. Thirst is a common complaint. The skin may feel cold or clammy. Without immediate treatment, multiple body systems will be affected and respiratory failure or renal failure may result. Figure 58.1 shows common symptoms of a client in shock.

The central problem in most types of shock is the inability of the cardiovascular system to send sufficient blood to the vital organs, with the heart and brain being affected early in the progression of the condition. Assessing the client's cardiovascular status will often give important indications for a diagnosis of shock. Blood pressure is usually low and cardiac output is diminished. Heart rate may be rapid with a weak pulse. Breathing is usually rapid and shallow. Figure 58.2 illustrates the physiological changes that occur during circulatory shock.

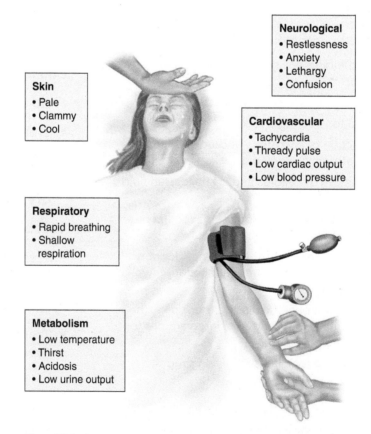

Skin
• Pale
• Clammy
• Cool

Neurological
• Restlessness
• Anxiety
• Lethargy
• Confusion

Cardiovascular
• Tachycardia
• Thready pulse
• Low cardiac output
• Low blood pressure

Respiratory
• Rapid breathing
• Shallow respiration

Metabolism
• Low temperature
• Thirst
• Acidosis
• Low urine output

Figure 58.1 Symptoms of shock.

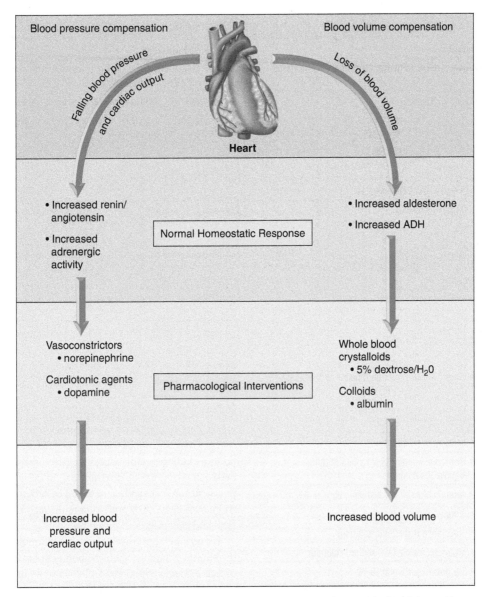

Figure 58.2 Physiological changes during circulatory shock and pharmacological intervention.

Causes of Shock

58.2 Shock is often classified by the underlying pathological process or by the organ system that is primarily affected. Types of shock include cardiogenic, hypovolemic, neurogenic, septic, and anaphylactic.

Shock is often classified by naming the underlying pathological process or organ system causing the condition. Table 58.1 lists the different types of shock and their primary causes.

Diagnosis of shock is rarely based on nonspecific symptoms. A careful medical history may give the nurse valuable clues as to what type of shock may be present. For example, obvious trauma or bleeding would suggest **hypovolemic shock**, related to volume depletion. If trauma to the brain or spinal cord is evident,

neurogenic shock, a type of distributive shock caused by a sudden loss of nerve impulse communication, may be suspected. A history of heart disease would suggest **cardiogenic shock**, which is caused by a loss of adequate cardiac output due to pump failure. A recent infection may indicate **septic shock**, a type of distributive shock caused by the presence of bacteria and toxins in the blood. A history of allergy with a sudden onset of symptoms following food or drug intake may suggest **anaphylactic shock**, the most severe type I allergic response.

FLUID REPLACEMENT AGENTS

Certain agents are used to replace blood or other fluids lost during hypovolemic shock. Fluid replacement therapy includes blood, blood products, colloids, and crystalloids, as shown in Table 58.2.

TABLE 58.1 Common Types of Shock

Type of Shock	Definition	Underlying Pathology
Cardiogenic	Failure of the heart to pump sufficient blood to tissues	Left heart failure, myocardial ischemia, myocardial infarction, dysrhythmias, pulmonary embolism, myocardial or pericardial infection
Hypovolemic	Loss of blood volume	Hemorrhage, burns, profuse sweating, excessive urination, vomiting, diarrhea
Neurogenic	Vasodilation due to overstimulation of the parasympathetic or understimulation of the sympathetic nervous systems	Trauma to spinal cord or medulla, severe emotional stress or pain, drugs that depress the central nervous system
Septic	Multiple organ dysfunction as a result of pathogenic organisms in the blood resulting in vasodilation and changes in permeability of capillaries; often a precursor to acute respiratory distress syndrome and disseminated intravascular coagulation	Widespread inflammatory response to bacterial, fungal, or parasitic infection
Anaphylactic	Acute allergic reaction	Severe reaction to allergen such as penicillin, nuts, shellfish, or animal proteins

TABLE 58.2 Fluid Replacement Agents

Agent	Examples
Blood products	• whole blood
	• plasma protein fraction
	• fresh frozen plasma
	• packed red blood cells
Colloids	• plasma protein fraction (Plasmanate, Plasma-Plex, Plasmatein, PPF, Protenate)
	• dextran 40 (Gentran 40, Hyskon, Rheomacrodex) or dextran 70 (Macrodex)
	• hetastarch (Hespan)
	• **Pr** normal human serum albumin (Albuminar, Alburex, Plasbumin)
Crystalloids	• normal saline (0.9% sodium chloride)
	• lactated Ringer's solution
	• Plasmalyte (hypertonic solution)
	• hypertonic saline (3% sodium chloride)
	• 5% dextrose in water (D_5W)

NCLEX Success Tips

Plasma protein fraction is a blood derivative that supplies colloids to the blood and expands plasma volume. It is used to treat clients who are in shock.

Hypertonic dextrose solutions are used in total parenteral nutrition (TPN). Hypertonic dextrose solutions are used to meet the body's calorie demands in a volume of fluid that will not overload the cardiovascular system.

Colloids are plasma expanders and blood products and are not used in TPN.

Treatment Priorities for Shock

58.3 The initial treatment of shock involves administration of basic life support and replacement of lost fluid. Whole blood may be indicated in cases of massive hemorrhage.

Shock is treated as a medical emergency, and the first goal is to maintain basic life support. Rapid identification of the underlying cause, followed by aggressive treatment, is essential since the client's condition may deteriorate rapidly without specific emergency measures. The initial nursing interventions consist of keeping the client quiet and warm and offering psychological support and reassurance. Maintaining the ABCs of life support—airway, breathing, and circulation—to sustain normal blood pressure is critical. The client is immediately connected to a cardiac monitor and a pulse oximeter is applied. Blood pressure readings are taken on the opposite arm of the pulse oximeter since peripheral vasoconstriction with the inflation of the cuff will alter oximetry readings. Unless contraindicated, oxygen is administered at 15 L/minute via a non-rebreather mask. Neurological status and level of consciousness are monitored.

Hypovolemic shock can be triggered by a number of conditions, including hemorrhage, extensive burns, severe dehydration, persistent vomiting or diarrhea, and intensive diuretic therapy. If the client has lost significant blood or other body fluids, immediate maintenance of blood volume through the administration of fluid and electrolytes or blood products is essential.

Blood and blood products may be administered, depending on the clinical situation. Whole blood is indicated for the treatment of acute, massive blood loss (depletion of more than 30% of the total volume) when there is the need to replace plasma volume and supply red blood cells to increase the oxygen-carrying capacity. The administration of whole blood has been largely replaced with the use of blood components. A unit of whole blood can be separated into its specific constituents (red and white blood cells, platelets, plasma proteins, fresh frozen plasma, and globulins), which can be used to treat more than one client. The supply of blood products depends on human donors and requires careful crossmatching to ensure compatibility between the donor and the recipient. Whole blood, while carefully screened, has the potential to transmit serious infections such as hepatitis and human immunodeficiency virus (HIV).

Treating Shock with Crystalloids and Colloids

58.4 During hypovolemic shock, crystalloids replace lost fluids and electrolytes; colloids expand plasma volume and maintain blood pressure.

Because it is safer to administer only the needed components, rather than whole blood, other products are used to provide volume expansion and to sustain blood pressure. These are of two basic types: colloids and crystalloids. Colloid and crystalloid infusions are often used when up to one-third of an adult's blood volume has been lost.

Colloids are proteins or other large molecules that stay suspended in the blood for a long period because they are too large to cross membranes. While circulating, they draw water molecules from the cells and tissues into the blood vessels through their ability to increase **oncotic pressure**. Blood product colloids include normal human serum albumin, plasma protein fraction, and serum globulins. The non-blood product colloids are dextran (40, 70, and high molecular weight) and hetastarch. These agents are indicated to provide life-sustaining support following massive hemorrhage, for plasma exchange, and to treat shock, burns, acute liver failure, and neonatal hemolytic disease.

Crystalloids are intravenous (IV) solutions that contain electrolytes in concentrations resembling those of plasma. Unlike colloids, crystalloid solutions can readily leave the blood and enter cells. They are used to replace fluids that have been lost and to promote urine output. Common crystalloids include normal saline, hypertonic saline, lactated Ringer's solution, and 5% dextrose in water (D_5W).

Nursing Considerations

The role of the nurse in crystalloid and colloid therapy for shock involves careful monitoring of the client's condition and providing education as it relates to the prescribed drug regimen. Because of the ability of all colloids to pull fluid into the vascular space, circulatory overload is a serious adverse outcome.

Monitoring for blood pressure changes is essential; pressure may increase with a healthy heart or decrease if the heart fails with fluid overload. Lung sounds must also be monitored; crackles will be heard with pulmonary congestion. Pulse oximetry can be used to monitor for changes in oxygenation that may become evident before lung sounds change. Monitoring intake, output, and body weight will assist in assessing fluid retention or loss. These products are used with caution in lactation and pregnancy (category C).

Anaphylactic reactions may occur with the use of plasma protein fraction, dextran 75, dextran 70, and hetastarch. Signs and symptoms of an allergic response may include periorbital edema, urticaria, wheezing, and difficulty breathing. The use of dextran, a high-molecular-weight polysaccharide, is further limited because it can interfere with coagulation and platelet adhesion. Hetastarch, a synthetic starch that resembles human glycogen, can increase the prothrombin time, partial thromboplastin time, and bleeding time when given in large doses, thus limiting its use in conditions where normal clotting is essential. Clients with renal failure who are exhibiting anuria or oliguria are at great risk for fluid overload because of the fluid shift that will occur and their inability to rid the body of excess fluid through urination.

Client education as it relates to fluid replacement therapy should include goals, reasons for obtaining baseline data such as vital signs and tests for cardiac and renal function, and possible side effects. Instruct the client to immediately report difficulty breathing, wheezing, and itching, as they may indicate an allergic response. See Nursing Process Focus: Clients Receiving Fluid Replacement Therapy for more teaching points.

NURSING PROCESS FOCUS

Clients Receiving Fluid Replacement Therapy

Assessment	Potential Nursing Diagnoses/Identified Patterns
Prior to administration: • Obtain complete health history, including allergies, drug history, and possible drug interactions. • Assess lung sounds. • Obtain vital signs. • Assess level of consciousness. • Assess renal function (blood urea nitrogen [BUN] and creatinine).	• Adequate knowledge regarding drug therapy and adverse effects • Safety from physical injury related to adverse effects of drug therapy • Effective tissue perfusion • Fluid and electrolyte balance • Comfort

Planning: Client Goals and Expected Outcomes

The client will:

• Immediately report difficulty breathing
• Report itching or flushing
• Maintain urinary output of at least 50 mL/hour
• Have vital signs within normal range for client
• Experience a safe environment with no evidence of physical injury
• Demonstrate an understanding of drug therapy by accurately describing intended effects, side effects, and precautions

Implementation	
Interventions (Rationales)	**Client Education/Discharge Planning**
• Monitor respiratory status. (Effects of drugs and rapid infusion may result in fluid overload.) • Monitor intake and output for changes in renal function. • Monitor electrolytes. (Crystalloid drugs may cause hypernatremia and resulting fluid retention.) • Observe client for signs of allergic reactions. (Administration of blood and blood products could cause allergic reactions.) • Observe urine for changes in colour. (Adverse reaction to blood could cause hematuria.)	Instruct client to: • Report any signs of respiratory distress • Report changes in sensorium such as lightheadedness, drowsiness, or dizziness • Instruct client concerning rationale for Foley catheter insertion • Instruct client to report any evidence of edema Instruct client: • To report itching, rash, chills, and difficulty breathing • That frequent blood draws are necessary to monitor possible complications of drug administration • Instruct client to notify the healthcare provider if changes in urine colour occur

Evaluation of Outcome Criteria
Evaluate the effectiveness of drug therapy by confirming that client goals and expected outcomes have been met (see "Planning").

See Table 58.2 for a list of the drugs to which these nursing actions apply.

PROTOTYPE DRUG	**Normal Human Serum Albumin (Albuminar, Alburex, Plasbumin)**

Actions and Uses: Normal serum **albumin** is a protein extracted from whole blood, plasma, or placental human plasma that contains 96% albumin and 4% globulins and other proteins. Albumin naturally comprises about 60% of all blood proteins. Its normal functions are to maintain plasma osmotic pressure and to shuttle certain substances through the blood, including a substantial number of drug molecules. After extraction from blood or plasma, it is sterilized to remove possible contamination by the hepatitis viruses or HIV.

Administered IV, albumin increases the osmotic pressure of the blood and moves fluid from the tissues to the general circulation. It is used to restore plasma volume in hypovolemic shock or to restore blood proteins in clients with hypoproteinemia. It has an immediate onset of action and is available in concentrations of 5% and 25%.

Pharmacokinetics: Albumin is confined to the intravascular space, unless vascular permeability is increased. Its half-life is 2 to 3 weeks.

Administration Alerts:
• Higher concentrations must be infused more slowly because the risk for a large, rapid fluid shift is greater.
• Use a large gauge (16–20) IV cannula for administration of drug.
• Albumin is pregnancy category C.

Adverse Effects and Interactions: Because albumin is a natural blood product, allergic reactions are possible. However, coagulation factors, antibodies, and most other blood proteins have been removed; therefore, the incidence of allergic reactions from albumin is not high. Signs of allergy include fever, chills, rash, dyspnea, and possibly hypotension. Protein overload may occur if excessive albumin is infused.

No clinically significant drug interactions have been established.

VASOCONSTRICTORS

In some types of shock, the most serious medical challenge facing the client is hypotension, which may become so profound as to cause collapse of the circulatory system. Vasoconstrictors are drugs for maintaining blood pressure when fluid replacement agents have proven ineffective. These agents are shown in Table 58.3.

TABLE 58.3 Vasoconstrictors for Shock

Drug	Route and Adult Dose
Nonspecific Alpha- and Beta-Adrenergic Agonists	
Pr norepinephrine (Levophed)	IV, 8–12 µg/minute (titrate to desired response), then 2–4 µg/minute for maintenance
Specific Alpha-Adrenergic Agonists	
phenylephrine	(Use only when norepinephrine use is contraindicated) IV bolus, 100-500 µg/dose every 10-15 minutes as needed (initial dose should not exceed 500 µg); IV infusion, start with 100-180 µg/minute or 0.5 µg/kg/minute; titrate to desired response

Treating Shock with Vasoconstrictors

58.5 Vasoconstrictors are critical care drugs sometimes needed during severe shock to maintain blood pressure.

In the early stages of shock, the body compensates for the fall in blood pressure by increasing the activity of the sympathetic nervous system. This sympathetic activity results in vasoconstriction, thus raising blood pressure and increasing the rate and force of myocardial contraction. The purpose of these compensatory measures is to maintain blood flow to vital organs such as the heart and brain and to decrease flow to other organs, including the kidneys and liver.

The body's ability to compensate is limited, however, and profound hypotension may develop as shock progresses. In severe cases, fluid replacement agents alone are not effective at raising blood pressure and other medications are indicated. Historically, sympathomimetic vasoconstrictors have been used to stabilize blood pressure in clients who are in shock. When given intravenously, these drugs will immediately raise blood pressure. Because of side effects and potential organ damage due to the rapid and extreme vasoconstriction, these drugs are used as a last resort. These emergency drugs are considered critical care agents. Sympathomimetics used for shock include norepinephrine, isoproterenol, and phenylephrine. The basic pharmacology of the beta-adrenergic agonists, or sympathomimetics, is presented in Chapter 14.

Nursing Considerations

The role of the nurse in vasoconstrictor therapy for shock involves careful monitoring of the client's condition and providing education as it relates to the prescribed drug regimen. Prior to administration, assess for history of narrow-angle glaucoma and cardiovascular disease, and obtain an electrocardiogram (ECG) reading. Vasoconstrictors are contraindicated in clients with severe cardiovascular disease and narrow-angle glaucoma, as they may worsen these conditions. Assess blood pressure, pulse, and urine output.

In addition to many of the adverse effects described in the Prototype Drug box for norepinephrine (Levophed), other drugs in this class could cause additional side effects. Phenylephrine will cause necrosis of tissue if extravasation occurs. Ensure IV patency prior to beginning the infusion and observe the IV site during the entire infusion. Monitor blood pressure and titrate the drip if blood pressure is elevated. Urine output should be monitored because extreme vasoconstriction may lead to decreased renal perfusion.

Monitor the client for chest pain and ECG changes. Dosages are usually reduced if the heart rate exceeds 110 beats/minute. Monitor mental status, skin temperature of extremities, and colour of earlobes, nail beds, and lips.

Client education as it relates to vasoconstrictor therapy should include goals, reasons for obtaining baseline data such as vital signs and tests for cardiac function, and possible side effects. Explain to the client the use of medication and the rationale for frequent monitoring. Instruct the client to immediately report any pain or burning at the IV site. See Nursing Process Focus: Clients Receiving Adrenergic Therapy in Chapter 14 for the complete nursing process applied to caring for clients receiving beta-adrenergic agonists (sympathomimetics).

PROTOTYPE DRUG	Norepinephrine (Levophed)

Actions and Uses: Norepinephrine (NE) is an adrenergic that acts directly on alpha-adrenergic receptors in vascular smooth muscle to immediately raise blood pressure. It also stimulates beta$_1$ receptors in the heart, thus producing a positive inotropic response that increases cardiac output. The primary indications for NE are acute shock and cardiac arrest. NE is the vasopressor of choice for septic shock because research has demonstrated that it significantly decreases mortality.

Pharmacokinetics: NE is administered by IV infusion, with an onset of action within 2 minutes. It is widely distributed. It is metabolized by the liver and kidneys. Its half-life is 1 minute. Because its duration of action is only 1 to 2 minutes after the infusion is terminated, discontinuing the drug in the case of overdose may be sufficient.

Administration Alerts:
- Infusion is started only after patency of the IV is ensured. Monitor the infusion rate continuously.
- Phentolamine (OraVerse, Rogitine) should be available in case of extravasation.
- Do not abruptly discontinue infusion.
- Norepinephrine is pregnancy category C.

Adverse Effects and Interactions: NE is a powerful vasoconstrictor, so continuous monitoring of blood pressure is required to detect hypertension. NE should not be administered if hypertension is present. When first administered, reflex bradycardia is sometimes experienced. It also has the ability to produce various types of dysrhythmia. Monitor heart rate and rhythm. Blurred vision and photophobia are signs of overdose.

NE interacts with many drugs, including alpha and beta blockers, which may antagonize the drug's vasopressor effects. Conversely, ergot alkaloids and tricyclic antidepressants may potentiate vasopressor effects. Halothane (Fluothane), digoxin (Lanoxin, Toloxin), and cyclopropane may increase the risk of dysrhythmias.

CARDIOTONIC AGENTS

Cardiotonic drugs increase the force of contraction of the heart. In the treatment of shock, they are used to increase the cardiac output. The cardiotonic agents are listed in Table 58.4.

NCLEX Success Tips

Dopamine, a sympathomimetic drug, improves myocardial contractility and blood flow through vital organs by increasing perfusion pressure.

Dopamine administration requires continuous blood pressure monitoring with an invasive or noninvasive device. The nurse may titrate the IV infusion to maintain a systolic blood pressure of 90 mm Hg.

Administration of a pain medication concomitantly with dopamine hydrochloride during shock is not recommended in clients with low hemodynamic values.

TABLE 58.4 Cardiotonic Drugs for Shock

Drug	Route and Adult Dose
digoxin (Lanoxin, Toloxin) (see Chapter 54, page 691, for the Prototype Drug box)	IV, digitalizing dose 2.5–5 µg every 6 hours (q6h) for 24 hours; maintenance dose 0.125–0.5 mg every day (qd)
dobutamine (Dobutrex)	IV infusion, start with 0.5-1 µg/kg/minute; may also initiate at higher doses depending on severity of decompensation, then titrate to desired response; maintenance dose is 2–20 µg/kg/minute (max 40 µg/kg/minute)
Pr dopamine	IV infusion, 2-20 µg/kg/minute; titrate to desired response (max 50 µg/kg/minute); doses > 20 µg/kg/minute may not have a beneficial effect on blood pressure and may increase the risk of tachyarrhythmias

At medium doses (4 to 8 µg/kg/minute), dopamine slightly increases the heart rate and improves contractility to increase cardiac output and improve tissue perfusion. When given at low doses (0.5 to 3.0 µg/minute), dopamine increases renal perfusion by dilating the renal arteries and helps prevent renal shutdown and mesenteric blood flow. At high doses (8 to 10 µg/kg/minute), dopamine produces vasoconstriction, which is an undesirable effect.

Dopamine should NOT be initiated if the client is hypotensive from hypovolemia. Fluid volume assessment should always be done first. Volume replacement should be initiated in a hypovolemic client prior to starting an inotrope such as dopamine.

Vesicant medications such as dopamine should not be administered through a midline catheter, as extravasation of the medication can cause tissue damage.

After successful resuscitation, dopamine would be given as an infusion to increase cardiac output and maintain blood pressure.

Dobutamine (Dobutrex) is a vasoactive adrenergic that works by increasing myocardial contractility and stroke volume in order to increase the cardiac output in heart failure clients and those undergoing cardiopulmonary bypass surgery. A serious side effect of adrenergic drugs is the worsening of a pre-existing cardiac disorder.

Treating Shock with Cardiotonic Agents

58.6 Cardiotonic drugs are useful in reversing the decreased cardiac output that results from shock.

As shock progresses, the heart may begin to fail; cardiac output decreases, lowering the amount of blood reaching vital tissues and deepening the degree of shock. Cardiotonic drugs, also known as **inotropic agents**, have the potential to reverse the cardiac symptoms of shock by increasing the strength of myocardial contraction. Digoxin increases myocardial contractility and cardiac output, thus quickly bringing critical tissues their essential oxygen. Chapter 54 should be reviewed because digoxin and other medications prescribed for heart failure are sometimes used for the treatment of shock.

Dobutamine is a beta$_1$-adrenergic agonist that has value in the short-term treatment of certain types of shock due to its ability to cause the heart to beat more forcefully. Dobutamine is especially beneficial in cases where the primary cause of shock is related to heart failure, not hypovolemia. The resulting increase in cardiac output assists in maintaining blood flow to vital organs. Dobutamine has a half-life of only 2 minutes, and it is only given as an IV infusion.

Dopamine is both an alpha and beta receptor agonist. Dopamine is used at different dosage levels and will have different effects based on what receptors are most affected. It is primarily used in shock conditions to increase blood pressure by causing peripheral vasoconstriction (alpha$_1$ stimulation) and increasing the force of myocardial contraction (beta$_1$ stimulation). Dopamine has the potential to cause dysrhythmias.

Nursing Considerations

The role of the nurse in cardiotonic therapy for shock involves careful monitoring of the client's condition and providing education as it relates to the prescribed drug regimen. Prior to administration, assess for history of cardiovascular disease, and obtain an ECG. Blood pressure, pulse, urine output, and body weight should also be assessed.

Cardiotonic agents are contraindicated in clients with ventricular tachycardia, because they will worsen dysrhythmia, and in hypertrophic idiopathic subaortic stenosis, because increasing contractility will precipitate heart failure. Safe use during pregnancy and lactation has not been established (category C). They should be used cautiously in clients who are hypertensive since they increase blood pressure. With atrial fibrillation, a rapid ventricular response may increase heart rate excessively. Hypovolemia should be corrected with whole blood or plasma prior to the start of dopamine infusion.

Cardiotonic medications may be used separately or concurrently with other antishock agents. They are only given as a continuous infusion, and dosage is based on micrograms per kilogram per minute. Careful calculations must be done to arrive at the appropriate number of millilitres per hour in order to set the IV pump to deliver the correct dosage. IV pump technology is such that some will automate calculations, and most have the ability to deliver dosages to a tenth of a millilitre. The IV rate can be found by multiplying the ordered dose times the client's weight in kilograms times 60 (to get micrograms per hour), then dividing this amount by the concentration of the infusion (micrograms per millilitre). The result will be the millilitres per hour the client should receive. Weigh the client each morning. The client's dose is recalculated each day, based on that weight.

Clients should be connected to a cardiac monitor prior to and during the infusion of cardiotonic drugs. Monitor the client's blood pressure frequently. If a pressure monitoring catheter is in place, pulmonary wedge pressure and cardiac output should be assessed to keep these parameters within normal ranges. Initiate the IV in a large vein; a central line is preferable. Extravasation of dopamine can cause severe, localized vasoconstriction resulting in sloughing of tissue and tissue necrosis if not reversed with phentolamine injections at the site of the infiltration. If extravasation occurs, discontinue the IV, restart it in another site, and administer the antidote. If infiltration occurs, dobutamine can be irritating to the vein and surrounding tissues, although it causes less severe vasoconstriction than dopamine.

Monitor renal function closely, including urine output, BUN, and creatinine levels. With improved cardiac output, renal function should improve and urine output should increase. Low doses of dopamine increase renal perfusion and should enhance urine output. Foley catheters are frequently employed to ensure accurate measurement of urine output.

Client education as it relates to cardiotonic therapy should include goals, reasons for obtaining baseline data such as vital signs and tests for cardiac and renal function, and possible side effects. Advise the client that continuous cardiac monitoring will occur while receiving the medication. The following are additional points to include when teaching clients regarding cardiotonic agents:

- Report chest pain, difficulty breathing, palpitations, or headache.
- Immediately report burning or pain at IV site.
- Immediately report chest pain or numbness or tingling in the extremities.

See Nursing Process Focus: Clients Receiving Adrenergic Therapy in Chapter 14 for the complete nursing process applied to caring for clients receiving beta-adrenergic agonists.

PROTOTYPE DRUG	Dopamine

Actions and Uses: Dopamine is the immediate metabolic precursor to norepinephrine. While classified as a sympathomimetic, dopamine's mechanism of action is dependent on the dose. At low doses, the drug selectively stimulates dopaminergic receptors, especially in the kidneys, leading to vasodilation and an increased blood flow through the kidneys. This makes dopamine of particular value in treating hypovolemic and cardiogenic shock.

At higher doses, dopamine stimulates beta$_1$-adrenergic receptors, causing the heart to beat more forcefully and increasing cardiac output. Another beneficial effect of dopamine when given in higher doses is its ability to stimulate alpha-adrenergic receptors, thus causing vasoconstriction and raising blood pressure.

Pharmacokinetics: Dopamine is administered IV only. It is widely distributed but does not cross the blood-brain barrier. It is metabolized rapidly by the liver and kidneys. Its half-life is 2 minutes. Therefore, discontinuing the drug in the case of overdose may suffice.

Administration Alerts:
- Drug is given as a continuous infusion only.
- Ensure patency of the IV site prior to beginning infusion.
- Phentolamine is the antidote for extravasation of the drug and should be readily available.
- Dopamine is pregnancy category C.

Adverse Effects and Interactions: Because of its profound effects on the cardiovascular system, the nurse must continuously monitor clients who are receiving dopamine for signs of dysrhythmias and hypotension. Side effects are normally self-limiting because of the short half-life of the drug. Dopamine is a vesicant drug that can cause severe, irreversible damage if it escapes from the vein into surrounding tissues.

Dopamine interacts with many other drugs. Concurrent administration with monoamine oxidase inhibitors and ergot alkaloids increases alpha-adrenergic effects. Phenytoin (Dilantin) may decrease dopamine action. Beta blockers may antagonize cardiac effects. Alpha blockers antagonize peripheral vasoconstriction. Halothane increases the risk for hypertension and ventricular dysrhythmias.

CHAPTER

58 Understanding the Chapter

Key Concepts Summary

The numbered key concepts provide a succinct summary of the important points from the corresponding numbered section within the chapter. If any of these points are not clear, refer to the numbered section within the chapter for review.

58.1 Shock is a clinical syndrome characterized by the inability of the cardiovascular system to pump enough blood to meet the metabolic needs of the tissues.

58.2 Shock is often classified by the underlying pathological process or by the organ system that is primarily affected. Types of shock include cardiogenic, hypovolemic, neurogenic, septic, and anaphylactic.

58.3 The initial treatment of shock involves administration of basic life support and replacement of lost fluid. Whole blood may be indicated in cases of massive hemorrhage.

58.4 During hypovolemic shock, crystalloids replace lost fluids and electrolytes; colloids expand plasma volume and maintain blood pressure.

58.5 Vasoconstrictors are critical care drugs sometimes needed during severe shock to maintain blood pressure.

58.6 Cardiotonic drugs are useful in reversing the decreased cardiac output that results from shock.

Chapter 58 Scenario

Ms. Pauline is a 42-year-old stay-at-home mom. She was hit by drunk driver this morning while riding her bicycle. She was found unresponsive at the site of the accident, when bystanders called 911. On arrival at the emergency department, her respirations were shallow, pulse was 56 but weak and thready, and blood pressure was initially unobtainable and later 84/40 mm Hg. Her skin is cool, pale, and dry, and her pupils are unequal and slightly reactive. Her external injuries include scalp lacerations and a contused wound in the abdomen, which is distended with hypoactive bowel sounds. She is suspected of having hypovolemic shock. She is placed on spinal precautions, oxygen 4 L/minute, and fluid replacement.

Critical Thinking Questions

1. Pauline was placed on a norepinephrine drip for cardiogenic shock. Why is this client on this medication? When and how should the norepinephrine drip be discontinued?

2. The healthcare provider orders 3 L of 0.9% normal saline (NS) for Pauline's vomiting and diarrhea. Is this an appropriate IV solution for this client? Why or why not?

3. Pauline was placed on a drip of 5% dextrose in water running at 150 mL/hour. Is the IV solution appropriate for this client? Why or why not?

See Answers to Critical Thinking Questions in Appendix B.

NCLEX Practice Questions

1 A client is receiving dopamine for treatment of shock. Which action should the nurse take?

a. Continuously monitor blood pressure.

b. Evaluate arterial blood gases at least every 2 hours.

c. Continuously monitor the client's heart rate.

d. Administer pain medication concurrently.

2 The nurse knows that the major clinical use of dobutamine is to

a. Increase cardiac output

b. Treat hypertension

c. Treat hypotension

d. Prevent sinus bradycardia

3 A client returns to an intensive care unit after coronary artery bypass graft surgery, which was complicated by prolonged cardiopulmonary bypass and hypotension. After 3 hours in the unit, the client's condition stabilizes. However, the urine output has decreased despite adequate filling pressures. The nurse expects the physician to add which drug, at which flow rate, to the client's regimen?

a. Dopamine, 3 µg/kg/minute

b. Dobutamine, 10 µg/kg/minute

c. Norepinephrine, 8 µg/minute

d. Epinephrine, 4 µg/kg/minute

4 Before administering digoxin, the nurse reviews information about the drug. She learns that after digoxin is metabolized, the body eliminates remaining digoxin as unchanged drug by way of the

a. Feces

b. Kidneys

c. Lungs

d. Skin

5 The nurse should teach the client that signs of digoxin toxicity include

a. Elevated blood pressure

b. Visual disturbances, such as seeing yellow spots

c. Increased appetite

d. A rash over the chest and back

See Answers to NCLEX Practice Questions in Appendix A.

UNIT

12

Pharmacology of Neoplastic Disorders

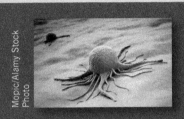

Mopic/Alamy Stock Photo

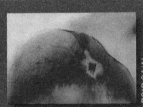

BSIP SA/Alamy Stock Photo

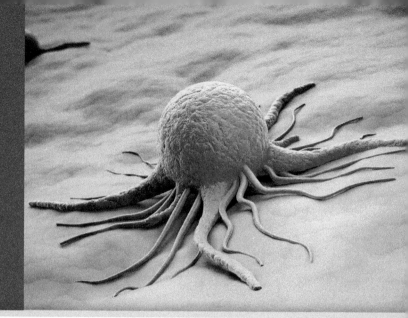

CHAPTER

59

Basic Principles of Antineoplastic Therapy

LEARNING OUTCOMES

After reading this chapter, the student should be able to:

1. Compare and contrast the differences between normal cells and cancer cells.

2. Identify etiological factors associated with an increased incidence of cancer.

3. Construct a table categorizing the major primary and secondary means of cancer prevention.

4. Compare and contrast the following goals of chemotherapy: cure, control, palliation, prophylaxis, adjuvant therapy, and neoadjuvant therapy.

5. Explain the purposes of staging and grading cancers.

6. Explain the significance of growth fraction and the cell cycle to the success of chemotherapy.

7. Assess the ability of antineoplastic drugs to achieve a total cancer cure based on the cell kill hypothesis.

8. Explain how special chemotherapy protocols increase the effectiveness of therapy.

9. Discuss the types of toxicity and adverse effects of chemotherapeutic agents on the various organ systems.

CHAPTER OUTLINE

▸ Characteristics of Cancer

▸ Etiology of Cancer

▸ Goals of Chemotherapy

▸ Staging and Grading of Cancer

▸ The Cell Cycle and Growth Fraction

▸ Cell Kill Hypothesis

▸ Improving the Success of Chemotherapy

▸ Toxicity of Antineoplastic Agents

KEY TERMS

adjuvant chemotherapy, 753

alopecia, 760

angiogenesis, 752

cachexia, 759

cancer, 751

carcinogens, 752

cell kill hypothesis, 756

chemotherapy, 753

emetic potential, 759

grading, 754

growth fraction, 755

metastasis, 752

mucositis, 759

nadir, 758

neoadjuvant chemotherapy, 753

neoplasm, 751

oncogenes, 752

palliation, 753

peripherally inserted central
   catheter (PICC) line, 757

sclerosing, 757

staging, 754

telomerase, 752

telomeres, 752

tumour, 751

vesicants, 760

Cancer is one of the most feared diseases in society for a number of valid reasons. In Canada, cancer has become the number one cause of mortality. It is often silent, producing no symptoms until it reaches an advanced stage. Cancer may strike at an early age, even during infancy, to deprive clients of a normal lifespan. Perhaps worst of all, the medical treatment of cancer often cannot offer a cure, and progression to death is sometimes slow, painful, and psychologically difficult for clients and their loved ones.

Despite its feared status, many successes have been made in the diagnosis and treatment of cancer. Modern treatment methods result in a cure for nearly two of every three people and the 5-year survival rate has steadily increased for most types of cancer. This chapter examines the basic principles of cancer therapy. Chapter 60 examines the medications used to treat cancer.

Characteristics of Cancer

59.1 Cancer is characterized by rapid, uncontrolled growth of cells that eventually invade normal tissues and metastasize.

The word **neoplasm** is often used interchangeably with **tumour**. Tumours may be benign or malignant. Whereas benign tumours are usually slow growing, remain localized, and rarely cause death, malignant tumours are rapidly growing, invasive, and will kill the host if left untreated. Malignant tumours are classified as carcinomas or sarcomas. Examples of various types of benign and malignant tumours are listed in Table 59.1.

Cancer or carcinoma is a disease characterized by abnormal, uncontrolled cell division. Cell division is a normal process that occurs extensively in most body tissues from conception to late childhood. At some point in time, whether it occurs during fetal life, childhood, or adulthood, the degree of cell division in every tissue must be controlled.

Each cell in the body has the ability to regulate its growth (proliferation) by turning specific genes on and off. For example, growth-promoting genes can be turned on when it is necessary to replace worn-out cells, as in the case of blood cells, skin cells, and the epithelial lining of the digestive tract. Growth suppressor genes are responsible for slowing the duplication rate and can completely shut down replication, as in the case of muscle cells and most neurons cells. If the suppressor genes become damaged or mutated and do not slow down or stop cell growth, the cells will undergo abnormal proliferation. Because of the critical importance of cell growth to life, it is likely that each cell has multiple genes that regulate division, all of which are responsive to various chemical signals or messages originating from both inside and outside the cell.

Cancer is thought to result from damage to the genes controlling cell growth. Once damaged, cells may become unresponsive to the chemical signals that normally check growth. The cancer cells lose their normal functions, dividing rapidly and invading surrounding tissues. Unlike most normal cells, cancerous cells are

TABLE 59.1 Classification and Naming of Tumours

Name	Description	Examples
Benign tumour	Slow growing; does not metastasize and rarely requires drug treatment	Adenoma, papilloma, lipoma, osteoma, meningioma
Carcinoma	Cancer of epithelial tissue; most common type of malignant neoplasm; grows rapidly and metastasizes	Malignant melanoma, renal cell carcinoma, adenocarcinoma, hepatocellular carcinoma
Glioma	Cancer of glial (interstitial) cells in the brain, spinal cord, and pineal gland	Telangiectatic glioma, brainstem glioma, posterior pituitary gland, or retina
Leukemia	Cancer of the blood-forming cells in bone marrow; may be acute or chronic	Myelocytic leukemia, lymphocytic leukemia
Lymphoma	Cancer of lymphoid tissue	Hodgkin's disease, lymphoblastic lymphoma
Sarcoma	Cancer of connective tissue; grows extremely rapidly and metastasizes early in the progression of the disease	Osteogenic sarcoma, fibrosarcoma, Kaposi's sarcoma, angiosarcoma

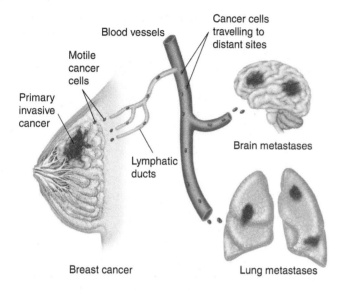

Figure 59.1 Invasion and metastasis by cancer cells.

TABLE 59.2 Common Chemical Carcinogens	
Agent	**Type of Cancer**
Alcohol	Liver
Arsenic	Skin and lung
Asbestos	Lung
Benzene	Leukemia
Nickel	Lung and nasal
Polycyclic aromatic hydrocarbons	Lung and skin
Tobacco substances	Lung
Vinyl chloride	Liver

able to move to other places in the body. The abnormal cells often travel to distant sites where they populate new tumours, a process called **metastasis**. Figure 59.1 illustrates some characteristics of cancer cells.

Each time a cell divides, it loses a small amount of deoxyribonucleic acid (DNA) at the end of each chromosome. These regions of "extra" repetitive DNA, called **telomeres**, serve to protect the vital sequences of DNA from being destroyed. Normal cells are able to undergo mitosis 50 to 60 times before the cell loses the protective telomeres. Certain human stem cells contain the enzyme **telomerase**, which can lengthen the DNA chains and allow continued replication. Interestingly, this enzyme is not produced in mature cells, which dooms the cells to eventual death.

Cancer cells are different from normal cells in that they do not die as quickly and can divide and form new cancer cells indefinitely. One explanation for this difference is that most cancer cells produce large amounts of telomerase, which continues to add pieces to the telomeres so that the cell can continue to divide. It is believed that the cancer cell begins to produce telomerase soon after it has mutated and that this may be an important factor in the progression to cancer.

To divide rapidly (and indefinitely) tumour cells need an adequate supply of nutrients. Solid tumours need to create a new capillary network to "feed" themselves. The process of **angiogenesis**, which is the formation of new blood vessels, is controlled by a cascade of events similar to blood coagulation. Some factors that are secreted by cells promote angiogenesis, whereas others inhibit it. Cancer cells appear to have the ability to control angiogenesis and to establish their own blood supply, which not only brings in nutrients but also provides an "escape route" during metastasis.

Etiology of Cancer

59.2 The etiology of cancer may be chemical, physical, or biological.

Numerous environmental factors have been found to cause cancer or to be associated with a higher risk for developing the disease. These factors are known as **carcinogens**. Many chemical carcinogens have been identified. Chemicals in tobacco smoke are thought to be responsible for about one-third of all cancers and 85% of all new cases of lung cancer in Canada. Chemicals such as asbestos and benzene have been associated with a higher incidence of cancer in the workplace. In some cases, the actual site of the cancer may be distant from the entry location, as with bladder cancer caused by the inhalation of certain industrial chemicals. Some known chemical carcinogens are listed in Table 59.2.

A number of physical factors are also associated with cancer. For example, exposure to large amounts of x-rays is associated with a higher risk for leukemia. Ultraviolet (UV) light from the sun is a known cause of skin cancer.

Viruses are associated with about 15% of all human cancers. Examples include herpes simplex types 1 and 2, Epstein-Barr virus, human papillomavirus (HPV), cytomegalovirus, and human T-lymphotrophic viruses. In February 2007, the National Advisory Committee on Immunization (NACI)—the expert committee that advises the Public Health Agency of Canada on immunization—recommended that females between 9 and 26 years of age be given the HPV vaccine to prevent cervical cancer caused by HPV.

Factors that suppress the immune system, such as human immunodeficiency virus (HIV) or drugs given after transplant surgery, may encourage the growth of cancer cells.

Some cancers have a strong genetic component. The fact that close relatives may acquire the same type of cancer suggests that certain genes may predispose close relatives to the condition. These abnormal genes somehow interact with chemical, physical, and biological agents to promote cancer formation. **Oncogenes** normally promote cell growth. When mutated, they can lead to cancer. Other genes, called tumour suppressor genes, may inhibit the formation of tumours. If these suppressor genes contain a mutation, cancer may result. Damage to the tumour suppressor gene known as p53 is associated with cancers of the breast, lung, brain, colon, and bone.

Although the formation of cancer has a genetic component, it also has a strong environmental component. Adopting healthy lifestyle habits may reduce the risk for developing cancer. Proper nutrition, avoiding chemical and physical risks, and keeping regular health checkups can help to prevent cancer from developing into a fatal disease. The following are lifestyle factors regarding cancer prevention or diagnosis to include when teaching clients about cancer prevention:

- Eliminate tobacco use and exposure to secondhand smoke.
- Limit or eliminate consumption of alcohol.
- Reduce fat in the diet, particularly from animal sources.
- Choose most foods from plant sources; increase fibre in the diet.
- Exercise regularly and keep body weight within recommended guidelines.
- Self-examine your body monthly for abnormal lumps and skin lesions.
- When exposed to direct sun, use skin lotions with the highest SPF (sun protection factor) value.
- Have periodic diagnostic testing performed at recommended intervals.
- Women should have periodic mammograms, as directed by their healthcare provider.
- Men should have a digital rectal prostate examination and a prostate-specific antigen test annually after age 50.
- Have a fecal occult blood test (FOBT) and flexible sigmoidoscopy performed at age 50, with FOBT annually after age 50.
- Women who are sexually active or have reached age 18 should have an annual Pap test and pelvic examination.
- Females and males between 9 and 26 years of age may be given the HPV vaccine to prevent cervical cancer caused by HPV.

The American Cancer Society recommends using the following acronym to help people remember what to look for when self-assessing for cancer:

Caution

C: Change in bowel or bladder habits

A: A sore that does not heal

U: Unusual bleeding or discharge

T: Thickening or lump in the breast or elsewhere

I: Indigestion or difficulty swallowing

O: Obvious change in a wart or mole

N: Nagging cough or hoarseness

Goals of Chemotherapy

59.3 The three primary goals of chemotherapy are cure, control, and palliation.

Pharmacotherapy of cancer is sometimes referred to as simply **chemotherapy**. Transported through the blood, drugs have the potential to reach cancer cells in virtually any location. Certain chemotherapeutic drugs are specifically designed to be able to cross the blood-brain barrier to reach brain tumours. Others are instilled directly into body cavities such as the urinary bladder to bring the highest dose possible to the cancer cells without producing systemic adverse effects. Chemotherapy has three general goals: cure, control, and palliation.

When diagnosed with cancer, the primary goal desired by most clients is to achieve a complete cure; that is, permanent removal of all cancer cells from the body. The possibility for cure is much greater if a cancer is identified and treated when the tumour is small and localized to a well-defined region. The 5-year survival rates for nearly all types of cancers have increased in the past 2 decades due to improved detection and more effective therapies. Examples in which chemotherapy has been used successfully as curative treatment include Hodgkin's lymphoma, certain leukemias, and choriocarcinoma.

When cancer has progressed and cure is not possible, a second goal of chemotherapy is to control or manage the disease. Although the cancer is not eliminated, preventing the growth and spread of the tumour may extend a client's life. Essentially, the cancer is managed as a chronic disease, such as hypertension or diabetes.

In its advanced stages, cure or control of the cancer may not be achievable. For these clients, chemotherapy is used as **palliation**. Chemotherapy drugs are administered to reduce the size of the tumour, easing the severity of pain and other tumour symptoms and thus improving the client's quality of life. Examples of advanced cancers for which palliation is frequently used include osteosarcoma, pancreatic cancer, and Kaposi's sarcoma.

Chemotherapy may be used alone or in combination with other treatment modalities such as surgery or radiation therapy. Surgery is especially useful for removing solid tumours that are localized. Surgery lowers the number of cancer cells in the body so that radiation therapy and pharmacotherapy can be more successful. When only a portion of the tumour is removed, it is referred to as *debulking*. Surgery is not an option for tumours of blood cells or when it would not be expected to extend a client's lifespan or improve the quality of life.

Approximately 50% of clients with cancer receive radiation therapy as part of their treatment. Radiation therapy is most successful and produces the fewest adverse effects for cancers that are localized when high doses of ionizing radiation can be aimed directly at the tumour and be confined to a small area. Radiation treatments are frequently prescribed postoperatively to kill cancer cells that may remain following an operation. Radiation is sometimes given as palliation for inoperable cancers to shrink the size of a tumour that may be pressing on vital organs and to relieve pain, difficulty breathing, or difficulty swallowing.

Adjuvant chemotherapy is the administration of antineoplastic drugs after surgery or radiation therapy. The purpose of adjuvant chemotherapy is to rid the body of any cancerous cells that were not removed during the surgery or to treat any micrometastases that may be developing.

Neoadjuvant chemotherapy is the administration of antineoplastic drugs before surgery or radiation therapy with the goal of shrinking a large tumour to a more manageable size. This may also be done if the tumour has invaded vital tissue around it, such as may happen with brain tumours. Shrinking the tumour preoperatively results in less surgical invasion when removing the tumour.

In a few cases, drugs are given as chemoprophylaxis with the goal of preventing cancer from occurring in clients who are at high risk for developing tumours. For example, clients with a close family history of breast cancer who have had a primary breast cancer removed may receive tamoxifen (Nolvadex), even if there is no evidence of metastases. Tamoxifen has been shown to prevent the recurrence of breast cancer in these clients. Chemoprophylaxis of cancer is uncommon because most of these drugs have potentially serious adverse effects.

Staging and Grading of Cancer

59.4 Cancers are described by their stage and grade.

Staging and grading must be done to determine the extent to which a cancer has invaded the body. These processes are performed on the initial diagnosis of cancer to determine the best course of therapy and predict client outcomes.

Staging is the process of determining where the cancer is located and the extent of its invasion. Staging helps the healthcare provider to more accurately communicate the prognosis of the disease with the client and helps to determine the best course of treatment.

During the staging of solid tumours, diagnostic testing determines the size of the tumour, whether the tumour has invaded surrounding tissue, the involvement of lymph nodes, and the presence or absence of metastasis (Table 59.3). The client's disease is assigned numerical values for the tumour (T), node (N), and metastasis (M). Once these are determined, an overall stage is assigned: I, II, III, or IV. Stage I is assigned to cancers that are the least invasive and have the best prognosis. Stage IV is assigned to the cancer that is the most aggressive and has the poorest prognosis.

Once a cancer is staged, the level does not change even if the cancer progresses. For example, if a cancer is staged as level II on diagnosis, the cancer will always be referred to as a stage II cancer even if it spreads to other sites. At this point, it may receive a qualifier, such as stage II *with metastasis* or stage II *recurrent*. Statistics regarding cancer survival and treatment are based on the initial stage at which the cancer was diagnosed.

Grading is a process that examines potential cancer cells under a microscope and compares their appearance to normal parent cells. Normal cells are highly differentiated: They have developed, become fully mature, look like the parent cell, and carry on the functions of the parent cell. For example, it is very easy to distinguish a liver cell from a muscle cell or a nerve cell microscopically. When a normal cell becomes cancerous, however, it gradually changes and becomes less differentiated in both structure and function. Once fully undifferentiated, the cancer cell will look very different from the parent cell from which it came and will not carry on the functions of the parent cell.

In the grading process, if the biopsy cells appear differentiated and very similar to the parent cells, the tumour is classified as a grade 1 (G1) and has the best prognosis. G4 cells are grossly abnormal and clearly different from normal cells. Clients with these malignant and aggressive cells have the worst prognosis.

Grading has certain limitations. For instance, solid tumours often contain many different types of cells that vary in appearance from near normal to grossly abnormal. One part of the tumour may have cells consistent with G2, whereas other parts of the same tumour may have cells consistent with G4. Unlike staging, grading may change over time as the tumour evolves.

The Cell Cycle and Growth Fraction

59.5 Many antineoplastic drugs are more effective when given at specific stages of the cell cycle and in tumours with a high growth fraction.

Both normal and cancerous cells go through a sequence of events known as the cell cycle, which is illustrated in Figure 59.2. Knowledge of the cell cycle is important to understanding the effectiveness of anticancer drugs.

In simplest terms, a cell is either performing its daily functions or it is undergoing cell division. There are certain cellular activities that occur in between these two basic functions of the cell that allow its life cycle to be divided into five stages or phases.

Stage G_0. Although sometimes called the resting stage, G_0 is the phase during which cells conduct their everyday activities such as metabolism, impulse conduction, contraction, or secretion. A cell may enter its G_0 phase at any point in the cycle and remain there for extended periods, depending on the specific

TABLE 59.3 Staging of Cancer*	
T Category: Describes the primary tumour.	
TX	Primary tumour cannot be assessed
T0	No evidence of primary tumour
T1	Tumour is confined to the primary area
T3–T4	Tumour has invaded areas surrounding the primary tumour
N Category: Describes whether the cancer has spread to lymph nodes.	
NX	Nearby lymph nodes cannot be assessed
N0	No regional lymph nodes metastasis
N1–N3	Primary tumour has spread to regional lymph nodes
M Category: Describes whether distant metastases are present.	
MX	Distant metastases cannot be assessed
M0	No distant metastases were found
M1	Distant metastases are present

*The exact staging of a tumour varies somewhat with each specific type of cancer. Most have multiple subcategories to better define the tumour.

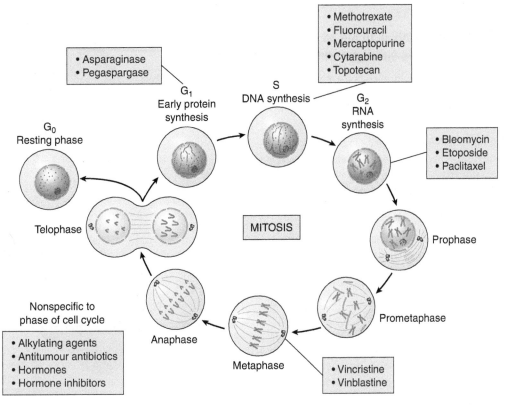

Figure 59.2 Antineoplastic agents and the cell cycle.

tissue and surrounding cellular signals. Cells spend most of their lifetime in the G_0 phase.

Stage G_1 (Gap 1). If a cell receives a signal to divide, it leaves the G_0 phase and enters the G_1 phase, during which it synthesizes the ribonucleic acid (RNA), proteins, and other components needed to duplicate its DNA.

Stage S (Synthesis). During the S phase the cell duplicates its DNA.

Stage G_2 (Gap 2). During the G_2 or premitotic phase the cell makes additional proteins and the spindle apparatus that are necessary for cell division or mitosis.

Stage M (Mitosis). The cell undergoes mitosis, which includes prophase, metaphase, anaphase, and telophase. Following mitosis in the M phase, the cell has split into two identical cells that will either start the process over at the G_1 phase or enter the G_0 phase, depending on the needs of the body. This is the briefest stage of the cell cycle.

The actions of some antineoplastics are specific to certain phases of the cell cycle, whereas others are mostly independent of the cell cycle. Cell cycle–specific drugs kill the most cancer cells when they are administered in divided but frequent doses. Cell cycle–specific drugs are most effective in treating hematological malignancies and other cancers that have a relatively large proportion of cells proliferating at any given point in time. Examples include mitotic inhibitors such as vincristine, which affect cells in the M phase, and antimetabolites such as fluorouracil, which are most effective against cells during the S phase. In general, cell cycle–specific drugs are not effective against tumours that have a large percentage of resting cells.

Cell cycle–nonspecific drugs can kill cancer cells in any stage of the cell cycle, including the G_0 resting phase. Often these drugs are incorporated into resting cancer cells and have no effects until the cells attempt to divide. These drugs act relatively slowly and are given intermittently to give normal cells an opportunity to recover. The effects of alkylating agents such as cyclophosphamide (Procytox), antitumour antibiotics, and hormonal therapies are generally independent of the phases of the cell cycle.

The **growth fraction** is a measure of the number of cells undergoing mitosis in a tissue. It is a ratio of the number of replicating cells to the number of resting cells. Antineoplastic drugs are more toxic to tissues and tumours with high growth fractions. For example, certain leukemias and lymphomas have a high growth fraction and therefore have a greater antineoplastic success rate. Solid tumours such as breast and lung cancer generally have a low growth fraction; therefore, they are less sensitive to antineoplastic agents. Because certain normal tissues, such as hair follicles, bone marrow, and the gastrointestinal (GI) epithelium, also have high growth fractions, they are sensitive to the effects of the antineoplastics.

With large solid tumours, a high percentage of the cells have entered the G_0 phase, causing the tumour to have a lower growth fraction. Chemotherapeutic drugs are not as effective against cells that are in the G_0 phase. To improve the success of chemotherapeutic drugs, the tumour may be debulked. When a tumour is debulked, a portion is removed surgically, causing the remaining cells to move into the active phases of mitosis. Once the cells enter into mitosis, the chemotherapeutic drugs can more effectively kill the cancer cells.

Cell Kill Hypothesis

59.6 The goal of chemotherapy is to kill as many cancer cells as possible while sparing normal cells.

Measurement of the success of chemotherapy is dependent on the therapeutic goal. If the desirable outcome is a total cure, success is measured by how long the client remains cancer free following treatment. If the goal is palliation, success is measured by the degree to which the client's quality of life is improved. Because chemotherapy is often prolonged and physically challenging, it is crucial that the client understand the goals of treatment and how they will be measured. In cases of palliation, the client must weigh whether the adverse effects associated with treatment are worth the anticipated increase in the quality of life.

Clients who are undergoing chemotherapy usually receive several rounds of treatment spaced over a designated time, usually several weeks or months. This is because each round of chemotherapy kills a set percentage of cancer cells, usually those that are rapidly dividing at the time of treatment. Subsequent rounds kill additional cells. Another reason is that the chemotherapy always damages normal cells and can cause serious adverse effects. Clients need time to recover between treatments. For example, neutrophils are especially sensitive to chemotherapy and the clients' absolute neutrophil count will usually plummet after a therapy session. Intervals between treatments allow the body to make more neutrophils so that body defences are able to fight infections.

The **cell kill hypothesis** is a theoretical model that predicts the ability of antineoplastic drugs to eliminate cancer cells. This hypothesis predicts that a drug will kill a certain percentage, rather than a constant number, of cancer cells. Why is this important?

Theoretically, every single cell in a malignant tumour must be eliminated from the body to cure a client. Leaving even a single malignant cell could result in regrowth of the tumour. However, eliminating every cancer cell is a very difficult task. As an example, consider that a small, 1-cm breast tumour may already contain 1 billion cancer cells before it can be detected during a manual examination. A drug that is able to kill 99% of these cells would be considered a very effective drug indeed. Yet even with this fantastic achievement, 10 million cancer cells would remain, any one of which could potentially cause the tumour to return and kill the client. The relationship between cell kill and chemotherapy is illustrated in Figure 59.3. It is likely that no antineoplastic drug (or combination of drugs) has the ability to kill 100% of the tumour cells. However, the large burden of cancer cells may be lowered sufficiently to permit the client's immune system to control or eliminate the remaining cancer cells. Because the immune system is able to eliminate only a relatively small number of cancer cells, it is imperative that as many cancerous cells as possible be eliminated during treatment. This example reinforces the need to diagnose and treat tumours at an early stage when the number of cancer cells is smaller.

Because of their rapid cell division, tumour cells express a high mutation rate, which continually changes their genetic structure, resulting in a more heterogenous mass as the tumour grows. Essentially, the tumour becomes a mass of hundreds of different types of cancer cells with different growth rates and physiological properties. Administration of an antineoplastic drug may kill only a small portion of the tumour, leaving some clones unaffected and able to repopulate the tumour with resistant cells. The appearance

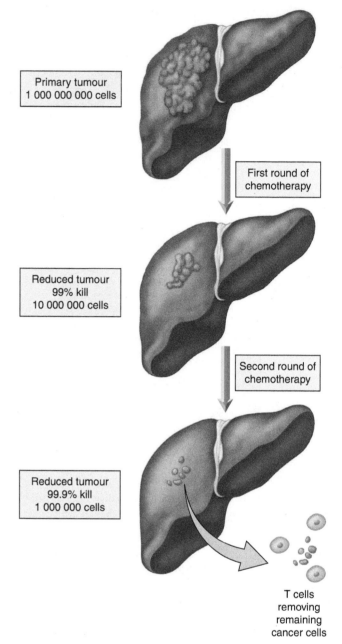

Primary tumour
1 000 000 000 cells

First round of chemotherapy

Reduced tumour
99% kill
10 000 000 cells

Second round of chemotherapy

Reduced tumour
99.9% kill
1 000 000 cells

T cells removing remaining cancer cells

Figure 59.3 Cell kill and chemotherapy.

of cancer cells that are resistant to antineoplastic drugs complicates the chances for a pharmacological cure because a therapy that was very successful in reducing the tumour mass at the start of chemotherapy may become less effective over time.

Improving the Success of Chemotherapy

59.7 Use of multiple drugs and intermittent dosing are strategies that allow for greater success of chemotherapy.

As has been seen throughout this text, the majority of pharmacotherapy is conducted with a single drug given in a constant amount over a specified time period. For most indications, the use of multiple drugs increases the expense of treatment and can cause additional adverse effects. Cancer chemotherapy is an important exception: the concurrent use of multiple drugs, combined with intermittent dosing, results in improved client outcomes.

Combination Chemotherapy

Chemotherapy is conducted using established protocols that are specific to the type of cancer and its stage. A cancer treatment protocol describes the specific combination of antineoplastics that will be given, their doses, and the cycles in which they will be administered. Using multiple drugs affects the different stages of the cancer cell's life cycle and attacks the various clones within the tumour via several mechanisms of action, thus increasing the percentage of cell kill. Combination chemotherapy also allows for lower dosages of each individual agent, thereby reducing toxicity and slowing the development of resistance. Examples of established protocols using combination therapy include cyclo-phosphamide-methotrexate-fluorouracil for breast cancer and cyclophosphamide-adriamycin-vincristine for lung cancer. Each type of cancer has its own individual protocol, which was established through clinical trials. These protocols are being refined and revised continually based on current research.

Dosing Schedules

Most chemotherapeutic medications are administered intermittently using specific dosing schedules that have been determined through research to increase the effectiveness of the antineoplastic agents. For example, some of the anticancer drugs are given as a single dose or perhaps as several doses over a few days. A few weeks may pass before the next series of doses begins. This gives normal cells time to recover from the adverse effects of the drugs and allows tumour cells that may not have been replicating at the time of the first dose to begin dividing and become more sensitive to the next round of chemotherapy. Sometimes the optimum dosing schedule must be delayed until the client sufficiently recovers from the drug toxicities, especially bone marrow suppression. Delays or reductions in the planned dosages are likely to negatively affect treatment outcomes. The specific dosing schedule chosen depends on the type of tumour, stage of the disease, and overall condition of the client.

Route of Administration

Antineoplastic agents are available for administration by virtually any route. Whenever possible, the oral (PO) route is used because it is most acceptable to the client and eliminates risks associated with intravenous (IV) administration, such as phlebitis or tissue necrosis. Antineoplastics may be given locally by topical application to the lesion or through direct instillation into the tumour region. Regional administration causes less systemic toxicity. The most common route for delivering antineoplastics is via the venous system.

Oral The PO route is the easiest, most convenient, and least expensive route for chemotherapy administration. Clients can self-administer their PO chemotherapy medications at home. One problem associated with PO administration is the inconsistency of absorption. Chemotherapeutic agents that are administered PO produce many of the same adverse reactions as the injectable agents, and the client and caregivers must be aware of these. They must also be taught safe handling and disposal of these drugs. Examples of antineoplastics available as PO preparations include

methotrexate, mercaptopurine (Purinethol), cyclophosphamide, and melphalan (Alkeran).

Intravenous IV is the most common route for delivery of chemotherapy agents. One advantage to the IV route is that a constant and consistent serum level of the drug can be obtained by fine adjustments to the infusion rate. A disadvantage is that **sclerosing**, or abnormal tissue hardening of the veins, may occur during prolonged administration. Another disadvantage to the client is that chemotherapy administration is done in a cancer centre, healthcare provider's office, or some other place away from the client's home. This may require many kilometres of commuting and present a hardship to the client and family. In addition, travelling out of the home may expose the client to viruses and other infectious agents, which can be hazardous to those with diminished immune function. In some geographic areas, an oncology nurse will come to the client's home and administer the chemotherapy.

Administration of chemotherapeutic agents can be done through a centrally located access device such as a Groshong catheter, which is inserted by being tunnelled under the skin on the chest into a major vein for long-term medication instillation, or through a peripheral vein via a **peripherally inserted central catheter (PICC) line**. A PICC line is a central catheter that is threaded into the vena cava for administration of chemotherapy. The advantages of a central line are that it is less likely to infiltrate and it is inserted in a large vein, which is less likely to become irritated during chemotherapy. A disadvantage of a central line is that it increases the client's risk for acquiring an infection.

Because IV administration requires a free-flowing IV in a large vein, it is imperative that the nurse constantly assesses the insertion site of the IV for signs of infiltration or phlebitis. Some antineoplastics can cause extreme cellular damage if the solution is allowed to enter surrounding tissues. Because of the potential for tissue damage, most antineoplastics are not administered by the intramuscular (IM) or subcutaneous routes. Examples of IV antineoplastics are carmustine (BiCNU), cisplatin, doxorubicin (Adriamycin), and mitomycin (Mutamycin).

Intrathecal Some antineoplastic medications may be delivered intrathecally into the subarachnoid space of the spinal cord. In intrathecal administration, the drug bypasses the blood-brain barrier and circulates with the cerebrospinal fluid (CSF) to expose central nervous system tumours to high concentrations of the drug. A specially trained individual must conduct the procedure because it requires a lumbar puncture or surgical placement of a reservoir or implanted pump for drug delivery. An advantage to intrathecal administration is that it provides a consistent drug level in the CSF. Potential adverse effects include headaches, confusion, lethargy, seizures, nausea, or vomiting, all of which are signs of increased intracranial pressure.

Intra-arterial Occasionally the healthcare provider may choose to administer chemotherapeutic medications through an artery. Intra-arterial administration requires a surgical procedure for catheter placement and, often, special x-ray techniques. In most cases, a catheter is passed via the femoral or brachial artery so that its end lies close to the blood supply of the tumour. Injection delivers a high dose of drug directly to the tumour site. Although the drug subsequently distributes via the circulation to other tissues, the tumour area receives the highest dose.

Intraperitoneal Intraperitoneal administration via a catheter or port is used to deliver antineoplastic drugs directly to intra-abdominal metastases. The drug is slowly absorbed into the systemic circulation, or it may be drained out of the peritoneum via a catheter after a few hours of treatment. A disadvantage of this method is that it requires the placing of a Tenckhoff catheter, which is a specialized catheter. One end placed into the peritoneum and the other end with an external port provides an access area into which medication is instilled.

Intravesicular The intravesicular route instills high doses of antineoplastics into the urinary bladder via a Foley catheter to treat tumours of the bladder mucosa. Only small amounts of the drugs are absorbed systemically. The client retains the drug for a specified period, after which it is voided or removed via catheter.

Toxicity of Antineoplastic Agents

59.8 Serious toxicity limits therapy with most antineoplastic agents.

Although cancer cells are clearly abnormal in structure and function, much of their physiology is identical to that of normal cells. Because it is difficult to kill cancer cells selectively without profoundly affecting normal cells, all antineoplastic drugs have the potential to cause serious toxicity. These drugs are often pushed to their maximum dosages to obtain the greatest tumour cell kill. These high dosages always result in adverse effects in the client, some of which are listed in Table 59.4. Because antineoplastic agents primarily affect cells with a high growth fraction, normal cells that are replicating, such as cells in the hair follicles, GI tract, and hematological system, are most susceptible to adverse effects.

Hematological System

Erythrocytes, leukocytes, and platelets have relatively short lifespans and must be continually replaced by hematopoietic stem cells residing in the bone marrow. Stem cells may be destroyed by antineoplastic agents, resulting in bone marrow suppression (myelosuppression). Myelosuppression is the most common dose-limiting adverse effect of chemotherapy and the one that most often causes discontinuation or delays of chemotherapy. Severe bone marrow suppression is a contraindication to therapy with most antineoplastic drugs.

Chemotherapy causes erythrocyte, leukocyte, and platelet counts to decrease until they reach their lowest value, known as the **nadir**. Clients are most susceptible to the symptoms, such as anemia, infections, or bleeding, during the nadir. Following the nadir, blood counts begin their recovery back to normal values. The nadir is specific for each chemotherapeutic agent and for each type of blood cell. For example, antimetabolites produce rapid nadirs for neutrophils in 7 to 14 days after the initiation of chemotherapy, with recovery within 7 to 21 days following the nadir. Other agents such as the nitrosoureas produce a delayed nadir for neutrophils at 26 to 63 days, with recovery at 35 to 89 days after the nadir.

Neutrophils are the type of white blood cells (WBCs) most affected by chemotherapy. This is primarily because the normal lifespan of a neutrophil is only 7 to 12 hours, and without continual replacement by stem cells the number of circulating neutrophils quickly falls. A client is diagnosed with neutropenia when the neutrophil count is less than 1500 cells/mL. Clients are very susceptible to infections while they are neutropenic. Many times clients who are neutropenic are placed in reverse isolation to protect them from exposure to any infections from family members or healthcare providers. Even an infection from a mild cold could be fatal to clients with extremely low neutrophil counts. If a client who is neutropenic and receiving chemotherapy acquires an infection, an increase in WBCs may not be evident. If a client who is neutropenic does develop a fever, this may be an indication of sepsis, and antibiotics are indicated.

Medications such as colony-stimulating factors (filgrastim [Neupogen] and sargramostim [Leukine]) are sometimes administered to accelerate recovery of suppressed bone marrow cells and to increase the WBC count. The administration of these drugs shortens the time of neutropenia, thus lowering the risk of opportunistic infections and allowing the client to maintain an optimum chemotherapy dosing schedule. Filgrastim is presented as a prototype drug in Chapter 57.

Because the lifespan of a platelet is only 7 to 8 days, these blood elements require constant replenishment by bone marrow stem cells. A client is diagnosed with thrombocytopenia when the platelet count is less than 100 000 per millilitre of blood. Chemotherapy is often delayed if this occurs. In clients who are receiving chemotherapy, thrombocytopenia usually occurs concurrently with neutropenia. Thrombocytopenia can cause the client to exhibit abnormal bleeding, with symptoms ranging from bruising to petechiae to serious hemorrhage. Bleeding precautions must be implemented if the platelet count falls below 50 000 per millilitre

TABLE 59.4 Examples of Adverse Effects of Anticancer Drugs

Common Expected Adverse Effects	Drug-Specific Adverse Effects	Dose-Limiting Adverse Effects
Nausea and vomiting	Fetal malformations (pemetrexed, methotrexate, mercaptopurine)	Bone marrow suppression
Stomatitis	Peripheral-sensory neuropathy (cisplatin)	Acute renal failure
Anorexia	Sterility (mechlorethamine)	Pulmonary fibrosis
Alopecia	Cardiotoxicity (doxorubicin, daunorubicin)	Diarrhea
Immunosuppression		
Fatigue		

of blood. To prevent the platelet count from decreasing to a harmful level, platelet infusions may be necessary. Oprelvekin (Neumega) is a thrombopoietic growth factor that may be administered to increase platelet production.

Because erythrocytes have a longer lifespan (90 to 120 days) than neutrophils or platelets, reductions in red blood cells (RBCs), or anemia, occur later in the course of chemotherapy. Hemoglobin carries oxygen to all tissues in the body; therefore, anemia may affect every system in the body. An infusion of RBCs may be required to increase a client's RBC count and hemoglobin value. A medication that the nurse may administer to help increase the number of RBCs is epoetin alfa (Epogen, Eprex), which is presented as a prototype in Chapter 57. When assessing for anemia, it should be remembered that the etiology may be the result of non-chemotherapy–related causes, such as bleeding, iron deficiency, or kidney damage.

Gastrointestinal Tract

The vomiting centre in the medulla is triggered by many antineoplastics. Acute nausea and vomiting often begin within minutes of chemotherapy administration and may last for 24 hours. Delayed nausea and vomiting begin 24 hours after chemotherapy and may continue for up to 6 days. Anticipatory nausea and vomiting may occur before chemotherapy because the client may be expecting an unpleasant experience. Antineoplastics are sometimes classified by their **emetic potential**. Before starting therapy with the highest emetic potential agents, clients may be pre-treated with antiemetic drugs such as ondansetron (Zofran), prochlorperazine (Stemetil), or lorazepam (Ativan). It is not uncommon to administer several different antiemetic medications that have several modes of action. Antiemetic medications are presented in detail in Chapter 35.

NCLEX Success Tip

Antiemetics work best when given continuously rather than as needed and should be administered 30 to 60 minutes before the initiation of chemotherapy to effectively counteract nausea.

The epithelial lining of the GI tract is very sensitive to the effects of chemotherapeutic agents. The GI mucosa commonly becomes inflamed, a condition known as **mucositis**. Consequences of mucositis include painful ulcerations in the mouth and esophagus, difficulty eating or swallowing, GI bleeding, intestinal infections, or severe diarrhea. Some research has shown that eating popsicles during chemotherapy infusions can decrease the severity of mucositis. The nurse may also instruct the client to eat a bland diet and to use a soft toothbrush for oral care. Some healthcare providers may order a "medical cocktail," which may include lidocaine viscous (Xylocaine), liquid diphenhydramine (Benedryl), and sucralfate to decrease the pain associated with the mucositis. The client should also be instructed to report any signs of thrush, which is an oral yeast infection.

Most clients who are receiving antineoplastics experience anorexia, usually due to a combination of nausea, vomiting, and mucositis. At times the client's appetite is decreased such that tube feedings or parenteral feedings may be indicated. The body needs sufficient nutrients and calories for normal cells to repopulate and for repair of body tissues. When assessing for anorexia, it should be remembered that this symptom may be the result of direct

effects from the tumour itself or from associated psychological changes such as depression or anxiety.

The client may experience constipation or diarrhea depending on the specific drugs administered. Some chemotherapeutic medications damage the intestinal lining, inhibiting the reabsorption of fluids and producing loose stools. Replacement of fluids and electrolytes as well as treatment with an antidiarrheal drug may be indicated. Some chemotherapeutic medications decrease the motility of the GI tract, resulting in greater reabsorption of fluids, which leads to constipation. When assessing for constipation, it should be remembered that other common reasons for this symptom include therapy with opioid analgesics and inadequate water and fibre intake.

Many clients with cancer experience a general wasting of muscle and other tissues referred to as **cachexia**. Cachexia may be caused by toxic effects from the cancer itself or from its treatment. Symptoms from the chemotherapy such as anorexia, mucositis, nausea, and vomiting may contribute to cachexia, but other non-GI factors such as serious chronic pain, depression, and fatigue also contribute.

Cardiopulmonary System

Some of the chemotherapeutic medications can be toxic to the heart and lungs. For example, doxorubicin (Adriamycin) is specifically known for its cardiotoxicity and the nurse should monitor the client for any changes in the electrocardiogram (ECG) and assess for any signs of heart failure. This adverse effect can be serious enough to later cause the client to need cardiac monitoring or a heart transplant. A cardioprotective drug such as dexrazoxane (Zinecard) is administered just prior to a doxorubicin infusion to prevent permanent heart damage.

Bleomycin (Blenoxane) is specifically known for causing pneumonitis in clients. Nursing care of the client who is receiving bleomycin should include monitoring the client's pulse oximeter and respiratory status. Auscultating crackles in the lung fields may be a sign of a developing pneumonitis. Chest x-rays may be necessary two to three times per week to assess for lung changes.

Urinary System

Some of the chemotherapeutic medications can exhibit considerable nephrotoxicity. For example, cisplatin can lead to kidney failure if the dosage limit is exceeded. When administering chemotherapeutic agents that are nephrotoxic, the nurse should closely monitor intake and output and urine dipstick results for RBCs. The client should remain well hydrated during the treatment to help prevent renal damage. Diuretics may be administered to help balance the intake and output of the client. In addition, the drug mesna is administered to prevent hemorrhagic cystitis during chemotherapy with cyclophosphamide or ifosfamide (Ifex).

Reproductive System

Some antineoplastics, particularly the alkylating agents, affect the gonads and have been associated with infertility in both males and females. If a woman is pregnant while receiving treatment, the fetus may be severely damaged due to the high growth fraction of the fetus's cells or it may be killed during the treatment. Sexually active male and female clients should be instructed to use reliable contraception while receiving chemotherapy and for 3 to 6 months following treatment.

Antineoplastic medications are more likely to cause permanent sterility in men than in women. Some clients choose to have their sperm or eggs harvested prior to treatment in case the chemotherapy does affect their fertility.

Many hospitals have protocols specifying that female nurses and pharmacists not handle chemotherapeutic agents if they are pregnant or are trying to become pregnant due to the toxic effects that the chemotherapy may have on the fetus.

Nervous System

Several chemotherapeutic agents are toxic to the nervous system. For instance, vincristine may cause muscle weakness and peripheral neuritis. It is important for the nurse to assess the client's neurological status frequently when administering this medication. Clients should also be informed of the potential adverse effects so that they may inform the nurse of any tingling or pain in their extremities or if changes occur in muscle strength.

Cisplatin has been known to cause hearing loss and deafness in some clients. The nurse should assess the client's hearing throughout the course of treatment and document any changes noted in the client's ability to hear.

Skin and Soft Tissue

Many antineoplastics are classified as **vesicants**, agents that can cause serious tissue injury if they escape from an artery or vein during an infusion or injection. Extravasation or infiltration from an injection site can produce severe tissue and nerve damage, local infection, and even loss of a limb. If a nurse is concerned that a peripheral IV is no longer working properly, the IV should not be used for chemotherapy administration. Although rare, extravasation can still occur with a central line, so the nurse should continue to frequently assess the insertion site of a central line while administering chemotherapy. Rapid treatment of extravasation is necessary to limit tissue damage, and certain antineoplastics have specific antidotes.

Other Effects

Fatigue is a common complaint during chemotherapy. The precise cause of the fatigue is often difficult to determine. If the client has anemia, the lack of hemoglobin to carry oxygen to the tissue can cause the client to feel fatigued. The client may be experiencing anxiety or depression due to the diagnosis of cancer, which may lead to sleep deprivation. The process of cellular regeneration after chemotherapy treatments may also cause feelings of fatigue. A nutritional consultation may be helpful in determining if the fatigue has a nutritional origin. Coping strategies for dealing with stress and scheduled periods of rest may benefit the client.

CONNECTIONS ◖ **Special Considerations**

◀ **General Guidelines for Extravasation**

- Stop infusion immediately.
- Leave the cannula in place to enable aspiration of infiltrated drug and administration of antidote through the cannula.
- Elevate limb to reduce swelling.
- Do not apply pressure.
- Follow agency policies regarding further interventions.
- Cold compresses applied for 20 minutes may be recommended to reduce tissue injury.
- Warm compresses may be recommended for alkaloid extravasation to increase blood flow to the area and enhance drug absorption.

Source: Oncology Nursing Society. (2014). *Chemotherapy and biotherapy guidelines and recommendations for practice* (4th ed.). Pittsburgh, PA: Oncology Nursing Society.

Hair follicles are damaged by many chemotherapeutic agents, resulting in hair loss or **alopecia**. Hair loss usually begins within 1 to 2 weeks of the first treatment, and regrowth may take 3 to 5 months after the last chemotherapeutic treatment. The potential for alopecia should be discussed with clients before treatment begins so that they may choose to wear a hat, bandana, wig, or other accessory.

One of the ironies of chemotherapy is that the medications that are given to kill the cancer may cause a secondary cancer to develop elsewhere in the body. This is not a common adverse effect, but it has been clearly demonstrated in clients. The secondary malignancy usually occurs many years after the initial cancer; therefore, this adverse effect is of most concern to children being treated with chemotherapy. It is estimated that pediatric cancer survivors have a 10 to 20 times greater risk than other children for developing a secondary malignancy. The most common secondary malignancy is nonlymphocytic leukemia.

Hyperuricemia is most frequently associated with chemotherapy for lymphomas and leukemias due to the rapid cell kill. A client is diagnosed with hyperuricemia when uric acid levels in the blood are elevated, which can lead to renal failure if the uric crystals deposit in the renal tubules. Signs of hyperuricemia are nausea, vomiting, and oliguria. Keeping the client well hydrated helps to preserve renal function by flushing microscopic crystals out of the kidney before they have a chance to form larger crystals. The nurse who is caring for a client who is suspected of developing or has been diagnosed with hyperuricemia should monitor the client's intake and output closely.

CHAPTER
59 Understanding the Chapter

Key Concepts Summary

The numbered key concepts provide a succinct summary of the important points from the corresponding numbered section within the chapter. If any of these points are not clear, refer to the numbered section within the chapter for review.

59.1 Cancer is characterized by rapid, uncontrolled growth of cells that eventually invade normal tissues and metastasize.

59.2 The etiology of cancer may be chemical, physical, or biological.

59.3 The three primary goals of chemotherapy are cure, control, and palliation.

59.4 Cancers are described by their stage and grade.

59.5 Many antineoplastic drugs are more effective when given at specific stages of the cell cycle and in tumours with a high growth fraction.

59.6 The goal of chemotherapy is to kill as many cancer cells as possible while sparing normal cells.

59.7 Use of multiple drugs and intermittent dosing are strategies that allow for greater success of chemotherapy.

59.8 Serious toxicity limits therapy with most antineoplastic agents.

Chapter 59 Scenario

Cheryl Ogen is a 39-year-old client who is employed as a kindergarten teacher. She has been married for 15 years and has never had any children. Her medical history confirms that both her mother and her maternal grandmother died from breast cancer. Now Cheryl has been diagnosed with breast cancer. She is admitted to the hospital for tumour resection and chemotherapy. Cheryl's breast cancer is stage T1, N0, M0, and G2. Cheryl has undergone the lumpectomy with regional lymph node biopsy and is now about to begin chemotherapy.

Critical Thinking Questions

1. Cheryl would like to know why she is receiving chemotherapy after the surgeon has removed the cancerous tumour. What would you tell her?

2. Why is it important to understand the staging and grading system used with cancer? How would you interpret the staging and grading of Cheryl's cancer?

3. Identify some of the hematological changes that Cheryl may experience while receiving chemotherapy.

See Answers to Critical Thinking Questions in Appendix B.

NCLEX Practice Questions

1 The healthcare provider has written in the client's chart that the cancer is at stage I. The nurse knows that the implications for this staging are that

a. The cancer is advanced and the client has a poor prognosis.

b. The cancerous cells are only moderately differentiated from the parent cells.

c. The cancer has been detected at an early stage.

d. The tumour is large and invading surrounding tissue.

2 Which of the following statements by a client undergoing chemotherapy would be of concern to the nurse? Select all that apply.

a. "I attended a meeting of a cancer support group this week."

b. "My husband and I are planning a short trip next week."

c. "I try to eat six small meals plus two protein shakes each day."

d. "I am taking my 15-month-old granddaughter to the pediatrician next week for her baby shots."

e. "I am going to go shopping at the mall next week."

3 The nurse determines that the client understands an important principle of chemotherapy when the client makes which statement?

a. "The use of multiple chemotherapy drugs affects different stages of the cancer cell's life cycle."

b. "Staging describes the process of determining how responsive the cancer is to the prescribed chemotherapy."

c. "Antineoplastic drugs kill the entire tumour, including the clones, and prevent repopulation."

d. "Combination chemotherapy requires higher dosages of each individual agent and increases toxicity."

4 The nurse is collaborating with the interdisciplinary team regarding the care of a client with a brain tumour. The nurse knows that the most common reason subsequent rounds of chemotherapy may be delayed is due to which condition?

a. Myelosuppression

b. Alopecia

c. Mucositis

d. Cachexia

5 A client with cancer is started on a chemotherapeutic agent that is a known vesicant. The nurse performs which priority activity related to this drug?

a. Monitoring the client's response to antinausea drugs

b. Monitoring the client's intake of calcium-rich foods

c. Monitoring the client's respiratory status for cough

d. Monitoring the client's IV port site for redness, swelling, and pain

See Answers to NCLEX Practice Questions in Appendix A.

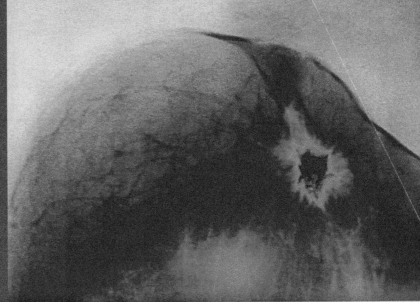

BSIP SA/Alamy Stock Photo

CHAPTER 60

Pharmacotherapy of Neoplasia

LEARNING OUTCOMES

After reading this chapter, the student should be able to:

1. Identify the three primary therapies for cancer.

2. Explain the therapeutic action of each class of antineoplastic (anticancer) drug in relation to the differences between normal cells and cancer cells.

3. Explain the significance of the rate of cancer cell growth and the cell cycle to the success of chemotherapy.

4. Explain how combination therapy and special dosing protocols increase the effectiveness of chemotherapy.

5. Discuss the role of the nurse in reducing risk of cancer through client teaching.

6. For each of the drug classes listed in Prototype Drugs, identify a representative drug and explain its mechanism of action, therapeutic effects, and important adverse effects.

7. Describe and explain, based on pharmacological principles, the rationale for nursing assessment, planning, and interventions for clients who are receiving drug therapy for cancer.

8. Discuss safety precautions when handling and administering antineoplastics.

9. Discuss interventions in the event of infiltration of vesicant drugs.

10. Use the nursing process to care for clients who are receiving drug therapy for cancer.

CHAPTER OUTLINE

▸ Treatment of Cancer: Surgery, Radiation Therapy, and Chemotherapy

▸ Antineoplastic Agents

▸ Alkylating Agents

  ▸ Pharmacotherapy with Alkylating Agents

▸ Antimetabolites

  ▸ Pharmacotherapy with Antimetabolites

▸ Antitumour Antibiotics

  ▸ Pharmacotherapy with Antitumour Antibiotics

▸ Plant-Derived Antineoplastic Agents

  ▸ Pharmacotherapy with Plant-Derived Antineoplastic Agents

Many successes have been made in the diagnosis, understanding, and treatment of cancer. Some types of cancer are now curable, and therapies may give the client a longer, symptom-free life. This chapter examines the role of drugs in the treatment of cancer. Medications used to treat this disease are called anticancer drugs, antineoplastics, or cancer chemotherapy drugs.

Treatment of Cancer: Surgery, Radiation Therapy, and Chemotherapy

60.1 Cancer may be treated using surgery, radiation therapy, and chemotherapy.

There is a much greater possibility of a cure if cancer is treated in its early stages, when the **tumour** is small and localized to a single area. Once the cancer has spread to distant sites, curing it is much more difficult; therefore, it is important to diagnose the disease as early as possible. In an attempt to remove every cancer cell, three treatment approaches are used: surgery, radiation therapy, and chemotherapy.

Surgery is performed to remove a tumour that is localized to one area or when the tumour is pressing on nerves, the airway, or other vital tissues. Surgery lowers the number of cancer cells in the body so that radiation and pharmacotherapy can be more successful. Surgery is not an option for tumours of blood cells or when it would not be expected to extend a client's lifespan or to improve the quality of life.

Radiation therapy is an effective non-surgical way to kill tumour cells; approximately 50% of clients with cancer receive radiation therapy as part of their treatment. High doses of ionizing radiation are aimed directly at the tumour and are confined to this area to the maximum extent possible. Radiation treatments may follow surgery to kill any cancer cells left behind following the operation. Radiation is sometimes given as **palliation** for inoperable cancers to shrink the size of a tumour that may be pressing on vital organs or to relieve pain, difficulty breathing, or difficulty swallowing.

Pharmacotherapy of cancer is called **chemotherapy**. Because drugs are transported through the blood, they have the potential to reach cancer cells in virtually every location in the body.

Some drugs can pass across the blood-brain barrier to treat brain tumours. Others are instilled directly into body cavities, such as the urinary bladder, to deliver the highest dose possible to the cancer cells without producing systemic side effects.

Anticancer drugs are sometimes given, in concert with surgery and radiation, to attempt a total cure or complete eradication of all tumour cells from the body. In other cases, the cancer is too advanced to expect a cure, and antineoplastic agents are given for palliation to reduce the size of the tumour. Palliation eases the severity of pain or discomfort and may extend the client's lifespan or improve quality of life. In a few cases, drugs are given as prophylaxis, with the goal of preventing cancer from occurring in clients at high risk for developing tumours.

Antineoplastic Agents

60.2 Serious toxicity—including thrombocytopenia; anemia; leukopenia; alopecia; and severe nausea, vomiting, and diarrhea—limits therapy with most antineoplastic agents.

Drugs used in cancer chemotherapy come from diverse pharmacological and chemical classes. Antineoplastics have been extracted from plants and bacteria, as well as created entirely in the laboratory. Some of the drug classes attack vital cellular macromolecules, such as DNA and proteins, while others interfere with vital metabolic pathways of rapidly growing cells. The common theme among all antineoplastic agents is that they kill or at least stop the growth of cancer cells.

Classification of the various antineoplastics is quite variable, as some of these drugs kill cancer cells by several different mechanisms and have characteristics from more than one class of drug. Furthermore, the mechanisms by which some antineoplastics act are not completely understood. A simple method of classifying this complex group of drugs includes the following seven categories:

1. Alkylating agents
2. Antimetabolites
3. Antitumour antibiotics

4. Hormones and hormone antagonists that have antineoplastic activity

5. Natural products that have antineoplastic activity

6. Biological response modifiers and targeted therapies

7. Miscellaneous anticancer drugs

ALKYLATING AGENTS

The first alkylating agents, the **nitrogen mustards**, were developed in secrecy as chemical warfare agents during World War II. Although the drugs in this class have quite different chemical structures, all share the common characteristic of forming bonds, or linkages, with DNA, a process called **alkylation**. Figure 60.1 illustrates the process of alkylation.

Pharmacotherapy with Alkylating Agents

60.3 Alkylating agents act by changing the structure of DNA in cancer cells. Some have a very broad spectrum of clinical activity.

Alkylation changes the shape of the DNA double helix and prevents the nucleic acid from completing normal cell division. Each alkylating agent attaches to DNA in a different manner; however, they collectively have the effect of killing or at least slowing the replication of tumour cells. Although the process of alkylation occurs independently of the cell cycle, the killing action does not occur until the cell begins to divide. The alkylating agents have a broad spectrum and are used against many types of malignancies. They are some of the most widely used antineoplastic drugs. These agents are listed in Table 60.1.

NCLEX Success Tips

Clients with nephrotic syndrome who are sensitive to steroids or have frequent relapses are candidates for therapy with cyclophosphamide (Procytox). Common adverse effects of this drug include decreased white blood cell (WBC) count, increased susceptibility to infections, cystitis (from bladder irritation when the drug accumulates in the bladder before excretion), and possibly hair loss and sterility.

Cystitis is a potential adverse effect of cyclophosphamide. The client should be monitored for pain on urination and hematuria.

An aminoglycoside may cause nephrotoxicity and ototoxicity when given concomitantly with cisplatin.

Blood cells are particularly sensitive to alkylating agents, and bone marrow suppression is the most important adverse effect of this class. Within days after administration, declines in erythrocytes, leukocytes, and platelets may be measured. Damaging

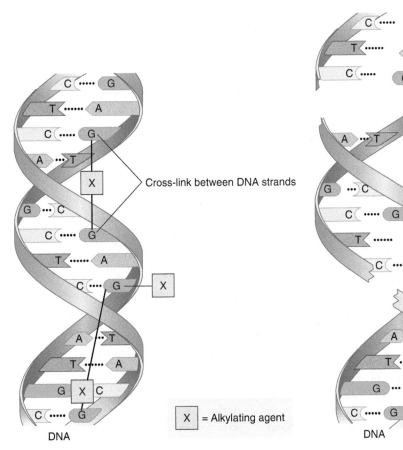

(a) Alkylation occuring during G₀ (resting) phase of cell cycle

Cross-link between DNA strands

X = Alkylating agent

DNA

(b) Strand breaks occuring when DNA replicates during S phase of cell cycle

DNA

Figure 60.1 Mechanism of action of the alkylating agents.

TABLE 60.1 Alkylating Agents

Drug	Route and Adult Dose
Nitrogen Mustards	
chlorambucil (Leukeran)	Chronic lymphocytic leukemia (CLL): Orally (PO), 0.15 mg/kg/day until WBC is 10 000/mm^3; interrupt treatment for 4 weeks, then resume at 0.1 mg/kg/day until desired response is achieved (generally 2 years) Hodgkin lymphoma: PO, 0.2 mg/kg/day for 4–8 weeks; for maintenance reduce dose or administer intermittently
Pr cyclophosphamide (Procytox)	PO, 1–5 mg/kg/day; IV, 40-50 mg/kg in divided doses over 2-5 days, or 10-15 mg/kg every 7-10 days, or 3-5 mg/kg twice weekly
estramustine (Emcyt)	PO, 14 mg/kg/day (typical range is 10–16 mg/kg/day) in 3-4 divided doses
ifosfamide (Ifex)	Intravenous (IV), 1.2 g/m^2 every day (qd) for 5 consecutive days every 3 weeks or after hematologic recovery
mechlorethamine (Mustargen)	IV, 6 mg/m^2 on days 1 and 8 of a 28-day cycle; malignant effusion, intracavitary, 0.4 mg/kg as a single dose
melphalan (Alkeran)	PO, 6 mg qd for 2–3 weeks
Nitrosoureas	
carmustine (BiCNU, Gliadel)	IV, 150-200 mg/m^2 every 6 weeks (q6wk) or 75-100 mg/m^2/day for 2 days q6wk
lomustine (CeeNU)	PO, 130 mg/m^2 as a single dose q6wk
streptozocin (Zanosar)	IV, 500 mg/m^2 for 5 consecutive days q6wk until max benefit or unacceptable toxicity is reached
Miscellaneous Alkylating Agents	
busulfan (Myleran, Busulfex)	PO, 4–8 mg/day
carboplatin	IV, 360 mg/m^2 once every 4 weeks (q4wk)
cisplatin	Bladder cancer: IV, 50-70 mg/m^2 q3wk-q4wk; ovarian cancer, metastatic: IV, 75-100 mg/m^2 q4wk; testicular cancer, metastatic: IV, 20 mg/m^2/day for 5 days repeated q3wk
dacarbazine	Hodgkin lymphoma, ABVD regimen: IV, 375 mg/m^2 on days 1 and 15 q4wk; metastatic malignant melanoma: IV, 250 mg/m^2 over 30 minutes qd on days 1 to 5 q3wk
temozolomide (Temodal)	PO/IV, start with 150 mg/m^2 qd for 5 consecutive days of a 28-day treatment cycle

effects on the epithelial cells lining the gastrointestinal (GI) tract are also common with alkylating agents.

Nursing Considerations

The role of the nurse in alkylating agent therapy involves careful monitoring of the client's condition and providing education as it relates to the prescribed drug treatment. Before starting any form of chemotherapy, assess baseline vital signs, complete blood count (CBC), and the client's overall health status, including renal and liver function, intake and output, and body weight. Alkylating agents must be administered with caution to clients with hepatic or renal impairment, recent steroid therapy, leukopenia, or thrombocytopenia.

Alkylating agents are highly toxic to tissues with a rapid growth rate. Bone marrow depression occurs because these agents kill normal hematopoietic cells. These drugs may cause injury to the GI mucosa and hair follicles. Mustard agents may cause skin eruptions such as blistering. Alkylating agents may depress spermatogenesis and oocyte production, and secondary leukemias are frequently associated with this class of drugs. Platinum alkylating agents (e.g., cisplatin) may cause high-frequency hearing loss.

Remain alert to the possible development of blood dyscrasias by observing the client for signs and symptoms such as bruising or bleeding and by closely monitoring the CBC with differential and platelet count. Clients of childbearing age should be informed of the potential adverse impact on fertility. Cyclophosphamide also diminishes sex drive. Clients should be encouraged to frankly discuss sexual issues with the nurse, especially regarding options to preserve fertility.

Alkylating agents range from pregnancy category D (streptozocin [Zanosar], cyclophosphamide) to category X (estramustine [Emcyt]). Both females and males should be counselled to abstain from coitus or to use reliable contraception during therapy and for 4 months thereafter. The nurse can assist the client in choosing an appropriate method for the client's cultural background, lifestyle, and health.

Client education as it relates to alkylating agents should include therapeutic goals; reasons for obtaining baseline data such as vital signs, blood work, and tests for cardiac and renal disorders; and possible side effects. The following are important points to include when teaching clients regarding alkylating agents:

- Sterility and amenorrhea may occur in clients on mechlorethamine or cyclophosphamide therapy, but these are reversible once therapy is discontinued.
- Obtain routine hearing screenings during therapy.
- Report any buzzing, ringing, or tingling sensation in the ears, or decreased hearing.
- Immediately report the following: tachycardia, fever, chills, sore throat, dyspnea, gout, kidney stones, skin rashes.

Refer to Nursing Process Focus: Clients Receiving Antineoplastic Therapy at the end of this chapter for additional teaching points.

PROTOTYPE DRUG **Cyclophosphamide (Procytox)**

Actions and Uses: Cyclophosphamide is a commonly prescribed nitrogen mustard. It is used alone, or in combination with other drugs, against a wide variety of cancers, including Hodgkin's disease, lymphoma, multiple myeloma, breast cancer, and ovarian cancer. Cyclophosphamide acts by attaching to DNA and disrupting replication, particularly in rapidly dividing cells. It is one of only a few anticancer drugs that are well absorbed when given orally. Because of its potent immunosuppressive properties, it has been used for certain non-neoplastic disorders such as prevention of transplant rejection and severe rheumatoid arthritis.

Administration Alerts:

- Dilute prior to IV administration.
- Monitor platelet count prior to intramuscular (IM) administration; if low, hold dose.
- To avoid GI upset, take with meals or divide doses.
- Cyclophosphamide is pregnancy category D.

Pharmacokinetics: Cyclophosphamide is administered IV or PO. It is well absorbed from the GI tract. The inactive parent drug is metabolized into active drug in the liver. It is widely distributed, crosses the placenta, and enters breast milk, and some drug crosses the blood-brain barrier. About 30% is excreted unchanged in urine. Half-life is 4 to 6.5 hours.

Adverse Effects and Interactions: The powerful immunosuppressant effects of cyclophosphamide peak 1 to 2 days after administration. Leukocyte counts sometimes serve as a guide to dosage adjustments during therapy. Thrombocytopenia is common, though less severe than with many other alkylating agents. Nausea, vomiting, anorexia, and diarrhea are frequently experienced. Cyclophosphamide damages hair follicles to cause **alopecia**, though this effect is usually reversible. Several metabolites of cyclophosphamide may cause hemorrhagic cystitis if the urine becomes concentrated; clients should be advised to maintain high fluid intake during therapy. Unlike other nitrogen mustards, cyclophosphamide exhibits little neurotoxicity.

Cyclophosphamide interacts with many drugs. For example, immunosuppressant agents used concurrently may increase risk for infections and further development of **neoplasms**. There is an increased chance of bone marrow toxicity if cyclophosphamide is used concurrently with allopurinol (Zyloprim). If anticoagulants are used concurrently, increased anticoagulant effects may occur, leading to hemorrhage.

If used concurrently with digoxin (Lanoxin, Toloxin), decreased serum levels of digoxin occur. Concurrent use with insulin may lead to increased hypoglycemia. Phenobarbital (Phenobarb), phenytoin (Dilantin), or glucocorticoids used concurrently may lead to an increased rate of cyclophosphamide metabolism by the liver. Thiazide diuretics used concurrently lead to increased possibility of leukopenia.

Use with caution with herbal supplements, such as echinacea, which is an immune stimulator and may interfere with the drug's immunosuppressant effects.

ANTIMETABOLITES

Antimetabolites are drugs that are chemically similar to essential building blocks of the cell. They are structurally similar to certain critical cell molecules. They interfere with aspects of the nutrient or nucleic acid metabolism of rapidly growing tumour cells.

Pharmacotherapy with Antimetabolites

60.4 Antimetabolites act by disrupting critical pathways in cancer cells, such as folate or DNA metabolism.

Rapidly growing cancer cells require large quantities of nutrients and other chemicals to construct proteins and nucleic acids. When cancer cells treated with antimetabolites attempt to synthesize proteins, RNA, or DNA, they use the antimetabolites instead of normal cellular precursors. By disrupting metabolic pathways in this manner, antimetabolites can kill cancer cells or slow their growth. These agents are prescribed for leukemias and solid tumours and are listed in Table 60.2.

Some antimetabolites become incorporated into the DNA of cancer cells and interfere with DNA replication and function. Others inhibit the enzymes that synthesize the vital components of the cell. All antimetabolites are cell cycle specific, with most of them affecting the S phase, although some can act during any of the active phases of the cell cycle. The three classes of antimetabolites are the folic acid analogues, the purine analogues, and the pyrimidine analogues.

The purine and pyrimidine analogues resemble the natural precursors for nucleic acid biosynthesis. For example, the pyrimidine analogue fluorouracil is able to block the formation of thymidylate, an essential chemical needed to make DNA; it is used in treating various solid tumours. After becoming activated and incorporated into DNA, cytarabine (Cytosar) blocks DNA synthesis; it is an important drug in forcing remission of acute myelocytic leukemia. Figure 60.2 illustrates the structural similarities of some antimetabolites to their natural counterparts.

NCLEX Success Tip

Antimetabolites act during the S phase of the cell cycle, contributing to cell destruction or preventing cell replication. They're most effective against rapidly proliferating cancers. Meiotic inhibitors interfere with cell division or mitosis during the M phase of the cell cycle. Meiotic spindle poisons are cell cycle specific in the M phase. Alkylating agents affect all rapidly proliferating cells by interfering with DNA; they may kill dividing cells in all phases of the cell cycle and may also kill nondividing cells. Antitumour antibiotics are cell cycle nonspecific; they interfere with DNA synthesis by binding with the DNA. They also prevent ribonucleic acid synthesis. Other cell cycle–nonspecific drugs include nitrosoureas and hormonal agents. Drugs that are cell cycle specific in the S phase include topoisomerase I inhibitors and antimetabolites.

TABLE 60.2 Antimetabolites

Drug	Route and Adult Dose
Folic Acid Antagonist	
Pr methotrexate	PO, 10–30 mg/day for 5 days; may repeat for 3-5 courses
Pyrimidine Analogs	
capecitabine (Xeloda)	PO, 1250 mg/m² twice daily (bid) for 2 weeks; then every 21 days
cytarabine (Cytosar)	IV, 100 mg/m²/day continuous infusion for 7 days, or 200 mg/m²/day continuous infusion (as 100 mg/m² over 12 hours every 12 hours) for 7 days
fluorouracil	IV, 12 mg/kg qd for 4 consecutive days
gemcitabine (Gemzar)	IV, 1000–1250 mg/m² over 30 minutes on specific days within the cycle every 21-28 days
Purine Analogues	
cladribine	IV, 0.09 mg/kg/day as a continuous infusion for 7 days for 1 cycle
fludarabine (Fludara)	IV, 25 mg/m² qd for 5 days every 28 days; PO, 40 mg/m² qd for 5 days every 28 days
mercaptopurine (Purinethol)	PO, 1.5–2.5 mg/kg qd
thioguanine (Lanvis)	PO, 2 mg/kg qd for 4 weeks

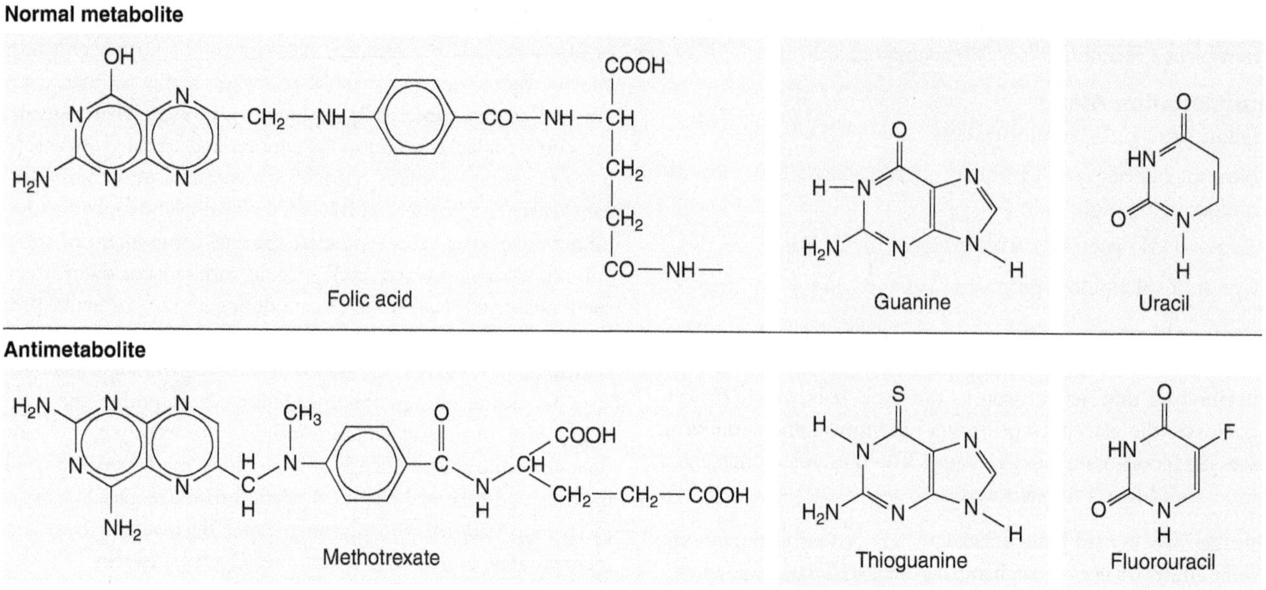

Normal metabolite

Antimetabolite

Figure 60.2 Structural similarities between antimetabolites and their natural counterparts.

Nursing Considerations

The role of the nurse in antimetabolite therapy involves careful monitoring of the client's condition and providing education as it relates to the prescribed drug treatment. Before initiating chemotherapy, assess baseline vital signs, CBC, and the client's overall health status, including renal and liver function, intake and output, and body weight.

Many antimetabolites are contraindicated in pregnancy; for example, methotrexate is a category X drug and pregnancy should be avoided for at least 6 months following termination of therapy. Further contraindications include hepatic, cardiac, and renal insufficiency; myelosuppression; and blood dyscrasias. Clients with peptic ulcer, ulcerative colitis, or poor nutritional status should be monitored closely. Antimetabolites cause many of the adverse effects common to other antineoplastics, including alopecia, fatigue, nausea, vomiting, diarrhea, bone marrow depression, and blood dyscrasias. These drugs may also cause photosensitivity and idiosyncratic pneumonitis.

Observe the client for signs and symptoms of respiratory infection, including shortness of breath, cough, fever, and especially rash or chest pain (pleurisy). Viral infections such as those from herpesviruses, including varicella-zoster, can be especially virulent when experienced during antimetabolite therapy. Immunizations, especially attenuated vaccines, should be avoided during this time due to drug-induced impaired immunity. Clients should be encouraged to regularly practise deep breathing, if necessary, with the aid of an incentive spirometer.

Client education as it relates to antimetabolites should include goals of therapy; reasons for obtaining baseline data such as vital signs, tests for immune, lung, and renal disorders, and blood work; and possible side effects. The following are important points to include when teaching clients regarding antimetabolites:

- Avoid immunizations and people with active infections.
- Regularly practise deep-breathing exercises.

- Eliminate or reduce respiratory irritants in the environment such as secondhand tobacco smoke and aerosol cosmetics (e.g., hair spray and deodorant).
- Immediately report the following: shortness of breath, chest pain, cough, fever, rash, dizziness, bruising, or bleeding.

Refer to Nursing Process Focus: Clients Receiving Antineoplastic Therapy at the end of this chapter for additional teaching points.

NCLEX Success Tips

Because some over-the-counter (OTC) vitamin supplements contain folic acid, the nurse should instruct the client to avoid self-medication with vitamins while taking methotrexate, a folic acid antagonist. Because methotrexate is hepatotoxic, the nurse should instruct the client to avoid drinking alcohol, which could increase the risk for hepatotoxicity. Methotrexate is a chemotherapy that can cause bone marrow depression and increases the risk for infection. The nurse should teach the client to perform meticulous mouth care to minimize the risk of infection. Contraception should be used during methotrexate therapy and for 8 weeks after the therapy has been discontinued because of its effect on mitosis. Methotrexate is teratogenic.

PROTOTYPE DRUG | Methotrexate

Actions and Uses: Methotrexate inhibits folic acid (vitamin B_9) metabolism. By blocking the synthesis of folic acid, methotrexate is able to inhibit replication, particularly in rapidly dividing cells. It is prescribed alone or in combination with other drugs for choriocarcinoma, osteogenic sarcoma, leukemias, head and neck cancers, breast carcinoma, and lung carcinoma. It is occasionally used to treat non-neoplastic disorders such as severe psoriasis and rheumatoid arthritis that have not responded to other medications.

Administration Alerts:
- Avoid skin exposure to the drug. Avoid inhaling drug particles.
- Dilute prior to IV administration.
- Methotrexate is pregnancy category X.

Pharmacokinetics: Methotrexate is administered IV or PO. It is well absorbed from the GI tract. It is widely distributed, crosses the placenta, and enters breast milk. Subtherapeutic amounts cross the blood-brain barrier. It is excreted mostly unchanged in urine. Half-life increases with dose and ranges from 3 to 15 hours.

Adverse Effects and Interactions: The adverse effects of methotrexate appear primarily in rapidly dividing tissues such as the GI epithelium and stem cells in the bone marrow. A potent immunosuppressant, methotrexate can result in fatal bone marrow toxicity at high doses. Leucovorin, a reduced form of folic acid, is sometimes administered with methotrexate to "rescue" normal cells or protect against severe bone marrow damage. Urine may be alkalinized to help protect the kidneys from toxicity. Hemorrhage and bruising are often observed due to low platelet counts. Nausea, vomiting, and anorexia are common. Although rare, pulmonary toxicity may develop and be quite serious.

Methotrexate interacts with several drugs. Bone marrow suppressants such as chemotherapeutic agents or radiation therapy may cause increased effects; the client will require a lower dose of methotrexate.

In concurrent use with nonsteroidal anti-inflammatory drugs (NSAIDs), methotrexate may lead to severe methotrexate toxicity. Acetylsalicylic acid (ASA [Aspirin]) may interfere with excretion of methotrexate, leading to increased serum levels and toxicity. Concurrent administration with live oral vaccine may result in decreased antibody response and increased adverse reactions to the vaccine.

Use with caution with herbal supplements, such as echinacea, which may interfere with the drug's immunosuppressant effects.

ANTITUMOUR ANTIBIOTICS

The antitumour antibiotics class of drug contains antibiotics, obtained from bacteria, that have the ability to kill cancer cells. They are not widely used but are very effective against certain tumours.

Pharmacotherapy with Antitumour Antibiotics

60.5 Due to their cytotoxicity, a few antibiotics are used to treat cancer by inhibiting cell growth. They have a narrow spectrum of clinical activity.

Antitumour properties have been identified in a number of substances isolated from microorganisms. These chemicals are more cytotoxic than the traditional antibiotics, and their use is restricted to treating a few specific types of cancer. For example, the only indication for idarubicin (Idamycin) is acute myelogenous leukemia. The antitumour antibiotics are listed in Table 60.3.

NCLEX Success Tip

Dactinomycin (Cosmegen) causes nausea and vomiting. Oral fluids are encouraged, and antiemetics are given to prevent dehydration.

The antitumour antibiotics bind to DNA and affect its function by a mechanism similar to that of the alkylating agents. Because of this, their general actions and side effects are similar to those of the alkylating agents. Unlike the alkylating agents, however, the antitumour antibiotics must be administered intravenously or through direct instillation via a catheter into a body cavity.

The antitumour antibiotics are divided into two groups: anthracyclines and nonanthracyclines. The anthracyclines include doxorubicin (Adriamycin), daunorubicin (Cerubidine), epirubicin (Ellence), idarubicin, and mitoxantrone. The anthracyclines are closely related in structure, and all exhibit cardiotoxicity, a major limiting adverse effect. Cardiotoxicity may occur within minutes of administration, or it may be delayed for months or years after chemotherapy has been completed. The nonanthracyclines, which include bleomycin (Blenoxane), dactinomycin, and mitomycin (Mutamycin), tend to cause less cardiotoxicity than the anthracyclines.

Nursing Considerations

The role of the nurse in antitumour antibiotic therapy involves careful monitoring of the client's condition and providing education as it relates to the prescribed drug treatment. Before initiating

TABLE 60.3 Antitumour Antibiotics

Drug	Route and Adult Dose
bleomycin (Blenoxane)	IV, 0.25–0.5 units/kg every 4–7 days (q4–7d)
dactinomycin (Cosmegen)	IV, 12-15 µg/kg/day for 5 days; dose intensity per 2-week cycle should not exceed 15 µg/kg/day for 5 days or 400-600 µg/m^2/day for 5 days
daunorubicin (Cerubidine)	IV, 30–60 mg/m^2 qd for 3–5 days
Pr doxorubicin (Adriamycin)	IV, 60–75 mg/m^2 as single dose at 21-day intervals or 30 mg/m^2 on each of 3 consecutive days (max: total cumulative dose 550 mg/m^2)
idarubicin (Idamycin)	IV, 8–12 mg/m^2 qd for 3 days
mitomycin (Mutamycin)	IV, 20 mg/m^2 q6wk-q8wk
mitoxantrone	IV, 12 mg/m^2 qd for 3 days
valrubicin (Valtaxin)	Intrabladder instillation, 800 mg every week (qwk) for 6 weeks

chemotherapy, assess the CBC and the client's overall health status, including renal and liver function, intake and output, and body weight. Interview the client regarding any history of allergy prior to initiating therapy. Vital signs, including auscultation of heart and chest sounds, and a baseline electrocardiogram (ECG) should be obtained to rule out signs of cardiac abnormality or heart failure. Also assess for pregnancy and lactation, as antitumour antibiotics range from pregnancy category D (dactinomycin and valrubicin [Valtaxin]) to category D (bleomycin, daunorubicin, all others).

Antitumour antibiotics require cautious use in many clients. These drugs produce the same general cytotoxic effects as other antineoplastics, including alopecia, fatigue, nausea, vomiting, diarrhea, bone marrow suppression, and blood dyscrasias. As antibiotics, the risk for hypersensitivity reactions such as life-threatening angioedema exists. Antitumour antibiotics can be damaging to the myocardium; therefore, they should be used with extreme caution, if at all, in clients with cardiac disease. Doxorubicin should be used cautiously if the client has received cyclophosphamide, pelvic radiation, or radiation therapy to areas surrounding the heart or has a history of atopic dermatitis. Other effects include hyperpigmentation of the mucosa and nail beds, particularly among African Canadians, and changes in the rectal mucosa. For this reason, suppositories and the taking of rectal temperature are contraindicated.

The nurse must be extremely cautious when administering antitumour antibiotics. Doxorubicin is easily absorbed through the skin and by inhalation and may cause fetal death or birth defects as well as liver disease. Therefore, wear protective clothing (gloves, mask, and apron) when preparing the drug.

Client education as it relates to antitumour antibiotics should include goals; reasons for obtaining baseline data such as vital signs, blood work, ECG, and other cardiac tests; and possible side effects. The following are important points to include when teaching clients regarding antitumour antibiotics:

- Proper attention to good oral hygiene is important. Changes in the colour of the mucosa can make it difficult to distinguish the degree of tissue oxygenation or the severity of mouth sores. Inform the dentist of antitumour antibiotic therapy.
- Avoid using OTC rectal drugs, such as for hemorrhoids, and taking rectal temperature.
- Seek emergency medical treatment for signs of severe allergic reaction or possible heart attack, such as shortness of breath, thick tongue, throat tightness or facial swelling, rash, palpitations, and chest, arm, or back pain.
- Immediately report headache, dizziness, or rectal bleeding.

Refer to Nursing Process Focus: Clients Receiving Antineoplastic Therapy at the end of this chapter for additional teaching points.

NCLEX Success Tip

Doxorubicin primary side effects are cardiac changes (including left ventricular failure and arrhythmias), complete hair loss within 3 to 4 weeks of receiving the drug, hepatic impairment, and red discoloration of the urine.

PROTOTYPE DRUG **Doxorubicin (Adriamycin)**

Actions and Uses: Doxorubicin attaches to DNA, distorting its double helical structure and preventing DNA synthesis. It is only administered by IV infusion. Doxorubicin is one of the broader spectrum cytotoxic antibiotics, prescribed for solid tumours of the lung, breast, ovary, and bladder and for various leukemias and lymphomas. It is structurally similar to daunorubicin.

A novel delivery method has been developed for both doxorubicin and daunorubicin. The drug is enclosed in small lipid sacs, or vesicles, called **liposomes**. The liposomal vesicle is designed to open and release the antitumour antibiotic when it reaches a cancer cell. The goal is to deliver a higher concentration of drug to the cancer cells, while sparing normal cells. An additional advantage is that liposomal doxorubicin has a half-life of 50 to 60 hours, which is about twice that of regular doxorubicin. The primary indication for this delivery method is AIDS-related Kaposi's sarcoma.

Pharmacokinetics: Since doxorubicin is administered IV, bioavailability is 100%. Doxorubicin is widely distributed but does not cross the blood-brain barrier. Tissue binding is extensive. It is mostly metabolized in the liver. Doxorubicin is mostly excreted in bile. Half-life is about 17 hours.

Administration Alerts:
- Extravasation from an injection site can cause severe pain and extensive tissue damage.
- For infants and children, verify concentration and rate of IV infusion with the physician.
- Avoid skin contact with the drug. If exposure occurs, wash thoroughly with soap and water.
- Doxorubicin is pregnancy category D.

Adverse Effects and Interactions: The most serious concern, which sometimes limits doxorubicin therapy, is cardiotoxicity. Acute effects include dysrhythmias; delayed effects may include irreversible heart failure. Like many of the anticancer drugs, doxorubicin may profoundly lower blood cell counts. Acute nausea and vomiting are common and often require antiemetic therapy. Complete, though reversible, hair loss occurs in most clients. It may cause the soles of feet, palms of hands, and nail beds to darken.

Doxorubicin interacts with many drugs. For example, if digoxin is taken concurrently, the client will have decreased serum digoxin levels. Phenobarbital taken concurrently leads to increased plasma clearance of doxorubicin and decreased effectiveness. Concurrent use of phenytoin may lead to decreased phenytoin level and possible seizure activity. Hepatotoxicity may occur if mercaptopurine is taken concurrently. Concurrent use of verapamil (Isoptin) may increase serum doxorubicin levels, leading to doxorubicin toxicity.

Use with caution with herbal supplements. For example, green tea may enhance the antitumour activity of doxorubicin.

PLANT-DERIVED ANTINEOPLASTIC AGENTS

Plants have been a valuable source of antineoplastic agents. These agents act by preventing cell division.

Pharmacotherapy with Plant-Derived Antineoplastic Agents

60.6 Some plant extracts that kill cancer cells by preventing cell division have been isolated.

Agents with antineoplastic activity have been isolated from a number of plants, including the common periwinkle (*Vinca rosea*), Pacific yew (*Taxus brevifolia*), mayapple (*Podophyllum peltatum*), and the Chinese tree *Camptotheca acuminata*. Although structurally different, medications in this class have the common ability to affect cell division; therefore, some of them are called mitotic inhibitors. The plant-derived drugs are listed in Table 60.4.

The **vinca alkaloids** vincristine and vinblastine are older drugs derived from the periwinkle plant. More than 100 alkaloids have been isolated from the periwinkle, and their properties were described in folklore in several regions of the world long before their modern medical uses were discovered. Despite being derived from the same plant, vincristine, vinblastine, and the semisynthetic vinorelbine exhibit different effects and toxicity profiles.

The **taxoids**, which include paclitaxel (Taxol) and docetaxel (Taxotere), were originally isolated from the bark of the Pacific yew, which is an evergreen found in forests throughout the western United States. More than 19 different taxane alkaloids have been isolated from the tree and several are being investigated for potential antineoplastic activity. Paclitaxel is used for metastatic ovarian and breast cancer and for Kaposi's sarcoma. Unlabelled uses include many other cancers. A semi-synthetic product of paclitaxel, docetaxel is claimed to have greater antitumour properties with lower toxicity. Bone marrow toxicity is usually the dose-limiting factor for the taxoids. Like the vinca alkaloids, the taxoids are mitotic inhibitors.

North American First Nations described uses of the mayapple (or wild mandrake) long before podophyllotoxin, the active ingredient in the plant, was isolated. As a botanical, podophyllum has been used as an antidote for snakebites, a cathartic, and a topical treatment for warts. Teniposide (Vumon) and etoposide (VePesid) are semi-synthetic products of podophyllotoxin. These agents act by inhibiting **topoisomerase I**, an enzyme that helps to repair DNA damage. By binding in a complex with topoisomerase and DNA, these antineoplastics cause strand breaks that accumulate and cause permanent damage to the DNA. Etoposide is used for refractory testicular carcinoma, small oat-cell carcinoma of the lung, and choriocarcinoma. Teniposide is used only for refractory acute lymphoblastic leukemia in children. Bone marrow toxicity is the primary dose-limiting side effect.

Other recently isolated topoisomerase I inhibitors include topotecan and irinotecan. These agents are called **camptothecins** because they were first isolated from *Camptotheca acuminata,* a tree native to China. The camptothecins are only administered intravenously, and their use is limited. Topotecan (Hycamtin) is used for metastatic ovarian cancer and small-cell lung cancer after failure of initial chemotherapy. Irinotecan (Camptosar) is indicated for metastatic cancer of the colon or rectum. Like many other cytotoxic natural products, bone marrow suppression is the dose-limiting toxicity for the camptothecins.

Nursing Considerations

The role of the nurse in plant-derived antineoplastic therapy involves careful monitoring of the client's condition and providing education as it relates to the prescribed drug treatment. Before initiating chemotherapy, assess baseline vital signs, CBC, and the client's overall health status, including renal and liver function, intake and output, and body weight.

Because natural plant extracts may produce allergic reactions in susceptible individuals, interview the client regarding any allergy to plants or flowers, including herbs and foods, which may provide clues to possible hypersensitivity to these drugs. Infusion hypersensitivity is an adverse reaction that may be ameliorated by steroid therapy. Vincristine may produce acute bronchospasm and skin rashes. Inquire about pregnancy and lactation, as many of these agents are contraindicated in pregnancy. Vincristine is contraindicated in clients with obstructive jaundice and those with demyelinating forms of Charcot-Marie-Tooth disease.

These drugs produce many of the same cytotoxic effects as other antineoplastics, including alopecia, fatigue, nausea, vomiting,

TABLE 60.4 Plant-Derived Antineoplastic Agents	
Drug	**Route and Adult Dose**
Vinca Alkaloids	
vinblastine	IV, 3.7–18.5 mg/m^2 qwk
Pr vincristine	IV, 1.4 mg/m^2 qwk (max 2 mg/m^2)
vinorelbine (Navelbine)	IV, 30 mg/m^2 qwk
Taxoids	
docetaxel (Taxotere)	IV, 60–100 mg/m^2 every 3 weeks (q3wk)
paclitaxel (Taxol)	IV, 135–175 mg/m^2 q3wk
Topoisomerase Inhibitors	
etoposide (VePesid)	IV, 35-100 mg/m^2 qd for 5 days; PO, due to poor bioavailability, oral doses should be twice the IV dose
teniposide (Vumon)	IV, 165 mg/m^2 every 3–4 days (q3–4d) for 4 weeks
irinotecan (Camptosar)	IV, 125 mg/m^2 qwk for 6 weeks
topotecan (Hycamtin)	IV, 0.75–1.5 mg/m^2 qd for 3–5 days every 21 days

diarrhea, bone marrow suppression, and blood dyscrasias. Plant-derived antineoplastics should also be used cautiously in many pre-existing conditions, such as seizure disorders; vincristine may lower the seizure threshold. Vincristine should also be used cautiously in clients with leukopenia, neuromuscular disease, and hypertension. These agents may cause muscle weakness, peripheral neuropathy (including nerve pain), and paralytic ileus. Emphasize the need to establish a nutritional plan to combat constipation, including high fluid and fibre intake. Plant-derived antineoplastics can affect blood pressure, causing either hypotension or hypertension. Observe the client for symptoms such as headache, dizziness, and syncope. These drugs may produce severe mental depression; therefore, remain alert to the possibility of suicidal ideation. Referrals to a chaplain, mental health nurse, or social worker for spiritual or emotional care should be offered.

Client education as it relates to plant-derived antineoplastics should include goals; reasons for obtaining baseline data such as vital signs, blood work, and renal and liver function tests; and possible side effects. The following are important points to include when teaching clients regarding this class of drug:

- Seek emergency medical treatment for signs of severe allergic reaction: shortness of breath, thick tongue, throat tightness or difficulty swallowing, and rash.

- Seek medical treatment for severe convulsions or suicide risk, such as feelings of despair, verbalized suicide plan, or suicide attempt.

- Immediately report the following: muscle weakness; difficulty walking or talking; visual disturbances; stomach, bone, or joint pain; swelling, especially in the legs or ankles; rectal bleeding; or significant changes in bowel habits.

- Avoid using OTC suppositories and taking rectal temperature.

- Avoid activities that require physical stamina until effects of the drug are known.

- Obtain assistance with walking if weakness or staggering gait is a problem.

- Maintain good bowel habits, including adequate fluid and fibre intake.

Refer to Nursing Process Focus: Clients Receiving Antineoplastic Therapy at the end of this chapter for additional teaching points.

NCLEX Success Tip

Neurotoxicity is the primary adverse effect of vincristine, and it may manifest as blindness, which the client must report promptly. Neurotoxicity may also cause constipation, so the client should be encouraged to eat a high-residue (fibre) diet.

PROTOTYPE DRUG	Vincristine

Actions and Uses: Vincristine is a cell cycle–specific agent that affects rapidly growing cells by preventing their ability to complete mitosis. It is thought to exert this action by inhibiting microtubule formation in the mitotic spindle. Although it must be given intravenously, a major advantage of vincristine is that it

causes minimal immunosuppression. It has a wider spectrum of clinical activity than vinblastine and is usually prescribed in combination with other antineoplastics for the treatment of Hodgkin's disease, non-Hodgkin lymphomas, leukemias, Kaposi's sarcoma, Wilms' tumour, bladder carcinoma, and breast carcinoma.

Administration Alerts:

- Extravasation could result in serious tissue damage. Stop injection immediately if extravasation occurs. Apply local heat and inject hyaluronidase as ordered. No specific antidote is available. Observe site for sloughing.

- Avoid eye contact, which causes severe irritation and corneal changes.

- Vincristine is pregnancy category D.

Pharmacokinetics: Since vincristine is administered IV, bioavailability is 100%. It is widely and rapidly distributed. Tissue binding is extensive. Excretion is biliary with fecal elimination. Half-life is 10 to 38 hours.

Adverse Effects and Interactions: The most serious limiting adverse effects of vincristine relate to nervous system toxicity. Children are particularly susceptible. Symptoms include numbness and tingling in the limbs, muscular weakness, loss of neural reflexes, and pain. Paralytic ileus may occur in young children. Severe constipation is common. Reversible alopecia occurs in most clients.

Vincristine interacts with many drugs. For example, asparaginase (Kidrolase) used concurrently with or before vincristine may cause increased neurotoxicity secondary to decreased hepatic clearance of vincristine. Doxorubicin or prednisone may increase bone marrow depression. Calcium channel blockers may increase vincristine accumulation in cells. Concurrent use of digoxin may decrease digoxin levels, so the client may need an increased digoxin dose. When vincristine is given with methotrexate, the client may need lower doses of methotrexate. Vincristine may decrease serum phenytoin levels, leading to increased seizure activity.

ANTITUMOUR HORMONES AND HORMONE ANTAGONISTS

Hormones significantly affect the growth of some tumours. Use of natural or synthetic hormones or their antagonists as antineoplastic agents is a strategy used to slow the growth of hormone-dependent tumours.

Pharmacotherapy with Antitumour Hormones and Hormone Antagonists

60.7 Some hormones and hormone antagonists are non-cytotoxic agents that are effective against reproductive-related tumours such as breast, prostate, and uterine. They are less cytotoxic than other antineoplastics.

A number of hormones are used in cancer chemotherapy, including glucocorticoids, estrogens, and androgens. In addition, several hormone antagonists have been found to exhibit antitumour activity. The mechanism of hormone antineoplastic activity is largely unknown. It is likely, however, that these antitumour properties are independent of their normal hormone mechanisms since the doses used in cancer chemotherapy are magnitudes larger than the amount normally present in the body. Only the antitumour properties of these hormones are discussed in this section; for other indications and actions, the student should refer to other chapters in this text. The antitumour hormones and hormone antagonists are listed in Table 60.5.

In general, the hormones and hormone antagonists act by blocking the substances that are essential for tumour growth. Because these drugs are not cytotoxic, they produce few of the life-threatening toxic effects of antineoplastics from other classes. They can, however, produce significant adverse effects when given at high doses for prolonged periods. Because they rarely produce cancer cures when used singly, these drugs are normally given for palliation. There are four general classes of hormone antagonists:

- Selective estrogen receptor modifiers
- Aromatase inhibitors
- Gonadotropin-releasing hormone analogues
- Androgen receptor blockers

Selective Estrogen Receptor Modifiers

Estrogen is a hormone produced by the ovary and the adrenal gland that has profound metabolic actions on many organs. Estrogen produces its actions throughout the body by activating estrogen receptors (ERs). Estrogen receptors are overexpressed in many breast cancers, which are known as ER-positive tumours. Estrogen promotes the growth of ER-positive breast tumours.

Selective estrogen receptor modifiers (SERMs) are drugs that act to either activate or inhibit the ER. SERMs have the ability to activate ERs in some tissues (such as bone), while blocking ERs in other tissues (such as breast). SERMs that block ERs have an anti-estrogen effect that slows tumour growth of ER-positive breast cancer. Tamoxifen (Nolvadex) is the most widely prescribed SERM and serves as the prototype for antineoplastic hormones.

Aromatase Inhibitors

Aromatase is the enzyme that catalyzes the last step in the synthesis of estrogen. During this step, aromatase converts androgens (testosterone and androstenedione) to estrogens (estradiol) in the peripheral tissues such as fat and muscle. Blocking this step will reduce the levels of estrogen in the blood, starving ER-dependent tumours of a major growth stimulus.

The aromatase inhibitors cannot prevent estradiol formation in the ovary, which is the primary site of estrogen synthesis in premenopausal women. Because of this, the drug is only effective in postmenopausal women, who secrete almost no estrogen from their ovaries.

Gonadotropin-Releasing Hormone Analogues

Gonadotropin-releasing hormone (GnRH) analogues mimic the actions of endogenous GnRH and provide feedback to the pituitary

TABLE 60.5 Hormone and Hormone Antagonists Used for Neoplasia

Drug	Route and Adult Dose
Hormones	
dexamethasone (Dexasone)	PO/IM/IV, 0.075–9 mg/day in divided doses q6h–q12h
ethinyl estradiol (Estrace)	PO, for treatment of breast cancer: 10 mg tid; for palliation of prostate cancer: 1–2 mg tid
medroxyprogesterone (Provera, Medroxy) (see Chapter 31, page 373, for the Prototype Drug box)	IM, 400–1000 mg/week ; PO, 200–400 mg/day
megestrol (Megace)	PO, 40–160 mg bid–qid
prednisone (see Chapter 42, page 499, for the Prototype Drug box)	PO, 10–100 mg/m^2 qd
testosterone (see Chapter 32, page 382, for the Prototype Drug box)	IM, 200–400 mg every 2–4 weeks (q2–4wk)
Hormone Antagonists	
anastrozole (Arimidex)	PO, 1 mg qd
bicalutamide (Casodex)	PO, 50 mg qd
exemestane (Aromasin)	PO, 25 mg qd after a meal
flutamide (Euflex)	PO, 250 mg tid
fulvestrant (Faslodex)	IM, start with 500 mg on days 1, 15, and 29; maintenance 500 mg monthly
goserelin (Zoladex)	Subcutaneous (SC), 3.6 mg every 28 days (q28d)
letrozole (Femara)	PO, 2.5 mg qd
leuprolide (Eligard, Lupron)	IM (Lupron depot) or SC (Eligard), 7.5 mg monthly, or 22.5 mg every 3 months, or 30 mg every 4 months, or 45 mg every 6 months
nilutamide (Anandron)	PO, 300 mg/day for 30 days, then 150 mg qd
Pr tamoxifen (Nolvadex)	PO, 20 mg qd for 5 years

gland. Initially, the effect is to increase the production of interstitial cell-stimulating hormone (ICSH), which increases the secretion of testosterone by the testes. ICSH is also known as follicle-stimulating hormone. With continued therapy, the pituitary becomes insensitive to the effects of GnRH, and the production of testosterone falls. In fact, testosterone secretion declines to near zero levels such that treatment with a GnRH analogue is considered a type of chemical or pharmacological castration. All are approved for the management of prostate cancer. The loss of testosterone "starves" prostate cancer cells of the hormone essential for their growth. Some drugs in this class are also approved to treat endometriosis and uterine leiomyomata and for the palliative treatment of advanced breast cancer. The GnRH analogues are administered by the IM route or SC implants. All GnRH analogues are pregnancy category X drugs and contraindicated during pregnancy.

Androgen Receptor Blockers

Growth of prostatic carcinoma is usually androgen dependent. The androgen receptor blockers prevent testosterone and other androgens from reaching their receptors on cancer cells, thus depriving the cells of an important growth promoter. Drugs in this group are all administered PO and are used only to treat prostate cancer. They have an additive or synergistic effect when used in combination with GnRH analogues.

The primary adrenocortical hormones used in chemotherapy are dexamethasone (Dexasone) and prednisone. Because of their natural ability to suppress lymphocytes, the principal value of the glucocorticoids is in the treatment of lymphomas, Hodgkin's disease, and leukemias. They are sometimes given to reduce the nausea, weight loss, and tissue inflammation caused by other antineoplastics. Prolonged use can result in symptoms of Cushing's disease.

The sex hormones are used to treat tumours that contain specific hormone receptors. Two androgens, fluoxymesterone and testolactone, are used for breast cancer in postmenopausal women. The estrogen ethinyl estradiol (Estrace) is used to treat metastatic breast cancer and prostate cancer. The progestins medroxyprogesterone (Provera, Medroxy) and megestrol (Megace) are used to treat endometrial cancer.

Hormone inhibitors include the antiandrogens bicalutamide (Casodex), nilutamide (Anandron), and flutamide (Euflex), which are prescribed for advanced prostate cancer. Antiestrogens include tamoxifen and anastrozole (Arimidex), which are indicated for breast cancer. Anastrozole, letrozole (Femara), and exemestane (Aromasin) are called **aromatase inhibitors** because they block the enzyme aromatase, which normally converts adrenal androgen to estradiol. Aromatase inhibitors can reduce plasma estrogen levels by as much as 95%, and they are used in postmenopausal women with advanced breast cancer whose disease has progressed beyond tamoxifen therapy.

Nursing Considerations

The role of the nurse in antitumour hormone and hormone antagonist therapy involves careful monitoring of the client's condition and providing education as it relates to the prescribed drug treatment. Before initiating chemotherapy, assess baseline vital signs, CBC, and the client's overall health status, including renal and liver function, intake and output, and body weight. Assess for pregnancy and breastfeeding, as both are contraindicated with the antitumour hormones and hormone antagonists.

Therapy that uses hormones other than tamoxifen may be palliative rather than curative; it is important that both the client and the family understand this limitation before beginning chemotherapy. They must understand that while the client may appear to be improving, the cancer is likely continuing to worsen.

One of the most common yet distressing side effects of sex hormone therapy is the development of cross-gender secondary sexual characteristics, such as gynecomastia in males and hirsutism in females. Fertility is sometimes affected. Discuss these effects frankly with the client and offer support and simple interventions to increase self-esteem. The nurse may discuss clothing options to disguise gynecomastia or methods of facial hair removal, such as waxes or depilatories.

The use of glucocorticoids may increase the risk for sexually transmitted infections and other infections by suppressing the immune response. Glucocorticoid therapy may cause swelling, weight gain, redistribution of body fat (Cushing's syndrome), and hyperglycemia. Discuss body image concerns and nutritional strategies to increase energy and limit weight gain. Weight gain remains a concern for a number of cancer clients—especially in the early phases of the disease. In some cases, cancer clients who are experiencing cachexia may benefit from glucocorticoid-induced weight gain. Glucocorticoids should be administered with caution to clients with diabetes mellitus. Obtain results of laboratory blood tests, including serum glucose, hormone levels, and electrolytes.

Client education as it relates to hormone therapy for cancer should include therapeutic goals; reasons for obtaining baseline data such as vital signs and tests for cardiac, renal, and endocrine function; and possible side effects. Instruct the diabetic client to monitor blood glucose more frequently; the client may need adjustments in antidiabetic medications. Instruct the client to report serum blood glucose readings as ordered by the healthcare provider (e.g., "less than 4 mmol/L or more than 11 mmol/L").

The following are other important points to include when teaching clients regarding hormonal therapy for cancer:

- Immediately report the following: shortness of breath, chest pain, difficulty with urination (too much, too little, pain, or irritation), excessive thirst, bleeding or injuries, sore throat, fever, and other signs of infection.
- Avoid persons with active infections.
- Practise excellent oral hygiene and skin care.

Refer to Nursing Process Focus: Clients Receiving Antineoplastic Therapy at the end of this chapter for additional teaching points.

NCLEX Success Tip

Tamoxifen is an estrogen blocker used to treat premenopausal and postmenopausal breast cancer. Tamoxifen is also used to prevent breast cancer in certain women who are at high risk of developing breast cancer. The drug causes hot flashes as an adverse effect.

PROTOTYPE DRUG	Tamoxifen (Nolvadex)

Actions and Uses: Tamoxifen is given orally and is a drug of choice for treating metastatic breast cancer. It is sometimes classified as a SERM. Tamoxifen is effective against breast tumours that require estrogen for their growth. These susceptible cancer cells are known as ER positive. While it blocks estrogen receptors on breast cancer cells, tamoxifen actually activates estrogen receptors in other parts of the body. This results in typical estrogen-like effects such as reduced low-density lipoprotein levels and increased bone mineral density. The drug is unique among antineoplastics because it is given not only to clients with breast cancer but also to high-risk clients to prevent the disease. Few if any other antineoplastics are given prophylactically, due to their toxicity.

Pharmacokinetics: Tamoxifen is well absorbed after oral administration. It is widely distributed. It is mostly metabolized by the liver and mostly excreted in feces. Half-life is 7 days.

Administration Alerts:

• Give with food or fluids to decrease GI irritation.

• Do not crush or chew the drug.

• Avoid antacid for 1 to 2 hours following PO dosage of tamoxifen.

• Tamoxifen is pregnancy category D.

Adverse Effects and Interactions: Other than nausea and vomiting, tamoxifen produces little of the serious toxicity observed with other antineoplastics. Of concern, however, is the association of tamoxifen therapy with an increased risk for endometrial cancer and thromboembolic disease. Hot flashes, fluid retention, and vaginal discharge are relatively common. Clients who experience abnormal vaginal bleeding or menstrual irregularities during therapy should be evaluated promptly. Tamoxifen causes initial "tumour flare"—an idiosyncratic increase in tumour size—but this is an expected therapeutic event.

Tamoxifen interacts with several other drugs. For example, anticoagulants taken concurrently may increase the risk for bleeding. Concurrent use with cytotoxic agents may increase the risk for thromboembolism.

BIOLOGICAL RESPONSE MODIFIERS AND MISCELLANEOUS ANTINEOPLASTICS

Biological response modifiers approach cancer treatment from a different perspective than other chemotherapeutic agents. Rather than being cytotoxic to cancer cells, they stimulate the client's own immune system to fight the cancer.

Pharmacotherapy with Biological Response Modifiers and Miscellaneous Antineoplastics

60.8 Biological response modifiers have been found to be effective against tumours by stimulating the client's immune system.

Certain anticancer drugs act through mechanisms other than those previously described. For example, asparaginase deprives cancer cells of asparagine, an essential amino acid; it is used for acute lymphocytic leukemia. Mitotane (Lysodren), similar to the insecticide DDT (dichlorodiphenyltrichloroethane), poisons cancer cells by forming links to proteins; it is used for advanced adrenocortical cancer. One of the newest antineoplastics, imatinib (Gleevec), inhibits the enzyme tyrosine kinase; it is currently used in chronic myeloid leukemia and shows promise for treating other cancers. These agents are listed in Table 60.6.

Biological response modifiers are a relatively new class of medications that do not kill tumour cells directly but instead stimulate the body's immune system. When given concurrently with other antineoplastics, biological response modifiers help to limit the severe immunosuppressive effects caused by other agents.

TABLE 60.6 Biological Response Modifiers and Miscellaneous Antineoplastics

Drug	Route and Adult Dose
alemtuzumab (Mabcampath)	IV, 3–30 mg three times a week
altretamine (Hexalen)	PO, 260 mg/m²/day in 4 divided doses for 14 or 21 days of a 28-day cycle
arsenic trioxide (Trisenox)	IV, 0.15 mg/kg qd (max 60 doses)
asparaginase (Kidrolase)	IM/IV, 200–1000 units/kg/day for 28 consecutive days
bortezomib (Velcade)	IV/SC, 1.3 mg/m² on days 1, 4, 8, 11, 22, 25, 29, and 32 of a 42-day treatment cycle for 4 cycles
gefitinib (Iressa)	PO, 250 mg qd
hydroxyurea (Hydrea)	PO, 20–30 mg/kg qd
imatinib mesylate (Gleevec)	PO, 400–600 mg qd
interferon alfa-2 (Intron A) (see Chapter 40, page 478, for the Prototype Drug box)	SC/IM, 2–3 million units qd for leukemia; increase to 36 million units qd for Kaposi's sarcoma
mitotane (Lysodren)	PO, start with 2–6 g/day in 3–4 divided doses
procarbazine (Matulane)	PO, 2–4 mg/kg qd
rituximab (Rituxan)	IV, 375 mg/m² on cycle day 1 then 500 mg/m² on day 1 (every 28 days) of cycles 2–6
trastuzumab (Herceptin)	IV, 4 mg/kg as a single dose, then 2 mg/kg qwk
tositumomab (Bexxar)	IV, 450 mg over 60 minutes
zoledronic acid (Zometa)	IV, 4 mg over at least 15 minutes

Refer to Chapter 40 for additional information on the biological response modifiers and the prototype drugs in this class.

Cytokines that act as biological response modifiers include the following:

- Interferons are natural proteins produced by T cells in response to viral infection and other antigens. They bind to specific receptors on cancer cell membranes and suppress cell division, enhance the phagocytic activity of macrophages, and promote the cytotoxic activity of T lymphocytes. Peginterferon alfa-2a (Pegasys) and interferon alfa-2b (Intron A) are approved to treat hairy cell leukemia, chronic myelogenous leukemia, Kaposi's sarcoma, and chronic hepatitis B and C.

- Interleukin 2 activates cytotoxic T lymphocytes and promotes other actions of the immune response. Marketed as aldesleukin (Proleukin), this drug is indicated only for metastatic renal cell carcinoma.

- **Hematopoietic growth factors** promote the formation of specific blood cells. These drugs enhance the ability of the immune system to respond and reduce some of the myelosuppression caused by antineoplastic medications. Hematopoietic growth factors include epoetin alfa (Epogen, Eprex), filgrastim (Neupogen), and sargramostim (Leukine).

Research into the mechanisms of cancer formation has allowed scientists to identify specific proteins (antigens) on the surface of cancer cells that are not present in normal cells. Different types of cancer cells exhibit different antigens. For example, cells in a brain tumour would have different antigens than those in a pancreatic tumour. Indeed, a single type of tumour in a client may contain cancer cells with varied surface antigens. A **targeted therapy** is an antineoplastic drug that has been specially engineered to attack these cancer antigens.

Monoclonal antibodies (MABs) are biological response modifiers that are a type of targeted therapy. Once the MAB binds to its specific antigen, the cancer cell is either killed directly by the drug or is marked for destruction by other cells of the immune response. For example, rituximab (Rituxan) is an MAB that binds to CD20, a surface protein present on premature B lymphocytes involved in certain leukemias and lymphomas.

CONNECTIONS Lifespan Considerations

◀ Chemotherapy in Older Adults

Older adults have a higher incidence of most types of cancer. This could be a result of a greater accumulation of carcinogenic effects over time and age-related reduction in immune system function.

Due to age-related changes, such as decreasing mobility of the myeloid cells from the bone marrow to bloodstream, elderly clients with cancer are not likely to respond as effectively to stress that would normally trigger hematopoiesis. This results in greater susceptibility to bone marrow suppression. Client teaching of older adults and their caregivers should include the following:

- Elderly clients who are receiving chemotherapy drugs may experience toxic effects from the binding of the drugs to red blood cells at a higher rate due to normal age-related factors of fewer circulating red blood cells. Inform the client to report and monitor any bleeding or bruising and to avoid all ASA products.
- For reduction of neutropenia and prevention of infection, instruct the client in the importance of monitoring temperature daily and avoiding antipyretics to reduce fever before calling the healthcare provider. Instruct the client to avoid crowds and people with respiratory infections. The client and caregivers should be instructed to use frequent handwashing to prevent the transmission of pathogens.
- Because older adults often have deficient nutritional intake, teach the client and caregivers regarding healthy food choices and assess for the client's ability to swallow food and medications.
- Because constipation may occur, encourage the client to obtain adequate fluid intake and to increase dietary fibre by eating whole grains and leafy vegetables.

Once bound, rituximab lyses the tumour cells. As is typical of MABs, the action of rituximab is very specific: it was designed to affect only cells with the CD20 protein, in this case tumour B cells. The key point about MABs is that the tumour cells must possess the specific protein receptor; otherwise, the MAB will be ineffective.

NURSING PROCESS FOCUS

Clients Receiving Antineoplastic Therapy

Assessment	Potential Nursing Diagnoses/Identified Patterns
Prior to administration: • Obtain complete health history, including laboratory values such as platelets, hematocrit (Hct), leukocyte count, liver and kidney function tests, and serum electrolytes. • Obtain drug history to determine possible drug interactions and allergies. • Assess neurological status, including mood and/or sensory impairment. • Assess for history or presence of herpes zoster or chickenpox. (Immunosuppressive effects of cyclophosphamide and vincristine can cause life-threatening exacerbations.)	• Need for knowledge regarding drug therapy and adverse effects • Risk for inadequate nutrition related to drug side effects • Risk for tissue injury related to extravasation • Risk for infection related to impaired immune system • Fatigue related to side effects of drug • Emotional needs related to cancer diagnosis and treatment

---

Planning: Client Goals and Expected Outcomes

The client will:

- Experience a reduction in tumour mass and/or progression of abnormal cell growth
- Experience a safe environment with no evidence of physical injury
- Demonstrate an understanding of the drug's action by accurately describing drug side effects, precautions, and therapeutic goals

---

Implementation

Interventions (Rationales)	Client Education/Discharge Planning
• Monitor haematological and immune status. • Observe for signs and symptoms of myelosuppression. (This could be indicative of overdose.) • Monitor CBC and temperature. • Collect stool samples for guaiac testing of occult blood. (Antineoplastics may cause anemia.) • Monitor cardiorespiratory status. • Monitor vital signs and chest/heart sounds. (Cyclophosphamide may cause myopericarditis and lung fibrosis. Doxorubicin may cause sinus tachycardia, cardiac depression, and delayed onset congestive heart failure [CHF].) • Observe ECG for T-wave flattening, ST depression, and voltage reduction. • Monitor for shortness of breath and pitting edema. • Monitor renal status, urinary output, intake and output, and daily weights. (Cyclophosphamide may cause renal toxicity and/or hemorrhagic cystitis. Vincristine and methotrexate increase uric acid levels, contributing to renal calculi and gout. Vincristine may also cause water retention and highly concentrated urine.) • Monitor GI status and nutrition. Administer antiemetics 30 to 45 minutes prior to antineoplastic administration or at the first sign of nausea. (Profound nausea, dry heaves, and/or vomiting are common with antineoplastic therapy. Dry mouth can also occur.) • Monitor for constipation. (Ileus or constipation and fecal impaction may occur with vincristine use, especially among older adults.) • Monitor neurological and sensory status. (Antineoplastics may cause peripheral neuropathy and mental depression. Vincristine may cause ataxia and hand/foot drop. Tamoxifen may cause photophobia and decreased vision. Such neurological changes may be irreversible.) • Monitor genitourinary status. (Antineoplastic agents, including hormones, and especially tamoxifen, may alter menstrual cycles in women and may produce impotence in men. Tamoxifen increases the risk for endometrial cancer.) • Monitor for hypersensitivity and other adverse reactions. • Monitor hair and skin status. (Alopecia is associated with most chemotherapy and may be a sign of overdosage. Methotrexate can cause a variety of skin eruptions.) • Monitor for conjunctivitis. (Doxorubicin may cause conjunctivitis.) • Monitor liver function tests. (Antineoplastics are metabolized by the liver, increasing the risk for hepatotoxicity.) • Administer with caution to clients with diabetes mellitus. (Hypoglycemia may occur secondary to combination of cyclophosphamide and insulin.)	Instruct client to: • Immediately report profound fatigue, fever, sore throat, epigastric pain, coffee-grounds vomit, bruising, tarry stools, or frank bleeding • Abstain from taking ASA unless prescribed • Avoid persons with active infections • Monitor vital signs (especially temperature) daily, ensuring proper use of home equipment • Anticipate fatigue and balance daily activities to prevent exhaustion • Avoid activities requiring mental alertness and physical strength until effects of the drug are known Instruct client: • To immediately report dyspnea; chest, arm, neck, or back pain; tachycardia; cough; frothy sputum; swelling; or activity intolerance • To maintain a regular schedule of ECGs as advised by the healthcare provider • That heart changes may be a sign of drug toxicity; heart failure (HF) may not appear for up to 6 months after completion of doxorubicin therapy Instruct client: • To immediately report the following: changes in thirst or the colour, quantity, and character of urine (e.g., "cloudy," with odour or sediment); joint, abdominal, flank, or lower back pain; difficult urination; and weight gain • That doxorubicin will turn urine red-brown for 1 to 2 days after administration; blood in the urine may occur several months after cyclophosphamide has been discontinued • To consume 3 L of fluid on the day before treatment and daily for 72 hours after (when client has no prescribed fluid restriction) Instruct client to: • Report loss of appetite, nausea/vomiting, diarrhea, mouth redness, soreness, or ulcers • Consume frequent small meals, drink plenty of cold liquids; avoid strong odours and spicy foods to control nausea • Examine mouth daily for changes • Use a soft toothbrush; avoid toothpicks Instruct client to: • Report changes in bowel habits • Increase activity, fibre, and fluids to reduce constipation Instruct client to: • Report changes in skin colour, vision, and hearing; numbness or tingling; staggering gait; or depressed mood; obtain no-self-harm contract • Limit sun exposure; wear sunscreen, sunglasses, and long sleeves when outdoors Instruct client to: • Report changes in menstruation, sexual functioning, and/or vaginal discharge

(continued)

Implementation	
Interventions (Rationales)	**Client Education/Discharge Planning**
	• Recognize the risk of endometrial cancer before giving tamoxifen
	• Instruct client to immediately report chest or throat tightness, difficulty swallowing, swelling (especially facial), abdominal pain, headache, or dizziness
	Instruct client to:
	• Immediately report desquamation of skin on hands and feet, rash, pruritus, acne, or boils
	• Wear a cold gel cap during chemotherapy to minimize hair loss
	• Instruct client or caregiver to immediately report eye redness, stickiness, pain, or weeping
	Instruct client to:
	• Report jaundice, abdominal pain, tenderness or bloating, or change in stool colour
	• Adhere to laboratory testing for serum blood level tests of liver enzymes as directed
	Instruct client to:
	• Report signs and symptoms of hypoglycemia (e.g., sudden weakness, tremors)
	• Monitor blood glucose daily; consult the healthcare provider regarding reportable results (e.g., less than 4 mmol/L)

Evaluation of Outcome Criteria

Evaluate the effectiveness of drug therapy by confirming that client goals and expected outcomes have been met (see "Planning").

See Tables 60.1 through 60.6 for lists of drugs to which these nursing actions apply.

CHAPTER

60 Understanding the Chapter

Key Concepts Summary

The numbered key concepts provide a succinct summary of the important points from the corresponding numbered section within the chapter. If any of these points are not clear, refer to the numbered section within the chapter for review.

60.1 Cancer may be treated using surgery, radiation therapy, and chemotherapy.

60.2 Serious toxicity—including thrombocytopenia; anemia; leukopenia; alopecia; and severe nausea, vomiting, and diarrhea—limits therapy with most antineoplastic agents.

60.3 Alkylating agents act by changing the structure of DNA in cancer cells. Some have a very broad spectrum of clinical activity.

60.4 Antimetabolites act by disrupting critical pathways in cancer cells, such as folate or DNA metabolism.

60.5 Due to their cytotoxicity, a few antibiotics are used to treat cancer by inhibiting cell growth. They have a narrow spectrum of clinical activity.

60.6 Some plant extracts that kill cancer cells by preventing cell division have been isolated.

60.7 Some hormones and hormone antagonists are noncytotoxic agents that are effective against reproductive-related tumours such as breast, prostate, and uterine. They are less cytotoxic than other antineoplastics.

60.8 Biological response modifiers have been found to be effective against tumours by stimulating the client's immune system.

Chapter 60 Scenario

Zack is a 12-year-old boy who had been in good health with no significant medical history until 6 months ago. At that time he began to experience episodic migraine-like headaches. Because of a paternal family history of migraines, Zack was evaluated for possible antimigraine therapy if the headaches continued. After 3 months of increasing severity of the headaches, he was diagnosed with a brain tumour by computed tomography (CT) scan. Zack underwent craniotomy for evacuation of a malignant tumour and began chemotherapy 1 month after surgery, prior to planned radiation therapy treatments. He has completed one cycle of chemotherapy over 2 months and will have a second cycle prior to radiation. He visits the oncology clinic today for evaluation prior to his second round of chemotherapy.

Physical examination on this clinic visit reveals a pleasant young male in no obvious distress. Zack weighs 43.6 kg (96 lb) and is 157.5 cm (62 inches) in height. Blood pressure (BP) is 92/40 mm Hg, pulse rate is 92 beats/minute, respirations are 24 breaths/minute, and temperature is 37.1°C (98.8°F). Zack denies having any pain and his neurological exam is unremarkable except for diminished patellar deep tendon reflexes (DTRs), graded at 1 (decreased but present; normal of 2). His white blood cell (WBC) count is 3420/mm^3, absolute neutrophil count (ANC) is 1800, hemoglobin (Hgb) is 13 g/dL, Hct is 36.5%, and platelet count is 225 000.

CBC is within the range expected postchemotherapy. Zack will be hospitalized for approximately 2 days for administration of cyclophosphamide (Procytox), carboplatin, and vincristine and will continue to receive doses of vincristine as an outpatient and start etoposide (VePesid) in several weeks. Because he experienced significant nausea and vomiting with the last round of chemotherapy, he will also be given ondansetron (Zofran) regularly with supplemental corticosteroids IV as needed.

Critical Thinking Questions

1. Why are four antineoplastic drugs used for Zack? What is the pharmacological classification of each of the drugs used?

2. What overlapping toxicities might Zack experience with these drugs? Considering his physical assessment findings today, what system toxicities would be of most concern?

3. Fifteen days after the start of the second cycle of chemotherapy, Zack experiences his nadir. At this time his WBC count is 340/mm^3, ANC is 98, Hgb is 9.3 g/dL, Hct is 25.7%, and platelet count is 55 000. Zack has been receiving filgrastim (Neupogen) SC since discharge and will continue until the WBC count begins to rise. Considering these laboratory values, what would be of most concern to the oncology team? What teaching should Zack and his family receive?

See Answers to Critical Thinking Questions in Appendix B.

NCLEX Practice Questions

1 The nurse is preparing to administer cyclophosphamide (Procytox) and knows that the client will experience a nadir in approximately 9 to 14 days. Which laboratory value(s) will indicate to the nurse that the client has reached the nadir?

a. Blood urea nitrogen and creatinine

b. White blood cell count and absolute neutrophil count

c. Ionized calcium

d. Serum albumin

2 A client has been receiving vincristine as one of the drugs in a chemotherapy regimen. Which important findings will the nurse monitor to prevent or limit the main dose-related toxicity for this client? Select all that apply.

a. Numbness of the hands or feet

b. Angina and dysrhythmias

c. Constipation

d. Diminished reflexes

e. Dyspnea and pleuritis

3 The nurse is caring for a client who is receiving tamoxifen for treatment of breast cancer. The nurse will teach the client that postchemotherapy monitoring will be necessary to detect or treat which drug-associated adverse effect?

a. Paralytic ileus

b. Alopecia

c. Pulmonary fibrosis

d. Endometrial cancer

4 A client with acute lymphoblastic leukemia has started therapy with doxorubicin (Adriamycin). The nurse will assist the client with which important intervention during the course of this treatment?

a. Performing active or assisted range-of-motion exercises to maintain strength

b. Participating in relaxation therapy to control pain

c. Using daily mouth rinses as prescribed

d. Maintaining bed rest during treatment

5 A client will be continuing to take methotrexate for treatment of osteosarcoma. Which OTC drugs will the nurse teach the client not to take concurrently with methotrexate?

a. Nonsteroidal anti-inflammatory drug pain relievers

b. Antihistamines

c. Laxatives

d. Cough suppressants

See Answers to NCLEX Practice Questions in Appendix A.

UNIT

13

Additional Drug Classes

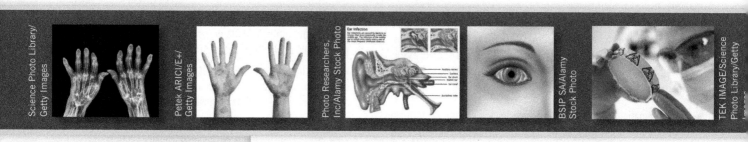

Science Photo Library/
Getty Images

Petek ARICI/E+/
Getty Images

Photo Researchers,
Inc/Alamy Stock Photo

BSIP SA/Alamy
Stock Photo

TEK IMAGE/Science
Photo Library/Getty
Images

PROTOTYPE DRUGS

**CALCIUM SUPPLE-
MENTS AND VITA-
MIN D THERAPY**
Pr *calcium
gluconate*
Pr *calcitriol (Calci-
jex, Rocaltrol)*
**BONE RESORPTION
INHIBITORS**
Hormonal Agents
Pr *raloxifene
(Evista)*

Bisphosphonates
Pr *etidronate diso-
dium (Didronel)*
**DISEASE-MODIFYING
DRUGS OF IMPOR-
TANCE FOR RHEUMA-
TOID ARTHRITIS**
Pr *hydroxychloro-
quine sulfate
(Plaquenil)*
**URIC ACID
INHIBITORS**
Pr *colchicine*

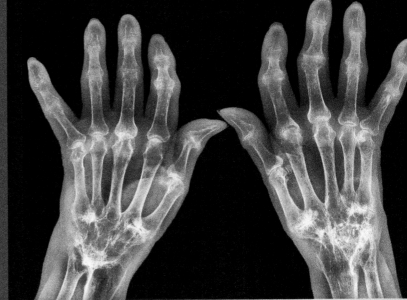

Science Photo Library/Getty Images

CHAPTER

61 Pharmacotherapy of Bone and Joint Disorders

LEARNING OUTCOMES

After reading this chapter, the student should be able to:

1. Identify important signs and symptoms of disorders associated with an imbalance of calcium, vitamin D, parathyroid hormone, and calcitonin.

2. Explain the therapeutic action of each class of drug used for bone and joint disorders in relation to the pathophysiology of the disorder.

3. Describe the nurse's role in the pharmacological management of disorders caused by calcium and vitamin D deficiency.

4. Describe the nurse's role, including client teaching, regarding the use of non-pharmacological therapies to prevent and treat bone and joint disorders.

5. For each of the drug classes listed in Prototype Drugs, identify a representative drug and explain its mechanism of action, therapeutic effects, and important adverse effects.

6. Describe and explain, based on pharmacological principles, the rationale for nursing assessment, planning, and interventions for clients with bone and joint disorders.

7. Use the nursing process to care for clients who are receiving drug therapy for bone and joint disorders.

CHAPTER OUTLINE

▶ Normal Calcium Physiology and Vitamin D

▶ Calcium-Related Disorders

　▶ Pharmacotherapy of Hypocalcemia

　▶ Pharmacotherapy of Osteomalacia

　▶ Pharmacotherapy of Osteoporosis

　▶ Pharmacotherapy of Paget's Disease

▶ Joint Disorders

　▶ Pharmacotherapy of Arthritis

　▶ Pharmacotherapy of Gout

The skeletal system and joints are at the core of body movement. Disorders associated with bones and joints may affect a client's ability to fulfill daily activities and lead to immobility. In addition, the skeletal system serves as the primary repository of calcium, one of the body's most important minerals. This chapter focuses on the pharmacotherapy of important skeletal disorders such as osteomalacia, osteoporosis, arthritis, and gout. The importance of calcium balance and the action of vitamin D are stressed as they relate to the proper structure and function of bones.

Normal Calcium Physiology and Vitamin D

61.1 Adequate levels of calcium in the body are necessary to properly transmit nerve impulses, to prevent muscle spasms, and to provide stability and movement. Adequate levels of vitamin D, parathyroid hormone, and calcitonin are also necessary for these functions.

One of the most important minerals in the body responsible for bone formation is calcium. Calcium balance is critical to the proper functioning of the nervous, muscular, skeletal, and cardiovascular systems. In the nervous system, calcium ions influence the release of neurotransmitters and the excitability of all neurons. Contraction is dependent on calcium ion movement in skeletal, smooth, and cardiac muscle cells. Calcium is important for the normal functioning of other body processes such as blood coagulation by converting prothrombin into thrombin and in activating enzymes that catalyze many essential chemical reactions.

Calcium is the major cation for the structure of the bones and teeth. Total body content of calcium is about 1200 g, or approximately 2% of the total body weight. More than 99% of that calcium is in the skeletal system and is bound as a hard matrix known as hydroxyapatite crystals. Only about 1% of the calcium in bone is rapidly exchangeable with blood calcium; the remaining calcium is more stable and slowly exchanged.

Levels of calcium in the blood are controlled by two endocrine glands: the parathyroid glands, which secrete parathyroid hormone (PTH), and the thyroid gland, which secretes calcitonin, as shown in Figure 61.1.

PTH stimulates bone cells called osteoclasts. These cells accelerate the process of **bone resorption**, a demineralization process that breaks down bone into its mineral components. Once bone is broken down, or resorbed, calcium becomes available to be transported and used elsewhere in the body. The opposite of this process is **bone deposition**, which is bone building. This process, which removes calcium from the blood, is stimulated by the hormone calcitonin.

PTH and calcitonin control calcium homeostasis in the body by influencing three major targets: bones, kidneys, and the gastrointestinal (GI) tract. The GI tract is mainly influenced by PTH and vitamin D. Vitamin D and calcium metabolism are intimately related: calcium disorders are often associated with vitamin D disorders.

Vitamin D is unique among vitamins in that the body is able to synthesize it from precursor molecules. In the skin, the inactive form of vitamin D, called **cholecalciferol**, is synthesized from cholesterol. Exposure of the skin to ultraviolet light increases the level of cholecalciferol in the blood. Sunlight exposure during Canadian winters is not adequate to prevent the occurrence of vitamin D deficiency, as evidenced by the high incidence of childhood rickets seen prior to the introduction of mandatory fortification of milk with vitamin D. Recent reports suggest that vitamin D levels in Canadians are still less than optimal (see References for this chapter for additional information). Cholecalciferol can be obtained from dietary products such as milk and other foods fortified with vitamin D. Figure 61.2 illustrates the metabolism of vitamin D.

Following its absorption or formation, cholecalciferol is converted to an intermediate vitamin form called **calcifediol**. Enzymes in the kidneys metabolize calcifediol to **calcitriol**, the active form of vitamin D. PTH stimulates the formation of calcitriol at the level of the kidneys. Clients with extensive kidney disease are unable to adequately synthesize calcitriol.

The primary function of calcitriol is to increase calcium absorption from the GI tract. Dietary calcium is absorbed more efficiently in the presence of active vitamin D and PTH, resulting in higher serum levels of calcium. Calcium is then transported from the blood to bone, muscle, and other tissues.

The importance of proper calcium balance in the body cannot be overstated. Calcium ion influences the excitability of all neurons. When calcium concentrations are too high (hypercalcemia), sodium permeability decreases across cell membranes. This is a dangerous state because nerve conduction depends on the proper influx of sodium into cells. When calcium levels in the bloodstream are too low (hypocalcemia), cell membranes become hyperexcitable. If this situation becomes severe, convulsions or muscle spasms may result. Calcium is also important for the normal functioning of other body processes such as blood coagulation and muscle contraction.

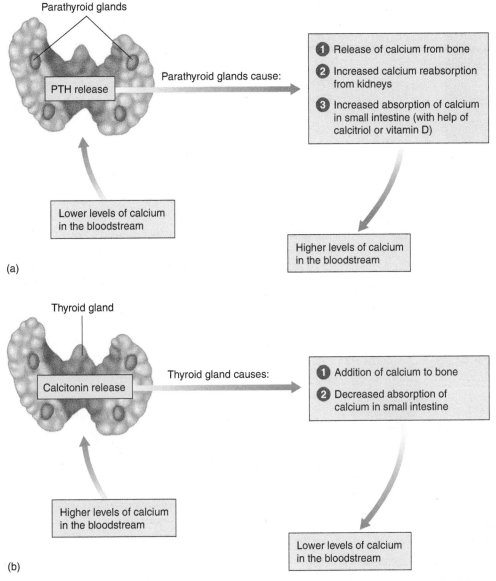

Figure 61.1 Regulation of calcium in the bloodstream: (a) parathyroid glands release parathyroid hormone (PTH); (b) thyroid gland releases calcitonin.

CALCIUM-RELATED DISORDERS

Diseases and conditions of calcium and vitamin D metabolism include hypocalcemia, osteomalacia, osteoporosis, and Paget's disease. Therapies for calcium disorders include calcium supplements, vitamin D supplements, bisphosphonates, and several miscellaneous agents.

Pharmacotherapy of Hypocalcemia

61.2 Hypocalcemia is a serious condition that requires immediate therapy with calcium supplements, often concurrently with vitamin D.

Hypocalcemia is not a disease but a sign of underlying pathology; therefore, diagnosis of the cause of hypocalcemia is essential.

One common cause is hyposecretion of PTH, as occurs when the thyroid and parathyroid glands are diseased or surgically removed. Digestive-related malabsorption disorders and vitamin D deficiencies also result in hypocalcemia. When taking a medical history, the nurse should assess for inadequate intake of calcium-containing foods.

Symptoms of hypocalcemia are those of nerve and muscle excitability. Muscle twitching, tremor, or cramping may be evident. Numbness and tingling of the extremities may occur, and convulsions are possible. Confusion and abnormal behaviour may be observed. Severe hypocalcemia requires intravenous (IV) administration of calcium salts, whereas less severe hypocalcemia can often be reversed with dietary modification or calcium supplements.

Increasing the consumption of calcium-rich foods, especially dairy products, fortified orange juice, cereals, and green leafy vegetables, may be sufficient to restore calcium balance

Sources of Vitamin D

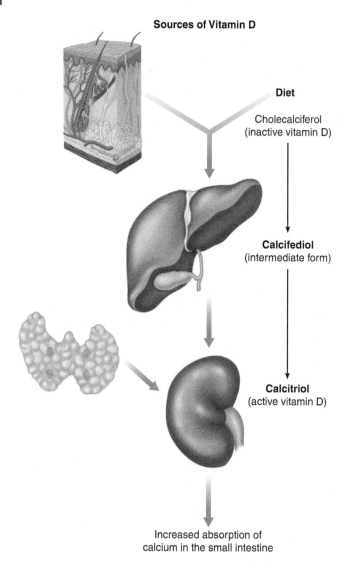

Diet

Cholecalciferol
(inactive vitamin D)

Calcifediol
(intermediate form)

Calcitriol
(active vitamin D)

Increased absorption of
calcium in the small intestine

Figure 61.2 Pathway of vitamin D activation and action.

when hypocalcemia is mild and non–life threatening. If dietary modification is not practical or adequate, calcium supplements are available over the counter (OTC) or by prescription. Calcium supplements often contain vitamin D to increase absorption.

The two major forms of calcium are complexed and elemental. Most calcium supplements are in the form of complexed calcium. These products are often compared on the basis of their ability to release elemental calcium into the bloodstream. The greater the ability of complexed calcium to release elemental calcium, the more potent the supplement.

Nursing Considerations

The role of the nurse in calcium supplement therapy involves careful monitoring of the client's condition and providing education as it relates to the prescribed drug treatment. Assess for signs and symptoms of calcium imbalance. For hypercalcemia, assess for drowsiness, lethargy, weakness, headache, anorexia, nausea, vomiting, thirst, and increased urination. Hypocalcemia

signs and symptoms to assess for include facial twitching, muscle spasms, paresthesias, and seizures. Obtain baseline and periodic vital signs, serum calcium levels, and electrocardiogram (ECG) to determine the effectiveness of the medication. Obtain a thorough health history, including dietary patterns; exercise patterns; bone health; pregnancy; medical conditions; and OTC, herbal, and prescribed medications. Calcium supplements are contraindicated in clients with hypercalcemia, digitalis toxicity, dysrhythmias, or renal calculi.

Client education as it relates to calcium supplements should include goals, reasons for obtaining baseline data, and possible side effects. The following are important points the nurse should include when teaching clients and caregivers about these supplements:

- Report signs or symptoms of hypercalcemia: drowsiness, lethargy, weakness, headache, anorexia, nausea and vomiting, increased urination, and thirst.
- Report signs or symptoms of hypocalcemia: seizures, muscle spasms, facial twitching, or paresthesias.
- Report side effects of medication such as nausea, vomiting, constipation, and difficulty urinating.
- Take safety precautions to prevent falling and fractures.
- Participate in active and passive range-of-motion exercises, as tolerated.
- Consume calcium-rich foods, including milk and dairy products, dark green vegetables, soybeans, and canned fish with bones, such as salmon.
- Avoid excessive intake of zinc-rich foods, such as nuts, legumes, seeds, sprouts, and tofu, as zinc decreases calcium absorption.
- Avoid taking antacids that contain calcium and avoid consuming calcium-fortified juices or foods without first notifying the healthcare provider.

PROTOTYPE DRUG	Calcium Gluconate

Actions and Uses: Calcium gluconate and other calcium compounds are used to correct hypocalcemia and treat osteoporosis and Paget's disease. The objective of calcium therapy is to return serum calcium levels to normal. People at high risk for developing these conditions include postmenopausal women, those with little physical activity over a prolonged period, and clients who are taking certain medications such as corticosteroids, immunosuppressive drugs, and some antiseizure medications. Calcium gluconate is available in tablets, powder, or as a 10% solution for IV injection.

Pharmacokinetics: Calcium gluconate is mostly excreted in the feces. It has an unknown half-life.

Administration Alerts:

- Give oral calcium supplements with meals or within 1 hour following meals.
- If administering IV, inject slowly to avoid cardiac abnormalities.
- Calcium gluconate is pregnancy category C.

Adverse Effects and Interactions: The most common adverse effects of calcium gluconate are constipation and hypercalcemia, brought on by taking too much of this supplement. Symptoms include drowsiness, lethargy, weakness, headache, anorexia, nausea and vomiting, increased urination, and thirst. IV administration of calcium may cause hypotension, bradycardia, dysrhythmias, and cardiac arrest.

Concurrent use of cardiac glycosides increases the risk of dysrhythmia. Magnesium may compete for GI absorption. Calcium decreases the absorption of tetracyclines.

Pharmacotherapy of Osteomalacia

61.3 Pharmacotherapy of osteomalacia (softening of bones) includes calcium and vitamin D supplements.

Osteomalacia, referred to as rickets in children, is a disorder characterized by softening of bones without alteration of basic bone structure. The cause of osteomalacia and rickets is a lack

NURSING PROCESS FOCUS

Clients Receiving Calcium Supplements

Assessment	Potential Nursing Diagnoses/Identified Patterns
Prior to administration: • Obtain complete health history, including allergies, drug history, and possible drug interactions. • Assess baseline ECG. • Assess baseline vital signs, especially apical pulse for rate and rhythm, and blood pressure. • Assess lab work, including complete blood count (CBC) and electrolytes, especially calcium.	• Risk for injury related to loss of bone mass and side effects of drug • Need for knowledge regarding drug therapy • Need for knowledge regarding sources of calcium and vitamin D

Planning: Client Goals and Expected Outcomes

The client will:

• Have normal serum calcium levels (adult: 2.05–2.55 mmol/L; children: 2.10–2.75 mmol/L, depending on specific age)
• Demonstrate an understanding of the drug's action by accurately describing drug side effects and precautions and measures to take to decrease any side effects
• Immediately report side effects and adverse reactions

Implementation

Interventions (Rationales)	Client Education/Discharge Planning
• Monitor electrolytes throughout therapy. (Calcium and phosphorus levels tend to vary inversely. Low magnesium levels tend to coexist with low calcium levels.) • Monitor for signs and symptoms of hypercalcemia. (Overtreatment may lead to excessive serum calcium levels.) • Initiate seizure precautions for clients at risk for hypocalcemia. (Low calcium levels may cause seizures.) • Monitor for musculoskeletal difficulties. (Calcium gluconate is used to treat osteoporosis, rickets, and osteomalacia.) • Monitor intake and output. Use cautiously in client with renal insufficiency. (Calcium is excreted by the kidneys.) • Monitor cardiac functioning. (Possible side effects include short QT wave, heart block, hypotension, dysrhythmia, or cardiac arrest with IV administration.) • Monitor injection site during IV administration for infiltration. (Extravasation may lead to necrosis.) • Monitor diet. (Consuming calcium-rich foods may increase effect of drug. Consuming foods rich in zinc may decrease calcium absorption.)	• Teach client importance of routine laboratory studies, so that deviations from normal can be corrected immediately • Instruct client to report signs or symptoms of hypercalcemia: drowsiness, lethargy, weakness, headache, anorexia, nausea and vomiting, increased urination, and thirst • Teach client to be aware of signs of hypocalcemia, such as seizures, muscle spasms, facial twitching, and paresthesias Instruct client to: • Take special precautions to prevent fractures • Report episodes of sudden pain, joints out of alignment, or inability to assume normal positioning • Instruct client to report any difficulty in urination and to measure intake and output • Inform client to recognize and report palpitations or shortness of breath to the healthcare provider • Instruct client to report any pain at IV site • Advise client to consume calcium-rich foods and avoid zinc-rich foods

Evaluation of Outcome Criteria

Evaluate the effectiveness of drug therapy by confirming that client goals and expected outcomes have been met (see "Planning").

of vitamin D and calcium in the diet, usually as a result of kidney failure or malabsorption of calcium from the GI tract. Signs and symptoms include hypocalcemia, muscle weakness, muscle spasms, and diffuse bone pain, especially in the hip area. Clients may also experience pain in the arms, legs, and spinal column. Classic signs of rickets in children include bowlegs and a pigeon breast. Children may also develop a slight fever and become restless at night.

Tests performed to verify osteomalacia include bone biopsy; bone radiographs; computed tomography (CT) scan of the vertebral column; and determination of serum calcium, phosphate, and vitamin D levels. Many of these tests are routine for bone disorders and are performed as needed to determine the extent of bone health.

In extreme cases, surgical correction of disfigured limbs may be required. Drug therapy for children and adults consists of calcium supplements and vitamin D. A summary of drugs used for these conditions is provided in Table 61.1.

NCLEX Success Tips

Clients with hypoparathyroidism are ordered daily supplements of vitamin D along with calcium because calcium absorption from the small intestine depends on vitamin D.

PTH stimulates the kidneys to reabsorb calcium and excrete phosphate. It also stimulates the kidneys to convert vitamin D to its active form, 1,25-dihydroxyvitamin D.

A diet with adequate amounts of vitamin D aids in the regulation, absorption, and use of calcium and phosphorus, which are needed for the normal calcification of bone. Instruct the client that moderate intake of alcohol has no known negative effects on bone density; however, excessive alcohol intake does reduce bone density. Figs, broccoli, and almonds are very good sources of calcium. Swimming, biking, and other non-weight-bearing exercises do not maintain bone mass, whereas walking and running are weight-bearing exercises and do maintain bone mass.

Clients receiving vitamin D are instructed to report GI upset and metallic taste because these are early signs and symptoms of vitamin D toxicity.

Vitamin D toxicity can cause headache, weakness, renal insufficiency, renal calculi, hypertension, arrhythmias, muscle pain, and conjunctivitis.

Symptoms of vitamin A toxicity include dry skin, hair loss, and inflamed mucous membranes.

Vitamin B_3 (niacin, nicotinic acid) may cause flushing and orthostatic hypotension due to vasodilation.

Vitamin B_6 (pyridoxine) toxicity may cause sensory neuropathy and difficulty maintaining balance.

Inactive, intermediate, and active forms of vitamin D are also available as medications. The biological activity of 40 IU of vitamin D equals that of 1 µg of ergocalciferol or cholecalciferol. The amount of vitamin D a client needs will often vary depending on the amount of sunlight exposure. Growing children and adolescents require adequate calcium and vitamin D for strong bones and teeth. For adults under age 50 without osteoporosis or conditions affecting vitamin D absorption, the average recommended intake is 400 to 1000 IU/day. For adults over age 50, supplements of between 800 and 2000 IU/day are recommended. Because vitamin D is needed to absorb calcium from the GI tract, many supplements combine vitamin D and calcium into a single tablet.

Nursing Considerations

The role of the nurse in vitamin D therapy involves careful monitoring of the client's condition and providing education as it relates to the prescribed drug regimen. Obtain a history of current medications and fat-soluble vitamin intake. Liver function should be assessed because liver impairment can lead to accumulation of this lipid-soluble vitamin and toxicity. Assess sclera, skin pigment, bowel movements, and laboratory results for evidence of liver dysfunction. Because high levels of vitamin D may cause renal impairment, urinalysis and renal test results should be monitored. Calcium, phosphate, and magnesium levels may be altered by vitamin D therapy and also should be monitored. Assess for adverse effects of vitamin D therapy, such as hypercalcemia, headache, weakness, dry mouth, thirst, increased urination, and muscle or bone pain.

Client education as it relates to vitamin D supplements should include goals, reasons for obtaining baseline data, and possible side effects. The following are important points to include when teaching clients and caregivers about vitamin D:

- Consume dietary sources of vitamin D such as fortified milk. Children and pregnant women often require extra dietary vitamin D.

- Take vitamin D exactly as directed because too much may cause toxic levels.

- Report signs of excess vitamin D, such as fatigue, weakness, nausea, vomiting, and changes in colour or amount of urine.

- Exposure to sunlight for 20 minutes a day may supply enough vitamin D to prevent disease.

- Avoid alcohol and other hepatotoxic drugs.

- Report any changes in medications or supplements to the healthcare provider.

TABLE 61.1 Calcium Supplements and Vitamin D Therapy

Drug	Route and Adult Dose
Calcium Supplements (all doses in terms of elemental calcium)	
calcium acetate	Orally (PO), start with 1334 mg with each meal; can be increased gradually
calcium carbonate (Caltrate, Os-Cal, Tums)	PO, 500 mg to 4 g daily in 1–3 divided doses
calcium chloride	IV, 200–1000 mg every day (qd) to every 3 days (q3d)
calcium citrate (Citracal)	PO, 500–1000 mg twice a day (bid)
Pr calcium gluconate	PO, 1–2 g bid to four times a day (qid)
	IV, 4.5–16 mEq
calcium lactate	PO, 325 mg–1.3 g tid with meals
calcium phosphate tribasic	PO, 1 mL bid–tid
Vitamin D Supplements	
Pr calcitriol (Calcijex, Rocaltrol)	PO, 0.25 µg qd; can increase up to 0.5 to 1 µg/daily
cholecalciferol (Vitamin D_3)	PO, 400–1000 IU/day for adults under age 50 without osteoporosis or conditions affecting vitamin D absorption; 800–2000 IU/day for adults over 50
ergocalciferol (Vitamin D_2)	PO/intramuscular (IM), 25–125 µg/day for 6–12 weeks

| PROTOTYPE DRUG | Calcitriol (Calcijex, Rocaltrol) |

Actions and Uses: Calcitriol is the active form of vitamin D, available in both oral and IV formulations. It promotes the intestinal absorption of calcium and elevates serum levels of calcium. This medication is used in cases when clients have impaired kidney function or have hypoparathyroidism. Calcitriol reduces bone resorption and is useful in treating rickets. The effectiveness of calcitriol depends on the client receiving an adequate amount of calcium; therefore, it is usually prescribed in combination with calcium supplements.

Pharmacokinetics: Calcitriol has an onset of action of 2 to 6 hours, a peak action in 10 to 12 hours, and a duration of action of 3 to 5 days. It is excreted mainly in feces. Its half-life is 3 to 6 hours.

Administration Alerts:

- Protect capsules from light and heat.
- Withhold calcitriol and calcium supplement and notify the healthcare provider if hypercalcemia develops.
- Calcitriol is pregnancy category C.

Adverse Effects and Interactions: Common side effects include hypercalcemia, headache, weakness, dry mouth, thirst, increased urination, and muscle or bone pain. Thiazide diuretics may enhance effects of vitamin D, causing hypercalcemia. Too much vitamin D may cause dysrhythmia in clients who are receiving cardiac glycosides. Magnesium supplements should not be given concurrently due to increased risk for hypermagnesemia.

Pharmacotherapy of Osteoporosis

61.4 Pharmacotherapy of osteoporosis includes bisphosphonates, estrogen modulator drugs, and calcitonin.

Osteoporosis is the most common metabolic bone disease, affecting about 1.4 million Canadians. This disorder is usually asymptomatic until the bones become brittle enough to fracture or for a vertebra to collapse. In some cases, a lack of dietary calcium and vitamin D contribute to bone deterioration. In other cases, osteoporosis is due to disrupted bone homeostasis. Simply stated, bone resorption outpaces bone deposition, and clients develop weak bones. The following are risk factors for osteoporosis:

- Postmenopause
- Family history of osteoporosis and age over 60 years
- Caucasian or Asian descent
- Testosterone deficiency
- High alcohol or caffeine consumption
- Inadequate intake of vitamin D or calcium

- Anorexia nervosa
- Tobacco use
- Physical inactivity
- Drugs that lower serum calcium levels, such as some anticonvulsants

The most common risk factor associated with the development of osteoporosis is the onset of menopause. When women reach menopause, estrogen secretion declines and bones become weak and fragile. One theory to explain this occurrence is that normal levels of estrogen may limit the lifespan of osteoclasts, the bone cells that resorb bone. When estrogen levels decrease, osteoclast activity is no longer controlled, and bone demineralization is accelerated, resulting in loss of bone density. In women with osteoporosis, fractures often occur in the hips, wrists, forearms, or spine. The metabolism of calcium in osteoporosis is illustrated in Figure 61.3.

Many drug therapies are available for osteoporosis. These include calcium and vitamin D therapy, estrogen replacement therapy, estrogen receptor modulators, statins, slow-release sodium fluoride, bisphosphonates, and calcitonin. Many of these drug classes are also used for other bone disorders or conditions

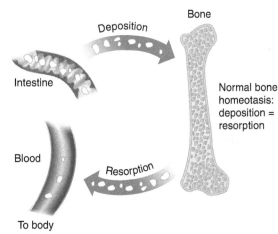

(a) Normal calcium intake

(b) Low calcium intake

Figure 61.3 Calcium metabolism in osteoporosis.

TABLE 61.2   Bone Resorption Inhibitor Drugs

Drug	Route and Adult Dose
Hormonal Agents	
calcitonin—salmon (Calcimar, Fortical, Miacalcin)	IM/subcutaneous (SC), 4 units q12h; may increase up to 8 units q12h Postmenopausal osteoporosis: SC/IM, 100 units/day; intranasal, 200 units (1 spray) in each nostril qd Paget's disease: SC/IM, 100 IU qd
Pr raloxifene (Evista)	PO, 60 mg qd
Bisphosphonates	
alendronate (Fosamax)	Osteoporosis treatment: PO, 10 mg qd or 70 mg once a week Osteoporosis prevention: PO, 5 mg qd or 35 mg once a week Paget's disease: PO, 40 mg qd for 6 months
Pr etidronate (Didronel)	Paget's disease: PO, 5–10 mg/kg qd for 6 months or 11–20 mg/kg qd for 3 months
pamidronate (Aredia)	IV, 60–90 mg in 1000 mL normal saline (NS) or 5% dextrose in water (D₅W) over 2–24 hours
risedronate (Actonel)	Paget's disease: 30 mg qd for 2 months; osteoporosis prevention, 5 mg qd or 35 mg once a week; osteoporosis treatment, 5 mg qd or 35 mg once a week or 150 mg once a month

unrelated to the skeletal system. Select drugs for osteoporosis are listed in Table 61.2.

NCLEX Success Tips

Raloxifene (Evista) is an estrogen-receptor modulator that increases bone mineral density without stimulating the endometrium. The drug is useful in preventing osteoporosis in postmenopausal women. This drug is contraindicated for women who smoke cigarettes or who have a history of venous thrombosis. One of its adverse effects is increased headaches.

Clients are instructed to take alendronate (Fosamax) on arising, preferably 30 minutes before food, with a full glass of water. Because the medication can cause severe oesophageal irritation, the client must be instructed to stay upright for 30 minutes after administration.

Educate the client that taking alendronate with food or juice significantly reduces absorption.

Hormone Replacement Therapy

Until recently, hormone replacement therapy (HRT) with estrogen was one of the most common treatments for osteoporosis in postmenopausal women. HRT is very effective at preventing fractures due to osteoporosis. Because of increased risks for uterine cancer, thromboembolic disease, breast cancer, and other chronic disorders associated with estrogen and progesterone in combination, the use of HRT in treating osteoporosis is no longer recommended. Additional information on HRT and the effects of estrogen may be found in Chapter 31.

Calcitonin

Calcitonin is a hormone secreted by the thyroid gland in response to elevated serum calcium. As a drug, it is approved for the treatment of osteoporosis in women who are more than 5 years postmenopause. It is available by nasal spray or SC injection. Calcitonin

(Calcimar, Fortical, Miacalcin) increases bone density and reduces the risk for vertebral fractures. Side effects are generally minor; the nasal formulation may irritate the nasal mucosa, and allergies are possible. Parenteral forms are rarely used because they may produce nausea and vomiting. In addition to treating osteoporosis, calcitonin is indicated for Paget's disease and hypercalcemia. Because calcitonin is less effective for osteoporosis than other therapies, it is considered a second-line treatment.

Selective Estrogen Receptor Modulators

Selective estrogen receptor modulators (SERMs) are a relatively new class of drug used in the prevention and treatment of osteoporosis. SERMs bind to estrogen receptors and may be estrogen agonists or antagonists, depending on the specific drug and the tissue involved. For example, raloxifene blocks estrogen receptors in the uterus and breast; therefore, it has no estrogen-like proliferative effects on these tissues that might promote cancer. Raloxifene does, however, decrease bone resorption, thus increasing bone density and reducing the risk for fractures. Like estrogen, it has a cholesterol-lowering effect. Another SERM, tamoxifen (Nolvadex), is used to treat breast cancer (see Chapter 60).

Nursing Considerations

The role of the nurse in drug therapy with hormones and SERMs involves careful monitoring of the client's condition and providing education as it relates to the prescribed drug regimen. The nurse should carefully evaluate and monitor clients who are taking this class of medication and obtain a thorough health history. The nurse should also obtain a history of medications and a complete physical examination, including liver function studies and a bone scan to determine the progression of the disease and to establish baseline data. Annual checkups and periodic bone density scans should be repeated throughout therapy to determine the effectiveness of the drug. Raloxifene is a pregnancy category X drug and is therefore contraindicated in pregnant clients.

Clients with a known history of thromboembolism or who are pregnant or lactating, taking HRT, or premenopausal should not take these drugs. SERMs should be used carefully when taking the following drugs: diazepam (Valium), diazoxide (Proglycem), ibuprofen (Motrin, Advil), indomethacin (Indocin), and naproxen (Aleve, Naprosyn).

Client education as it relates to SERMs should include goals, reasons for obtaining baseline data, and possible side effects. The following are important points the nurse should include when teaching clients and caregivers about SERMs:

- Report side effects that may indicate thromboembolic disease, especially sudden chest pain, dyspnea, pain in calves, and swelling in the legs.
- Consume supplements of calcium and vitamin D as directed by the healthcare provider.
- Participate in active weight-bearing exercises such as stair climbing or lifting weights.
- Avoid prolonged periods of immobility.
- Take special safety precautions to prevent falling and fractures.
- Discuss the possibility of using a "hip protector" to prevent hip fractures caused by accidental falls.

◀ The Impact of Ethnicity and Lifestyle on Osteoporosis

Women of Caucasian and Asian descent have a higher incidence of osteoporosis than those of African descent, although postmenopausal women are at the highest risk in all ethnic groups. It is important to remember that men also can develop this disease.

Even though medications are available to halt bone deterioration, prevention by establishing and maintaining a healthy lifestyle is the key to conquering osteoporosis. During childhood and adolescence, the focus should be on building bone mass. Children should be encouraged to eat foods that are high in calcium and vitamin D, exercise regularly, and avoid smoking and excessive use of alcohol.

During adulthood, the focus should be on maintaining bone mass and continuing healthy eating and exercise habits. Vitamin supplements may be taken on the advice of the healthcare provider. Post-menopausal women should focus on preventing bone loss. In addition to a healthy lifestyle, bone density tests should be done, and the possibility of taking medication to prevent or treat osteoporosis should be discussed with the healthcare provider.

PROTOTYPE DRUG | **Raloxifene (Evista)**

Actions and Uses: Raloxifene is a SERM. It decreases bone resorption and increases bone mass and density by acting through the estrogen receptor. Raloxifene is primarily used for the prevention of osteoporosis in postmenopausal women. This drug also reduces serum total cholesterol and low-density lipoprotein without lowering high-density lipoprotein or triglycerides.

Pharmacokinetics: Because raloxifene undergoes extensive first-pass metabolism in the liver, its bioavailability is about 2%. It is eliminated mainly in feces. Its half-life is 28 to 33 hours.

Administration Alerts:

- Drug may be taken with or without food.
- Raloxifene is pregnancy category X.

Adverse Effects and Interactions: Common side effects are hot flashes, migraine headache, flu-like symptoms, endometrial disorder, breast pain, and vaginal bleeding. Clients should not take cholesterol-lowering drugs or estrogen replacement therapy concurrently with this medication.

Warfarin (Coumadin) use may lead to decreased prothrombin time. Decreased raloxifene absorption will result from concurrent use of ampicillin or cholestyramine (Questran, Olestyr). Use of raloxifene with other highly protein-bound drugs (e.g., ibuprofen, indomethacin, diazepam) may interfere with binding sites.

Bisphosphonates

The most common drug class for osteoporosis is the **bisphosphonates**. These drugs are structural analogues of pyrophosphate, a natural substance that inhibits bone resorption. Bisphosphonates inhibit bone resorption by suppressing osteoclast activity, thus

increasing bone density and reducing the incidence of fractures by about 50%. Adverse effects include GI problems such as nausea, vomiting, abdominal pain, and esophageal irritation. Because these drugs are poorly absorbed, they should be taken on an empty stomach. Recent studies suggest that once-weekly dosing may give the same bone density benefits as daily dosing, due to the extended duration of drug action.

Denosumab (Proloa) is a nonoclonal antibody that is made to target and destroy only certain cells in the body. It is given parenterally to increase bone mass in patients with a high risk of bone fracture following certain cancer treatments. Prolia can also be used in patients with osteoporosis when bisphosphonates are not indicated.

Nursing Considerations

The role of the nurse in bisphosphonate drug therapy involves careful monitoring of the client's condition and providing education as it relates to the prescribed drug treatment. Obtain a thorough history to determine risk factors (especially a history of fractures), GI conditions, and current medications and dietary supplements. Pre-existing vitamin D deficiency or hypocalcemia should be corrected with supplements before initiating bisphosphonate therapy. A complete physical examination should include CBC, pH, chemistry panel, renal and liver function studies, vital signs, and bone density studies such as a dual x-ray absorptiometry to establish baseline data. Several months of bisphosphonate therapy are required to obtain desired effects.

These drugs are contraindicated in pregnant or lactating clients and in clients with colitis and severe renal disease. Bisphosphonates should be used cautiously in children, as safety and efficacy in children have not yet been established.

Client education as it relates to bisphosphonates should include goals, reasons for obtaining baseline data, and possible side effects. The following are important points the nurse should include when teaching clients and caregivers about bisphosphonates:

- Immediately report seizures, muscle spasms, facial twitching, and paresthesias.
- Report difficulty urinating, decreased urination, darkened urine, nausea, vomiting, diarrhea, or bone pain.
- Take medication on an empty stomach 2 hours before eating. Take with a full glass of plain water and sit upright for at least 30 minutes after the drug is taken to promote proper absorption.
- Consume calcium-rich foods, such as milk and milk products, dark green vegetables, canned fish with bones (such as salmon), and soybeans.
- Report pain, warmth, inflammation, or decreased movement in joints.
- Participate in light exercise and range-of-motion exercises, as possible.
- Store medication as recommended by the manufacturer and out of the reach of children.

PROTOTYPE DRUG | **Etidronate (Didronel)**

Actions and Uses: Bisphosphonates are a common treatment for postmenopausal osteoporosis. Etidronate is available in oral and IV forms and has the capability of strengthening bones

NURSING PROCESS FOCUS

Clients Receiving Bisphosphonates

Assessment	Potential Nursing Diagnoses/Identified Patterns
Prior to administration: • Obtain complete health history, including allergies, drug history, and possible drug interactions. • Assess for the presence or history of pathological fractures, hypocalcemia, and hypercalcemia. • Assess nutritional status. • Obtain lab work, including CBC, pH, electrolytes, renal function studies (blood urea nitrogen [BUN], creatinine, uric acid), and serum calcium and phosphorus.	• Need for knowledge regarding drug therapy • Risk for fluid imbalance • Risk for fractures • Nausea related to side effects of drug • Bone pain related to adverse drug reaction • Reduced adherence because therapeutic response may take 1–3 months

Planning: Client Goals and Expected Outcomes

The client will:

• Demonstrate decreased progression of osteoporosis or Paget's disease
• Demonstrate decreased risk for pathological fractures
• Remain free of side effects or adverse reactions
• Demonstrate understanding of dietary needs and modifications
• Maintain adequate fluid volume

Implementation

Interventions (Rationales)	Client Education/Discharge Planning
• Monitor for pathological fractures and bone pain. (Drug may cause defective mineralization of newly formed bone.) • Monitor for GI side effects. (There may be problems with absorption if client has persistent nausea or diarrhea.) • Monitor calcium lab values: serum calcium levels should be 2.05–2.55 mmol/L. (Through inhibition of bone resorption, drug causes blood levels of calcium to fall.) • Monitor kidney function, especially creatinine level. (Etidronate cannot be used in clients whose creatinine is >442 mmol/L.) • Monitor BUN, vitamin D, urinalysis, and serum phosphate and magnesium levels. • Monitor dietary habits. (Diet must have adequate amounts of vitamin D, calcium, and phosphate.) • Monitor adherence with recommended regimen. (Client may discontinue drug due to apparent lack of response.)	• Instruct client to report any sudden bone or joint pain, inability to correctly position self, or swelling over bone or joint • Advise client that new-onset nausea or diarrhea may be a symptom of adverse reaction and to report immediately Advise client to: • Have lab studies performed prior to beginning bisphosphonate therapy and periodically during therapy • Report symptoms of hypocalcemia (muscle spasms, facial grimacing, convulsions, irritability, depression, psychoses) • Report symptoms of hypercalcemia (increased bone pain, anorexia, nausea/vomiting, constipation, thirst, lethargy, fatigue, confusion, depression) • Instruct client to report any urinary changes, such as decreased urine production or increased urination • Advise client to include good food sources of vitamin D, calcium, and phosphate, including dairy products and green leafy vegetables Advise client: • That therapy should continue for 6 months maximum, but full therapeutic response may take 1–3 months • That effects continue for several months after drug is discontinued • To avoid vitamins, mineral supplements, antacids, and high-calcium products within 2 hours of taking bisphosphonates

Evaluation of Outcome Criteria

Evaluate the effectiveness of drug therapy by confirming that client goals and expected outcomes have been met (see "Planning").

See Table 61.2 under "Bisphosphonates" for a list of drugs to which these nursing actions apply.

with continued use by slowing bone resorption. Effects begin 1 to 3 months after therapy starts and may continue for months after therapy is stopped. This drug lowers serum alkaline phosphatase, the enzyme associated with bone turnover, without major adverse effects. Etidronate is also used for Paget's disease and to treat hypercalcemia due to malignancy.

Pharmacokinetics: Systemic absorption of oral etidronate is about 3%. Of the absorbed etidronate, about 50% is distributed to bone compartments and slowly eliminated. Etidronate is excreted unchanged in urine and feces. Its half-life is 1 to 6 hours.

Administration Alerts:
- Take drug on an empty stomach 2 hours before a meal.
- Etidronate is pregnancy category C.

Adverse Effects and Interactions: Common side effects of etidronate are diarrhea, nausea, vomiting, esophageal irritation, metallic or altered taste perception, hair loss, bone pain, and leg cramps. Pathological fractures may occur if the drug is taken for longer than 3 months.

Calcium supplements may decrease absorption of etidronate; therefore, concomitant use should be avoided. Food-drug interactions are common. Milk and other dairy products and medications such as calcium, iron, antacids, and mineral supplements must be reviewed before beginning bisphosphonate therapy because they have the potential to decrease the effectiveness of bisphosphonates.

Pharmacotherapy of Paget's Disease

61.5 Pharmacotherapy of clients with Paget's disease includes bisphosphonates and calcitonin.

Paget's disease, or osteitis deformans, is a chronic, progressive condition characterized by enlarged and abnormal bones. With this disorder, the processes of bone resorption and bone formation occur at a high rate. Excessive bone turnover causes the new bone to be weak and brittle; deformity and fractures may result. The client may be asymptomatic or have only vague, nonspecific complaints for many years. Symptoms include pain of the hips and femurs, joint inflammation, headaches, facial pain, and hearing loss if bones around the ear cavity are affected. Nerves along the spinal column may be pinched due to compression between the vertebrae.

Paget's disease is sometimes confused with osteoporosis because some of the symptoms are similar. In fact, medical treatments for osteoporosis are similar to those for Paget's disease. The cause of Paget's disease, however, is quite different. The enzyme alkaline phosphatase is elevated in the blood because of the extensive bone turnover, and the disease is usually confirmed by early detection of this enzyme in the blood. Calcium is also liberated because of its close association with phosphate. If diagnosed early enough, symptoms can be treated successfully. If the diagnosis is made late in the progression of the disease, permanent skeletal abnormalities may develop and other disorders may appear, including arthritis, kidney stones, and heart disease.

Bisphosphonates are the drugs of choice for the pharmacotherapy of Paget's disease. Therapy is usually cyclical, with bisphosphonates administered until serum alkaline phosphatase levels return to normal, followed by several months without the drugs. When serum alkaline phosphatase becomes elevated, therapy begins again. The pharmacological goals are to slow the rate of bone reabsorption and encourage the deposition of strong bone. Calcitonin nasal spray is used as an option for clients who cannot tolerate bisphosphonates. Surgery may be indicated in cases of severe bone deformity, degenerative arthritis, or fracture. Clients with Paget's disease should maintain adequate intake of calcium and vitamin D on a daily basis.

JOINT DISORDERS

Joint conditions such as osteoarthritis, rheumatoid arthritis, and gout are frequent indications for pharmacotherapy. **Osteoarthritis (OA)** is a degenerative, age-onset disease characterized by the wearing away of cartilage at articular joint surfaces. It is the most common type of arthritis and the second most common cause of disability in Canada, affecting between 3 and 4 million persons. Weight-bearing joints such as the knee, vertebral column, and hip are most commonly affected. The hands are also affected because they are frequently used. OA may be classified as idiopathic or secondary. Idiopathic OA, the most common type, has no known cause but is associated with increasing age. The causes of secondary OA include trauma, mechanical stress, inflammation of the joint structures, neurological disorders, use of certain medications, and joint instability. Excessive weight contributes to the development of OA, particularly in the knee and hip. Other risk factors associated with OA include decreased estrogen in menopausal women, excessive growth hormone, and increased PTH.

As cartilage thins in the affected joints, there is less padding and eventually the underlying bone is exposed. The bone thickens in the exposed areas, forming bone spurs and cysts that narrow the joint space. As these growths enlarge, small pieces may break off, leading to inflammation of the synovial membrane and a loss of lubricating fluid. This leads to further pain, inflammation, and destruction of the synovial membrane lining the joint. The affected joint becomes unstable and more susceptible to injury, with partial joint dislocations and other deformities that are common in advanced disease being seen.

The onset of OA is usually gradual, with pain and stiffness in one or more joints being the first manifestations. The client with OA typically describes a deep, aching, localized pain, which is usually aggravated by movement and relieved by rest. Pain at night may be accompanied by paresthesias. As the disease advances, the range of motion of the joint decreases; this is often accompanied by complaints of progressive pain. Bone enlargement can increase joint size; flexion contractures contribute to joint instability. It is important to note that OA is not accompanied by the degree of inflammation associated with other forms of arthritis. The joints of a client with OA are characteristically hard and cool to palpation. The diagnosis of OA is typically made using a detailed history and physical examination. Routine x-rays may be useful in determining structural joint changes.

Nonpharmacological therapies are an essential component of OA management. Walking, non-impact aerobics, and passive range-of-motion exercises are important to maintain joint flexibility. Improving muscle strength, especially of the quadriceps muscle, will help clients to improve their ability to perform activities of daily living. Bracing may help to keep joints positioned correctly and to relieve pain. Knowledge of proper body mechanics and posture may offer some benefit. Clients who are obese should consider a weight loss program, especially if weight-bearing joints such as the hip and knee are affected. Weight loss has been associated with decreased pain and disability. Surgical procedures such as joint replacement and reconstructive surgery may become necessary when other methods are ineffective.

Rheumatoid arthritis (RA) is a systemic, autoimmune disorder characterized by disfigurement and inflammation of multiple joints that occurs at an earlier age than osteoarthritis. It is characterized by disfigurement and inflammation of multiple joints. RA is less common than OA in Canada. Typically RA occurs at an earlier age than OA, with the incidence of RA increasing up to age 70. It is important to differentiate between the two types of arthritis because the treatments vary greatly.

In RA, **autoantibodies** known as rheumatoid factors attack the person's tissues, activating complement and drawing leukocytes into the area, where they attack the cells of the synovial membranes and blood. Inflammation first occurs in the synovial membranes, which line joint cavities, and then progresses to the surrounding articular cartilage. The damaged synovial membrane swells and the persistent inflammation spreads and damages the surrounding blood vessels, ligaments, and tendons. The swelling also causes hemorrhage, coagulation, and deposits of fibrin within the joints. This ultimately leads to scar tissue formation that immobilizes the joint.

The exact cause of RA is not known, but it is likely a combination of environmental and genetic factors. Female reproductive hormones may influence the development of RA because it affects women three to five times more frequently than it does men. Infectious organisms, such as the Epstein-Barr virus, may play a role in a person developing the autoimmune processes seen with RA.

The course of RA is variable, and the rate at which joint deformities develop is not consistent. Disease progression is typically fastest during the first 6 years, slowing thereafter. The onset is typically insidious, although it may be acute if precipitated by a stressor, such as infection. The client with early RA typically experiences morning joint stiffness, swelling, pain, and generalized fatigue. The joints may be slightly reddened, warm, and tender to palpation. The pattern of joints involved is usually symmetrical. The upper extremity joints are often involved, beginning with the hands and wrists, as are the joints of the toes, ankles, and knees. As the disease worsens, the morning stiffness can extend several hours into the day and occur with any periods of prolonged rest. The persistent inflammation causes deformities of the joints and the supporting ligaments, tendons, and muscles, making activity painful. Muscle weakness and decreased range of motion may be apparent. Most or all synovial joints are eventually affected.

Joint manifestations in RA typically precede systemic manifestations, which are associated with advancing disease. Extreme fatigue, anorexia, weight loss, anemia, and low-grade fever are common. Rheumatoid nodules may develop in the subcutaneous tissue of the forearm, toes, and fingers and in the viscera surrounding the heart, lungs, dura, and intestinal tract. Inflammation of the blood vessels can result in vasculitis. Respiratory complications,

CONNECTIONS Natural Therapies

◀ Glucosamine and Chondroitin for Osteoarthritis

Glucosamine sulfate and chondroitin sulfate are available individually or in combination as OTC natural health products used for osteoarthritis. Glucosamine is a natural substance that is an important building block of cartilage. With aging, glucosamine is lost with the natural thinning of cartilage. As cartilage wears down, joints lose their normal cushioning ability, resulting in the pain and inflammation of osteoarthritis. Some studies have shown glucosamine sulfate to be more effective than a placebo in reducing mild arthritis and joint pain. It is purported to promote cartilage repair in the joints. Chondroitin sulfate is also purported to promote cartilage repair. It is a natural substance that forms part of the matrix between cartilage cells. These products are considered relatively safe with few side effects. Recent research suggests that glucosamine combined with chondroitin may be effective only for moderate to severe OA pain (Clegg et al., 2006). More research regarding efficacy is needed.

including pleurisy, pneumonitis, and fibrosis, are common, as are cardiac complications such as pericarditis and myocarditis.

Diagnosis of RA is based on the client's history, physical examination, and diagnostic tests. Laboratory tests that are helpful in supporting a diagnosis of RA include elevations in the serum rheumatoid factor, erythrocyte sedimentation rate, antinuclear antibody titres, and serum immunoglobulin levels. Routine x-rays are used to determine the degree of structural joint damage.

Like OA, non-pharmacological therapies are an essential component of RA management. Range-of-motion and joint and muscle strengthening exercises are important if the client is to continue performing normal activities of daily living. Psychological counselling may help the client to deal with a potentially debilitating disease. Braces, splints, canes, and walkers can assist in ambulation. Loss of excess weight can help to take the stress off of inflamed joints. Proper rest helps to reduce pain.

Gout is a metabolic disorder that is a form of acute arthritis characterized by joint pain caused by the accumulation of uric acid in the bloodstream or joint cavities. Because joint pain is common to all three disorders, analgesics and anti-inflammatory drugs are important components of pharmacotherapy. A few additional drugs are specific to the particular joint pathology.

Pharmacotherapy of Arthritis

61.6 For osteoarthritis, the main drug therapy is pain medication that includes NSAIDs (ASA, acetaminophen, COX-2 inhibitors) or stronger analgesics. Drug therapy for rheumatoid arthritis may include NSAIDs, glucocorticoids, immunosuppressants, and disease-modifying drugs.

Arthritis is a general term meaning inflammation of a joint. There are several types of arthritis, each of which has somewhat different

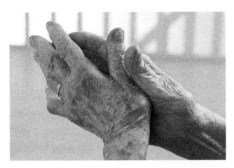

Figure 61.4 The hand of a client with osteoarthritis.
Source: Courtesy of JPC-PROD/Shutterstock

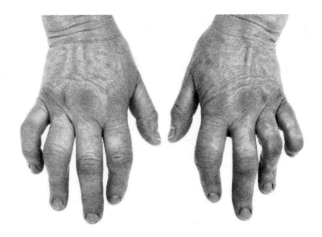

Figure 61.5 The hands of a client with rheumatoid arthritis.
Source: Adam J/Shutterstock

characteristics based on the etiology. OA, the most common type, is due to wear and tear of the cartilage of weight-bearing joints, including knees, hips, and spine. Symptoms of OA include localized pain and stiffness, joint and bone enlargement, and limitations in movement. OA is not accompanied by the degree of inflammation associated with other forms of arthritis. Many consider OA to be a normal part of the aging process. The hand of a client with OA is shown in Figure 61.4.

The goals of pharmacotherapy for OA include reduction of pain and inflammation. Topical medications (capsaicin cream and balms), nonsteroidal anti-inflammatory drugs (NSAIDs; including acetylsalicylic acid [ASA (Aspirin)], acetaminophen [Tylenol], and cyclooxygenase-2 [COX-2] inhibitors), and tramadol (Ultram, Tridural, Ralivia) are of value for treatment of pain associated with OA. Celecoxib (Celebrex) is presently the only COX-2 inhibitor approved by Health Canada because of the cardiovascular risk associated with this drug class. In acute cases, intra-articular glucocorticoids may be used on a temporary basis. Although these drugs help to relieve symptoms, they do not cure the disorder. The actions of NSAIDs are described in Chapter 42.

A newer type of drug therapy for clients with moderate OA who do not respond adequately to analgesics is sodium hyaluronate, a chemical normally found in high amounts within synovial fluid. Sodium hyaluronate is injected directly into the knee joint to replace the body's natural hyaluronic acid that deteriorated due to the inflammation of OA. Treatment consists of one injection per week for 3 to 5 weeks. By coating the articulating cartilage surface, sodium hyaluronate helps to provide a barrier, thus preventing friction and further inflammation of the joint. Information given to the client prior to administration should include side effects, such as pain and/or swelling at the injection site, and the advice to avoid any strenuous activity for approximately 48 hours after injection.

RA, the second most common form of arthritis, occurs at an earlier age than OA and has an autoimmune etiology. As discussed, autoantibodies called *rheumatoid factors* activate complement and draw leukocytes into the area, where they attack normal cells. This results in persistent injury and the formation of inflammatory fluid within the joints. Joint capsules, tendons, ligaments, and skeletal muscles may also be affected. Unlike OA, which causes local pain in affected joints, clients with RA may develop systemic manifestations that include infections, pulmonary disease, pericarditis, abnormal numbers of blood cells, and symptoms of metabolic dysfunction such as fatigue, anorexia, and weakness. The hands of a client with RA are shown in Figure 61.5.

Pharmacotherapy for relief of RA symptoms includes the same classes of analgesics and anti-inflammatory drugs used for OA. Glucocorticoids may be used for acute RA flare-ups because of their potent anti-inflammatory action.

Disease-modifying antirheumatic drugs (DMARDs) may be used to slow the progression of RA. DMARDs include drugs from several classes. Research has shown that hydroxychloroquine (Plaquenil), sulfasalazine (Salazopyrin), and methotrexate may reduce mortality when therapy is started early in the course of the disease. D-penicillamine, gold salts, and immunosuppressants such as leflunomide (Arava), azathioprine (Imuran), cyclosporine (Sandimmune, Neoral), and cyclophosphamide (Procytox) may also be used, although they may produce more toxic effects. Newer agents that inhibit the inflammatory process and produce more tolerable side effects include etanercept (Enbrel), infliximab (Remicade), and anakinra (Kineret). Several months may be required before maximum therapeutic effects are achieved. Because many of these drugs can be toxic, clients should be closely monitored. Adverse effects vary depending on the type of drug. These agents are listed in Table 61.3.

TABLE 61.3   Disease-Modifying Drugs for Rheumatoid Arthritis

Drug	Route and Adult Dose
azathioprine (Imuran)	PO, start with 1 mg/kg/day (50–100 mg) qd or divided into 2 doses (max 2.5 mg/kg/day)
gold sodium thiomalate (Myochrysine)	IM, 10 mg week 1, 25 mg week 2, then 25–50 mg/week to a cumulative dose of 1 g
Pr hydroxychloroquine (Plaquenil)	PO, 200–600 mg qd
leflunomide (Arava)	PO, loading dose 100 mg/day for 3 days; maintenance dose 10–20 mg qd
methotrexate (see Chapter 60, page 768, for the Prototype Drug box)	PO, 2.5–5 mg every 12 hours (q12h) for three doses each week or 7.5 mg once/week
sulfasalazine (Salazopyrin)	PO, start with 0.5–1 g qd; increase weekly to maintenance dose of 2 g/day in two divided doses (max 3 g/day)

NCLEX Success Tips

Sulfasalazine can cause gastrointestinal distress and is best taken after meals and in equally divided doses. During sulfasalazine therapy, the nurse should instruct the client to have adequate fluid intake of at least 8 glasses per day to prevent crystalluria and stone formation.

Sulfasalazine gives alkaline urine an orange-yellow colour, but it is not necessary to stop the drug when this occurs.

In long-term sulfasalazine therapy, the client becomes at risk of folic acid deficiency. The client can take folic acid supplements, but the nurse should also encourage the client to increase the intake of folic acid in his or her diet. Green leafy vegetables are a good source of folic acid.

Non-pharmacological therapies for relief of arthritic pain are common. The use of non-impact and passive range-of-motion exercises to maintain flexibility along with rest is encouraged. Splinting may help to keep joints positioned correctly and relieve pain. Other therapies commonly used to relieve pain and discomfort include thermal therapies, meditation, visualization, distraction techniques, and massage therapy. Knowledge of proper body mechanics and posturing may offer some benefit. Physical and occupational therapists are usually active in helping clients to minimize pain through these approaches. Surgical techniques such as joint replacement and reconstructive surgery may become necessary when other methods are ineffective.

NCLEX Success Tip

The client must undergo ophthalmological examination before therapy is begun and at 6-month intervals because of the possibility of an irreversible retinal degeneration caused by deposits of hydroxychloroquine in the layers of the retina.

PROTOTYPE DRUG	**Hydroxychloroquine (Plaquenil)**

Actions and Uses: Hydroxychloroquine is prescribed for RA and systemic lupus erythematosus in clients who have not responded well to other anti-inflammatory drugs. This agent relieves the severe inflammation characteristic of these disorders. For full effectiveness, hydroxychloroquine is most often prescribed with salicylates and glucocorticoids. This drug is also used for the prophylaxis and treatment of malaria (see Chapter 45).

Pharmacokinetics: Hydroxychloroquine is mainly metabolized in the liver. About 25% is excreted unchanged in urine. Its half-life is 32 to 50 days.

Administration Alerts:

- Take the drug at the same time every day.
- Administer with milk to decrease GI upset.
- Store the drug in a safe place, as it is very toxic to children.
- Hydroxychloroquine is pregnancy category D.

Adverse Effects and Interactions: Adverse symptoms include blurred vision, dizziness, itchiness, GI disturbances, loss of hair, headache, and mood and mental changes. Hydroxychloroquine has possible ocular effects that include blurred vision, photophobia, diminished ability to read, and blacked-out areas in the visual field.

Antacids with aluminum and magnesium may prevent absorption. This drug interferes with the client's response to rabies vaccine. Hydroxychloroquine may increase the risk for liver toxicity when administered with hepatotoxic drugs; alcohol use should be eliminated during therapy. It also may lead to increased digoxin (Lanoxin, Toloxin) levels.

Pharmacotherapy of Gout

61.7 Gout is characterized by a buildup of uric acid in either the blood or the joint cavities. Drug therapy includes agents that inhibit uric acid buildup or enhance its excretion.

Gout results from an accumulation of uric acid crystals that occurs because of increased metabolism of DNA or RNA or the reduced excretion of uric acid by the kidneys. Uric acid is the final breakdown product of DNA and RNA metabolism. One metabolic step that is important to the pharmacotherapy of this disease is the conversion of hypoxanthine to uric acid by the enzyme xanthine oxidase. An elevated blood level of uric acid is called hyperuricemia.

Gout may be classified as primary or secondary. Primary gout, caused by genetic errors in uric acid metabolism, is most commonly observed in Pacific Islanders. Secondary gout is caused by diseases or drugs that increase the metabolic turnover of nucleic acids or that interfere with uric acid excretion. Examples of drugs that may cause gout include thiazide diuretics, ASA, cyclosporine, and alcohol (when ingested on a chronic basis). Conditions that can cause secondary gout include diabetic ketoacidosis, kidney failure, and diseases associated with rapid cell turnover, such as leukemia, hemolytic anemia, and polycythemia.

Acute gouty arthritis occurs when needle-shaped uric acid crystals accumulate in joints, resulting in red, swollen, and inflamed tissue. Attacks have a sudden onset, often occur at night, and may be triggered by diet, injury, or other stresses. Gouty arthritis most often occurs in the big toes, heels, ankles, wrists, fingers, knees, and elbows. Of the clients with gout, 90% are men.

The goals of gout pharmacotherapy are twofold: termination of acute attacks and prevention of future attacks. NSAIDs are the drugs of choice for treating the pain and inflammation of acute attacks. Indomethacin is an NSAID that has been widely used for acute gout, although a COX-2 inhibitor may also be prescribed.

Prophylaxis of gout includes avoidance of foods and drugs that increase uric acid accumulation and worsen gout and treatment with antigout medications. Clients should avoid high-purine foods such as meat, legumes, alcoholic beverages, mushrooms, and oatmeal because nucleic acids will be formed when they are metabolized. Prophylaxis therapy includes drugs that lower serum uric acid. Allopurinol (Zyloprim) blocks xanthine oxidase, thus inhibiting the formation of uric acid. Prophylactic therapy is used for clients who suffer frequent and acute gout attacks. Drugs for gout are listed in Table 61.4.

TABLE 61.4 Uric Acid-Inhibiting Drugs for Gout and Gouty Arthritis

Drug	Route and Adult Dose
allopurinol (Zyloprim)	PO, 100 mg qd; may increase by 100 mg/week (max 800 mg/day)
Pr colchicine	Flare treatment: PO, start with 1.2 mg at the first sign of flare followed in 1 hour with a single 0.6 mg dose (max 1.8 mg within 1 hour); do not repeat treatment for at least 3 days; wait at least 12 hours to resume prophylactic dose Prophylaxis: PO, 0.6 mg qd-bid (max 1.2 mg/day)
probenecid (Benuryl)	PO, 250 mg bid for 1 week; then 500 mg bid (max 3 g/day)

NCLEX Success Tips

Allopurinol is used to treat renal stones composed of uric acid. Destruction of malignant cells during chemotherapy produces large amounts of uric acid. The client's kidneys may not be able to eliminate the uric acid, and tubular obstruction from the crystals could result in renal failure and uremia. Allopurinol interrupts the process of purine breakdown and uric acid synthesis, leading to decreases in uric acid excretion through the kidneys. The drug's effectiveness is assessed by evaluating for a decreased serum uric acid concentration.

Allopurinol must be taken consistently to be effective in the treatment of gout. The nurse should instruct the client to take the drug after meals to avoid gastrointestinal distress and to drink 3000 mL/day to avoid the development of renal calculi.

Adverse effects of allopurinol include drowsiness, maculopapular rash, anemia, abdominal pain, nausea, vomiting, and bone marrow depression.

The nurse should instruct the client to report rashes and unusual bleeding or bruising.

The uric acid inhibitors such as colchicine and allopurinol are also used for acute gout. Uric acid inhibitors block the accumulation of uric acid within the blood or of uric acid crystals within the joints. When uric acid accumulation is blocked, symptoms associated with gout diminish. About 80% of the clients who use uric acid inhibitors experience GI complaints such as abdominal cramping, nausea, vomiting, and/or diarrhea. These agents are summarized in Table 61.4. Glucocorticoids are useful for the short-term therapy of acute gout, particularly when the symptoms are in a single joint and the medication is delivered intra-articularly.

Nursing Considerations

The role of the nurse in drug therapy with antigout agents involves careful monitoring of the client's condition and providing education as it relates to the prescribed drug regimen. The nurse should carefully evaluate and monitor clients who are taking this class of drug and obtain a thorough health history. The nurse should obtain a drug history and a complete physical examination, including the following laboratory studies: CBC, platelets, liver and renal function studies, uric acid levels, and urinalysis. Vital signs should also be taken to establish baseline data. These tests should be repeated throughout the treatment to assess the effectiveness of the drug.

Clients with known hypersensitivity; pregnancy; or severe GI, renal, hepatic, or cardiac disease should not take antigout agents. These drugs should be used carefully in children and cautiously in clients who have blood dyscrasias or mild liver disease.

Client education as it relates to antigout drugs should include goals, reasons for obtaining baseline data, and possible side effects. The following are important points the nurse should include when teaching clients and caregivers regarding antigout agents:

- Take the medication exactly as ordered.
- Report side effects such as rash, headache, anorexia, lower back pain, pain on urination, hematuria, and decrease in urinary output to the healthcare provider.
- Increase fluid intake to 3 to 4 L/day.
- Decrease or eliminate alcohol consumption; alcohol increases uric acid levels.
- Limit foods that will cause the urine to be more alkaline, such as milk, fruits, carbonated drinks, most vegetables, molasses, and baking soda, in order to decrease the chance of stone formation.
- Avoid taking ASA and large doses of vitamin C; they enhance stone formation.
- Use effective birth control during drug therapy and notify the healthcare provider of any suspicion of pregnancy.

NCLEX Success Tip

Gout is a disease caused by urate crystal deposits in the joints and characterized by joint inflammation. Clients are prescribed colchicine to reduce these deposits and thus ease joint inflammation. The nurse should monitor the client for diarrhea, which is an adverse reaction associated with colchicine. The nurse should instruct the client to report diarrhea in order to ask the physician to reduce the dosage of colchicine. Although acetylsalicylic acid reduces joint inflammation and pain in clients with osteoarthritis and rheumatoid arthritis, it isn't indicated for gout because it has no effect on urate crystal formation.

PROTOTYPE DRUG | **Colchicine**

Actions and Uses: Colchicine is a natural product obtained from the autumn crocus, which is found in Canada and the United States. Colchicine reduces inflammation associated with gouty arthritis by inhibiting the synthesis of microtubules, which are subcellular structures responsible for helping white blood cells to infiltrate an area. Although colchicine has no analgesic properties, the reduction in inflammation may lead to pain reduction. Colchicine may be taken to prevent or treat acute gout, sometimes in combination with other uric acid–inhibiting agents.

Pharmacokinetics: Colchicine has an unknown onset and peaks in 0.5 to 2 hours. Its half-life is 20 minutes.

Administration Alerts:

- Take drug on an empty stomach, when symptoms first appear.
- Colchicine is pregnancy category C. Parenteral doses must not be given to pregnant women.

Adverse Effects and Interactions: Side effects such as nausea, vomiting, diarrhea, and GI upset are more likely to occur at the beginning of therapy. These side effects are related to disruption of microtubules that are responsible for cell proliferation. Colchicine may also directly interfere with the absorption of vitamin B_{12}.

Colchicine interacts with many drugs. For example, NSAIDs may increase GI symptoms, and cyclosporine may increase bone marrow suppression. Erythromycin (Eryc) may increase colchicine levels. Loop diuretics may decrease colchicine effects. Alcohol and products that contain alcohol may cause skin rashes and increase liver damage. Effects of CNS depressants may be increased.

NURSING PROCESS FOCUS

Clients Receiving Colchicine

Assessment	Potential Nursing Diagnoses/Identified Patterns
Prior to administration: • Obtain complete health history, including allergies, drug history, and possible drug interactions. • Obtain baseline vital signs. • Obtain lab work, including CBC, platelets, uric acid levels, renal and liver function tests, and urinalysis.	• Need for knowledge regarding drug therapy • Activity intolerance related to joint pain • Altered body image related to joint swelling

Planning: Client Goals and Expected Outcomes

The client will:
• Report a decrease in pain and an increase in function of affected joints
• Demonstrate an understanding of the drug's action by accurately describing drug side effects and precautions and measures to take to decrease any side effects
• Report side effects and adverse reactions

Implementation

Interventions (Rationales)	Client Education/Discharge Planning
• Monitor lab results throughout therapy. (Agranulocytosis and thrombocytopenia may occur.) Perform Coombs test for hemolytic anemia. • Monitor for signs of toxicity. • Monitor for signs of renal impairment such as oliguria. Record intake and output. • Ensure that medication is administered correctly. • Monitor for pain and mobility. (This is used to assess effectiveness of medication.)	• Teach client the importance of routine lab studies, so that deviations from normal can be corrected immediately • Instruct client to report weakness, abdominal pain, nausea, and/or diarrhea • Instruct client to report a decrease in urinary output and to increase fluid intake to 3–4 L/day • Inform client to take medication on an empty stomach. Medication should be taken at first sign of gout attack • Inform client to report an increase or decrease in discomfort and swelling

Evaluation of Outcome Criteria

Evaluate the effectiveness of drug therapy by confirming that client goals and expected outcomes have been met (see "Planning").

CHAPTER
61   Understanding the Chapter

Key Concepts Summary

The numbered key concepts provide a succinct summary of the important points from the corresponding numbered section within the chapter. If any of these points are not clear, refer to the numbered section within the chapter for review.

61.1 Adequate levels of calcium in the body are necessary to properly transmit nerve impulses, to prevent muscle spasms, and to provide stability and movement. Adequate levels of vitamin D, parathyroid hormone, and calcitonin are also necessary for these functions.

61.2 Hypocalcemia is a serious condition that requires immediate therapy with calcium supplements, often concurrently with vitamin D.

61.3 Pharmacotherapy of osteomalacia (softening of bones) includes calcium and vitamin D supplements.

61.4 Pharmacotherapy of osteoporosis includes bisphosphonates, estrogen modulator drugs, and calcitonin.

61.5 Pharmacotherapy of clients with Paget's disease includes bisphosphonates and calcitonin.

61.6 For osteoarthritis, the main drug therapy is pain medication that includes NSAIDs (ASA, acetaminophen, COX-2 inhibitors) or stronger analgesics. Drug therapy for rheumatoid arthritis may include NSAIDs, glucocorticoids, immunosuppressants, and disease-modifying drugs.

61.7 Gout is characterized by a buildup of uric acid in either the blood or the joint cavities. Drug therapy includes agents that inhibit uric acid buildup or enhance its excretion.

Chapter 61 Scenario

Darlene Coleman is a 65-year-old woman who is generally in good health. She has an annual check-up visit with her gynecologist. While assessing Darlene's vital signs, height, and weight, the nurse notes a significant deviation from the data recorded during last year's visit. The client has lost 2.5 cm (1 in.) in height during the last year. The nurse then shares this information with Darlene. The client states, "I have always been short. You should see my mother, who is much shorter than I am. But lately, my clothes just don't seem to fit. I haven't lost any weight, but my pant legs drag on the ground. Is it possible that I'm actually getting shorter?"

Critical Thinking Questions

1. As the nurse, how would you respond to the client's statement?
2. As you talk with Darlene, she asks you, "Is there any way to slow my declining height?" What could you recommend?

See Answers to Critical Thinking Questions in Appendix B.

NCLEX Practice Questions

1 A client who has been prescribed alendronate (Fosamax) demonstrates an understanding of how to correctly take the medication when stating,

a. "I will take my medication prior to eating my lunch or dinner."

b. "I will take my medication immediately before bedtime or at 9 p.m."

c. "I will take my medication with a full glass of water 30 minutes before breakfast."

d. "I should lie flat for at least 30 minutes after I take this medication."

2 Which of the following symptoms would alert the nurse to the possibility of the development of toxicity to methotrexate?

a. Headache, dizziness, and blurred vision

b. Hematuria, hiccoughs, and jaundice

c. Stomatitis, constipation, and dyspepsia

d. Jaundice, ascites, and edema formation

3 A client asks the nurse to explain how colchicine works. The nurse would base her response on which physiological principle?

   a. It increases the deposits of uric acid in the synovial spaces of the joints.

   b. It reduces the pain associated with joint inflammation from gouty arthritis.

   c. It prevents the accumulation of uric acid crystals in the joints.

   d. It increases renal excretion of uric acid crystals.

4 Which laboratory findings would the nurse monitor to determine whether pharmacotherapy is helping a client taking calcium supplementation for osteomalacia?

   a. Increasing serum calcium and increasing phosphate levels

   b. Increasing serum calcium and decreasing phosphate levels

   c. Decreasing serum calcium and increasing phosphate levels

   d. Decreasing serum calcium and decreasing phosphate levels

5 Which assessment findings in a client who is receiving calcitriol (Rocaltrol) should the nurse immediately report to the prescriber?

   a. Muscle weakness, nausea, and vomiting

   b. Diarrhea, abdominal pain, and stomatitis

   c. Bone pain, joint stiffness, and fever

   d. Photosensitivity, tinnitus, and bone pain

See Answers to NCLEX Practice Questions in Appendix A.

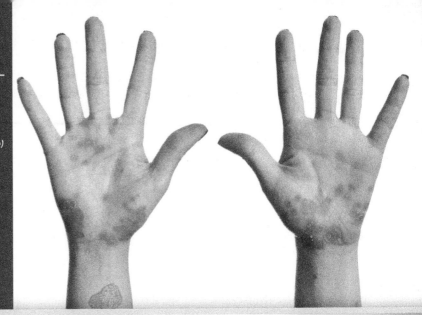

Petek ARICI/E+/Getty Images

62 Pharmacotherapy of Dermatological Disorders

LEARNING OUTCOMES

After reading this chapter, the student should be able to:

1. Identify drug classes used for treating skin disorders.

2. Explain the therapeutic action of drug therapies used for bacterial, fungal, or viral infections; mite and lice infestations; sunburn; acne vulgaris; rosacea; dermatitis; and psoriasis in relation to the pathophysiology of the disorders.

3. Describe the nurse's role in the pharmacological management of clients receiving drugs for skin disorders.

4. For each of the drug classes listed in Prototype Drugs, identify a representative drug and explain its mechanism of action, therapeutic effects, and important adverse effects.

5. Describe and explain, based on pharmacological principles, the rationale for nursing assessment, planning, and interventions for clients who are receiving drug therapy for skin disorders.

6. Use the nursing process to care for clients who are receiving drug therapy for skin disorders.

CHAPTER OUTLINE

▶ Structure and Function of the Skin

▶ Causes of Skin Disorders

▶ Skin Infections

  ▶ Pharmacotherapy of Bacterial, Fungal, and Viral Skin Infections

▶ Skin Parasites

  ▶ Pharmacotherapy with Scabicides and Pediculicides

▶ Sunburn and Minor Burns

  ▶ Pharmacotherapy of Sunburn and Minor Skin Irritation

▶ Acne and Rosacea

  ▶ Pharmacotherapy of Acne and Acne-Related Disorders

KEY TERMS

The integumentary system consists of the skin, hair, nails, sweat glands, and oil glands. The largest and most visible of all organs, the skin normally provides an effective barrier between the outside environment and the body's internal organs, helps to regulate body temperature, and assists in maintaining fluid and electrolyte balance. At times, however, external conditions become too extreme or conditions within the body change, resulting in unhealthy skin. When this occurs, pharmacotherapy may be used to improve the skin's condition. This chapter examines pharmacotherapy for a broad scope of skin disorders.

Structure and Function of the Skin

62.1 Three layers of skin—epidermis, dermis, and subcutaneous layer—provide effective barrier defences for the body.

To understand the actions of drugs used for skin disorders, it is necessary to have a thorough understanding of skin structure. The skin is composed of three primary layers: the epidermis, dermis, and subcutaneous layer. The epidermis is the visible, outermost layer that comprises only about 5% of the skin depth. The middle layer is the dermis, or cutis, which comprises about 95% of the entire skin thickness. The subcutaneous layer lies beneath the dermis. The subcutaneous layer is sometimes considered to be separate from the skin and not one of its layers. The anatomy of the skin is illustrated in Figure 62.1.

Each layer of skin is distinct in form and function. Drugs to treat the skin may be injected or applied topically (see Chapter 9). The epidermis has either four or five sublayers, depending on its location on the body. From the innermost to outermost, the five layers of skin are as follows: stratum basale (also referred to as the stratum germinativum), stratum spinosum, stratum granulosum, stratum lucidum, and the strongest layer, stratum corneum. The stratum corneum is referred to as the horny layer because of the abundance of the protein keratin. Keratin is also found in the hair, hooves, and horns of many mammals. Keratin forms a barrier to repel bacteria and foreign matter, and most substances cannot penetrate it. The largest amount of keratin is found in those areas subject to mechanical stress—for example, the soles of the feet and the palms of the hands.

The innermost sublayer of the epidermis, the stratum basale, continuously supplies the epidermis with new cells as older superficial cells are damaged or lost through normal sloughing. Over their lifetime, these newly created cells migrate from the stratum basale to the outermost layers of the skin. As these cells are pushed to the surface, they are flattened and covered with a water-insoluble material that forms a protective seal. The average time it takes for a cell to move from the stratum basale to the body surface is about 3 weeks. Specialized cells within the deeper layers of the epidermis, called melanocytes, secrete the dark pigment melanin, which offers a degree of protection from the sun's ultraviolet rays. The number and type of melanocytes determine the pigment of the skin. The more melanin, the darker the skin colour. In areas where the melanocytes are destroyed, there are milk-white areas of depigmented skin referred to as **vitiligo**.

The second primary layer of skin, the dermis, consists of dense, irregular connective tissue. The dermis provides a foundation for the epidermis and accessory structures such as hair and nails. Most receptor nerve endings, oil glands, sweat glands, and blood vessels are found within the dermis.

Beneath the dermis is the subcutaneous layer, or hypodermis, that consists mainly of adipose tissue that cushions, insulates, and provides a source of energy for the body. The amount of subcutaneous tissue varies in an individual and is determined by nutritional status, age, and heredity.

Causes of Skin Disorders

62.2 Skin disorders that may benefit from pharmacotherapy are acne, sunburns, infections, dermatitis, and psoriasis.

Of the various skin disorders, some have vague, generalized signs and symptoms and others have specific and easily identifiable causes. **Pruritus**, or itching, is a general condition associated with dry, scaly skin, or it may be a symptom of mite or lice infestation. Inflammation, a characteristic of burns and other traumatic disorders, occurs when damage to the skin is extensive. Local **erythema**, or redness, accompanies inflammation and many other skin disorders. Trauma to deeper tissues may cause additional symptoms such as bleeding, bruises, and infections.

Skin disorders may be grouped into three general categories: infectious, inflammatory, and neoplastic. A summary of these disorders is given in Table 62.1. Bacterial, fungal, viral, and parasitic infections of the skin are relatively common and are frequent

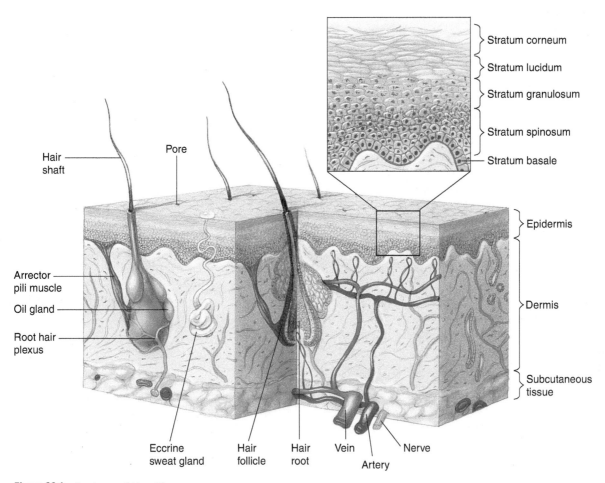

Hair shaft

Pore

Stratum corneum

Stratum lucidum

Stratum granulosum

Stratum spinosum

Stratum basale

Epidermis

Dermis

Subcutaneous tissue

Arrector pili muscle

Oil gland

Root hair plexus

Eccrine sweat gland

Hair follicle

Hair root

Vein

Artery

Nerve

Figure 62.1   Anatomy of the skin.

TABLE 62.1   Classification of Skin Disorders

Type	Examples
Infectious	Bacterial infections such as boils, impetigo, infected hair follicles; fungal infections such as ringworm, athlete's foot, jock itch, nail infection; parasitic infections such as mosquito bites, ticks, mites, lice; viral infections such as cold sores, fever blisters (herpes simplex), chickenpox, warts, shingles (herpes zoster), measles (rubeola), and German measles (rubella)
Inflammatory	Injury and exposure to the sun such as sunburn and other environmental stresses; disorders marked by a combination of overactive glands, increased hormone production, and/or infection such as acne, blackheads, whiteheads, rosacea; disorders marked by itching, cracking, and discomfort such as eczema (atopic dermatitis), other forms of dermatitis (contact dermatitis, seborrheic dermatitis, stasis dermatitis), and psoriasis
Neoplastic	Several types of skin cancer: squamous cell carcinoma, basal cell carcinoma, and malignant melanoma; malignant melanoma is the most dangerous; benign neoplasms include keratosis and keratoacanthoma

targets of anti-infective pharmacotherapy. Inflammatory disorders encompass a broad range of pathology that includes acne, burns, eczema, dermatitis, and psoriasis. Pharmacotherapy of inflammatory skin disorders includes many of the agents discussed in Chapter 42, such as glucocorticoids. Neoplastic disease includes malignant melanoma and basal cell carcinoma, which are treated with the therapies described in Chapter 60.

Not all skin disorders are localized to the skin. Skin disorders may indicate the presence of underlying systemic conditions associated with other organ systems. If skin conditions are noted, a complete history and physical assessment is needed to identify potential systemic causes such as liver or renal impairment, primary or metastatic tumours, recent injury, or poor nutritional status. During client assessment, the nurse must observe for skin abnormalities, including the colour, size, type, and character of any lesions. Skin turgor and moisture are examined for signs of possible dehydration. The relationship between the integumentary system and other body systems is depicted in Figure 62.2. Common symptoms associated with a range of conditions are shown in Table 62.2.

Although there are many skin disorders, some warrant only localized or short-term pharmacotherapy. Examples include lice

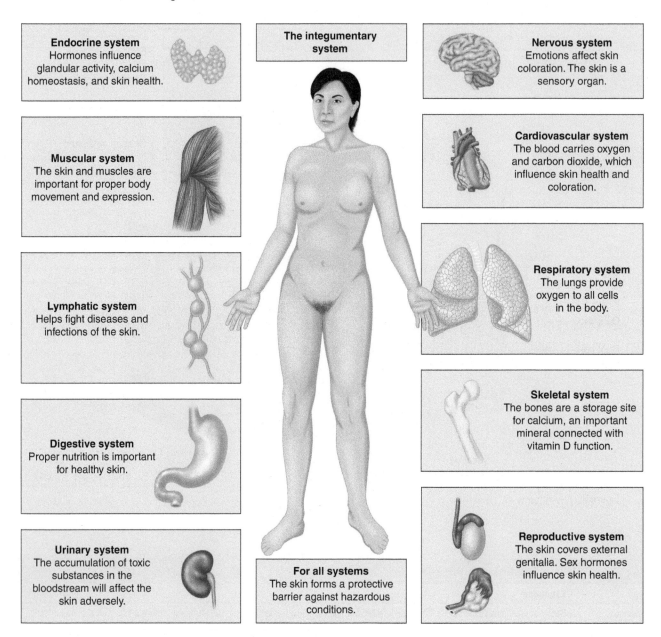

Endocrine system
Hormones influence glandular activity, calcium homeostasis, and skin health.

The integumentary system

Nervous system
Emotions affect skin coloration. The skin is a sensory organ.

Muscular system
The skin and muscles are important for proper body movement and expression.

Cardiovascular system
The blood carries oxygen and carbon dioxide, which influence skin health and coloration.

Lymphatic system
Helps fight diseases and infections of the skin.

Respiratory system
The lungs provide oxygen to all cells in the body.

Digestive system
Proper nutrition is important for healthy skin.

Skeletal system
The bones are a storage site for calcium, an important mineral connected with vitamin D function.

Urinary system
The accumulation of toxic substances in the bloodstream will affect the skin adversely.

For all systems
The skin forms a protective barrier against hazardous conditions.

Reproductive system
The skin covers external genitalia. Sex hormones influence skin health.

Figure 62.2 Interrelationships of the integumentary system with other body systems.

TABLE 62.2 Signs and Symptoms Associated with Changing Health, Age, or Weakened Immune System

Sign	Description
Discoloration of the skin	Discoloration is often a sign of an underlying medical disorder (for example, anemia, cyanoisis, fever, jaundice, and Addison's disease); some medications have photosensitive properties, making the skin sensitive to the sun and causing erythema.
Delicate skin, wrinkles, and hair loss	Many degenerative changes occur in the skin; some are found in elderly clients; others are genetically related (fragile epidermis, wrinkles, reduced activity of oil and sweat glands, male pattern baldness, poor blood circulation); hair loss may also be linked to medical procedures—for example, radiation and chemotherapy.
Seborrhea/oily skin and bumps	This condition is usually associated with younger clients; examples include cradle cap in infants and an oily face, chest, arms, and back in teenagers and young adults; pustules, cysts, papules, and nodules represent lesions connected with oily skin.
Scales, patches, and itchy areas	Some symptoms may be related to a combination of genetics, stress, and immunity; other symptoms are due to a fast turnover of skin cells; some symptoms develop for unknown reasons.
Warts, skin marks, and moles	Some skin marks are congenital; others are acquired or may be linked to environmental factors.
Tumours	Tumours may be genetic or may occur because of exposure to harmful agents or conditions.

infestation, sunburn with minor irritation, and acne. Eczema, dermatitis, and psoriasis are more serious disorders that require extensive and sometimes prolonged therapy.

SKIN INFECTIONS

Normally, the skin has a diverse population of microorganisms and flora that includes viruses, fungi, and bacteria. Intact skin provides an effective barrier against infection from these organisms. The skin is very dry, and keratin is a poor energy source for microbes. Although perspiration often provides a moist environment, its high salt content discourages microbial growth. Furthermore, the outer layer is continually being sloughed off, and the microorganisms go with it.

Pharmacotherapy of Bacterial, Fungal, and Viral Skin Infections

62.3 When the skin integrity is compromised, bacteria, viruses, and fungi can gain entrance and cause infections. Anti-infective therapy may be indicated.

Bacterial skin diseases can occur when the skin is punctured or cut or when the outer layer is abraded through trauma or removed through severe burns. Some bacteria also infect hair follicles. The two most common bacterial infections of the skin are caused by *Staphylococcus* and *Streptococcus*, which are normal skin inhabitants. *Staphylococcus aureus* is responsible for furuncles, carbuncles, and abscesses of the skin. Both *S. aureus* and *Streptococcus pyogenes* can cause impetigo, a skin disorder that commonly occurs in school-aged children.

Although many skin bacterial infections are self-limiting, others may be serious enough to require pharmacotherapy. When possible, pharmacotherapy uses topical agents applied directly to the site of infection. Topical agents offer the advantage of causing fewer side effects, and many are available over the counter (OTC) for self-treatment. If the infection is deep within the skin, affects large regions of the body, or has the potential to become systemic, then oral or parenteral therapy is indicated. Chapter 44 provides a complete discussion of antibiotic therapy. Some of the more common topical antibiotics include the following:

- Bacitracin ointment
- Chloramphenicol cream (Chloromycetin)
- Erythromycin ointment (Erysol)
- Gentamicin cream and ointment (Garamycin)
- Neomycin cream and ointment
- Tetracycline

Fungal infections of the skin or nails commonly occur in dark areas covered by clothing, such as tinea pedis (athlete's foot) and tinea cruris (jock itch). Tinea capitis (ringworm of the scalp) and tinea unguium (onycholysis of the nails) are also common. These pathogens generally are responsive to therapy with topical antifungal agents. More serious fungal infections of the skin and mucous membranes, such as *Candida albicans* infections that occur in immunocompromised clients, require systemic antifungals (see Chapter 45).

Some viral infections of the skin are considered diseases of childhood and are usually self-limiting. These include varicella (chickenpox), rubeola (measles), and rubella (German measles). Treatment of these infections is directed at controlling symptoms such as pruritus and preventing spread and scarring from skin lesions. Viral infections of the skin in adults include herpes zoster (shingles) and herpes simplex (cold sores and genital lesions). Pharmacotherapy of severe viral skin lesions may include antiviral therapy with acyclovir, as discussed in Chapter 46.

NCLEX Success Tips

Petroleum jelly is thought to smother lice. Lindaine and other pediculicides should not be applied to the face or close to the eyes.

The instillation of erythromycin (Eryc) into the neonate's eyes provides prophylaxis for ophthalmia neonatorum, or neonatal blindness caused by gonorrhea in the mother. Erythromycin is also effective in the prevention of infection and conjunctivitis from chlamydia trachomatis. The medication may result in redness of the neonate's eyes, but this redness will eventually disappear.

Erythromycin ointment is not effective in treating neonatal chorioretinitis from cytomegalovirus.

Tetracycline should be avoided in children younger than age 8 because it may cause enamel hypoplasia and permanent yellowish-grey to brownish tooth discoloration.

The nurse should put on gloves and clean the eyes before administering erythromycin ophthalmic ointment. The nurse should open the eyes by putting a thumb and finger at the corner of each lid and gently pressing on the periorbital ridges. Afterward the nurse should apply a 1- to 2-cm (0.4- to 0.7-in.) ribbon of ointment to the lower conjunctival sac of each eye, spreading the ointment from the inner canthus to the outer canthus. After 1 minute, the nurse should wipe the excess ointment from the eye.

SKIN PARASITES

Common skin parasites include mites and lice. Scabies is an eruption of the skin caused by the female mite *Sarcoptes scabiei*, which burrows into the skin to lay eggs that hatch after about 5 days. Scabies mites are barely visible without magnification and are smaller than lice. Scabies lesions most commonly occur between the fingers, on the extremities, in the axillary and gluteal folds, around the trunk, and in the pubic area, as shown in Figure 62.3. The major symptom is intense itching; vigorous scratching may lead to secondary infections. Scabies is readily spread through contact with upholstery and shared bed and bath linens.

Lice are small parasites ranging from 1 to 4 mm in length. They are readily spread by infected clothing or close personal contact. They require human blood for survival and will die within 24 hours without the blood of a human host. Lice (singular = louse) often infest the pubic area or the scalp and lay eggs, referred to as **nits**, which attach to body hairs. Head lice are *Pediculus capitis*, body lice are *Pediculus corpus*, and pubic lice are *Phthirus pubis*. *P. capitis*, the most common type in Canada, are shown in Figure 62.4. The pubic louse is referred to as a crab louse because it looks like a tiny crab when viewed under the microscope. Individuals with pubic lice will sometimes say that they have "crabs." Pubic lice may produce sky-blue macules on the inner thighs or lower abdomen. The bite of the louse and the release of saliva into the wound lead to intense itching, followed by vigorous scratching. Secondary infections can result from scratching.

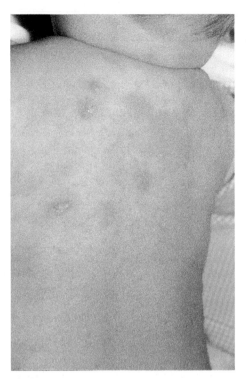

Figure 62.3 Scabies.
Source: Courtesy of Dr. Jason L. Smith.

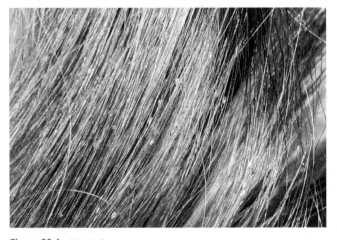

Figure 62.4 Head lice.
Source: Courtesy of Dr. Jason L. Smith.

Pharmacotherapy with Scabicides and Pediculicides

62.4 Scabicides and pediculicides are used to treat parasitic mite and lice infestations, respectively.

Scabicides are drugs that kill mites, and **pediculicides** are drugs that kill lice. Some drugs are effective against both types of parasite. The choice of drug may depend on where the infestation is located, as well as other factors such as age, pregnancy, or breastfeeding.

The traditional drug of choice for both mites and lice is permethrin (Nix, Kwellada-P). Permethrin is absorbed directly into lice, mites, and their eggs, producing seizures, paralysis, and death of the parasites. Permethrin, a combination scabicide/pediculicide, is available as a cream or lotion. All scabicides and pediculicides must be used strictly as directed because their excessive use can cause serious systemic effects and/or skin irritation, although some are safer than others. Drugs for the treatment of lice or mites must not be applied to the mouth, open skin lesions, or eyes, as this will cause severe irritation.

To ensure the effectiveness of pharmacotherapy, clients should inspect hair shafts after treatment, checking for nits by combing with a fine-toothed comb after the hair is dry. This must be conducted daily for at least 1 week after treatment. Some strains of lice and mites have become resistant to common medications, adding to the importance of checking the client several times during the post-application period to be sure that all parasites have been killed. Because nits may be present in bedding, carpets, combs, brushes, seams of clothing, and upholstery, all material coming in close contact with the client must be washed in hot water or treated with medication.

Nursing Considerations

The role of the nurse in scabicide and pediculicide therapy involves careful monitoring of the client's condition and providing education as it relates to the prescribed drug regimen. Before applying a scabicide or pediculicide, the nurse should assess the client's skin and hair, examining for signs of lice, nits, or scabies to verify the need for the medication. Lice may not be obvious on the body but may be found in seams of clothing that contact the axilla, neckline, groin, or beltline. Assess the skin for abrasions, cuts, rashes, and inflammation to determine areas that might be prone to irritation from the medication or increased absorption.

Obtain a complete history, including when the condition began; what treatment, if any, has already been tried (including OTC and home remedies); client allergies; and whether anyone in the family has a similar infestation. Assess the client for history of epilepsy, as these drugs can lower the seizure threshold in some clients.

Assess females of childbearing age to determine if the client is pregnant or nursing. Scabicides and pediculicides are used with caution in these clients, and precautions should be taken to protect the nursing infant. Permethrin is contraindicated in premature infants and should not be applied to children younger than 2 months of age due to increased risk of central nervous system (CNS) toxicity. Children and older adults may need reduced dosages. Instructions for applying these drugs must be carefully followed. If overapplied, wrongly applied, or accidentally ingested, the client may experience headaches; nausea or vomiting; irritation of the nose, ears, or throat; dizziness; tremors; restlessness; or convulsions.

Wear gloves when applying permethrin. Lesions should be cleansed with antibacterial soap and tepid water three times a day to promote healing and reduce chances of secondary infection. The skin should be dried before applying medication.

Client education as it relates to scabicides and pediculicides should include goals, reasons for obtaining baseline data, and possible side effects. The following are important points to include when teaching clients regarding scabicides and pediculicides:

- Keep medication out of the reach of children, as it is toxic if swallowed or inhaled.

- If breastfeeding, use another source of milk for a minimum of 4 days after using permethrin or similar drugs.

- Keep room humidity neither low nor high in order to reduce itching.

- Prevent re-infestation from household animals by frequently bathing pets and making sure that their bedding is washed in hot water or sprayed with a pediculicide or scabicide.

- If the child is in daycare, notify caregivers of treatment so that other infected children may be identified.

See Nursing Process Focus: Clients Receiving Permethrin for specific points the nurse should include when teaching clients regarding this drug.

NURSING PROCESS FOCUS

Clients Receiving Permethrin

Assessment	Potential Nursing Diagnoses/Identified Patterns
Prior to administration: • Obtain complete health history including allergies, drug history, and possible drug interactions. • Assess vital signs. • Assess skin for presence of lice and/or mite infestation, skin lesions, raw or inflamed skin, and open cuts. • Obtain history of seizure disorders. • Obtain client's age. • Assess pregnancy and lactation status. • Obtain social history of close contacts, including household members and sexual partners.	• Adequate knowledge regarding drug therapy and adverse effects • Psychosocial support may be needed to help reduce embarrassment and promote adherence to treatment • Risk for impaired skin integrity related to lesions and itching • Need for knowledge about ways to reduce risk of re-infestation • Need for knowledge of environmental modifications to reduce risk of re-infestation, reduce itch, and promote comfort

Planning: Client Goals and Expected Outcomes

- Client and significant others will be free of lice or mites and experience no re-infestation.
- Client will express an understanding of how lice and mites are spread; proper administration of permethrin; necessary household hygiene; and the need to notify household members, sexual partners, and other close contacts such as classmates of the infestation.
- Skin will be intact and free of secondary infection and/or irritation.
- Client will demonstrate an understanding of the drug therapy by accurately describing the drug's intended effects, usage, side effects, and precautions.

Implementation

Interventions (Rationales)	Client Teaching/Discharge Planning
• Monitor for presence of lice or mites. (This determines the effectiveness of drug therapy.) • Apply permethrin properly. (Proper application is critical to elimination of infestation.) • Inform client and caregivers about proper care of clothing and equipment. (Contaminated articles can cause re-infestation.)	Instruct client and caregiver to: • Examine for nits on hair shafts and for lice on skin and clothes; inner thigh areas and the seams of clothes that come in contact with axilla, neckline, or beltline may harbour lice • Examine for mites between the fingers, on the extremities, in the axillary and gluteal folds, around the trunk, and in the pubic area Instruct client and caregiver: • To wear gloves during application, especially if applying permethrin to more than one person, or if pregnant • That all skin lotions, creams, and oil-based hair products should be removed completely prior to application by scrubbing the whole body well with soap and water and drying the skin • To apply permethrin to clean and dry affected body area as directed • That eyelashes can be treated with the application of petroleum jelly twice a day for 8 days followed by combing to remove nits • To use a fine-tooth comb to comb affected hair following permethrin application to the hair and scalp and to treat all household members and sexual contacts simultaneously • To re-check affected hair or skin daily for 1 week after treatment Instruct client and caregiver to: • Wash all bedding and clothing in hot water and dry-clean all non-washable items that came in close contact with client • Clean combs and brushes with permethrin and rinse thoroughly

Evaluation of Outcome Criteria

Evaluate the effectiveness of drug therapy by confirming that client goals and expected outcomes have been met (see "Planning").

PROTOTYPE DRUG | **1%–5% Permethrin (Nix, Kwellada-P)**

Actions and Uses: Permethrin is marketed as a cream or lotion for mites and head lice. Permethrin cream or lotion takes longer to produce its effect, but each product is slightly different, so it is important to read the labels on each individual product because each might have slightly varying directions. Clients should be aware that penetration of the skin with mites causes itching, which lasts up to 2 or 3 weeks even after the parasites have been killed. Permethrin kills mites and lice by overstimulating their nervous system.

Treatment may be reapplied in 24 hours when there is evidence of live lice or in 7 days for continued evidence that live mites are present.

Pharmacokinetics: Although systemic absorption of permethrin is not desired, 10% of the drug (more if skin is damaged from itching) may be absorbed. The minimal amount of permethrin that is systemically absorbed is rapidly cleaved into inactive metabolites by skin esterases and ultimately excreted in the urine.

Administration Alerts:
• Do not use for premature infants and children less than 2 months of age.

• Do not use on areas of skin that have abrasions, rash, or inflammation.
• Excessive application may cause dangerous CNS toxicity.
• Permethrin is pregnancy category B.

Adverse Effects and Interactions: Adverse effects are generally mild, such as transient itching and redness, but may uncommonly include burning, stinging, rash, and numbness.

No clinically significant interactions have been established.

SUNBURN AND MINOR BURNS

Burns are a unique type of stress that may affect all layers of the skin. Minor, first-degree burns affect only the outer layers of the epidermis, are characterized by redness, and are analogous to sunburn. Sunburn results from overexposure to ultraviolet light, and it is associated with light skin complexions, prolonged exposure to the sun during the more hazardous hours of the day (10 a.m. until 4 p.m.), and lack of protective clothing when outdoors. Non-pharmacological approaches to sunburn prevention include the appropriate use of sunscreens and sufficient clothing. Chronic sun exposure can result in serious conditions, including cataracts and skin cancer.

Pharmacotherapy of Sunburn and Minor Skin Irritation

62.5 The pharmacotherapy of sunburn includes the symptomatic relief of pain using soothing lotions, topical anesthetics, and analgesics.

The best treatment for sunburn is prevention. Clients must be reminded of the acute and chronic hazards of exposure to direct sunlight. Liberal application of a lotion or oil with a very high sun protection factor (SPF) to areas of skin directly exposed to sunlight is strongly recommended.

The symptoms of sunburn include erythema, intense pain, nausea, vomiting, chills, and headache. These symptoms usually resolve within a matter of hours or days, depending on the severity of the exposure. Once sunburn has occurred, medications can only alleviate the symptoms; they do not speed recovery time.

Treatment for sunburn consists of addressing symptoms with soothing lotions, rest, prevention of dehydration, and topical anesthetic agents, if needed. Treatment is usually done on an outpatient basis. Topical anesthetics for minor burns include lidocaine (Xylocaine, Lidoderm, Betacaine), dibucaine (Nupercainal), and tetracaine (Pontocaine). Aloe vera and vitamin E are popular natural therapies for minor skin irritations and burns. These agents may also provide relief from minor pain due to insect bites and pruritus. In more severe cases, oral analgesics such as acetylsalicylic acid (ASA [Aspirin]) or ibuprofen (Advil, Motrin) may be indicated.

Nursing Considerations

The role of the nurse in drug therapy for sunburn and minor skin irritation involves careful monitoring of the client's condition and providing education as it relates to the prescribed drug regimen. Obtain a drug history, including allergies. When clients present with sunburn, assess the location, body surface area, and extent of injury (erythema, blistering, edema). Assess for weakness, fever, chills, and shock if sunburn is severe. Assess whether any home remedies or OTC medications were used to treat the sunburn. Obtain sunburn and tanning history, including the amount of time the client usually spends in the sun, how easily the client tends to burn, and the SPF rating of sunscreen products if used.

Topical anesthetics are contraindicated in areas of serious burns or infection. Topical lidocaine may cause a hypersensitivity reaction. For clients who are using the medication for the first time, a trial application on a small area of skin should be conducted to check for allergy. If no adverse reaction has occurred after 30 to 60 minutes, the medication may be applied to the entire area of mild to moderate sunburn.

Client education as it relates to topical, regional anesthetics should include goals, reasons for obtaining baseline data such as vital signs, and possible side effects. It is important that nurses educate clients about the safe use of topical regional anesthetic agents, appropriate treatment of sunburn, and prevention of overexposure to the sun. The following are important points to include when teaching clients about topical regional anesthetics:

- Apply topical products as directed.
- Avoid applying medication to open or infected skin.
- Drink plenty of water to avoid dehydration.

- If severe pain persists, notify the healthcare provider.
- Prevent sunburn by wearing a hat and protective clothing and by using sunscreens with an SPF of at least 15.
- Refrigerate topical lotions so that they soothe and cool the skin when applied.

PROTOTYPE DRUG | **Lidocaine (Xylocaine, Lidoderm, Betacaine)**

Actions and Uses: Lidocaine is a local anesthetic that provides temporary relief from pain and discomfort in cases of sunburn, pruritus, minor wounds, and insect bites. Its pharmacological action is to cause local anesthesia of skin receptor nerve endings by inhibiting transport of sodium ions across neuronal membranes. Preparations are also available to treat specific areas such as the ear, mouth, throat, and rectal and genital areas.

Pharmacokinetics: About 3% of topical lidocaine is absorbed systemically, so it is important to use as directed and not to exceed the maximum dose. Lidocaine is extensively metabolized by the liver, and only 10% is excreted in urine. Its half-life is 1.5 to 2 hours.

Administration Alerts:
- Lidocaine should not be used for treatment of clients with open lesions, traumatized mucosal areas, or a history of sensitivity to local anesthetics.
- Clients should use preparations only in areas of the body for which the medication is intended.
- Topical lidocaine is pregnancy category B.

Adverse Effects and Interactions: Topical lidocaine has a low toxicity when used as directed. Lidocaine gel or spray when applied to mucous membranes is rapidly absorbed, and overdose can cause neurological or cardiac toxicity. Allergic reactions and anaphylaxis are rare.

Lidocaine may interfere with the activity of some antibacterial sulfonamides.

ACNE AND ROSACEA

Acne vulgaris is a common condition that affects 80% of adolescents. Although acne occurs most often in teenagers, it is not unusual to find clients older than 30 years of age with acne. This condition in adults is referred to as mature acne or acne tardive. Acne vulgaris is more common in males but tends to persist longer in females.

The etiology of acne vulgaris is unknown, although factors associated with this condition include **seborrhea**, the overproduction of sebum by oil glands, and abnormal formation of keratin that blocks oil glands. The bacterium *Propionibacterium acnes* grows within oil gland openings and changes sebum to an acidic and irritating substance. As a result, small inflamed bumps appear on the surface of the skin. Other factors associated with acne include androgens, which stimulate sebaceous gland activity, and lower than normal production of linoleic acid in the sebum.

Acne lesions include open and closed **comedones**. Blackheads, or open comedones, occur when sebum has plugged the oil gland, causing it to become black because of the presence of

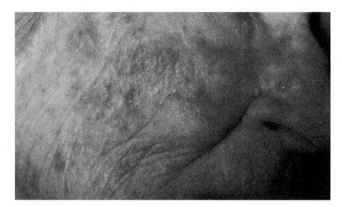

Figure 62.5 Rosacea.
Source: Courtesy of Dr. Jason L. Smith.

melanin granules. Whiteheads, or closed comedones, develop just beneath the surface of the skin and appear white rather than black.

Rosacea is another skin disorder with lesions that affect mainly the face. Unlike acne, which most commonly affects teenagers, rosacea is a progressive disorder with an onset between 30 and 50 years of age. Rosacea is characterized by small papules or inflammatory bumps without pus that swell, thicken, and become painful, as shown in Figure 62.5. The face takes on a reddened or flushed appearance, particularly around the nose and cheek area. With time, the redness becomes more permanent and lesions resembling acne appear. The soft tissues of the nose may thicken, giving the nose a reddened, bullous, irregular swelling called **rhinophyma**.

Rosacea is exacerbated by factors such as sunlight, stress, increased temperature, and agents that dilate facial blood vessels, including alcohol, spicy foods, skin care products, and warm beverages. It affects more women than men, although men more often develop rhinophyma.

Pharmacotherapy of Acne and Acne-Related Disorders

62.6 The pharmacotherapy of acne includes treatment with benzoyl peroxide, retinoids, and antibiotics. Therapies for rosacea include retinoids and metronidazole.

Medications used for acne and related disorders are available OTC and by prescription. Because of their increased toxicity, prescription agents are reserved for severe, persistent cases. These drugs are shown in Table 62.3.

Benzoyl peroxide (Benzac) is the most common topical OTC medication for acne. Benzoyl peroxide has a **keratolytic** effect, which helps to dry out and shed the outer layer of the epidermis. Other effects include possible sebum-suppressing action and antimicrobial activity that lasts up to 48 hours following application. This medication may be dispensed as a topical lotion, cream, or gel and is available in various percent concentrations. Other keratolytic agents used for severe acne include resorcinol (Resinol), salicylic acid, and sulfur.

NCLEX Success Tips

Acne is an inflammation of the sebaceous glands that results in excessive production of sebum. Washing the face with mild soap and water keeps the sebaceous glands from becoming plugged by removing fatty acids from the skin. The nurse should encourage the client to avoid frequent washing and to avoid squeezing the eruptions, as this can lead to rupture of these glands, spreading the sebum, causing further inflammation, and sometimes spreading infection if the ruptured gland was infected. The nurse should teach the client that applying vitamin E to the lesions does not decrease inflammation and, in fact, may obstruct the ducts due to the greasiness of the preparation. The client should be instructed to apply isotretinoin at night and to avoid sun exposure, which can result in sunburn and an increased risk of skin cancer. Sunscreen with a sun protection factor (SPF) of at least 15 should be applied before the client gets exposed to the sun.

TABLE 62.3 Drugs for Acne and Acne-Related Disorders

Drug	Remarks
OTC Agent	
benzoyl peroxide (Benzac)	Sometimes combined with tetracycline, erythromycin, or clindamycin in severe cases to fight bacterial infection (these combination agents are only available by prescription)
Prescription Agents (Topical)	
adapalene (Differin)	Retinoid-like compound used to treat acne formation
azelaic acid (Finacea)	For mild to moderate inflammatory acne
sulfacetamide	For sensitive skin; sometimes combined with sulfur to promote peeling, as in the condition rosacea; also used for conjunctivitis
tretinoin (Retin-A, Stieva-A)	To prevent clogging of pore follicles; also used for the treatment of acute promyelocytic leukemia and wrinkles
Prescription Agents (Oral)	
estradiol	Oral contraceptives are sometimes used for acne; combination drugs may be helpful—for example, ethinyl estradiol plus norgestimate (Ortho Tri-Cyclen)
doxycycline (Vibramycin)	Antibiotic; refer to Chapter 44
Pr isotretinoin (Accutane)	For acne with cysts or acne formed in small, rounded masses; pregnancy category X
tetracycline	Antibiotic; refer to Chapter 44 for the Prototype Drug box (page 529)

Women of childbearing age must meet certain criteria to be prescribed the medication because isotretinoin (Accutane) increases the risks of birth defects. Physicians and nurses should monitor clients closely for signs of depression. It is not enough to use a single form of birth control after initiating the drug. Women of childbearing age must use two forms of effective birth control for 2 months before, during, and 1 month after taking the medication.

Instruct the client that isotretinoin may cause muscle aches, and extreme exercise should be avoided.

Doxycycline (Vibramycin) is contraindicated in pregnancy because it can stain the teeth of the developing fetus if given during the last half of pregnancy.

Retinoids are newer agents, usually by prescription only, that are effective against severe acne. Tretinoin is a vitamin A derivative with an irritant action that decreases comedone formation and increases extrusion of comedones from the skin. Another use of tretinoin is for wrinkle removal. Topically applied tretinoin is minimally absorbed into the body. Other retinoids include isotretinoin, which is an oral medication and vitamin A metabolite that aids in reducing the size of sebaceous glands, thereby decreasing oil production and the occurrence of clogged pores. Isotretinoin is not recommended during pregnancy because of possible harmful effects to the fetus. A common reaction to retinoids is sensitivity to sunlight. Additional retinoid-like agents and related compounds used to treat acne include the following prescription medications: adapalene (Differin), azelaic acid (Finacea), and sulfacetamide.

Antibiotics are sometimes used in combination with acne medications to lessen the severe redness and inflammation associated with the disorder. Doxycycline and tetracycline have been the traditional antibiotics used in acne therapy.

Ethinyl estradiol is an estrogen commonly found in oral contraceptives that is also used to help clear the skin of acne. For the actions and contraindications of this and related hormones, see Chapter 31.

Pharmacotherapy for rosacea includes a number of drugs given for acne vulgaris, including isotretinoin, topical azelaic acid 20% cream, sulfacetamide preparations, and systemic antibiotics. In addition, clients with rosacea may be prescribed metronidazole 0.75% to 1% topical preparation, an antibacterial, and an antiprotozoal preparation. Crotamiton 10% cream (Eurax) or lotion may also be prescribed if hair follicle mites are present. In addition to medications, some clients have vascular or carbon dioxide laser surgery for rhinophyma.

Nursing Considerations

The role of the nurse in drug therapy for acne-related disorders includes careful monitoring of the client's condition and providing education as it relates to the prescribed drug regimen. The nurse working with teenagers with acne first needs to establish rapport since many clients may be embarrassed or have an altered body image or self-esteem disturbance because of the acne. Establishing rapport early will help the nurse when obtaining the health history and physical assessment. The nurse should record when the acne began, what treatments have been tried, and with what success. Most acne sufferers will have attempted many OTC therapies before seeing a healthcare provider for a prescription drug, and they may continue to use these preparations in addition to new prescriptions. Because some medications prescribed for acne are not recommended for the pregnant client, the nurse should ask women of childbearing age their pregnancy status.

The nurse should wear gloves when examining the skin. As with all dermatological conditions, the nurse should have the client undress in order to observe as much of the skin surface as possible. The acne on exposed areas such as the face may present somewhat differently than acne on the back or elsewhere. In some instances, clients are not aware of the extent of their skin disorder.

Isotretinoin is contraindicated in clients with a history of severe depression and suicidal ideation, and clients should sign a consent regarding understanding of suicide risks prior to treatment. Concurrent use of isotretinoin and carbamazepine (Tegretol) will decrease blood levels of carbamazepine, which may lead to increased seizure activity. Concurrent use of isotretinoin and hypoglycemic agents may lead to loss of glycemic control as well as increased risk for cardiovascular disease, secondary to elevated triglyceride levels.

A patch test should be done before the acne drug is used for the first time. When applying ointment, lotion, or cream to the skin, cleanse and completely dry the skin and apply the medication to a small area to test for sensitivity. A very small amount of topical medication, about the size of a pea, is enough to cover the face adequately. Topical medication should not be applied to the eyes, mouth, or mucous membranes.

Because isotretinoin may cause severe birth defects or spontaneous abortions, female clients must have a negative pregnancy test result within 2 weeks of beginning treatment. Tetracycline or minocycline (Minocin) use may increase the risk for pseudotumour cerebri, manifested by headache, papilledema, and decreased vision.

Client education as it relates to drugs used to treat acne should include goals, reasons for obtaining baseline data, and possible side effects. Client teaching and understanding is vital to the proper use of acne drugs. The following are the important points

CONNECTIONS Natural Therapies

◀ Burdock Root for Acne and Eczema

Burdock root, *Arctium lappa*, comes from a thick, flowering plant sometimes found on the roadsides of Britain and North America. It contains several active substances such as bitter glycosides and flavonoids, and it has a range of potential actions in the body: anti-infective, diuretic, mild laxative, and skin detoxifier. It is sometimes described as an attacker of skin disorders from within because it fights bacterial infections, reduces inflammation, and treats some stages of eczema, particularly the dry and scaling phases. Some claim that it is also effective against boils and sores.

Burdock root is considered safe, having few side effects or drug interactions. It contains 50% inulin, a fibre widely distributed in vegetables and fruits, and it is consumed as a regular part of the daily diet in many Asian countries. In many cases, burdock root is combined with other natural products for a wider range of effectiveness. Such products include sarsaparilla (*Smilax officinalis*), yellow dock (*Rumex crispus*), licorice root (*Glycyrrhiza glabra*), echinacea (*Echinacea purpurea*), and dandelion (*Taraxacum officinale*).

the nurse should include when teaching clients about drugs used for the treatment of acne:

- Inform the healthcare provider of all OTC medications used for acne.
- Use acne medications correctly and for the prescribed length of time.

- Avoid foods that seem to make acne worse. Keep a food log to determine which foods tend to worsen the condition.
- Avoid products that will irritate the skin, such as cologne, perfumes, and other alcohol-based products.
- If severe skin irritation or inflammation develops during therapy, discontinue use and call the healthcare provider.

NURSING PROCESS FOCUS

Clients Receiving Isotretinoin (Accutane)

Assessment	Potential Nursing Diagnoses/Identified Patterns
Prior to administration: • Obtain complete health history, including allergies, drug history, and possible drug interactions. • Obtain pregnancy and lactation status. • Assess for history of psychiatric disorders. • Assess vital signs to obtain baseline information.	• Need for knowledge regarding drug therapy and adverse effects • Psychosocial body image adjustment related to presence of acne and possible worsening of symptoms after treatment begins • Risk for impaired skin integrity related to inflammation, redness, and scaling, secondary to treatment • Decisional conflict related to desire for pregnancy and necessity of preventing pregnancy during therapy with isotretinoin • Difficulty adhering to therapy related to length of treatment time • Failure to use effective contraception

Planning: Client Goals and Expected Outcomes

The client will:

- Experience decreased acne, without side effects or adverse reactions
- Demonstrate acceptance of body image
- Demonstrate an understanding of the drug therapy by accurately describing the drug's intended effects, side effects, and precautions

Implementation

Interventions (Rationales)	Client Education/Discharge Planning
• Monitor laboratory studies during treatment, including blood glucose. • Discuss potential adverse reactions to drug therapy. (Understanding of drug effects is important for adherence.) • Monitor for cardiovascular problems. (Use isotretinoin with caution in clients with heart block, especially if client is also taking a beta blocker.) • Monitor emotional health. (Client may become depressed secondary to acne itself, length of treatment, possibility of worsening symptoms at beginning of treatment, changed body image, or drug itself.) • Monitor complete blood count (CBC), blood lipid levels, glucose levels, liver function tests, eye exam, gastrointestinal (GI) status, urinalysis. • Monitor for vision changes. (Corneal opacities and/or cataracts may develop as a result of isotretinoin use. Dryness of eyes during treatment is common. Night vision may be diminished during treatment.) • Monitor alcohol use. (Alcohol use with isotretinoin leads to increased triglyceride levels.) • Monitor skin problems. (This will determine the effectiveness of drug therapy.) • Monitor for side effects.	• Instruct client on importance of laboratory studies prior to therapy and periodically during therapy and of doing home blood glucose monitoring if diabetic Instruct client: • To use two forms of reliable birth control for 1 month before beginning treatment, during treatment, and for 1 month following completion of treatment • Not to donate blood during treatment and for a minimum of 4 weeks after completion of treatment; isotretinoin in donated blood could cause fetal damage if given to a pregnant woman • To talk with pediatrician about alternative methods of feeding if breastfeeding • To avoid use of vitamin A products • Discuss with client the importance of complete disclosure regarding medical history and medications. Instruct client: • To report signs of depression immediately and discontinue isotretinoin • Regarding signs and symptoms of depression • To report any feelings of suicide ideation • Teach client the importance of a complete workup prior to starting isotretinoin therapy and periodically during course of treatment. Instruct client: • To report any decreased vision and discontinue use of isotretinoin • To avoid driving at night if possible • That use of artificial tears may relieve dry eyes • That use of contact lenses may need to be discontinued during therapy

Advise client to:

- Eliminate or greatly reduce alcohol use, including alcohol-containing preparations such as mouthwashes and OTC medications
- Read labels for alcohol content

Advise client:

- That acne may worsen during beginning of treatment
- To monitor skin for improvement in 4–8 weeks; if no improvement is noted, contact the primary healthcare provider
- Instruct client to be aware of and to report headache (especially if accompanied by nausea and vomiting), fatigue, depression, lethargy, severe diarrhea, rectal bleeding, abdominal pain, dry mouth, hematuria, proteinuria, liver dysfunction (jaundice, pruritus, dark urine)

Evaluation of Outcome Criteria

Evaluate the effectiveness of drug therapy by confirming that client goals and expected outcomes have been met (see "Planning").

PROTOTYPE DRUG | **Isotretinoin (Accutane)**

Actions and Uses: The principal action of isotretinoin is regulation of skin growth and turnover. As cells from the stratum germinativum grow toward the skin's surface, skin cells are lost from the stratum pore openings, and their replacement is slowed. Isotretinoin also decreases oil production by reducing the size and number of oil glands. Symptoms take 4 to 8 weeks to improve, and maximum therapeutic benefit may take 5 to 6 months. This drug is most often used in cases of cystic acne or severe keratinization disorders.

Pharmacokinetics: Isotretinoin is metabolized by the liver. It is excreted in urine and feces. Its half-life is 21 hours.

Administration Alerts:

- Do not use this drug in clients with a history of severe depression and suicidal ideation.
- Take with meals to minimize GI distress.
- Isotretinoin is pregnancy category X.

Adverse Effects and Interactions: Isotretinoin is a toxic metabolite of retinol, or vitamin A. Common adverse effects are conjunctivitis, dry mouth, inflammation of the lip, dry nose, nosebleed, increased serum concentrations of triglycerides (by 50% to 70%), bone and joint pain, and photosensitivity. Liver function, serum glucose, and serum triglyceride tests should be performed when taking isotretinoin.

Isotretinoin interacts with vitamin A supplements, which increase toxicity. In addition, tetracycline or minocycline use may increase risk for pseudotumour cerebri. Concurrent use of hypoglycemic agents may lead to loss of glycemic control as well as increased risk for cardiovascular disease, secondary to elevated triglyceride levels. Concurrent use with carbamazepine will decrease blood levels of carbamazepine, which may lead to increased seizure activity.

DERMATITIS

Dermatitis is an inflammatory skin disorder characterized by local redness, pain, and pruritus. Intense scratching may lead to **excoriation**,

scratches that break the skin surface and fill with blood or serous fluid to form crusty scales. Dermatitis may be acute or chronic.

Atopic dermatitis, or **eczema**, is a chronic, inflammatory skin disorder with a genetic predisposition. Clients who present with eczema will often have a family history of asthma and hay fever as well as allergies to a variety of irritants such as cosmetics, lotions, soaps, pollens, food, and dust. About 75% of clients with atopic dermatitis will have had an initial onset before 1 year of age. In those babies predisposed to eczema, breastfeeding seems to offer protection, as it is rare for a breastfed child to develop eczema before the introduction of other foods. In infants and small children, lesions usually begin on the face and scalp, then progress to other parts of the body. A frequent and prominent symptom in infants is the appearance of red cheeks.

Contact dermatitis can be caused by a hypersensitivity response resulting from exposure to specific natural or synthetic allergens, such as plants, chemicals, latex, drugs, metals, or foreign proteins. Accompanying the allergic reaction may be various degrees of cracking, bleeding, or small blisters.

Seborrheic dermatitis is sometimes seen in newborns and in teenagers after puberty. It is characterized by yellowish, oily, crusted patches of skin that appear in areas of the face, scalp, chest, back, or pubic area. Bacterial infection or dandruff may accompany these symptoms.

Stasis dermatitis, a condition found primarily in the lower extremities, results from poor venous circulation. Redness and scaling may be observed in areas where venous circulation is impaired or where deep venous blood clots have formed.

Pharmacotherapy of Dermatitis

62.7 The most effective treatment for dermatitis is topical glucocorticoids.

Pharmacotherapy of dermatitis is symptomatic and involves lotions and ointments to control itching and skin flaking. Antihistamines may be used to control inflammation, and analgesics or topical anesthetics may be prescribed for pain relief.

TABLE 62.4 Topical Glucocorticoids for Dermatitis and Related Symptoms

Generic Name	Trade Names
Highest Level of Potency	
betamethasone	Diprosone, Valisone, Betaderm
clobetasol	Dermovate, Clobex
Middle Level of Potency	
amcinonide	Cyclocort, Amcort
desoximetasone	Topicort
fluocinonide	Lidex
halcinonide	Halog
mometasone	Elocom
triamcinolone	Kenalog, Oracort, Triaderm
Lower Level of Potency	
fluocinolone	Synalar, Derma-Smoothe
fluticasone	Flonase
hydrocortisone	Westcort, Hyderm, HydroVal, EmoCort
Lowest Level of Potency	
desonide	Desocort, Tridesilon
dexamethasone	Dexasone

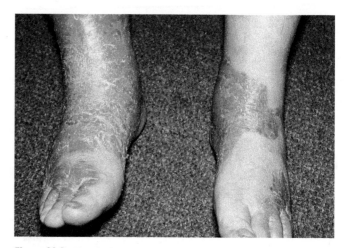

Figure 62.6 Psoriasis.
Source: Courtesy of Dr. Jason L. Smith.

PSORIASIS

Psoriasis is a chronic, non-infectious, inflammatory disorder characterized by red, raised patches of skin covered with flaky, thick, silver scales called plaques, as shown in Figure 62.6. These plaques shed the scales, which are sometimes greyish. The reason for the appearance of plaques is an extremely fast skin cell turnover rate, with skin cells reaching the surface in 4 to 7 days instead of the usual 14 days. Plaques are ultimately shed from the surface, while the underlying skin becomes inflamed and irritated.

The various forms of psoriasis are described in Table 62.5. Lesion size varies, but the shape tends to be round. Lesions are usually discovered on the scalp, elbows, knees, extensor surfaces of the arms and legs, sacrum, and occasionally around the nails. The etiology of psoriasis is unknown, but about 50% of cases involve a family history of the disorder. One theory of causation is that psoriasis is an autoimmune condition. In psoriasis, certain overactive immune cells release cytokines that cause the increased production of skin cells.

Topical glucocorticoids are the most effective treatment for dermatitis. As shown in Table 62.4, there are many formulations of glucocorticoids available in different potencies. Creams, lotions, solutions, gels, and pads are specially formulated to penetrate deep into the skin layers for relief of local inflammation, burning, and itching. Long-term glucocorticoid use, however, may lead to irritation, redness, and thinning of the skin membranes. If absorption occurs, topical glucocorticoids may produce undesirable systemic effects including adrenal insufficiency, mood changes, serum imbalances, and bone defects, as discussed in Chapter 30.

TABLE 62.5 Types of Psoriasis

Form of Psoriasis	Description of Form	Most Common Location of Lesions	Comments
Guttate (drop-like) or eruptive psoriasis	Lesions smaller than those of psoriasis vulgaris	Upper trunk and extremities	More common in early-onset psoriasis; can appear and resolve spontaneously a few weeks following a streptococcal respiratory infection
Psoriasis annularis	Ring-shaped lesions with clear centres		Rare
Psoriatic arthritis	Resembles rheumatoid arthritis	Fingers and toes at distal interphalangeal joints; can affect skin and nails	About 20% of clients with psoriasis also have arthritis
Psoriasis vulgaris	Lesions are papules that form into erythematous plaques with thick, silver or grey plaques, which bleed when removed; plaques in dark-skinned individuals often appear purple	Skin over scalp, elbows, and knees; lesions possible anywhere on the body	Most common form; requires long-term, specialized management
Psoriatic erythrodema or exfoliative psoriasis	Generalized scaling; erythema without lesions	All body surfaces	
Pustular psoriasis	Eruption of pustules; presence of fever	Trunk and extremities; can appear on palms, soles, and nail beds	

Pharmacotherapy of Psoriasis

62.8 Both topical and systemic drugs, including glucocorticoids, immunomodulators, and methotrexate, are used to treat psoriasis.

A number of prescription and OTC drugs are available for the treatment of psoriasis, including both topical and systemic agents, as shown in Table 62.6. A primary treatment is topical glucocorticoids, such as betamethasone (Diprosone, Valisone, Betaderm) ointment, lotion, or cream and hydrocortisone acetate cream or ointment. Topical glucocorticoids reduce the inflammation associated with fast skin turnover.

Another class of preparations is the topical immunomodulators (TIMs), which are agents that suppress the immune system. One example is tacrolimus ointment. Other agents applied topically are retinoid-like compounds such as calcipotriene (Dovonex), a synthetic vitamin D ointment, cream, or scalp solution; and tazarotene (Tazorac), a vitamin A derivative gel or cream. These drugs provide the same benefits as topical glucocorticoids but exhibit a lower incidence of adverse effects. Calcipotriene may produce hypercalcemia if applied over large areas of the body or used in higher doses than recommended. This drug is usually not used on an extended basis.

The most often prescribed systemic drug for severe psoriasis is methotrexate. Methotrexate is used in the treatment of a variety of disorders, including carcinomas and rheumatoid arthritis, in addition to psoriasis. Methotrexate is discussed as a prototype drug in Chapter 60. Other systemic drugs for psoriasis include acitretin and etretinate. These drugs are taken orally to inhibit excessive skin cell growth.

Other drugs used for different disorders, but that provide relief of severe psoriatic symptoms, are hydroxyurea and cyclosporine (Sandimmune, Neoral). Hydroxyurea is a sickle cell anemia drug. Cyclosporine is an immunosuppressive agent that is presented as a prototype drug in Chapter 40. In addition, etanercept and infliximab, which are approved for other autoimmune conditions, have been found to improve symptoms of psoriasis. Etanercept (Enbrel) and infliximab (Remicade) are tumour necrosis factor blockers.

Other skin therapy techniques may be used with or without additional psoriasis medications. These include various forms of tar treatment (coal tar) and anthralin (Anthranol), which are applied to the skin's surface. Tar and anthralin inhibit DNA synthesis and arrest abnormal cell growth.

Phototherapy with ultraviolet B (UVB) and ultraviolet A (UVA) is used in cases of severe psoriasis. UVB therapy is less hazardous than UVA therapy. UVB has a wavelength similar to sunlight, and it reduces widespread lesions that normally resist topical treatments. With close supervision, this type of phototherapy can be administered at home. Keratolytic pastes are often applied between treatments. The second type of phototherapy is referred to as PUVA because **psoralens** are often administered in conjunction with the phototherapy. Psoralens are oral or topical agents that, when exposed to UV light, produce a photosensitive reaction. This reaction reduces the number of lesions, but unpleasant side effects such as headache, nausea, and skin sensitivity still occur, limiting the effectiveness of this therapy. Immunosuppressant drugs such as cyclosporine are not used in conjunction with PUVA therapy because they increase the risk for skin cancer.

TABLE 62.6 Drugs for Psoriasis and Related Disorders

Drug	Route and Adult Dose
Topical Medications	
calcipotriene (Dovonex)	Topically to lesions every day (qd) or twice a day (bid)
tazarotene (Tazorac)	Acne: apply thin film to clean dry area qd Plaque psoriasis: apply thin film qd in the evening
Systemic Medications	
acitretin (Soriatane)	Orally (PO), 10–50 mg qd with the main meal
cyclosporine (Neoral, Sandimmune)	PO, 1.25 mg/kg bid (max 5 mg/kg/day)
hydroxyurea (Hydrea)	PO, 15 mg/kg/day
methotrexate (see Chapter 60, page 768, for the Prototype Drug box)	PO, 2.5–5 mg bid for three doses each week (max 25–30 mg/week) Intramuscular/intravenous (IM/IV), 10–30 mg/week

CHAPTER 62

Understanding the Chapter

Key Concepts Summary

The numbered key concepts provide a succinct summary of the important points from the corresponding numbered section within the chapter. If any of these points are not clear, refer to the numbered section within the chapter for review.

62.1 Three layers of skin—epidermis, dermis, and subcutaneous layer—provide effective barrier defences for the body.

62.2 Skin disorders that may benefit from pharmacotherapy are acne, sunburns, infections, dermatitis, and psoriasis.

62.3 When the skin integrity is compromised, bacteria, viruses, and fungi can gain entrance and cause infections. Anti-infective therapy may be indicated.

62.4 Scabicides and pediculicides are used to treat parasitic mite and lice infestations, respectively.

62.5 The pharmacotherapy of sunburn includes the symptomatic relief of pain using soothing lotions, topical anesthetics, and analgesics.

62.6 The pharmacotherapy of acne includes treatment with benzoyl peroxide, retinoids, and antibiotics. Therapies for rosacea include retinoids and metronidazole.

62.7 The most effective treatment for dermatitis is topical glucocorticoids.

62.8 Both topical and systemic drugs, including glucocorticoids, immunomodulators, and methotrexate, are used to treat psoriasis.

Chapter 62 Scenario

Danny McBride is a 17-year-old high school student in his senior year. He is active in lacrosse and baseball but is finding that his skin is breaking out more often lately and is becoming discouraged at the increase in breakouts. He feels that his skin condition has started to affect his social life, and his parents make an appointment for him with a dermatologist. The healthcare provider diagnoses Danny's skin condition as acne vulgaris and prescribes tretinoin (Retin-A).

Critical Thinking Questions

1. What would you tell Danny about his condition? Include what acne is, who is prone to develop it, and what methods of treatment have been found to be beneficial.

2. What are some reasons why Danny's acne outbreaks may have increased at this time?

3. What will you teach Danny about the application of tretinoin and adverse effects that may occur?

See Answers to Critical Thinking Questions in Appendix B.

NCLEX Practice Questions

1 An important inclusion in a teaching plan prepared for a client who is taking permethrin (Nix) is that

   a. Permethrin can be applied after body lotion is applied.

   b. All body hair, including eyelashes and eyebrows, can be treated with permethrin.

   c. Lice cannot live outside the body.

   d. In addition to hair shafts, the inner thigh areas, gluteal folds, and pubic areas should be examined for lice.

2 A client is being treated with a course of topical desoximetasone (Topicort) for atopic dermatitis. In planning teaching for this client, which adverse effects will the nurse anticipate?

   a. Burning and stinging of the skin in the affected area

   b. Development of localized pruritus and hives

   c. Hair loss in the application area

   d. Worsening of acne vulgaris

3 The client reports using benzoyl peroxide + clindamycin (Benzaclin) for treatment of acne. The nurse notes that the action of this drug includes which of the following? Select all that apply.

a. Sebum suppression

b. Antimicrobial effect

c. Keratolytic effect

d. Microdermal abrasion

e. Sunscreen activity

4 A client has been prescribed topical tretinoin (Retin-A) for treatment of acne unresponsive to over-the-counter products. What essential information should the nurse include in the client's teaching?

a. Wash the face thoroughly three times per day with an antiacne soap while using this medication.

b. Plan to expose the involved skin areas to sunlight for a minimum of 15 minutes each day.

c. Use only mild soaps and warm water, and pat the skin dry to avoid excessive irritation.

d. Alternate the topical tretinoin with benzoyl peroxide on an every-other-day rotation for best results.

5 Benzocaine (Anbesol) has been recommended to a 17-year-old client for treatment of a mild sunburn. What should the client be taught about using this product?

a. It may be used on superficial and partial-thickness sunburns.

b. Warming the lotion under warm water will prevent a chilled sensation when it's applied.

c. A small area of skin should be tested to assess for allergy if the drug has not been used before.

d. Cover the treated area with a light dressing of plastic wrap to keep it from rubbing off.

See Answers to NCLEX Practice Questions in Appendix A.

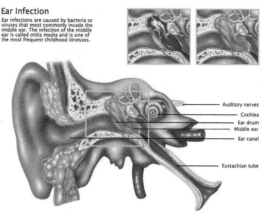

Ear Infection
Ear infections are caused by bacteria or viruses that most commonly invade the middle ear. The infection of the middle ear is called otitis media and is one of the most frequent childhood illnesses.

Auditory nerves
Cochlea
Ear drum
Middle ear
Ear canal
Eustachian tube

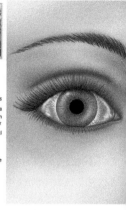

Photo Researchers, Inc/Alamy Stock Photo

BSIP SA/Alamy Stock Pho

CHAPTER

63

Pharmacotherapy of Eye and Ear Disorders

LEARNING OUTCOMES

After reading this chapter, the student should be able to:

1. Identify drug classes used for treating eye and ear disorders.

2. Explain the therapeutic action of drug therapies used for glaucoma and other eye and ear disorders in relation to the pathophysiology of the disorders.

3. For each of the drug classes listed in Prototype Drugs, identify a representative drug and explain its mechanism of action, therapeutic effects, and important adverse effects.

4. Explain the two major mechanisms by which drugs reduce intraocular pressure.

5. Describe the nurse's role in the pharmacological management of clients who are receiving drugs for eye and ear disorders.

6. Describe and explain, based on pharmacological principles, the rationale for nursing assessment, planning, and interventions for clients who are receiving drug therapy for eye and ear disorders.

7. Use the nursing process to care for clients who are receiving drug therapy for eye and ear disorders.

CHAPTER OUTLINE

▶ Anatomy of the Eye

▶ Glaucoma
  ▶ Types of Glaucoma
  ▶ General Treatment of Glaucoma
  ▶ Pharmacotherapy of Glaucoma

▶ Pharmacotherapy for Eye Exams and Minor Eye Conditions

▶ Ear Conditions
  ▶ Pharmacotherapy with Otic Preparations

Eyes and ears are vulnerable to a variety of conditions, many of which can be prevented, controlled, or reversed with proper treatment. The first part of this chapter covers various drugs used for the treatment of glaucoma. Drugs used routinely by ophthalmic healthcare providers are also discussed. The remaining part of the chapter presents drugs used for the treatment of ear disorders, including infections, inflammation, and the buildup of earwax.

Anatomy of the Eye

63.1 Knowledge of basic eye anatomy is fundamental for an understanding of eye disorders and pharmacotherapy.

A simple scratch to the eye can cause the client almost unbearable discomfort as well as concern about the effect that the damage may have on vision. Some eye disorders may be more bearable but extremely dangerous—including glaucoma, a leading cause of blindness. A firm knowledge of basic eye anatomy, shown in Figures 63.1 and 63.2, is required to understand eye disorders and

their pharmacotherapy. A fluid called **aqueous humour** is found in the anterior cavity of the eye. The anterior cavity has two divisions, the anterior chamber, which extends from the cornea to the iris, and the posterior chamber, which lies between the iris and the lens. The aqueous humour originates in the posterior chamber from a muscular structure called the ciliary body.

Aqueous humour helps to retain the shape of the eye, and it circulates to bring nutrients to the area and remove wastes. From its origin in the ciliary body, the aqueous humour flows through the pupil and into the anterior chamber. Within the anterior chamber and around the periphery is a network of spongy connective tissue, or trabecular meshwork, which contains an opening called the canal of Schlemm. The aqueous humour drains into the canal of Schlemm and out of the anterior chamber into the venous system, thus completing its circulation. Under normal circumstances, the rate of aqueous humour production is equal to its outflow, thus maintaining intraocular pressure (IOP) within a normal range. Interference with either the production or the outflow of aqueous humour can lead to an increase in IOP.

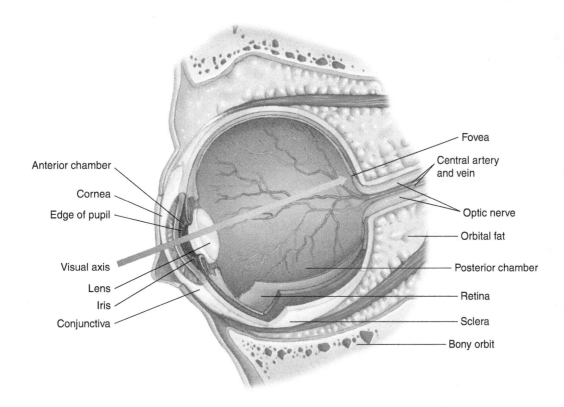

Figure 63.1 Internal structures of the eye.
Pearson Education.

GLAUCOMA

Glaucoma occurs when the IOP becomes high enough to cause optic nerve damage, leading to visual field loss and possibly advancing to blindness. Although the median IOP in the population is 15 to 16 mm Hg, this pressure varies greatly with age, daily activities, and even time of day. As a rule, IOP consistently above 21 mm Hg is considered abnormal. Many clients, however, tolerate IOP in the mid to high 20s without damage to the optic nerve. IOP above 30 mm Hg requires treatment because it is associated with permanent vision changes. Some clients of Asian descent may experience glaucoma at "normal" IOP values, below 21 mm Hg.

Glaucoma often exists as a primary condition without an identifiable cause. In some cases, glaucoma is associated with genetic factors; it can be congenital in infants and children. Glaucoma can also be secondary to eye trauma, infection, diabetes, inflammation, hemorrhage, tumour, high blood pressure, or cataracts. Some medications may contribute to the development or progression of glaucoma, including the long-term use of topical or oral glucocorticoids and some antihypertensives, antihistamines, and antidepressants. Glaucoma is the leading cause of *preventable* blindness in Canada.

Types of Glaucoma

63.2 Glaucoma develops because the flow of aqueous humour in the anterior eye cavity becomes disrupted, leading to increasing intraocular pressure. Two principal types of glaucoma are closed-angle glaucoma and open-angle glaucoma.

Diagnosis of glaucoma is sometimes difficult because it often occurs without symptoms. **Tonometry** is an ophthalmic technique that tests for glaucoma by measuring IOP. Other routine refractory and visual field tests may uncover signs of glaucoma. One problem with diagnosis is that clients with glaucoma typically do not experience symptoms and therefore do not schedule regular eye exams. In some cases, glaucoma occurs so gradually that clients do not notice a problem until late in the disease process.

As shown in Figure 63.2, the two principal types of glaucoma are **closed-angle glaucoma** and **open-angle glaucoma**. Both disorders result from the same problem: an increase of aqueous humour in the anterior cavity. This increase is caused either by excessive production of aqueous humour or by a blockage of its outflow. In either case, IOP increases, leading to progressive damage to the optic nerve. As degeneration of the optic nerve is occurring, the client will first notice a loss of visual field, then a loss of central visual acuity, and lastly total blindness. Major differences between closed-angle and open-angle glaucoma include how quickly the IOP develops and whether there is narrowing of the anterior chamber angle between the iris and cornea.

Closed-angle glaucoma, also called acute glaucoma or narrow-angle glaucoma, is uncommon. The incidence is higher in older adults and in persons of Asian descent. This acute type of glaucoma is usually unilateral and caused by stress, impact injury, or medications. Pressure inside the anterior chamber increases suddenly, with the iris being pushed over the area where the aqueous

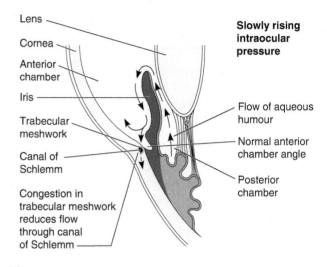

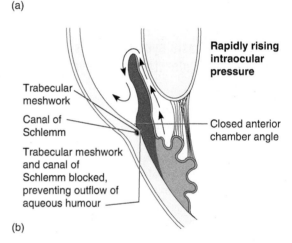

Figure 63.2 Forms of primary adult glaucoma: (a) in chronic open-angle glaucoma, the anterior chamber angle remains open, but drainage of aqueous humour through the canal of Schlemm is impaired; (b) in acute closed-angle glaucoma, the angle of the iris and anterior chamber narrows, obstructing the outflow of aqueous humour.

humour normally drains. The displacement of the iris is due in part to the dilation of the pupil or accommodation of the lens, causing the narrowed angle to close. Signs and symptoms, caused by acute obstruction of the outflow of aqueous humour from the eye, include intense headaches, difficulty concentrating, bloodshot eyes, blurred vision, and a bulging iris. Closed-angle glaucoma constitutes an emergency situation.

Open-angle glaucoma, or chronic simple glaucoma, is the most common type, accounting for 90% of the cases. It is usually bilateral, and IOP develops slowly, over a period of years. It is called "open-angle" because the iris does not cover the trabecular meshwork. Clients may be asymptomatic.

General Treatment of Glaucoma

63.3 General therapy of glaucoma may require laser surgery to correct the underlying pathology.

All of the approaches to glaucoma therapy are directed to the goal of increasing the circulation of aqueous humour that has been reduced (in the case of chronic, open-angle glaucoma) or prevented (in the case of acute, closed-angle glaucoma). In cases of acute, closed-angle glaucoma, surgery such as gonioplasty, laser iridotomy, and peripheral iridectomy may be performed to return the iris back to its original position. In gonioplasty, an argon laser burns the periphery of the iris. When the burn scars heal, tension is created that draws the iris away from the cornea, thus widening the angle. Iridectomy involves the laser creation of a number of small perforations in the iris, which allow the aqueous humour to drain through the normal pathway. Iridectomy involves removal of a small section of the iris to increase the flow of aqueous humour. Although surgery is often performed in acute, closed-angle glaucoma, the majority of cases of open-angle glaucoma are treated with medication.

Pharmacotherapy of Glaucoma

63.4 Drugs used for glaucoma decrease IOP by increasing the outflow of aqueous humour or by decreasing the formation of aqueous humour.

Pharmacotherapy for glaucoma works by one of two mechanisms: increasing the outflow of aqueous humour at the canal of Schlemm or decreasing the formation of aqueous humour at the ciliary body. Many agents for glaucoma act by affecting the autonomic nervous system (see Chapter 12). Agents for glaucoma, as shown in Table 63.1, include cholinergic agonists, non-selective adrenergics, prostaglandins, beta-adrenergic blockers, alpha$_2$-adrenergic agonists, carbonic anhydrase inhibitors, and osmotic diuretics.

NCLEX Success Tips

Carbachol (Miostat) reduces intraocular pressure during ophthalmological procedures; topical carbachol is used to treat open-angle and closed-angle glaucoma.

The abbreviation "gtt" stands for drop, "OU" signifies both eyes while "OD" and "OS" stand for right eye and left eye, respectively.

When administering pilocarpine (Isopto Carpine) eye drops, the nurse should apply pressure on the inner canthus to prevent systemic absorption of the drug. Flushing the client's eye with normal saline solution after administering eye drops is contraindicated because it will wash the drug out of the eye, rendering treatment ineffective.

The client should look up while the nurse instills the eye drops. The client does not need to keep both eyes open while the nurse administers the drug. The nurse should encourage the client to gently blink his or her eyes after the eye drops have been instilled. Using a tissue to wipe the eyes could remove some of the medication, decreasing its efficacy.

TABLE 63.1 Selected Drugs for Glaucoma

Drug	Route and Adult Dose
Cholinergic Agonists	
carbachol (Miostat) pilocarpine (Isopto Carpine)	1–2 drops 0.75%–3% solution in lower conjunctival sac up to three times a day (tid) Elevated intraocular pressure: 1 drop in the affected eye up to four times a day (qid) Glaucoma (acute angle closure): 1 drop 1% or 2% solution into the affected eye up to tid
Non-Selective Adrenergics	
dipivefrin (Propine)	1 drop 0.1% solution twice a day (bid)
Prostaglandins	
bimatoprost (Lumigan) **Pr** latanoprost (Xalatan)	1 drop 0.03% solution every day (qd) in the evening 1 drop (0.005%) solution qd in the evening
Beta-Adrenergic Blockers	
betaxolol (Betoptic) carteolol levobunolol (Betagan) metipranolol **Pr** timolol (Timoptic)	1-2 drops into affected eye bid 1 drop 1% solution bid 1–2 drops 0.25%–0.5% solution qd–bid 1 drop 0.3% solution bid 1–2 drops of 0.25%–0.5% solution qd–bid; gel (salve), apply qd
Alpha$_2$-Adrenergic Agonists	
apraclonidine (Iopidine) brimonidine (Alphagan)	1-2 drops into affected eye tid 0.15%: 1 drop in affected eye tid (approx every 8 hours [q8h]); 0.2%: 1 drop in affected eye bid (approx q12h)
Carbonic Anhydrase Inhibitors	
acetazolamide (Diamox) brinzolamide (Azopt) methazolamide	Orally (PO), 250 mg qd–qid 1 drop 1% solution tid PO, 50–100 mg bid or tid
Osmotic Diuretics	
isosorbide mannitol (Osmitrol)	PO, 1–3 g/kg bid–qid Intravenous (IV), 1.5–2 mg/kg as a 15%–25% solution over 30–60 minutes

Cholinergic Agonists

Drugs that activate cholinergic receptors in the eye produce constriction of the pupil, known as **miosis**, and contraction of the ciliary muscle. These agents are sometimes called **miotics**. These actions change the trabecular meshwork to allow greater outflow of aqueous humour and a lowering of the IOP. Agents such as carbachol and pilocarpine act *directly* on cholinergic receptors. Demecarium, echothiophate, isoflurophate, and physostigmine act *indirectly* by blocking acetylcholinesterase (AchE), the enzyme responsible for breaking down the neurotransmitter acetylcholine. The indirect-acting AchE inhibitors produce essentially the same effects as direct-acting drugs, except that they have a longer duration of action. Because of greater toxicity and longer action, these drugs are normally used only in clients with open-angle glaucoma who do not respond to other agents. The cholinergic agonists are applied topically to the eye. The antidote for serious drug toxicity from cholinergic agonists is atropine or pralidoxime chloride.

Non-Selective Adrenergics

Adrenergics (sympathomimetics) activate the sympathetic nervous system. Dipivefrin (Propine) is a non-selective adrenergic administered topically for open-angle glaucoma. Epinephrine produces mydriasis (pupil dilation) and increases the outflow of aqueous humour, resulting in a lower IOP. Dipivefrin is converted to epinephrine in the eye. Should epinephrine reach the systemic circulation, it increases blood pressure and heart rate.

Prostaglandins

Latanoprost (Xalatan) is a prostaglandin analogue available as a 0.005% eye drop solution, which decreases aqueous humour formation and increases outflow in open-angle glaucoma. Latanoprost is presented in this chapter as a prototype drug. Another prostaglandin used in the treatment of glaucoma is bimatoprost (Lumigan). The main side effect of these medications is heightened pigmentation, usually a brown colour of the iris in clients with lighter coloured eyes. These drugs cause cycloplegia, local irritation, and stinging of the eyes. Because of these effects, prostaglandins are normally administered just before bedtime.

Beta-Adrenergic Blockers

Beta-adrenergic blockers are drugs of choice for open-angle glaucoma. These include betaxolol (Betoptic), carteolol, levobunolol (Betagan), metipranolol, and timolol (Timoptic). These drugs act by decreasing the production of aqueous humour, thus reducing IOP. They generally produce fewer ocular adverse effects than cholinergic or adrenergic agonists. The topical administration of beta blockers for glaucoma treatment does not result in significant systemic absorption. Should absorption occur, however, systemic side effects may include bronchoconstriction, bradycardia, and hypotension.

Alpha₂-Adrenergic Agonists

Alpha₂-adrenergic agonists are prescribed less frequently than the other antiglaucoma medications. These drugs include apraclonidine, which is used for short-term therapy, and brimonidine, which is approved for long-term therapy. These drugs produce minimal cardiovascular and pulmonary side effects. The most significant side effects are headache, drowsiness, dry mucosal membranes, blurred vision, and irritated eyelids.

Carbonic Anhydrase Inhibitors

Carbonic anhydrase inhibitors may be administered topically or systemically to reduce IOP in cases of open-angle glaucoma. They act by decreasing the production of aqueous humour. Usually these medications are used as a second choice if beta blockers have not produced therapeutic results. Examples include acetazolamide (Diamox), brinzolamide (Azopt), dichlorphenamide, dorzolamide (Trusopt), and methazolamide. Clients must be cautioned when taking these medications because they contain sulfur and may cause an allergic reaction. Because these drugs are diuretics and can reduce IOP quickly, serum electrolytes should be monitored during treatment.

Osmotic Diuretics

Osmotic diuretics, like Mannitol (Osmitrol), are occasionally used in cases of eye surgery or acute, closed-angle glaucoma. Because they have the ability to quickly reduce plasma volume (see Chapter 53), they are effective in reducing the formation of aqueous humour. Side effects include headache, tremors, dizziness, dry mouth, fluid and electrolyte imbalances, and thrombophlebitis or venous clot formation near the site of IV administration.

Nursing Considerations

The role of the nurse in drug therapy for glaucoma involves careful monitoring of the client's condition and providing education as it relates to the prescribed drug regimen. The initial assessment of a client with glaucoma includes a general health history to determine past and current medical problems and medications. The nurse should determine if the client has a history of second- or third-degree heart block, bradycardia, heart failure, or chronic obstructive pulmonary disease (COPD). Antiglaucoma agents that affect the autonomic nervous system may be contraindicated for clients with these conditions because of possible drug absorption into the systemic circulation.

Several preparations used in glaucoma have a potential risk for cardiorespiratory side effects that will occur if the medication is systemically absorbed. Prior to starting drug therapy, baseline blood pressure and pulse should be established. When a beta blocker is used, the client should be taught how to check pulse and blood pressure before medication administration. The nurse should review the parameters of the pulse and blood pressure with the client and family members and establish guidelines when the healthcare provider should be notified. Because the safety of ophthalmic beta blocker preparations during pregnancy or lactation has not been established, the nurse should obtain information concerning the possibility of pregnancy or breastfeeding.

A key factor in preventing further ocular pathology is client adherence with the medication regimen. The nurse should determine any factors that could decrease adherence, such as insufficient financial resources, lack of knowledge, lack of dexterity or skill in inserting eye drops, or forgetting the dosing schedule. Fear and anxiety about potential blindness and disability may also be evident in the client who is diagnosed with glaucoma. It is crucial that the nurse allow the client to verbalize feelings and provide emotional support to the client and family. An explanation of how the disease can be controlled may facilitate adherence as well as alleviate the client's anxiety.

Client education as it relates to drugs to treat glaucoma should include goals, reasons for obtaining baseline data such as vital signs and tests for cardiac and respiratory function, possible side effects, and safe administration of eye medications.

Frequently the person with glaucoma is elderly, so a caregiver will administer the eye drops or gels. The nurse should review the proper method for administering eye medications outlined in Chapter 9. The following are the important points the nurse should include when teaching clients and caregivers regarding ophthalmic solutions used in glaucoma therapy:

- The client is at risk for falls and accidents secondary to decreased vision. Assess for environmental hazards and simple methods to ensure safety.

- Visual difficulty is often worse immediately following instillation of eye drops, as vision may be blurred. Remain still until the blurring diminishes.

- Report side effects, including eye irritation, conjunctival edema, burning, stinging, redness, blurred vision, pain, irritation, itching, sensation of foreign body in the eye, photophobia, and visual disturbances.

- Remove contact lenses before instilling drops and wait at least 15 minutes before reinserting them to allow the medication sufficient contact time with the eye.

- Report any reactions to the medication as well as any possibility of pregnancy.

See Nursing Process Focus: Clients Receiving Ophthalmic Solutions for Glaucoma for additional client teaching points.

CONNECTIONS Lifespan Considerations

◀ Ophthalmic Drugs in the Home Setting

Older adults may live alone or with family or friends. Ophthalmic drugs often need to be used at home. The ability of the aging individual to safely administer ophthalmic drugs in the home setting should be assessed. Return demonstration by the client may be critical for the nurse to assess the older adult's dexterity and skill in self-administering eye medications. If needed, seek reasonable alternatives, such as help from a neighbour, family member, or caregiver.

Teaching is critical for positive outcomes in this population. The older adult needs to understand that touching or rubbing the eye can result in infection or damage to the eye. Because vision may already be compromised, the older adult may experience blurred vision that should clear in a reasonable time after using ophthalmic drugs. Caution older adults about trying to drive or even ambulate until this unclear vision improves. In addition, diminished vision puts the older adult at increased risk for falls. The nurse can assess the home and make suggestions to improve safety.

Care should be taken to label eye medicines to indicate which is for the left eye and which is for the right eye. Scheduling medications around a routine, such as meals, also may help the older adult to remember to take the ophthalmic medications as prescribed, increasing the adherence necessary for healing.

Medications should be stored safely out of reach of children.

PROTOTYPE DRUG   Latanoprost (Xalatan)

Actions and Uses: Latanoprost is a prostaglandin analogue believed to reduce IOP by increasing the outflow of aqueous humour. The recommended dose is one drop in the affected eye(s) in the evening. It is used to treat open-angle glaucoma and elevated IOP.

Administration Alerts:

- Remove contact lens before instilling eye drops. Do not reinsert contact lens for 15 minutes.

- Avoid touching the eye or eyelashes with any part of the eyedropper to avoid contamination from one area to another.

- Wait 5 minutes before or after instillation of a different eye prescription to administer eye drops.

- Latanoprost is pregnancy category C.

Pharmacokinetics: Latanoprost is absorbed through the cornea. Onset of action is 3 to 4 hours. It is metabolized to its active form in the cornea, reaching its peak effect in about 12 hours. It is excreted by the kidneys.

Adverse Effects and Interactions: Adverse effects include ocular symptoms such as conjunctival edema, tearing, dryness, burning, pain, irritation, itching, sensation of foreign body in the eye, photophobia, and/or visual disturbances. The eyelashes on the treated eye may grow, thicken, and/or darken. Pigmentation changes may occur in the iris of the treated eye and in the periocular skin. The most common systemic side effect is a flu-like upper respiratory infection. Rash, asthenia, or headache may occur.

Latanoprost interacts with thimerosal: if mixed with eye drops containing thimerosal, precipitation may occur.

NURSING PROCESS FOCUS

Clients Receiving Ophthalmic Solutions for Glaucoma

Assessment	Potential Nursing Diagnoses/Identified Patterns
Prior to drug administration: • Obtain complete health history, including allergies, drug history, and possible drug interactions. • Obtain complete physical examination, focusing on visual acuity and visual field assessments. • Assess for the presence or history of ocular pain.	• Risk for injury if vision is impaired • Self-care challenges if vision is impaired • Pain related to disease process • Need for knowledge regarding drug therapy

---

Planning: Client Goals and Expected Outcomes

The client will:

- Exhibit no progression of visual impairment
- Demonstrate an understanding of the disease process
- Safely function within own environment without injury
- Report absence of pain
- Demonstrate an understanding of the drug by accurately describing the drug's purpose, action, side effects, and precautions

---

Implementation

Interventions (Rationales)	Client Education/Discharge Planning
• Monitor visual acuity, blurred vision, papillary reactions, extraocular movements, and ocular pain.	• Instruct client to report changes in vision and headache
• Monitor the client for specific contraindications to prescribed drug. (There are many physiological conditions in which ophthalmic solutions may be contraindicated.)	• Instruct client to inform healthcare provider of all health-related problems and prescribed medications
• Remove contact lenses before administration of ophthalmic solutions.	• Instruct client to remove contact lenses prior to administering eye drops and wait 15 minutes before reinsertion
• Administer ophthalmic solutions using proper technique.	Instruct client in the proper administration of eye drops:
• Monitor for ocular reaction to the drug such as conjunctivitis and lid reactions.	• Wash hands prior to eye drop administration
• Assess IOP readings. (These are used to determine effectiveness of drug therapy.)	• Avoid touching the tip of the container to the eye, which may contaminate the solution
• Monitor colour of iris and periorbital tissue of treated eye.	• Administer the eye drop in the conjunctival sac
• Monitor for systemic absorption of ophthalmic preparations. (Ophthalmic drugs for glaucoma can cause serious cardiovascular and respiratory complications if the drug is systemically absorbed.)	• Apply pressure over the lacrimal sac for 1 minute
	• Wait 5 minutes before administering other ophthalmic solutions
• Monitor and adjust environmental lighting to aid in client's comfort. (People who have glaucoma are sensitive to excessive light, especially extreme sunlight.)	• Schedule glaucoma medications around daily routines such as waking, mealtimes, and bedtime to lessen the chance of missed doses
• Encourage compliance with treatment regimen.	• Instruct client to report itching, drainage, ocular pain, or other ocular abnormalities
	• Instruct client that IOP readings will be done prior to beginning treatment and periodically during treatment
	Instruct client that:
	• More brown colour may appear in the iris and in the periorbital tissue of treated eye
	• Any pigmentation changes develop over months to years
	• Instruct client to immediately report palpitations, chest pain, shortness of breath, and irregularities in pulse
	Instruct client to:
	• Adjust environmental lighting as needed to enhance vision or reduce ocular pain
	• Wear darkened glasses as needed
	Instruct client:
	• To adhere to medication schedule for eye drop administration
	• About the importance of regular follow-up care with ophthalmologist

---

Evaluation of Outcome Criteria

Evaluate the effectiveness of drug therapy by confirming that client goals and expected outcomes have been met (see "Planning").

See Table 63.1 for a list of drugs to which these nursing actions apply.

PROTOTYPE DRUG	Timolol (Timoptic)

Actions and Uses: Timolol is a non-selective beta-adrenergic blocker available as a 0.25% or 0.5% ophthalmic solution. Timolol reduces elevated IOP in chronic, open-angle glaucoma by reducing the formation of aqueous humour. The usual dose is one drop in the affected eye(s) twice a day. Timoptic XE allows for once-a-day dosing. Treatment may require 2 to 4 weeks for maximum therapeutic effect. It is also available in tablets, which are prescribed to treat mild hypertension.

Pharmacokinetics: Onset of action is 30 minutes. It reaches peak effect in about 1 to 2 hours. Duration of action is 24 hours.

Administration Alerts:

- Proper administration lessens the danger of the drug being absorbed systemically, which can mask symptoms of hypoglycemia.
- Timolol is pregnancy category C.

Adverse Effects and Interactions: The most common side effects are local burning and stinging upon instillation. In most clients, there is no significant systemic absorption to cause adverse effects as long as timolol is applied correctly. If significant systemic absorption occurs, however, drug interactions could occur. Anticholinergics, nitrates, reserpine, methyldopa, and/or verapamil (Isoptin) use could lead to increased hypotension and bradycardia. Indomethacin and thyroid hormone use could lead to decreased antihypertensive effects of timolol. Epinephrine (Adrenalin) use could lead to hypertension followed by severe bradycardia. Theophylline (Theolair, Uniphyl) use could lead to decreased bronchodilation.

Pharmacotherapy for Eye Exams and Minor Eye Conditions

63.5 Mydriatic (pupil-dilating) drugs and cycloplegic (ciliary muscle–relaxing) drugs are routinely used for eye examinations.

Some drugs are specifically designed to enhance eye examinations during ophthalmic procedures. **Cycloplegic drugs** paralyze the ciliary muscles and prevent the lens from moving during assessment. **Mydriatic drugs** dilate the pupils to allow better observation of retinal structures. These agents include anticholinergics, such as atropine (Isopto Atropine) and tropicamide (Mydriacyl, Diotrope), and adrenergics such as phenylephrine (Mydfrin). Cycloplegics cause severe blurred vision and a loss of near vision. Mydriatics cause intense photophobia and pain in response to bright light.

Anticholinergic mydriatics can worsen glaucoma by impairing aqueous humour outflow and thereby increasing IOP. In addition, anticholinergics have the potential to produce central side effects such as confusion, unsteadiness, or drowsiness. Examples of cycloplegic, mydriatic, and lubricant drugs are listed in Table 63.2.

Mydriatics cause intense photophobia and pain in response to bright light. Mydriatics can worsen glaucoma by impairing aqueous

TABLE 63.2   Drugs for Mydriasis, Cycloplegia, and Lubrication of the Eye

Drug	Route and Adult Dose
Mydriatics: Adrenergics	
phenylephrine (Mydfrin)	1 drop 2.5% or 10% solution every 3 minutes as needed (PRN) (max 3 drops per eye)
Cycloplegics: Anticholinergics	
atropine (Isopto Atropine)	Mydriasis, cycloplegia: 1–2 drops 1% solution 1 hour before procedure; uveitis: 1 to 2 drops 1% solution up to qid
cyclopentolate (Cyclogyl, Diopentolate)	Mydriasis, cycloplegia: 1–2 drops 0.5%, 1%, or 2% solution; may repeat in 5–10 minutes
homatropine	Refraction: 1–2 drops 2% or 5% solution in affected eye; may repeat in 5–10 minutes if necessary; uveitis: 1–2 drops 2% or 5% solution in affected eye q3h-q4h
scopolamine hydrobromide (Isopto Hyoscine)	1–2 drops 0.25% solution 1 hour before eye exam
tropicamide (Mydriacyl, Diotrope)	1–2 drops 0.5%–1% solution before eye exam
Lubricants	
lanolin alcohol (Lacri-Lube)	Apply a thin film to the inside of the eyelid
naphazoline (Albalon, Clear Eyes, Refresh Redness)	1–2 drops into conjunctival sac q3h-q4h PRN
oxymetazoline HCl (Visine)	1–2 drops 0.025% solution qid
polyvinyl alcohol (Tears Natural)	1–2 drops PRN
tetrahydrozoline HCl (Visine)	1–2 drops 0.05% solution up to qid

humour outflow and thereby increasing IOP. In addition, strong concentrations of anticholinergics have the potential to have systemic effects on the central nervous system (CNS) and cause confusion, unsteadiness, or drowsiness. Cycloplegics can cause severe blurred vision and loss of near vision. Scopolamine (Isopto Hyoscine), an anticholinergic often used to prevent motion sickness, can cause blurred vision due to cycloplegia, as well as angle-closure glaucoma attacks. The response to mydriatics and cycloplegics can last from 3 hours up to several days. The client should be taught to wear sunglasses and that the ability to drive, read, and perform visual tasks may be affected during treatment.

Diagnostic agents are used to help locate lesions or foreign bodies within the eye and to provide some local anesthesia. Fluorescein sodium (Fluorescite) is a dye used in assessing the cornea and fitting contact lenses. Scratches may turn bright green; foreign bodies are surrounded by a green halo. Areas where the conjunctiva is damaged show an orange-yellow discoloration. Fluorescein sodium with benoxinate (Fluress) adds local anesthesia, making it useful for the identification and removal of foreign bodies from the cornea.

Local anesthetic agents are used to prevent the pain associated with diagnostic and surgical procedures, suturing and removal of foreign bodies, and ocular injections. The agents used include proparacaine (Alcaine, Ophthaine) and tetracaine. Application consists of one to two drops applied to the affected eye. Anesthesia typically occurs within 20 seconds and lasts for 10 to 20 minutes. Adverse effects of their use include local irritation, including conjunctivitis. Systemic effects are rarer, but CNS excitation has been known to occur. The nurse must be careful to protect the client's eye from injury while anesthetized, or corneal damage may occur.

NCLEX Success Tips

Instilled in the eye, phenylephrine acts as a mydriatic agent, causing the pupil to dilate. It also constricts small blood vessels in the eye.

Atropine causes pupil dilation. This action is contraindicated for the client with glaucoma because it increases intraocular pressure. If the client with glaucoma is scheduled for surgery, the client should be reminded to resume taking all medications for glaucoma immediately after surgery.

If atropine is absorbed systematically, it can cause tachycardia, palpitations, flushing, dry skin, ataxia, confusion, and dry mouth. To minimize systemic absorption, the client should apply digital pressure over the punctum at the inner canthus for 2 to 3 minutes after instilling the drops.

Drugs for minor irritation and dryness come from a broad range of classes, including antimicrobials, local anesthetics, glucocorticoids, and nonsteroidal anti-inflammatory drugs. In each case, a range of drug preparations, including drops, salves, optical inserts, and injectable formulations, may be used. Some agents only provide lubrication to the eye's surface, whereas others are designed to penetrate and affect a specific area of the eye.

EAR CONDITIONS

The ear has two major sensory functions: hearing and maintenance of equilibrium and balance. As shown in Figure 63.3, three

CONNECTIONS | Natural Therapies

◀ **Bilberry for Eye Health**

Bilberry (*Vaccinium myrtillus*), a plant whose leaves and fruit are used medicinally, is found in central and northern Europe, Asia, and North America. It has been shown in clinical studies to increase conjunctival capillary resistance in clients with diabetic retinopathy, thereby providing protection against hemorrhage of the retina. Bilberry contains anthocyanosides, which have a collagen-stabilizing effect. Increased synthesis of connective tissue (including collagen) is one of the contributing factors that may lead to blindness caused by diabetic retinopathy. Bilberry has also been used to reduce eye inflammation and improve night vision. It may be taken as a tea to treat nonspecific diarrhea and topically to treat inflammation of the mucous membranes of the mouth and throat.

structural areas—the outer ear, middle ear, and inner ear—carry out these functions.

Otitis, inflammation of the ear, most often occurs in the outer and middle ear compartments. **External otitis**, commonly called swimmer's ear, is inflammation of the outer ear that is most often associated with water exposure. **Otitis media**, inflammation of the middle ear, is most often associated with upper respiratory infections, allergies, or auditory tube irritation. Of all ear infections, the most difficult ones to treat are inner ear infections. **Mastoiditis**, or inflammation of the mastoid sinus, can be a serious problem because if left untreated it can result in hearing loss.

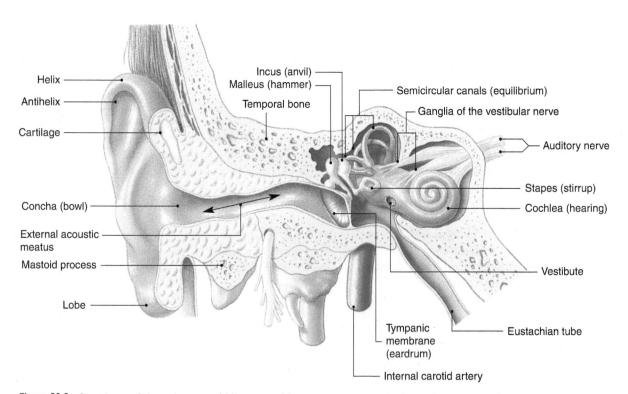

Helix — Antihelix — Cartilage — Concha (bowl) — External acoustic meatus — Mastoid process — Lobe — Incus (anvil) — Malleus (hammer) — Temporal bone — Semicircular canals (equilibrium) — Ganglia of the vestibular nerve — Auditory nerve — Stapes (stirrup) — Cochlea (hearing) — Vestibute — Eustachian tube — Tympanic membrane (eardrum) — Internal carotid artery

Figure 63.3 Structures of the outer ear, middle ear, and inner ear.

Pharmacotherapy with Otic Preparations

63.6 Otic preparations treat infections, inflammation, and earwax buildup.

The basic treatment for ear infections is topical antibiotics in the form of eardrops. Chloramphenicol (Chloromycetin) is the most commonly used topical otic antibiotic. Systemic antibiotics may be needed in cases where outer ear infections are extensive or in clients with middle or inner ear infections.

In cases of otitis media, drugs for pain, edema, and itching may also be necessary. Glucocorticoids are often combined with antibiotics or other drugs when inflammation is present. Examples of these drugs are listed in Table 63.3.

Mastoiditis is frequently the result of chronic or reoccurring bacterial otitis media. The infection moves into the bone and surrounding structures of the middle ear. Antibiotics are usually given for a trial period. If the antibiotics are not effective and symptoms persist, surgery such as mastoidectomy or meatoplasty may be indicated.

Cerumen (earwax) softeners are also used for proper ear health. When cerumen accumulates, it narrows the ear canal and may interfere with hearing. This is especially true for older clients and may be part of the changes associated with aging. Healthcare providers who work with older adults should be trained to take appropriate measures when removing impacted cerumen. This procedure usually involves instillation of an earwax softener and then a gentle lavage of the wax-impacted ear with tepid water using an asepto-type syringe to gently insert the water. An instrument called an ear loop may be used to help remove earwax, but it should be used only by healthcare providers who are skilled in using it. Nurses should advise clients not to perform earwax removal, especially in children, due to the potential for damage to the eardrum.

Nursing Considerations

The role of the nurse in drug therapy with otic preparations involves careful monitoring of the client's condition and providing education as it relates to the prescribed drug regimen. Before any of the otic preparations are administered, the nurse should assess the client's baseline hearing and auditory status. The nurse should assess the client's symptoms and any current medical conditions. Because the structure of the inner ear changes according to the client's age, the nurse should have a thorough understanding of the anatomy of the ear.

The nurse should obtain information regarding hypersensitivity to hydrocortisone, neomycin sulfate, or polymyxin B. The use of these medications is contraindicated in the presence of perforated eardrum. Chloramphenicol eardrops are contraindicated in hypersensitivity and eardrum perforation. Side effects include burning, redness, rash, swelling, and other signs of topical irritation.

When instilling otic preparations, the ear should be thoroughly cleansed and the cerumen removed through irrigation. The nurse should review the proper method for administering otic medications outlined in Chapter 9. Eardrops should be warmed to body temperature before instillation (but not higher than body temperature). The nurse should administer wax emulsifiers according to the manufacturer's guidelines or healthcare provider's orders.

Client education as it relates to otic preparations should include goals, reasons for obtaining baseline data such as hearing and auditory tests, and possible side effects. The following are important points the nurse should include when teaching clients regarding otic preparations:

- Lie down while instilling chloramphenicol drops since dizziness may occur. Also, do not touch the dropper to the ear.
- Administer eardrops at body temperature by running warm water over the bottle.
- With adults and children older than 3 years, the pinna should be held up and back during instillation. With children younger than 3 years of age, the pinna should be gently pulled down and back during instillation.
- Massage the area around the ear gently after instillation to promote thorough administration to the ear canal.
- Lie on the opposite side of the affected ear for 5 minutes after instillation.

TABLE 63.3 Otic Preparations	
Drug	**Route and Adult Dose**
acetic acid and hydrocortisone	3 to 5 drops q4h–qid for 24 hours, then 5 drops tid–qid
aluminum sulfate and calcium acetate	2 drops 2% solution tid–qid
benzocaine and antipyrine (Auralgan)	Fill ear canal with solution tid for 2 or 3 days
carbamide peroxide	5-10 drops bid for up to 4 days
ciprofloxacin hydrochloride and hydrocortisone	3 drops of the suspension instilled into ear bid for 7 days
polymixin B, neomycin, and hydrocortisone (Cortisporin)	4 drops in ear tid–qid
triethanolamine polypeptide oleate 10% condensate (Cerumenex)	Fill ear canal with solution; wait 10–20 minutes

CHAPTER

63   Understanding the Chapter

Key Concepts Summary

The numbered key concepts provide a succinct summary of the important points from the corresponding numbered section within the chapter. If any of these points are not clear, refer to the numbered section within the chapter for review.

63.1 Knowledge of basic eye anatomy is fundamental for an understanding of eye disorders and pharmacotherapy.

63.2 Glaucoma develops because the flow of aqueous humour in the anterior eye cavity becomes disrupted, leading to increasing intraocular pressure. Two principal types of glaucoma are closed-angle glaucoma and open-angle glaucoma.

63.3 General therapy of glaucoma may require laser surgery to correct the underlying pathology.

63.4 Drugs used for glaucoma decrease IOP by increasing the outflow of aqueous humour or by decreasing the formation of aqueous humour.

63.5 Mydriatic (pupil-dilating) drugs and cycloplegic (ciliary muscle–relaxing) drugs are routinely used for eye examinations.

63.6 Otic preparations treat infections, inflammation, and earwax buildup.

Chapter 63 Scenario

Therese Duclos is 65 years old. She visits her ophthalmologist with reports of blurry vision and not being able to see well at night while driving. Her health history includes adult-onset diabetes for the past 10 years and osteoporosis since age 55. Her medical regimen includes diet control for the diabetes and risedronate (Actonel) monthly. She denies any injury to her eyes and last had an eye checkup 1 year ago.

Critical Thinking Questions

1. What factors are present in Therese's health history that you identify as predisposing conditions for the development of primary open-angle glaucoma?

2. Therese needs to learn the proper administration of eye drops. What teaching would you provide to ensure that the skill will be performed correctly?

3. What would be possible effects from systemic absorption if the client were taking beta-adrenergic drops (e.g., timolol, carteolol)? Prostaglandin drops (e.g., latanoprost, bimatoprost)? Cholinergic agonists (e.g., carbachol, pilocarpine)?

See Answers to Critical Thinking Questions in Appendix B.

NCLEX Practice Questions

1 The nurse is teaching a client about a new eye drop prescription for timolol (Timoptic) for treatment of open-angle glaucoma. The client has a history of seasonal allergies and hypertension. What is an important administration technique to stress for this client?

a. Take any eye drops for allergies 5 minutes before administering the timolol drops.

b. Do not use the timolol drops while concurrently taking allergy medication.

c. The timolol drops may temporarily worsen seasonal allergies.

d. Gently put pressure on the inner canthus (tear duct) for 1 minute after instilling the timolol drop.

2 The nurse is providing health teaching to a client who has been prescribed latanoprost (Xalatan) for open-angle glaucoma. While harmless, the nurse would caution the client about which potential nonocular effects of the drug? Select all that apply.

a. Darkening and thickening of the upper eyelid

b. Darkening and thickening of eyelashes

c. A lightening of iris colour and a slight darkening of the sclera

d. A slight darkening of the iris colour

e. A permanent bluish tint to the conjunctiva

3 Pilocarpine (Isopto Carpine) has been ordered for a client with closed-angle glaucoma who has not responded well to other drugs. Pilocarpine causes _____, which stretches the trabecular meshwork, allowing a greater outflow of aqueous humour and lowering intraocular pressure.

4 The nurse is teaching a 25-year-old client about the administration of ciprofloxacin with hydrocortisone for otitis. In which order will the nurse instruct the client to use the drug?

a. Gently massage the area in front of the ear.

b. Pull the earlobe upward and back.

c. Allow the drop to fall into the ear canal, flowing down the side.

d. Remain with the treated ear in an uppermost position for 5 minutes.

5 The nurse is teaching a client with otitis about a prescription for polymyxin B, neomycin, with hydrocortisone. The client should be instructed to immediately report which symptom?

a. Mild itching in the outer ear canal

b. Gradually decreasing pain

c. Slight dizziness after instilling the eardrop

d. Increasing pain, particularly in the area around the ear

See Answers to NCLEX Practice Questions in Appendix A.

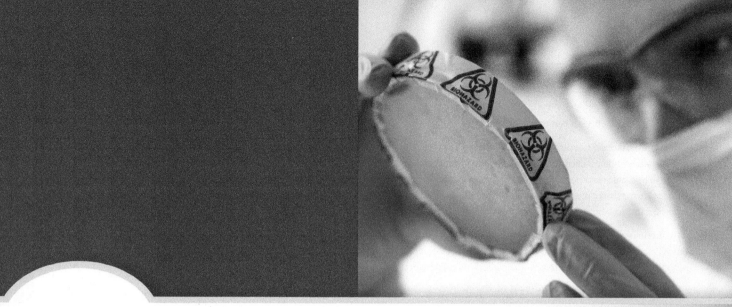

TEK IMAGE/Science Photo Library/Getty Images

CHAPTER

64 Toxicology, Bioterrorism, and Emergency Preparedness

LEARNING OUTCOMES

After reading this chapter, the student should be able to:

1. Explain why drugs are important in the context of toxicity and emergency preparedness.

2. Describe common causes of toxicity and the meaning of exposure.

3. Discuss the role of the nurse in the prevention and management of poisoning.

4. Discuss the role of the nurse in preparing for and responding to a bioterrorist act.

5. Identify the purpose and components of the National Emergency Stockpile System (NESS).

6. Explain the threat of anthrax contamination and how anthrax is transmitted.

7. Discuss the clinical manifestations and treatment of anthrax exposure.

8. Identify specific viruses that most likely would be used in a bioterrorist act.

9. Explain the advantages and disadvantages of vaccination as a means of preventing illness due to bioterrorist acts.

10. Provide examples of chemical agents that might be used in a bioterrorism act, and describe their treatments.

11. Describe the symptoms of acute radiation exposure and the role of potassium iodide (KI) in preventing thyroid cancer.

CHAPTER OUTLINE

▶ Preventing and Controlling Toxicity
  ▶ Toxicology
  ▶ Management of Poisoning
  ▶ Effectiveness of Activated Charcoal in Poisoning

▶ Emergency Preparedness
  ▶ The Nature of Bioterrorism
  ▶ Role of the Nurse in Emergency Preparedness
  ▶ National Emergency Stockpile System

▶ Agents Used in Bioterrorism
  ▶ Biological Agents
  ▶ Viruses
  ▶ Toxic Chemical and Physical Agents
  ▶ Ionizing Radiation

Emergency preparedness is the ability to respond swiftly and effectively to an unexpected event that may affect human health. The unexpected event may be a natural disaster caused by severe weather, an accidental chemical spill, or a purposeful terrorist attack on the public. It is also important that nursing students are aware that some naturally occurring and manufactured substances can produce harmful effects on human health and that special services and drugs are available to help counter these effects. Drugs are the most powerful tools available for counteracting toxicity and for preventing or controlling global disease outbreaks and the effects of bioterrorist acts. If medical personnel cannot identify, isolate, or treat the causes of global diseases, a major incident could easily overwhelm healthcare resources and produce a catastrophic loss of life. Drugs are a major component of emergency preparedness plans. This chapter discusses the role of pharmacology in the prevention and treatment of toxicity and diseases or conditions that might develop in the context of a biological, chemical, or nuclear attack.

PREVENTING AND CONTROLLING TOXICITY

Poisoning ranks as the third most frequent type of injury, after falls and motor vehicle collisions, that leads to hospitalization in Canada. Sources of toxicity or poisoning are numerous and include plants, household and industrial chemicals, drugs, and agents that may be used for bioterrorism. Nurses play key roles in preventing and minimizing harm from toxicity.

Toxicology

64.1 Poisoning is the third most frequent type of injury that leads to hospitalization in Canada. Drugs are the most common cause in all poisonings.

The Canadian Network of Toxicology Centres defines **toxicology** as the study of the harmful effects of naturally occurring and human-made substances on living organisms. Any substance can be toxic. **Exposure** occurs when a harmful substance enters the body through the skin, lungs, or gastrointestinal (GI) tract. Substances that are poorly absorbed reduce exposure. Substances that are stored in tissues prolong exposure. In general, the higher the dose and the longer the exposure to a potentially toxic substance, the greater the chance of an adverse effect. Carbon monoxide, arsenic, rattlesnake venom, botulinum toxin,

and pesticides are some familiar sources of toxicity (poisoning). Many foods, beverages, drugs, and nutritional supplements have ingredients that can be toxic in large quantities. For example, vitamin A is an essential nutrient, but it can cause birth defects when taken at high doses during pregnancy. Health Canada is responsible for maintaining an adequate and safe food supply for Canadians and controlling exposure to toxins. Health Canada regulates the use of additives to prolong the shelf-life of foods, use of fertilizers and pesticides to protect crops, and use of growth stimulants and antibiotics to promote health and efficient growth in animals. Foods labels must indicate ingredients and additives. Drug labels must include directions for use. Products that may be hazardous must have clear warning labels.

Toxicity may be classified as acute or chronic. **Acute toxicity** refers to the rapid development of symptoms following short-term exposure (less than 24 hours) to a harmful substance. An example is nausea and vomiting following inhalation of bleach fumes. **Chronic toxicity** occurs following long-term repeated exposure to a harmful substance, with cumulative effects. A substance may produce both acute and chronic toxicity. Mechanisms of toxicity include disruption of nerve impulses, disruption of the body's ability to transport or use oxygen, damage to the immune system, and impairment of organ function. These effects may include reversible or irreversible physiological injury, disease, cancer, genetic damage or mutation, birth defects, or death. Individuals may differ in terms of their resistance (or susceptibility) to toxins. Nutrition, age, body mass, immune function, respiratory function, genetics, and other factors may affect susceptibility in humans. For example, clients with asthma may be more susceptible to toxins that affect respiration. Infants have less well developed immune systems and may be more susceptible to toxins from infectious agents. Developing fetuses are susceptible to environmental toxins such as drugs or alcohol taken during pregnancy. The Canadian Congenital Anomalies Surveillance Network was established in 2002 to monitor rates of birth defects across Canada.

Antidotes refer to substances used to reduce the effects of toxins. It is often difficult to identify a particular causative substance because individuals may be exposed to multiple substances that interact in different ways. Substances that when combined are less toxic than either would be individually are referred to as having antagonistic effects. Antagonistic substances may be used as antidotes for one another. When no specific antidote is available, activated charcoal may be used to bind drugs and poisons within the GI tract so that they are expelled in the feces. Examples of some common sources of toxicity and their antidotes are presented in Table 64.1.

TABLE 64.1 Specific Antidotes

Poison	Antidote
acetaminophen (Tylenol)	acetylcysteine (Mucomyst)
anticholinergic drugs	physostigmine (Antilirium)
benzodiazepines	flumazenil (Romazicon)
beta-adrenergic blockers	glucagon
calcium channel blockers	calcium, IV insulin in high doses with IV glucose
carbamates	atropine, pralidoxime (Protopam)
digoxin (Lanoxin, Toloxin)	digoxin immune Fab (Digibind)
ethylene glycol (antifreeze, brake fluid, coolants)	ethanol, fomepizole (Antizol)
heavy metals	chelating drugs
iron	deferoxamine (Desferal)
isoniazid (INH)	pyridoxine (vitamin B_6)
methanol	ethanol, fomepizole (Antizol)
methemoglobin-forming drugs (some local anesthetics, nitrates, nitrites, phenacetin, sulfonamides)	methylene blue
opioids	naloxone (Narcan)
organophosphates	atropine, pralidoxime (Protopam)
tricyclic antidepressants	sodium bicarbonate

NCLEX Success Tips

Acetylcysteine (Mucomyst) tastes like rotten eggs and is often diluted by mixing it with a flavoured drink such as cola. Use of a straw is recommended to minimize discomfort from taste. The nebulizer form of this medication is used for pneumonia, not for acetaminophen (Tylenol) overdose. The medication should not be mixed with food and is not administered intravenously.

During a hypoglycemic reaction, it is recommended that a layperson administer glucagon, an antihypoglycemic agent, to raise the blood glucose level quickly in a client who can't ingest an oral carbohydrate. Glucagon is a normal body protein that interacts adversely with oral anticoagulants, increasing their anticoagulant effects.

Seizures are the most common serious adverse effect of using flumazenil (Romazicon) to reverse benzodiazepine overdose. The effect is magnified if the client has a combined tricyclic antidepressant and benzodiazepine overdose.

Flumazenil must be given in small quantities, such as 0.2 mg over 15 to 30 seconds, but never as a bolus. Flumazenil may be given undiluted in incremental doses. Adverse effects of flumazenil may include shivering and hypotension. The nurse should monitor the client's level of consciousness while recovering from sedation. Flumazenil must be given through a free-flowing IV line in a large vein because extravasation causes local irritation.

Naloxone (Narcan) is an opioid-reversal agent used to reverse the effects of acute opioid overdose and is the drug of choice for reversal of opioid-induced respiratory depression.

Disulfiram (Antabuse) does not block the effects of alcohol, but blocks the breakdown of alcohol in the blood, which produces marked discomfort, such as throbbing headache, flushing, and nausea and vomiting. As such, it curbs the impulsiveness of the problem drinker. Disulfiram does not decrease cravings for alcohol.

Activated charcoal binds with the ingested drug to inhibit or decrease its absorption. Giving a client activated charcoal won't promote vomiting or stimulate bowel motility, and it doesn't neutralize the drug. After administering appropriate stomach lavage, the nurse should give the client activated charcoal every 4 hours for 24 hours.

The **Canadian Association of Poison Control Centres (CAPCC)** was established in 1982 to provide a centralized forum for information exchange among Canadian poison control centres. Provinces, territories, and regional jurisdictions have poison control and drug information centres that can be accessed by phone 24 hours a day. Centres are often staffed primarily with specially educated nurses and pharmacists who consult as needed with pharmaceutical companies, toxicologists, and physicians with expertise in toxicology and overdose management. The centres guide both laypersons and healthcare professionals in the event of chemical, herbal, or drug toxicity. The centres provide current, evidence-based advice about poisons and drugs specific to the caller's situation (either the layperson or the healthcare provider). About 70% of poison exposures can be managed at home safely and cost effectively. Surveillance data are collected. Nurses should be knowledgeable about their local poison advisory centres. The CAPCC website maintains links to poison centres in Canada.

Priorities for treatment of poisoned clients are maintenance of airway, breathing, and circulation. The next priorities are to reduce absorption and action of the toxic substance by administering an antidote or activated charcoal. The use of syrup of ipecac to induce vomiting is often not recommended, as significant quantities of the ingested substance may not be vomited or may already have passed through the stomach. There is an added risk that the client may lose consciousness and aspirate vomit during ipecac therapy.

The role of the nurse includes prevention of harm from toxins. Nurses should know the antidotes that are available for each medication the client receives. The antidotes should be readily available in case toxicity occurs. Clients should be informed about proper use and safe storage of medicines, household cleaners, and other substances. The following are important points to include when teaching clients and families about prevention of toxicity:

- Immediately report known or suspected exposure to toxins to the local poison control centre for guidance and referral.
- Immediately report confusion, shortness of breath, chest congestion, heart palpitations, or other signs of adverse reaction.
- Store medications in their original containers and out of reach of children.
- Select products in containers with child-resistant safety caps.
- Read warning labels and follow directions when using medicines and household or industrial products.
- Ensure that contact information for the local poison and drug advisory centre is readily accessible.

Management of Poisoning

64.2 The general management of poisoning includes contacting the poison control centre or emergency medical services as soon as possible.

The general management of poisoning includes contacting the poison control centre or emergency medical services as soon as possible. Virtually any chemical may cause poisoning if taken in excessive amounts. The body has a remarkable capacity to tolerate a wide variety of chemicals and has physiological mechanisms to detoxify and rapidly eliminate many of them. Toxicity results when the body's abilities for detoxification and excretion are exceeded. Toxic effects may appear immediately or they may appear decades after the initial exposure.

Medications are the most frequently involved substances in poisonings for all age groups. Household cleaning compounds comprise a second large group responsible for poisonings, with cosmetics being close behind them. Although exposure to poisons may occur by any route, ingestion accounts for more than 75% of all poisoning cases. Swallowing dangerous substances is common among children with curious minds who naturally put strange substances into their mouths. Most poisonings present with low levels of toxicity, but some can result in fatalities, such as the ingestion of gun-bluing agents used to maintain the colour of gun barrels. Signs and symptoms of ingested poisons include abdominal cramping or stomach pain; nausea; vomiting; diarrhea; sleepiness or loss of consciousness; bottles or containers of poisons close by; or odour, stains, or burns around the oral cavity.

Poisoning from medications may be unintentional or intentional (suicide). Acetaminophen is a common toxin because so many analgesic medications contain this drug. Although legal for adults, alcohol is a potential poison and its abuse is a major health problem in Canada. Ingestion of alcohol, along with certain prescribed medications, amphetamines, hallucinogens, barbiturates, tranquilizers, opiates, or inhaled substances such as solvents or glue can create life-threatening situations. Whether the overdose of alcohol is intentional or unintentional, the result is the same. Symptoms of drug overdose include confusion, elevated heart rate, drowsiness, enlarged or dilated pupils, and hallucinations. Other medications that cause frequent poisonings include iron, calcium channel blockers, and tricyclic antidepressants.

When a specific antidote is available, it is administered as soon as the poisoning is diagnosed (see Table 64.1). In the vast majority of poisoning cases, there is no specific antidote. General therapies such as activated charcoal, peritoneal dialysis, and gastric lavage have only limited effectiveness. In some cases, they are totally ineffective. Emergency physicians and nurses are generally faced with treating individual symptoms either because the poison is unknown or because there is no antidote. The strategy for treatment of acute poisoning consists of five general principles:

- *Topical decontamination.* Removal of contaminated clothing, flushing of the skin or eyes
- *Prevention of absorption.* Administration of adsorbents (activated charcoal), whole bowel irrigation, induction of vomiting, and gastric lavage
- *Neutralization.* Administration of acids or bases
- *Increase in the rate of excretion.* Administration of diuretics, peritoneal or extracorporeal dialysis, and ion trapping
- *Antidotes and symptomatic therapy.* Administration of specific antidotes and support of vital functions

Treatment for ingested poisons depends on the age of the client, the physical size of the client, and the time between swallowing and presenting for medical intervention. Any information about the poisoning that can be obtained from the client, family, or caregiver can be helpful, such as the type of poison that was swallowed, when it was ingested, and how much was swallowed.

The following are some specific interventions for managing the client who has been poisoned by ingestion:

- Do not implement the package instructions for poisoning without consulting the CAPCC or an appropriate healthcare provider. Preferred therapy may have changed since the packaging was printed.
- Contact the poison control centre if the poisoning is the result of taking too much medication or the wrong medication being taken.
- Provide fresh air to the person if the poison was inhaled.
- Remove contaminated clothes if the poison came in contact with the person's skin. Take care not to spread contamination from the poisoned clothes to the surrounding environment. Flush the skin with water for 15 to 20 minutes to dilute or remove the poison.
- Rinse the eyes with running water for 15 to 20 minutes if contacted by poison.
- Do not induce vomiting by gagging or tickling the back of the throat.
- Do not give ipecac syrup. Though once considered a routine procedure, this method of poison management is now considered ineffective. Discourage parents from keeping ipecac syrup in the home. There is no evidence that syrup of ipecac actually helps to improve the outcome in poisoning cases. Furthermore, the administration of syrup of ipecac can delay the administration of more effective treatments, such as activated charcoal or antidotes.
- Do not give milk or water unless directed to do so by the poison centre. Though once thought to dilute the poison, fluids can liquefy dry poison and send it more rapidly to the small intestine. The exception to this is caustic or corrosive poisons.

Effectiveness of Activated Charcoal in Poisoning

64.3 Activated charcoal is effective at adsorbing (binding) most poisons if administered within 60 minutes of ingestion.

Activated charcoal has been used as an adsorbent for acute poisoning for almost 200 years. Although activated charcoal is effective in the treatment of many poisons, it is not beneficial when given to individuals with lithium, iron, or cyanide poisoning or strong acid or alkali ingestion.

PROTOTYPE DRUG Activated Charcoal

Actions and Uses: Activated charcoal consists of organic material such as coal, wood, or vegetables that has been carbonized, reduced, and dried to a charcoal-like substance. It is then activated by exposing it to steam, carbon dioxide, or other oxidizing chemicals at extremely high temperatures. The activation drives off impurities and reduces the particle size so that the surface area of the charcoal is very large.

Pharmacokinetics: This drug effectively adsorbs toxins in the intestinal tract, thus preventing their systemic absorption. Adsorption is the process of a drug physically binding to the charcoal. As a general-purpose emergency antidote, it is used in the treatment of poisonings of most drugs and chemicals.

Administration Alerts:

- To be most effective, the charcoal should be administered within 1 hour of oral ingestion of a poison.
- Normally, a single dose is administered, although some poisons benefit from multiple doses of charcoal.
- The general dosage is 5 to 10 times the estimated weight of the poison ingested.
- Activated charcoal can also be used off-label to adsorb intestinal gases in the treatment of dyspepsia, flatulence, and distention. It is sometimes used topically as a deodorant for foul-smelling wounds and ulcers.

EMERGENCY PREPAREDNESS

Bioterrorist activities and threats and the emergence of new infectious diseases such as severe acute respiratory syndrome (SARS) have led to widespread changes in emergency preparedness planning. Nurses play key roles in planning for such incidents.

The Nature of Bioterrorism

64.4 Bioterrorism is the deliberate use of a biological, chemical, or physical agent to cause panic and mass casualties. The health aspects of biological and chemical agents have become important public issues.

Prior to the September 11, 2001, terrorist attacks on the United States, the attention of healthcare providers regarding disease outbreaks was mainly focused on the spread of traditional infectious diseases. These included possible epidemics caused by influenza, tuberculosis, cholera, and human immunodeficiency virus (HIV). Table 64.2 shows the 10 most dangerous infectious diseases ranked according to which caused the most deaths worldwide in the year 2000. Other diseases such as food poisoning and sexually transmitted infections were also common, though considered less important because they produced fewer fatalities.

The aftermath of the September 11, 2001, attacks prompted the healthcare community to expand its awareness of outbreaks and treatments to include bioterrorism and the health effects of biological and chemical weapons. **Bioterrorism** may be defined as the intentional use of infectious biological agents, chemical substances, or radiation to cause widespread harm or illness. The public has become more aware of the threat of bioterrorism because such agencies as the World Health Organization (WHO), Centre for Emergency Preparedness and Response of the Public Health Agency of Canada, and Centers for Disease Control and Prevention (CDC) in the United States have stepped up efforts to inform, educate, and prepare the public for disease outbreaks of a less traditional nature.

TABLE 64.2   The 10 Most Dangerous Infectious Diseases in the World, 2000

Disease	Cause	Target	Deaths per Year (millions)
Influenza	*Haemophilus influenzae*	Respiratory system	3.7
Tuberculosis	*Mycobacterium tuberculosis*	Lungs	2.9
Cholera	*Vibrio cholerae*	Digestive tract	2.5
Acquired immune deficiency syndrome (AIDS)	HIV	Immune system	2.3
Malaria	*Plasmodium falciparum*	Blood	1.5
Measles	Rubeola virus	Lungs and meninges	0.96
Hepatitis B	Hepatitis B virus (HBV)	Liver	0.605
Whooping cough	*Bordetella pertussis*	Respiratory system	0.41
Tetanus	*Clostridium tetani*	Entire body (infections)	0.275
Dengue fever	Flavivirus	Entire body (fever)	0.14

Based on World Health Organization data, www.ac-reunion.fr/pedagogie/anglaislp/OurFood/General_bacteriology.html

The goals of a bioterrorist are to create widespread public panic and cause as many casualties as possible. There is no shortage of agents that can be used for this purpose. Indeed, some of these agents are easily obtainable and require little or no specialized knowledge to disseminate. Areas of greatest concern include acutely infectious diseases such as anthrax, smallpox, plague, and hemorrhagic viruses; incapacitating chemicals such as nerve gas, cyanide, and chlorinated agents; and physical threats such as nuclear bombs and radiation. Biological threats have been categorized based on their potential impact on public health, as shown in Table 64.3.

Role of the Nurse in Emergency Preparedness

64.5 Nurses play key roles in emergency preparedness, including providing education, resources, diagnosis and treatment, and planning.

Emergency preparedness includes all activities, such as plans, procedures, contact lists, and exercises, undertaken in anticipation of a likely emergency. The goal of these preparedness activities is to make sure that the Public Health Agency of Canada, with the support of Health Canada, is ready and able to respond quickly and effectively in the event of an emergency. Emergency preparedness is not a new concept. For more than 40 years, accredited hospitals have been required to develop disaster plans and to conduct

TABLE 64.3   Categories of Infectious Agents

Category	Description	Examples
A	Agents that can be easily disseminated or transmitted person to person; cause high mortality, with potential for major public health impact; might cause public panic and social disruption; require special action for public health preparedness	*Bacillus anthracis* (anthrax) *Clostridium botulinum* toxin (botulism) *Francisella tularensis* (tularemia) *Variola major* (smallpox) Viral hemorrhagic fevers such as Marburg and Ebola *Yersinia pestis* (plague)
B	Agents that are moderately easy to disseminate; cause moderate morbidity and low mortality; require specific enhancements of CDC's diagnostic capacity and enhanced disease surveillance	*Brucella* species (brucellosis) *Burkholderia mallei* (glanders) *Burkholderia pseudomallei* (melioidosis) *Chlamydia psittaci* (psittacosis) *Coxiella burnetii* (Q fever) Epsilon toxin of *Clostridium perfringens* Food safety threats such as *Salmonella* and *Escherichia coli* Ricin toxin from *Ricinus communis* *Staphylococcus* enterotoxin B Viral encephalitis Water safety threats such as *Vibrio cholerae* and *Cryptosporidium parvum*
C	Emerging pathogens that could be engineered for mass dissemination in the future because of their availability, ease of production and dissemination, and potential for high morbidity and mortality rates and major health impacts	Hantaviruses Multidrug-resistant tuberculosis *Nipah virus* (NiV) Tick-borne encephalitis viruses Yellow fever

Based on Centers for Disease Control and Prevention, www.bt.cdc.gov/Agent/agentlist.asp.

periodic emergency drills to determine readiness. Originally, disaster plans and training focused on natural disasters such as tornados, hurricanes, and floods or on accidents such as explosions that could cause multiple casualties. More recently, bioterrorism and virulent infectious organisms have been included as possible scenarios in disaster preparedness.

In the past few decades, infectious diseases have re-emerged as a growing threat to global health security. Both newer diseases, such as SARS and bovine spongiform encephalopathy (BSE), and older ones, such as tuberculosis and influenza, have had serious impacts on Canada and the world. Increases in antimicrobial resistance, in diseases transmitted from animals to humans, and in international trade and travel all compound the public health threat posed by infectious diseases. The WHO establishes the International Health Regulations and leads international cooperation to ensure maximum security against the international spread of infectious diseases. Emergency preparedness includes more than responding to the immediate casualties caused by a disaster: it also considers how an agency's healthcare delivery system will shift during a crisis and how it will return to normal operations following the incident. The expanded focus also includes how the individual healthcare agency will coordinate its efforts with community resources, such as other hospitals and public health agencies. National, provincial, territorial, and local agencies have revised their emergency preparedness guidelines in an attempt to more rationally plan for possible bioterrorist acts.

Planning for bioterrorist acts requires close cooperation among all healthcare professionals. Nurses are central to the effort. Because a bioterrorist incident may occur in any community without advance warning, nurses must be prepared to respond immediately. The Canadian Nurses Association (CNA) works with the Public Health Agency of Canada's Centre for Emergency Preparedness to combine expertise for a more effective response to emergency situations and to define nurses' role in a national emergency response plan. The CNA is a member of the International Council of Nurses, which published a position statement titled "Nurses and Disaster Preparedness" (2001) that provides information pertinent to global nursing issues, such as coping with terrorism and disaster preparedness. The following elements underscore the key roles of nurses in meeting the challenges of a potential bioterrorist event:

- *Education.* Nurses must maintain a current knowledge and understanding of emergency management relating to bioterrorist activities.

- *Resources.* Nurses must maintain a current listing of health and law enforcement contacts and resources in their local community that would assist in the event of bioterrorist activity.

- *Diagnosis and treatment.* Nurses must be aware of the early signs and symptoms of chemical and biological agents, and their immediate treatment.

- *Planning.* Nurses should be involved in developing emergency management plans.

National Emergency Stockpile System

64.6 The National Emergency Stockpile System is used to rapidly deploy medical necessities to communities that are experiencing a chemical or biological attack.

Should a chemical or biological attack occur, it would likely be rapid and unexpected and produce multiple casualties. Although planning for such an event is an important part of emergency preparedness, individual healthcare agencies and local communities could easily be overwhelmed by such a crisis. Shortages of needed drugs, medical equipment, and supplies would be expected.

The Public Health Agency of Canada maintains a $300 million **National Emergency Stockpile System (NESS)** to quickly provide emergency supplies to provinces and territories when requested. The system consists of a central depot in Ottawa, as well as eight other warehouses and 1300 pre-positioned supply centres (under the combined management of the provinces and federal government) strategically located across Canada. It includes 165 mobile hospitals, with 200 beds in each, ready to be set up in buildings such as schools and community centres. The NESS contains everything that you would expect to find in a hospital, from blankets to a supply of pharmaceuticals and a range of antibiotics. A 24-hour response capability is maintained. The Agency assesses and refurbishes stockpile units and distributes medical and pharmaceutical supplies at the request of provinces. The NESS has been used to support a number of emergencies, both in Canada and internationally.

The stockpiling of antibiotics and vaccines by local hospitals, clinics, or individuals for the purpose of preparing for a bioterrorist act is not recommended. Pharmaceuticals have a finite lifespan, and keeping large stores of drugs can be costly. Furthermore, stockpiling could cause drug shortages and prevent the delivery of these pharmaceuticals to communities where they may be needed most.

AGENTS USED IN BIOTERRORISM

Bioterrorists could potentially use any biological, chemical, or physical agent to cause widespread panic and serious illness. Knowing which agents are most likely to be used in an incident helps nurses to plan and implement emergency preparedness policies.

Biological Agents

64.7 Biological agents such as anthrax, botulism, and pneumonic plague can enter the body through ingestion, through inhalation, or by the cutaneous route. Antibiotic therapy can be successful if given prophylactically or within a short time after exposure.

One of the first threats following the terrorist attacks of September 11, 2001, was **anthrax**. In fall 2001, five people died as a result of exposure to anthrax, presumably due to purposeful, bioterrorist actions. At least 13 U.S. citizens were infected, several

governmental employees were threatened, and the U.S. Postal Service was interrupted for several weeks. There was initial concern that anthrax outbreaks might disrupt many other essential operations throughout the country.

Anthrax is caused by the bacterium *Bacillus anthracis*, which normally affects domestic and wild animals. A wide variety of hoofed animals are affected by the disease, including cattle, sheep, goats, horses, donkeys, pigs, bison, antelopes, elephants, and lions. If transmitted to humans by exposure to an open wound, through contaminated food, or by inhalation, *B. anthracis* can cause serious damage to body tissues. Symptoms of anthrax infection usually appear 1 to 6 days after exposure. Depending on how the bacterium is transmitted, specific types of anthrax "poisoning" may be observed, each characterized by hallmark symptoms. Clinical manifestations of anthrax are summarized in Table 64.4.

NCLEX Success Tip

Anthrax is treated with antibiotics, and the client must continue the prescription for 60 days, even if symptoms do not persist. The client may have skin lesions at the point of contact, with macula or papule formation; the eschar will fall off in 1 to 2 weeks. Clients with anthrax are not contagious and do not need to follow isolation procedures at home.

B. anthracis causes disease by the emission of two types of toxin: edema toxin and lethal toxin. These toxins cause necrosis and accumulation of exudate, which produces pain, swelling, and restriction of activity, the general symptoms associated with almost every form of anthrax. Another component, the anthrax binding receptor, allows the bacterium to bind to human cells and act as a "doorway" for both types of toxins to enter.

Further ensuring its chance to spread, *B. anthracis* is spore forming. Anthrax spores can remain viable in soil for hundreds, and perhaps thousands, of years. Anthrax spores are resistant to drying, heat, and some harsh chemicals. These spores are the main cause for public health concern because they are responsible for

TABLE 64.4	Clinical Manifestations of Anthrax	
Type	**Description**	**Symptoms**
Cutaneous anthrax	Most common but least complicated form of anthrax; almost always curable if treated within the first few weeks of exposure; results from direct contact of contaminated products with an open wound or cut	Small skin lesions develop and turn into black scabs; inoculation takes less than 1 week; cannot be spread by person-to-person contact
Gastrointestinal anthrax	Rare form of anthrax; without treatment, can be lethal in up to 50% of cases; results from eating anthrax-contaminated food, usually meat	Sore throat, difficulty swallowing, cramping, diarrhea, and abdominal swelling
Inhalation anthrax	Least common but most dangerous form of anthrax; can be successfully treated if identified within the first few days after exposure; results from inhaling anthrax spores	Initially fatigue and fever for several days, followed by persistent cough and shortness of breath; without treatment, death can result within 4–6 days

producing inhalation anthrax, the most dangerous form of the disease. After entry into the lungs, *B. anthracis* spores are ingested by macrophages and carried to lymphoid tissue, resulting in tissue necrosis, swelling, and hemorrhage. One of the main body areas affected is the mediastinum, which is a potential site for tissue injury and fluid accumulation. Meningitis is also a common pathology. If treatment is delayed, inhalation anthrax is lethal in almost every case.

B. anthracis is found in contaminated animal products such as wool, hair, dander, and bonemeal, but it can also be packaged in other forms, making it transmissible through the air or by direct contact. Terrorists have delivered it in the form of a fine powder, making it less obvious to detect. The powder can be inconspicuously spread on virtually any surface, making it a serious concern for public safety.

The antibiotic ciprofloxacin (Cipro) has traditionally been used for anthrax prophylaxis and treatment. For prophylaxis, the usual dosage is 500 mg by mouth (PO, *per os*) every 12 hours for 60 days. If exposure has been confirmed, ciprofloxacin should be immediately administered intravenously at a usual dose of 400 mg every 12 hours. Other antibiotics, including penicillin, vancomycin (Vancocin), ampicillin, erythromycin (Eryc), tetracycline, and doxycycline (Vibramycin), are also effective against anthrax.

Many members of the public have become intensely concerned about bioterrorism threats and have asked their healthcare provider to provide them with ciprofloxacin. The public should be discouraged from seeking the prophylactic use of antibiotics in cases where anthrax exposure has not been confirmed. Indiscriminate, unnecessary use of antibiotics can be expensive, cause significant side effects, and promote the appearance of resistant bacterial strains. Refer to Chapter 44 to review the precautions and guidelines regarding the appropriate use of antibiotics.

Although anthrax immunization (vaccination) has been in use for 30 years, it has not been widely used because of the extremely low incidence of this disease. The vaccine has been prepared from proteins from the anthrax bacterium, dubbed "protective antigens." Anthrax vaccine works in the same way as other vaccines, by causing the body to make protective antibodies and thus preventing the onset of disease and symptoms. Immunization for anthrax consists of three subcutaneous (SC) injections given 2 weeks apart, followed by three additional SC injections given at 6, 12, and 18 months. Annual booster injections of the vaccine are recommended. At this time, vaccination is recommended only for select populations: laboratory personnel who work with anthrax, military personnel deployed to high-risk areas, and those who deal with animal products imported from areas with a high incidence of the disease.

There is an ongoing controversy regarding the safety of the anthrax vaccine and whether it is truly effective in preventing the disease. Until these issues are resolved, the use of anthrax immunization will likely remain limited to select groups. Vaccines and the immune response are discussed in more detail in Chapters 39, 40, and 41.

Botulism is caused by *Clostridium botulinum*, an organism that secretes a potent toxin that paralyzes the muscles after a person is poisoned. Respiratory failure and paralysis may force a client to be on a ventilator for weeks or months. As a biological weapon, botulism could be transmitted in air, food, or water. Treatment includes immediate administration of an antitoxin and assisted ventilation until clients are able to function independently. The antitoxin should be given as soon as possible and never delayed pending the microbiological testing.

Pneumonic plague is a life-threatening infectious lung disease that occurs after breathing *Yersinia pestis*, a bacterium found on rodents and their fleas that is responsible for the bubonic plague. It is highly contagious and can be deadly if untreated within 24 hours of contact. As a biological agent, *Y. pestis* could be spread by aerosol over the population. Within 1 to 6 days of exposure, the client would be infectious to everyone he or she has come in contact with during that time. This makes the plague difficult to contain. Symptoms include fever and weakness, rapid development of pneumonia, chest pain with shortness of breath, cough, and bloody sputum. Without immediate treatment, respiratory failure will result, followed by shock and death. Treatment with antibiotics must occur within 24 hours and last for at least 7 days to prevent death from the infection. The primary antibiotic for *Y. pestis* infection is doxycycline 100 mg twice a day or ciprofloxacin 500 mg twice a day for 7 days.

Caused by the organism *Francisella tularensis*, **tularemia** is a serious infectious disease found in rodents, rabbits, and hares. According to the Public Health Agency of Canada, 289 cases and 12 deaths were reported in Canada between 1940 and 1981. *F. tularensis* is one of the most infectious bacteria known and survives at low temperatures for weeks in hay, straw, moist soil, or the bodies of decaying animals. As a biological weapon, the most casualties would occur with aerosol release in an area of high population, causing hemorrhagic inflammation of the respiratory airway. Treatment includes IV therapy with streptomycin as the drug of choice, with parenteral gentamicin (Garamycin) being an alternative. Aminoglycosides should be used for 10 days. Tetracyclines and chloramphenicol can be used for at least 14 days but have a higher rate of relapse and treatment failure. In mass casualty incidents, oral doxycycline for 14 to 21 days and ciprofloxacin for 10 days are preferred for adults and children.

Viruses

64.8 Viruses such as polio, smallpox, and the hemorrhagic fever viruses are potential biological weapons. If available, vaccines are the best treatments.

In 2002, the public was astounded as researchers in the United States announced that they had "built" a poliovirus, a threat considered essentially eradicated from the Western Hemisphere in 1994. Polio persists among infants and children in areas with contaminated drinking water or food, mainly in underdeveloped regions of India, Pakistan, Afghanistan, western and central Africa, and the Dominican Republic. International travel can expose Canadians to infectious diseases, like polio, that are not frequently seen in North America.

The current concern regarding polio is that bioterrorists will culture the poliovirus and release it into regions where people have not been vaccinated. An even more dangerous threat is that a mutated strain, for which there is no effective vaccine, might be developed. Because the genetic code of the poliovirus is small (around 7500 base pairs), it can be manufactured in a relatively simple laboratory. Once the virus is isolated, hundreds of different mutant strains could be produced in a very short time.

In addition to polio, smallpox is considered a potential bioterrorism hazard. Smallpox was eradicated from the planet in the 1970s, but the variola virus that causes this disease is harboured in research labs in different countries. Much of its genetic code (200 000 base pairs) has been sequenced and is public information. The disease is spread person to person as an aerosol or droplets or by contact with contaminated objects such as clothing or bedding. Only a few viral particles are needed to cause infection. If released into an unvaccinated population, as many as one in three could die from the virus.

There are no effective therapies for treating people infected by most types of viruses that could be used in a bioterrorist attack. For some viruses, however, it is possible to create a vaccine. The WHO does not recommend systematic vaccination against smallpox because the disease has already been eradicated. However, the WHO and many countries, including Canada, are stockpiling smallpox vaccine with which to combat new epidemics resulting from bioterrorist activity, if necessary. The variola vaccine provides a high level of protection if given prior to exposure or up to 3 days afterwards. Re-vaccination may extend immunity for 10 to 20 years or more. Since mass vaccination in Canada ended in 1972, most people in Canada have little or no immunity to the virus that causes smallpox. As a result, people at high risk for infection in a bioterrorist attack—certain healthcare workers, public health personnel, and members of the military—are being vaccinated. Contraindications to receiving the smallpox vaccine include atopic dermatitis or eczema, altered immune states (e.g., HIV, acquired immune deficiency syndrome [AIDS], leukemia, lymphoma, taking immunosuppressive drugs), pregnancy, breastfeeding, and allergy to any component of the vaccine.

One suggestion has been that multiple vaccines be created, mass produced, and stockpiled to meet the challenges of a terrorist attack. Another suggestion has called for mass vaccination of the public, or at least those healthcare providers and law enforcement employees who might be exposed to infected members of the public; however, vaccines have side effects, some of which are quite serious. In addition, terrorists with some knowledge of genetic structure could create a modified strain of the virus that renders existing vaccines totally ineffective. It appears, then, that mass vaccination is not an appropriate solution until research can produce safer and more effective vaccines.

Toxic Chemical and Physical Agents

64.9 Chemicals and neurotoxins are potential bioterrorist threats for which specific antidotes are not always available.

Chemical warfare agents have been used since World War I, but few drug antidotes exist today. Many treatments provide minimal help, other than to relieve some symptoms and provide comfort following exposure. Whether a chemical is released by terrorists, enemy military, or industry in a chemical accident, the result is

the same: a hazardous chemical that may harm the health of the public is released into the environment. The CDC has classified hazardous chemicals into categories that include:

- *Biotoxins.* Poisons from plants or animals
- *Vesicants and blister agents.* Severely blister the skin, respiratory tract, or eyes on contact
- *Blood agents.* Poisons that are absorbed into the circulation
- *Acids and caustics.* Chemicals that burn the eyes, skin, or lining of the respiratory tract on contact
- *Pulmonary and choking agents.* Chemicals that irritate the lung and cause swelling and choking
- *Incapacitating agents.* Chemicals that alter consciousness, making it difficult for the client to think clearly
- *Long-acting anticoagulants.* Chemicals that produce uncontrolled bleeding by preventing clotting
- *Metals.* Agents that are metallic poisons
- *Nerve agents.* Poisons that impair nervous system functioning
- *Organic solvents.* Chemicals that damage living tissue by dissolving fats and oils
- *Tear gas or mace.* Used for riot or crowd control by law enforcement or for self-defence; irritates the eyes and the respiratory tract, resulting in incapacitation
- *Toxic alcohols.* Chemicals that damage vital organs such as the heart, kidneys, and nervous system
- *Vomiting agents.* Chemicals that induce nausea and vomiting.

Most chemical agents used in warfare were created to cause mass casualties; others were designed to cause so much discomfort that soldiers would be too weak to continue fighting. Potential chemicals that could be used in a terrorist act include nerve gases, blood agents, choking and vomiting agents, and those that cause severe blistering. Table 64.5 provides a summary of selected chemical agents and known antidotes and first-aid treatments.

The category of main pharmacological significance is **nerve agents**. Exposure to these acutely toxic chemicals can cause convulsions and loss of consciousness within seconds and respiratory failure within minutes. Almost all signs of exposure to nerve gas agents relate to overstimulation of the neurotransmitter acetylcholine (Ach) at both central and peripheral sites throughout the body.

Acetylcholine is normally degraded in the synaptic space by the enzyme acetylcholinesterase (AchE). Nerve agents block AchE, increasing the action of Ach in the synaptic space; therefore, all symptoms of nerve gas exposure, such as salivation, increased sweating, muscle twitching, involuntary urination and defecation, confusion, convulsions, and death, are the direct result of Ach overstimulation. To remedy this condition, Mark I injector kits that contain the anticholinergic drug atropine and a related antidote are available in cases where nerve agent release is expected. Atropine blocks the attachment of Ach to receptor sites and prevents the overstimulation caused by the nerve agent. Neurotransmitters, synapses, and autonomic receptors are discussed in detail in Chapter 12.

TABLE 64.5 Chemical Warfare Agents and Treatments

Category	Signs of Exposure	Antidotes/First Aid
Nerve Agents		
tabun or GA (liquid) sarin or GB (gaseous liquid) soman or GD (liquid) VX (gaseous liquid)	Depending on the nerve agent, symptoms may be slow to appear and cumulative depending on exposure time: miosis, runny nose, difficulty breathing, excessive salivation, nausea, vomiting, cramping, involuntary urination and defecation, twitching and jerking of muscles, headaches, confusion, convulsion, coma, death	Nerve agent antidote and Mark I injector kits with atropine are available. Flush eyes immediately with water. Apply sodium bicarbonate or 5% liquid bleach solution to the skin. Vomiting should not be induced.
Blood Agents		
hydrogen cyanide (liquid) cyanogen chloride (gas)	Red eyes, flushing of the skin, nausea, headaches, weakness, hypoxic convulsions, death Loss of appetite, irritation of the respiratory tract, pulmonary edema, death	Flush eyes and wash skin with water. For inhalation of mist, oxygen and amyl nitrate may be given. For ingestion of cyanide liquid, 1% sodium thiosulfate may be given to induce vomiting. Oxygen and amyl nitrate may be given. Give client milk or water. Do not induce vomiting.
Choking/Vomiting Agents		
phosgene (gas) Adamsite or DM (crystalline compound dispensed in aerosol)	Dizziness, burning eyes, thirst, throat irritation, chills, respiratory and circulatory failure, cyanosis, frostbite-type lesions Irritating to the eyes and respiratory tract, tightness of the chest, nausea, and vomiting	Provide fresh air. Administer oxygen. Flush eyes with normal saline or water. Keep client warm and calm. Rinse nose and throat with saline, water, or 10% solution of sodium bicarbonate. Treat the skin with borated talcum powder.
Blister/Vesicant Agents		
phosgene oxime (crystalline compound or liquid) mustard-lewisite mixture or HL nitrogen mustard: HN-1, HN-2, HN-3 sulfur mustard agents	Destruction of mucous membranes, eye tissue, and skin (subcutaneous edema), followed by scab formation Irritating to the eyes, nasal membranes, and lungs; nausea and vomiting; formation of blisters on the skin; cytotoxic reactions in hematopoietic tissues including bone marrow, lymph nodes, spleen, and endocrine glands	Flush affected area with copious amounts of water. If ingested, do not induce vomiting. Flush affected area with water. Treat the skin with 5% solution of sodium hypochlorite or household bleach. Give milk to drink. Do not induce vomiting. Skin contact with lewisite may be treated with 10% solution of sodium carbonate.

Based on Chemical Fact Sheets, U.S. Army Center for Health Promotion and Preventative Medicine, http://chemistry.about.com/gi/dynamic/offsite.htm?site=http%3A%2F%2Fchppm-www.apgea.army.mil%2Fdts%2Fdtchemfs.htm.

Ionizing Radiation

64.10 Potassium iodide may be used to block the effects of acute radiation exposure on the thyroid gland, but it is not effective for protecting other organs.

In addition to biological and chemical weapons, it is possible that bioterrorists could develop nuclear bombs capable of mass destruction. In such a scenario, the greatest number of casualties would occur due to the physical blast itself. However, survivors could be exposed to high levels of **ionizing radiation** from hundreds of different radioisotopes created by the nuclear explosion. Some of these radioisotopes emit large amounts of radiation and persist in the environment for years. As was the case in the 1986 Chernobyl nuclear accident in Ukraine, the resulting radioisotopes could travel by wind currents to land thousands of kilometres away from the initial explosion. Smaller scale radiation exposure could occur through terrorist attacks on nuclear power plants or by the release of solid or liquid radioactive materials into public areas.

The acute effects of ionizing radiation have been well documented and depend primarily on the dose of radiation received. **Acute radiation syndrome**, sometimes called radiation sickness, can occur within hours or days after extreme doses. Immediate symptoms are nausea, vomiting, and diarrhea. Later symptoms include weight loss, anorexia, fatigue, and bone marrow suppression. Clients who survive the acute exposure are at high risk for developing various cancers, particularly leukemia.

Symptoms of nuclear and radiation exposure remain some of the most difficult to treat pharmacologically. Apart from the symptomatic treatment of radiation sickness, taking potassium iodide (KI) tablets after an incident is the only recognized therapy specifically designed for radiation exposure. Following a nuclear explosion, one of the resultant radioisotopes is iodine-131 (I-131). Because iodine naturally concentrates in the thyroid gland, I-131 will immediately enter the thyroid and damage thyroid cells. For example, following the Chernobyl nuclear disaster, the incidence of thyroid cancer in Ukraine jumped from 4 to 6 cases per million people to 45 cases per million. If taken prior to, or immediately following, a nuclear incident, KI can prevent up to 100% of the radioactive iodine from entering the thyroid gland. It is effective even if taken 3 to 4 hours after radiation exposure. Generally, a single 130-mg dose is necessary.

Unfortunately, KI only protects the thyroid gland from I-131. It has no protective effects on other body tissues, and it offers no protection against the dozens of other harmful radioisotopes generated by a nuclear blast. Like vaccines and antibiotics, the stockpiling of KI by local healthcare agencies or individuals is not recommended. Of interest, I-131 is also a medication used to shrink the size of overactive thyroid glands. Thyroid medications are presented in Chapter 29.

CHAPTER 64

Understanding the Chapter

Key Concepts Summary

The numbered key concepts provide a succinct summary of the important points from the corresponding numbered section within the chapter. If any of these points are not clear, refer to the numbered section within the chapter for review.

64.1 Poisoning is the third most frequent type of injury that leads to hospitalization in Canada. Drugs are the most common cause in all poisonings.

64.2 The general management of poisoning includes contacting the poison control centre or emergency medical services as soon as possible.

64.3 Activated charcoal is effective at adsorbing (binding) most poisons if administered within 60 minutes of ingestion.

64.4 Bioterrorism is the deliberate use of a biological, chemical, or physical agent to cause panic and mass casualties. The health aspects of biological and chemical agents have become important public issues.

64.5 Nurses play key roles in emergency preparedness, including providing education, resources, diagnosis and treatment, and planning.

64.6 The National Emergency Stockpile System is used to rapidly deploy medical necessities to communities that are experiencing a chemical or biological attack.

64.7 Biological agents such as anthrax, botulism, and pneumonic plague can enter the body through ingestion, through inhalation, or by the cutaneous route. Antibiotic therapy can be successful if given prophylactically or within a short time after exposure.

64.8 Viruses such as polio, smallpox, and the hemorrhagic fever viruses are potential biological weapons. If available, vaccines are the best treatments.

64.9 Chemicals and neurotoxins are potential bioterrorist threats for which specific antidotes are not always available.

64.10 Potassium iodide may be used to block the effects of acute radiation exposure on the thyroid gland, but it is not effective for protecting other organs.

Chapter 64 Scenario

As an emergency department nurse in a busy urban hospital, Carol Boler participates in frequent emergency practice drills to be prepared for mass casualty events and acts of bioterrorism. Although there have been no incidents yet, she knows that with a military base nearby, there is a chance that such an incident could occur. She is working with unit staff to plan a series of staff education meetings to discuss bioterrorism threats.

Critical Thinking Questions

1. When discussing the bioterrorism threat with a group of staff nurses, which information regarding smallpox should be included?

2. Identify the nursing assessments and interventions that the nurse should initiate when a client is exposed to anthrax.

3. Discuss the mode of transmission and symptoms associated with *Y. pestis* exposure.

See Answers to Critical Thinking Questions in Appendix B.

NCLEX Practice Questions

1 A client is suspected of being exposed to ionizing radiation. Which nursing intervention would have the greatest priority?

   a. Providing supportive care for nausea, vomiting, and diarrhea

   b. Limiting the client's exposure to ultraviolet light

   c. Avoiding contamination of self through limited exposure to the client

   d. Administering antiradiation medications as indicated

2 The nurse has received a telephone call from an anxious mother of an 18-month-old child. In a panicked voice, the mother states, "I just discovered that my baby has swallowed an unknown amount of household cleanser." Which instruction would be appropriate for the nurse to give?

   a. "Consult the package instructions for information concerning poisoning."

   b. "Force your child to vomit using a mixture of warm water and raw eggs."

   c. "Call 911 to take your child immediately to the nearest emergency department or healthcare agency."

   d. "If your child develops seizures or difficulty breathing, call the healthcare provider."

3 Activated charcoal is ordered for a client who accidently overdosed on prescription medications. The nurse would question the order for a client with which condition?

   a. Acute hepatitis and cirrhosis

   b. Impairment of renal function

   c. Decreased level of consciousness

   d. Anxiety and nervousness

4 The nurse knows that the mechanism of action for chelating therapy is

   a. Removal of positively charged metals

   b. Deactivation of chemical reaction

   c. Increased liver metabolism

   d. Decreased glomerular filtration

5 Which of the preadministration assessment parameters would the nurse consider before administering edetate calcium disodium to a client?

   a. Bowel sounds

   b. Urinary output

   c. Visual acuity

   d. Skin turgor

See Answers to NCLEX Practice Questions in Appendix A.

Appendix A

Answers to Chapter Review

Chapter 1

1 Answer: b Rationale: Health Canada requires that drug manufacturers demonstrate both the safety and the effectiveness of pharmaceutical products. Options a, c, and d are incorrect. All drugs have potential reactions and adverse effects. Many factors determine the cost of a drug and newly approved drugs may be the most expensive and not fully covered by healthcare insurance plans. Not all drugs have been tested in diverse populations and women, minority ethnic groups, children, and older adults are often underrepresented in drug research studies. Cognitive Level: Applying; Client Need: Safe and Effective Care Environment; Nursing Process: Implementation

2 Answer: b Rationale: Phase 2 of the clinical investigation relies on studying clients with the disease to be treated. Options a, c, and d are incorrect. Phase 1 studies use small groups of healthy subjects. Phase 3 studies use large numbers of subjects with the condition being treated by the drug. Phase 4 is considered post-marketing surveillance after the drug has been approved. Cognitive Level: Applying; Client Need: Safe and Effective Care Environment; Nursing Process: Implementation

3 Answer: b Rationale: Most drug testing occurs using adult, Caucasian males, which may limit the generalization of the results to other populations. Options a, c, and d are incorrect. Drug testing is seldom performed on children, women, or older adults. Although many drugs are tested using animals, effectiveness in animals does not always verify that the drug will be effective in humans. Cognitive Level: Applying; Client Need: Safe and Effective Care Environment; Nursing Process: Implementation

4 Answer: d Rationale: Telephone orders are not permissible under federal law for Schedule II controlled substances. Options a, b, and c are incorrect. Refill prescriptions are usually not any more or less expensive than the original prescription. The number of listeners is irrelevant. Prescriptions are not confirmed or verified by the RCMP. Cognitive Level: Applying; Client Need: Safe and Effective Care Environment; Nursing Process: Implementation

5 Answer: a Rationale: The more likely a drug's potential for abuse and dependency, the stricter the regulation to control access to the substance. Options b, c, and d are incorrect. The cost and production difficulty do not influence the degree of regulation. Adverse effects and drug or food interactions do not dictate the level of regulatory control. The length of time taken to confirm that a drug is effective does not affect the degree of regulation. Cognitive Level: Applying; Client Need: Safe and Effective Care Environment; Nursing Process: Implementation

Chapter 2

1 Answer: c Rationale: Indications are the conditions for which a particular drug is approved. Options a, b, and d are incorrect. A description of how a drug works on its target organs and cells is called the mechanism of action. The dosage is the amount of the drug that is given. The conditions whereby the drug should be avoided are contraindications. Cognitive Level: Applying; Client Need: Safe and Effective Care Environment; Nursing Process: Implementation

2 Answer: c Rationale: Trade names or proprietary names are designed to help the client remember the name of the drug. Options a, b, and d are incorrect. The chemical name refers to the chemical substances that comprise the drug. A drug's generic name is its International Nonproprietary Name, and each drug has only one generic name. There is no category that is referred to as "standard" in the categories of drug names. Cognitive Level: Applying; Client Need: Physiological Integrity; Nursing Process: Assessment

3 Answer: a Rationale: Drugs are only tools that are part of the overall therapeutic treatment plan. Other treatment options and the nurse–client relationship are also important to the care of the client as an individual. Options b, c, and d are incorrect. Drug therapy alone is usually insufficient to correct and cure human illness. Nurses play a major role in the drug therapy of clients by administering, educating, monitoring, and assessing the response to drugs. Too much reliance on drug therapy can diminish the importance of the nurse–client relationship. Cognitive Level: Applying; Client Need: Physiological Integrity; Nursing Process: Implementation

4 Answer: b Rationale: Antihypertensive indicates the therapeutic classification of the drug by describing its usefulness in lowering blood pressure. Options a, c, and d are incorrect. Beta-adrenergic antagonists, diuretics, and calcium channel blockers all focus on how the drug works, rather than on what therapeutic effects occur. Cognitive Level: Applying; Client Need: Physiological Integrity; Nursing Process: Implementation

5 Answer: d Rationale: Motrin and Advil are trade names for the generic drug ibuprofen. Options a, b, and c are incorrect. No error is noted because "ibuprofen" is the generic name for Advil and Motrin, both trade names. Each drug has only one generic name but may have different trade names, depending on the company that manufactures the drug. Cognitive Level: Applying; Client Need: Health Promotion and Maintenance; Nursing Process: Implementation

Chapter 3

1 Answer: b Rationale: Although taking a larger dose of a medication usually results in a greater therapeutic response, the response also depends on the drug's plasma concentration. If a toxic level is reached from too large a dose, the drug will have adverse effects instead of a better therapeutic response. Options a, c, and d are incorrect because they are true statements. The liquid form of a drug will be absorbed faster than its tablet form. Food decreases the absorption rate of most drugs. Clients should always consult a healthcare provider if unexpected adverse effects develop. Cognitive Level: Applying; Client Need: Physiological Integrity; Nursing Process: Evaluation

2 Answer: a Rationale: Infants do not develop a mature microsomal enzyme system until they are a year old and therefore do not metabolize drugs very efficiently. Options b, c, and d are incorrect. Pregnancy does not significantly affect drug metabolism. The concern with pregnant clients is primarily focused on alterations in distribution due to the fetal–placental barrier. The presence of kidney stones would not influence drug metabolism. Hypertension is not a factor that directly results in abnormal metabolism. Cognitive Level: Applying; Client Need: Physiological Integrity; Nursing Process: Implementation

3 Answer: c Rationale: Peristalsis is the wavelike muscular contraction of the gastrointestinal tract that propels stomach and intestinal content through the system. An increase in this activity would decrease the time that drugs would remain in the GI system and therefore decrease absorption. Options a, b, and d are incorrect. Excretion for most drugs occurs mostly through the kidneys, lungs, and glands. Peristalsis would not reduce excretions of medications. A delay in peristalsis would prolong absorption time, and peristalsis is not involved in the distribution of drugs to their target sites. Cognitive Level: Applying; Client Need: Physiological Integrity; Nursing Process: Evaluation

4 Answer: c Rationale: Inhaled drugs produce an immediate therapeutic response. Options a, b, and d are incorrect. Inhaled medication can be used at any time during the day and is not restricted to the morning. Doses for inhaled drugs are small compared to orally ingested medications, and because these drugs go directly to the lung surface area and are readily absorbed, very little of the substance is lost due to metabolism. Cognitive Level: Applying; Client Need: Physiological Integrity; Nursing Process: Evaluation

5 Answer: d Rationale: The length of time a drug concentration remains in the therapeutic range is its duration of action. Clients with hepatic impairment do not effectively metabolize drugs, which increases the duration of action. Options a, b, and c are incorrect. In clients with hepatic disease, the duration of action most likely will increase since drug metabolism is impaired. Although the duration of action is extended, the effects of the drug are not improved. Cognitive Level: Applying; Client Need: Physiological Integrity; Nursing Process: Evaluation

Chapter 4

1 Answer: a, b, c, e Rationale: One of the critical determinants of the effectiveness of drug therapy is a physical examination. Nurses will use assessment skills to ascertain whether the drug is being effective. In many cases, a client's vital signs may indicate the effectiveness of a drug such as a decrease in body temperature, a change in blood pressure and pulse, or improved respiratory status. The effects of many drugs are monitored by diagnostic laboratory values such as white blood cell counts, cultures, and various electrolyte values. *Efficacy* is the term that describes the ability of a drug to produce the desired therapeutic effect. Option d is incorrect. The dosage time does not directly evaluate the effectiveness of drug therapy. Cognitive Level: Applying; Client Need: Physiological Integrity; Nursing Process: Implementation

2 Answer: a Rationale: Therapeutic index is the ratio between therapeutic dose of a drug and the toxic dose and is used as a measure of the relative safety of the drug. The higher the therapeutic index, the greater the safety of the drug. Options b, c, and d are incorrect. A drug may be labelled "dangerous" for many reasons other than the therapeutic index, including potential for abuse. The higher the therapeutic index, the less risk of drug toxicity. A high degree of safety does not signify the degree of effectiveness. Cognitive Level: Applying; Client Need: Physiological Integrity; Nursing Process: Assessment

3 Answer: a Rationale: A dose-response curve is a graphic representation that shows the relation between the amount of a drug administered and the extent of response it produces. Options b, c, and d are incorrect. A dose-response curve does not illustrate the toxic effects related to a drug or any specific population or graphically present the duration of action of a drug. Serum drug levels must be measured to determine the peak serum drug level. It is unique to each client and the dose-response curve only represents a maximum (toxic) dose level. Cognitive Level: Applying; Client Need: Physiological Integrity; Nursing Process: Assessment

4 Answer: b Rationale: Antagonists bind to receptors and block the effects of an endogenous chemical or another drug by competing with receptor binding sites or inhibiting the drug effect. As an antagonist, benztropine (Cogentin) would block the effects of neostigmine (Prostigmin) and the neostigmine would exhibit a lesser effect. Options a, c, and d are incorrect. A drug that produces an effect after binding with a receptor is an agonist. Cognitive Level: Analyzing; Client Need: Physiological Integrity; Nursing Process: Implementation

5 Answer: a Rationale: Potency is a reflection of a drug's ability to bind to a receptor. Options b, c, and d are incorrect. Efficacy and the affinity of a drug to bind to a receptor are separate variables from potency. Metabolism is a function of pharmacokinetics, not pharmacodynamics. First-pass effect is a phenomenon that occurs during enteral absorption and does not affect drug affinity. Cognitive Level: Applying; Client Need: Safe and Effective Care Environment; Nursing Process: Implementation

Chapter 6

1 Answer: b Rationale: It is recommended that all drugs be avoided as much as possible during pregnancy due to the potential effect on the fetus or infant. Options a, c, and d are incorrect. Drugs that are available OTC may also be hazardous and may affect the unborn fetus and nursing infant. Drugs used for treating medical conditions such as asthma, hypertension, diabetes, and epilepsy should be continued throughout pregnancy after review by the healthcare provider for the safety of both mother and infant. There must be close monitoring during this time. In such cases the benefits may outweigh the risks. The woman should consult with her healthcare provider regarding any drugs taken during pregnancy and lactation. Cognitive Level: Applying; Client Need: Physiological Integrity; Nursing Process: Implementation

2 Answer: d Rationale: Drugs in category X are clearly contraindicated because they pose serious risk to the fetus. Options a, b, and c are incorrect. Category A drugs are safe for the pregnant woman because they demonstrate

no risk of injury to the unborn fetus. Category B consists of drugs that may be given to the mother during pregnancy. Drugs in category C represent those for which there is insufficient evidence that the drug is either safe or dangerous to the fetus, and these drugs will be evaluated by the provider to determine if the benefit outweighs the risk. Cognitive Level: Applying; Client Need: Physiological Integrity; Nursing Process: Implementation

3 Answer: a Rationale: Although multiple factors affect the transfer of drugs across the placenta, highly lipid-soluble drugs will cross the placental barrier more easily than water-soluble drugs. Options b, c, and d are incorrect. Small molecules such as alcohol easily cross the placental barrier, whereas larger molecules are slower to cross. When drugs are highly protein bound, they are too large to cross the placental membrane. Cognitive Level: Applying; Client Need: Health Promotion and Maintenance; Nursing Process: Implementation

4 Answer: a Rationale: Weeks 1–2 of the first trimester are known as the preimplantation phase. Before implantation, the developing embryo has not yet established a blood supply with the mother. This is sometimes called the "all-or-none" period because exposure to a teratogen either causes death of the embryo or has no effect. Drugs are less likely to cause congenital malformations during this period because the baby's organ systems have not yet begun to form. Options b, c, and d are incorrect because the embryonic period is 3 to 8 weeks postconception. During the embryonic period there is rapid development of internal structures and maximum sensitivity to teratogens. Teratogenic agents taken during this phase can lead to structural malformation and spontaneous abortion. The specific abnormality depends on which organ is forming at the time of exposure. Cognitive Level: Analyzing; Client Need: Physiological Integrity; Nursing Process: Planning

5 Answer: a, c, d, e Rationale: OTC drugs are generally safe when taken as directed but any drug taken by the mother should be discussed with the healthcare provider first. Lowering the dose will not alter the safety profile of an unsafe OTC drug. Medications are found in breast milk and may be ingested by the infant. The provider will review any prescription medications the mother is taking and will plan for alternatives if any are unsafe during breastfeeding. The form of the medication does not affect the passage of the drug into the breast milk. Option b is incorrect. It is true that the higher the dose, the more likely it is that the drug will enter the breast milk and the client has understood that part of the teaching. Cognitive Level: Analyzing; Client Need: Health Promotion and Maintenance; Nursing Process: Evaluation

Chapter 7

1 Answer: b Rationale: The statement reflects an attempt to understand the client holistically. The nurse understands that multiple contributing factors may contribute to illness and involving the client helps elicit possible factors. Options a, c, and d are incorrect. Tylenol should not be recommended initially because it may not address the possible causative factors related to the headaches. Monitoring the client's pupil response to light, although eventually appropriate, should not be performed initially. An ophthalmology referral may be inevitable; however, making such a referral should be done after ruling out other possible sources of the headaches. Cognitive Level: Applying; Client Need: Health Promotion and Maintenance; Nursing Process: Implementation

2 Answer: c Rationale: Factors associated with a drug's expense and the client's ability to purchase or access needed medication are considered psychosocial variables that may influence adherence to drug therapy. Options a, b, and d are incorrect. Unpleasant taste or medications that are difficult to swallow may hinder client adherence; however, the problem is physiological rather than psychosocial. Liver damage (hepatotoxicity) is also a physiological factor. Cognitive Level: Analyzing; Client Need: Health Promotion and Maintenance; Nursing Process: Evaluation

3 Answer: b Rationale: Cultural beliefs refer to the cumulative ideas of knowledge, experiences, values, attitudes, meanings, and roles acquired by a group of people. A preference for traditional healers, such as a shaman, reflects these beliefs. Options a, c, and d are incorrect. Ethnicity is a population of human beings whose members identify with each other on the basis of either common genealogy or common ancestry. Genetic polymorphisms are changes in enzyme structure and DNA function that occur within a specific subset of the population. A health-related bias is a prejudice or a sense of preference for one particular point of view and is not specifically culturally related. Cognitive

Level: Analyzing; Client Need: Health Promotion and Maintenance; Nursing Process: Evaluation

4 Answer: a, b, c, d Rationale: All of these factors—fat-to-muscle ratio, cerebral blood flow, limited drug research on women, and health beliefs—may be considered gender factors that influence pharmacotherapy. Option e is incorrect. Dietary considerations are a potential ethnic or cultural consideration. Cognitive Level: Applying; Client Need: Physiological Integrity; Nursing Process: Evaluation

5 Answer: d Rationale: Drug response is unique to each individual. The nurse should observe the responses and exercise caution with all medications. Options a, b, and c are incorrect. Client self-report may not be a reliable method, and the client may not have taken a particular drug before. Learning more about genetic effects on pharmacotherapy is important, but each client response is unique. Other clients' responses to a drug will not help predict the response in another client and there are many genetic variations, even within racial groups. Cognitive Level: Applying; Client Need: Physiological Integrity; Nursing Process: Implementation

Chapter 8

1 Answer: a Rationale: Collecting additional information will provide the prescriber with knowledge about the type and severity of the reaction to that specific drug and will assist in determining the appropriateness of the order. Options b, c, and d are incorrect. The nurse should gather additional information from the client or family member before notifying the prescriber. A medication is never administered to a client when allergic sensitivity is suspected until further investigation into the type and severity of the reaction has been completed. Although documentation of the event may be in the client's medical record, the reaction may not have been documented or may have occurred after the last healthcare visit. Cognitive Level: Applying; Client Need: Physiological Integrity; Nursing Process: Implementation

2 Answer: a Rationale: As the dose increases, the risk for adverse effects also increases. The client should be closely observed for the onset of adverse effects whenever the dose of the drug is increased. Options b, c, and d are incorrect. Although adverse effects are sometimes noted after the first dose, they may occur at any time during drug administration. Although some adverse effects are common when a drug is given PO, others are more common when given by other routes, such as IV or IM. The timing of medication is not a factor associated with dose-related adverse effects. Cognitive Level: Applying; Client Need: Physiological Integrity; Nursing Process: Implementation

3 Answer: d Rationale: Promoting adequate hydration may significantly reduce the risk of renal damage produced by drug therapies. Options a, b, and c are incorrect. Avoiding direct sunlight is appropriate teaching to provide to clients receiving drugs that cause photosensitivity or phototoxicity. The consumption of potassium-enriched foods will not reduce the risk of drug-induced nephrotoxicity, nor will avoiding alcohol consumption. Cognitive Level: Applying; Client Need: Physiological Integrity; Nursing Process: Implementation

4 Answer: b Rationale: The function of the bone marrow is to produce blood cells. When drugs cause bone marrow toxicity, the condition manifests as a decrease in all blood cell types. Options a, c, and d are incorrect. Muscle and bone pain are most often associated with muscle toxicity. Bone marrow toxicity is not related to a decline in an individual's range of motion. Liver enzymes are not typically affected by bone marrow toxicity. Cognitive Level: Applying; Client Need: Physiological Integrity; Nursing Process: Evaluation

5 Answer: c Rationale: The presence of right upper quadrant pain and anorexia are early symptoms often associated with drug-induced liver damage. Options a, b, and d are incorrect. Black, "furry" tongue or infections elsewhere are not related to liver damage. A sudden drop in BP is orthostatic hypotension. Unusual and uncontrolled movements are neurologic-related effects. Cognitive Level: Analyzing; Client Need: Physiological Integrity; Nursing Process: Evaluation

Chapter 9

1 Answer: c Rationale: The safest practice is to contact the prescriber to evaluate the client's swallowing reflex or prescribe the same medications with different routes of administration. Options a, b, and c are incorrect.

Repositioning the client does not ensure safety of the airway. Medications in the liquid form are more likely to be aspirated due to their thin consistency, which makes them difficult to control in the mouth. Crushing the medication may be contraindicated, especially for extended-release forms, and does not address the intactness of the swallowing reflex. Cognitive Level: Analyzing; Client Need: Physiological Integrity; Nursing Process: Implementation

2 Answer: a Rationale: Swallowing the tablet leads to early disintegration of its content and neutralizes its action. Options b, c, and d are incorrect. Elevation of the head of the bed does not have a direct impact on the pharmacodynamics of sublingual nitroglycerin. Keeping the tablet between the gums and the cheek is the buccal route, not the sublingual route as prescribed. Drinking water will dilute the medication and push it through the GI system, minimizing its therapeutic effect. Cognitive Level: Applying; Client Need: Physiological Integrity; Nursing Process: Implementation

3 Answer: c Rationale: The most accurate answer is that the order is to be given only once at a specified time. Options a, b, and d are incorrect. Single orders must be administered during a specific time frame to ensure consistent and adequate therapeutic levels in the blood. Stat orders are given immediately. Administering an additional dose can put the client at risk for overdose. Cognitive Level: Applying; Client Need: Physiological Integrity; Nursing Process: Implementation

4 Answer: c Rationale: The eyes are very susceptible to infection and medication administered via the ophthalmic route must be sterile to minimize the introduction of bacteria. Options a, b, and d are incorrect. The GI system is not sterile, so medications administered as oral solutions should be clean. The vaginal environment is clean, not sterile, thus medications administered via this route do not need to be sterile. The nasal cavity is not sterile, so medications administered via this route should be clean. Cognitive Level: Applying; Client Need: Physiological Integrity; Nursing Process: Implementation

5 Answer: c Rationale: Allowing 5 minutes to ensure absorption of the medication will minimize interaction and provide better efficacy of the medication. Immediately applying other eye drops may lead to inadvertent drug interaction and possible crystallization or inactivation of the administered drugs. There is no need to contact the healthcare provider or to wait 2 hours between medications. Cognitive Level: Analyzing; Client Need: Physiological Integrity; Nursing Process: Implementation

Chapter 10

1 Answer: d Rationale: When medication orders are given via telephone, it is critical for the nurse to repeat the order verbatim to the prescriber. Options a, b, and c are incorrect. Whenever possible it is best for the prescriber to write an order for medication, but this is not always possible. It is correct for the nurse to attempt to comfort the client using a number of nursing interventions for pain. However, the nurse is required to consult the prescriber when a change in the client's status occurs, regardless of the time. The nurse is responsible for contacting the prescriber and it is the nurse who can relay clinical findings and assessment. Cognitive Level: Applying; Client Need: Safe and Effective Care Environment; Nursing Process: Planning

2 Answer: a Rationale: Whenever a medication order is unclear, the nurse should always contact the prescriber, and then have the order rewritten to prevent errors. Options b, c, and d are incorrect. Having another nurse read the order will not necessarily ensure that the dosage is correct for the client's condition. Whereas the pharmacist or a drug guide may provide the nurse with the usual dose for most clients, they do not take into consideration the client's weight, disease condition, and other variables that influence the drug's pharmacokinetic and pharmacodynamic actions. Cognitive Level: Applying; client Need: Safe and Effective Care Environment; Nursing Process: Implementation

3 Answer: b Rationale: Pharmacies maintain records of medication dispensed to individuals. If a pharmacist can conduct a medication reconciliation by reviewing the client's drug history on each subsequent visit, serious potential drug–drug interactions may be identified. Options a, c, and d are incorrect. Insisting on acquiring a brand name drug rather than a generic does not ensure the safety of a medication. For safety reasons, drugs are dispensed in containers that are sometimes difficult to open. Unless there is a specific reason (such as impaired hand dexterity), medications should be stored in their original safety bottles. Information found on the Internet may vary in quality and may be provided by non–healthcare-related sources. When in doubt, the prescriber or pharmacist can provide the most accurate information about expected effects. Cognitive Level: Applying; Client Need: Health Promotion and Maintenance; Nursing Process: Implementation

4 Answer: c   Rationale: The nurse should always validate a questionable order when a client or a family member verbalizes concern. Options a, b, and d are incorrect. Medications purchased by a clinical agency vary in appearance depending on the manufacturer from which the drug is purchased. The nurse should withhold the medication and then confirm that it is the correct drug as ordered before administering. If a client questions a change in medication or procedure, the nurse should verify the order and obtain validation from the prescriber. Cognitive Level: Applying; Client Need: Safe and Effective Care Environment; Nursing Process: Implementation

5 Answer: c   Rationale: Returning when the client is available ensures that the client takes the medication and offers opportunity for the nurse to assess for effects or provide teaching related to the medication. Options a, b, and d are incorrect. A nurse must ensure that the client takes the medication. By leaving the medication at the bedside or with visitors, the nurse will not know with certainty that the client took the medication. When a client refuses a medication, the nurse should document reasons for the refusal so that appropriate follow-up may be carried out. In this situation, the client did not refuse the medication but was not available to take it at that moment. Cognitive Level: Applying; Client Need: Safe and Effective Care Environment; Nursing Process: Implementation

Chapter 11

1 Answer: a   Rationale: Although CAM medications have been used for thousands of years, many of these substances lack adequate scientific clinical studies to verify their effectiveness. Most healthcare providers are hesitant to recommend a substance that has questionable effectiveness. Options b, c, and d are incorrect. CAM has a rich history of use over thousands of years in treating certain diseases and conditions. To imply that all alternative therapies are nothing more than fable is incorrect. There is no evidence that response to CAM therapies is related to the placebo effect. In many cases the CAM therapy may be less expensive than prescription medications. Cognitive Level: Applying; Client Need: Safe and Effective Care Environment; Nursing Process: Implementation

2 Answer: c   Rationale: It is best to advise the client to take small amounts of a new supplement to determine any initial intolerance. Options a, b, and d are incorrect. Doubling dosages can be extremely dangerous and is seldom, if ever, advisable. There is no indication that fluid intake should be reduced with echinacea. Allergic reactions are possible with natural supplements. Clients should be taught to read the label carefully and avoid any supplement that contains any known allergy-provoking substances. Cognitive Level: Applying; Client Need: Physiological Integrity; Nursing Process: Implementation

3 Answer: a   Rationale: Older adults with hepatic disease are at higher risk for developing serious drug reactions when taking herbal supplements. Options b, c, and d are incorrect. Clients with cardiac irregularities, pneumonia, or acne may require traditional medications and should be encouraged to consult their healthcare provider. If the client prefers to use CAM, this can also be discussed with the provider at the time of the healthcare visit. Cognitive Level: Applying; Client Need: Physiological Integrity; Nursing Process: Evaluation

4 Answer: a, b, c, e   Rationale: Herbal supplements can be found in almost every supermarket, pharmacy, and health food store. Due to aggressive marketing, herbal supplements are also extremely popular. Most herbal supplements are less expensive than prescribed medications and are therefore more appealing to individuals for whom cost is a critical issue. Older clients may also seek therapeutic alternatives for chronic health conditions. Option d is incorrect. Natural substances are not necessarily safer than synthetic products and do not undergo the same rigorous testing as synthetic products. Cognitive Level: Applying; Client Need: Safe and Effective Care Environment; Nursing Process: Implementation

5 Answer: d   Rationale: Changes in liver or kidney function in the older adult may lead to changes in metabolism or excretion for herbal as well as synthetic medications. Options a, b, and c are incorrect. Older adults are no more likely to have difficulty taking herbal medications or to spend more money on these products than the younger adult population. These difficulties are client specific at any age. Due to aggressive marketing campaigns by the herbal and dietary supplement industry, all age groups are as likely to hold unrealistic expectations for herbal products. Cognitive Level: Applying; Client Need: Physiological Integrity; Nursing Process: Evaluation

Chapter 13

1 Answer: a   Rationale: Muscarinic agonists may cause reflex tachycardia, which is precipitated by a drop in the client's blood pressure. When this occurs, the baroreceptors recognize the decline in pressure and alert the medulla to increase the heart rate as a compensatory mechanism. Options b, c, and d are incorrect. Although the heart rate increases, muscarinic agonists do not directly affect the sinoatrial node. Hypertension is not a problem with this drug therapy; however, hypotension may occur. Muscarinic agents stimulate bronchial smooth muscles; however, this does not affect the heart rate. Cognitive Level: Applying; Client Need: Physiological Integrity; Nursing Process: Implementation

2 Answer: d   Rationale: Bethanechol (Duvoid) works on the muscles needed for urination by increasing ureteral peristalsis and promoting urinary bladder elimination. Options a, b, and c are incorrect. Bethanechol does not cause changes to urinary structures, nor does it increase urine production or renal blood flow. Cognitive Level: Applying; Client Need: Physiological Integrity; Nursing Process: Implementation

3 Answer: a, b, c, e   Rationale: Common adverse effects of bethanechol include abdominal discomfort, sweating, flushed skin, and blurred vision. Option d is incorrect because bethanechol increases GI peristalsis and promotes bowel evacuation. Cognitive Level: Analyzing; Client Need: Physiological Integrity; Nursing Process: Evaluation

4 Answer: c   Rationale: Because of the potential for bronchoconstriction, clients with COPD should be treated cautiously with cholinergic agonists. Options a, b, and d are incorrect. Neostigmine (Prostigmin) is used to reduce postoperative abdominal distention. Urinary retention may also be relieved with the administration of neostigmine. Neostigmine may be used to reverse the effects of non-depolarizing muscle relaxants. Cognitive Level: Applying; Client Need: Physiological Integrity; Nursing Process: Evaluation

5 Answer: a   Rationale: If the heart rate falls below 60 beats/minute or other established parameter, the nurse should notify the prescriber. Atropine may be ordered to restore heart rate. Options b, c, and d are incorrect. Miosis and increased salivation are expected adverse effects of this drug therapy. A respiratory rate of 16 is normal, so there is no need to notify the prescriber. Cognitive Level: Analyzing; Client Need: Physiological Integrity; Nursing Process: Evaluation

Chapter 14

1 Answer: a   Rationale: Phenylephrine causes vasoconstriction, reducing the swelling in the nasal passages. Options b, c, and d are incorrect. The drug does not destroy organisms or coat nasal passages. Whereas some drugs may be swallowed via the nasopharynx, localized action is predominant, and excessive drug use and swallowing may result in adverse effects. Cognitive Level: Applying; Client Need: Physiological Integrity; Nursing Process: Implementation

2 Answer: a, b, d   Rationale: Adrenergic agonist nasal sprays should not be shared among individuals due to the risk for spreading infection. Individuals should be taught the dangers of using adrenergic nasal sprays for longer than 3 days. These medications can cause increased blood pressure, increased heart rate, and insomnia. Habitual use of nasal adrenergic drugs can also cause rebound congestion as well as necrosis of the nasal mucosa due to the severe vasoconstriction caused by the drug. Due to the CNS stimulation, nasal adrenergic agents are not indicated in children and infants. Options c and e are incorrect. The drug causes CNS stimulation rather than depression. People with diabetes must use caution when using adrenergic drugs and must monitor their blood glucose levels more frequently for hyperglycemia. They are also at higher risk for adverse cardiac effects. Cognitive Level: Applying; Client Need: Health Promotion and Maintenance; Nursing Process: Implementation

3 Answer: d   Rationale: Epinephrine (Adrenalin) is used during anaphylaxis to prevent hypotension and bronchoconstriction. Options a, b, and c are incorrect because the administration of epinephrine for anaphylaxis does not prevent the formation of histamine or antibodies in response to an invading antigen nor does it affect white blood cell function. Cognitive Level: Applying; Client Need: Physiological Integrity; Nursing Process: Evaluation

4 Answer: a Rationale: When beta$_2$-adrenergic agonists such as salbutamol (Ventolin) are taken too close to bedtime, the client may experience insomnia. Options b, c, and d are incorrect because all adrenergic agonists act as stimulators, and urticaria and tinnitus are not adverse effects associated with this drug therapy. Cognitive Level: Applying; Client Need: Physiological Integrity; Nursing Process: Evaluation

5 Answer: a, d Rationale: The nurse should consult with the prescriber when adrenergic drugs are prescribed for individuals with hyperthyroid disease or dysrhythmias. The medication will further increase the already overactive metabolic system in hyperthyroidism and may increase the risk for dysrhythmias due to the cardiac stimulation caused by these medications. Options b, c, and e are incorrect. These are therapeutic indications for the administration of adrenergic agonists. Cognitive Level: Analyzing; Client Need: Physiological Integrity; Nursing Process: Implementation

Chapter 16

1 Answer: c Rationale: Ataxia, weakness, restlessness, dizziness, and other motor problems can occur with lorazepam. Options a, b, and d are incorrect. These are not adverse effects associated with lorazepam. Cognitive Level: Applying; Client Need: Physiological Integrity; Nursing Process: Implementation

2 Answer: d Rationale: Sleeping for 7 hours is the desired effect of temazepam (Restoril). Options a, b, and c are incorrect. The client should experience periods of sleep lasting longer than 3 hours and should obtain a full night's sleep. The client will be taking temazepam to assist with insomnia, not to treat anxiety related to everyday stress or to help control panic attacks. Cognitive Level: Applying; Client Need: Physiological Integrity; Nursing Process: Evaluation

3 Answer: c Rationale: This medication must be gradually reduced, not abruptly terminated. Abrupt termination may cause withdrawal symptoms (nausea, vomiting, abdominal cramps, diaphoresis, confusion, tremors, seizures). Options a, b, and d are incorrect. These are appropriate statements, and indicate that the client understands the teaching. Cognitive Level: Analyzing; Client Need: Health Promotion and Maintenance; Nursing Process: Evaluation

4 Answer: b Rationale: Panic disorder is not an appropriate use for phenobarbital (Phenobarb). Options a, c, and d are incorrect. Treatment of status epilepticus, use prior to diagnostic testing, and use prior to receiving general anesthesia are all appropriate for phenobarbital. Cognitive Level: Applying; Client Need: Physiological Integrity; Nursing Process: Implementation

5 Answer: a Rationale: Smoking enhances the metabolism of benzodiazepines, so the medication is broken down and removed from the body more quickly if the client is a smoker. Therefore, a smoker may require a larger dose of a benzodiazepine to get the same effect as that of a nonsmoker. Options b, c, and d are incorrect. A smaller or half dose, or a single extra dose, may not adequately help relieve the client's symptoms. Cognitive Level: Applying; Client Need: Physiological Integrity; Nursing Process: Implementation

Chapter 17

1 Answer: a Rationale: Imipramine (Impril) should not be used by clients with seizure disorders because it lowers the seizure threshold. Options b, c, and d are incorrect. Imipramine is a drug that is effective in treating depression and is one of only two drugs approved for enuresis (bedwetting) in children. Like other TCAs, imipramine has a number of off-label indications. These include the adjuvant treatment of cancer or neuropathic pain. Cognitive Level: Applying; Client Need: Physiological Integrity; Nursing Process: Implementation

2 Answer: c Rationale: Full therapeutic effects of fluoxetine may take up to 1 month. Options a, b, and d are incorrect. Normal water and sodium intake do not affect fluoxetine (Prozac). The client cannot take an MAOI or other CNS depressant concurrently. The use of other drugs or CNS depressants such as alcohol could increase the risk for adverse effects or increased depression. Cognitive Level: Analyzing; Client Need: Physiological Integrity; Nursing Process: Evaluation

3 Answer: a, b Rationale: Persistent GI upset and confusion are signs of elevated lithium levels between 1.5 and 2, which signify early toxicity. Options c, d, and e are incorrect. Polyuria is an adverse effect that may occur in early therapy but is not associated with early toxicity. Convulsions may occur at serum levels above 2.5 but not in early stages of toxicity. Ataxia is also not a sign of early lithium toxicity. Cognitive Level: Analyzing; Client Need: Physiological Integrity; Nursing Process: Evaluation

4 Answer: a Rationale: The client taking lithium (Carbolith, Lithane) must be conscious of maintaining normal sodium intake. Because lithium is a salt, if sodium intake is low the body will replace the sodium with lithium, leading to lithium toxicity. Options b, c, and d are incorrect. The client taking lithium must have regular blood studies, and toxicity is a very real concern; hence the necessity for routine blood studies. Women should refrain from breastfeeding while taking lithium. Cognitive Level: Analyzing; Client Need: Physiological Integrity; Nursing Process: Evaluation

5 Answer: b, c Rationale: Fluoxetine (Prozac) causes weight loss in some clients, while other clients experience weight gain or fluctuations in weight. A healthy diet and adequate exercise will help maintain normal weight while on this drug. While rare, an increased risk for suicide has been noted in clients up to age 24, and the client should be carefully monitored, especially during the early initiation of therapy. Options a, d, and e are incorrect. Fluoxetine may cause insomnia but not sedation. Abrupt withdrawal of fluoxetine may lead to withdrawal symptoms. If the drug needs to be discontinued, gradually tapering the dose is recommended. Fluoxetine is not known to cause excessive thirst. Cognitive Level: Analyzing; Client Need: Physiological Integrity; Nursing Process: Evaluation

Chapter 18

1 Answer: d Rationale: ADHD drugs are Schedule II through IV drugs that require tight controls. Because they can be abused, they should be kept under lock and tightly monitored with only the minimal number of doses kept at the school as per school policy. Options a, b, and c are incorrect. Keeping the drug in a lunch bag may lead to the child forgetting to take it or to other children taking the drug. Because it is a highly regulated drug, additional prescriptions or dosages are not allowed under the Schedule because they could result in the misuse of the drug by people other than the student for whom it is prescribed. Cognitive Level: Applying; Client Need: Health Promotion and Maintenance; Nursing Process: Implementation

2 Answer: b Rationale: Atomoxetine (Strattera) should decrease hyperactivity. Options a, c, and d are incorrect. Atomoxetine should increase attention, not decrease it. Mydriasis and elevated liver enzymes are adverse effects associated with atomoxetine; they are not therapeutic effects. Cognitive Level: Applying; Client Need: Health Promotion and Maintenance; Nursing Process: Evaluation

3 Answer: a Rationale: Chlorpromazine is the preferred drug to assist in counteracting amphetamine overdosage. It has strong alpha-adrenergic blocking actions that treat the effects of amphetamine. Options b, c, and d are incorrect. Phenytoin (Dilantin) is an antiepileptic drug; propofol (Diprivan) is a nonbarbiturate sedative–hypnotic; and dexamethasone (Dexasone) is a corticosteroid. None of these drugs would counteract the effects of an amphetamine overdose. Cognitive Level: Applying; Client Need: Physiological Integrity; Nursing Process: Planning

4 Answer: c Rationale: Atomoxetine (Strattera) has been linked to suicidal ideations and an increased risk for suicide. These symptoms should be reported immediately to the family or caregiver for assessment and treatment by the healthcare provider. Options a, b, and d are incorrect. The need for drug withdrawal will be determined by the provider after assessing the client. The drug may take up to 4 weeks to achieve maximum therapeutic effects, but this client is experiencing an adverse effect linked to the drug. Caffeine will not counteract depressive effects and may increase the risk for CNS adverse effects. Cognitive Level: Analyzing; Client Need: Psychosocial Integrity; Nursing Process: Evaluation

5 Answer: c Rationale: Taking the medication before late afternoon ensures that peak drug activity will occur during waking hours. Options a, b, and d are incorrect. Drinking wine with dinner should not have a noticeable effect on sleep unless taken directly before bedtime when the metabolism of the alcohol may actually diminish sleep as the blood glucose rises and falls. Chocolate contains caffeine, and also sugar, which may cause additional wakefulness. Decaffeinated coffee will limit the intake of the additional stimulant of caffeine but will not significantly improve the client's sleep if the methylphenidate is taken later in the afternoon or evening. Cognitive Level: Applying; Client Need: Health Promotion and Maintenance; Nursing Process: Implementation

Chapter 19

1 Answer: d   Rationale: Antipsychotic medications treat the symptoms associated with mental illness but do not cure these disorders. Without the medication, the symptoms will return. Options a, b, and c are incorrect. These are not symptoms associated with abrupt withdrawal of an antipsychotic medication. Cognitive Level: Analyzing; Client Need: Physiological Integrity; Nursing Process: Evaluation

2 Answer: b   Rationale: Acute dystonia, or severe muscle spasms, especially of the back, neck, face, or tongue, may appear within hours or days of the first dose of a phenothiazine and should be reported immediately. Options a, c, and d are incorrect. Social withdrawal is a symptom of the disease, and slowed activity may occur as a result of the medication. However, the client's body will become adjusted to the medication in a short time period and it will disappear. Tardive dyskinesias occurs late in therapy and is more common in the older adult. The phenothiazine medications usually cause adverse effects even when taken as prescribed. Cognitive Level: Analyzing; Client Need: Physiological Integrity; Nursing Process: Implementation

3 Answer: a   Rationale: Benztropine (Cogentin) is classified as an autonomic nervous system drug and an anticholinergic. It suppresses tremor and rigidity by decreasing the excess cholinergic effect associated with dopamine deficiency. Options b, c, and d are incorrect. Diazepam (Valium) and lorazepam (Ativan) are antianxiety medications that will not improve the client's symptoms. Haloperidol (Haldol) is an antipsychotic medication that may cause these symptoms. Cognitive Level: Analyzing; Client Need: Physiological Integrity; Nursing Process: Planning

4 Answer: b, d   Rationale: EPS occurs frequently, especially at the beginning of therapy with haloperidol (Haldol). A person with Parkinson's disease, seizure disorders, alcoholism, or severe mental depression should not take haloperidol because they are all disorders that affect the CNS. Dementia, seizures, depression, and severe CNS depression are known to occur with the use of haloperidol in these clients. Options a, c, and e are incorrect. Haloperidol and antacids may be given simultaneously; there are no known interactions between these two medications. Haloperidol must be taken as ordered, on a regular schedule. Taking the drug prn will not reduce symptoms of psychosis because it takes several weeks of regular administration before therapeutic levels are reached. Sustained-release medications should never be crushed. If the client cannot take the medication, another form should be used. Cognitive Level: Applying; Client Need: Physiological Integrity; Nursing Process: Implementation

5 Answer: d   Rationale: The client taking risperidone (Risperdal) or any antipsychotic medication should refrain from consuming alcohol. Concurrent use of alcohol with antipsychotic medications will increase CNS depression. Because there is an increased risk for hyperglycemia or diabetes in clients taking risperidone, alcohol should also be avoided because it may affect blood sugar levels. Options a, b, and c are incorrect. Weight gain may occur, and obtaining a weekly weight will help the client track any gain. Increasing fluids and fibre may help to limit GI adverse effects. Hypotension is related to adverse reactions the client may experience and must be monitored and reported if it occurs. Cognitive Level: Analyzing; Client Need: Physiological Integrity; Nursing Process: Evaluation

Chapter 20

1 Answer: b   Rationale: Benztropine (Cogentin), a cholinergic antagonist, is frequently used as combination therapy with other antiparkinson drugs to decrease tremors. Options a, c, and d are incorrect. Amantadine (Symmetrel) acts to increase dopamine's release, but only as long as dopamine is available. Haloperidol (Haldol) is a phenothiazine antipsychotic that may lead to pseudoparkinsonism in many persons. Donepezil (Aricept) prolongs the time between diagnosis and the institutionalization of the client with Alzheimer's disease and is not used for Parkinson's disease. Cognitive Level: Analyzing; Client Need: Physiological Integrity; Nursing Process: Implementation

2 Answer: c   Rationale: Being independent with ADLs shows an improvement in physical abilities. Options a, b, and d are incorrect. Drowsiness is a common adverse effect of antiparkinson medications. Anorexia or loss of appetite is a common adverse effect, not an expected therapeutic effect. Itchy skin is not directly related to Parkinson's disease symptoms or to the medications used. Cognitive Level: Applying; Client Need: Health Promotion and Maintenance; Nursing Process: Evaluation

3 Answer: c   Rationale: It is important that the caregivers understand that there is no cure for AD, but that the medication may delay the worsening of

symptoms. Options a, b, and d are incorrect. The medication should be given continuously and not only when the symptoms are present. The client may become constipated but does not require emergency treatment. The drug may cause bradycardia or atrial fibrillation and the pulse rate should be checked weekly, but it is not necessary to take the client's vital signs before each dose of medication. Cognitive Level: Applying; Client Need: Health Promotion and Maintenance; Nursing Process: Evaluation

4 Answer: d   Rationale: Potentially life-threatening cardiac dysrhythmias, including atrial fibrillation and sinus bradycardia, are possible adverse effects associated with donepezil (Aricept). Options a, b, c, and e are incorrect. Donepezil is given once a day, not four times a day. It may cause diarrhea, rather than constipation, and does not cause vision difficulties. Donepezil is available by prescription only and cannot be purchased over the counter. Cognitive Level: Applying; Client Need: Physiological Integrity; Nursing Process: Planning

5 Answer: a, b, d   Rationale: Flu-like symptoms with general malaise, body aches, fever, and headache are common. Insomnia and rashes may also occur and may be treated symptomatically after conferral with the provider. Options c and e are incorrect. Depression should never be ignored and should be reported immediately. Significant pain with darkening or blackening of the skin at the injection site indicates that tissue necrosis may be occurring and requires prompt treatment. Cognitive Level: Analyzing; Client Need: Psychosocial Integrity; Nursing Process: Evaluation

Chapter 21

1 Answer: c   Rationale: GI effects such as nausea, anorexia, and abdominal pain are common with ethosuximide (Zarontin). Because the client is still growing, improper nutrition may affect normal growth. Monitoring height and weight weekly will assist in tracking normal growth. Options a, b, and d are incorrect. Physical activity will not affect the drug's metabolism and activity is normal and needed for healthy growth and development. Ethosuximide is not known to cause bone loss or dehydration. Cognitive Level: Applying; Client Need: Health Promotion and Maintenance; Nursing Process: Planning

2 Answer: d   Rationale: Oxcarbazepine is excreted by the kidneys, and renal function laboratory studies will be monitored to detect adverse renal effects. Because hyponatremia may develop during treatment, serum sodium levels should also be monitored. Options a, b, and c are incorrect. Oxcarbazepine does not affect CBC, platelets, sedimentation rate, or albumin or serum glucose levels. Cognitive Level: Applying; Client Need: Physiological Integrity; Nursing Process: Planning

3 Answer: d   Rationale: Sedation and an increased risk for falls are associated with carbamazepine. Options a, b, and c are incorrect. Carbamazepine (Tegretol) is used off-label to treat dementia with aggressiveness and agitation. The drug is not associated with insomnia and has not been demonstrated to increase the risk for stroke. Cognitive Level: Applying; Client Need: Physiological Integrity; Nursing Process: Implementation

4 Answer: b   Rationale: Slurred speech, diplopia, sedation, and dyspnea are symptoms of gabapentin (Neurontin) overdose. Options a, c, and d are incorrect. Seizure activity is likely to recur if the drug is stopped abruptly. Neither grapefruit juice nor smoking is known to affect drug level. Cognitive Level: Analyzing; Client Need: Physiological Integrity; Nursing Process: Evaluation

5 Answer: a   Rationale: High doses of phenytoin (Dilantin) can cause nystagmus, confusion, ataxia, coma, and seizures and the dosage should be reduced. Options b, c, and d are incorrect. Increasing or maintaining the same dose will continue or exacerbate the symptoms of toxicity. The drug should not be discontinued abruptly because seizure activity may occur. Cognitive Level: Analyzing; Client Need: Physiological Integrity; Nursing Process: Planning

Chapter 22

1 Answer: a, d, e   Rationale: Cyclobenzaprine (Flexeril) may cause tachycardia, and any palpitations or rapid heart rate should be reported. Drowsiness may also occur, and driving or other hazardous activities should be avoided until the effects of the drug are known. Swelling of the face or tongue may occur and must be reported immediately to the provider. Options b and c are incorrect. Clients with severe muscle spasms are encouraged to rest affected muscle groups until acute spasms subside. Cyclobenzaprine may cause dry mouth, and alcohol-based mouth rinses may exacerbate the condition. Cognitive Level: Applying; Client Need: Physiological Integrity; Nursing Process: Planning

2 Answer: c   Rationale: Abruptly discontinuing baclofen (Lioresal) may result in fever, seizures, rebound spasticity, and hallucinations. Options a, b, and d are incorrect. Baclofen may cause weakness, and like other muscle relaxants and antispasmodics, may cause constipation. Being cautious with activities and increasing fluid and fibre intake will help to limit the adverse effects caused by baclofen. It may take several months before the full effects of baclofen are reached. Cognitive Level: Analyzing; Client Need: Physiological Integrity; Nursing Process: Evaluation

3 Answer: b   Rationale: Capsaicin should be applied to the site of pain with a gloved hand to prevent irritation of the skin on the hands and to avoid introducing the capsaicin to the eyes or other parts of the body not under treatment. Options a, c, and d are incorrect. Capsaicin should only be applied to the site of pain, not proximal or distal to the pain. If capsaicin begins to irritate and cause redness and inflammation, it should be discontinued. Capsaicin should not be applied with a bare hand. Cognitive Level: Applying; Client Need: Physiological Integrity; Nursing Process: Implementation

4 Answer: b   Rationale: Dysphagia, blurred vision, and ptosis are all symptoms of possible botulism toxicity and should be reported immediately. Options a, c, and d are incorrect. Fever, aches, and chills are not anticipated adverse effects of this drug, and while they should be evaluated, they do not require immediate reporting. Moderate levels of muscle weakness may occur after the drug is administered, and strengthening exercises may be needed on the affected side. Continuous muscle spasms and pain should not occur because the drug blocks muscle contraction. Cognitive Level: Analyzing; Client Need: Physiological Integrity; Nursing Process: Evaluation

5 Answer: b, c, e   Rationale: Dantrolene (Dantrium) may cause hepatotoxicity with the greatest risk occurring in women over age 35. Estrogen taken concurrently with dantrolene may increase this risk. The drug may cause xerostomia, and sucking on hard candy or sipping water or ice chips may relieve the dryness. Options a and d are incorrect. Fluids and fibre may also help diarrhea, but dantrolene may cause diarrhea, not constipation. Dantrolene may cause photosensitivity, so clients taking the drug should avoid direct exposure to the sun. Cognitive Level: Applying; Client Need: Health Promotion and Maintenance; Nursing Process: Implementation

Chapter 23

1 Answer: a, c, d, e   Rationale: Common adverse effects of opioids include respiratory depression, urinary retention, constipation, and nausea. Option b is incorrect. Hypotension, not hypertension, is an adverse effect of opioids. Cognitive Level: Analyzing; Client Need: Physiological Integrity; Nursing Process: Evaluation

2 Answer: d   Rationale: Opioids decrease peristalsis, and bowel surgery may produce a temporary cessation of peristalsis (paralytic ileus). Both lead to constipation. Once bowel function has returned enough for the client to start eating, constipation is still likely and needs to be prevented by increased dietary fibre and fluids as well as taking a stool softener. Options a, b, and c are incorrect. Respiratory depression and urinary retention are not likely after several days with decreasing opioid use. Addiction is not a concern in the treatment of acute pain in this scenario. Cognitive Level: Applying; Client Need: Physiological Integrity; Nursing Process: Planning

3 Answer: c   Rationale: Chest pain is a serious adverse effect of sumatriptan (Imitrex) and needs to be differentiated from angina, which can also be caused by the drug. Options a, b, and d are incorrect. The client should not use the drug again until being evaluated by the provider and should report the chest pain immediately. Reclining in a quiet room with cold packs is a non-drug treatment for migraines, but reporting the chest pain is most important at this time. Cognitive Level: Applying; Client Need: Physiological Integrity; Nursing Process: Implementation

4 Answer: b   Rationale: The client is describing neuropathic pain, which is most likely to respond to the adjuvant analgesic gabapentin, an antiseizure drug used for neuropathic pain. Options a, c, and d are incorrect. Non-opioids such as ibuprofen (Advil, Motrin), or opioids such as methadone (Metadol), are less effective at relieving pain that is of neurological origin. Naloxone (Narcan)

is an opioid antagonist and will not relieve the client's pain. Cognitive Level: Applying; Client Need: Physiological Integrity; Nursing Process: Planning

5 Answer: d   Rationale: Older adult client are at highest risk for hypotension, respiratory depression, and increased incidence of adverse CNS effects such as confusion. Options a, b, and c are incorrect. Most 23-year-old clients can tolerate opioids without adverse effects. Individuals who suffer from traumatic injury may receive narcotic analgesia. However, caution should be taken if the individual has also experienced any type of head injury. Opioids are often used with individuals who suffer MI. No adverse effects such as hypotension or respiratory depression are usually present if the dose is appropriate for the size of the client. Cognitive Level: Analyzing; Client Need: Physiological Integrity; Nursing Process: Evaluation

Chapter 24

1 Answer: b   Rationale: In stage 2, the client becomes excitable with hyperactivity and irregular heart and respiratory rates. Options a, c, and d are incorrect. In stage 1, the client loses general sensation but remains awake. In stage 3, the client's skeletal muscles become relaxed, and delirium stabilizes. In stage 4, the client has paralysis of the medulla with possible adverse effects on respiratory and cardiac function. Cognitive Level: Analyzing; Client Need: Physiological Integrity; Nursing Process: Evaluation

2 Answer: a   Rationale: Clients who have an allergy to eggs or soy products may have an allergic reaction to the propofol emulsion, which contains these products. Options b, c, and d are incorrect. Clients with allergies to iodine, kidney disease, or Addison's disease may be administered propofol (Diprivan) cautiously. Cognitive Level: Analyzing; Client Need: Physiological Integrity; Nursing Process: Implementation

3 Answer: d   Rationale: Anxiety, excitement, and combativeness are signs that the dose of nitrous oxide is high and the client is exhibiting signs of the second stage of anesthesia. Lowering the dose may reduce these symptoms. Options a, b, and c are incorrect. The dose of nitrous oxide would be lowered, not increased. Propofol would cause additional CNS depression and is not advised. Succinylcholine (Quelicin) is a neuromuscular blocking agent that will increase the risk for significant respiratory adverse effects due to its muscle-paralyzing actions. Cognitive Level: Analyzing; Client Need: Physiological Integrity; Nursing Process: Planning

4 Answer: c   Rationale: Ketamine (Ketalar) produces dissociation anesthesia, which is a feeling of being separated from the environment. Options a, b, and d are incorrect because anxiety and dry mouth are not significant adverse effects of ketamine. Ketamine may cause decreased energy. Cognitive Level: Applying; Client Need: Physiological Integrity; Nursing Process: Evaluation

5 Answer: a   Rationale: Epinephrine is administered with lidocaine (Xylocaine) to increase the duration of the anesthetic action at the site by causing vasoconstriction, keeping the anesthetic localized. Options b, c, and d are incorrect because epinephrine will cause vasoconstriction, not vasodilation at the site; may increase blood pressure if the drug enters the systemic circulation; and neither lidocaine nor epinephrine has any antibacterial properties. Cognitive Level: Applying; Client Need: Physiological Integrity; Nursing Process: Evaluation

Chapter 25

1 Answer: a   Rationale: Addiction is not a problem for the majority of clients who receive narcotic analgesia in the postoperative period. The nurse should administer the dose to treat the pain. Options b, c, and d are incorrect. Reviewing the client's past medical history is an important assessment that should guide nursing practice, but a client's past tendencies toward substance abuse are not appropriate criteria to consider in the nurse's decision to treat the pain with analgesia. Pain is best treated in the early stage. If a nurse waits to treat pain until it becomes intolerable, the client may require a higher dose of the analgesia. There is no evidence that clients request medication when it is not needed. Cognitive Level: Applying; Client Need: Physiological Integrity; Nursing Process: Implementation

2 Answer: c   Rationale: Clients with a substance use disorder tend to revert back to drug-seeking behaviour when they return to the company of other substance abusers. Options a, b, and d are incorrect. A good support system can be extremely beneficial when an individual is attempting to withdraw from physiologically and psychologically addictive substances. Clients with substance use disorder may experience the desire to use drugs long after the drug has physiologically cleared the body. Generally speaking, individuals who share a common experience will be perceived as being most helpful to an individual undergoing the same or similar experience. Cognitive Level: Analyzing; Client Need: Health Promotion and Maintenance; Nursing Process: Evaluation

3 Answer: a, d, e Rationale: Varenicline (Champix) doses are increased over an 8-day period and maintained for 12 to 24 weeks, reducing withdrawal symptoms and craving for smoking. Serious dermatological reactions have been noted and any unusual skin reactions or angioedema should be reported to the provider immediately and the drug stopped. Varenicline carries a black box warning for serious neuropsychiatric events, and any changes in behaviour, depression, hostility, or thoughts of suicide should be immediately reported. Options b and c are incorrect. Varenicline activates nicotinic acetylcholine receptors in the brain and blocks nicotine from reaching the receptors. It does not prevent nicotine's harmful effects on body systems from occurring. It has several adverse effects, including serious dermatological and neuropsychiatric effects. Cognitive Level: Applying; Client Need: Physiological Integrity; Nursing Process: Evaluation

4 Answer: b Rationale: Sedatives cause a profound suppression of the respiratory system through direct action with the CNS. Clients who have experienced an overdose of sedatives are at high risk for respiratory arrest. Options a, c, and d are incorrect. Sedatives do not typically cause any type of stimulation. Long-term effects of overdose will most likely manifest through liver and kidney dysfunction, but the immediate need is to determine the current status of the client. Level of consciousness is one of the assessments to be made with a client receiving sedatives, but the nurse would expect a decrease in consciousness with an overdose of sedatives. Cognitive Level: Applying; Client Need: Physiological Integrity; Nursing Process: Assessment

5 Answer: d Rationale: Typical symptoms of heroin withdrawal include chills, dilated pupils, diarrhea, runny nose, muscle spasms, goose bumps, abdominal pain, sweating, and agitation. Options a, b, and c are incorrect. Heroin is an opiate that depresses the CNS, and the client may exhibit hyperactive behaviour during withdrawal. Dermatological effects are not common during heroin withdrawal. Paranoia, delusions, or hallucinations are more typical effects. Cognitive Level: Applying; Client Need: Physiological Integrity; Nursing Process: Evaluation

Chapter 27

1 Answer: b Rationale: GH cannot be given PO; it can only be administered subcutaneously by injections. Options a, c, and d are incorrect. A lack of GH is not associated with mental retardation. Children whose epiphyseal plates have closed are not candidates for GH therapy; therefore, most adolescents would see minimal gain in height. Periodic testing for blood hormone levels is required during therapy. Cognitive Level: Applying; Client Need: Physiological Integrity; Nursing Process: Planning

2 Answer: a, b, c Rationale: GH increases the length and width of long bones; promotes organ, muscle, and connective tissue growth; and increases the synthesis of proteins. Options d and e are incorrect. GH may cause an increase in serum glucose levels, not a decrease. It may improve and decrease fat deposits around the abdomen and improve lipid levels. Cognitive Level: Applying; Client Need: Physiological Integrity; Nursing Process: Evaluation

3 Answer: c Rationale: Clients on desmopressin (DDAVP, Nocdurna) need to obtain a daily weight and should monitor for the presence of any peripheral edema. Options a, b, and d are incorrect. Desmopressin must be given in regular doses for continued therapeutic effects. Increasing the dosage may cause an increased risk for vasoconstriction and other adverse effects. Leg cramping when walking may indicate adverse peripheral vascular effects and should be assessed by the provider. Taking NSAIDs concurrently may increase the antidiuretic effect, leading to adverse effects. Cognitive Level: Applying; Client Need: Health Promotion and Maintenance; Nursing Process: Planning

4 Answer: a Rationale: Octreotide (Sandostatin) prolongs intestinal transit time and stimulates reabsorption of fluids and electrolytes from the GI tract. These effects would have the therapeutic action of decreasing diarrhea related to the cancer or treatment. Options b, c, and d are incorrect. Octreotide will not slow cancer growth or metastasis or improve lean body mass or fat deposits. Hypoglycemia and hyperglycemia are possible adverse effects of octreotide, not therapeutic effects. Cognitive Level: Analyzing; Client Need: Physiological Integrity; Nursing Process: Evaluation

5 Answer: d Rationale: Vasopressin (Pressyn) is a potent vasoconstrictor and may precipitate angina or myocardial infarction. Options a, b, and c are incorrect. Glaucoma, COPD, or alcoholism would not be contraindications for this drug. Cognitive Level: Applying; Client Need: Physiological Integrity; Nursing Process: Assessment

Chapter 28

1 Answer: b Rationale: Insulin peaks are the times of maximum insulin use with the greatest risk for hypoglycemia. Options a, c, and d are incorrect. Because the risk for hypoglycemia is highest at peak serum insulin levels, exercise or additional insulin may increase the risk further. Insulin schedules for the client are developed by the provider and the client should not self-select a schedule for insulin use. Cognitive Level: Applying; Client Need: Physiological Integrity; Nursing Process: Implementation

2 Answer: b, c, e Rationale: The blood glucose level should be checked prior to administering most types of insulin. Because lispro (Humalog) is a rapid-acting insulin, the nurse should ensure that a meal is available and that the client will be able to eat shortly after receiving a dose. If signs of hypoglycemia are present, the insulin dose should be held and the client treated for hypoglycemia. The provider should be notified. Options a and d are incorrect. Urine testing for glucose and ketones does not give exact information, and clients vary on the degree to which glucose and ketones will "spill" into the urine. While a check of the pulse or blood pressure may be included in routine vital signs or to further assess symptoms of hypoglycemia, they do not provide information directly pertinent to the administration of insulin. Cognitive Level: Applying; Client Need: Physiological Integrity; Nursing Process: Implementation

3 Answer: c Rationale: A serious adverse effect of metformin (Glucophage) is the risk for developing lactic acidosis. Renal insufficiency and failure, excess alcohol use, and IV contrast agents increase the risk for lactic acidosis and are contraindications to the use of metformin. Options a, b, and d are incorrect. Hypoglycemia, GI distress, and weight loss are common adverse effects to most oral antidiabetic drugs and are not specific to metformin. Cognitive Level: Analyzing; Client Need: Physiological Integrity; Nursing Process: Evaluation

4 Answer: b Rationale: It can take several weeks for rosiglitazone (Avandia) to provide full therapeutic effects, so the appropriate response would be to give it more time to reach effectiveness. Options a, c, and d are incorrect. It is not within a nurse's scope of practice to prescribe additional drugs or change the dosage. The healthcare provider should be consulted about any change to the Client's drug regimen. Cognitive Level: Applying; Client Need: Health Promotion and Maintenance; Nursing Process: Implementation

5 Answer: d Rationale: Glucagon injections can be repeated if one dose is not effective. Hypoglycemia is a medical emergency, and because this woman has not fully recovered, medical attention is needed. Options a, b, and c are incorrect. The client is still experiencing symptoms of hypoglycemia, and continued treatment is indicated. Because she is still groggy and disoriented, it would not be safe to give this client anything by mouth. Cognitive Level: Applying; Client Need: Physiological Integrity; Nursing Process: Implementation

Chapter 29

1 Answer: d Rationale: The administration of too much levothyroxine (Synthroid) may cause hyperthyroidism, characterized by nervousness, palpitations, weight loss, diarrhea, and muscle tremors. Before altering the dosage, thyroid function studies will be performed to verify this condition. Options a, b, and c are incorrect. Nervousness, palpitations, and tremors are not symptoms of hypothyroidism or normal thyroid states. While these symptoms may occur with diabetes and hyperglycemia, other symptoms would dominate and would be noted before these symptoms occurred. Cognitive Level: Analyzing; Client Need: Physiological Integrity; Nursing Process: Evaluation

2 Answer: c, d, e Rationale: A euthyroid (normal) state is indicated by a return to normal performance of ADLs without fatigue, normalizing cholesterol levels, and vital signs within normal limits with a pulse rate between 60 and 100 beats/minute. Options a and b are incorrect. Constipation and weight gain are symptoms of hypothyroidism. Decreased blinking and exophthalmos are symptoms of hyperthyroidism. Cognitive Level: Applying; Client Need: Physiological Integrity; Nursing Process: Evaluation

3 Answer: a Rationale: Low-grade fever, sore throat, and chills are symptoms of a possible infection. Because propylthiouracil (PTU) may cause agranulocytosis, these symptoms should be reported to the provider. Options b, c, and d are incorrect. Increased appetite and caloric intake signal a return to a more euthyroid state. Tinnitus, altered taste, thickened saliva, insomnia, nightmares, and night sweats are not effects usually associated with propylthiouracil and if they occur, other causes should be investigated. Cognitive Level: Analyzing; Client Need: Physiological Integrity; Nursing Process: Implementation

4 Answer: c Rationale: A heart rate of 110 beats/minute would cause the nurse to hold the scheduled dose of levothyroxine, because it could indicate too high a level of thyroid hormone. Options a, b, and d are incorrect. A low level of thyroid hormone could cause weight gain or decreased blood pressure. These are symptoms of hypothyroidism and would not cause the nurse to hold the medication. An elevated temperature without other signs of hyperthyroidism would not warrant withholding the medication. Cognitive Level: Analyzing; Client Need: Physiological Integrity; Nursing Process: Implementation

5 Answer: b Rationale: The high levels of iodine found in potassium iodide solution will inhibit the synthesis and release of thyroid hormone. The effectiveness decreases over time so it is only used short term before more definitive treatment can be accomplished. Options a, c, and d are incorrect. Iodine deficiency is rare and does not cause symptoms of hyperthyroidism, the indication for the client's potassium iodide solution. High-dose iodine is not always used prior to thyroid surgery and the thyroidectomy is not related to a loss of iodine. High doses of iodine will not prevent diabetes. Cognitive Level: Applying; Client Need: Physiological Integrity; Nursing Process: Implementation

Chapter 30

1 Answer: a, c, e Rationale: Edema, eye pain or vision changes, and abdominal pain are symptoms of possible adverse effects from the methylprednisolone (Medrol Dosepak). Options b and d are incorrect. Tinnitus is not an adverse effect commonly associated with methylprednisolone and if it occurs, other causes should be investigated. Dizziness upon standing indicates possible *hypo*tension. *Hyper*tension is a possible adverse effect from methylprednisolone. Cognitive Level: Analyzing; Client Need: Physiological Integrity; Nursing Process: Implementation

2 Answer: a Rationale: An irregular heart rate and rhythm is a symptom of hypokalemia. Hydrocortisone (Cortef) given concurrently with diuretics such as thiazides, which cause loss of potassium, increases the risk of hypokalemia. Options b, c, and d are incorrect. While these are common adverse effects of hydrocortisone, they do not require immediate attention. Cognitive Level: Analyzing; Client Need: Physiological Integrity; Nursing Process: Evaluation

3 Answer: a, b Rationale: Weight-bearing exercise three to four times weekly and increased dietary intake of calcium and vitamin D may help to prevent bone loss and osteoporosis. Options c, d, and e are incorrect. Remaining sedentary is not advisable and may increase the risk for osteoporosis and other adverse effects such as thrombophlebitis. Increased fluid intake and avoidance of alcohol are advised, but carbonated sodas should also be avoided because they have been linked to an increased risk of osteoporosis. While a bisphosphonate may be needed if bone density studies indicate the development of osteoporosis, it is not necessarily required at this time. Cognitive Level: Applying; Client Need: Health Promotion and Maintenance; Nursing Process: Implementation

4 Answer: d Rationale: The client should obtain a daily weight, ideally at the same time each day to assess for excessive fluid retention. Fludrocortisone (Florinef) is a mineralocorticoid and may cause fluid retention, edema, and hypertension. Options a, b, and c are incorrect. Abdominal pain and changes to the stool colour may indicate GI bleeding, which is an adverse effect associated with glucocorticoids. Increased lipid levels and mood changes are also associated with glucocorticoids. Cognitive Level: Applying; Client Need: Physiological Integrity; Nursing Process: Implementation

5 Answer: c Rationale: The client is experiencing symptoms of acute adrenal insufficiency related to the inability to take the prescribed drug for several days and will require immediate IV administration of hydrocortisone. Options a, b, and d are incorrect. Fludrocortisone is a mineralocorticoid and is not indicated in this emergency situation. Ketoconazole (Nizoral) and metyrapone (Metopirone) have antiadrenal effects and would worsen the situation. Cognitive Level: Analyzing; Client Need: Physiological Integrity; Nursing Process: Planning

Chapter 31

1 Answer: b, c, d Rationale: A history of thromboembolic conditions, breast cancer, or hyperlipidemia may be contraindications for the use of HRT for this client and will require further assessment by the healthcare provider before prescribing conjugated estrogen. Options a and e are incorrect. Because conjugated estrogen is metabolized through the P450 pathways and the drug may have hepatic effects, women with diabetes may need to more closely monitor their blood glucose to ensure that their diabetes medications are effective, but this is not considered a contraindication to the drug. A past history of cesarean section is also not a contraindication. Cognitive Level: Analyzing; Client Need: Physiological Integrity; Nursing Process: Assessment

2 Answer: c Rationale: Regular contractions increasing in occurrence indicate that the oxytocin (Pitocin) is exerting a therapeutic effect. Options a, b, and d are incorrect. Control of postpartum hemorrhage is a therapeutic effect of oxytocin but would not be considered a therapeutic effect during labour. Sustained contractions are an adverse effect of oxytocin and immediate intervention is needed to prevent serious injury to the mother or baby should they occur. Oxytocin stimulates the milk letdown reflex in nursing, but this would not be considered a therapeutic effect during labour. Cognitive Level: Analyzing; Client Need: Physiological Integrity; Nursing Process: Evaluation

3 Answer: d Rationale: Clomiphene (Clomid) is given over six ovulatory-menstrual cycles in increasing doses with hCG added as needed. If no pregnancy has occurred after six cycles, other treatment options will be considered. Options a, b, and c are incorrect. The drug will not be continued for 1 year if pregnancy has not occurred, and the dosage may be increased after each cycle. Clomiphene is a category X drug and should be stopped if pregnancy occurs. Cognitive Level: Applying; Client Need: Health Promotion and Maintenance; Nursing Process: Implementation

4 Answer: c Rationale: Medroxyprogesterone (Provera) is known to decrease bone density over time. The client should be taught to report any bone, joint, or musculoskeletal pain and to report any difficulty or pain with movement or ambulation. Options a, b, and d are incorrect. Insomnia or sleep difficulty and mouth, eye, or vaginal dryness are not related adverse effects. The drug may cause breakthrough spotting between menstrual cycles, but this is a common effect and does not require evaluation unless the bleeding is heavy or continuous. Cognitive Level: Analyzing; Client Need: Physiological Integrity; Nursing Process: Implementation

5 Answer: b Rationale: The standard treatment with clomiphene is to begin with a low dose for 5 days beginning on the fifth day of the menstrual cycle. Options a, c, and d are incorrect. Starting therapy on the first day of the menstrual cycle would not be as effective in stimulating ovulation because this usually occurs closer to mid-cycle. Because women experience menstrual periods of varying length, starting the drug on the "last day" would vary, and the drug might be started sooner or later than the recommended fifth day of the menstrual cycle. Many women do not know when ovulation occurs to be able to take it based on an ovulatory cycle and there is likelihood that this client is not experiencing ovulation. Cognitive Level: Applying; Client Need: Health Promotion and Maintenance; Nursing Process: Implementation

Chapter 32

1 Answer: b Rationale: Primary hypogonadism results in clients with normal pituitary function and testes that are either diseased or unresponsive to FSH and LH. A primary goal of therapy would be an increased sperm count with an increase in male masculinization. Options a, c, and d are incorrect. Testosterone (Testoderm) should not affect RBC count. Administering testosterone to the client will not increase FSH or LH levels. Cognitive Level: Applying; Client Need: Physiological Integrity; Nursing Process: Evaluation

2 Answer: a Rationale: The use of nitrates is contraindicated with sildenafil because dangerous hypotension may result. Options b, c, and d are incorrect. A history of diabetes would not be of concern and may be an indication for treatment if ED occurs. An allergy to penicillin products is not a contraindication for use of sildenafil (Viagra). There are no expected adverse reactions with sildenafil and the use of antiulcer medication. Cognitive Level: Applying; Client Need: Physiological Integrity; Nursing Process: Assessment

3 Answer: b, c, e Rationale: Women and children should avoid skin contact with areas where testosterone gels or creams have been applied to avoid drug absorption. Testosterones may trigger sodium and water retention and a weight gain of 2 kg (5 lb) or more per week should be reported to the provider. They may also increase blood lipid levels. Therefore, the client should follow a low-fat diet and have periodic blood lipid level assessments. Options a and d are incorrect. Testosterone gel should be applied to the upper arms, shoulders, or abdomen and never to the scrotum, perineal area, or on broken or irritated skin. Showering or swimming should be avoided for several hours after application to allow drug absorption, but a wait of 12 to 14 hours is excessive. Cognitive Level: Applying; Client Need: Physiological Integrity; Nursing Process: Implementation

4 Answer: b   Rationale: For sildenafil to be effective, the ED must be physiological in nature. It is not effective if the dysfunction has solely psychological origins and therefore does not always cause an erection. Options a, c, and d are incorrect. Sildenafil simply enhances, rather than causes, an erection. Prolonged use does not result in less intense feelings over time. Use of sildenafil by men will not have effects on female sexual function. Cognitive Level: Applying; Client Need: Health Promotion and Maintenance; Nursing Process: Implementation

5 Answer: a, b, d   Rationale: Finasteride (Proscar) promotes shrinkage of enlarged prostates and subsequently helps restore urinary function. Women should avoid handling crushed medication because it may be absorbed through the skin and have teratogenic effects. Maximum benefit may take 6 to 12 months to be achieved. Options c and e are incorrect. Dizziness is a possible adverse effect but significant dizziness or orthostatic hypotension should not occur and should be reported to the healthcare provider. Finasteride does not affect vision. Cognitive Level: Applying; Client Need: Physiological Integrity; Nursing Process: Implementation

Chapter 34

1 Answer: b   Rationale: Magnesium compounds, especially in higher doses, often cause diarrhea. Options a, c, and d are incorrect. Aluminum compounds and calcium compounds may cause constipation. Sodium compounds may cause flatulence. Cognitive Level: Applying; Client Need: Physiological Integrity; Nursing Process: Evaluation

2 Answer: a, b, d, e   Rationale: Symptoms of GERD include dysphagia, dyspepsia, nausea, belching, heartburn, and chest pain. Option c is incorrect. The nurse would not expect a decrease in the client's appetite due to this medication. Cognitive Level: Applying; Client Need: Physiological Integrity; Nursing Process: Evaluation

3 Answer: c   Rationale: The proton pump is activated by food intake. Therefore, administering it about 20 to 30 minutes before the first major meal of the day allows peak serum levels to coincide with when the maximum levels of pumps are activated, allowing maximum efficiency of the PPI. Options a, b, and d are incorrect. The proton pumps are less active at night, in the fasting state, or between meals. Cognitive Level: Applying; Client Need: Physiological Integrity; Nursing Process: Planning

4 Answer: b   Rationale: Blood dyscrasias have been reported, especially neutropenia and thrombocytopenia, with long-term use. Periodic blood counts should be performed. Options a, c, and d are incorrect. Ranitidine (Zantac) does not cause photophobia and skin irritations. Dyspnea and productive cough are not expected adverse effects for this medication. Ranitidine is not known to cause these symptoms. Cognitive Level: Applying; Client Need: Physiological Integrity; Nursing Process: Planning

5 Answer: c   Rationale: Antibiotics have no role in the treatment of GERD, although certain antibiotics are used in treating PUD to eradicate the *H. pylori* organism. Options a, b, and d are incorrect. H₂-receptor antagonists and PPIs are used routinely to relieve symptoms of GERD. Over-the-counter antacids provide intermittent relief for mild cases. Cognitive Level: Applying; Client Need: Physiological Integrity; Nursing Process: Implementation

Chapter 35

1 Answer: c   Rationale: Diphenoxylate with atropine (Lomotil) is given for diarrhea. The client should report a decrease in the number of loose, watery stools after administration. Options a, b, and d are incorrect. Although diphenoxylate with atropine may decrease abdominal cramping and gas as a result of slowed peristalsis, it is not the main therapeutic effect desired from this drug. Slowing peristalsis may cause a decrease in bowel sounds rather than an increase. Cognitive Level: Analyzing; Client Need: Physiological Integrity; Nursing Process: Evaluation

2 Answer: d   Rationale: Ondansetron (Zofran) is known to prolong the QT interval and may cause cardiac dysrhythmias. Options a, b, and c are

incorrect. An allergy to soy or soy products, chronic constipation, or glaucoma does not present contraindications to the drugs. Cognitive Level: Analyzing; Client Need: Physiological Integrity; Nursing Process: Evaluation

3 Answer: a   Rationale: The enzymes in pancrelipase (Pancreaze) come from pork. If the client is allergic to or has religious restrictions on pork, the drug is contraindicated. Options b, c, and d are incorrect. Pancrelipase is not contraindicated for individuals with hypertension or coronary artery disease. Pancrelipase is not an iodine-based agent. There is no expected cross-sensitivity. Cognitive Level: Applying; Client Need: Physiological Integrity; Nursing Process: Implementation

4 Answer: d   Rationale: Because magnesium hydroxide (Milk of Magnesia) will stimulate peristalsis, it is important that the nurse assess for bowel sounds before giving the drug. If blockage or an ileus is suspected, the drug should be held and the provider notified. Options a, b, and c are incorrect. Blood pressure is an important vital sign to monitor postoperatively, but the magnesium hydroxide should not have direct effects. The dosage of the opioid drug and the client's ability to ambulate to the bathroom will not affect the drug's use or action. Cognitive Level: Applying; Client Need: Physiological Integrity; Nursing Process: Assessment

5 Answer: a, c   Rationale: The nurse should explore possible causes for the diarrhea with the mother before making a recommendation because if diarrhea is caused by infections, slowing motility may allow the infection to increase. Salicylates, including bismuth subsalicylate (Pepto-Bismol), are contraindicated in children under the age of 19 because of an increased risk for Reye's syndrome. Options b, d, and e are incorrect. Activity level and weight are important growth and development parameters to assess but are unrelated to the drug's use. The school schedule would not have a direct impact on which drug is recommended. Cognitive Level: Applying; Client Need: Physiological Integrity; Nursing Process: Implementation

Chapter 36

1 Answer: d   Rationale: Orlistat (Xenical) is a pregnancy category X drug and should not be used if the client is pregnant or there is a possibility of pregnancy. Options a, b, and c are incorrect. Orlistat is used for short-term treatment of obesity, and the presence of extreme obesity may be an indication for the drug. The drug is used cautiously in clients with diabetes and hypertension, but neither is an absolute contraindication for the drug. Careful monitoring will be required if either of these conditions exist. Cognitive Level: Applying; Client Need: Physiological Integrity; Nursing Process: Assessment

2 Answer: d   Rationale: Typically, orlistat is taken just prior to meals containing fats so that the drug can inhibit lipase and thus the absorption of lipids in the meal. Options a, b, and c are incorrect. Orlistat is taken throughout the day with each meal. It does not decrease appetite; it interferes with the absorption of fat in the diet. Although exercise is a part of the treatment plan for obesity, orlistat does not have to be administered before exercise. Cognitive Level: Applying; Client Need: Health Promotion and Maintenance; Nursing Process: Implementation

3 Answer: d   Rationale: Intake of the proper amount and type of vitamins and nutrients is important in a healthy weight loss program. Because orlistat interferes with lipid absorption, the client should be taught to supplement the diet with a product that contains all essential fat-soluble vitamins. The supplement should be taken at least 2 hours before or after the orlistat. Options a, b, and c are incorrect. While increasing fluid intake may assist in a weight loss program, diet soda may contain sodium, citric acid, or other ingredients not necessary to a balanced diet. Orlistat does not cause photosensitivity, and additional sunscreen is not needed. Orlistat does not cause orthostatic hypotension, and no dizziness should be noted when rising from a lying or sitting position. Cognitive Level: Applying; Client Need: Health Promotion and Maintenance; Nursing Process: Implementation

4 Answer: a   Rationale: Flatus and oily stools are adverse effects that are often troubling to the client. The nurse should inform the client that these often occur when taking orlistat. Options b, c, and d are incorrect. Heartburn and dyspepsia (indigestion), constipation, and nausea and vomiting are not common adverse effects associated with orlistat. Cognitive Level: Applying; Client Need: Physiological Integrity; Nursing Process: Implementation

5 Answer: a, b, c   Rationale: Body weight, body mass index (BMI), and waist circumference are all indicators used to assess levels of obesity. Options d and e are incorrect. A treadmill test assesses physical fitness, not necessarily obesity. Buoyancy analysis is not a test used to determine the degree of obesity.

Cognitive Level: Applying; Client Need: Physiological Integrity; Nursing Process: Assessment

Chapter 37

1 Answer: b Rationale: Oral contraceptives may increase the serum levels of vitamin A. Options a, c, and d are incorrect. Vitamins D and E are also fat-soluble vitamins and may be taken along with vitamin A. Mineral oil may decrease the fat-soluble vitamins, including vitamin A. Antibiotics are not known to have an effect on the serum levels of vitamin A. Cognitive Level: Applying; Client Need: Physiological Integrity; Nursing Process: Assessment

2 Answer: d Rationale: Pyridoxine (vitamin B_6) may reverse or antagonize the effects of antiparkinson drugs. Options a, b, and c are incorrect. INH, oral contraceptives, and hydralazine (Apresoline) may increase the need for pyridoxine. Cognitive Level: Applying; Client Need: Physiological Integrity; Nursing Process: Assessment

3 Answer: c Rationale: Muscle cramping and spasms may be early signs of hypocalcemia. Options a, b, and d are incorrect. Night blindness is a sign of possible vitamin A deficiency. Anemia may indicate an iron deficiency. Bleeding abnormalities may signal a deficiency in vitamin K. Cognitive Level: Analyzing; Client Need: Physiological Integrity; Nursing Process: Evaluation

4 Answer: c Rationale: A client receiving enteral feedings can be at risk for dehydration caused by an inadequate intake of free water. It is important to irrigate the tube with water as ordered, or per protocol (before and after an intermittent feeding or medication, or every 4 to 6 hours for continuous feedings), and to include additional free water throughout the day unless contraindicated. Options a, b, and d are incorrect. Daily weights are important to track fluid balance, but they do not maintain fluid balance. The NG tube should be irrigated more than just once a day. While assessment of the skin around a PEG tube site is important, it will not indicate the client's fluid balance. This client is receiving the feeding via an NG tube, which is passed through the nose. Cognitive Level: Applying; Client Need: Physiological Integrity; Nursing Process: Assessment

5 Answer: d Rationale: 10% dextrose in water contains the highest concentration of glucose and should be hung until the new TPN bag is available. The solution selected should minimize the risk for hypoglycemia. Options a, b, and c are incorrect. They will not be effective in preventing hypoglycemia. Cognitive Level: Applying; Client Need: Physiological Integrity; Nursing Process: Implementation

Chapter 38

1 Answer: a Rationale: A quick-acting inhaled beta agonist such as salbutamol (Ventolin) is used to abort bronchospasm. Options b, c, and d are incorrect. Beclomethasone (QVAR), ipratropium (Atrovent), and zafirlukast (Accolate) are drugs used to prevent and control bronchospastic attacks and will not cause bronchodilation quickly enough to abort an attack. Cognitive Level: Applying; Client Need: Physiological Integrity; Nursing Process: Implementation

2 Answer: c Rationale: Corticosteroids can decrease the beneficial oral flora that will allow for an overgrowth of fungal infections such as *Candida*. Rinsing the mouth removes any corticosteroid drug deposited there and prevents it from being swallowed, decreasing the likelihood of systemic absorption. Options a, b, and d are incorrect. Inhaled corticosteroids such as beclomethasone do not cause tachycardia, nervousness, or tremors, and caffeine does not need to be avoided while the drug is used. Cognitive Level: Applying; Client Need: Health Promotion and Maintenance; Nursing Process: Implementation

3 Answer: a Rationale: Bronchodilators such as salbutamol may have an adverse effect on heart rate elevation and palpitations related to dosage. Options b, c, and d are incorrect. Bronchodilators do not decrease the immune response or increase alertness. While some bronchodilators have been known to cause unexpected problems and paradoxical bronchospasm, this is uncommon. Cognitive Level: Applying; Client Need: Physiological Integrity; Nursing Process: Implementation

4 Answer: a, b Rationale: Because corticosteroids such as beclomethasone decrease the immune response, the risk for infections is increased. Corticosteroids also increase blood glucose, thus increasing the possibility of hyperglycemia. Options c, d, and e are incorrect. Corticosteroids do not cause urinary retention, do not increase the likelihood of tachycardia, and do not cause

photophobia. Cognitive Level: Applying; Client Need: Physiological Integrity; Nursing Process: Assessment

5 Answer: c Rationale: Some clients have difficulty mastering the coordination between inhalation and activation of the medication. In these instances, a spacer will hold the medication cloud so that this is not a concern. The spacer has additional advantages because it results in more effective delivery of the drug to the site of action and less drug deposition in the mouth and oropharynx. However, note that spacers are only available for use with MDI inhalers. Options a, b, and d are incorrect. Additional practice may help in the long term, but it is not the priority for an immediate solution to the problem and may only serve to frustrate the client further. The healthcare provider would not need to be contacted because the client has difficulty learning, provided that a solution is readily available. Substitution of an oral form of the drug is not within the nursing scope of practice. Cognitive Level: Analyzing; Client Need: Health Promotion and Maintenance; Nursing Process: Planning

Chapter 40

1 Answer: a Rationale: Interferon alpha-2b (Intron A) causes flu-like symptoms in up to 50% of clients receiving the drug. Options b, c, and d are incorrect. While depression with suicidal thoughts has been reported, it is not a common effect. Hypotension or hypertension, edema, fluid volume overload, tachycardia, and renal insufficiency are not adverse effects commonly associated with this drug. Cognitive Level: Analyzing; Client Need: Physiological Integrity; Nursing Process: Assessment

2 Answer: b Rationale: The client's high fever (39.4°C) and chills are indicative of an infectious process. The use of two immunosuppressant drugs (i.e., basiliximab [Simulect] and cyclosporine [Sandimmune]) increases the risk for infection related to the additional immunosuppressant effects. Options a, c, and d are incorrect. Basiliximab has fewer significant adverse effects than other monoclonal antibodies; however, GI effects (nausea, vomiting, abdominal pain) are common and anaphylaxis has been reported. Capillary leak syndrome is a condition in which fluid and protein leak out of tiny blood vessels and flow into surrounding tissue. This complication is not associated with basiliximab administration. Graft-versus-host rejection is a type of transplant rejection, and androgen insensitivity is a genetically linked syndrome. Both are unrelated to the drug. Cognitive Level: Analyzing; Client Need: Physiological Integrity; Nursing Process: Assessment

3 Answer: b Rationale: Cyclosporine is toxic to bone marrow although less so than other immunosuppressants. A decrease in WBCs to below 4000/mm^3 should be reported to the provider. Options a, c, and d are incorrect. Cyclosporine does not cause an elevation in RBCs. The provider should be notified if platelet counts drop below 75 000/mm^3, but a count of 100 000/mm^3 is within acceptable limits. A creatinine level of less than 1 mg/100 mL is within normal limits. Cognitive Level: Applying; Client Need: Physiological Integrity; Nursing Process: Assessment

4 Answer: c Rationale: Azathioprine (Imuran) should be used with extreme caution in clients with a previous history of varicella zoster (chickenpox, shingles) because the immunosuppression may cause the virus to reactivate and cause a serious infection. Options a, b, and d are incorrect. Benign prostatic hyperplasia and cataracts are not contraindications for the drug. Azathioprine may be used as a treatment for severe RA. Cognitive Level: Applying; Client Need: Physiological Integrity; Nursing Process: Assessment

5 Answer: d Rationale: Tacrolimus (Prograf) is a potent immunosuppressant and clients should decrease their risk for infection by taking precautions such as avoiding raw fruits and vegetables that may harbour pathogens on the skin or inside, and by eating only fully cooked meats after the heat of cooking has destroyed pathogens. Options a, b, and c are incorrect. Aspirin may increase GI irritation, placing the client at risk for GI infections gaining entry through the inflamed mucosa. Physical activity is important to overall health, but this drug has no direct connection with weight gain. Tacrolimus is not known to have significant cardiac effects, although hypertension is a possible adverse effect and the blood pressure should be monitored. Cognitive Level: Applying; Client Need: Health Promotion and Maintenance; Nursing Process: Planning

Chapter 41

1 Answer: b Rationale: A parent's preconceived ideas or reservations about accepting vaccinations will be most influential on whether the infant receives the scheduled injections. This also presents an excellent teaching opportunity for the nurse to answer questions, allay any fears the mother may have, and teach post-vaccine care. Options a, c, and d are incorrect. An allergy history will be taken, but unless the infant has demonstrated an allergy to the components in the vaccine, allergies to other medications will not necessarily increase the risk for reaction, nor will the parents' allergies increase the risk. Nurses working with pediatric clients should be knowledgeable about the recommended schedule and, when in doubt, verify the necessary immunizations needed. Cognitive Level: Analyzing; Client Need: Physiological Integrity; Nursing Process: Assessment

2 Answer: c Rationale: The MMR vaccination is an attenuated (live) virus and there is a slight risk that the virus could be transmitted to the child's father because he is immunocompromised from the chemotherapy. The nurse would check with the provider about delaying the vaccine until the father is finished with the chemotherapy. Options a, b, and d are incorrect. The nurse would teach the mother the signs of reaction and when to report them, and the family can safely go out of town if health care is available at their destination. Although additional teaching may be required to allay the mother's fears of reaction, the mother's reaction to MMR will not necessarily result in a reaction in the child. As long as the brother's immune system is healthy, he should not have any adverse effects from his sister's MMR because of his cold. Cognitive Level: Applying; Client Need: Physiological Integrity; Nursing Process: Implementation

3 Answer: d Rationale: Acetaminophen (Tylenol) or ibuprofen (Advil) is an appropriate analgesic to treat the soreness that occurs post–tetanus toxoid vaccination. Options a, b, and c are incorrect. There is no requirement to keep the arm still; in fact, motion may help disperse the medication and help it to absorb. There is no need to restrict fluids or to avoid crowds with a toxoid vaccination. Cognitive Level: Analyzing; Client Need: Health Promotion and Maintenance; Nursing Process: Evaluation

4 Answer: c Rationale: Known hypersensitivity to yeast is an absolute contraindication for hepatitis B vaccine. Options a, b, and d are incorrect. Smoking and hypertension are not contraindications for the vaccine and present an opportunity for health teaching. Hepatitis B is only available by injection and the nurse would explore methods to help the client be less fearful of the injection prior to administration. Cognitive Level: Analyzing; Client Need: Physiological Integrity; Nursing Process: Assessment

5 Answer: a Rationale: Hypersensitivity reactions are likely to occur within the first 20 minutes of administration. The nurse should closely monitor the client's vital signs during the initial period. Options b, c, and d are incorrect. RhoGAM does not cause thrombocytopenia or anemia or increase liver enzymes. There is no need for a low-saturated-fat, low-cholesterol diet after receiving Rh₀ immune globulin, and RhoGAM does not cause a cough. Cognitive Level: Applying; Client Need: Physiological Integrity; Nursing Process: Implementation

Chapter 42

1 Answer: b Rationale: Acetaminophen (Tylenol) overdose is treated with PO or IV acetylcysteine (Mucomyst). For maximum effectiveness, the antidote should be administered within 8 hours of acetaminophen ingestion. Options a, c, and d are incorrect. The administration of 1000 mL per hour of normal saline IV would place the client at risk for fluid volume overload. The client will not require cardioversion to treat acetaminophen poisoning. The client's hepatic enzymes will be assessed; however, these enzymes only provide information as to the extent of liver damage. They do not treat acute acetaminophen overdose; they merely monitor for the effectiveness of the treatment and any effects of the overdose itself. Cognitive Level: Applying; Client Need: Physiological Integrity; Nursing Process: Planning

2 Answer: c Rationale: Acetaminophen is the drug of choice for reduction of fever in the event the client has a hypersensitivity to aspirin. Options a, b, and d are incorrect. A client who has hypersensitivity to aspirin should not be administered ibuprofen (Motrin, Advil) or celecoxib (Celebrex) due to the risk of hypersensitivity with the NSAIDs. Ketorolac is not administered for reduction of fever; it is administered for pain control. Cognitive Level: Applying; Client Need: Physiological Integrity; Nursing Process: Planning

3 Answer: d Rationale: Ibuprofen should be discontinued 7 to 14 days before surgery to reduce the risk for bleeding. Options a, b, and c are incorrect. Ibuprofen should not be continued until surgery and the client should continue her anti-inflammatory agent until 7 to 14 days before surgery to maintain its antiarthritis effects. Cognitive Level: Applying; Client Need: Physiological Integrity; Nursing Process: Implementation

4 Answer: a Rationale: Acetaminophen is metabolized in the liver. The client with cirrhosis of the liver has impaired liver function and should not receive acetaminophen for pain or fever reduction. Options b, c, and d are incorrect. A client who has COPD, has breast cancer, or is taking warfarin (Coumadin) (exercise caution when warfarin and acetaminophen are combined together as it can affect the INR) can be administered with acetaminophen for fever and analgesia. Cognitive Level: Applying; Client Need: Physiological Integrity; Nursing Process: Implementation

5 Answer: a, b, c, d Rationale: A client who is experiencing toxic effects from aspirin (acetylsalicylic acid) may experience tinnitus, hyperventilation, GI bleeding, or decreased urine output related to renal impairment. Option e is incorrect. A client with salicylate toxicity does not tend to experience peripheral neuropathy. Cognitive Level: Analyzing; Client Need: Physiological Integrity; Nursing Process: Evaluation

Chapter 44

1 Answer: c Rationale: Ampicillin may decrease the effectiveness of oral contraceptives, and the client should be instructed to use a barrier method to avoid unwanted pregnancies while on the antibiotic and until the next cycle of oral contraceptives is started. Options a, b, and d are incorrect. The combination of ampicillin and oral contraceptives will not increase the risk for adverse effects related to the antibiotic. Oral contraceptive effectiveness may be reduced during ampicillin therapy, and ampicillin will not create serious toxicity related to the use of oral contraceptives. Cognitive Level: Applying; Client Need: Health Promotion and Maintenance; Nursing Process: Implementation

2 Answer: c Rationale: Ototoxicity is associated with serum concentrations of vancomycin (Vancocin) above 60 to 80 μg/mL and manifests with tinnitus, dizziness, or balance and coordination effects. Options a, b, and d are incorrect. Redness of the ears, itching of the ears, and ocular pain are not symptoms related to ototoxicity caused by vancomycin. Cognitive Level: Analyzing; Client Need: Physiological Integrity; Nursing Process: Evaluation

3 Answer: b Rationale: A vaginal yeast infection with discharge may be a symptom of a superinfection. Superinfection is a possible adverse effect associated with all antibiotics and particularly with fungal and viral infections. Options a, c, and d are incorrect. A hypersensitivity reaction is not usually manifested by vaginal discharge. The symptoms associated with PMC are significant GI effects. Vaginal discharge is not a symptom of antibiotic toxicity. Cognitive Level: Applying; Client Need: Physiological Integrity; Nursing Process: Evaluation

4 Answer: d Rationale: Watery diarrhea containing mucus, blood, or pus is symptomatic of *Clostridium difficile*–associated diarrhea and must be monitored closely for progressing to PMC; both are adverse effects related to antibiotic use. Options a, b, and c are incorrect. These symptoms are not related to peptic ulcers, malabsorption, or hypersensitivity reactions. Cognitive Level: Analyzing; Client Need: Physiological Integrity; Nursing Process: Evaluation

5 Answer: a Rationale: Ampicillin should be taken on an empty stomach to ensure adequate absorption. Options b, c, and d are incorrect. A black and furry tongue is the symptom of an oral superinfection and should be reported. The client should be taught to take the full prescription even if the symptoms subside. Clients should never take two doses because this will place them at risk for toxicity. Cognitive Level: Analyzing; Client Need: Health Promotion and Maintenance; Nursing Process: Evaluation

Chapter 45

1 Answer: b, c, d Rationale: When administered too rapidly, amphotericin B (Fungizone) may cause hypotension, hypokalemia, and shock. Options a and e are incorrect. Amphotericin is not known to cause laryngeal spasms or hypoglycemia. Cognitive Level: Analyzing; Client Need: Physiological Integrity; Nursing Process: Evaluation

2 Answer: a Rationale: Clients who take fluconazole (Diflucan) may experience nausea, vomiting, and diarrhea. Nutritional intake is especially important to maintain optimum health in a client with AIDS. Keeping a food diary will assist the provider in determining overall calorie and fluid intake.

Antinausea medication may be helpful if nausea or vomiting is severe. Options b, c, and d are incorrect. Loss of muscle mass is not related to fluconazole therapy. The decision to wear a high-filtration mask is not related to fluconazole, and clients on this drug do not need to avoid fat-based soaps. Allowing adequate air circulation to body areas will help prevent surface fungal infections but is not required as part of fluconazole therapy. Cognitive Level: Applying; Client Need: Physiological Integrity; Nursing Process: Implementation

3 Answer: a, b Rationale: Unless otherwise directed by the provider, small amounts of water after a feeding will rinse the mouth of milk proteins and sugars that can provide an ideal medium for *Candida* to grow. The suspension should be applied to all surfaces of the mouth and tongue, by syringe or applicator, and the infant should swallow the remainder to treat possible GI *Candida*. Options c, d, and e are incorrect. Nystatin suspension does not require chilling before administration. The suspension should not be added to formula or given before feedings and should be administered after feedings so that it can be retained in the mouth to treat the area of infection. Cognitive Level: Applying; Client Need: Physiological Integrity; Nursing Process: Implementation

4 Answer: d Rationale: Nails grow very slowly and lengthy treatment may be required to adequately treat the infection. Options a, b, and c are incorrect. The infection will be evaluated during the treatment period but it will take many months to adequately treat the infection. Purchasing more pills at one time does not necessarily reduce the cost of the prescription. Toxic doses are never administered, even to shorten treatment cycles. Cognitive Level: Applying; Client Need: Health Promotion and Maintenance; Nursing Process: Implementation

5 Answer: c Rationale: Amphotericin B can cause a number of serious adverse effects including fever, chills, and headache. Pretreatment with corticosteroids, antihistamines, and antipyretics may reduce the severity of these distressing adverse effects. Options a, b, and d are incorrect. Pretreatment does not enhance the effectiveness of this antifungal agent. The by-products of amphotericin are not affected by the pretreatment of the client, and pretreatment does not affect the half-life of the drug. Cognitive Level: Applying; Client Need: Physiological Integrity; Nursing Process: Planning

Chapter 46

1 Answer: a Rationale: Acyclovir (Zovirax) is associated with renal toxicity, especially when given IV. The drug should be administered IV over a minimum of 1 hour and increased fluid intake encouraged throughout the day to prevent adverse renal effects. Options b, c, and d are incorrect. Acyclovir is not associated with an increased risk for fungal infections or eye discomfort. Itching and skin irritation may occur with topical use but if it occurs with IV drug administration, drug allergy should be questioned and the administration stopped until evaluated. Cognitive Level: Applying; Client Need: Physiological Integrity; Nursing Process: Implementation

2 Answer: a Rationale: Individuals with herpes must understand that transferring the virus remains a possibility even if drug therapies are used. Options b, c, and d are incorrect. Clients with herpes lesions should gently cleanse affected areas with soap and water three to four times daily and dry well prior to application of the topical medication. With application of medication to the genitals, the client should wear loose-fitting clothes over affected areas for comfort. For best results, the client should be instructed to start the antiviral therapy as soon as possible after the onset of signs and symptoms. Cognitive Level: Applying; Client Need: Health Promotion and Maintenance; Nursing Process: Evaluation

3 Answer: b, c, e Rationale: Amantadine (Symmetrel) is associated with renal toxicity, possible severe CNS effects including seizures, psychosis and suicidal ideation, and peripheral edema and heart failure. Options a and d are incorrect. Amantadine is not known to interfere or affect the white blood cell or platelet count. Potassium and sodium levels are not affected by amantadine. Cognitive Level: Applying; Client Need: Physiological Integrity; Nursing Process: Assessment

4 Answer: b Rationale: Tenofovir (Viread) is known to cause lactic acidosis. Symptoms such as anxiety, fatigue, nausea, vomiting, palpitations, lethargy, rapid breathing and heart rate, weakness, chest pain or tightening, hypotension, or shortness of breath should be immediately reported to the provider. Options a, c, and d are incorrect. Tenofovir is not associated with systemic yeast infections, heart failure, or ventricular dysrhythmias. Cognitive Level: Applying; Client Need: Physiological Integrity; Nursing Process: Implementation

5 Answer: d Rationale: Ribavirin (Ibavyr) is associated with an increased risk for hemolytic anemia. Increased fatigue, dizziness, headache, abdominal

pain, pallor, and chest pain are associated with this anemia. Options a, b, and c are incorrect. Respiratory, dermatological, or neurological adverse effects may occur but are not as severe as the hemolytic anemia associated with this drug. Cognitive Level: Analyzing; Client Need: Physiological Integrity; Nursing Process: Evaluation

Chapter 47

1 Answer: b Rationale: This is a false statement. No vaccine currently exists to provide immunity to this disease, although testing is ongoing. Options a, c, and d are incorrect. The client should be informed that therapy for HIV will require lifelong treatment since there is not a cure. Since treatment is often complex and lifelong, whenever possible the client should be taught how to adjust the daily schedule so as to not interfere with ADLs. With recent advances in pharmacotherapy for HIV infection, many individuals are able to live symptom-free lives. Cognitive Level: Applying; Client Need: Health Promotion and Maintenance; Nursing Process: Evaluation

2 Answer: d Rationale: Lactic acidosis is known to occur with all NRTIs, although the risk with emtricitabine (Emtriva) is less than that of some drugs. It is one of the preferred drugs for initial HIV therapy. Options a, b, and c are incorrect. Ventricular cardiac dysrhythmias, pulmonary fibrosis, and necrotic bowel syndrome are not associated with emtricitabine. Cognitive Level: Applying; Client Need: Physiological Integrity; Nursing Process: Evaluation

3 Answer: c Rationale: Myelosuppression is the declining ability of the bone marrow to produce blood cells such as platelets, red blood cells, and white blood cells. Options a, b, and d are incorrect. Myelosuppression is not reflected in an increase in the serum blood urea nitrogen level. Myelosuppression causes a decrease in white blood cells rather than an increase. A decline in blood pressure is not indicative of myelosuppression. Cognitive Level: Analyzing; Client Need: Physiological Integrity; Nursing Process: Evaluation

4 Answer: a, b, c Rationale: Clients receiving antiretroviral therapy are immunocompromised and should avoid sources of infection such as crowds and individuals who have infections. The client should be instructed to notify the healthcare provider at the first sign of a rash. Several antiretroviral medications may cause Stevens–Johnson syndrome, a dermatological adverse effect that can be fatal. Current research has shown that HAART, especially when started early in HIV infection, significantly reduces viral load, reducing the chance of transmission. Transmission is still possible and infection control measures should still be practised. Options d and e are incorrect. Total discontinuation of medication is not recommended because viral load increases when drug therapy is discontinued. Some herbal supplements, such as St. John's wort, interfere with antiretroviral therapy. Cognitive Level: Applying; Client Need: Health Promotion and Maintenance; Nursing Process: Planning

5 Answer: d Rationale: Tenofovir (Viread) is known to lower bone mineral density, which may increase the risk for osteopenia or bone fractures. The client should alert the chiropractor to this drug and possible risk before beginning any treatments. Options a, b, and c are incorrect. Many clients will turn to alternative therapy when faced with HIV infection. These activities provide the client with a sense of control and comfort and should be supported as long as they are not contraindicated with the prescribed drug therapy. Yoga, guided imagery, massage therapy, meditation, and journalling are low-impact alternative therapies that may be tried. Cognitive Level: Applying; Client Need: Health Promotion and Maintenance; Nursing Process: Planning

Chapter 49

1 Answer: a Rationale: Rhabdomyolysis is a serious adverse effect of the statins. Early signs include unexplained fatigue or muscle weakness, pain in joints or muscles, and an increase in CK level. Options b, c, and d are incorrect. The weakness, fatigue, and pain that the client is experiencing are not symptoms of renal failure or hepatic insufficiency. In rheumatoid arthritis, pain is often present but tends to be greatest in the mornings and associated with red, hot, swollen joints. Cognitive Level: Analyzing; Client Need: Physiological Integrity; Nursing Process: Evaluation

2 Answer: b Rationale: One of the most serious adverse effects of cholestyramine (Questran) is obstruction of the GI tract. Options a, c, and d are incorrect. Cholestyramine does not cause orange urine, sore throat, and fever, or affect capillary refill. Cognitive Level: Applying; Client Need: Physiological Integrity; Nursing Process: Planning

3 Answer: a   Rationale: Although there are few contraindications to using bile acid sequestrants such as colestipol (Colestid), they should be used cautiously in clients with GI disorders such as peptic ulcer disease. Options b, c, and d are incorrect. MI is not a contraindication for the use of bile acid sequestrants. Bile acid sequestrant agents do not affect serum sodium levels, and clients allergic to foods high in tyramine may be prescribed bile acid sequestrants. Cognitive Level: Applying; Client Need: Physiological Integrity; Nursing Process: Implementation

4 Answer: b, c   Rationale: Intense flushing and hot flashes occur in almost every client who is taking niacin. Tingling of the extremities may also occur. Options a, d, and e are incorrect. Neither fever and chills nor dry mucous membranes are associated adverse effects of niacin therapy. Niacin may cause an *increase* in fasting blood glucose, especially in people with diabetes. Cognitive Level: Analyzing; Client Need: Physiological Integrity; Nursing Process: Evaluation

5 Answer: a, d, e   Rationale: Fibric acid agents (fibrates) such as gemfibrozil (Lopid) may cause or worsen gallbladder disease and may enhance the hypoglycemic effects of antidiabetes drugs. Because it is excreted through the kidneys, it may be used cautiously in clients with renal impairment, but the order should be validated with the provider before giving if the client has a history of renal impairment. Options b and c are incorrect. Angina and hypertension may indicate the existence of atherosclerosis and arteriosclerosis, both of which are indications for a lipid-lowering drug. Cognitive Level: Applying; Client Need: Physiological Integrity; Nursing Process: Implementation

Chapter 50

1 Answer: c   Rationale: Clients should be taught to remove the old ointment before applying the next dose. Options a, b, and d are incorrect. Nitroglycerin should be kept at room temperature, not in the refrigerator. Clients should take the medication before chest pain becomes severe. Nitroglycerin can be applied to any skin surface. However, absorption is decreased when applied to hairy areas, soles of feet, and palms. Cognitive Level: Applying; Client Need: Health Promotion and Maintenance; Nursing Process: Implementation

2 Answer: d   Rationale: A decline in blood pressure is an expected adverse effect. The nurse should always assess the blood pressure prior to and 5 minutes after administering nitroglycerin. Options a, b, and c are incorrect. Photosensitivity, vomiting, and diarrhea are not expected adverse effects. Nitroglycerin will cause a decline in blood pressure, not an increase. Cognitive Level: Applying; Client Need: Physiological Integrity; Nursing Process: Planning

3 Answer: d   Rationale: Skin irritation due to the nitroglycerin patch can occur if the same site is used repeatedly. Options a, b, and c are incorrect. Clients should be instructed to rotate the site of application when using nitroglycerin patch. Repeated use of the same application site may actually decrease absorption. Rebound phenomenon is not an expected occurrence with nitroglycerin. Cognitive Level: Applying; Client Need: Health Promotion and Maintenance; Nursing Process: Implementation

4 Answer: a   Rationale: Atenolol (Tenormin) increases blood flow to the myocardium, thereby increasing oxygen supply by reducing the heart rate and decreasing the contractility. Options b, c, and d are incorrect. Atenolol is a beta-adrenergic antagonist, which decreases heart rate. This drug does not affect the sodium channels. Although this drug reduces blood pressure, the mechanism of action is not by blocking the alpha$_2$ receptors. Cognitive Level: Applying; Client Need: Physiological Integrity; Nursing Process: Implementation

5 Answer: a, c   Rationale: Verapamil (Isoptin) decreases blood pressure and heart rate. The administration of this drug may cause significant hypotension and bradycardia in some clients. Options b, d, and e are incorrect. Verapamil may be used to treat fast heart rates and hypertension in addition to angina. Tinnitus and hearing loss are not adverse effects associated with verapamil. Cognitive Level: Analyzing; Client Need: Physiological Integrity; Nursing Process: Evaluation

Chapter 51

1 Answer: a   Rationale: Hot baths and showers, prolonged standing in one position, and strenuous exercise may enhance orthostatic hypotension. Options b, c, and d are incorrect. Methyldopa does not discolour the urine. Bloating and weight gain are not typical adverse effects of methyldopa, and methyldopa can be taken without food. Cognitive Level: Applying; Client Need: Physiological Integrity; Nursing Process: Implementation

2 Answer: d   Rationale: Orthostatic hypotension is a common adverse effect of vasodilators such as hydralazine (Apresoline). Options a, b, and c are incorrect. Hydralazine does not typically cause atelectasis. Crystalluria is not an adverse effect of hydralazine and it does not cause photosensitivity. Cognitive Level: Applying; Client Need: Physiological Integrity; Nursing Process: Planning

3 Answer: a   Rationale: Clients who have recently been prescribed hydralazine may experience dizziness initially and should be instructed not to engage in activities that may be hazardous. Options b, c, and d are incorrect. Clients should always consult their healthcare providers before discontinuing antihypertensive medications. Clients should report dizziness to the healthcare provider and should not adjust the dosage until the etiology of the problem is determined. Clients on this drug have no restriction on air travel. Cognitive Level: Analyzing; Client Need: Health Promotion and Maintenance; Nursing Process: Evaluation

4 Answer: d   Rationale: The nurse will titrate (adjust) the rate of infusion based on the client's blood pressure. Options a, b, and c are incorrect. Listening for bowel sounds in the client with hypertensive crisis is not a nursing priority. Urine specific gravity and glucose levels may be obtained but are not associated with hypertensive crisis or the administration of this drug. Observing skin pressure points is a nursing intervention that does not directly relate to hypertensive crisis or nitroprusside (Nipride) therapy. Cognitive Level: Applying; Client Need: Physiological Integrity; Nursing Process: Implementation

5 Answer: b, c, d   Rationale: New guidelines in the JNC-8 report recommend ACEIs or ARBs, CCBs, and thiazide diuretics as primary treatment options for most clients. Options a and e are incorrect. Beta blockers may still be used for some clients but are no longer recommended for primary treatment of hypertension. Direct-acting vasodilators are used to treat hypertensive crisis and for clients who have not responded adequately to other antihypertensive drugs. Cognitive Level: Analyzing; Client Need: Physiological Integrity; Nursing Process: Planning

Chapter 52

1 Answer: b   Rationale: As a diuretic, furosemide (Lasix) may dramatically reduce the client's circulating blood volume, thus producing episodes of orthostatic hypotension. Clients may minimize this effect by rising slowly from sitting or lying positions. Options a, c, and d are incorrect. Cabbage, cauliflower, and kale are high in vitamin K, but furosemide does not require restricted consumption of these foods. Monitoring pulse rate during administration of furosemide for reflex tachycardia secondary to hypotension is advised, but it is not required that it be taken before the dose or for 1 full minute. Due to the potential for significant diuresis, fluids should not be restricted unless ordered by the healthcare provider. Cognitive Level: Applying; Client Need: Physiological Integrity; Nursing Process: Implementation

2 Answer: c   Rationale: Muscle cramps and weakness may indicate hypokalemia and should be reported to the healthcare provider. Options a, b, and d are incorrect. Many clients taking diuretic therapy are instructed to monitor the intake of both sodium and water to maintain adequate but not excessive amounts. Clients should ingest foods high in potassium, not vitamin K. Thiazide diuretics and antihypertensive drugs are not known to cause sleepiness when taken together. Cognitive Level: Applying; Client Need: Physiological Integrity; Nursing Process: Implementation

3 Answer: a   Rationale: Spironolactone (Aldactone) is a potassium-sparing diuretic and may cause hyperkalemia. Options b, c, and d are incorrect. This drug does not have a direct effect on magnesium and does not cause hypokalemia. It does not have calcium-binding effects. Cognitive Level: Applying; Client Need: Physiological Integrity; Nursing Process: Assessment

4 Answer: d   Rationale: In the early stages of the administration of mannitol (Osmitrol), fluid is drawn into extracellular spaces and vascular compartments. Pulmonary and peripheral edema may occur, and increased intracranial pressure may also occur along with an early change in level of consciousness. Options a, b, and c are incorrect. Keeping a urinal or bedpan nearby; monitoring electrolytes, including potassium; and recording I&O and daily weight are important nursing interventions but are not the main nursing priority in the early administration of mannitol. Cognitive Level: Applying; Client Need: Physiological Integrity; Nursing Process: Implementation

5 Answer: a   Rationale: Clients receiving acetazolamide (Diamox) are at risk for metabolic acidosis due to excess bicarbonate loss. Options b, c, and d are incorrect. Metabolic alkalosis is characterized by a deficit of bicarbonate and is not an adverse effect of acetazolamide. Acetazolamide does not cause respiratory acidosis. Respiratory alkalosis is also not an expected adverse effect of acetazolamide. Cognitive Level: Analyzing; Client Need: Physiological Integrity; Nursing Process: Evaluation

Chapter 53

1 Answer: a Rationale: The serum pH is a measure of alkalinity or acidity in the blood. The administration of bicarbonate neutralizes acidic conditions and causes the client's serum to become more alkaline. Options b, c, and d are incorrect. Changes in the pH can affect the ability of RBCs to release oxygen, but administration of sodium bicarbonate will not influence the number of circulating RBCs. The liver does not metabolize sodium bicarbonate; it is naturally occurring in the body and does not metabolize. Liver function tests are not indicators of the drug's effectiveness. Although sodium bicarbonate excretion occurs in the kidneys, the blood urea nitrogen level will not reflect the effectiveness of this drug. Cognitive Level: Applying; Client Need: Physiological Integrity; Nursing Process: Evaluation

2 Answer: b Rationale: Liquid preparations are very irritating to the gastric mucosa and should always be diluted with juice or water. Options a, c, and d are incorrect. Salt substitutes are high in potassium and should be avoided by clients on potassium supplementation. Symptoms such as weakness or fatigue may be the first indicators of potassium imbalances. The GI secretions are rich in potassium. Episodes of persistent vomiting may lead to hypokalemia and should be reported to the healthcare provider. Cognitive Level: Applying; Client Need: Physiological Integrity; Nursing Process: Evaluation

3 Answer: b Rationale: This solution is often used to dilute (reconstitute) powdered forms of drugs that are intended to be given parenterally. Options a, c, and d are incorrect. This solution can cause hyperglycemia in the client with diabetes due to the dextrose content. D_5W is considered a crystalloid solution. One litre of this solution supplies only 170 calories, which is not enough to supply the metabolic nutritional needs of adult clients. Cognitive Level: Applying; Client Need: Physiological Integrity; Nursing Process: Implementation

4 Answer: d Rationale: Magnesium sulfate toxicity may cause significant neuromuscular depression as noted by changes in level of consciousness and diminished deep tendon reflexes. Options a, b, and c are incorrect. Pupillary constriction to bright light is a normal physiological response. The nurse should notify the prescriber when the client develops chest congestion and coughing, but they are not directly associated with magnesium sulfate toxicity. Elevated blood pressure is common in pre-eclampsia, but it is not associated with magnesium toxicity. Cognitive Level: Applying; Client Need: Physiological Integrity; Nursing Process: Implementation

5 Answer: a, c, d Rationale: Normal serum albumin is a product derived from blood. Although rare, transfusion reactions can still occur with normal serum albumin. Albumin causes intercellular and interstitial fluid to move into the intravascular compartment. This movement of fluid will cause increases in the client's blood pressure and heart rate. The nurse should monitor the client for fluid overload with this solution. As the circulating fluid volume is corrected, the client's urinary output will increase. Options b and e are incorrect. Clients receiving normal serum albumin typically do not have any dietary restrictions while receiving this solution. Serum albumin is not administered for potassium imbalances. Cognitive Level: Applying; Client Need: Physiological Integrity; Nursing Process: Planning

Chapter 54

1 Answer: b Rationale: ACE inhibitors such as enalapril (Vasotec) lower peripheral resistance through the inhibition of angiotensin II formation, and reduce blood volume through inhibition of aldosterone secretion. This reduces arterial blood pressure, decreasing afterload and increasing cardiac output. Options a, c, and d are incorrect. Enalapril is not a positive inotropic agent and does not strengthen the force of myocardial contraction. It does not slow heart rate (negative chronotropic and dromotropic effects) and it does not have diuretic effects. Cognitive Level: Analyzing; Client Need: Physiological Integrity; Nursing Process: Evaluation

2 Answer: b Rationale: The client will be taught to take the pulse daily and to contact the prescriber if the pulse rate is less than 60 or greater than 100 beats per minute. Options a, c, and d are incorrect. The medication

should be taken at the same time each day, but preferably after the client has been active for a period of time (mid-morning). Typically, the pulse rate will be lower in the morning before the client rises. Digoxin (Lanoxin) should be withheld if the pulse rate is below 60 beats per minute. A high-fibre diet may decrease the absorption of digoxin, and the drug should not be taken along with meals high in fibre. Furthermore, foods high in calcium may create hypercalcemia, which will potentiate the possibility of digoxin toxicity. Cognitive Level: Applying; Client Need: Health Promotion and Maintenance; Nursing Process: Implementation

3 Answer: d Rationale: Hydralazine with isosorbide may cause hypotension with reflex tachycardia, resulting in dizziness and rapid heart rate. Options a, b, and c are incorrect. Hydralazine with isosorbide does not cause confusion, agitation, bleeding, or tingling of the extremities. If these occur, other causes should be investigated. Cognitive Level: Analyzing; Client Need: Physiological Integrity; Nursing Process: Evaluation

4 Answer: a Rationale: Beta-adrenergic blockers such as carvedilol (Coreg) must be started at 1/10 to 1/20 of a usual dose and gradually increased to a target dosage. Options b, c, and d are incorrect. Because lower dosages are required, a higher loading dose will not be given, and beta-adrenergic blockers are often combined with ACE inhibitors, although dosage will not be directly related to the ACE inhibitor. While caution is required if beta-adrenergic blockers are used to treat HF, they are an important drug group used to treat HF. Cognitive Level: Applying; Client Need: Physiological Integrity; Nursing Process: Implementation

5 Answer: a, b, d Rationale: Beta-adrenergic blockers require gradual increases in dosage amount approximately every 2 weeks to a target dosage. Significant improvement may not be noticed in early therapy and the client may feel worse during initiation of therapy. Overall, however, the therapy has been proven to reduce the number of HF-related hospitalizations and mortalities. Options c and e are incorrect. Beta-adrenergic blocker therapy may require alterations in dosage for other cardiac drugs but not all drugs will be affected. Lifestyle changes may be advisable in HF but are not necessarily directly related to beta-adrenergic blocker use. Cognitive Level: Applying; Client Need: Health Promotion and Maintenance; Nursing Process: Planning

Chapter 55

1 Answer: d Rationale: Procainamide (Procan) should be avoided in clients suffering from severe HF since this drug can worsen the condition. Options a, b, and c are incorrect. Ventricular tachycardia, paroxysmal atrial tachycardia, and atrial fibrillation are indications for the use of procainamide. Cognitive Level: Applying; Client Need: Physiological Integrity; Nursing Process: Implementation

2 Answer: c Rationale: Early signs of lidocaine toxicity include CNS effects such as paresthesias, drowsiness, confusion, anxiety, or tremors. Options a, b, and d are incorrect. Decreased platelet levels are not related to the administration of lidocaine (Xylocaine). Unless the client experiences hypotension, there is no need to routinely keep the client supine. Although coughing and deep breathing are effective nursing strategies to maintain pulmonary function, they are not pertinent for the administration of IV lidocaine. Cognitive Level: Applying; Client Need: Physiological Integrity; Nursing Process: Implementation

3 Answer: c Rationale: The therapeutic goal of verapamil (Isoptin) is to stabilize the dysrhythmia by slowing the conduction. While the atrial dysrhythmia may continue, the rate should return to a normal range (e.g., 60–100 in an adult). Options a, b, and d are incorrect. Verapamil may cause hypotension, but as an adverse rather than a therapeutic effect. It should not cause increases in potassium levels or reduction in urine output. Cognitive Level: Analyzing; Client Need: Physiological Integrity; Nursing Process: Evaluation

4 Answer: c Rationale: Beta blockers such as propranolol (Inderal) are negative inotropic drugs and reduce myocardial contractility. In clients with existing HF, this may result in less cardiac output and worsening of symptoms. Options a, b, and d are incorrect. Propranolol does not cause sodium retention and its adverse effects include hypotension rather than hypertension. It may cause bronchoconstriction because it is a nonselective beta-adrenergic antagonist (blocker), but this effect does not worsen HF. It warrants caution or is contraindicated in clients with COPD and other respiratory conditions. Cognitive Level: Analyzing; Client Need: Physiological Integrity; Nursing Process: Evaluation

5 Answer: c Rationale: An adverse effect associated with amiodarone (Cordarone) is photosensitivity. The client should be instructed to avoid direct sunlight, wear protective clothing, and use adequate sunscreen lotions of SPF 15 or higher.

Options a, b, and d are incorrect. Amiodarone is not known to cause immunosuppression or to interact with oral contraceptives. Increased bleeding tendencies are not an adverse effect of amiodarone. Cognitive Level: Applying; Client Need: Health Promotion and Maintenance; Nursing Process: Implementation

Chapter 56

1 Answer: a Rationale: An activated partial thromboplastin time (aPTT) is the appropriate laboratory value that should be monitored with heparin infusions. When the client is receiving this drug, the results should be 1.5 to 2 times that client's baseline, or 60 to 80 seconds. Options b, c, and d are incorrect. A prothrombin time or INR is used to monitor the effectiveness of warfarin (Coumadin). Platelets are not affected by anticoagulants and are therefore not used in the monitoring of these drugs. Cognitive Level: Analyzing; Client Need: Physiological Integrity; Nursing Process: Evaluation

2 Answer: a, b, c Rationale: The client should be taught proper injection technique, including the need to inject the heparin into the deep subcutaneous fat layer. A soft toothbrush should be used for oral hygiene. Puncture wounds or cuts will require longer than normal pressure held at the site to stop bleeding—15 minutes or longer. Options d and e are incorrect. Dental flossing should be avoided while the client is receiving anticoagulants. The flossing can cause gum irritation and excessive bleeding. Aspirin has antiplatelet effects and concurrent use may increase the risk for bleeding or hemorrhage. Cognitive Level: Applying; Client Need: Health Promotion and Maintenance; Nursing Process: Planning

3 Answer: c Rationale: Many drugs such as aspirin and ibuprofen (Motrin) have strong anticoagulant effects. When the client on warfarin takes these drugs, the increased risk for bleeding can be hazardous. Options a, b, and d are incorrect. Drugs such as aspirin and ibuprofen do not neutralize the effect of an anticoagulant. Anticoagulants do not influence the half-life of any drugs. The pain associated with arthritis is not worsened by the combination of these drugs. Cognitive Level: Applying; Client Need: Physiological Integrity; Nursing Process: Implementation

4 Answer: a Rationale: Clopidogrel (Plavix) is an antiplatelet drug used to prevent blood clots from forming inside arteries by inhibiting platelet aggregation. Options b, c, and d are incorrect. Heparin is an anticoagulant that blocks the formation of blood clots by activating antithrombin III. Warfarin is a vitamin K antagonist used to prevent the blood from clotting. The drug alteplase (Activase) is a tissue plasminogen activator that dissolves fibrin clots. Cognitive Level: Applying; Client Need: Physiological Integrity; Nursing Process: Implementation

5 Answer: a, c, d, e Rationale: Ginger, garlic, and green tea may all increase the risk for bleeding. Dabigatran (Pradaxa) may be used for DVT. The drug is contraindicated in clients with gastritis because of the increased risk for bleeding. Option b is incorrect. Vitamin B_{12} does not enhance the response of dabigatran. Cognitive Level: Applying; Client Need: Physiological Integrity; Nursing Process: Planning

Chapter 57

1 Answer: b Rationale: The client who receives epoetin alfa (Epogen, Eprex) has anemia. This reduction in RBCs produces cellular oxygen deficiency, which causes severe fatigue and weakness. Clients receiving this drug should be taught to take scheduled rest periods to avoid overexertion. Options a, c, and d are incorrect. Avoiding fresh fruits and vegetables or uncooked meat would be instructions more appropriate for an individual with neutropenia. Limiting exposure to direct sunlight and using sunscreen would be appropriate instructions for a client who is receiving a drug that causes photosensitivity, but epoetin alfa is not associated with this adverse effect. Clients with anemia are not necessarily thrombocytopenic and do not routinely need to avoid activities that may cause injury. Cognitive Level: Applying; Client Need: Health Promotion and Maintenance; Nursing Process: Planning

2 Answer: c Rationale: Filgrastim (Neupogen) increases WBC counts. The nurse would monitor for effectiveness by examining this laboratory value. Options a, b, and d are incorrect. Epoetin alfa is the drug that increases RBC count. Oprelvekin (Neumega) may be given to increase platelet levels. Reticulocytes are immature RBCs and mean cell volume is a measure of the volume of RBCs. Cognitive Level: Analyzing; Client Need: Physiological Integrity; Nursing Process: Evaluation

3 Answer: d Rationale: Oprelvekin does not affect iron levels and there would be no reason to instruct the client to increase dietary intake of it.

Options a, b, and c are incorrect. Oprelvekin is used to stimulate the production of platelets in clients who are at risk for severe thrombocytopenia. Oprelvekin may cause severe fluid retention that may lead to pulmonary edema, pericardial effusion, and ascites. Clients should monitor weight gain and report significant increases to the healthcare provider. Visual impairment, including blurred vision, papilledema, and optic neuropathy, may occur with oprelvekin, and vision changes should be reported. Cognitive Level: Analyzing; Client Need: Physiological Integrity; Nursing Process: Evaluation

4 Answer: a Rationale: Clients who regularly consume large amounts of alcohol often suffer from a nutritional deficit of vitamin B_{12}, which can manifest as abnormal neurological symptoms. Options b, c, and d are incorrect. Alcohol interferes with folate metabolism in the liver, but lack of folate does not cause destruction of vitamin B_{12}. Pernicious anemia is caused by a lack of intrinsic factor, a substance needed to absorb vitamin B_{12} from the GI tract, which may lead to anemia, not neutropenia. Vitamin B_{12} is a water-soluble vitamin and is not stored in the body. Cognitive Level: Applying; Client Need: Physiological Integrity; Nursing Process: Implementation

5 Answer: a, b, c Rationale: Ferrous preparations bind to many substances including food and other drugs. To ensure complete absorption of the drug, iron supplements should be taken 1 hour before or 2 hours after eating. Liquid iron preparations are often given to children. Such preparations should be given with a straw to prevent contact with the teeth, which can produce staining. After swallowing, the client should be instructed to brush the teeth or thoroughly rinse the mouth to prevent staining. The client should be informed that iron preparations can cause dark tarry-like or green-tinged stools and may cause constipation. When clients take iron preparations, increased fibre and water intake are measures to take to decrease constipation. Options d and e are incorrect. Vitamin C increases the absorption of iron preparations, not vitamin E. Caffeinated beverages inhibit the absorption of this drug. Cognitive Level: Applying; Client Need: Physiological Integrity; Nursing Process: Planning

Chapter 58

1 Answer: a Rationale: In a case of shock, dopamine is given to increase the blood pressure in order to maintain peripheral perfusion. Therefore, monitoring blood pressure gives an indication of its therapeutic effect. Options b, c, and d are incorrect. Evaluating the arterial blood gases does not indicate the action of dopamine. Although it is important to monitor the heart rate, since dopamine increases it, the primary indication in a case of shock is to maintain adequate blood pressure and ensure peripheral perfusion. Option d is not related to the mechanism of action of dopamine. Cognitive Level: Analyzing; Client Need: Physiological Integrity; Nursing Process: Implementation

2 Answer: a Rationale: Dobutamine (Dobutrex) is a beta$_1$-adrenergic agonist used to treat heart failure by increasing the cardiac output. Options b, c, and d are incorrect. Dobutamine increases blood pressure because it increases cardiac output. Although dobutamine can increase blood pressure, the primary indication in patients with heart failure is to increase cardiac input. Although dobutamine can increase heart rate due to its direct action on beta$_1$ receptors in the heart, the major indication for its administration is to increase cardiac output. Cognitive Level: Understanding; Client Need: Physiological Integrity; Nursing Process: Evaluation

3 Answer: a Rationale: At low doses (3 µg/kg/minute), dopamine selectively stimulates dopaminergic receptors, especially in the kidneys, leading to vasodilation and an increased blood flow through the kidneys. Therefore, dopamine increase renal perfusion and should enhance urine output. Options b, c, and d are incorrect. While dobutamine can increase renal perfusion by increasing cardiac output, dopamine has better selective and direct action effect on the kidneys. Norepinephrine (Levophed) can cause severe vasoconstriction of the renal arteries, thus decreasing urine output. Epinephrine can cause severe vasoconstriction of the renal arteries; therefore, it can potentially decrease renal perfusion and urine output. Cognitive Level: Applying; Client Need: Physiological Integrity; Nursing Process: Implementation

4 Answer: b Rationale: The kidneys are the major organ for digoxin (Lanoxin, Toloxin) elimination. Options a, c, and d are incorrect. Digoxin is eliminated from the body in the urine, not in feces, through breathing, or through the skin. Cognitive Level: Applying; Client Need: Physiological Integrity; Nursing Process: Implementation

5 Answer: b Rationale: Visual disturbances, such as seeing yellow spots, can be an early symptom of digoxin toxicity. Options a, c, and d are incorrect.

Decreased blood pressure, not elevated blood pressure, is associated with digoxin toxicity. Digoxin toxicity can cause nausea and decrease appetite, not increase it. Rash over the chest and back is not related to digoxin toxicity. Cognitive Level: Applying; Client Need: Physiological Integrity; Nursing Process: Implementation

Chapter 59

1 Answer: c   Rationale: Stage 1 suggests that the tumour is relatively small in size, has not invaded the surrounding tissue, and has not been detected in surrounding lymph nodes; thus it has been detected at an early stage. Options a, b, and d are incorrect. Stage 1 is the earliest staging and has the best prognosis. Cell differentiation refers to grading of cancer cells, not staging of cancer cells. Stage 1 suggests that the tumour is small and has not begun to invade surrounding tissue. Cognitive Level: Analyzing; Client Need: Physiological Integrity; Nursing Process: Evaluation

2 Answer: d, e   Rationale: Clients and family members should avoid receiving live virus vaccination or exposure to chickenpox. Varicella (chickenpox) vaccination is usually given to children between the age of 12 and 18 months and the client should not care for her granddaughter if immunization with live virus vaccines is planned. The client should also avoid crowds, especially in enclosed areas, to minimize the risk for infection. Options a, b, and c are incorrect. Attending a support group, maintaining normal activities when possible, and eating small, frequent meals with sufficient protein are routine care measures during chemotherapy. Cognitive Level: Analyzing; Client Need: Physiological Integrity; Nursing Process: Evaluation

3 Answer: a   Rationale: The use of multiple drugs affects different stages of the cancer cell's life cycle and attacks the various clones within the tumour via several mechanisms of action, thus increasing the percentage of cell kill. Combination chemotherapy also allows lower dosages of each individual agent, thus reducing toxicity and slowing the development of resistance. Options b, c, and d are incorrect. Staging describes the process of determining the extent of cancer in the body and where the cancer is located. Antineoplastic drugs may kill only a small portion of the tumour, leaving some clones unaffected and able to repopulate the tumour with resistant cells. Combination chemotherapy also allows lower dosages of each individual agent, thus reducing toxicity and slowing the development of resistance. Cognitive Level: Applying; Client Need: Physiological Integrity; Nursing Process: Evaluation

4 Answer: a   Rationale: Myelosuppression is the most common dose-limiting adverse effect of chemotherapy and the one that most often causes discontinuation or delays of chemotherapy. Options b, c, and d are incorrect. Although alopecia may be distressing for the client, its presence does not determine when the next round of chemotherapy can be administered. Mucositis is not a reason that subsequent rounds of chemotherapy should be delayed. Cachexia is the physical wasting with loss of weight and muscle mass caused by disease. Although it is considered, it is not the most common reason for delaying chemotherapy. Cognitive Level: Applying; Client Need: Physiological Integrity; Nursing Process: Planning

5 Answer: d   Rationale: Many antineoplastics are classified as vesicant agents that can cause serious tissue injury if they leak into the surrounding tissue from an artery or vein during an infusion or injection. The nurse should closely monitor the infusion site for swelling and pain. Options a, b, and c are incorrect. Vesicants do not necessarily cause nausea. It would be inappropriate for the nurse to monitor the client's intake of calcium-rich foods because this is not related to receiving a chemotherapy classified as a vesicant. Respiratory status is not related to the administration of a vesicant-type chemotherapy agent. Cognitive Level: Applying; Client Need: Physiological Integrity; Nursing Process: Implementation

Chapter 60

1 Answer: b   Rationale: The nadir indicates that myelosuppression has occurred and is indicated by decreased blood cell counts. WBC and ANC are sensitive indicators of the nadir. Options a, c, and d are incorrect. BUN, creatinine, ionized calcium, and serum albumin are not indicators of the nadir and myelosuppression. Cognitive Level: Analyzing; Client Need: Physiological Integrity; Nursing Process: Evaluation

2 Answer: a, c, d   Rationale: The main dose-limiting toxicity to occur with vincristine is neurotoxicity. Numbness of the hands and feet, constipation

related to decreased peristalsis, and diminished reflexes are all signs of neurotoxicity. Options b and e are incorrect. Cardiac and pulmonary toxicities are not associated with vincristine. Cognitive Level: Analyzing; Client Need: Physiological Integrity; Nursing Process: Evaluation

3 Answer: d   Rationale: Tamoxifen (Nolvadex) is associated with an increased risk for endometrial cancer and monitoring will be necessary to detect early changes that may indicate that this adverse effect has occurred. Options a, b, and c are incorrect. Paralytic ileus and pulmonary fibrosis are not associated with tamoxifen. Alopecia is a common adverse effect of many chemotherapy drugs but will not require long-term monitoring. Cognitive Level: Applying; Client Need: Physiological Integrity; Nursing Process: Implementation

4 Answer: c   Rationale: As with many chemotherapy drugs, doxorubicin (Adriamycin) is associated with mucositis. Daily mouth rinses will be prescribed to decrease the risk for opportunistic infections from yeast and mouth bacteria. Options a, b, and d are incorrect. Performing active or assisted range-of-motion is an important intervention associated with drugs that cause neurotoxicities. Controlling pain is associated with chemotherapy that may cause pain as an adverse effect. Maintaining bedrest is not related to the use of chemotherapy but may be required for other reasons. Cognitive Level: Applying; Client Need: Physiological Integrity; Nursing Process: Implementation

5 Answer: a   Rationale: NSAIDs may cause severe and fatal myelosuppression when taken concurrently with methotrexate. Options b, c, and d are incorrect. Antihistamines, laxatives, and cough suppressants may be used with methotrexate. However, the provider should be consulted if they are needed because symptoms associated with these drugs may indicate a more serious condition that requires additional treatment. Cognitive Level: Applying; Client Need: Physiological Integrity; Nursing Process: Implementation

Chapter 61

1 Answer: c   Rationale: Alendronate (Fosamax) may cause severe GI adverse effects. To decrease this risk, particularly for esophageal irritation, and to promote the absorption of the medication, alendronate should be taken with a full glass of water after rising in the morning. The client should not eat or drink anything or lie down for 30 minutes after administration. Options a, b, and d are incorrect. The medication should be taken before breakfast, not before lunch or at bedtime. The client should not lie down after taking alendronate for at least 30 minutes, preferably longer. Cognitive Level: Applying; Client Need: Health Promotion and Maintenance; Nursing Process: Evaluation

2 Answer: a   Rationale: Headache, dizziness, and blurred vision are all early symptoms of toxicity to methotrexate. Options b, c, and d are incorrect. Hematuria, jaundice, and ascites are not associated with the use of methotrexate. While stomatitis may occur, constipation would be unrelated to methotrexate. Cognitive Level: Analyzing; Client Need: Physiological Integrity; Nursing Process: Evaluation

3 Answer: b   Rationale: Colchicine prevents the migration of neutrophils (WBCs) into the area of inflammation caused by uric acid crystals, reducing further inflammation and relieving the symptoms of gout and gouty arthritis. Options a, c, and d are incorrect. Colchicine does not increase uric acid deposits in the synovial spaces of the joints, prevent accumulation of uric acid crystals in the joints, or increase renal excretion of uric acid crystals. Clients feel better from decreased inflammation secondary to fewer uric acid crystal deposits. Renal excretion of uric acid is not a mechanism of action of colchicine. Cognitive Level: Applying; Client Need: Physiological Integrity; Nursing Process: Implementation

4 Answer: a   Rationale: The client with osteomalacia has low serum calcium and low phosphate levels. An indicator that replacement therapy is achieving therapeutic benefits would be increasing serum calcium and phosphate levels. Options b, c, and d are incorrect. Increasing or decreasing actions of the serum calcium and phosphate levels are incorrectly stated. Cognitive Level: Analyzing; Client Need: Physiological Integrity; Nursing Process: Evaluation

5 Answer: a   Rationale: Vitamin D toxicity may occur in the client receiving calcitriol. Symptoms to assess include muscle weakness, fatigue, nausea, vomiting, and changes in the colour or amount of urine. Options b, c, and d are incorrect. Diarrhea, stomatitis, and photosensitivity are not symptoms that would be associated with the effects of vitamin D therapy. Bone pain and fever are symptoms of vitamin D deficiency. Cognitive Level: Analyzing; Client Need: Physiological Integrity; Nursing Process: Evaluation

Chapter 62

1 Answer: d   Rationale: Lice and nits can live in areas of the body other than the hair on the client's head. Options a, b, and c are incorrect. Permethrin (Nix) should not be applied after body lotions and should not be used on eyelashes or eyebrows. Lice can survive for up to 24 to 48 hours on inanimate objects. Cognitive Level: Applying; Client Need: Health Promotion and Maintenance; Nursing Process: Implementation

2 Answer: a   Rationale: Clients taking topical corticosteroids for the treatment of atopic dermatitis may expect to experience a degree of burning and stinging of the skin in the affected area. Options b, c, and d are incorrect. Localized pruritus and hives, a loss of hair in the application area, or a worsening of acne vulgaris are not symptoms that would be related specifically to the effects of therapy. Cognitive Level: Applying; Client Need: Physiological Integrity; Nursing Process: Assessment

3 Answer: a, b, c   Rationale: Benzoyl peroxide suppresses sebum production and has antimicrobial action against the bacteria that cause acne. It also has a keratolytic effect, drying and encouraging more rapid cell turnover in the outer layer of the epidermis. Options d and e are incorrect. Microdermal abrasion is not a primary mechanism of action of the drug and benzoyl peroxide does not have sunscreening activity. Cognitive Level: Applying; Client Need: Physiological Integrity; Nursing Process: Evaluation

4 Answer: c   Rationale: Tretinoin (Retin-A) may cause dryness, irritation, and erythema. Mild soaps, gentle cleansing, warm but not hot water, and gentle drying should be used while tretinoin therapy is used. Options a, b, and d are incorrect. Antiacne soaps often contain compounds that dry and desquamate the skin and may cause further irritation. Sunscreens with an SPF of 15 and coverings should be used while on tretinoin to avoid sunburn. Alternating tretinoin with benzoyl peroxide may cause excessive dryness and irritation and increase the risk for adverse effects. Cognitive Level: Applying; Client Need: Health Promotion and Maintenance; Nursing Process: Implementation

5 Answer: c   Rationale: A small test area should be used if benzocaine (Anbesol) has not been used before to assess for allergy. If no symptoms are noted within 30 to 60 minutes, it may be used on a wider area. Options a, b, and d are incorrect. Benzocaine should not be used on partial-thickness burns because of the risk for open blistered areas. The solution should not be warmed to avoid further heat and damage to the area of the burn. The burn should not be covered with plastic wrap to avoid heat trapping, potentially increasing the damage. Cognitive Level: Applying; Client Need: Health Promotion and Maintenance; Nursing Process: Implementation

Chapter 63

1 Answer: d   Rationale: Timolol (Timoptic) is a beta-adrenergic blocker. To prevent swallowing and systemic absorption, pressure is to be applied to the inner canthus of the eye for 1 minute after instilling the drop. Options a, b, and c are incorrect. No other eye drops or ointments should be used when taking timolol or other drops for glaucoma without the approval of the provider. Eye solutions for allergies may contain adrenergic drugs that may worsen glaucoma. Timolol is not contraindicated during seasonal allergies. It is not known to worsen seasonal allergies although it may cause bronchoconstriction in the sensitive individual or if swallowed and systemic effects occur. Cognitive Level: Applying; Client Need: Physiological Integrity; Nursing Process: Planning

2 Answer: a, b, d   Rationale: Latanoprost (Xalatan) may cause thickening and darkening of the eyelashes and upper eyelid and may cause darkening of the iris, especially noticeable in clients with light eye colours. Options c and e are incorrect. Latanoprost will not cause lightening of the iris or darkening of the sclera or a permanent bluish tint to the conjunctiva. Cognitive Level: Applying; Client Need: Physiological Integrity; Nursing Process: Implementation

3 Answer: Pilocarpine (Isopto Carpine) causes miosis, which stretches the trabecular meshwork, allowing greater outflow of aqueous humour and

decreasing the IOP. Cognitive Level: Applying; Client Need: Physiological Integrity; Nursing Process: Implementation

4 Answer: b, c, a, d   Rationale: The ear should be pulled gently upward and back and the drop instilled, allowing it to flow down the side of the canal. Dropping the solution directly on the tympanic membrane may cause dizziness or nausea. The area in front of the ear (the tragus) should be gently massaged. The client should remain in a side-lying position or with the treated ear uppermost for 5 minutes to allow complete absorption of the solution. If needed, a dry cotton ball may be placed in the outer ear area to prevent leakage of solution. Cognitive Level: Applying; Client Need: Health Promotion and Maintenance; Nursing Process: Implementation

5 Answer: d   Rationale: Increasing pain, particularly around the ear area, may indicate worsening infection or mastoiditis and should be immediately reported. Options a, b, and c are incorrect. Mild itching and irritation may occur, but severe itching or swelling should be reported. Gradually decreasing pain is a therapeutic effect as the infection clears. Dizziness may occur if the eardrop is instilled directly onto the tympanic membrane. Cognitive Level: Applying; Client Need: Physiological Integrity; Nursing Process: Planning

Chapter 64

1 Answer: a   Rationale: No antidote or specific treatment exists for radiation poisoning. Supportive therapy for the associated symptoms is the only treatment available. Options b, c, and d are incorrect. Ultraviolet light does not affect individuals who experience radiation poisoning. An individual with radiation toxicity is incapable of contaminating other individuals. No antiradiation medications exist. Cognitive Level: Applying; Client Need: Physiological Integrity; Nursing Process: Implementation

2 Answer: c   Rationale: Time is a critical factor in acute poisonings. The emergency should be called into 911 and the rescue squad should transport the child to the nearest healthcare facility immediately. Options a, b, and d are incorrect. Instructions for poisoning may have changed since the packaging was printed. Based on the information provided in the question, the nurse does not know what chemicals the child has ingested. Forced vomiting is contraindicated for most poisonings. Waiting for the child to develop seizures or shortness of breath is too late since the development of these symptoms most likely represents a toxic level of the poison. Cognitive Level: Applying; Client Need: Physiological Integrity; Nursing Process: Implementation

3 Answer: c   Rationale: Clients with decreased sensorium are at high risk for pulmonary aspiration. Activated charcoal should only be given to these clients if the airway is maintained with an endotracheal tube. Options a, b, and d are incorrect. Activated charcoal is not absorbed in the GI tract and therefore would not be contraindicated in clients with liver pathology. Activated charcoal is eliminated in the feces and therefore would not be contraindicated in clients with renal impairment. Anxiety and nervousness are not reasons to withhold the administration of activated charcoal. Cognitive Level: Applying; Client Need: Physiological Integrity; Nursing Process: Assessment

4 Answer: a   Rationale: Chelating agents capture the toxic metal through a bonding process. The kidneys remove both the chelator and the metal bound to it from the body. Options b, c, and d are incorrect. A chelator binds heavy metals but does not deactivate any chemical reactions. Chelation therapy is not involved in metabolism. Glomerular filtration is not affected by chelation therapy. Cognitive Level: Applying; Client Need: Physiological Integrity; Nursing Process: Assessment

5 Answer: b   Rationale: Edetate calcium disodium may produce renal damage that may be reduced by ensuring adequate diuresis before therapy begins. Options a, c, and d are incorrect. Bowel function is not a critical parameter to consider prior to giving this drug. Edetate calcium disodium administration is not based on visual acuity. Skin integrity is not a critical parameter to consider prior to giving edetate calcium disodium. Cognitive Level: Applying; Client Need: Physiological Integrity; Nursing Process: Assessment

Appendix B

Suggested Answers to Critical Thinking Questions in Chapter Scenarios

Chapter 1

1 Many people think that OTC drugs are harmless. Any drug can have dangerous properties if taken inappropriately, and adverse effects can vary from person to person. OTC drugs may produce toxic results if not used as directed. Also, the use of OTC drugs may prevent individuals from seeking health care when needed. OTC drugs should be used as a temporary measure for minor problems. Individuals who use OTC drugs for recurrent and persistent problems should see a healthcare provider.

2 Some advantages of OTC medications are (1) Time—These drugs are available when the client wants and needs them. They also do not require a visit to a healthcare provider. (2) Cost—In many cases, OTC drugs are reasonably priced. Many prescription medications are costly and may create financial hardship for individuals who have limited resources. (3) Easy administration—Most OTC medications are created so that the administration is fairly simple and does not require any advanced knowledge of human physiology. (4) Readily accessible—OTC medications are sold in a variety of places from grocery stores to vending machines.

The disadvantages of OTC drugs are (1) Improper use—Some individuals take OTC medications in improper amounts and frequencies. OTC medications should be used only as described in the directions. (2) Self-diagnosis—When clients diagnose themselves, the potential for misdiagnosis of serious and life-threatening illnesses occurs. Using OTC medications is not a substitute for physical examination and care by a healthcare provider when the health problem is persistent. (3) Delay in seeking appropriate health care—When health problems are persistent or intense in nature, individuals should seek medical care. Individuals with conditions such as chest pain, chronic cough, or abdominal pain who prolong seeking medical care by taking OTC medications may increase the risk for disability and mortality.

3 Gertrude can obtain correct information about OTC drugs by talking to a pharmacist or healthcare provider. Most pharmacists and healthcare providers will be happy to talk with individuals about possible drug-drug interactions, adverse effects, and contraindications for OTC medications.

Chapter 2

1 The therapeutic classification describes what the drug is treating. These drugs are often identified by the prefix *anti-*, such as antiseizure, anti-inflammatory, and antihypertensive. The pharmacological classification describes how the drug acts within the body. A drug's pharmacological classification is more specific than its therapeutic classification.

2 A barbiturate is the pharmacological classification for a major sedative. A macrolide is the pharmacological classification for a major type of antibiotic. Although the words *birth control pills* don't begin with *anti-*, this classification describes what the drug is being used for (anticonception). Laxatives, folic acid antagonists, and antianginals are examples of therapeutic classifications of these drug groups. Laxatives are substances that loosen stools and increase the frequency of bowel movements. Folic acid antagonists interfere with the action of folic acid in the body and produce symptoms of folic acid deficiency. Antianginals are drugs used in the treatment of angina pectoris, a symptom of ischemic heart disease.

3 A prototype is a member of a category that best represents the group as a whole. A prototype is representative of a group, classification, or category. By learning a prototype drug, students can apply their knowledge of the actions and adverse effects of other drugs in the same class.

4 The nurse is a critical member of the healthcare team and has tremendous responsibility for a client's drug therapy. The nurse not only administers medication but also closely monitors the client for the desired outcome and adverse effects. Nurses provide clients with essential drug-related education.

Chapter 3

1 Mr. Kessler's deteriorating condition will affect drug metabolism in several ways. First, the condition of diabetes is an alteration in metabolism and therefore the nurse must always consider that drug therapies given to a diabetic client may be influenced by this pathology. In addition, Mr. Kessler's condition is likely to be complicated by heart disease and hepatic malfunction. When perfusion to the liver is less than optimal, it can disturb the hepatic metabolism of drugs and nutrients. Another consideration regarding metabolism involves Mr. Kessler's lifestyle and ultimately his hepatic function with his habitual use of alcohol. Chronic alcohol abuse is destructive to the liver.

2 The client has pre-existing kidney disease and requires renal dialysis. Remember that pathological states such as kidney disease can increase the duration and intensity of drug action when drugs are not excreted as expected. The nurse must be particularly vigilant in monitoring the client for signs of drug toxicity.

3 Both IV and inhalation routes of administration allow the drug to be immediately absorbed and circulated to the target organs. Therapeutic responses to drugs given by these routes are frequently rapid in onset, as are toxic effects. Although these are the preferred routes of administration for this client, the nurse must not forget that the client has other factors that will affect both the metabolism and the excretion of these drugs.

4 When it is desirable to achieve the target plasma level rapidly, a loading dose (also known as a bolus dose) is necessary. This large dose of medication is used to achieve the therapeutic range quickly. Since the client is critically ill, there is no time to wait several days for the desired therapeutic action as the drug level gradually reaches a therapeutic range. He will be given maintenance doses to maintain a steady plasma level of the drug.

Chapter 4

1 Potency refers to the amount of drug (usually expressed in milligrams) needed to produce an effect. Efficacy refers to the potential maximum therapeutic response that a drug can produce.

2 In most cases, efficacy is more important than potency. When judging the relative merits of drugs for a client, other factors should be considered, such as adverse effects, potential toxicity, duration of effect (which determines the number of doses needed each day), and cost.

3 Comparison of drugs is not always a simple process. Generally, higher doses produce more intense adverse effects. However, when two drugs are compared, one cannot assume that the drug with the lower dose produces fewer adverse effects.

Chapter 5

1 The purpose of the question is to encourage use of communication skills required for the assessment phase of the nursing process. It is recommended that students consult a nursing diagnosis handbook to support their answers.

The nurse would need to determine that the client's poor eating habits are related to a non-therapeutic environment. One might be tempted to make this initial judgment due to the mother's appearance. Instead, the nurse should determine if other indicators of nonadherence exist; for example, unused medications, missed medical appointments, and other signs of progression of the disease process may suggest nonadherence. The nurse should also determine if the financial cost of therapy is affecting adherence. He or she should also evaluate the type and quality of diabetic education that the client and her mother received.

The nurse should use open-ended questions to encourage the client's mother to verbalize her concerns about her daughter's diagnosis and wellbeing. He or she should determine if the client's mother has unrealistic expectations about her daughter's ability to manage her disease process (i.e., diet, medications, and exercise).

2 Depending on what system of nursing diagnoses is being used, the instructor could modify this question. The question also assumes that the student has a basic understanding of the pathophysiology of diabetes and the use of the subcutaneous insulin pumps.

Typical client needs would include the following:

- Support in coping with a complex self-care treatment plan
- Sufficient knowledge of the condition and medication to manage the treatment plan safely and effectively
- Nutritional information
- Information to reduce risk for infection
- Body image disturbances
- Self-concept disturbances (the client is 13 years old)

3 Accountability is the act of being professionally responsible and accountable for one's behaviour. The client has a right to information about drug therapy, including the name of the drug and its purpose, action, and potential side effects. The nurse is the professional who is responsible for client and family education. Failing to teach can affect the client's ability to safely self-administer medications and may affect adherence to pharmacological therapy. The nurse should routinely integrate teaching as a critical part of drug administration.

Chapter 6

1 Once it has been established that Ms. David is indeed pregnant, the nurse's first concern is to talk with her about the pregnancy and any concerns she may have. She may be very happy, be ambivalent, or not wish to continue the pregnancy. If she plans to continue the pregnancy, the nurse should consider the antiseizure medications, or any other medications she may be taking, including the herbal products she has mentioned. A thorough drug history should be taken at this time, if it was not included in an earlier assessment. The healthcare provider will use the information to assist in determining whether the benefits of taking the drug outweigh the risks to the fetus and to consider alternative strategies.

2 At this early stage of pregnancy, the nurse would provide Ms. David with necessary prenatal teaching regarding caring for herself and her baby during pregnancy. She should be taught to avoid all medications and herbal supplements unless prescribed by the healthcare provider and to discuss any concerns regarding her current medications with her provider. Once the nurse has established a rapport with Ms. David, a discussion about the effects that smoking, illicit drugs, or alcohol would have on the developing baby should occur and, if necessary, strategies to help her avoid these substances should be developed. If Ms. David requires any medications during her pregnancy, the healthcare provider will make any adjustments necessary so that the effects on the developing baby are minimized as much as possible. The nurse would teach Ms. David that it is important that she continue with the prescribed drug regimen as directed by her provider to keep both her and the developing baby healthy.

3 The established pregnancy categories are A, B, C, D, and X, according to the risk assigned. Category A consists of drugs that have failed to demonstrate a risk to the fetus in the first trimester or subsequent trimesters. Category B indicates that there is not enough information to determine the risk the drug has to the fetus. Category C indicates that animal studies have revealed adverse fetal effects but that no controlled studies in women have been done, or that no studies in women or animals are available. With category D drugs, there is clear evidence of human fetal risk, but the benefits derived from use in pregnant women should be weighed against the risks. Category X includes drugs that have clearly demonstrated fetal abnormalities, and the risk of using the drug in a pregnant woman clearly outweighs any benefit except when the life of the mother is at risk.

4 Nicotine and smoking nearly double a woman's risk for having a low-birth-weight baby. Low birth weight can result from poor growth before birth, preterm delivery, or a combination of both.

Chapter 7

1 It is critical that nurses strive to understand the client's cultural beliefs about health and the attainment of wellness. The nurse must remain nonjudgmental about cultural practices that may seem unusual or different from their own. Open communication will establish a rapport with the client and will allow the nurse to better understand the client's beliefs and practices. If clients experience prejudicial criticism from healthcare providers, they are likely to be selective in what they are willing to talk about. When this communication breakdown occurs, an increased risk for potentially harmful drug interactions between conventional and non-conventional healthcare practices may occur.

2 Most clients are willing to share their cultural beliefs and practices. Often the nurse can engage the client in casual conversation, which may reveal valuable information. In addition, reference materials found in libraries and on the Internet may also provide further information about specific cultural beliefs or practices.

3 It is impossible for healthcare providers to totally understand all cultures. Cultural competence is an ongoing process for all healthcare providers. Providers who support holistic health will clearly understand and respect the cultural differences of their clients. The opportunity to work with a variety of clients from all cultures increases this competence, as does a willingness to be open to learning about other cultures.

Chapter 8

1 There are several steps a nurse can take to help Elizabeth minimize adverse drug effects. First, electronic health records allow a summary list of multiple medical diagnoses and medications to be created. For institutions that still use paper documents, including clinics that treat lower socioeconomic clients, nurses may consider proposing that a "medical summary page," which could include medical diagnoses, hospital admissions, and prescribed drug therapies, be added to the medical record.

Second, Elizabeth should be advised to carry a list of her medications at all times. When clients are on multiple medications, it is easy to forget one or two when asked about drug therapies. Listing the purpose and dosage of each medication would also be helpful for Elizabeth and the healthcare provider. The nurse could assist Elizabeth if she is unable to do this herself or encourage her family's participation. The nurse should review the list with Elizabeth each time she comes to the clinic.

Elizabeth should be taught to report any symptoms or feelings that "just don't seem right." In addition, the nurse should encourage her to become more assertive when healthcare providers suggest a new drug. Assure Elizabeth that it is acceptable to question providers about her health and her drug therapy.

Learning all of her drugs and their potential adverse effects may be overwhelming for Elizabeth. The nurse can assist her with ongoing education related to her drug therapy at each office visit or with follow-up telephone calls.

2 Several conditions make Elizabeth more susceptible to a drug reaction. The aging process makes the metabolism and excretion of drugs less predictable. In addition, as the number of drugs a client takes increases, so does the risk for adverse drug reactions. Alterations in pharmacokinetics will influence the reactions expected from a given drug. The speed of absorption (specifically, of enteral drugs) may enhance or reduce the effect of a drug. The distribution of a drug can be altered through modification in protein binding and may produce an unpredicted reaction. Elizabeth has also experienced a stroke, suggesting that vascular changes that could affect the distribution of her medications or hepatic and renal blood flow (thus metabolism and excretion) may be present.

3 Pharmacokinetics is the movement of drugs from the point of administration to the target cell. Drug reactions can affect each element of pharmacokinetics. Drug-drug reactions that increase or decrease gastric motility may influence absorption time for enteral drugs. Examples include laxatives and antacids. In addition, when drugs compete for binding ability to plasma proteins or change the pH of the plasma, drug distribution can be altered.

Any drug-generated modification in hepatic enzymes has the ability to cause a drug-drug interaction. Lastly, if a drug changes the rate of renal filtration, a drug interaction may occur.

4 An additive effect occurs when two drugs from a similar therapeutic class generate a combined response. A synergistic effect is the interaction of two or more drugs so that their combined effect is greater than the sum of their individual effects. An antagonistic effect is described as the interaction of two or more drugs that produces a reduced pharmacological response.

Chapter 9

1 Medication incidents continue to occur despite efforts to prevent errors and increase client safety. The nurse can prevent most errors by following the 10 rights and 3 checks of drug administration. However, errors can occur when the client takes drugs or herbal products that are not disclosed to the healthcare provider or when an incomplete drug history is obtained. Human errors include misspelling; ordering the wrong drug, dose, and route; entering a drug order in the wrong client's record; and incomplete or inaccurate assessment, such as failing to assess blood pressure before and at peak effect when a drug that lowers blood pressure is being administered. Other factors may include distractions, poor lighting, or other workplace factors.

2 When a client refuses to take a prescribed medication, the nurse should first attempt to discover the reason for the refusal. A common reason for refusal to take a prescribed medication is lack of knowledge regarding the intended effect of a drug, in which case specific information about the drug can be provided at the level the client is able to understand. Sometimes the refusal may be because of intolerable side effects, fear related to previous serious reaction, or allergy to a drug by the client or a family member.

3 IV route has the fastest onset of drug action because the drug is given directly into the bloodstream. With the oral, topical, IM, and SC routes, the drug must be absorbed through the capillary wall into the bloodstream and circulated to the site of action. Only oral drugs undergo the hepatic first-pass effect. The IM, SC, and IV routes require strict aseptic technique because the skin is penetrated.

Chapter 10

1 All members of the healthcare team are responsible for safe medication administration. The nurse failed to follow the standard routines designed to safeguard a client from medication errors. It is not usual for clients to forget some part of their health history, and healthcare professionals must always consider that client-generated information may not be totally accurate. The physician should have indicated the route of administration at the time the order was given, and the nurse failed to clarify the complete order before administration. Nurses should look up all unknown or unfamiliar drug orders in a pharmacology reference and consult the pharmacist if further clarification on administration techniques is needed. When any one part of the normal routine for drug administration is overlooked, medication errors can occur, sometimes with disastrous consequences.

2 First, the nurse must always be certain that the route of administration is clearly specified and never assume to know the route or dose of a medication. Second, when unfamiliar with a drug, the nurse should look it up in a drug handbook. Doing so would have alerted the nurse to a typical dose, possible adverse reactions to monitor, and the dilution required by the drug. It is virtually impossible to know everything about every drug. To ensure safety, the nurse must rely on quick resources, including consultation with the agency's pharmacist, to verify any unknowns. Lastly, reading a label or dilution guidelines is another step in the process of administration and must not be skipped.

3 The nurse can use multiple strategies to decrease the chances of medication error. The nurse always clarifies a medication order and never assumes dose or route. Drug references and the agency's pharmacist can be consulted. The nurse also learns to take into consideration environmental factors, such as noise or the stress of an emergency situation, and the impact they have on drug administration. In this scenario, the nurse may have been anxious about the stat order. Remember that *stat* means immediately but with all required procedures and caution included.

4 Healthcare facilities have taken multiple steps to reduce medication errors. In most hospitals, medications that require pre-mixing or pre-preparation are done within the hospital pharmacy. When this is not the case, the medication is packaged with the solution to be used for dilution. Regular updates and education by pharmacists, nurse educators, and unit staff can also assist all personnel involved in medication administration to prevent medication errors.

Chapter 11

1 Ginkgo is reported to have some major undesirable effects in individuals who are taking anticoagulants. This supplement will increase the time required for coagulation and therefore place the client at risk for bleeding. Although his vital signs do not indicate active bleeding, the bruises on his arms indicate that localized bleeding has occurred in the tissue.

2 Larry should stop taking the ginkgo immediately. Further doses of this supplement will exacerbate his potential for bleeding. Furthermore, the prescriber may inform the client to temporarily stop taking the anticoagulant until the risk for hemorrhage subsides. Larry should also be informed not to take any OTC medications that will increase his risk for bleeding. These OTC medications include aspirin and NSAIDs, such as ibuprofen (Motrin, Advil).

3 Many complementary and alternative therapies, if used correctly, are considered safe products and are gaining popularity. However, there are some risks involved in taking these preparations. Clients should be told that dietary supplements do not require testing prior to marketing and that safety does not need to be demonstrated by the manufacturer. Although dietary supplement labels must state that the product is not intended to diagnose, treat, cure, or prevent any disease, it is acceptable for the manufacturer to use statements such as "helps to promote a healthy immune system."

4 Larry's forgetfulness should not be minimized. Several abnormalities, including electrolyte disturbances, lack of mental stimulation, diet, and brain pathologies such as a microemboli from the episode of atrial fibrillation, can contribute to changes in a client's mental status. Larry should receive a diagnostic evaluation to rule out physiological reasons for his forgetfulness. There are also some psychosocial conditions that can influence a client's cognitive ability. The nurse should assess the client for sources of stress or anxiety. Appropriate referral is critical to assist the client with this problem.

Chapter 13

1 The nurse should inform the client to take the medication 1 hour before or 2 hours after meals to avoid nausea and vomiting. Dizziness, lightheadedness, or fainting may occur with bethanechol (Duvoid), especially when rising from a lying or sitting position. Clients who are receiving this medication should be instructed not to drive or engage in activities that require alertness until the effects of this drug have been determined and should be cautious in low-light conditions. The nurse would also want to explore Hilda's home situation and determine whether a caregiver is available to assist her and any home modifications (e.g., safety hazards that may cause tripping or falls) should be made. Some minor adverse effects of bethanechol include belching, stomach rumbling and mild cramps, salivation, diarrhea, and bladder urgency. All are attributable to the stimulation of the parasympathetic system. However, if the client experiences difficulty breathing, chest tightness, or pain, she should immediately contact her healthcare provider.

2 The nurse can help the client by providing these tips to help her remember to take her medication. The nurse might suggest the following:

- Place your medication next to something you use frequently or in plain sight.
- Post reminder notes on the refrigerator or the bathroom mirror.
- Ask a friend or a relative to remind you to take your medication.
- Take the medication at the same time every day.
- Set an alarm clock or watch to remind you when it is time to take the medication.
- Keep a medication diary or checklist so that you know when you have taken your pills each day.
- Carry your medication in your purse or pocket if you leave your house.
- If you accidentally miss a dose, take the missed dose as soon as you remember it. However, if it is almost time for the next dose, skip the missed dose and continue your regular dosing schedule. Do not take a double dose to make up for a missed one.

3 For this client, bethanechol is being prescribed to relieve urinary retention. The nurse should monitor the client's urinary system to determine the effectiveness of this drug therapy. If the therapy is not effective or the dose of the medication is insufficient, the client may complain of a sensation of being unable to empty the bladder even though she feels a strong urge to urinate. In addition, many people with acute urinary retention also feel pain in the lower abdomen (pelvis) or experience a small amount of urine leaking out of the bladder. If urinary retention is allowed to continue, the client may demonstrate symptoms of urinary tract infection, which include back pain, fever, and painful urination.

Chapter 14

1 Salbutamol (Ventolin) is a sympathomimetic drug that selectively stimulates beta$_2$-adrenergic receptors. The therapeutic responses associated with this drug are bronchodilation and vasodilation. Therefore, salbutamol (Ventolin) expands constricted bronchial tubes and enhances the passage of airflow into the lungs.

2 Salbutamol is used to relieve and prevent bronchospasms in clients with various obstructive diseases, such as asthma. The client is receiving the medication via the inhalation route because it is one of the fastest and most effective routes to administer respiratory medications. Administration of an adrenergic agonist by the parenteral or inhalation routes causes immediate relaxation of bronchial smooth muscle, resulting in bronchodilation.

3 Alexis is demonstrating typical adverse effects associated with the administration of an adrenergic agonist. These adverse effects include CNS stimulation, such as tremor, anxiety, and irritability. Tachycardia is another classic adverse effect related to this classification of medications.

Chapter 16

1 Seraphina and Joe have made plans for their retirement, and these plans are probably going to have to be changed or postponed. They may have financial concerns now. Raising teenagers is costly, and it will be difficult if their income is limited to Old Age Security and pensions. Seraphina feels resentful toward her grandchildren and also feels guilty for being resentful because she recognizes that they did not cause the situation.

2 The healthcare provider may order antianxiety medications, such as alprazolam (Xanax), buspirone (BuSpar), diazepam (Valium), or lorazepam (Ativan). All of these are administered PO. She may also be prescribed a medication such as zolpidem (Sublinox), which is used for short-term treatment of insomnia, while receiving psychotherapy for assistance in resolving her current difficulties.

3 Herbal remedies used by persons of the Latino culture influence the effects of traditional Western medicine. Herbs that are commonly used include kava, which promotes muscle relaxation and sleep and acts as an antidepressant. It may be used in combination with St. John's wort and valerian to promote relaxation. St. John's wort is used for mild depression. It is not effective for moderate to severe depression. If taken with a prescription antidepressant, St. John's wort may increase the risk for suicide. Valerian is a mild sedative and induces sleep. Its effects are similar to those of the benzodiazepines. Special care must be taken when combining herbs with prescription medications. They can enhance or decrease the actions of the medications. Seraphina must reveal to her healthcare provider all herbs she is taking so that the interactions between them and her ordered medications can be determined and further client teaching can be performed.

Chapter 17

1 The priority is for Jane to receive a complete physical and mental assessment. Any physical cause for the changes in Jane's behaviour must be ruled out. After this has been done, a mental status exam must be performed, with an emphasis on suicidal ideation.

2 Antidepressants are drugs used to enhance, elevate, or stabilize mood and are often beneficial in treating depression. Most antidepressants act by helping to restore normal neurotransmitter balances of primarily norepinephrine, serotonin, and to a lesser degree, dopamine.

3 To determine if antidepressants are achieving a therapeutic effect, the nurse can monitor the patient's interest in personal appearance and the performance of normal activities of daily living. In Jane's case, the clues that clearly demonstrate that her depression is improving will include a renewed interest in her personal appearance and in her children and their activities, a return to her normal day-to-day activities, and resumption of contact with friends and social activities.

Chapter 18

1 ADHD is characterized by inattention and hyperactivity. It is four times more common for males to present with inattention and inappropriate behaviour than it is for females. A child who is diagnosed with ADHD has difficulty completing tasks, is frequently loud, and interrupts others. Females with ADHD show less aggression but suffer from greater anxiety and mood swings. Jonathon is exhibiting the symptoms of ADHD and may be experiencing more difficulty now that he is in grade 2 and has more homework.

2 Amphetamine and dextroamphetamine (Dexedrine) may increase Jonathon's attention and alertness and assist him with his schoolwork by increasing his ability to focus on his class activities and lessons.

3 Jonathon and his parents should be taught that the drug should be taken in the morning to avoid nighttime insomnia. Because the drug causes anorexia, Jonathon should eat an adequate breakfast before the drug is taken. If anorexia at lunch is a problem, high-calorie, nutrient-dense foods can be packed in his lunch sack and an afternoon snack can be provided when he arrives home. Weekly weights should be taken and a record kept to show the healthcare provider to ensure that adequate growth is continuing. Insomnia, heart palpitations, excessive anxiety, or nervousness should be reported to the healthcare provider. The drug should be kept secured in the home, and if it is to be taken at school, the school's protocols for dosages and labelling should be followed.

Chapter 19

1 Many persons with schizophrenia feel normal when taking their medications as prescribed. These clients may come to believe that they no longer need the medications. George was functioning as any adult does—he went to work, he provided for his family, and he cared for his wife. Because he views all of these activities as "normal," he convinced himself he no longer has schizophrenia and stopped taking his medications.

2 There are many clues, probably subtle at first, then becoming more obvious. George exhibited a decline in personal hygiene and appearance and then quit his job without reason.

3 Sheri can assist George by working with him to develop a schedule for taking his medications and helping him to keep track on a calendar. Many psychiatric clients do not want anyone else to manage, or even assist them in managing, their medication regimen. Having Sheri help George in a matter-of-fact way that demonstrates interest in his health may decrease George's resistance. She may need to count his remaining medications to ensure that he is taking it as prescribed. She can intervene at the first sign of negative symptoms (decline in personal hygiene, decreased interest in usual activities, delusions, etc.). Other family members can tell Sheri if they notice anything unusual in George's behaviour or thought patterns. Sheri is the appropriate person to tell, because George will not want to admit that he has stopped taking his medication as ordered, or will not recognize that his behaviours or thoughts are abnormal.

Chapter 20

1 A complete physical examination is imperative, as is laboratory work to determine any electrolyte disturbances, diabetes, or other condition that may be present. A complete personal history, as well as a family history, to determine if any other close family members may have or have had AD is necessary. In addition, the assessment should include cognitive rating scale measurements and assessment of individual and family coping skills.

2 The healthcare provider will probably recommend that Mary begin taking one of the medications used to treat early AD, such as donepezil (Aricept). It will be recommended that she not be allowed to drive any longer. Other measures to ensure her safety and the safety of others should be taken, including making sure that she does not leave home alone, leave pots cooking on the stove, or leave water running in the sink or tub. A bedside commode may assist Mary with toileting if she has confusion or difficulty walking. Furniture, clothing, other belongings, and routines at home, including where items are stored and which people come into the home, must be kept as much the same as possible. This will assist Mary in maintaining some semblance of control over her life for as long as possible. As her disease progresses she will not be able to process new information, but she should be able to remember old information for a time.

3 Donepezil may cause some common adverse effects: headache, fatigue, insomnia, nausea, vomiting, diarrhea, anorexia, and abdominal pains. Other adverse effects include vertigo, depression, irritability, syncope, hypertension (remember that Mary has mild hypertension and takes an antihypertensive), dehydration, incontinence, and blurred vision. Robert will have to be alert for anorexia and encourage Mary to eat if she loses weight. If she is unable to sleep, she may begin to wander, so Robert may have to install better locks on the doors. She is already depressed at her diagnosis, so if the medication causes increased depression, suicidal ideation may appear. The family needs to be made aware that these agents do not stop progression of the disease, rather they delay progression (since there is no cure). Also, they should know that if the agent is to be stopped, they might not get back the cognitive gain they have received (cannot turn back time, rather slow progression of disease).

Chapter 21

1 Even with multiple medications, Jorge may continue to experience seizure activity. Jorge's family should be told that their primary concern is to protect him from injury. It is important for Jorge's mother to look closely at the home setting for potential hazards.

Here are just a few considerations:

- Pad sharp corners.
- Do not leave the client unattended in a bathtub or swimming pool.
- Avoid climbing activities high off the ground (rock or rope climbing).
- Avoid sleeping in the top bunk.
- Place screen guards around fireplaces.
- Wear a helmet and other protective gear when bicycling.
- Wear a medical alert bracelet (in case a seizure occurs when the mother is not around).

2 Jorge's mother should be instructed on the action, adverse effects, administration guidelines, and nursing implications regarding carbamazepine (Tegretol) and phenytoin (Dilantin). It is important that she understand that a medication dose should not be missed, and if it is, to administer it immediately. Instruct her that missing doses of antiepileptic medications could result in status epilepticus. Instruct her to keep using the same brand of phenytoin. Neither of the medications should be stopped abruptly.

Chapter 22

1 The back pain experienced by Andrew is a result of excessive use and local injury to the lower back at the lumbosacral region. Other possible causes of muscle spasm include hypocalcemia, debilitating neurological disorders, seizure disorders, and overmedication with antipsychotic agents. Muscle spasms are involuntary contractions of a muscle group or group of muscles. The muscles become tight with a fixed pattern of resistance, which results in diminished function.

2 Cyclobenzaprine (Flexeril) is used to relieve muscle spasms associated with acute and painful musculoskeletal disorders. It has been prescribed to relax the muscles of the lumbosacral region. It has the ability to promote skeletal muscle relaxation and thus decrease muscle spasms.

3 Cyclobenzaprine produces muscle relaxation and CNS depression. Andrew should be instructed to protect himself from injury, not engage in the operation of machinery while taking the medication, and not consume alcoholic beverages or mood-altering drugs. He should also be warned against taking OTC medications. He should be instructed on all adverse effects and advised to notify the prescriber if therapeutic effects do not occur within 2 to 3 weeks. Due to anticholinergic effects the client should be instructed to notify the provider for any difficulties in urination and to sip water or ice chips to relieve dry mouth.

Chapter 23

1 Given the complexity of Mr. Smith's situation, the best solution would be referral to the hospital pain management team (if one exists). In most instances, baseline opioid analgesics would be continued and acute surgical pain management would be superimposed on that baseline. The nurse caring for Mr. Smith after surgery should consider several interventions related to pain management. His age puts him at higher risk for hypotension, respiratory depression, and increased incidence of adverse CNS effects. The nurse would monitor for these problems and should consider supplemental interventions such as frequent repositioning, relaxation techniques, and distraction.

2 Depending on the type of documentation used in the agency, the nursing plan of care should include Acute and Chronic Pain as his first nursing diagnoses, with a brief note about his chronic pain history. An alert might be placed on the physical chart if electronic medical records are not used. Pain management should be included in all shift reporting, and if possible, the same nurses should be assigned to his care.

3 Hypotension, with unsafe ambulation, and constipation are the most likely adverse effects that Mr. Smith will experience from all opioids (very important to have a scheduled bowel protocol in place). In addition to monitoring vital signs, including respiratory rate and blood pressure, position changes should be made gradually and assisted ambulation would be necessary. A high-fibre diet would be started, with stool softeners and laxative as needed. Mr. Smith should walk three to four times a day for increasing distances. In addition, nausea would need to be assessed and managed if it occurs.

Chapter 24

1 Balanced anesthesia is the use of a combination of medications to produce general anesthesia. Balanced anesthetics provide for a rapid and smooth induction (beginning of anesthesia). The agents administered include neuromuscular blocking agents, short-acting barbiturates, opioids, and nitrous oxide. The purpose of the combination of these medications is to provide muscle relaxation and analgesia along with sedation and loss of sensation.

2 The main actions of nitrous oxide are analgesia and reduction in anxiety. Nitrous oxide suppresses the pain mechanism of the CNS. This agent has a low potency and does not produce loss of consciousness or profound skeletal muscle relaxation. Since nitrous oxide does not induce stage 3 surgical anesthesia it is commonly combined with other surgical anesthetic agents.

3 The client should be educated on the action and effect of balanced anesthesia and the agent to be used to induce and maintain anesthesia. Propofol (Diprivan) is administered to induce and maintain balanced anesthesia. The client will continue to receive the medication throughout the procedure, which will prevent her from awakening during surgery. The client should also be aware that the medication may cause shivering when she awakens. Inform her that she will be provided with warm blankets to ensure her comfort.

Chapter 25

1 J.C.'s substance use is classified as both a physical and a psychological dependence. Remember she said that when she is unable to acquire drugs, she feels sick with symptoms of trembling and diaphoresis. This would describe a physiological state that results in a withdrawal syndrome when addictive drug use is stopped. Her comments about needing drugs just to "get through the night" is characteristic of psychological dependence that is defined as a condition in which a person feels that he or she needs drugs in order to cope with problems.

2 Here are the drugs that J.C. reports using, along with the associated withdrawal symptoms:

Drug Reported	Withdrawal Symptoms
Alcohol	Tremors, anxiety, confusion, seizures
Heroin	Diaphoresis, agitation, dilated pupils (mydriasis), goose bumps (piloerection), tremors
Crack	Agitation, depression, intense craving for the drug, extreme fatigue
Valium	Rapid heartbeat, tremor, insomnia, sweating, irritability, anxiety, blurred vision, decreased concentration

It is critical that the nurse realize that clients with substance use disorder problems frequently underreport drug use and may not report all substances used or the amount of the drugs consumed.

3 Drug use can trigger serious complications during pregnancy and possibly damage the fetus. Heavy consumption of certain drugs such as alcohol, tobacco, heroin, and tranquilizers taken during pregnancy can lead to premature birth, low birth weight, and increased risk for stillbirth. It is usually advisable for a pregnant woman to stop using drugs during pregnancy. However, this is not always the case when heroin use is present, as sudden discontinuation of heroin during pregnancy can be dangerous to the fetus.

Some healthcare professionals believe that it is safer for the mother to continue using the drug until the baby is born.

4 Essential to dealing with a pregnant client with a substance use disorder is the development of a nonjudgmental attitude. The effect of the substance use on the unborn child evokes strong emotions with most people, including nurses. However, little can be accomplished if a client feels that the healthcare provider views him or her as evil or unworthy of health care. Obviously, J.C. needs a stabilizing force in her life. The nurse has a tremendous opportunity to assist this client to seek a healthy lifestyle that will be a positive influence for both mother and baby. A nurse who is open and willing to accept the client will have a greater chance of referring this client to critical resources.

5 J.C.'s life has all of the variables that trap her in a web of addiction. The drug factor in this case may include the quickness of the substance to relieve her psychological pain. The user factors involve her risk-taking behaviour (prostitution) and prior history of drug abuse. J.C.'s limited opportunities for education and for the development of healthy social norms put her at risk. Her peer influences were most likely individuals in similar living situations.

Chapter 27

1 Raj and his parents will need instruction on when, where, and how to give the injections, how to store the medication, and any signs or symptoms of adverse effects that should be reported. The medication will be given subcutaneously in the abdomen, anterior thigh, or buttocks, and the injection sites should be rotated with each injection.

Giving the injection in the evenings will help to mimic the body's own hormone rhythms. Raj may prefer to learn to give his own injections, and he should be included when teaching his parents. Teach the parents about the need for follow-up assessments of height, weight, bone age, and laboratory testing. Provide information on potential adverse effects, especially those that must be reported to the healthcare provider immediately, such as sudden weight gain, swelling, flank pain, or severe bone and joint pain.

2 It is important and appropriate to discuss with the parents their ability to afford this medication. Therapy will be expensive if medicine is not covered by insurance programs. Therapy is also long term, usually continuing for several years until closure of the epiphyseal plates and attainment of final adult height. In some cases, you might consider referring the family to a social worker who might be able to find other sources of funding, if necessary. It is also important to discuss the realistic effects of therapy: that the increases in height are often modest but still important to the overall well being of the client.

3 The adverse effects to discuss are hyperglycemia and insulin resistance, with the possibility of developing diabetes mellitus, hypothyroidism, and calcium-based kidney stones. Routine testing will monitor for these conditions. Other possible adverse effects are edema, headache, and hypertension. These usually resolve with continued treatment and dose adjustments. Other adverse effects are joint and bone pain, local pain at the injection site, and the rare possibility of developing antibodies to growth hormone.

Chapter 28

1 Oral antidiabetic drugs are often used in combination to better treat type 2 diabetes. Glyburide (Diabeta) stimulates the release of insulin and increases the sensitivity to insulin in peripheral tissues. Metformin (Glucophage) reduces blood glucose by reducing glycogenolysis and decreasing the intestinal reabsorption of glucose. Together they work by different mechanisms to lower blood glucose levels.

2 Ellen should take the drugs before her morning meal. If the metformin prescription is not an extended-release formulation, additional doses throughout the day, around mealtimes, may be required. Hypoglycemia is a possible adverse effect, particularly from the glyburide, and Ellen should be taught how to monitor her fingerstick blood glucose levels. Appropriate care when ill or if Ellen changes her exercise routine should also be discussed.

3 Clients with type 2 diabetes produce their own insulin but it is either insufficient to meet their body's needs or their body has developed a resistance to it. Providing oral drug therapy that assists Ellen's own insulin to work more efficiently is a goal of therapy for type 2 diabetes. While insulin may not be needed at this time, it may be needed in the future, particularly if illness or stress cause blood glucose levels to increase. Note that you *could* always start with insulin in a type 2 diabetic; however, oral therapy is always preferred to start with at the beginning.

4 Occasional small amounts of alcohol may be allowed, but Ellen should discuss this with her healthcare provider. Alcohol consumption increases the risk for hyperglycemia and hypoglycemia and it is known to produce disulfiram (Antabuse)-type reactions in clients who are taking glyburide. If the provider allows Ellen to drink an occasional glass of wine, she should be taught to consume the wine along with meals so that the food balances the alcohol consumption. She should also be taught the symptoms of a disulfiram-type reaction and to notify the provider if they occur.

Chapter 29

1 It is anticipated that Helen's laboratory reports may return with abnormal values consistent with hypothyroidism. Other possible testing the healthcare provider may order includes an ultrasound of her thyroid gland, a radioactive iodine uptake test, or a test for antithyroid antibodies.

2 Helen should take the levothyroxine (Synthroid, Eltroxin) in the morning on awakening and as close to the same time each morning as possible to mimic the body's own natural thyroid hormone rhythm. If she forgets to take a dose, she should take it as soon as she remembers it. If she is unable to take the drug for more than 1 day because of illness, she should contact the provider for further instructions. She also needs to be made aware that levothyroxine should be taken on an empty stomach and that she should not consume any food for at least an hour after taking it (as levothyroxine has many drug interactions as it binds to other molecules and becomes less effective).

3 Because the symptoms of hypothyroidism occur after the thyroid is no longer producing enough thyroid hormone, lifelong replacement therapy will be required.

4 Because replacing a hormone exogenously does not precisely mimic the body's own hormone levels, there may be times when Helen experiences symptoms of hyperthyroidism or the return of symptoms similar to the ones she experienced from hypothyroidism. Symptoms similar to what she experienced before do not need to be reported to the provider immediately unless they are significantly worse than previously experienced. If they continue for longer than a few days, she should inform the provider because a dosage adjustment may be required. Symptoms she should report to her provider immediately are those similar to hyperthyroidism. These include rapid heart rate, palpitations, headache, shortness of breath, anxiety, and intolerance to heat.

Chapter 30

1 Some questions that the nurse may ask Charlie to determine if any adverse effects are present are as follows: Have you experienced any sore throat, fever, or chills? (Immunosuppression) Have you noticed any cuts or scrapes that are not healing? (Immunosuppression) Are you experiencing any abdominal pain? (Peptic ulcer formation) Have you noticed any changes in your stool colour? (GI bleeding) Are you experiencing any hip, knee, or other pain? (Osteoporosis changes or fracture) Do you feel like your moods have changed lately, either positively or with irritability? (Behavioural changes) Have you noticed any changes in your vision? (Cataracts or open-angle glaucoma) Have you noticed any swelling or weight gain? (Edema or metabolic changes) Have you experienced any unusual or increasing muscle aches? (Myopathy)

2 As the nurse, you would want to teach Charlie that abrupt discontinuation of the medication may cause significant adverse effects. Withdrawal from corticosteroids, even from long-term inhaler use, may cause an exacerbation of disease symptoms. Depending on the frequency and length of time Charlie has used his inhaler, his adrenal glands may have slowed or stopped producing normal amounts of cortisol. If the medication is to be stopped, it should be done gradually under his healthcare provider's supervision.

3 Charlie is at risk for infection, especially since he is producing mucus along with the flare-up of his bronchitis, and he should avoid exposure to individuals who have active infections such as colds and influenza. He should increase his fluid intake to help reduce the thickness of his sputum and eat smaller, more frequent meals if dyspnea makes eating difficult. Adequate amounts of protein, along with carbohydrates and fats will maintain his health. Once Charlie returns to work, he should be cautious about work-related injuries to avoid skin infections or falls with a risk for fractures.

Chapter 31

1 Eileen is over 35 years of age and smokes cigarettes, both of which place her at greater risk for thromboembolic events related to hormone replacement therapy (HRT). The healthcare provider and Eileen will make the decision to place Eileen on HRT after discussing the therapy and considering other factors such as a previous history of thrombus or embolism, a personal and/or family history of cardiovascular disease, and her blood pressure and heart rate.

2 Eileen may be a candidate for HRT. Estrogen, progesterone, and testosterone decrease as a woman approaches menopause. She may also choose to take natural therapies such as black cohosh. Should Eileen choose to begin medication treatment, the aim would be to normalize the ratio between estrogen and progesterone. Testosterone is useful in elevating the woman's mood, sex drive, and energy. The overall goal is to restore balance between the hormones and to diminish the unpleasant symptoms of menopause. A likely drug is estrogen (Premarin).

3 Should this client choose to begin HRT, she will need to adjust her lifestyle. She should discontinue smoking, as smoking increases the risk for thromboembolic events. She should be particularly cautious to monitor for any unusual symptoms, such as headache, pain or warmth in her calf, or sudden chest pain, in the first year of drug therapy. She should reduce or completely discontinue her caffeine intake because estrogen and caffeine may lead to increased CNS stimulation, further accentuating her nervousness, anxiety, and insomnia. In addition, she should begin a regular exercise program that includes walking, which retards the chances for osteoporosis.

Chapter 32

1 Common contributing factors to the diagnosis of ED include recent divorce, a diagnosis of depression, job-related stress, use of antidepressants, and a history of hypertension.

2 A discussion with Mike is needed about the effects of tadalafil (Cialis). The combination of this drug with antidepressants and his antihypertensive, nifedipine, must be evaluated so as not to develop severe adverse effects, like severe hypertension. Instruct Mike on the correct administration of the drug and that its effects last for up to 36 hours. Encourage continued visits with the psychiatrist.

3 It is important to let Mike know about the differences between these drugs. Sildenafil (Viagra) has an onset of action that is relatively rapid, less than 1 hour, and its effects last for up to 4 hours. Tadalafil acts within 30 to 60 minutes and has a longer duration of action than sildenafil: up to 36 hours. The longer duration of tadalafil allows for more spontaneity of sexual activity. Contraindications include clients who take nitrates, and dosing can be prescribed every 72 hours. Tadalafil will produce less of a decrease in blood pressure than the other drugs in this class, making it safer for clients like Mike with hypertension who are already taking other medications for this condition. Sildenafil (including all other phosphodiesterase 5 inhibitors) is contraindicated in clients who are also taking nitrates, although Mike is not currently on a nitrate drug.

Chapter 34

1 Risk factors for the development of PUD include infection with *H. pylori*, use of NSAIDs (including ibuprofen or aspirin), smoking tobacco, alcohol use, serious illness, and genetic factors.

2 Antibiotics are used to eradicate *H. pylori*. Although Hugh is allergic to penicillin, other combinations of drugs to eradicate *H. pylori* are available; these may include combinations of the following: clarithromycin (Biaxin), tetracycline, metronidazole (Flagyl), and bismuth compounds. A proton pump inhibitor, which may further decrease bacterial load and suppress acid, also may be prescribed.

Client adherence is necessary to eradicate the organism. Clients must understand that they must complete the antibiotic regimen to fully treat the peptic ulcer and combat antibiotic resistance. They should be advised of adverse effects, including nausea, diarrhea, and headache.

3 In some clients with hypertension, the use of NSAIDs has been shown to worsen the effects of hypertension. The chief mechanism by which NSAIDs contribute to hypertension and decrease the effectiveness of antihypertensive drugs appears to be the inhibition of prostaglandin synthesis. This inhibition results in an increase in sodium reabsorption and water retention.

Chapter 35

1 Dicyclomine (Bentylol) is an antispasmodic that will relax smooth muscle and slow peristalsis. Loperamide (Imodium) is an antidiarrheal drug similar to diphenoxylate with atropine that slows peristalsis but without the analgesia or dependence effects. Both will slow peristalsis, reducing the abdominal cramping and diarrhea associated with IBS.

2 Dicyclomine and loperamide may cause drowsiness, dry mouth, and blurred vision. Kerry should take the drug at night before bed to ascertain if any adverse effects that might affect her classroom study or attendance occur. If dry mouth is a problem, Kerry could sip water during class, chew gum, or suck on hard candy. If her vision is affected, she may need to sit in the front of the classroom or return to Student Health Services to discuss possible options with the nurse practitioner.

3 Some clients experience relief of IBS symptoms from the use of fibre through diet or bulk-forming laxatives such as psyllium. For others, these remedies worsen the symptoms. During a weekend or break week, Kerry could try to introduce extra fibre into her diet and note the effects. Kerry should be taught to keep a diary to detect possible food triggers such as caffeine, wheat, or lactose. If stress seems to be a trigger, complementary and alternative therapies such as relaxation and biofeedback may be helpful.

Chapter 36

1 Diet drugs, both prescription and OTC, have had a rocky history. Early drugs were amphetamines or amphetamine-like substances with significant cardiovascular complications and addiction potential. More recently, the drugs fenfluramine and phentermine (Fen-Phen), phenylpropanolamine (PPA, Accutrim), and sibutramine (Meridia) have also been removed from the market because of cardiovascular adverse effects. Orlistat (Xenical) is a lipase inhibitor and has not been noted to have cardiovascular effects.

2 Orlistat is available in both non-prescription strength (the one Rosemary has seen in stores) and prescription strength. Before starting on orlistat, Rosemary should be screened for a past history of gallbladder disease, because the drug slows gallbladder contractions and can worsen cholestasis. Other medical causes for weight gain, such as hypothyroidism, should also be ruled out before Rosemary starts the drug. Orlistat is usually taken up to three times per day and should be taken with or within 1 hour of a meal containing fat. The drug may be skipped if the meal eaten does not contain some fats. Most of the adverse effects are GI in nature, including gas, oily and loose stools, urge to defecate and possible difficulty controlling bowel movements, stomach or rectal area pain, and headache. Rosemary may want to begin the drug on a Friday to determine what side effects she experiences over the weekend before returning to work.

1 Factors that may have contributed to Rosemary's weight gain include a sedentary lifestyle; a diet with high-calorie, low nutrient-dense foods; alcohol use; post-menopausal hormonal changes; and stress. Rosemary should be encouraged to make small changes in her daily eating and activity rather than large and sudden changes that may be more difficult to sustain. As the positive reinforcement from weight loss occurs, Rosemary may be able to make more substantial changes. She may find that keeping a refillable water bottle at her desk to increase her consumption of water throughout the day may be helpful, and the extra activity of refilling the bottle and restroom trips will increase her activity level. At her desk, Rosemary can take hourly "breaks" to stretch and move about, perhaps going up and down one flight of stairs each hour. Packing healthy snacks such as carrots, peppers, celery, unbuttered popcorn, or rice cakes the night before to take to work may help her to avoid high-calorie takeout lunches. Having packets of instant plain oatmeal or other cereals to microwave before work may cut down on trips to the local fast-food place. Using smaller plates and visualizing the plate with one-quarter protein source, one-quarter carbohydrates, and one-half vegetables and fruits may also offer a simple method to help her limit caloric intake at dinner. If Rosemary would like to continue her evening glass of wine, switching to a smaller glass will assist in limiting intake, as well as calories.

Chapter 37

1 Additional assessment data that would assist in determining Charlene's need for vitamin therapy would include her current diet, alcohol use, medication history, menstrual history (including especially heavy periods), recent weight loss plans or dieting, and the possibility of pregnancy.

2 Charlene should not take the prenatal vitamins without checking with her healthcare provider. Some vitamins degrade and become less effective if stored near heat or humidity. Prenatal vitamins also contain higher amounts of some vitamins and minerals that Charlene may not need. Depending on the possibility of pregnancy, a new prescription for prenatal vitamins may be required. Charlene should be increasing her folic acid content during pregnancy and also at any time where she is thinking of trying to conceive.

3 Charlene should be encouraged to seek dietary sources of vitamins and minerals with a wide variety of foods whenever possible. Depending on Charlene's history and assessment data gathered, a nutritional consult may be advisable. If she enjoys alcohol, she should be encouraged to limit her intake to a maximum of one glass per day. If symptoms continue, she should check with her provider about a more complete physical examination to detect other possible causes.

Chapter 38

1 Nathan's acute asthma attack began after competing in a swim meet in an indoor pool. Potential triggers for the attack include exercise, inhaled chlorine or other substances from the pool, and the possibility of moulds or other allergens in the indoor air. Nathan admits to missing his budesonide (Pulmicort) dose and is not sure about the monteleukast (Singular). The absence of these preventative medications may also have factored into his acute attack.

2 Nathan will be given oxygen therapy, and a nebulizer treatment with salbutamol (Ventolin) or other quick-acting beta agonist may also be used. If these fail to abort the attack, Nathan may require more aggressive therapy with epinephrine (Adrenalin) or isoproterenol (Isuprel), both of which are adrenergic drugs used to achieve rapid bronchodilation.

3 Because Nathan had forgotten to use his budesonide preventive inhaler and was not sure about taking the monteleukast, the nurse should explore the need for methods to remind Nathan to take his medications if this is a routine problem. Involving Nathan and his family in determining strategies will help to ensure adherence. A long-acting beta agonist inhaler such as salmeterol (Serevent) may be added to the routine to provide longer-term bronchodilation. Because allergens may have triggered the asthma attack, the provider may want to test Nathan for allergies. If allergy testing is ordered, the nurse will need to teach the rationale behind and methods used for the testing and check with the provider regarding any changes to Nathan's current drug regimen before testing is started. A short-term administration of oral corticosteroids may also be needed to reduce the inflammation from Nathan's recent attack. If changes to his other medications do not achieve the desired results, omalizumab (Xolair) may be added to Nathan's routine. Since omalizumab is given subcutaneously, it may be less desirable than inhalers or oral drugs and may be considered only if the other options have not had the desirable outcome.

Chapter 40

1 Normally, interferon is produced by body cells to fight infection and tumours. These substances are secreted by the lymphocytes and macrophages. It is thought that interferon, although unable to protect the infected cell, warns nearby cells of an impending infection. Interferons slow the spread of viral infections, enhance the activity of existing leukocytes, and increase phagocytosis and cytotoxic T-cell activity.

2 Common adverse effects of Intron A include flu-like symptoms, increased body temperature, feeling ill, fatigue, headache, muscle pain, convulsion, dizziness, hair thinning, and depression. The nurse can help the client to cope with these symptoms. Analgesics and antipyretics will help the client to feel better. Allowing the client to express feelings of depression may also be therapeutic and a referral to a mental health provider may be appropriate. The client should be informed that the adverse effects are short term and usually diminish as therapy progresses.

3 Carol will need to learn how to self-administer the injectable interferon. Many clients are fearful of self-administering injectable medications. The nurse will be instrumental in providing the client with information on injection techniques. In addition, Carol must be instructed to pace her daily activities to avoid overtiring herself. The nurse should assist this client to identify designated rest periods while performing activities of daily living. The client must also be encouraged to notify the healthcare provider promptly if symptoms of infection develop (sore throat, fever, vomiting, or diarrhea).

Chapter 41

1 It would be important to ask the parents the nature of Samantha's reaction to her first immunization. This should be compared to her office visit record, her immunization schedule, dosage, and the manufacturer's information to determine the cause of the reaction.

2 Minor adverse effects are frequently seen with the administration of vaccines and are effectively managed with good education. In addition, some minor adverse effects, such as inflammation, pain, and redness at the injection site, can be helped by pre-dosing acetaminophen (Tylenol) before the injections. Clarification of questions will also decrease the fear of the effects of the vaccine and increase adherence. Parental adherence to the recommended pediatric immunization schedule is very important for the health of the child.

3 It would be important to discuss the cause of the symptoms and the rationale for the administration of vaccines with Mr. and Mrs. Abbott. It would also be important to obtain information about their treatment of Samantha's symptoms and to provide them with education regarding the management of symptoms and potential adverse effects in both verbal and written forms.

Chapter 42

1 During acute inflammation, the inflammatory process begins as a response to the invasion of particulate matter, bacteria, or cell damage. Fever results from inflammatory chemical mediators or bacterial toxins.

2 Acetylsalicylic acid (ASA [Aspirin]) reduces fever by suppression of prostaglandins in the hypothalamus to lower the body temperature, and indirectly by causing peripheral vasodilation and sweating, helping to dissipate heat.

3 Joycee should not take the aspirin. The use of aspirin for fever in children and adolescents under the age of 19 has been associated with an increased risk of Reye's syndrome, a potentially fatal condition that causes increased pressure in the brain and liver and other organ damage. While it can occur at any age, it tends to occur most often in pediatric clients who have been administered aspirin in the presence of viral infections such as the flu or varicella.

4 Joycee should be told that aspirin is not an appropriate drug for her to take, considering that the symptoms suggest she may have the flu as well. If she cannot reach her parents about an acceptable alternative such as obtaining more ibuprofen, she should rest, drink additional fluids throughout the day, wear lightweight clothing but not so that she feels chilled, and not go to school today. To limit the spread of the flu or other viral infection she may have, she should stay home from school to avoid exposing her friends and classmates. If her fever continues or increases, or if she has additional symptoms, she should call her parents or contact you to assess her need for more definitive health care.

Chapter 44

1 Several factors may contribute to the client's wound infection. First, wet dressings are breeding sites for microorganisms since pathogens thrive in warm, moist, dark environments. Clients should be taught to change a wet dressing or return to the health facility for routine dressing changes. Second, older adult clients have an increased risk for infection due to age-related declines in immune function. Furthermore, proper wound healing is dependent on adequate nutrition. Many older adults fail to consume adequate amounts of nutrients, particularly proteins, needed for wound healing.

2 Laboratory studies for this client might include hematocrit, hemoglobin, and white blood cell counts. In addition, serum albumin levels may be evaluated. These laboratory values not only indicate the presence or degree of infection, but also may indicate the degree of nutritional impairment that contributes to poor wound healing. Most likely a specimen of the wound drainage will be sent to the laboratory for culture and sensitivity testing to determine the infecting organism as well as the specific antibiotic therapy that is indicated.

3 Ms. Dennison should be instructed about her prescribed medication, including potential adverse effects, when and how to take it in relation to meals and food, when to stop taking it, and indicators that would warrant seeking additional health care.

4 Cefazolin (Ancef) inhibits bacterial wall synthesis. It is bactericidal and exhibits a broad spectrum of bacterial coverage.

Chapter 45

1 *Candida albicans* can reproduce in large numbers in the mouth. Signs and symptoms include red- or white-coloured patches, slightly raised, on mucous membranes, tongue, mouth, and throat. Underneath the patches, the area is raw, may bleed, and can be painful. The throat may be sore and swallowing may be difficult. Taste may diminish.

2 Pathogenic fungi attack hosts with compromised immune systems. Conditions that can weaken the immune system include chemotherapy and corticosteroid use, which both apply to Sarah.

3 Sarah will most likely be given a topical suspension with an antifungal drug that will also be swallowed. She should be taught to remove her dentures before using the medication and to swish the solution around her mouth and then swallow. She should not drink water or rinse her mouth immediately after using the medication and should leave her dentures out overnight.

Chapter 46

1 Herpes simplex viruses are usually acquired through direct physical contact with an infected person. HSV may remain in a latent, asymptomatic, non-replicating state in sensory or autonomic nerve root ganglia for many years. Infection is lifelong. Immunosuppression, physical challenge, or emotional stress can promote active replication of the virus and reappearance of the characteristic lesions.

2 Antiviral agents are not routinely prescribed for prophylaxis due to the cost and potential adverse effects. Clients who experience particularly severe or recurrent episodes may receive low-dose antiviral agents.

3 Richard should apply the acyclovir (Zovirax) as soon as symptoms of a herpes infection appear. The medication should be applied to all sores every 3 hours (6 times a day) for 7 days, or as directed. Sometimes this medication causes burning, stinging, and redness. Cold sores are contagious at all stages and can spread to other people through kissing or sharing things that touch the lips, such as towels or utensils. Given the nature of his part-time job at a restaurant, Richard should use disposable gloves when applying the medication to avoid spreading the infection. Lastly, a healthy lifestyle may reduce the recurrence of cold sores. This would include a balanced diet, exercise, restful sleep, and managing emotional stress. Richard's university may have stress management and other support courses and services available that may be helpful.

Chapter 47

1 The primary concern with this hospitalization is the treatment of the secondary infection. Ryan will most likely be placed on antibiotics and antifungal medication first. Rarely is antiretroviral medication initiated until the presenting infection is treated and under control. The optimal time to start antiretroviral therapy depends on many factors, including the presentation of HIV symptoms, the viral load and CD4 cell counts, and the client's ability to accept the HIV diagnosis and willingness to comply with the therapy.

2 HIV infections occur when individuals are exposed to contaminated body fluids such as blood or semen. After the virus enters the body, it uses the host's own immune cells to replicate. Ryan's white blood cell count is diminished and may indicate his body's attempt to fight off an existing infection as well as the effect of the HIV virus. His HIV viral load is high, indicating that he has an active HIV infection, but his CD4 count (which counts the type of cell that the HIV virus uses to replicate) is still within an acceptable level. HIV is the infection with the human immunodeficiency virus, and AIDS is the very last stage of an overwhelming HIV infection that occurs as the host's immune system can no longer function. As diagnosed by his provider, Ryan has an HIV infection but does not currently have AIDS.

3 The antiretroviral drugs used to treat HIV infection will be required long term and require the client to be consistent with the treatment regimen to keep the infection from increasing or from being transmitted to others. There are many adverse effects of the drugs. The nurse and healthcare provider will provide specific instructions, ideally verbally and in written form, on administration needs, adverse effects, and when to notify the provider. As the nurse is discussing each medication, it should be kept in mind that a new diagnosis of HIV infection may be difficult for or devastating to the client. At this point in time, teaching may need to be brief and repeated several times, with written materials and follow-up teaching provided on subsequent office visits to ensure that the information is processed by Ryan.

Chapter 49

1 The etiology of hyperlipidemia may be inherited or acquired. Diets high in saturated fats, lack of exercise, smoking, and excessive alcohol intake may contribute significantly to hyperlipidemia and resulting cardiovascular diseases. However, genetics determines one's ability to metabolize lipids and contributes to high lipid levels in a substantial number of clients. For most clients, dyslipidemias are the result of a combination of genetic and environmental (lifestyle) factors.

2 The client should be taught the following health concepts related to lowering her LDL level:

- Maintain weight at an optimal level.
- Implement a medically supervised exercise plan.
- Reduce dietary saturated fats and cholesterol.
- Increase soluble fibre in the diet.
- Eliminate tobacco use.
- Eliminate alcohol use or consume no more than one 120-mL (4-oz) glass per day (for women; no more than two glasses per day for men).
- Monitor blood lipid levels regularly, as recommended by the physician.

3 Back pain, asthenia, hypersensitivity reaction, myalgia, headache, abdominal pain, constipation, diarrhea, dyspepsia, and flatulence are potential adverse effects.

Chapter 50

1 Heart cells require a steady supply of oxygen. When the supply is decreased or stopped, heart cells begin to die. The chest pain that Michael was experiencing is a symptom of the lack of adequate blood supply to his heart. The treatment is aimed at supplying the heart muscle with adequate oxygen-enriched blood.

2 Nitroglycerin (Nitro-Dur, Minitran, Nitrostat, Trinipatch) is a drug that dilates the blood vessels, both arteries and veins. This may result in some dilation of the coronary arteries, which will allow more blood to reach the oxygen-deprived myocardial tissue. In addition, nitroglycerin causes venous dilation, which decreases cardiac afterload and the oxygen demand of the myocardium. Together, the non-selective vasodilation is an attempt to restore the supply and demand balance to the myocardium.

3 Adverse effects associated with nitroglycerin infusions include hypotension, tachycardia, flushing, and headache.

4 IV nitroglycerin infusions are typically titrated (adjusted) based on the client's pain and other hemodynamic indicators, such as blood pressure and heart rate. Also, IV nitroglycerin must be administered using specialized IV tubing and should always be delivered via infusion pump.

Chapter 51

1 Elmer is on the right track. Although lifestyle changes aid in reducing high blood pressure, they take time. Plus, even with dietary changes, exercising, and smoking cessation, hypertension may still be present. Elmer needs to be informed that it is not unusual that controlling hypertension sometimes requires more than one medication, and that it may take some time to find the right combination to effectively treat his condition.

2 Hypertension is complex and may be caused by a series of physiological factors. It is not unusual for multiple medications to be prescribed before the right type and right dosage bring high blood pressure under control.

3 Elmer should be praised for his efforts. There is a good chance that his blood pressure reading would have been much higher had he not initiated the various lifestyle changes he did. Hypertension is a chronic disease that can cause some individuals to feel hopeless. Providing the client with support and encouragement is an important nursing intervention. It may be the determining factor in the client choosing to adhere to the therapeutic regimen.

Chapter 52

1 Loop diuretics act on the ascending loop of Henle in the kidney and are considered potent diuretics. They are primarily used in medicine to treat hypertension and edema, often due to congestive heart failure or renal insufficiency. Although all electrolytes may be lost due to diuretic therapy, it is potassium that is most severely lost and presents the greatest problem to clients who are receiving this drug.

Thiazide diuretics also deplete the body's potassium levels and cause the body to lose magnesium. It can cause hypokalemia, hyperuricemia, and hypercalcemia as well. Thiazides are used to lower blood pressure and are frequently used in combination with other drugs to treat hypertension.

Potassium-sparing diuretics do not promote the secretion of potassium into the urine. Watch out for hyperkalemia and instruct clients not to take additional potassium supplements. Potassium-sparing diuretics are also used as adjunctive therapy in the treatment of hypertension and congestive heart failure.

Osmotic diuretics work through the diffusion of fluid through semipermeable membranes by creating a shift in fluid from intercellular and interstitial areas to the intravascular space. Initially, due to the increase in circulating volume, the nurse should monitor the client for fluid overload. Because of shifting fluid volume, these diuretics may cause electrolytes to increase or decrease, and electrolyte levels should be monitored frequently.

2 Most diuretics potentially create a deficit of potassium. Hypokalemia predisposes the client to digoxin toxicity.

3 The client who is taking diuretics should be instructed to:

- Take the medication exactly as prescribed.
- Watch for electrolyte imbalances and dehydration and know the steps to prevent these from occurring.
- Weigh self weekly and report significant changes, such as weight gain of 1 kg (2 lb) in 24 hours, to the healthcare provider.
- Consult the prescriber before consuming OTC medications.
- Rise slowly to minimize orthostatic hypotension.

Chapter 53

1 Because Peggy has been in good health, an IV is not required to replace lost fluids but to serve as an IV route to administer other drugs during surgery. The dextrose 5% in water (D_5W) solution that Peggy is receiving will provide only minimal calories at the rate of 15 mL/hour and will not prevent dehydration. It is anticipated that Peggy will return home that afternoon and should be able to resume oral fluids soon thereafter. You would explain this to Peggy and also tell her that should additional fluids or drugs be required during or after surgery, they may be administered through her existing IV line.

2 The two main categories of IV fluids are colloids and crystalloids. Blood products is a third category but is not indicated in this scenario. Colloids are proteins, starches, or other large molecules that have the same effect as hypertonic solutions. Crystalloids are the most commonly used IV fluids and are

solutions that contain electrolytes or other agents, such as dextrose. Peggy has an order for dextrose 5% in water (D_5W), which is a crystalloid solution.

3 Dextrose 5% in water (D_5W) is an isotonic solution that will supply a small amount of calories through metabolism of the glucose and will provide this client with fluids and an IV route should drugs or additional fluids be required during or after surgery. The nurse should question Peggy about a possible history of diabetes or cardiac or renal conditions before administering the fluids and notify the provider if any of these are noted.

Chapter 54

1 The combination of digoxin (Lanoxin, Toloxin), furosemide (Lasix), and potassium supplementation is common. The purpose of the digoxin is to promote effective cardiac pumping and the improvement of cardiac output. The diuretic (furosemide) eliminates excessive body fluid and reduces the workload of the failing heart. The potassium supplement is prescribed to replace the loss of potassium caused by the diuretic.

2 Serum digoxin levels are blood tests to determine if the amount of the drug in the body will be therapeutic to treat Jim's heart condition. The blood should not be drawn for at least 6 to 12 hours after the last dose of digoxin. The patient should write down the time of the last dose.

3 Heart failure patients with normal renal function should be encouraged to consume foods that are rich in potassium, such as bananas, tomatoes, citrus fruits and juices, prunes, potatoes, and broccoli.

Chapter 55

1 The heart possesses a specialized system to control electrical impulses that are needed for cardiac contraction. Normally the impulse is initiated in a bundle of cells located in the right atrium, called the sinoatrial (SA) node. Once generated, the electrical impulse moves from cell to cell down through the heart until it reaches the atrioventricular (AV) node. This area is located in the middle of the heart, between the atrium and ventricles. After the AV node, the electrical impulses travel through a bundle of fibres that separate the right and left ventricles. The bundles are known as the bundle of His. Once the electrical impulse reaches the base of the ventricle (apex), it travels upward and spreads across both ventricles through the Purkinje fibres. Jada's diagnosis tells what part of the conduction is affected. Atrial fibrillation is a condition that occurs in the upper chambers of the heart. Fibrillation is a rapid uncoordinated twitching movement of the atrium that impairs cardiac function. This abnormality would be manifested by the lack of clear P waves on the ECG.

2 Amiodarone (Cordarone), when given IV, is usually only administered over 2 to 3 days to achieve a rapid therapeutic blood level. Afterwards, clients are often placed on the oral preparation of this drug. As you explain the mechanism of action to Jada, begin by saying that this drug helps to regulate the electrical condition system of the heart. It slows the rate at which the heart's electrical system recharges and prolongs the electrical phase during which the heart is electrically stimulated. This, in turn, helps to restore the normal heartbeat.

3 The client should understand that it is important to take amiodarone exactly as directed by the prescriber. And because amiodarone interacts with many other medications; it is important that no other medications are changed or altered without talking a pharmacist or doctor first. If a dose is missed, the client should take the missed dose as soon as it is remembered; however, never double the dose. In some clients, amiodarone causes dizziness, drowsiness, and blurred vision. Until the effects of the drug are fully known, the client should avoid driving or operating machinery. In addition, clients should check their pulse daily and report values lower than 60 beats/minute to the healthcare provider. Lastly, some clients who are receiving amiodarone may suffer from photosensitivity. They should be advised to protect their skin from ultraviolet rays and to wear sunglasses.

4 Jada needs to know that she should avoid grapefruit or grapefruit juice during treatment with amiodarone. Amiodarone can interact with grapefruit and grapefruit juice with dangerous effects.

Chapter 56

1 Atrial fibrillation is the rapid, uncoordinated firing of electrical impulses from multiple sites in the upper chambers of the heart. This condition causes ineffective cardiac contractions and the atria of the heart quiver instead of beating normally. When blood pools in parts of the atrium, subsequent to the poor pumping action, there is an increase in the risk that blood clots will form. Even small blood clots can cause strokes and heart attacks if they leave the heart and are released into the general circulation. Warfarin (Coumadin) reduces the chance that the clotting process will begin due to the pooling of blood.

2 While taking this medication, Lewis should contact the healthcare provider immediately if any bleeding or bruising occurs. Lewis should also be told not to take any prescriptions or OTC medications, such as aspirin, vitamins, or herbal preparations (especially those containing vitamin E or vitamin K), unless ordered by the healthcare provider. The reason for this is that many of these medications may interact with warfarin. If he forgets to take his medication, warn him not to try to catch up or double up on the dosage. He should contact his healthcare provider for instructions. Before starting any new medication or having a medical or surgical procedure, Lewis should talk with the healthcare provider.

3 Foods high in vitamin K, such as liver, broccoli, cabbage, cauliflower, spinach, lentils, chickpeas (garbanzo beans), turnip greens, soybean oil, seaweed, green tea, and herbal teas, can all affect warfarin. He should minimize his intake of these foods.

4 The effects of warfarin are evaluated using blood tests such as prothrombin time (PT) or international normalized ratio (INR). The INR is the ratio of a patient's prothrombin time to a normal (control) sample. Both blood tests measure how long it takes for blood to clot. The warfarin will be adjusted according to the time it takes for blood to clot. Normal INR is between 2 and 3.

Chapter 57

1 This drug is given when certain WBCs, called neutrophils, are below normal level. Neutrophils are the most plentiful type of WBC and are the primary infection-fighters. These cells are normally produced in the bone marrow. Filgrastim (Neupogen, Grastofil) stimulates the bone marrow to produce these cells, which will reduce the risk for infections.

2 Neutropenic clients must take multiple precautions to prevent contact with pathogenic organisms. Some of the precautions include avoiding crowds, people with known infections, or young children who have a higher risk for having an infection. Uncooked fruits and vegetables or undercooked meats are also possible sources of infection, and families or other caregivers should prepare these items and perform the cleanup afterwards. Careful and frequent handwashing is essential for neutropenic clients as well as for those caring for them. Clients who experience fever, sore throat, or flu-like symptoms should report them immediately to their healthcare provider. The need for complete isolation from others is usually not needed unless the cell counts are extremely low, in which case hospitalization for a short time may be necessary.

3 Some common adverse effects of filgrastim include bone pain, nausea, and swelling or redness at the injection site.

Chapter 58

1 A major action of this vasopressor medication is the positive inotropic action that it has on a damaged myocardium that is having difficulty maintaining a good cardiac output (and therefore blood pressure). The drip must be slowly tapered to a point at which the blood pressure is well maintained, normally a systolic blood pressure greater than 100. The nurse must never stop the vasopressor drip abruptly, as the client may become acutely hypotensive.

2 This isotonic solution is appropriate for the client. Based on history and assessment, the client is demonstrating signs of being hypovolemic (a heart rate of 122) and requires a solution that will meet the intracellular need. As the client responds to the fluid, the nurse expects to note a corresponding decrease in the heart rate and other symptoms (e.g., weakness, lethargy, and dry mouth).

3 This is not an appropriate IV solution for a head injury client. Once this IV solution is infused into the client, it is considered to be a hypotonic solution that moves fluids into the cells. A client with an increased intracranial pressure cannot tolerate an increase in fluid at the cellular level, as this may cause the brain to herniate and lead to death.

Chapter 59

1 Even though the surgeon has removed the large part of the tumour, if there is even one cancerous cell left it may repopulate. The goal of chemotherapy is to obtain a total cell kill of any cancerous cells that remain after the surgery before the cells have a chance to repopulate the cancer.

2 Staging and grading are important to understand because these systems are used to establish treatment and prognosis for the client with cancer. T1, N0, M0 tells us that the tumour is relatively small in size and not significantly invading surrounding tissues, no cancerous cells were found in the lymph nodes, and no metastases were found. G2 tells us that the cells are moderately differentiated and look somewhat like the parent cells. The staging and grading for Cheryl's cancer leads us to believe that she has a good prognosis.

3 Hematological changes that Cheryl may experience during chemotherapy are thrombocytopenia, neutropenia, and anemia. Thrombocytopenia is a platelet count of less than 100 000 per mL of blood. This can cause the client to exhibit abnormal bleeding. If the platelet count drops to less than 20 000 per mL of blood, the client may begin to bruise easily. The client may also exhibit petechiae or purpura. If the platelet count continues to decrease, the client may hemorrhage or die.

A client is diagnosed with neutropenia when the neutrophil count is less than 1500 cells. The chemotherapy may cause a decrease in all of the client's WBCs (leukopenia); however, the neutrophils are usually the type of WBCs that are affected the most. Cheryl's nadir must be calculated prior to administering any more chemotherapy.

A client is diagnosed with anemia when the RBC count drops below 4.2 million/mm^3 for men or 3.6/mm^3 for women, or when the hemoglobin count is less than 14 g/dL for men or 12 g/dL for women. Because hemoglobin carries oxygen to all tissues and major organs in the body, anemia may affect every system in the body.

Chapter 60

1 Using different drugs affects the different stages of the cancer's life cycle, allowing lower doses of each individual drug to be used, and possibly slowing the development of resistance to the drugs. Cyclophosphamide (Procytox) is an alkylating agent of the nitrogen mustard class. Carboplatin is also an alkylating agent, a platinum compound. Vincristine is a natural product, a vinca alkaloid, and etoposide (VePesid) is also a natural product of the topoisomerase inhibitor class.

2 There are often overlapping toxicities when multiple chemotherapy drugs are used that have similar adverse effects, most commonly bone marrow suppression. The chance for overlapping toxicities for Zack is also high for the neurological system (e.g., decreased deep tendon reflexes, peripheral neuropathies, weakness, and cranial nerve effects). All four drugs are likely to cause these adverse effects, and given Zack's diminished deep tendon reflexes at this clinic visit, he should be monitored closely for increasing motor effects such as clumsiness or difficulty holding heavy objects. Other overlapping toxicities from this group of drugs include effects on the cardiovascular or respiratory systems.

3 Zack is at great risk for infection. Any absolute neutrophil count of less than 500 is a concern, and scrupulous infection control measures should be taken. While neutropenic precautions may not be required at this time, extra care should be taken to avoid exposing Zack to any extra risk for infection. He should not have visitors with known infections and should avoid crowded indoor places. Previous teaching should be reviewed with Zack and his family, including that he should continue any mouth rinses ordered by the provider and should bathe daily with a mild soap and covering the PICC line insertion site as directed by the provider. Excellent handwashing should be performed by Zack and his family, especially prior to his filgrastim (Neupogen, Grastofil) injections. His PICC line care should be performed using aseptic technique. Any fever over 38.3°C (101°F) or three sequential temperatures over 38.1°C (100.5°F) taken 4 hours apart should be reported to the oncologist. Considering his age, this time may be very frustrating for Zack. The nurse could explore options to help Zack maintain contact with his friends, perhaps by synchronous online games, video conferencing, or chat sessions, until his WBC count increases. Also, with a platelet count of 55 000, he is at increased risk for bleeding. While his fatigue may prevent him from participating in activities that may cause direct injury (e.g., sports), he should be monitored for increased bruising, petechiae, or any obvious bleeding, such as nosebleeds. Zack and his family should be reminded that if bleeding occurs, prolonged pressure will be required to stop it and the healthcare provider should be notified.

Chapter 61

1 Osteoporosis is a condition in which the bone loses minerals and decreases in density, causing a subsequent loss in height. Her recent loss in height may explain why her pants seem longer, and you should explain the details of this condition to the client. Points to include are as follows:

- Risk factors: menopause, age over 60, family history of osteoporosis, Caucasian or Asian race, high alcohol intake, estrogen deficiency, smoking history, androgen deficiency, anorexia nervosa, low calcium or vitamin D intake, physical inactivity, and thin, lean body build.
- Signs and symptoms: fractures seen in the hips, wrists, forearms, or spine, and height loss.
- Diagnosis: height loss, bone fractures, and bone mineral density values.
- Treatments: Many drugs may be helpful. These include calcium and vitamin D, estrogen receptor modulators, statins, slow-release sodium fluoride, bisphosphonates, and calcitonin.

2 The nurse should encourage the client to participate in preventive measures, which include adequate intake of calcium and vitamin D according to age requirements; physical exercise; routine healthcare follow-up, especially to evaluate estrogen needs; use of OTC calcium supplements as recommended by a healthcare provider; and avoidance of alcohol.

Chapter 62

1 Acne vulgaris is a common skin condition in the teenage years. It is thought to occur as hair follicles become blocked and trapped sebum interacts with the bacterium *Propionibacterium acnes* in the hair follicle, causing inflammation and the classic papular acne lesion. It is especially common in puberty and adolescence and is associated with the rise in hormone levels at that time, although it may persist beyond the age of 30. Topical keratolytic drugs such as benzoyl peroxide (Benzac) may be used to help dry the skin and act as an antibacterial against *P. acnes*. Topical antibiotics may also be used. In severe cases, tretinoin (Retin-A, Stieva-A) may be required to adequately treat the condition.

2 Danny's increase in acne at this time may be linked to rising androgen levels as he progresses through puberty. Because he is active in outdoor sports, sweat, dust and dirt from athletic fields, and the use of sunscreen may also be aggravating the condition.

3 Danny should wash his face gently with a mild soap and water, especially after participating in sports practices or games. He should apply a thin layer of the tretinoin to the acne, avoiding the eye area. He should discontinue any benzoyl peroxide or other topical drugs while he is using the tretinoin to avoid excessive dryness. Tretinoin often causes local skin effects such as redness, peeling, or a temporary hyperpigmentation.

Danny should limit sun exposure to the treated areas and should consult with his healthcare provider about the use of sunscreens.

Chapter 63

1 Predisposing factors that Mrs. Duclos has include the fact that she is an older adult with a history of diabetes. Other general predisposing factors that

may not apply to Mrs. Duclos include African or Asian descent, genetic factors, congenital defects in infants and children, history of eye trauma, infection, inflammation, hemorrhage, tumours, or cataracts. Long-term use of topical corticosteroids, some antihypertensives, antihistamines, and antidepressants may also contribute to the development or progression of glaucoma. Risk factors associated with glaucoma include hypertension, migraine headaches, refractive disorders with a high degree of nearsightedness or farsightedness, and the normal aging process.

2 Wash hands prior to administering eye drops. Avoid touching the eye or eyelashes with any part of the eyedropper to avoid cross-contamination. Administer the eye drop solution into the conjunctival sac.

Apply gentle pressure over the lacrimal (tear) duct for 1 minute. Apply to only the affected eye(s). Ensure that only one drop is instilled unless ordered otherwise. Wait at least 5 minutes before instilling other eye drops. If indicated, refrigerate and protect the solution from light.

3 If eye drops for glaucoma are given frequently or if the tear duct is not held after administering the drop and the solution is swallowed, systemic effects may be observed. Adverse effects from beta-adrenergic blocker drops include angina, anxiety, bronchoconstriction, hypotension, and dysrhythmias. Systemic adverse effects from prostaglandin drops include respiratory infection, angina, and muscle or joint pain.

Cholinergic agonist drops may cause systemic adverse effects such as salivation, tachycardia, hypotension, bronchospasm, nausea, and vomiting.

Chapter 64

1 Because smallpox is caused by the variola virus, there is no specific treatment for smallpox disease. The only prevention is vaccination. The virus can be spread from one person to another by direct and prolonged face-to-face contact. Smallpox also can be spread through direct contact with infected bodily fluids or contaminated objects such as bedding or clothing. Exposure to smallpox is followed by an incubation period of 7 to 17 days, during which people do not have any symptoms. Initially, symptoms of smallpox include high fever, malaise, head and body aches, and sometimes vomiting. Often the development of a rash begins in the mouth. However, it quickly spreads to the face and moves to the arms and legs. Supportive care and infection control measures should be instituted for the client with smallpox.

2 The method of transmission affects the symptoms of anthrax contamination. The most common (cutaneous anthrax) and the most serious (inhalation anthrax) forms of anthrax are transmitted through open skin and inhalation. The nurse should examine the client's skin for open wounds that may be contaminated. Respiratory assessment and support is imperative for the client who may have contracted anthrax via respiratory exposure (inhalation). The CDC recommends that standard contact precautions be maintained for clients suspected of exposure to anthrax.

3 *Yersinia pestis* is a gram-negative anaerobic bacterium that causes a life-threatening condition known as pneumonic plague. The isolation of this disease is extremely difficult because it can be spread by aerosol. The person who has the disease would be infectious to everyone with whom he or she has come in contact within 1 to 6 days after exposure. If untreated, pneumonic plague will result in respiratory failure with subsequent shock and death. Bubonic plague, a more common form, results in enlarged, painful lymph nodes.

Glossary

A

A delta fibres nerves that transmit sensations of sharp pain

absence seizure seizure with a loss or reduction of normal activity, including staring and transient loss of responsiveness

absorption the process of moving a drug across body membranes

accessory organs of digestion include the salivary glands, liver, gallbladder, and pancreas

acetylcholine (Ach) primary neurotransmitter of the parasympathetic nervous system; also present at somatic neuromuscular junctions and at sympathetic preganglionic nerves

acetylcholinesterase (AchE) enzyme that degrades acetylcholine within the synaptic cleft, enhancing effects of the neurotransmitter

acetylcholinesterase (AchE) inhibitors indirect-acting cholinergic agonists that are nonselective and affect all acetylcholine (Ach) synapses

acidosis condition of having too much acid in the blood; plasma pH below 7.35

acne vulgaris condition characterized by small inflamed bumps that appear on the surface of the skin

acquired immune deficiency syndrome (AIDS) infection caused by the human immunodeficiency virus (HIV)

acquired resistance condition in which a microbe is no longer affected by a drug following anti-infective pharmacotherapy

acromegaly excessive growth hormone disorder in which bones become deformed

action potential electrical changes in the membrane of a muscle or nerve cell due to changes in membrane permeability

activated partial thromboplastin time (aPTT) blood test used to determine how long it takes clots to form, to regulate heparin dosage

active immunity resistance resulting from a previous exposure to an antigen

active transport the process by which molecules move across the cell membrane against a concentration or electrochemical gradient

acute gouty arthritis condition in which uric acid crystals accumulate in the joints of the big toes, ankles, wrists, fingers, knees, or elbows, resulting in red, swollen, or inflamed tissue

acute radiation syndrome life-threatening symptoms resulting from acute exposure to ionizing radiation, including nausea, vomiting, severe leukopenia, thrombocytopenia, anemia, and alopecia

acute retroviral syndrome symptoms during the initial phase of human immunodeficiency virus (HIV) infection

acute toxicity severe or sudden onset of poisoning

adaptive defences defences that are specific to certain threats; the immune response

addiction the continued use of a substance despite its negative health and social consequences

Addison's disease hyposecretion of glucocorticoids and aldosterone by the adrenal cortex

additive effect type of drug interaction in which two agents combine to produce a summation response

adherence taking a medication in the manner prescribed by the healthcare provider or, in the case of over-the-counter (OTC) drugs, following the instructions on the label

adjuvant chemotherapy administration of antineoplastic drugs *after* surgery or radiation therapy

adolescence period of life from 13 to 18 years of age

adrenal atrophy condition in which the adrenal cortex shrinks and stops secreting endogenous corticosteroids due to lack of stimulation by adrenocorticotropic hormone (ACTH)

adrenal crisis condition that occurs when corticosteroid medication is abruptly withdrawn

adrenergic relating to nerves that release norepinephrine or epinephrine

adrenergic agonists agents that activate adrenergic receptors in the sympathetic nervous system; also known as sympathomimetics

adrenergic antagonist drug that blocks the actions of the sympathetic nervous system

adrenergics class of antagonist drugs that block the actions of the sympathetic nervous system

adrenocortical insufficiency lack of adequate corticosteroid secretion by the adrenal cortex

adrenocorticotropic hormone (ACTH) hormone secreted by the anterior pituitary that stimulates the release of glucocorticoids by the adrenal cortex

adverse drug effect an undesirable and potentially harmful action caused by the administration of medication

adverse drug reaction (ADR) an undesired response to a drug

aerobic pertaining to an oxygen environment

aerosol suspension of minute liquid droplets or fine solid particles suspended in a gas

affinity chemical attraction that impels certain molecules to unite with others to form complexes

afterload pressure that must be overcome for the ventricles to eject blood from the heart

agonist drug that is capable of binding with receptors to induce a cellular response

akathisia inability to remain still; constantly moving

albumin protein that acts as a carrier molecule in the blood and helps to maintain blood volume and blood pressure

aldosterone hormone secreted by the adrenal cortex that increases sodium reabsorption in the distal tubule of the kidney

alimentary canal hollow tube in the digestive system that starts in the mouth and includes the esophagus, stomach, small intestine, and large intestine

alkalosis condition of having too many basic substances in the blood; plasma pH above 7.45

alkylation process by which certain chemicals attach to DNA and change its structure and function

allergic reaction acquired, hyperresponse of body defences to a foreign substance (allergen)

allergic rhinitis syndrome of sneezing, itchy throat, watery eyes, and nasal congestion resulting from exposure to antigens; also known as hay fever

alopecia hair loss

alpha (α) receptor type of subreceptor found in the sympathetic nervous system

alpha-adrenergic antagonists drugs that block alpha-adrenergic receptors in the sympathetic nervous system

Alzheimer's disease (AD) most common dementia, characterized by loss of memory, delusions, hallucinations, confusion, and loss of judgment

amide type of chemical linkage found in some local anesthetics involving carbon, nitrogen, and oxygen (-NH-CO-)

amyloid plaque abnormal protein fragments related to neuronal damage; a sign of Alzheimer's disease observed during autopsy

anabolic steroid compound resembling testosterone with hormonal activity; commonly abused by athletes

anaerobic pertaining to an environment without oxygen

analgesic drug used to reduce or eliminate pain

anaphylactic shock type of shock caused by an acute allergic reaction

anaphylaxis acute allergic response to an antigen that results in severe hypotension and may lead to life-threatening shock if untreated

anastomoses natural communication networks among the coronary arteries

androgen steroid sex hormone that promotes the appearance of masculine characteristics

anemia lack of adequate numbers of red blood cells or decreased oxygen-carrying capacity of the blood

angina pectoris acute chest pain upon physical or emotional exertion due to inadequate oxygen supply to the myocardium

angiogenesis the formation of new blood vessels

angiotensin II chemical released in response to falling blood pressure that causes vasoconstriction and release of aldosterone

angiotensin II receptor blocker (ARB) a drug that lowers blood pressure by selectively blocking angiotensin II from binding to its receptor, which causes vasodilatation

angiotensin-converting enzyme (ACE) enzyme responsible for converting angiotensin I to angiotensin II

anion negatively charged ion

anorexiant drug used to suppress appetite

antacid drug that neutralizes stomach acid

antagonist drug that blocks the response of another drug

antagonistic effect type of drug interaction in which adding a second drug results in a diminished pharmacological response

anterior pituitary gland (adenohypophysis) consists of glandular tissue that manufactures and secretes hormones that control major body functions and systems

anthrax a bacterial infection that can cause severe disease and high mortality in humans

antiadrenergic drug used to block adrenergic receptors in the sympathetic nervous system

antibiotic substance produced by a microorganism that inhibits or kills other microorganisms

antibody protein produced by the body in response to an antigen; used interchangeably with the term *immunoglobulin*

anticholinergic drug that blocks the actions of the parasympathetic nervous system

anticoagulant agent that inhibits the formation of blood clots

antidiuretic hormone (ADH) hormone produced by the hypothalamus and secreted by the posterior pituitary that stimulates the kidneys to conserve water

antidote a substance used to block the effects of another substance or drug

antiemetic drug that prevents vomiting

antifibrinolytic drug used to prevent and treat excessive bleeding from surgical sites

antigen foreign organism or substance that induces the formation of antibodies by the immune system

anti-infective general term for any medication that is effective against pathogens

antimicrobial (antibacterial) resistance the development of resistance by microbes to the effects of an antimicrobial drug

antipyretic drug that lowers body temperature

antiretroviral drug that is effective against retroviruses

antithrombin III protein that prevents abnormal clotting by inhibiting thrombin

antitussive drug used to suppress cough

anxiety state of apprehension and autonomic nervous system activation resulting from exposure to a non-specific or unknown cause

anxiolytic drug that relieves anxiety

apoprotein protein component of a lipoprotein

apothecary system of measurement older system of measurement using drams; rarely used

appetite a psychological response that drives food intake based on associations and memory

aqueous humour fluid that fills the anterior and posterior chambers of the eye

aromatase inhibitor hormone inhibitor that blocks the enzyme aromatase, which normally converts adrenal androgen to estradiol

ASAP order as soon as possible order, which should be available for administration to the client within 30 minutes of the written order

assessing appraisal of a client's condition that involves gathering and interpreting data

asthma chronic inflammatory disease of the lungs characterized by airway obstruction

astringent effect shrinkage of swollen mucous membranes or loosening of secretions and facilitation of drainage

atherosclerosis condition characterized by a buildup of fatty plaque and loss of elasticity of the walls of the arteries

atonic seizure very short–lasting seizure during which the client may stumble and fall for no apparent reason

atrial fibrillation rapid irregular heart rhythm originating in the atria of the heart

atrial natriuretic peptide (ANP) hormone secreted by specialized cells in the right atrium when large increases in blood volume produce excessive stretch on the atrial wall

atrial reflex causes the heart rate and cardiac output (CO) to increase until the backlog of venous blood (or intravenous fluid) is distributed throughout the body

atrioventricular bundle cardiac tissue that receives electrical impulses from the atrioventricular (AV) node and sends them to the bundle branches; also known as the *bundle of His*

atrioventricular (AV) node cardiac tissue that receives electrical impulses from the sinoatrial (SA) node and conveys them to the ventricles

attention deficit disorder (ADD) condition characterized by an inability to focus attention on a task for a sufficient length of time

attention deficit/hyperactivity disorder (ADHD) condition typically diagnosed in childhood and adolescence characterized by hyperactivity as well as attention, organization, and behaviour control issues

attenuated organisms that have been rendered less able to cause disease through the application of heat or chemicals from which effective vaccines can be developed

atypical antidepressant drug used to treat depression that has a mechanism of action that differs from traditional classes of antidepressants

atypical antipsychotic drug used to treat both the positive and the negative symptoms of psychosis or schizophrenia

aura sensory cue such as bright lights, smells, or tastes that precedes a migraine

autoantibody protein called *rheumatoid factor*, released by B lymphocytes, that tears down the body's own tissue

automaticity ability of certain myocardial cells to spontaneously generate an action potential

autonomic nervous system (ANS) portion of the peripheral nervous system that provides involuntary control over smooth muscle, cardiac muscle, and glands

azoles major class of drugs used to treat mycoses

azoospermia complete absence of sperm in ejaculate

azotemia accumulation of nitrogenous waste products in the kidneys that can result in death if untreated

B

bactericidal ability to kill bacteria

bacteriostatic ability to inhibit the growth of bacteria

balanced anesthesia use of multiple medications to rapidly induce unconsciousness, cause muscle relaxation, and maintain deep anesthesia

baroreceptor a collection of nerves located in the walls of the atria, aortic arch, vena cava, and carotid sinus that sense changes in blood pressure

Barrett's esophagus precancerous condition of the esophagus

basal metabolic rate resting rate of metabolism in the body

basal nuclei area of the brain responsible for starting and stopping synchronized motor activity such as leg and arm motions during walking; also called basal ganglia

baseline data client information that is gathered before pharmacotherapy is implemented

B cell lymphocyte responsible for humoral immunity

beneficence ethical principle of doing good

benign prostatic hyperplasia (BPH) non-malignant enlargement of the prostate gland

benzodiazepines major class of drugs used to treat anxiety disorders

beriberi deficiency of thiamine

beta-adrenergic antagonists drugs that block beta-adrenergic receptors; may be non-selective or selective; also called beta blockers

beta-lactam ring chemical structure found in most penicillins and some cephalosporins

beta-lactamase (penicillinase) enzyme present in certain bacteria that is able to inactivate many penicillins and some cephalosporins

beta (β) receptor type of subreceptor found in the sympathetic nervous system

bile acid resin drug that binds bile acids, thus lowering cholesterol

bioavailability ability of a drug to reach the bloodstream and its target tissues

biological response modifier substance that is able to enhance or stimulate the immune system

biologics substances that produce biological responses within the body; synthesized by cells of the human body, animal cells, or microorganisms

bioterrorism intentional use of infectious biological agents, chemical substances, or radiation to cause widespread harm or illness

biotransformation the process by which drug molecules are metabolized and prepared for excretion from the body

bipolar disorder (manic depression) syndrome characterized by extreme and opposite moods, such as euphoria and depression

bisphosphonates class of drugs that block bone resorption by inhibiting osteoclast activity

blood-brain barrier anatomical structure that prevents certain substances from gaining access to the brain

body mass index (BMI) measurement of obesity determined by dividing body weight (in kilograms) by the square of height (in metres)

body surface area (BSA) method method of calculating pediatric dosages using an estimate of the child's BSA

body weight method method of calculating pediatric dosages that requires a calculation of the number of milligrams of drug, based on the child's weight in kilograms (mg/kg)

bolus feedings method of enteral feeding that typically delivers 250 to 400 mL of formula every 4 to 6 hours via a syringe or funnel

bone deposition the process of depositing mineral components into bone; opposite of bone resorption

bone resorption the process of bone demineralization or the breaking down of bone into mineral components

boosters follow-up doses of vaccines that are required to provide prolonged protection

botanical plant extract used to treat or prevent illness

botulism condition caused by *Clostridium botulinum*, an organism that secretes a potent toxin that paralyzes the muscles after a person is poisoned

Bowman's capsule portion of the nephron that filters blood and receives the filtrate from the glomerulus

bradydysrhythmias disorders characterized by a heart rate of less than 60 beats/minute

bradykinesia difficulty initiating movement and controlling fine muscle movements

bradykinin chemical released by cells during inflammation that produces pain and side effects similar to those of histamine

brain attack *see* cerebrovascular accident (CVA)

broad-spectrum antibiotic anti-infective that is effective against many different gram-positive and gram-negative organisms

bronchospasm rapid constriction of the airways

buccal route administration method in which a tablet or capsule is placed in the oral cavity between the gum and the cheek

buffer chemical that helps to maintain normal body pH by neutralizing strong acids or bases

bundle branch electrical conduction pathway in the heart leading from the atrioventricular (AV) bundle and through the wall between the ventricles

C

C fibres nerves that transmit dull, poorly localized pain

cachexia general wasting of muscle and other tissue

calcifediol substance formed in the first step of vitamin D formation

calcineurin intracellular messenger molecule to which immunosuppressants bind

calcitonin hormone secreted by the thyroid gland that increases the deposition of calcium in bone

calcitriol substance that is transformed in the kidneys during the second step of the conversion of vitamin D to its active form

calcium channel blocker drug that blocks the flow of calcium ions into myocardial cells

calcium ion channel pathway in a plasma membrane through which calcium ions enter and leave

camptothecins class of antineoplastics that inhibit the enzyme topoisomerase

Canadian Association of Poison Control Centres (CAPCC) an organization that provides a centralized forum for communication, information, and exchange of ideas among Canadian poison control centres

cancer malignant disease characterized by rapidly growing, invasive cells that spread to other regions of the body and eventually kill the host

capsid protein coat that surrounds a virus

carbonic anhydrase enzyme that forms carbonic acid by combining carbon dioxide and water

carcinogens agents that cause cancer

cardiac output (CO) amount of blood pumped by a ventricle in 1 minute

cardiogenic shock type of shock caused when the heart is diseased such that it cannot maintain circulation to the tissues

cardiotonic drugs agents that increase the force of cardiac contraction; also called inotropic agents

cardioversion (defibrillation) conversion of fibrillation to a normal heart rhythm

carotenes class of yellow-red pigments that are precursors to vitamin A

catecholamines class of agents secreted in response to stress that include epinephrine, norepinephrine, and dopamine

cathartic substance that causes complete evacuation of the bowel

cation positively charged ion

CD4 receptor protein that accepts human immunodeficiency virus (HIV) and allows entry of HIV into the T4 lymphocyte

cell kill hypothesis theoretical model that predicts the ability of antineoplastic drugs to eliminate cancer cells

cell signalling the transfer of information from one cell to another

central nervous system (CNS) division of the nervous system consisting of the brain and spinal cord

central nervous system (CNS) stimulants agents that raise the general alertness level of the brain

central vein total parenteral nutrition the administration of enteral feeding solution through a central vein

cerebrovascular accident (CVA), also called *stroke* or *brain attack;* acute condition of a blood clot or bleeding in a vessel in the brain

chemical name strict chemical nomenclature used for naming drugs; established by the International Union of Pure and Applied Chemistry (IUPAC)

chemoreceptor collection of nerves located in the aortic arch and carotid sinus that sense changes in oxygen content, pH, or carbon dioxide levels in the blood

chemotherapy drug treatment of cancer

chief cell cell located in the mucosa of the stomach that secretes pepsinogen, an inactive form of the enzyme pepsin that chemically breaks down proteins

cholecalciferol vitamin D_3 formed in the skin by exposure to ultraviolet light

cholesterol a sterol that is synthesized in the liver and is a normal constituent of bile; it is an important precursor in the formation of steroid hormones

cholinergic relating to nerves that release acetylcholine

cholinergic agonists drugs and chemicals that increase the action of acetylcholine (Ach) at a cholinergic receptor; also called parasympathomimetics

cholinergic crisis caused by an overdosage with acetylcholinesterase (AchE) inhibitors or poisoning with organophosphate insecticides or toxic nerve gases; characterized by intense signs of parasympathetic stimulation such as miosis, nausea, vomiting, urinary incontinence, increased exocrine secretions, abdominal cramping, and diarrhea

cholinergics drugs that stimulate cholinergic receptors in the parasympathetic nervous system

chronic bronchitis recurrent disease of the lungs characterized by excess mucus production, inflammation, and coughing

chronic obstructive pulmonary disease (COPD) generic term used to describe several pulmonary conditions characterized by cough, mucus production, and impaired gas exchange

chronic toxicity poisoning that occurs during prolonged exposure to a substance

chyme semifluid, partly digested food that is passed from the stomach to the duodenum

circadian rhythm cyclic basis by which body temperature, blood pressure, hormone levels, and respiration all fluctuate throughout the 24-hour day

clinical trial testing of a new drug in selected clients

clonic spasm multiple, rapidly repeated muscular contractions

closed-angle glaucoma acute glaucoma that is caused by decreased outflow of aqueous humour from the anterior chamber

clotting factor substance contributing to the process of blood hemostasis

coagulation process of blood clotting

coagulation cascade complex series of steps to stop blood flow

colloid type of intravenous (IV) fluid consisting of large organic molecules that are unable to cross membranes

colony-stimulating factor (CSF) hormone that regulates the growth and maturation of specific white blood cell (WBC) populations

combination drug drug product with more than one active generic ingredient

comedone acne lesion that develops just beneath the surface of the skin (whitehead) or as a result of a plugged oil gland (blackhead)

Compendium of Pharmaceuticals and Specialties (CPS) a compilation of drug monographs that are prepared by pharmaceutical manufacturers

complement series of proteins involved in the nonspecific defence of the body that promote antigen destruction

complement system a cluster of 20 plasma proteins that combine in a specific sequence and order when an infection occurs

complementary and alternative medicine (CAM) system of medicine that considers the health of the whole person and promotes disease prevention

complementary and alternative therapies treatments considered outside the realm of conventional Western medicine

conjugate side chain that, during metabolism, makes drugs more water soluble and more easily excreted by the kidney

conjugation the direct transfer of small pieces of DNA from one bacterium to another

constipation infrequent passage of abnormally hard and dry stools

continuing order an order for a drug to be administered at prescribed intervals over a period of days or weeks

continuous infusion feedings enteral feedings delivered by an infusion pump at a slow rate over a 16- to 24-hour period

contractility the strength by which the myocardial fibres contract

controlled substance in the United States, a drug whose use is restricted by the Comprehensive Drug Abuse Prevention and Control Act; in Canada, a drug subject to guidelines outlined in Part III, Schedule G of the Canadian Food and Drugs Act

conventional (typical) antipsychotic a drug that is used to treat the positive symptoms of schizophrenia

convulsion uncontrolled muscle contractions or spasms that occur in the face, torso, arms, or legs

coronary arterial bypass graft (CABG) surgical procedure performed to restore blood flow to the myocardium by using a section of the saphenous vein or internal mammary artery to go around the obstructed coronary artery

coronary artery disease (CAD) narrowing of the coronary arteries, usually as a result of atherosclerosis

corpora cavernosa tissues in the penis that fill with blood during an erection

corpus luteum ruptured follicle that remains in the ovary after ovulation and secretes progestins

corpus striatum area of the brain responsible for unconscious muscle movement; a point of contact for neurons projecting from the substantia nigra

cretinism condition marked by profound mental retardation and impaired growth that results from untreated congenital hypothyroidism

Crohn's disease chronic inflammatory bowel disease affecting the ileum and sometimes the colon

cross-tolerance situation in which tolerance to one drug makes the client tolerant to another drug

crystalloid type of intravenous (IV) fluid resembling blood plasma minus proteins, which is capable of crossing membranes

culture set of beliefs, values, religious rituals, and customs shared by a group of people

culture and sensitivity (C&S) testing laboratory exam used to identify bacteria and to determine which antibiotic is most effective

Cushing's syndrome condition of having too much corticosteroid in the blood, caused by excessive secretion by the adrenal glands or by overdosage with corticosteroid medication

cyclic feedings enteral feedings that are commonly infused over 8 to 16 hours daily (day or night)

cyclooxygenase (COX-1, COX-2) key enzyme in the prostaglandin metabolic pathway that is blocked by acetylsalicylic acid (ASA) and other nonsteroidal anti-inflammatory drugs (NSAIDs)

cycloplegic drug drug that relaxes or temporarily paralyzes ciliary muscles and causes blurred vision

cytokine chemical produced by white blood cells, such as interleukins, leukotrienes, interferon, and tumour necrosis factor, that guides the immune response

D

deep vein thrombosis (DVT) the formation of a blood clot in a deep vein such as the femoral vein or the popliteal vein

defecation evacuation of the colon; bowel movement

delusion false idea or belief not founded in reality

dementia degenerative disorder characterized by progressive memory loss, confusion, and the inability to think or communicate effectively

dependence strong physiological or psychological need for a substance

depolarization reversal of the plasma membrane charge such that the inside is made less negative

depression disorder characterized by depressed mood; lack of energy; sleep disturbances; abnormal eating patterns; and feelings of despair, guilt, and misery

dermatitis inflammatory condition of the skin characterized by itching and scaling

dermatophytic characteristic of a superficial fungal infection

designer drug substance produced in a laboratory and intended to mimic the effects of other psychoactive controlled substances

desmopressin (DDAVP) synthetic hormone that is similar to the natural human (antidiuretic hormone) vasopressin often used to reduce urine output

diabetes insipidus condition characterized by excessive urination due to lack of secretion of antidiuretic hormone

diabetic ketoacidosis (DKA) type of metabolic acidosis due to an excess of ketone bodies; most often occurring when diabetes mellitus is uncontrolled

diagnosing the process of identifying clients' needs or problems based on analysis of assessment findings

diarrhea abnormal frequency and liquidity of bowel movements

diastolic blood pressure blood pressure during the relaxation phase of heart activity

dietary fibre ingested substance that is neither digested nor absorbed that contributes to the fecal mass

dietary reference intakes (DRIs) the nutrient values that guide decision making on nutrition policies and programs to promote the health of Canadians

diffusion the tendency of molecules to move from a region of high concentration to a region of lower concentration

digestion the process by which the body breaks down ingested food into small molecules that can be absorbed

digestive system body system consisting of the alimentary canal and the accessory organs

directly observed therapy (DOT) requires that a healthcare provider directly observe the client swallowing the pills, whether it is in the hospital, office, or home care setting

distal tubule portion of the nephron that collects filtrate from the loop of Henle

distribution the process of transporting drugs throughout the body

diuretic substance that increases urine output

dopamine chemical precursor in the synthesis of norepinephrine; classified as a catecholamine

dopamine D_2 receptor receptor for dopamine in the basal nuclei of the brain that is associated with schizophrenia and antipsychotic drugs

dopamine system stabilizers (DSSs) drugs that exhibit both antagonist and partial agonist activities on dopamine receptors

dose-response relationship the way a client responds to varying doses of a drug

downregulation the process by which cells make fewer receptors on their surface

drug general term for any substance capable of producing biological responses in the body

drug allergies a hyperresponse of body defences to a particular drug that may result in a diverse range of client symptoms

Drug Identification Number (DIN) a unique number located on the label of a prescription or over-the-counter drug product that has been evaluated by the Therapeutic Products Directorate (TPD) and approved for sale in Canada

drug interaction occurs when a medication interacts with another substance such as another drug, a dietary supplement, an herbal product, or food that is taken concurrently with the medication, and the drug's actions are affected

drug misuse improper use of drugs that includes overuse, underuse, or, in some cases, erratic use

Drug Product Database a database maintained by Health Canada that contains product and company information on drug products marketed in Canada

drug-protein complex drug bound reversibly to plasma proteins, particularly albumin, that makes the drug unavailable for distribution to body tissues

dry powder inhaler (DPI) device used to convert a solid drug to a fine powder for the purpose of inhalation

dumping syndrome the result of a sudden influx of enteral feeding into the gastrointestinal (GI) tract and the creation of a high osmotic gradient within the small intestine

duodenum first section of the small intestine

dwarfism a growth hormone deficiency disorder in children associated with normal birth length followed by a slowing of the growth rate

dysentery severe diarrhea that may include bleeding

dysfunctional uterine bleeding hemorrhage that occurs at abnormal times or in excessive quantity during the menstrual cycle

dyslipidemia abnormal (excess or deficient) levels of lipoproteins in the blood

dysrhythmia abnormality in cardiac rhythm

dystonia severe muscle spasms, particularly of the back, neck, tongue, and face; characterized by abnormal tension starting in one area of the body and progressing to other areas

E

ectopic foci/pacemakers cardiac tissue outside the normal cardiac conduction pathway that generates action potentials

eczema skin disorder with unexplained symptoms of inflammation, itching, and scaling; also called *atopic dermatitis*

efficacy ability of a drug to produce a desired response

electrocardiogram (ECG, EKG) device that records the electrical activity of the heart

electroconvulsive therapy (ECT) treatment used to treat serious and life-threatening mood disorders in clients who are unresponsive to pharmacotherapy

electroencephalogram (EEG) diagnostic test that records brain waves through electrodes attached to the scalp

electrolytes charged substances in the blood such as sodium, potassium, calcium, chloride, and phosphate

embolus blood clot carried in the bloodstream

emergency preparedness the ability to respond quickly and effectively to an unexpected event that may affect human health

emesis vomiting

emetic drug used to induce vomiting

emetic potential usually applied to antineoplastic agents; degree to which an agent is likely to trigger the vomiting centre in the medulla, resulting in nausea and vomiting

emphysema terminal lung disease characterized by permanent dilation of the alveoli

endocrine system body system that consists of various glands that secrete hormones

endogenous opioid chemical produced naturally within the body that decreases or eliminates pain; closely resembles the actions of morphine

endometriosis presence of endometrial tissue in non-uterine locations such as the pelvis and ovaries; common cause of infertility

endorphins a group of neurotransmitters that function as endogenous opioids or natural pain modifiers in the central nervous system (CNS)

endothelium inner lining of a blood vessel

endotoxins harmful non-proteins that are part of the normal cell wall of gram-negative bacteria

enteral nutrition nutrients supplied orally or by feeding tube

enteral route administration method in which drugs are given orally, including through nasogastric or gastrostomy tubes

enteric-coated having a hard, waxy coating designed to dissolve in the alkaline environment of the small intestine

enteric nervous system (ENS) network of neurons in the submucosa of the alimentary canal that has sensory and motor functions that regulate the gastrointestinal (GI) tract

enteroendocrine cells cells that secrete hormones that modify the digestive processes

enterohepatic recirculation recycling of drugs and other substances by the circulation of bile through the intestine and liver

enzyme induction process in which a drug changes the function of the hepatic microsomal enzymes and increases metabolic activity in the liver

epilepsy disorder of the central nervous system (CNS) characterized by seizures and/or convulsions

ergocalciferol activated form of vitamin D

ergosterol lipid substance in fungal cell membranes

erythema redness associated with skin irritation

erythrocytic stage phase in malaria during which infected red blood cells rupture, releasing merozoites and causing fever and chills

erythropoietin hormone secreted by the kidney that regulates the process of red blood cell formation, or erythropoiesis

esophageal reflux backward flow of stomach contents into the esophagus

ester type of chemical linkage found in some local anesthetics involving carbon and oxygen (-CO-O-)

estrogen class of steroid sex hormone secreted by the ovary

estrogen replacement therapy (ERT) a treatment for women who are post-menopausal or whose ovaries have been damaged or removed that involves taking the hormone estrogen on a regular basis to replace their own

ethics branch of philosophy that deals with distinguishing between right and wrong and the moral consequences of human actions

ethnic having a common history and similar genetic heritage

euphoria an intense sense of happiness and well-being

evaluating systematic, objective assessment of the effectiveness and impact of interventions

excoriation condition in which scratches that break the skin surface fill with blood or serous fluid to form crusty scales

excretion process of removing substances from the body

exocrine glands that excrete hormones to the epithelial surface

exophthalmos an outward bulging of the eyes

exotoxins proteins released by bacteria into surrounding tissues that have the ability to inactivate or kill host cells

expectorant drug used to increase bronchial secretions

exposure contact with an agent that is able to cause disease or injury such as a microbe, a chemical, or the radioactive source

external otitis inflammation of the outer ear; commonly called *swimmer's ear*

extracellular fluid (ECF) compartment body fluid lying outside of cells, which includes plasma and interstitial fluid

extrapyramidal signs (EPs) symptoms of acute dystonia, akathisia, parkinsonism, and tardive dyskinesia often caused by antipsychotic drugs

extrapyramidal system part of the central nervous system (CNS) that controls locomotion, complex muscular movements, and posture

extrinsic pathway activated in response to injury when blood leaks out of a vessel and enters tissue spaces; the pathway takes several seconds to complete

F

fat-soluble vitamins group of vitamins stored in the liver and fatty tissue that includes vitamins A, D, E, and K

febrile seizure tonic-clonic motor activity lasting 1 to 2 minutes with rapid return of consciousness that occurs in conjunction with elevated body temperature

ferritin one of two protein complexes that maintains iron stores inside cells (hemosiderin is the other protein complex)

fetal-placental barrier special anatomical structure that inhibits many chemicals and drugs from entering the fetus

fibrin insoluble protein formed from fibrinogen by the action of thrombin in the blood clotting process

fibrinogen blood protein that is converted to fibrin by the action of thrombin in the blood coagulation process

fibrinolysis removal of a blood clot

fight-or-flight response characteristic set of signs and symptoms produced when the sympathetic nervous system is activated

filtrate fluid in the nephron that was filtered by Bowman's capsule

first-dose phenomenon serious orthostatic hypotension that occurs with the initial doses of alpha$_1$-adrenergic blockers

first-pass effect mechanism whereby drugs are absorbed across the intestinal wall and enter the hepatic portal circulation

folic acid (folate) B vitamin that is a coenzyme in protein and nucleic acid metabolism

follicle-stimulating hormone (FSH) hormone secreted by the anterior pituitary gland that regulates sperm or egg production

follicular cell cell in the thyroid gland that secretes thyroid hormone

formulary list of drugs and drug recipes commonly used by pharmacists

Frank-Starling law the greater the degree of stretch on the myocardial fibres, the greater will be the force by which they contract

frequency distribution curve graphical representation that illustrates inter-individual variability in responses to drugs

fungi kingdom of organisms that includes mushrooms, yeasts, and moulds

G

gamma-aminobutyric acid (GABA) neurotransmitter in the central nervous system (CNS)

ganglion collection of neuron cell bodies located outside the central nervous system (CNS)

gastroesophageal reflux disease (GERD) condition characterized by regurgitation of stomach contents into the esophagus

gate control theory proposes a gating mechanism for the transmission of pain in the spinal cord

general anesthesia medically induced condition of unconsciousness and loss of sensation throughout the entire body

generalized anxiety disorder (GAD) difficult to control, excessive anxiety that lasts 6 months or more, focuses on a variety of life events, and interferes with normal day-to-day functions

generalized seizure seizure that travels throughout the entire brain

generic name non-proprietary name of a drug assigned by the government

genetic polymorphism change in enzyme structure and function due to mutation of the encoding gene

glaucoma a group of eye diseases characterized by increased intraocular pressure, leading to atrophy of the optic nerve and possibly blindness

glomerular filtration rate (GFR) the volume of water filtered through the Bowman's capsules per minute

glucagon pancreatic hormone that acts to increase blood glucose levels

glucocorticoids class of hormones secreted by the adrenal cortex that help the body to respond to stress

gluconeogenesis the production of new glucose from non-carbohydrate molecules

glutamate amino acid that is the most common neurotransmitter in the central nervous system (CNS)

glycogenolysis the process of glycogen breaking down

glycoprotein IIb/IIIa enzyme that binds fibrinogen and von Willebrand's factor to begin platelet aggregation and blood coagulation

goal any object or objective that the client or nurse seeks to attain or achieve

goiter refers to an increase in the size of the thyroid gland

gonadocorticoids sex hormones secreted by the adrenal cortex

gonadotropin-releasing hormone (GnRH) a hormone secreted by the hypothalamus that stimulates the secretion of follicle-stimulating hormone (FSH) and luteinizing hormone (LH)

gout metabolic disorder characterized by the accumulation of uric acid in the bloodstream or joint cavities

graded dose-response relationship between the client's response and different doses of a drug

grading process that examines potential cancer cells under a microscope and compares their appearance to normal parent cells

gram negative describes bacteria that do not retain a purple stain because they have an outer envelope

gram positive describes bacteria that stain purple because they have no outer envelope

Graves' disease syndrome caused by hypersecretion of thyroid hormone

growth fraction ratio of the number of replicating cells to resting cells in a tumour

growth hormone (GH) hormone that is produced and secreted by the anterior pituitary gland; also called somatotropin or somatropin

H

H⁺,K⁺-ATPase enzyme responsible for pumping acid to the mucosal surface of the stomach

H₁ receptor site located on smooth muscle cells in the bronchial tree and blood vessels that is stimulated by histamine to produce bronchodilation and vasodilation

H₂ receptor site located on cells of the digestive system that is stimulated by histamine to produce gastric acid

H₂-receptor antagonist drug that inhibits the effects of histamine at its receptors in the gastrointestinal (GI) tract

hallucination seeing, hearing, or feeling something that is not real

Hashimoto's thyroiditis an autoimmune disorder that is the most common cause of hypothyroidism

Health Canada federal department responsible for helping the people of Canada to maintain and improve their health

health care–associated infections (HAIs) infections acquired in a healthcare setting that are often resistant to common antibiotics

heart failure (HF) disease in which the heart muscle cannot contract with sufficient force to meet the body's metabolic needs

Helicobacter pylori bacterium associated with a large percentage of peptic ulcer disease

helminth type of flat, round, or segmented worm

hematopoiesis production and maturation of blood cells that occurs in red bone marrow; also called hemopoiesis

hematopoietic growth factors drugs that promote the formation of specific blood cells and enhance the ability of the immune system to reduce some of the myelosuppression caused by antineoplastic medications

hemophilia hereditary lack of a specific blood clotting factor

hemopoiesis process of blood cell production, which begins with primitive stem cells that reside in bone marrow

hemorrhagic stroke type of stroke caused by bleeding from a blood vessel in the brain

hemosiderin one of two protein complexes that maintains iron stores inside cells (ferritin is the other protein complex)

hemostasis the slowing or stopping of blood flow

hepatic microsomal enzyme system as it relates to pharmacotherapy, liver enzymes that inactivate drugs and accelerate their excretion; sometimes called the P450 system

hepatic portal system a network of venous vessels that collects blood draining from the stomach, small intestine, and most of the large intestine

hepatitis viral infection of the liver

herb plant with a soft stem that is used for healing or as a seasoning

high-alert medications drugs that have a high risk for causing significant harm to the client when used in error

high-density lipoprotein (HDL) lipid-carrying particle in the blood that contains high amounts of protein and lower amounts of cholesterol; considered to be "good" cholesterol

highly active antiretroviral therapy (HAART) drug therapy for human immunodeficiency virus (HIV) infection that includes high doses of multiple medications that are given concurrently

hippocampus part of the limbic system of the brain that is responsible for learning and memory

histamine chemical released by mast cells in response to an antigen that causes dilation of blood vessels, bronchoconstriction, tissue swelling, and itching

HIV-AIDS acronym for human immunodeficiency virus–acquired immune deficiency syndrome; characterized by profound immunosuppression that leads to opportunistic infections and malignancies not commonly found in clients with functioning immune defences

HMG-CoA reductase primary enzyme in the biochemical pathway for the synthesis of cholesterol

holistic viewing a person as an integrated biological, psychosocial, cultural, communicating whole, existing and functioning within the communal environment

hormone chemical secreted by endocrine glands that acts as a chemical messenger to affect homeostasis

hormone replacement therapy (HRT) drug therapy consisting of estrogen and progestin combinations that is used to treat symptoms associated with menopause

host flora normal microorganisms found in or on a client

household system of measurement older system of measurement using teaspoons, tablespoons, and cups

human immunodeficiency virus (HIV) the causative agent for acquired immune deficiency syndrome (AIDS)

hyperaldosteronism excessive secretion of aldosterone

hypercholesterolemia high levels of cholesterol in the blood

hyperemia increase in blood supply to a body part or tissue space causing swelling, redness, and pain

hyperglycemic effect the tendency of a drug or substance to cause an increase in blood glucose

hyperkalemia high potassium level in the blood

hyperlipidemia excess amount of lipids in the blood

hypernatremia high sodium level in the blood

hyperosmolar nonketotic coma (HNKC) life-threatening metabolic condition that occurs in people with type 2 diabetes

hypertension (HTN) high blood pressure

hypervitaminosis excess intake of vitamins

hypnotic drug that causes sleep

hypoaldosteronism lack of adequate aldosterone secretion

hypoglycemic effect the tendency of a drug or substance to cause a decrease in blood glucose

hypogonadism below normal secretion of the steroid sex hormones

hypokalemia low potassium level in the blood

hypomania characterized by the same symptoms as bipolar disorder, but they are less severe and do not cause impaired functioning

hyponatremia low sodium level in the blood

hypovolemic shock type of shock caused by loss of fluids such as occurs during hemorrhage, extensive burns, or severe vomiting or diarrhea

I

idiosyncratic response unpredictable and unexplained drug reaction

ileum third portion of the small intestine extending from the jejunum to the ileocecal valve

immunity ability to resist injury and infections

immunization process of disease prevention in which the body produces its own antibodies in response to initial exposure to antigens

immunomodulator general term referring to any drug or therapy that affects body defences

immunostimulants drugs that increase the ability of the immune system to fight infection and disease

immunosuppressant any drug, chemical, or physical agent that lowers the immune defence mechanisms of the body

implementing the step of the nursing process in which actual client care is provided

impotence inability to obtain or sustain an erection; also called *erectile dysfunction*

incubation period following the first exposure to an antigen, the time needed for the body to process the antigen and mount an effective response

indications the medical conditions for which a drug is approved

infancy period of childhood under the age of 1 year

infertility inability to become pregnant after at least 1 year of frequent, unprotected intercourse

inflammation nonspecific body defence that occurs in response to an injury or antigen

inflammatory bowel disease (IBD) disease characterized by the presence of ulcers in the distal portion of the small intestine (Crohn's disease) or mucosal erosions in the large intestine (ulcerative colitis)

influenza common viral infection; often called *flu*

ingestion the process of taking food into the body by mouth

innate body defences those defences that are present even before an infection occurs and that provide the first line of protection from pathogens

inotropic drug agent used to change the force of cardiac contractions; positive inotropes strengthen the force of the cardiac contractions, whereas negative inotropes weaken the force of cardiac contractions

inotropic agent drug or chemical that changes the force of contraction of the heart

insomnia inability to fall asleep or stay asleep

insulin pancreatic hormone that acts to decrease blood glucose levels

insulin resistance the condition in which normal amounts of insulin are inadequate to produce a normal insulin response from fat, muscle, and liver cells

insulin-like growth factor (IGF) a family of peptides that promote cartilage and bone growth

integrase an enzyme unique to human immunodeficiency virus (HIV) that incorporates the viral DNA into the host's chromosomes

interferon (IFN) type of cytokine secreted by T cells in response to antigens to protect uninfected cells

interleukin (IL) type of cytokine synthesized by lymphocytes, monocytes, macrophages, and certain other cells that enhances the capabilities of the immune system

intermittent claudication (IC) condition caused by insufficient blood flow to skeletal muscles in the lower limbs, resulting in ischemia of skeletal muscles and severe pain on walking, especially in calf muscles

intermittent feedings enteral feedings that are administered every 3 to 6 hours

International System of Units (SI) an internationally standardized system of units of measurement

intracellular fluid (ICF) compartment body fluid that is inside cells; accounts for about two-thirds of the total body water

intracellular parasite infectious microbe that lives inside host cells

intradermal (ID) administration method that delivers the drug into the dermis layer of the skin

intramuscular (IM) administration method that delivers the drug into specific muscles

intravenous (IV) administration method that delivers the drugs and fluids directly into the bloodstream

intrinsic factor chemical substance secreted by the parietal cells in the stomach that is essential for the absorption of vitamin B_{12}

intrinsic pathway coagulation pathway activated in response to injury; it takes several minutes to complete

invasiveness the ability of a pathogen to grow extremely rapidly and cause direct damage to surrounding tissues by virtue of sheer numbers

ionizing radiation radiation that is highly penetrating and can cause serious biological effects

irritable bowel syndrome (IBS) inflammatory disease of the small or large intestine, characterized by intense abdominal cramping and diarrhea

islets of Langerhans cell clusters in the pancreas responsible for the secretion of insulin and glucagon

K

kappa receptor type of opioid receptor

keratolytic action that promotes shedding of old skin

keto acid acidic waste product of lipid metabolism that lowers the pH of the blood

L

laxative drug that promotes defecation

lecithin phospholipid that is an important component of cell membranes

leprosy a chronic infection caused by *Mycobacterium leprae*

leukotriene chemical mediator of inflammation stored and released by mast cells with effects similar to those of histamine

libido interest in sexual activity

ligand any chemical that binds to a specific receptor site

limbic system area of the brain responsible for emotion, learning, memory, motivation, and mood

lipoatrophy decrease of subcutaneous fat at an insulin injection site, resulting in an indenture

lipodystrophy a disorder in which fat is redistributed in specific areas in the body

lipoprotein substance carrying lipids in the bloodstream that is composed of proteins bound to fat

liposome small sac of lipid designed to carry drugs inside it

loading dose comparatively large dose given at the beginning of treatment to rapidly obtain the therapeutic effect of a drug

local anesthesia loss of sensation to a limited part of the body without loss of consciousness

loop of Henle portion of the nephron between the proximal and distal tubules

low-density lipoprotein (LDL) lipid-carrying particle that contains relatively low amounts of protein and high amounts of cholesterol; considered to be "bad" cholesterol

low-molecular-weight heparin (LMWH) drug closely resembling heparin that inhibits blood clotting

luteinizing hormone (LH) secreted by the pituitary gland, triggers ovulation in the female and stimulates sperm production in the male

lymph nodes the principal lymphoid organs in the body

lymphatic system consists of a network of cells, vessels, and tissues that provide immune surveillance

M

macromineral inorganic compound needed by the body in amounts of 100 mg or more daily

maintenance dose dose that keeps the plasma drug concentration continuously in the therapeutic range

major depressive disorder a depressed mood lasting for a minimum of 2 weeks that is present for most of the day, every day, or almost every day

malaria tropical disease characterized by severe fever and chills caused by the protozoan *Plasmodium*

mania condition characterized by an expressive, impulsive, excitable, and overreactive nature

margin of safety (MOS) the amount of drug that is lethal to 1% of animals (LD1) divided by the amount of drug that produces a therapeutic effect in 99% of the animals (ED99)

mast cell connective tissue cell located in tissue spaces that releases histamine following injury

mastoiditis inflammation of the mastoid sinus

mechanism of action how a drug exerts its effects

median effective dose (ED_{50}) dose required to produce a specific therapeutic response in 50% of a group of people

median lethal dose (LD_{50}) often determined in preclinical trials, the dose of drug that will be lethal in 50% of a group of animals

median toxicity dose (TD_{50}) dose that will produce a given toxicity in 50% of a group of people

medication drug that is considered medically therapeutic

medication administration record (MAR) documentation of all pharmacotherapies received by the client

medication error any preventable event that may cause or lead to inappropriate medication use or client harm while the medication is in the control of the healthcare provider, client, or consumer

menopause period of time when females stop secreting estrogen and menstrual cycles cease

merozoite a body formed by segmentation and breaking up of a schizont that is capable of invading other corpuscles

metabolism total of all biochemical reactions in the body

metastasis travel of cancer cells from their original site to distant tissue

metered dose inhaler (MDI) device used to deliver a precise amount of drug to the respiratory system

methadone maintenance treatment of opioid dependence by using methadone

methylxanthine chemical derivative of caffeine

metric system most common system of drug measurement that uses grams and litres

microbial antagonism condition of various host flora in competition with each other for physical space and nutrients that helps to protect the host from being overrun by pathogenic organisms

micromineral (trace mineral) inorganic compound needed by the body in amounts of 20 mg or less daily

middle adulthood period of life from 40 to 65 years of age

migraine severe headache often preceded by auras that may include nausea and vomiting

milk-alkali syndrome syndrome caused by the administration of calcium carbonate antacids with milk or food containing vitamin D; symptoms include headache, urinary frequency, anorexia, nausea, and fatigue

mineralocorticoids hormones secreted by the adrenal glands that affect the secretion of sodium and water

minimum effective concentration amount of drug required to produce a therapeutic effect

miosis constriction of the pupil

miotic drug that causes pupil constriction

mitochondrial toxicity specific type of adverse effects resulting from a drug's toxic actions on mitochondria

monitored anesthesia care (MAC) use of sedatives, analgesics, and other low-dose drugs that allow clients to remain responsive and breathe without assistance

monoamine oxidase (MAO) enzyme that destroys norepinephrine in the nerve terminal

monoamine oxidase (MAO) inhibitor drug inhibiting monoamine oxidase, an enzyme that terminates the actions of neurotransmitters such as dopamine, norepinephrine, epinephrine, and serotonin

monoclonal antibody antibody produced by a single B cell that targets a single type of cell or receptor

mood disorder condition characterized by changes in mood such as clinical depression, emotional swings, or manic depression

mood stabilizer drug that moderates mood that is used to treat bipolar disorder and mania

mu receptor type of opioid receptor

mucolytic drug used to loosen thick mucus

mucosa inner lining of the alimentary canal that provides a surface area for the various acids, bases, and enzymes to break down food

mucositis inflammation of the epithelial lining of the digestive tract

muscarinic type of cholinergic receptor found in smooth muscle, cardiac muscle, and glands

muscarinic agonist drug that is selective for muscarinic receptors

muscarinic antagonists drugs that block receptors at cholinergic synapses in the parasympathetic nervous system and at a few target organs in the sympathetic nervous system

muscle spasm involuntary contractions of a muscle or group of muscles that become tightened, develop a fixed pattern of resistance, and result in a diminished level of functioning

mutation permanent, inheritable change to DNA

myasthenia gravis motor disorder caused by a destruction of nicotinic receptors on skeletal muscles and characterized by profound muscular fatigue

myasthenic crisis extreme muscular weakness and symptoms similar to those of cholinergic crisis; caused by abrupt discontinuation of medication for myasthenia gravis

mycoses diseases caused by fungi

mydriatic drug drug that causes pupil dilation

myocardial infarction (MI) ischemia and necrosis of cardiac muscle caused by a blood clot blocking a portion of a coronary artery

myocardial ischemia lack of blood supply to the myocardium due to a constriction or obstruction of a blood vessel

myocardium the muscular layer of the heart, responsible for its physical pumping action

myoclonic seizure seizure characterized by brief, sudden contractions of a group of muscles

myxedema condition caused by insufficient secretion of thyroid hormone

myxedema coma a life-threatening end-stage condition of hypothyroidism

N

nadir the lowest concentration of blood cells found after taking a drug that suppresses the bone marrow

narcotic natural or synthetic drug related to morphine; may be used as a broader legal term referring to hallucinogens, central nervous system (CNS) stimulants, marijuana, and other illegal drugs

narrow-spectrum antibiotic anti-infective that is effective against only one or a small number of organisms

National Emergency Stockpile System (NESS) the program within the Public Health Agency of Canada responsible for maintaining sufficient quantities of supplies to alleviate pain and suffering and to save the lives of Canadians and others affected by natural and human-caused disasters

natural health product (NHP) a product that does not require a prescription and is a vitamin, mineral, herbal remedy, homeopathic medicine, traditional Chinese medicine, or other traditional medicine; a probiotic; or another product such as an amino acid or essential fatty acid

nausea uncomfortable wave-like sensation that precedes vomiting

nebulizer device used to convert liquid drugs into a fine mist for the purpose of inhalation

negative feedback regulatory mechanism in homeostasis in which the first hormone in a pathway is shut off by the last hormone or product in the pathway

negative symptoms in schizophrenia, symptoms that subtract from normal behaviour, including a lack of interest, motivation, responsiveness, or pleasure in daily activities

neoadjuvant chemotherapy the administration of antineoplastic drugs before surgery or radiation therapy with the goal of shrinking a large tumour to a more manageable size

neoplasm tumour

nephron structural and functional unit of the kidney

nerve agent chemical used in warfare or by bioterrorists that can affect the central nervous system (CNS) and cause death

neurofibrillary tangle bundle of nerve fibres found in the brain of clients with Alzheimer's disease on autopsy

neurogenic shock type of shock resulting from brain or spinal cord injury

neuroleptic a drug that is also called antipsychotic and is used to treat psychosis

neuroleptic malignant syndrome (NMS) potentially fatal condition caused by certain antipsychotic medications characterized by an extremely high body temperature, drowsiness, changing blood pressure, irregular heartbeat, and muscle rigidity

neuromuscular blocker drug used to cause total muscle relaxation

neuron the primary functional cell in all portions of the nervous system; its purpose is to communicate messages through conduction of an action potential

neuropathic pain pain caused by injury to nerves and typically described as burning, shooting, or numbness

neurotransmitter a substance that, when released from the axon terminal of a presynaptic neuron, is capable of inhibiting or exciting a target cell

New Drug Submission (NDS) an application made by a drug manufacturer to Health Canada to authorize a safe, efficacious, and high-quality drug

nicotinic type of cholinergic receptor found in ganglia of both the sympathetic and the parasympathetic nervous systems

nicotinic agonist drug that selectively activates nicotinic receptors

nicotinic antagonists drugs that block receptors at cholinergic synapses in the ganglia or in the somatic nervous system at the neuromuscular junction

nit egg of the louse parasite

nitrogen mustard alkylating agent used to treat a variety of tumours

nociceptor receptor connected with nerves that receive and transmit pain signals to the spinal cord and brain

nociceptor pain pain caused by injury to tissues, producing either somatic pain (sharp, localized sensations) or visceral pain (described as generalized dull pain, throbbing, or aching)

nomogram chart used to plot a child's height and weight to determine body surface area

non-maleficence ethical obligation to not harm the client

non–rapid eye movement (NREM) sleep phase of sleep during which respirations slow, heart rate and blood pressure decrease, oxygen consumption by muscles decreases, and urine formation decreases

nonspecific cellular response drug action that is independent of cellular receptors and not associated with other mechanisms, such as changing the permeability of cellular membranes, depressing membrane excitability, or altering the activity of cellular pumps

norepinephrine (NE) primary neurotransmitter in the sympathetic nervous system

nosocomial infection infection acquired in a healthcare setting such as a hospital, physician's office, or nursing home

Notice of Compliance (NOC) certifies that a drug complies with the *Food and Drugs Act* and *Regulations* and may be marketed in Canada

nursing diagnosis clinical-based judgment about the client and his or her response to health and illness

O

objective data information gathered through physical assessment, laboratory tests, and other diagnostic sources

obsessive-compulsive disorder (OCD) recurrent, intrusive thoughts or repetitive behaviours that interfere with normal activities or relationships

octreotide a synthetic hormone intended to mimic the function of the human somatostatin hormone; as such, it inhibits the release of growth hormone, glucagon, and insulin

older adulthood period of life over age 65

oligospermia presence of less than 20 million sperm in an ejaculate

oncogene gene responsible for the conversion of normal cells into cancer cells

oncotic pressure a form of osmotic pressure exerted by proteins in blood plasma that tends to pull water into the circulatory system

open-angle glaucoma chronic, simple glaucoma caused by hindered outflow of aqueous humour from the anterior chamber of the eye

opiate substance closely related to morphine extracted from the poppy plant

opioid substance obtained from the unripe seeds of the poppy plant; natural or synthetic morphine-like substance

orthostatic hypotension fall in blood pressure that occurs when changing position from recumbent to upright

osmolality number of dissolved particles or solutes in 1 kg (1 L) of water

osmosis process by which water moves from areas of low solute concentration (low osmolality) to areas of high solute concentration (high osmolality)

osmotic pressure creates a force that moves substances between body compartments or across a membrane

osteoarthritis (OA) disorder characterized by degeneration of joints, particularly the fingers, spine, hips, and knees

osteomalacia rickets in children; caused by vitamin D deficiency and characterized by softening of the bones without alteration of basic bone structure

osteoporosis condition in which bones lose mass and become brittle and susceptible to fracture

otitis media inflammation of the middle ear

ototoxity drug-induced hearing impairment

outcome objective measure of goals

ovulation release of an egg by the ovary

oxytocics agents used to stimulate uterine contractions

P

Paget's disease disorder of bone formation and resorption characterized by weak, enlarged, and deformed bones

palliation form of cancer chemotherapy intended to alleviate symptoms rather than cure the disease

pancreatitis inflammation of the pancreas that may be acute or chronic

panic disorder anxiety disorder characterized by intense feelings of immediate apprehension, fearfulness, terror, or impending doom accompanied by increased autonomic nervous system activity

parafollicular cell cell in the thyroid gland that secretes calcitonin

paranoia having an extreme suspicion and delusion that one is being followed and that others are trying to inflict harm

parasympathetic nervous system portion of the autonomic nervous system that is active during periods of rest and that results in the rest or relaxation response

parenteral nutrition nutrients administered via a route other than ingestion

parenteral route administration method in which the drug is delivered via a needle into the skin layers

parietal cell cell in the stomach mucosa that secretes hydrochloric acid

parkinsonism symptoms of tremor, muscle rigidity, stooped posture, and a shuffling gait

paroxysmal supraventricular tachycardia (PSVT) occurs when episodes of atrial tachycardia alternate with periods of normal rhythm; also called paroxysmal atrial tachycardia (PAT)

partial agonist medication that produces a weaker, or less efficacious, response than an agonist

partial (focal) seizure seizure that starts on one side of the brain and travels a short distance before stopping

partial parenteral nutrition a parenteral solution that lacks an essential element, usually fats or lipids

passive immunity immune defence that lasts 2 to 3 weeks; obtained by administering antibodies

passive transport the movement of molecules from high to low concentration with no energy input

patent protection a guaranteed period of market exclusivity given to the manufacturer of a new drug

pathogen organism capable of causing disease

pathogenicity ability of an organism to cause disease in humans

pediculicide medication that kills lice

pegylation process that attaches polyethylene glycol (PEG) to an interferon to extend its pharmacological activity

pellagra deficiency of niacin

penicillin-binding protein a protein that binds penicillin

peptic ulcer erosion of the mucosa in the alimentary canal, most commonly in the stomach and duodenum

peptidoglycan substance containing sugars bound to peptides that is only found in bacteria

percutaneous transluminal coronary angioplasty (PTCA) procedure by which a balloon-shaped catheter is used to compress fatty plaque against an arterial wall for the purpose of restoring normal blood flow

perfusion blood flow through a tissue or organ

peripheral edema swelling in the limbs, particularly the feet and ankles, due to an accumulation of interstitial fluid

peripheral nervous system division of the nervous system containing all nervous tissue outside the central nervous system (CNS), including the autonomic nervous system

peripheral resistance amount of friction encountered by blood as it travels through the vessels

peripheral vein total parenteral nutrition delivery system used when a central venous line cannot be accessed or when it is not appropriate for the client

peripherally inserted central catheter (PICC) line a central catheter that is threaded into the vena cava for administration of chemotherapy

peristalsis involuntary wave-like contraction of smooth muscle lining the alimentary canal

pernicious (megaloblastic) anemia type of anemia usually caused by lack of secretion of intrinsic factor

pH measure of the acidity or alkalinity of a solution

phagocytes cells that engulf and destroy pathogens and other foreign substances

pharmacodynamics study of how the body responds to drugs

pharmacogenetics area of pharmacology that examines the role of genetics in drug response

pharmacokinetics study of how drugs are handled by the body

pharmacological classification method for organizing drugs on the basis of their mechanism of action

pharmacology study of medicines; discipline pertaining to how drugs improve or maintain health

pharmacotherapy (pharmacotherapeutics) treatment or prevention of disease by means of drugs

pheochromocytoma a tumour, usually benign, arising from the adrenal medulla that is characterized by excessive secretion of catecholamines

phobia fearful feelings attached to a situation or object such as snakes, spiders, crowds, or heights

phosphodiesterase enzyme in muscle cells that cleaves phosphodiester bonds; its inhibition increases myocardial contractility

phospholipid type of lipid that contains two fatty acids, a phosphate group, and a chemical backbone of glycerol

physical dependence condition of experiencing unpleasant withdrawal symptoms when a substance is discontinued

placenta organ that allows for nutrition and gas exchange between the mother and fetus

planning linking strategies, or interventions, to established goals and outcomes

plaque fatty material that builds up in the lining of blood vessels and may lead to hypertension, stroke, myocardial infarction, or angina

plasma cell cell derived from B lymphocytes that produces antibodies

plasma half-life ($t_{1/2}$) length of time required for a drug to decrease its concentration in the plasma by one-half after administration

plasmin enzyme formed from plasminogen that dissolves blood clots

plasminogen protein that prevents fibrin clot formation; precursor of plasmin

pneumonic plague life-threatening infectious lung disease that occurs after breathing *Yersinia pestis*, a bacterium found on rodents and their fleas that is responsible for the bubonic plague

polyclonal antibodies contain a wide mixture of different antibodies that attack the T cells or T-cell receptors

polyene antifungal class of drugs containing amphotericin B and nystatin

polypharmacy the taking of multiple drugs concurrently

positive symptoms in schizophrenia, symptoms that add on to normal behaviour, including hallucinations, delusions, and a disorganized thought or speech pattern

post-antibiotic effect antimicrobial activity that continues for a time after discontinuation of a drug

posterior pituitary gland (neurohypophysis) consists of nervous tissue and is an extension of the hypothalamus that secretes antidiuretic hormone and oxytocin

postsynaptic neuron in a synapse, the nerve that has receptors for the neurotransmitter

post-traumatic stress disorder (PTSD) type of anxiety that develops in response to re-experiencing a previous life event that was psychologically traumatic

potassium ion channel pathway in a plasma membrane through which potassium ions enter and leave

potency strength of a drug at a specified concentration or dose

preclinical investigation procedure implemented after a drug has been licensed for public use, designed to provide information on use and on occurrence of side effects

preload degree of stretch of the cardiac muscle fibres just before they contract

prenatal preceding birth

preschool child child from 3 to 5 years of age

presynaptic neuron nerve that releases the neurotransmitter into the synaptic cleft when stimulated by an action potential

PRN order (Latin: *pro re nata*) order for medication to be administered as required by the client's condition

prodrug drug that becomes more active after it is metabolized

progesterone hormone secreted by the corpus luteum and placenta that is responsible for building up the uterine lining in the second half of the menstrual cycle and during pregnancy

prostaglandins class of local hormones that promote local inflammation and pain when released by cells in the body

protease viral enzyme that is responsible for the final assembly of the human immunodeficiency virus (HIV) virions

prothrombin blood protein that is converted to thrombin in blood coagulation

prothrombin activator enzyme in the coagulation cascade that converts prothrombin to thrombin; also called *prothrombinase*

prothrombin time (PT) blood test used to determine the time needed for plasma to clot for the regulation of warfarin dosage

proton pump inhibitor drug that inhibits the enzyme H^+,K^+-ATPase

prototype drug well-understood model drug to which other drugs in a pharmacological class may be compared

protozoan single-celled animal

provirus stage of a virus in which the viral DNA integrates into the host chromosome

provitamin inactive chemical that is converted to a vitamin in the body

proximal tubule portion of the nephron that collects filtrate from Bowman's capsule

pruritus itching associated with dry, scaly skin

pseudomembranous colitis (PMC) caused by *Clostridium difficile*, a rare though potentially severe disorder resulting from therapy with tetracyclines and other classes of antibiotics

pseudo-parkinsonism symptoms of parkinsonism that are drug induced

psoralen drug used along with phototherapy for the treatment of psoriasis and other severe skin disorders

psychedelic substance that alters perception of reality

psychological dependence intense craving for a drug that drives people to continue drug abuse

psychology science that deals with normal and abnormal mental processes and their impact on behaviour

psychosis a mental disorder in which there is a loss of contact with reality

pulmonary embolism condition that occurs when a venous clot dislodges, migrates to the pulmonary vessels, and blocks arterial circulation to the lungs

Purkinje fibres electrical conduction pathway leading from the bundle branches to all portions of the ventricles

R

rapid eye movement (REM) sleep stage of sleep characterized by quick, scanning movements of the eyes

Raynaud's disease vasospasms of vessels serving the fingers and toes that can lead to intermittent pain and cyanosis of the digits

reabsorption movement of filtered substances from the kidney tubule back into the blood

rebound congestion condition of hypersecretion of mucus following use of intranasal sympathomimetics

rebound insomnia increased sleeplessness that occurs when long-term antianxiety or hypnotic medication is discontinued

receptor structural component of a cell to which a drug binds in a dose-related manner to produce a response

red-man syndrome rash on the upper body caused by certain anti-infectives

reflex tachycardia temporary increase in heart rate that occurs when blood pressure falls

refractory period time during which the myocardial cells rest and are not able to contract

regional anesthesia similar to local anesthesia except that it encompasses a larger body area, such as an entire limb

renal failure occurs when the kidneys are no longer able to adequately filter and excrete urine and serum creatinine levels increase

renin-angiotensin-aldosterone system (RAAS) series of enzymatic steps by which the body raises blood pressure

replacement therapy hormones administered to clients who are unable to secrete sufficient quantities of their own endogenous hormones

repolarization return of a negative resting membrane potential to the cell

respiration exchange of oxygen and carbon dioxide in the lungs; also the process of deriving energy from metabolic reactions

rest-and-digest response signs and symptoms produced when the parasympathetic nervous system is activated

reticular activating system (RAS) part of the brain responsible for sleeping and wakefulness and for performing an alerting function for the cerebral cortex; includes the reticular formation, hypothalamus, and part of the thalamus

reticular formation portion of the brain affecting awareness and wakefulness

retinoid compound resembling vitamin A used in the treatment of severe acne and psoriasis

reverse cholesterol transport process by which cholesterol is transported away from body tissues to the liver

reverse transcriptase viral enzyme that converts RNA to DNA

Reye's syndrome potentially fatal complication of infection associated with acetylsalicylic acid (ASA) use in children

rhabdomyolysis breakdown of muscle fibres usually due to muscle trauma or ischemia

rheumatoid arthritis (RA) systemic autoimmune disorder characterized by inflammation of multiple joints

rhinophyma reddened, bulbous, irregular swelling of the nose

risk–benefit ratio determination of whether the risks from a drug outweigh the potential benefits received by taking the medication

rosacea chronic skin disorder characterized by clusters of papules on the face

S

salicylism poisoning due to acetylsalicylic acid (ASA) and ASA-like drugs

scabicide drug that kills scabies mites

schizoaffective disorder psychosis with symptoms of both schizophrenia and mood disorders

schizophrenia psychosis characterized by abnormal thoughts and thought processes, withdrawal from other people and the outside environment, and apparent preoccupation with one's own mental state

school-aged child child from 6 to 12 years of age

sclerosing abnormal tissue hardening of the veins

scurvy deficiency of vitamin C

seborrhea skin condition characterized by overactivity of oil glands

second messenger chemical in a cascade of biochemical events that initiates a drug's action by either stimulating or inhibiting a normal activity of the cell

secretion in the kidney, movement of substances from the blood into the tubule after filtration has occurred

sedative substance that depresses the central nervous system (CNS) to cause drowsiness or sleep

sedative-hypnotic drug with the ability to produce a calming effect at lower doses while having the ability to induce sleep at higher doses

seizure symptom of epilepsy characterized by abnormal neuronal discharges within the brain

selective estrogen receptor modulator (SERM) drug that produces an action similar to estrogen in body tissues; used for the treatment of osteoporosis in postmenopausal women

selective serotonin reuptake inhibitor (SSRI) drug that selectively inhibits the reuptake of serotonin into nerve terminals; used mostly for depression

selective toxicity a desired feature of antibiotics; selectively attacking only the pathogenic bacteria makes them ideal and minimizes the host's adverse side effects; it depends on either the presence of a receptor required for drug attachment or inhibition of biochemical events essential to the bacteria but not to the host

septic shock type of shock caused by severe infection in the bloodstream

serotonin a natural neurotransmitter that is found in high concentrations in the hypothalamus, limbic system, medulla, and spinal cord

serotonin syndrome (SES) set of signs and symptoms associated with overmedication with antidepressants that includes altered mental status, fever, sweating, and lack of muscular coordination

shock condition in which there is inadequate blood flow to meet the body's metabolic needs

short stature height below the fifth percentile for age and gender, or more than two standard deviations below the mean (average) for age and gender

side effects types of drug effects that are less serious than adverse effects, are predictable, and may occur even at therapeutic doses

single order medication that is to be given only once, and at a specific time, such as a preoperative order

sinoatrial (SA) node pacemaker of the heart located in the wall of the right atrium that controls the basic heart rate

sinus rhythm number of beats per minute normally generated by the sinoatrial (SA) node

situational anxiety anxiety experienced by people faced with a stressful environment

sociology study of human behaviour within the context of groups and societies

sodium ion channel pathway in a plasma membrane through which sodium ions enter and leave

somatic nervous system division of the nervous system that provides voluntary control over skeletal muscle

somatostatin synonym for growth hormone inhibiting factor that is released from the hypothalamus

Somogyi phenomenon rapid decrease in blood glucose that stimulates the release of hormones (epinephrine, cortisol, glucagon), resulting in an elevated morning blood glucose

spasticity inability of opposing muscle groups to move in a coordinated manner

Special Access Program (SAP) Canadian program that provides for drugs that are not generally available to be used under certain conditions

specialty supplements non-herbal dietary products used to enhance a wide variety of body functions

spermicides agents that kill sperm

spirituality capacity to love, to convey compassion and empathy, to give and forgive, to enjoy life, and to find peace of mind and fulfillment in living

SSRI discontinuation syndrome symptoms that occur in some individuals when selective serotonin reuptake inhibitor (SSRI) therapy is stopped

stable angina type of angina that occurs in a predictable pattern, usually relieved by rest

staging the process of determining where a cancer is located and the extent of its invasion

standards of care skills and learning commonly possessed by members of a profession

standards of professional practice criteria established by a profession to guide safe and competent actions

standing order order written in advance of a situation that is to be carried out under specific circumstances

STAT order order for a medication that is needed immediately and is to be given only once

status epilepticus condition characterized by repeated seizures or one prolonged seizure attack that continues for at least 30 minutes

steatorrhea stool containing high content of fat, as occurs in some malabsorption syndromes

stem cell cell that resides in the bone marrow and is capable of maturing into any type of blood cell

steroid type of lipid that consists of four rings that comprises certain hormones and drugs

sterol nucleus ring structure common to all steroids

stroke *see* cerebrovascular accident (CVA)

stroke volume amount of blood pumped out by a ventricle in a single beat

subcutaneous (SC) administration method in which medication is delivered beneath the skin

subjective data information gathered regarding what a client states or perceives

sublingual (SL) administration method in which medication is placed under the tongue and allowed to dissolve slowly

substance abuse self-administration of a drug that does not conform to the medical or social norms of the client's given culture or society

substance P neurotransmitter within the spinal cord that is involved in the neural transmission of pain

substantia nigra region in the brain where dopamine is synthesized that is responsible for regulation of unconscious muscle movement

superinfection new infection caused by an organism different from the one causing the initial infection; usually a side effect of anti-infective therapy

supraventricular located above the ventricle

surgical anesthesia stage 3 of anesthesia, where most major surgery occurs

sustained-release tablets or capsules designed to dissolve slowly over an extended time

sympathetic nervous system portion of the autonomic system that is active during periods of stress and results in the fight-or-flight response

sympathomimetics drugs that activate adrenergic receptors in the sympathetic nervous system

synapse junction between two neurons consisting of a presynaptic nerve, a synaptic cleft, and a postsynaptic nerve

synaptic transmission process by which a neurotransmitter reaches receptors to regenerate the action potential

synergistic effect type of drug interaction in which two drugs produce an effect that is much greater than would be expected from simply adding the two individual drugs' responses

systolic blood pressure blood pressure during the contraction phase of heart activity

T

tachydysrhythmias disorders exhibiting a heart rate greater than 100 beats/minute

tardive dyskinesia unusual tongue and face movements such as lip-smacking and worm-like motions of the tongue that occur during pharmacotherapy with certain antipsychotics

target cells cells affected by hormones

targeted therapy drug that has been specifically engineered to attack cancer-specific antigens, such as those on cancer cells

taxoid antineoplastic drug obtained from the Pacific yew tree

T cell type of lymphocyte that is essential for the cell-mediated immune response

telomerase an enzyme contained in certain human stem cells that can lengthen the DNA chains and allow continued replication

telomeres regions in chromosomes that prevent the vital sequences of DNA from being destroyed each time a cell divides

10 rights of drug administration client's rights that the nurse must fulfill when administering medications; failure to meet these rights is a professional liability

tension headache common type of head pain caused by stress and relieved by non-narcotic analgesics

teratogen drug or other agent that causes developmental birth defects

tetrahydrocannabinol (THC) active chemical in marijuana

therapeutic classification method for organizing drugs on the basis of their clinical usefulness

therapeutic drug monitoring practice of monitoring plasma levels of drugs that have low safety profiles and using the data to predict drug action or toxicity

therapeutic index (TI) ratio of a drug's median lethal dose (LD_{50}) to its median effective dose (ED_{50})

therapeutic range dosage range or serum concentration that achieves the desired drug effects

therapeutics branch of medicine concerned with the treatment of disease and suffering

three checks of drug administration in conjunction with the 10 rights of drug administration, these ascertain client safety and drug effectiveness

threshold potential an action potential triggered by the membrane potential during myocardial electrical conduction

thrombin enzyme that causes clotting by converting the plasma fibrinogen to fibrin strands

thrombocytopenia reduction in the number of circulating platelets

thromboembolic disorder condition in which the client develops blood clots

thrombolytic drug used to dissolve existing blood clots

thrombopoietin hormone produced by the kidneys that controls megakaryocyte activity

thrombotic stroke type of stroke caused by a blood clot blocking an artery in the brain

thrombus blood clot obstructing a vessel

thyroid crisis a rare, life-threatening form of thyrotoxicosis; also called thyroid storm

thyroid storm a rare, life-threatening form of thyrotoxicosis; also called thyroid crisis

thyroid-stimulating hormone (TSH) hormone secreted by the anterior pituitary when stimulated by thyrotropin-releasing hormone

thyroid-stimulating immunoglobulins (TSI) stimulate the thyroid gland in Graves' disease

thyrotoxicosis an acute condition caused by very high levels of circulating thyroid hormone

thyrotropin-releasing hormone (TRH) hormone secreted by the hypothalamus when blood levels of thyroid hormone are low

thyroxine (T_4) thyroid hormone that is synthesized from the amino acid tyrosine and four atoms of iodine

thyroxine-binding globulin (TBG) a plasma protein produced in the liver

tissue plasminogen activator (tPA) natural enzyme and a drug that dissolves blood clots

tocolytic drug used to inhibit uterine contractions

tocopherol generic name for vitamin E

toddlerhood period of childhood from 1 to 3 years of age

tolerance process of adapting to a drug over a period of time and subsequently requiring higher doses to achieve the same effect

tonic spasm single, prolonged muscular contraction

tonic-clonic seizure seizure characterized by intense jerking motions and loss of consciousness

tonicity ability of a solution to cause a change in water movement across a membrane due to osmotic forces

tonometry technique for measuring intraocular tension and pressure

topoisomerase I enzyme that assists in the repair of DNA damage

torsades de pointes type of ventricular tachycardia that is characterized by rates between 200 and 250 beats/minute and "twisting of the points" of the QRS complex on the electrocardiogram (ECG)

total parenteral nutrition (TPN) nutrition provided through a peripheral or central vein

toxic concentration level of drug that will result in serious adverse effects

toxicology the study of poisoning

toxoid substance that has been chemically modified to remove its harmful nature but is still able to elicit an immune response in the body

trade (proprietary or brand) name name of a drug assigned by the manufacturer; also called the *brand name* or *product name*

transferrin protein complex that transports iron to the sites in the body where it is needed

transplant rejection reaction of the immune system in which it recognizes a transplanted tissue as being foreign and attacks it

tricyclic antidepressant (TCA) class of drugs used in the pharmacotherapy of depression

triglyceride type of lipid that contains three fatty acids and a chemical backbone of glycerol

triiodothyronine (T$_3$) thyroid hormone that is synthesized from the amino acid tyrosine and three atoms of iodine

tropic hormones ability of the anterior pituitary gland hormones to regulate the secretory actions of other endocrine glands

tubercle cavity-like lesion in the lung characteristic of infection by *Mycobacterium tuberculosis*

tularemia serious infectious disease found in rodents, rabbits, and hares that is caused by the organism *Francisella tularensis*

tumour abnormal swelling or mass

type 1 diabetes mellitus (DM) metabolic disease characterized by hyperglycemia and caused by a lack of secretion of insulin by the pancreas

type 2 diabetes mellitus (DM) chronic metabolic disease caused by insufficient secretion of insulin by the pancreas and a lack of sensitivity of insulin receptors

tyramine form of the amino acid tyrosine that is found in foods such as cheese, beer, wine, and yeast products

U

ulcerative colitis inflammatory bowel disease of the colon

undernutrition lack of adequate nutrition to meet the metabolic demands of the body

unit (U) one of anything

unstable angina severe angina that occurs frequently and is not relieved by rest

upregulation process by which cells create more receptors on their surface to capture hormone molecules

urinalysis diagnostic test that examines urine for the presence of blood cells, proteins, pH, specific gravity, ketones, glucose, and microorganisms

V

vaccination (immunization) using a vaccine or toxoid to prevent disease

variant angina chest pain that is caused by acute spasm of the coronary arteries rather than by physical or emotional exertion

vasomotor centre area of the medulla that controls baseline blood pressure

venous return the volume of blood returning to the heart from the veins

ventilation process by which air is moved into and out of the lungs

very-low–density lipoprotein (VLDL) lipid-carrying particle that is converted to low-density lipoprotein (LDL) in the liver

vesicants agents that can cause serious tissue injury if they escape from an artery or vein during an infusion or injection; many antineoplastics are vesicants

vestibular apparatus portion of the inner ear responsible for the sense of position

vinca alkaloid chemical obtained from the periwinkle plant that has antineoplastic activity

viral load a measurement of human immunodeficiency virus (HIV) RNA levels in the blood that provides an estimate of how rapidly the virus is replicating

virilization appearance of masculine secondary sex characteristics

virion virus particle capable of causing an infection

virulence severity of disease that a pathogen is able to cause

virus non-living particle containing nucleic acid that is able to cause disease

vitamin organic compound required by the body in small amounts

vitiligo milk-white areas of depigmented skin

vomiting centre area in the medulla that controls the vomiting reflex

von Willebrand's disease (vWD) decrease in quantity or quality of von Willebrand factor (vWF), which acts as a carrier of factor VIII and has a role in platelet aggregation

W

water-soluble vitamins group of vitamins stored briefly in the body and then excreted in the urine, including the C and B-complex vitamins

withdrawal physical signs of discomfort associated with the discontinuation of an abused substance

withdrawal syndrome symptoms that result when a client discontinues taking a substance upon which he or she was dependent

Y

young adulthood period of life from 18 to 40 years of age

Z

Zollinger-Ellison syndrome disorder of excess acid secretion in the stomach, resulting in peptic ulcer disease

Selected Bibliography and References

General References

Adams, M. P., Holland, L. N., Bostwick, P. M., & King, S. L. (2010). *Pharmacology for nurses: A pathophysiologic approach* (Canadian ed.). Toronto, ON: Pearson.

Adams, M. P., & Urban, C. (2016). *Pharmacology: Connections for nursing practice* (3rd ed.). Upper Saddle River, NJ: Pearson.

Beers, M. H., & Berkow, R. (Eds.). (2011). *Merck manual: Diagnoses and therapy* (19th ed.). Whitehouse Station, NJ: Merck & Co.

Bruntun, L., Chabner, A., & Knollmann, B. (Eds.). (2011). *Goodman & Gilman's the pharmacological basis of therapeutics* (12th ed.). New York, NY: McGraw-Hill.

Copstead, L. C., & Banasik, J. L. (2013). *Pathophysiology* (5th ed.). St. Louis, MO: Elsevier Canada.

Deglin, J. H., & Vallerand, A. H. (2015). *Davis's drug guide for nurses* (14th ed.). Philadelphia, PA: Davis.

Epocrates Online. (2016). https://online.epocrates.com/rxmain

Health Canada. (2016). *Drug product database.* Retrieved from http://www.hc-sc.gc.ca/dhp-mps/prodpharma/databasdon/index-eng.php

Health Canada. (2016). *MedEffect.* Retrieved from http://www.hc-sc.gc.ca/dhp-mps/medeff/index-eng.php

Herdman, T. H. (Ed.). (2012). *NANDA international nursing diagnoses: Definitions and classification, 2012–2014.* Oxford, UK: Wiley-Blackwell.

Hogan, M. (2012). *Comprehensive review for NCLEX-RN: Reviews & rationales* (2nd ed.). Upper Saddle River, NJ: Pearson Education.

Institute for Safe Medication Practices. (2016). ISMP Medication Safety Alert! Nurse Advise-ERR. Retrieved from http://www.ismp.org/NEWSLETTERS/nursing/default.aspx

Krogh, D. (2011). *Biology: A guide to the natural world* (5th ed.). Indianapolis, IN: Pearson Education.

Lippincott's NCLEX-RN PassPoint, powered by PrepU. (2013). http://www.lww.com/Product/9781469809359

Marieb, E. N., & Hoehn, K. (2014). *Human anatomy & physiology* (10th ed.). Upper Saddle River, NJ: Prentice Hall.

Mulvihill, M. L., Zelman, P., Holdaway, P., Tompary, E., & Turchany, J. (2006). *Human diseases: A systemic approach* (6th ed.). Upper Saddle River, NJ: Prentice Hall.

Neal, M. J. (2015). *Medical pharmacology at a glance* (8th ed.). Oxford, UK: Blackwell.

Silverhorn, D. U. (2015). *Human physiology: An integrated approach* (global ed.). San Francisco, CA: Benjamin Cummings.

Statistics Canada. (2016). http://www.statcan.gc.ca

Chapter 1: Introduction to Pharmacology and Drug Regulations in Canada

Canada. Controlled Drug and Substances Act, S.C. 1996, c. 19.

Canada. Government Organization Act, R.S.C. 2000, c. G-10.

Canada. Health Professions Act, R.S.C. 2000, c. H-7.

Canada. Regulations Amending the Marihuana Medical Access Regulations (2013). Retrieved from http://lois-laws.justice.gc.ca/eng/regulations/SOR-2013-119/index.html

Health Canada. (2005). *Meeting notes: Canada's research-based pharmaceutical companies (Rx&D) and the Therapeutic Products Directorate (TPD).* Retrieved from http://www.hc-sc.gc.ca/dhpmps/alt_formats/hpfb-dgpsa/pdf/prodpharma/2005-03-21_e.pdf

Health Canada. (2008). *Drug products.* Retrieved from http://www.hc-sc.gc.ca/dhp-mps/prodpharma/databasdon/index-eng.php

Marra, C. A., Lynd, L. D., Anis, A. H., & Esdaile, J. M. (2006). Approval process and access to prescription drugs in Canada. *Arthritis Care & Research, 55*(1), 9–11.

Rawson, N. S., & Kaitin, K. I. (2003). Canadian and US drug approval times and safety considerations. *Annals of Pharmacotherapy, 37*, 1403–1408.

Chapter 2: Drug Classes and Schedules in Canada

Brass, E. P. (2001). Drug therapy: Changing the status of drugs from prescription to over-the-counter availability. *New England Journal of Medicine, 345*, 810–816.

Canada. Controlled Drug and Substances Act, S.C. 1996, c. 19.

Canada. Regulations Amending the Marihuana Medical Access Regulations (2013). Retrieved from http://lois-laws.justice.gc.ca/eng/regulations/SOR-2013-119/index.html

Morgan, S., Grootendorst, P., Lexchin, J., Cunningham, C., & Greyson, D. (2011). The cost of drug development: A systematic review. *Health Policy, 100*, 4–17.

World Health Organization. (1997). *Guidelines on the use of international nonproprietary names (INNs) for pharmaceutical substances.* Retrieved from http://www.who.int/medicines/services/inn/en/

Chapter 3: Pharmacokinetics

Amur, S., Zineh, I., Abernethy, D. R., Huang, S., & Lesko, L. J. (2010). Pharmacogenomics and adverse drug reactions. *Personalized Medicine, 7*, 633–642. doi:10.2217/pme.10.63

Bauer, L. A. (2011). Clinical pharmacokinetics and pharmacodynamics. In J. T. DiPiro, R. L. Talbert, G. C. Yee, G. R. Matzke, B. G. Wells, & L. M. Posey (Eds.), *Pharmacotherapy: A pathophysiology approach* (8th ed., pp. 12–35). New York, NY: McGraw-Hill.

Buxton, I. L., & Benet, L. Z. (2011). Pharmacokinetics: The dynamics of drug absorption, distribution, action and elimination. In L. L. Brunton, B. A. Chabner, & B. C. Knollman (Eds.), *The pharmacological basis of therapeutics* (12th ed., pp. 17–40). New York, NY: McGraw-Hill.

Canadian Institute for Health Information (CIHI). (2011). *Adverse drug reaction–related hospitalizations among seniors, 2006 to 2011.* Retrieved from https://secure.cihi.ca/estore/productFamily.htm?locale=en&pf=PFC2128&lang=en&media=0

Hirani, J. J., Rathod, D. A., & Vadalia, K. R. (2009). Orally disintegrating tablets: A review. *Tropical Journal of Pharmaceutical Research, 8*, 161–172.

Monster, T. B. M., de Jong, P. E., & de Jong-van den Berg, L. T. W. (2003). Drug-induced renal function impairment: A population-based survey. *Pharmacoepidemiology and Drug Safety, 12*(2), 135–143.

Scott, G. N., & Elmer, G.W. (2002). Update on natural product–drug interactions. *American Journal of Health-System Pharmacy, 59*(4), 339–347.

Shargell, L., Yu, A., & Wu-Pong, S. (2012). *Applied biopharmaceutics & pharmacokinetics* (6th ed.). Blacklick, OH: McGraw-Hill.

Thames, G. (2004). Drug forum: Making pharmacokinetics clinically useful. *Gastroenterology Nursing, 27*(2), 74–75.

Chapter 4: Pharmacodynamics

Carter, S. M. (2012). *Glucose-6-phosphate dehydrogenase deficiency.* Retrieved from http://emedicine.medscape.com/article/200390-overview

Evans, W. E., & McLeod, H. (2003). Pharmacogenomics—Drug disposition, drug targets, and side effects. *New England Journal of Medicine, 348,* 538–549.

Gandhi, M., Aweeka, F., Greenblatt, R. M., & Blaschke, T. F. (2004). Sex differences in pharmacokinetics and pharmacodynamics. *Annual Review of Pharmacology and Toxicology, 44*(1), 499–523.

Neal, M. J. (2015). *Medical pharmacology at a glance* (8th ed.). Oxford, UK: Blackwell.

Weng, L., Zhang, L., Peng, Y., & Huang, R. S. (2013). Pharmacogenetics and pharmacogenomics: A bridge to individualized cancer therapy. *Pharmacogenomics, 14*(3), 15–24.

Chapter 5: The Nursing Process in Pharmacology

Carpenito, L. J. (2012). *Nursing diagnosis: Application to nursing practice* (14th ed.). Philadelphia, PA: Lippincott Williams and Wilkins.

College and Association of Registered Nurses of Alberta. (2015). *Medication administration: Guidelines for registered nurses.* Edmonton, AB: Author.

Gardner, P. (2003). *Nursing process in action.* New York, NY: Thompson Delmar Learning.

Hogan, M. A. (2013). *Nursing fundamentals: Reviews & rationales* (3rd ed.). Upper Saddle River, NJ: Prentice Hall.

Jahraus, D., Sokolosky, S., Thurston, N., & Guo, D. (2002). Evaluation of an education program for patients with breast cancer receiving radiation therapy. *Cancer Nursing, 24*(4), 266–275.

Kozier, B., Erb, G., Berman, A. J., Burke, K., Bouchal, D. S. R., & Hirst, S. P. (2003). *Fundamentals of nursing: The nature of nursing practice in Canada* (1st Canadian ed.). Toronto, ON: Pearson Education Canada.

North American Nursing Diagnosis Association. (2015). *Nursing diagnoses: Definitions and classification 2015–2017.* Philadelphia, PA: Wiley Blackwell.

Smith, S., Duell, D., Martin, B., Gonzalez, L., & Aebersold, M. (2016). *Clinical nursing skills: Basic to advanced skills* (9th ed.). Upper Saddle River, NJ: Pearson Education.

Chapter 6: Lifespan Considerations in Pharmacotherapy

Bánhidy, F., Lowry, R. B., & Czeize, A. E. (2005). Risk and benefit of drug use during pregnancy. *International Journal of Medical Science, 2,* 100–106.

Canadian Pediatric Society, Drug Therapy and Hazardous Substances Committee. (2003; reaffirmed 2006). Drug investigation for Canadian children: The role of the Canadian Pediatric Society. *Pediatrics & Child Health, 8*(4), 231–234.

Corsonello, A., Onder, G., Abbatecola, A. M., Guffanti, E. E., Gareri, P., & Lattanzio, F. (2012). Explicit criteria for potentially inappropriate medications to reduce the risk of adverse drug reactions in elderly people. *Drug Safety, 35*(Suppl. 1), 21–28.

Doherty, C., & McDonnell, C. (2012). Tenfold medication errors: 5 years' experience at a university-affiliated pediatric hospital. *Pediatrics, 129,* 916–924.

Food and Drug Administration. (2008). *Content and format of labeling for human prescription drug and biological products: Requirements for pregnancy and lactation labeling.* Retrieved from http://www.regulations.gov/#!documentDetail;D=FDA-2006-N-0515-0001

Friedman, J. M. (2006). ACE inhibitors and congenital anomalies. *New England Journal of Medicine, 354*(23), 2498–2500.

Giaginis, C., Theocharis, S., & Tsantili-Kakoulidou, A. (2012). Current toxological aspects on drug and chemical transport and metabolism across the human placental barrier. *Expert Opinion on Drug Metabolism & Toxicology, 8,* 1263–1275.

Gibson, P. (2003, February). Baby safe: Which drugs are safe in pregnancy? *The Canadian Journal of CME,* 67–76.

Grant, E., & Golightly, P. (2010). Safe use of medications in breastfeeding mothers. *Prescriber, 21,* 70–73.

Health Canada. (2004). *Canadian perinatal surveillance system.* Retrieved from http://www.phac-aspc.gc.ca/rhs-ssg/factshts/index-eng.php

Health Canada. (2013). *Congenital anomalies in Canada: A perinatal health surveillance report.* Retrieved from http://publications.gc.ca/site/eng/443924/publication.html

Health Canada. (2015). *Infant feeding.* Retrieved from http://www.hc-sc.gc.ca/fn-an/nutrition/infant-nourisson/index-eng.php

Holmes, L. B., Wyszynski, D. F., & Lieberman, E. (2004). The AED (antiepileptic drug) pregnancy registry: A 6-year experience. *Archives of Neurology, 61*(5), 673–678.

Isoherranen, N., & Thummel, K. E. (2013). Drug metabolism and transport during pregnancy: How does drug disposition change during pregnancy and what are the mechanisms that cause such changes? *Drug Metabolism and Disposition, 41,* 256–262.

Jeong, H. (2010). Altered drug metabolism during pregnancy: Hormonal regulation of drug-metabolizing enzymes. *Expert Opinion on Drug Metabolism & Toxicology, 6,* 689–699.

Kliegman, R. M., Stanton, B., St. Geme, J., Schor, N., & Behrman, R. E. (Eds.). (2011). *Nelson textbook of pediatrics* (19th ed.). Philadelphia, PA: W. B. Saunders.

Leipzig, R. M. (Ed.). (2003). *Drug prescribing for older adults: An evidence-based approach.* Philadelphia, PA: American College of Physicians.

Lo, W. Y., & Friedman, J. M. (2002). Teratogenicity of recently introduced medications in human pregnancy. *Obstetrics and Gynecology, 100*(3), 465–473.

Martin, M., Kohler, C., Kim, Y., Kratt, P., Schoenberger, Y., Litaker, M., … Pisu, M. (2010). Taking less than prescribed: Medication nonadherence and provider–patient relationships in lower-income, rural minority adults with hypertension. *Journal of Clinical Hypertension, 12,* 706–713.

Mitchell, A. A., Gilboa, S. M., Werler, M. M., Kelley, K. E., Louik, C., & Hernandez-Diaz, S. (2011). Medication use during pregnancy, with particular focus on prescription drugs: 1976–2008. *American Journal of Obstetrics and Gynecology, 205,* 51.e1-51.e8.

Mone, S. M., Gillman, M. W., Miller, T. L., Herman, E. H., & Lipshultz, S. E. (2004). Effects of environmental exposures on the cardiovascular system: Prenatal period through adolescence. *Pediatrics, 113*(4), 1058–1069.

Peters, S. L., Lind, J. N., Humphrey, J. R., Friedman, J. M., Honein, M. A., Tassinari, M. S., … Brousard, C. S. (2013). Safe lists for medication in pregnancy: Inadequate evidence base and inconsistent guidance from Web-based information, 2011. *Pharmacoepidemiology and Drug Safety, 22,* 324–328.

Rowe, H., Baker, T., & Hale, T. W. (2013). Maternal medication, drug use, and breastfeeding. *Pediatric Clinics of North America, 60,* 275–294.

Sehgal, V., Bajwa, S. J., Sehgal, R., Bajaj, A., Khaira, U., & Kresse, V. (2013). Polypharmacy and potentially inappropriate medication use as the precipitating factor in readmissions to the hospital. *Journal of Family Medicine and Primary Care, 2,* 194–199.

Spiers, M. V., Kutzik, D. M., & Lamar, M. (2004). Variation in medication understanding among the elderly. *American Journal of Health-System Pharmacy, 61*(4), 373–380.

U.S. Food and Drug Administration. (2013). *2013 safety alerts for human medical products, drugs and therapeutic biological products, medical devices, and special nutrition and cosmetic products.* Retrieved from http://www.fda.gov/Safety/MedWatch/SafetyInformation/SafetyAlertsforHumanMedicalProducts/ucm333878.htm

World Health Organization. (2002). *Breastfeeding and maternal medication: Recommendations for drugs in the eleventh WHO model list of essential drugs.* Retrieved from http://whqlibdoc.who.int/hq/2002/55732.pdf

Chapter 7: Individual, Psychosocial, and Cultural Influences on Drug Responses

Brody, H., & Hunt, L. M. (2006). Bidil: Assessing a race-based pharmaceutical. *Annals of Family Medicine, 4*(6), 482–483.

Burroughs, V., Maxey, R., Crawley, L., & Levy, R. (2002). *Cultural and genetic diversity in America: The need for individualized pharmaceutical treatment.* Washington, DC: National Pharmaceutical Council, National Pharmaceutical Association. Available online at http://www.npc-now.org/issues_productlist/PDF/culturaldiversity.

Canadian Language and Literacy Research Network. (2016). http://www.cllrnet.ca/

Canadian Nurses Association. (2006). *Toward 2020: Visions for nursing.* Ottawa, ON: Author.

Canadian Nurses Association. (2016). *Promoting culturally competent care.* Retrieved from https://www.cna-aiic.ca/~/media/cna/page-content/pdf-en/ps114_cultural_competence_2010_e.pdf?

Davidhizar, R. (2002). Strategies for providing culturally appropriate pharmaceutical care to the Hispanic patient. *Hospital Pharmacy, 37*(5), 505–510.

Goodwill, J. C. (1989). *Indian & Inuit nurses of Canada.* Retrieved from http://www.sicc.sk.ca/archive/saskindian/a89mar14.htm

Kudzma, E. C. (2001). Cultural competence: Cardiovascular medications. *Progress in Cardiovascular Nursing, 16*(4), 152–160, 169.

Spector, R. E. (2012). *Cultural diversity in health & illness* (8th ed.). Upper Saddle River, NJ: Pearson Education.

Statistics Canada. (2016). http://www.statscan.ca

Chapter 8: Drug Effects, Adverse Reactions, and Interactions

Bilyeu, K. M., Gumm, C. J., Fitzgerald, J. M., Fox, S. W., & Selig, P. (2011). Cultivating quality: Reducing the use of potentially inappropriate medications in older adults. *American Journal of Nursing, 111*(1), 47–52.

Boullata, J. I., & Armenti, V. T. (Eds). (2010). *Handbook of drug-nutrient interactions* (2nd ed.). New York, NY: Humana Press.

Chen, X. W., Sneed, K. B., Pan, S. Y., Cao, C., Kanwar, J. R., Chew, H., & Zhou, S. F. (2012). Herb–drug interactions and mechanistic and clinical considerations. *Current Drug Metabolism, 13,* 640–651.

George, E. L., Henneman, E. A., & Tasota, F. J. (2010). Nursing implications for prevention of adverse drug events in the intensive care unit. *Critical Care Medicine, 38*(Suppl. 6), S136–S144.

Jordan, S. (2011). Adverse events: Expecting too much of nurses and too little of nursing research. *Journal of Nursing Management, 19,* 287–292.

Magro, L., Moretti, U., & Leone, R. (2012). Epidemiology and characteristics of adverse drug reactions caused by drug–drug interactions. *Expert Opinion on Drug Safety, 11,* 83–94.

Posadzki, P., Watson, L., & Ernst, E. (2013). Herb–drug interactions: An overview of systematic reviews. *British Journal of Clinical Pharmacology, 75,* 603–618.

Pronsky, Z., & Crowe, S. R. (2012). *Food–medication interactions* (17th ed.). Pottstown, PA: Food Medication Interactions.

Tsai, H.-H., Lin, H.-W., Simon Pickard, A., Tsai, H.-Y., & Mahady, G. B. (2012). Evaluation of documented drug interactions and contraindications associated with herbs and dietary supplements: A systematic literature review. *International Journal of Clinical Practice, 66,* 1056–1078.

Valente, S., & Murray, L. P. (2011). Creative strategies to improve patient safety: Allergies and adverse drug reactions. *Journal for Nurses in Staff Development, 27*(1), E1–E5.

Chapter 9: Principles of Drug Administration

Armitage, G., & Knapman, H. (2003). Adverse events in drug administration: A literature review. *Journal of Nursing Management, 11*(2), 130–140.

Berman, A. J., Snyder, S., Kozier, B., & Erb, G. (2015). *Kozier & Erb's fundamentals of nursing concepts, process, and practice* (10th ed.). Upper Saddle River, NJ: Pearson Education.

Blais, K. K., & Hayes, J. (2015). *Professional nursing practice: Concepts and perspectives* (7th ed.). Upper Saddle River, NJ: Pearson Education.

College and Association of Registered Nurses of Alberta. (2014). *Medication administration: Guidelines for registered nurses.* Edmonton, AB: Author.

Khaldi, N., Miras, A., & Gromb, S. (2005). Toxic epidermal necrolysis and clarithromycin. *Canadian Journal of Clinical Pharmacology, 12*(3), e264–e268.

Koo, M. M., Krass, I., & Aslani, P. (2003). Factors influencing consumer use of written drug information. *Annals of Pharmacotherapy, 37*(2), 259–267.

Mitchell, J. F. (2006). *Oral dosage forms that should not be crushed.* Horsham, PA: Institute for Safe Medication Practices.

Nicholas, P., & Agius, C. (2005). Toward safer IV medication administration: The narrow safety margins of many IV medications make this route particularly dangerous. *American Journal of Nursing, 105*(Suppl. 3), 25–30.

Olsen, J. L., Giangrasso, A. P., & Shrimpton, D. M. (2015). *Medical dosage calculations* (11th ed.). Upper Saddle River, NJ: Pearson Education.

Smith, S., Duell, D., & Martin, B. (2016). *Clinical nursing skills: Basic to advanced skills* (9th ed.). Upper Saddle River, NJ: Pearson Education.

Zaybak, A., Günes, Ü. Y., Tamsel, S., Khorshid, L., & Eşer, I. (2007). Does obesity prevent the needle from reaching muscle in intramuscular injections? *Journal of Advanced Nursing, 58*(6), 552–556.

Chapter 10: Medication Incidents and Risk Reduction

Baker, G. R., Norton, P. G., Flintoft, V., Blais, R., Brown, A., Cox, J., … Tamblyn, R. (2004). The Canadian adverse events study: The incidence of adverse events among hospital patients in Canada. *Canadian Medical Association Journal, 170*(11), 1678–1686.

Barnsteiner, J. H. (2005). Medication reconciliation: Transfer of medication information across settings—Keeping it free from error. *American Journal of Nursing, 105*(Suppl. 3), 31–36.

Canadian Medication Incident Reporting and Prevention System (CMIRPS). (2016). http://www.cmirps-scdpim.ca/wp-content/uploads/2011/03/CMIRPS-Presentation.pdf

Canadian Nurses Association. (2008). *Code of ethics for registered nurses.* Retrieved from https://www.cna-aiic.ca/~/media/cna/page-content/pdf-fr/code-of-ethics-for-registered-nurses.pdf?la=en

Canadian Nurses Association. (2016). *CNA position statement on patient safety.* Retrieved from https://www.cna-aiic.ca/~/media/cna/page-content/pdf-en/8%20-%20ps70_patient-safety_en.pdf?la=en

Capital Health. (2013). *Briefing note: Prohibited abbreviations.* Retrieved from https://www.fraserhealth.ca/media/Medication-Quality-and-Safety-Initiatives-Report.pdf

College and Association of Registered Nurses of Alberta. (2013). *Practice standards for regulated members.* Retrieved from http://www.nurses.ab.ca/content/dam/carna/pdfs/DocumentList/Standards/PracticeStandards_CNA_Ethics_2008.pdf

Drug innovation and patient safety: The need for a new paradigm. Proceedings of a Satellite Symposium. (2006). *Canadian Journal of Clinical Pharmacology, 13*(Suppl. 1), e1–e49.

Fialová, D., & Onder, G. (2009). Medication errors in elderly people: Contributing factors and future perspectives. *British Journal of Clinical Pharmacology, 67*, 641–645.

Force, M. V., Deering, L., Hubbe, J., Anderson, M., Hagermann, B., Cooper-Hahn, M., & Peters, W. (2006). Effective strategies to increase reporting of medication errors in hospitals. *Journal of Nursing Administration, 36*(1), 34–41.

Health Canada. (2006). *MedEffect program.* Retrieved from http://www.hc-sc.gc.ca/dhp-mps/medeff/index-eng.php

Health Canada. (2016). *Canadian Adverse Drug Reaction Monitoring Program (CADRMP) guidelines for the voluntary reporting of suspected adverse reactions to health products by health professionals and consumers.* Retrieved from http://www.hc-sc.gc.ca/dhp-mps/medeff/databasdon/index-eng.php

Health Canada. (2016). *Canadian Medication Incident Reporting and Prevention System (CMIRPS).* Retrieved from http://www.ismp-canada.org/cmirps/

Hodgkinson, B., Koch, S., Nay, R., & Nichols, K. (2006). Strategies to reduce medication errors with reference to older adults. *International Journal of Evidence-Based Healthcare, 4*(1), 2–41.

Kaushal, R., Shojania, K. G., & Bates, D. W. (2003). Effects of computerized physician order entry and clinical decision support systems on medication safety: A systematic review. *Archives of Internal Medicine, 163*(12), 1409–1416.

Koper, D., Kamenski, G., Flamm, M., Böhmdorfer, B., & Sönnichsen, A. (2013). Frequency of medication errors in primary care patients with polypharmacy. *Family Practice, 30*, 313–319.

Levy, A., & MacLeod, S. (2005). Drug innovation and patient safety: The need for a new paradigm. *The Canadian Journal of Clinical Pharmacology, 13*(1), e1–e49.

Movement for Canadian Literacy. (2016). *Literacy in Canada: It's time for action.* Retrieved from https://archive.org/details/ERIC_ED533645

Nursinglabs. (2016). *10 rights of drug administration.* Retrieved from http://nurseslabs.com/10-rs-rights-of-drug-administration/

Walton, M. (2004). Creating a "no blame" culture: Have we got the balance right? *Quality and Safety in Health Care, 13*(3), 163–164.

Chapter 11: Complementary and Alternative Therapies and Their Roles in Pharmacotherapy in Canada

Anastasi, J. K., Chang, M., & Capilli, B. (2011). Herbal supplements: Talking with your patients. *The Journal for Nurse Practitioners, 7*, 29–35.

Barnes, J. (2012). Adverse drug reactions and pharmacovigilance of herbal medicines. In J. Talbott & J. K. Aronson (Eds.), *Stephens' detection and evaluation of adverse drug reactions: Principles and practice* (6th ed., pp. 645–683). Chichester, UK: John Wiley & Sons.

College and Association of Registered Nurses of Alberta. (2011). *Complementary and/or alternative therapy and natural health product: Standards for registered nurses.* Retrieved from http://www.nurses.ab.ca/content/dam/carna/pdfs/documentlist/standards/rn_compalt-therapy_jan2011.pdf.

Ebadi, M. (2006). *Pharmacodynamic basis of herbal medicine* (2nd ed.). Boca Raton, FL: CRC Press.

First Annual Complementary and Alternative Health Care and Paediatrics Forum. (2004). *Canadian Journal of Clinical Pharmacology, 11*(2), e245–e256.

Fontaine, K. L. (2011). *Complementary and alternative therapies for nursing practice* (3rd ed.). Upper Saddle River, NJ: Prentice Hall.

Harris, P. E., Cooper, K. L., Relton, C., & Thomas, K. J. (2012). Prevalence of complementary and alternative medicine (CAM) use by the general population: A systematic review and update. *The International Journal of Clinical Practice, 66*, 924–939.

Health Canada. (2016). *Natural and Non-prescription Health Products Directorate.* Retrieved from http://www.hc-sc.gc.ca/ahc-asc/branch-dirgen/hpfb-dgpsa/nhpd-dpsn/index-eng.php

Izzo, A., & Edzard, E. (2009). Interactions between herbal medicines and prescribed drugs: An updated systematic review. *Drugs, 69*, 1777–1798.

Statistics Canada. (2016). http://www.statscan.ca

Chapter 12: Brief Review of the Autonomic Nervous System and Neurotransmitters

Aronson, J. K. (2000). Where name and image meet: The argument for "adrenaline." *British Medical Journal, 320*, 506–509.

Krogh, D. (2011). *Biology: A guide to the natural world* (5th ed.). San Francisco, CA: Benjamin Cummings.

Martini, F. H., Nath, J. L., & Batholomew, E. F. (2012). *Fundamentals of human anatomy and physiology* (9th ed.). San Francisco, CA: Benjamin Cummings.

Parati, G., & Esler, M. (2012). The human sympathetic nervous system: Its relevance in hypertension and heart failure. *European Heart Journal, 33*, 1058–1066.

Silverthorn, D. U. (2010). *Human physiology: An integrated approach* (5th ed.). Upper Saddle River, NJ: Pearson/Benjamin Cummings.

Squire, L. R., Berg, D., Bloom, F. E., Du Lac, S., & Ghosh, A. (Eds.). (2012). *Fundamental neuroscience*. Waltham, MA: Academic Press.

Westfall, T. C., & Westfall, D. P. (2011). Neurotransmission: The autonomic and somatic motor nervous systems. In L. L. Brunton, B. A. Chabner, & B. C. Knollman (Eds.), *Goodman and Gilman's the pharmacological basis of therapeutics* (12th ed., pp. 171–218). New York, NY: McGraw-Hill.

Chapter 13: Pharmacotherapy with Cholinergic Agonists and Antagonists

Anderson, P. D. (2012). Emergency management of chemical weapons injuries. *Journal of Pharmacy Practice, 25*, 61–68.

Brown, J. H., & Laiken, N. (2011). Muscarinic receptor agonists and antagonists. In L. L. Brunton, B. A. Chabner, & B. C. Knollman (Eds.), *The pharmacological basis of therapeutics* (12th ed., pp. 219–238). New York, NY: McGraw-Hill.

Chaplin, S., & Hajek, P. (2010). Nicotine replacement therapy for smoking cessation. *Prescriber, 21*(19), 62–65.

Defilippi, J., & Crismon, M. L. (2003). Drug interactions with cholinesterase inhibitors. *Drugs & Aging, 20*(6), 437–444.

Diaz-Manera, J., Rojas Garcia, R., & Illa, I. (2012). Treatment strategies for myasthenia gravis: An update. *Expert Opinion on Pharmacotherapy, 13*, 1873–1883.

Drag, L. L., & Wright, S. (2012). Prescribing practices of anticholinergic medications and their association with cognition in an extended care setting. *Journal of Applied Gerontology, 31*, 239–259.

Ellsworth, P., & Kirshenbaum, E. (2010). Update on the pharmacologic management of overactive bladder: The present and the future. *Urologic Nursing, 30*(1), 29–39.

Herbison, P., Hay-Smith, J., Ellis, G., & Moore, K. (2003). Effectiveness of anticholinergic drugs compared with placebo in the treatment of overactive bladder: Systematic review. *British Medical Journal, 326*(7394), 841–844.

Hibbs, R. E., & Zambon, A. C. (2011). Agents acting at the neuromuscular junction and autonomic ganglia. In L. L. Brunton, B. A. Chabner, & B. C. Knollman (Eds.), *The pharmacological basis of therapeutics* (12th ed., pp. 255–276). New York, NY: McGraw-Hill.

Taylor, P. (2011). Anticholinesterase agents. In L. L. Brunton, B. A. Chabner, & B. C. Knollman (Eds.), *The pharmacological basis of therapeutics* (12th ed., pp. 239–254). New York, NY: McGraw-Hill.

Chapter 14: Pharmacotherapy with Adrenergic Agonists and Antagonists

Al-Gobari, M., El Khatib, C., Pillon, F., & Gueyffier, F. (2013). Beta-blockers for the prevention of sudden cardiac death in heart failure patients: A meta-analysis of randomized controlled trials. *BMC Cardiovascular Disorders, 13*, 52.

Bouchard, R., Weber, A. R., & Geiger, J. D. (2002). Informed decision-making on sympathomimetic use in sport and health. *Clinical Journal of Sports Medicine, 12*(4), 209–224.

Campbell, R. L., Manivannan, V., Hartz, M. F., & Sadosty, A. T. (2012). Epinephrine auto-injector pandemic. *Pediatric Emergency Care, 28*, 938–942.

Chen, J. M., Heran, B. S., Perez, M. I., & Wright, J. M. (2010). Blood pressure lowering efficacy of beta-blockers as second-line therapy for primary hypertension. *Cochrane Database of Systematic Reviews, 1*, CD007185.

Havel, C., Arrich, J., Losert, H., Gamper, G., Müllner, M., & Herkner, H. (2011). Vasopressors for hypotensive shock. *Cochrane Database of Systematic Reviews, 5*, CD003709.

McHugh, J., Pokhrel, P., Barber, K., & Guozhen, L. (2010). Beta-blockers in the management of cardiovascular diseases. *Osteopathic Family Physician, 2*, 131–138.

Ortega, V. E., & Peters, S. P. (2010). Beta-2 adrenergic agonists: Focus on safety and benefits versus risks. *Current Opinions in Pharmacology, 10*, 246–253.

Ruz, M. E., Lennie, T. A., & Moser, D. K. (2010). Effects of β-blockers and anxiety on complication rates after acute myocardial infarction. *American Journal of Critical Care, 20*, 67–74.

Self, T. H., Wallace, J. L., & Soberman, J. E. (2012). Cardioselective beta-blocker treatment of hypertension in patients with asthma: When do benefits outweigh risks? *Journal of Asthma, 49*, 947–951.

Stephens, S. (2010). State of the science: β-blockers and reduction of perioperative cardiac events. *Critical Care Nursing Clinics of North America, 22*(2), 209–215.

Westfall, T. C., & Westfall, D. P. (2011). Adrenergic agonists and antagonists. In L. L. Brunton, B. A. Chabner, & B. C. Knollman (Eds.), *The pharmacological basis of therapeutics* (12th ed., pp. 277–334). New York, NY: McGraw-Hill.

Wiysonge, C. S., Bradley, H. A., Volmink, J., Mayosi, B. M., Mbewu, A., & Opie, L. H. (2012). Beta-blockers for hypertension. *Cochrane Database of Systematic Reviews, 11*, CD002003.

Chapter 15: Brief Review of the Central Nervous System

Isik, A. T. (2010). Late onset Alzheimer's disease in older people. *Clinical Interventions in Aging, 5*, 307–311.

Krogh, D. (2011). *Biology: A guide to the natural world* (5th ed.). San Francisco, CA: Benjamin Cummings.

Marieb, E. N., & Hoehn, K. (2013). *Human anatomy and physiology* (9th ed.). San Francisco, CA: Benjamin Cummings.

Martini, F. H., Nath, J. L., & Bartholomew, E. F. (2012). *Fundamentals of human anatomy and physiology* (9th ed.). San Francisco, CA: Benjamin Cummings.

Silverthorn, D. U. (2012). *Human physiology: An integrated approach* (6th ed.). San Francisco, CA: Benjamin Cummings

Westfall, T. C., & Westfall, D. P. (2011). Neurotransmission: The autonomic and somatic motor nervous systems. In L. L. Brunton, B. A. Chabner, & B. C. Knollman (Eds.), *The pharmacological basis of therapeutics* (12th ed., pp. 171–218). New York, NY: McGraw-Hill.

Chapter 16: Pharmacotherapy of Anxiety and Sleep Disorders

Aventis Pharma Ltd. (2015). *Imovane: Tablets*. Retrieved from http://www.medsafe.govt.nz/profs/datasheet/i/imovanetab.pdf

Chandola, T., Ferrie, J. E., Perski, A., Akbaraly, T., & Marmot, M. G. (2010). The effect of short sleep duration on coronary heart disease risk is greatest among those with sleep disturbance: A prospective study from the Whitehall II cohort. *Sleep, 33*(6), 739–744.

Holcomb, S. S. (2006). Sedative hypnotics in older people with insomnia: Meta-analysis of risks and benefits. Recommendations for assessing insomnia. *Obstetrics & Gynecology, 107*(3), 736–737.

McClung, C. A. (2007). Circadian genes, rhythms and the biology of mood disorders. *Pharmacology & Therapeutics, 114*(2), 222–232.

Mihic, S. J., & Harris, R. A. (2011). Hypnotics and sedatives. In L. L. Brunton, B. A. Chabner, & B. C. Knollman (Eds.), *The pharmacological basis of therapeutics* (12th ed., pp. 457–480). New York, NY: McGraw-Hill.

Mistraletti, G., Donatelli, F., & Carli, F. (2005). Metabolic and endocrine effects of sedative agents. *Current Opinion in Critical Care, 11*(4), 312–317.

Morgan, K., Dixon, S., Mathers, N., Thompson, J., & Tomeny, M. (2004). Psychological treatment for insomnia in the regulation of long-term hypnotic drug use. *Health Technology Assessment, 8*(8), 1–68.

Pagel, J. F. (2005). Medications and their effects on sleep. *Primary Care Clinics in Office Practice, 32*, 491–509.

Reeve, K., & Balles, B. (2010). Insomnia in adults: Etiology and management. *Journal for Nurse Practitioners, 6*, 53–60. doi:10.1016/j.nurpra.2009.09.013

Roth, T., & Roehrs, T. (2010). Pharmacotherapy for insomnia. *Sleep Medicine Clinics, 5*, 529–539

Townsend-Roccichelli, J., Sanford, J. T., & VandeWaa, E. (2010). Managing sleep disorders in the elderly. *Nurse Practitioner, 35*(5), 30–37.

Yang, C. M., Spielman, A. J., & Glovinsky, P. (2006). Nonpharmacologic strategies in the management of insomnia. *Psychiatric Clinics of North America, 29*, 895–919.

Chapter 17: Pharmacotherapy of Emotional and Mood Disorders

Barbui, C., Esposito, E., & Cipriani, A. (2009). Selective serotonin reuptake inhibitors and risk of suicide: A systematic review of observational studies. *Canadian Medical Association Journal, 180*, 291–297.

DeBattista, C., Solvason, H. B., Poirier, J., Kendrick, E., & Schatzberg, A. F. (2003). A prospective trial of bupropion SR augmentation of partial and non-responders to serotonergic antidepressants. *Journal of Clinical Psychopharmacology, 23*(1), 27–30.

Furukawa, T. A., McGuire, H., & Barbui, C. (2002). Meta-analysis of effects and side effects of low dosage tricyclic antidepressants in depression: Systematic review. *British Medical Journal, 325*(7371), 991–1000.

Goodwin, F. K., & Goldstein, M. A. (2003). Optimizing lithium treatment in bipolar disorder: A review of the literature and clinical recommendations. *Journal of Psychiatric Practice, 9*(5), 333–343.

Hong Ng, C., Norman, T. R., Naing, K. O., Schweitzer, I., Kong Wai Ho, B., Fan, A., & Klimidis, S. (2006). A comparative study of sertraline dosages, plasma concentrations, efficacy and adverse reactions in Chinese versus Caucasian patients. *International Clinical Psychopharmacology, 21*(2), 87–92.

Janicak, P. (2002). *Research report: rTMS vs. ECT in depressed patients.* Chicago, IL: University of Illinois.

Leon, A. C., Solomon, D. A., Li, C., Fiedorowicz, J. G., Coryell, W. H., Endicott, J., & Keller, M. B. (2011). Antidepressants and risks of suicide and suicide attempts: A 27-year observational study. *The Journal of Clinical Psychiatry, 72*, 580–586.

Luca, A., Luca, M., & Caladra, C. (2013). Sleep disorders and depression: Brief review of literature, case report, and nonpharmacologic interventions for depression. *Clinical Interventions in Aging, 8*, 1033–1039.

Nelson, J. C., Mazure, C. M., Jatlow, P. I., Bowers Jr., M. B., & Price, L. H. (2004). Combining norepinephrine and serotonin reuptake inhibition mechanisms for treatment of depression: A double-blind, randomized study. *Biological Psychiatry, 55*, 296–300.

Rocha, F. L., Fuzikawa, C., Riera, R., & Hara, C. (2012). Combination of antidepressants in the treatment of major depressive disorder: A systematic review and meta-analysis. *Journal of Clinical Psychopharmacology, 32*, 278–281.

Serretti, A., Artioli, P., & Quartesan, R. (2005). Pharmacogenetics in the treatment of depression: Pharmacodynamic studies. *Pharmacogenetics & Genomics, 15*(2), 61–67.

Spector, R. E. (2012). *Cultural diversity in health and illness* (8th ed.). Upper Saddle River, NJ: Pearson Education.

Stahl, S. M. (2005). Antidepressant treatment of psychotic major depression: Potential role of the sigma receptor. *CNS Spectrums, 10*(4), 319–323.

Statistics Canada. (2014). *Canadian community health survey, 2014.* Retrieved from http://www.statcan.gc.ca/daily-quotidien/150617/dq150617b-eng.htm

Van Lieshout, R. J., & MacQueen, G. M. (2010). Efficacy and acceptability of mood stabilizers in the treatment of acute bipolar depression: Systematic review. *British Journal of Psychiatry 196*, 266–273.

Willner, P., Hale, A. S., & Argyropoulos, S. (2005). Dopaminergic mechanism of antidepressant action in depressed patients. *Journal of Affective Disorders, 86*(1), 37–45.

Yatham, L. N., Kennedy, S. H., O'Donovan, C., Parikh, S., MacQueen, G., McIntyre, R., … Gorman, C. P. (2005). Canadian Network for Mood and Anxiety Treatments (CANMAT) guidelines for the management of patients with bipolar disorder: Consensus and controversies. *Bipolar Disorders, 7*(Suppl. 3), 5–69.

Chapter 18: Central Nervous System Stimulants and Pharmacotherapy of Attention Deficit and Hyperactive Disorders

American Psychiatric Association. (2013). *Diagnostic and statistical manual of mental disorders* (5th ed.). Washington, DC: Author.

Charach, A., & Fernandez, R. (2013). Enhancing ADHD medication adherence: Challenges and opportunities. *Current Psychiatry Reports, 15*(7), 1–8.

Dopheide, J. A., & Pliszka, S. R. (2009). Attention-deficit–hyperactivity disorder: An update. *Pharmacotherapy, 29*, 656–679.

Elia, J., & Vetter, V. L. (2010). Cardiovascular effects for the treatment of attention-deficit hyperactivity disorder: What is known and how should it influence prescribing in children? *Pediatric Drugs, 12*, 165–175.

Evans, S. W., Brady, C. E., Harrison, J. R., Bunford, N., Kern, L, State, T., & Andrews, C. (2013). Measuring ADHD and ODD symptoms and impairment using high school teachers' ratings. *Journal of Clinical Child & Adolescent Psychology, 42*, 197–207.

March of Dimes. (2012). *Caffeine in pregnancy.* Retrieved from http://www.marchofdimes.com/pregnancy/caffeine-in-pregnancy.aspx

Ryan, J. B., Katsiyannis, A., & Hughes, E. M. (2011). Medication treatment for attention deficit hyperactivity disorder. *Theory into Practice, 50*(1), 52–60.

Schweitzer, J. B., & McBurnett, K. (2012). New directions for therapeutics in ADHD. *Neurotherapeutics, 9*, 487–489.

Sonuga-Barke, E. J., Brandeis, D., Cortese, S., Daley, D., Ferrin, M., Holtmann, M., … Sergeant, J. (2013). Nonpharmacological interventions for ADHD: Systematic review and meta-analyses of randomized controlled trials of dietary and psychological treatments. *American Journal of Psychiatry, 170*, 275–289.

Chapter 19: Pharmacotherapy of Psychoses

Ardizzone, I., Nardecchia, F., Marconi, A., Ferrara, M., & Carratelli, T. I. (2010). Antipsychotic medication in adolescents suffering from schizophrenia: A meta-analysis of randomized controlled trials. *Psychopharmacology Bulletin, 43*(2), 45–66.

Bailey, K. (2003). Aripiprazole: The newest antipsychotic agent for the treatment of schizophrenia. *Psychosocial Nursing and Mental Health Services, 41*(2), 14–18.

Health Canada. (2016). *Drug product database.* Retrieved from http://www.hc-sc.gc.ca/dhp-mps/prodpharma/databasdon/index-eng.php

Kneisl, C. R., Wilson, H. S., & Trigoboff, E. (2004). *Contemporary psychiatric-mental health nursing.* Upper Saddle River, NJ: Prentice Hall.

Mattal, A. K., Hill, J. L., & Lenroot, R. K. (2010). Treatment of early onset schizophrenia. *Current Opinion in Psychiatry, 23*, 304–310.

Meyer, J. M. (2011). Pharmacotherapy of psychosis and mania. In L. L. Brunton, B. A. Chabner, & B. C. Knollman (Eds.), *The pharmacological basis of therapeutics* (11th ed., pp. 417–457). New York, NY: McGraw-Hill.

Pringsheim, T., Panagiotopoulos, C., Davidson, J., & Ho, J. (2011). Evidence-based recommendations for monitoring safety of second generation antipsychotics in children and youth. *Journal of the Canadian Academy of Child and Adolescent Psychiatry, 20*(3), 218–233.

Ronsley, R., Rayter, M., Smith, D., Davidson, J., & Panagiotopoulos, C. (2012). Metabolic monitoring training program implementation in the community setting was associated with improved monitoring in second-generation antipsychotic-treated children. *Canadian Journal of Psychiatry, 57*(5), 292–299.

Chapter 20: Pharmacotherapy of Degenerative Diseases of the Nervous System

Alzheimer's disease fact sheet. Retrieved from http://www.alzheimers.org

Birks, J., Grimley-Evans, J., & Van Dongen, M. (2002). Ginkgo biloba for cognitive impairment and dementia. *Cochrane Database of Systematic Reviews, 4*, CD003120.

Brain-cell growth protein shows promise for Parkinson's in early human trial. Retrieved from http://www.parkinsons-foundation.org

Health Canada. (2016). *Drug product database.* Retrieved from http://www.hc-sc.gc.ca/dhp-mps/prodpharma/databasdon/index-eng.php

Hoozemans, J. J., Veerhuis, R., Rozemuller, J. M., & Eikelenboom, P. (2011). Soothing the inflamed brain: Effect of non-steroidal anti-inflammatory drugs on Alzheimer's disease. *CNS & Neurological Disorders Drug Targets, 10*(1), 57–67.

Miller, C. E., & Umhauer, M. A. (2011). Emerging oral therapies for multiple sclerosis. *Journal of Neuroscience Nursing, 43*, 3–14.

National Institute on Aging. (2015). *Alzheimer's disease: Unraveling the mystery.* Retrieved from https://www.nia.nih.gov/alzheimers/publication/alzheimers-disease-unraveling-mystery/preface

Ontaneda, D., Hyland, M., & Cohen, J. A. (2012). Multiple sclerosis: New insights in pathogenesis and novel therapeutics. *Annual Review of Medicine, 63*, 389–404.

Querfurth, H. W., & LaFerla, F. M. (2010). Alzheimer's disease. *New England Journal of Medicine, 362*, 329–344.

Richter, R., & Richter, B. (Eds.). (2014). *Alzheimer's disease: The physicians' guide to practical management.* New York, NY: Springer Science + Business Media.

Sacco, K. A., Bannon, K. L., & George, T. P. (2004). Nicotinic receptor mechanisms and cognition in normal states and neuropsychiatric disorders. *Journal of Psychopharmacology, 18*(4), 457–474.

Warren, S. A., Svenson, L. W., Metz, L. M., Schopflocher, D. P., & Warren, K. G. (2004). Prevalence of multiple sclerosis (MS) among First Nations people in Alberta, Canada: P03.063. *Neurology, 62*(7, Suppl. 5), A215–A216.

Chapter 21: Pharmacotherapy of Seizures

American Academy of Neurology. (2008). *Breastfeeding while taking seizure medicine does not appear to harm children.* Retrieved from https://www.aan.com/PressRoom/Home/PressRelease/603

Beghi, M., Savica, R., Beghi, E., Nobili, A., & Garattini, L. (2009). Utilization and costs of antiepileptic drugs in the elderly: Still an unsolved issue. *Drugs and Aging, 26*(2), 157–168.

Chong, D. J., & Bazil, C. W. (2010). Update on anticonvulsant drugs. *Current Neurology and Neuroscience Reports, 10*(4), 308–318.

Health Canada. (2016). *Drug product database.* Retrieved from http://www.hc-sc.gc.ca/dhp-mps/prodpharma/databasdon/index-eng.php

Ochoa, J. G., & Riche, W. (2013). *Antiepileptic drugs.* Retrieved from http://emedicine.medscape.com/article/1187334-overview

Pack, A. M., & Morrell, M. J. (2003). Treatment of women with epilepsy. *Seminars in Neurology, 22*(3), 289–298.

Verrotti, A., Loiacono, G., Coppola, G., Spalice, A., Mohn, A., & Chiarelli, F. (2011). Pharmacotherapy for children and adolescents with epilepsy. *Expert Opinion on Pharmacotherapy, 12*, 175–194.

Wyllie, E. (2015). *Wyllie's treatment of epilepsy: Principles and practice* (6th ed.). Philadelphia, PA: Wolters Kluwer.

Chapter 22: Pharmacotherapy of Muscle Spasms and Spasticity

Abel-Hamid, H. Z. (2013). *Cerebral palsy.* Retrieved from http://emedicine.medscape.com/article/1179555-overview#aw2aab6b2b2

Amatya, B., Khan, F., La Mantia, L., Demetrios, M., & Wade, D. T. (2013). Non-pharmacological interventions for spasticity in multiple sclerosis. *Cochrane Database of Systematic Reviews, 2*, CD009974.

Brashear, A., & Elovic, E. (2011). *Spasticity: Diagnosis and management.* New York, NY: Demos Medical.

Darlington, A. B. (2011). The Botox phenomenon. *Plastic Surgical Nursing, 30*, 22–26.

Dystonia Medical Research Foundation. (2003). *Botulism toxin injections.* Retrieved from http://www.dystonia-foundation.org/treatment/botox.asp

Dystonia Medical Research Foundation. (2003). *Dystonia defined.* Retrieved from http://www.dystonia-foundation.org/defined/

Health Canada. (2008). *Health Canada reviewing issue of distant toxin spread potentially associated with Botox and Botox Cosmetic.* Retrieved from http://healthycanadians.gc.ca/recall-alert-rappel-avis/hc-sc/2008/13271a-eng.php

Katzberg, H. D., Khan, A. H., & So, Y. T. (2010). Assessment: Symptomatic treatment for muscle cramps (an evidence-based review): Report of the Therapeutics and Technology Assessment Subcommittee of the American Academy of Neurology. *Neurology, 74*, 691–696.

Lemone, P., & Burke, K. (2012). *Medical surgical nursing: Critical thinking in client care* (5th ed.). Upper Saddle River, NJ: Pearson.

Van Beek, A. L., Lim, P. K., Gear, A. J., & Pritzker, M. R. (2007). Management of vasospastic disorders with botulinum toxin A. *Plastic and Reconstructive Surgery, 119,* 217–226.

Ward, A. B., Molenaers, G., Colosimo, C., & Berardelli, A. (2006). Clinical value of botulinum toxin in neurological indications. *European Journal of Neurology, 13*(Suppl. 4), 20–26.

Chapter 23: Pharmacotherapy of Pain and Migraine

Canadian Pain Society. (2007). *Pharmacological management of chronic neuropathic pain: Consensus statement and guidelines from the Canadian Pain Society.* Retrieved from http://pharmamgmtofcnp.pdf

Chaparro, L. E., Wiffen, P. J., Moore, R. A., & Gilron, I. (2012). Combination pharmacotherapy for the treatment of neuropathic pain in adults. *Cochrane Database of Systematic Reviews, 7,* CD008943.

Chawla, J. (2013). *Migraine headache.* Retrieved from http://emedicine.medscape.com/article/1142556-overview

Drenth, J. P. H., & Verheugt, F. W. A. (2007). Do COX-2 inhibitors give enough gastrointestinal protection? *Lancet, 369,* 439–440.

Gordon, A. (2012). The five pillars of pain management. *Pain Management, 2,* 335–344.

Holmer Pettersson, P., Hein, A., Owall, A., Anderson, R. E., & Jakobsson, J. G. (2005). Early bioavailability in day surgery: A comparison between orally, rectally, and intravenously administered paracetamol. *Ambulatory Surgery, 12*(1), 27.

Mayo Clinic. (2013). *Migraine: Alternative medicine.* Retrieved from http://www.mayoclinic.org/diseases-conditions/migraine-headache/basics/alternative-medicine/CON-20026358

McKeever, T. M., Lewis, S. A., Smit, H. A., Burney, P., Britton, J. R., & Cassano, P. A. (2005). The association of acetaminophen, aspirin, and ibuprofen with respiratory disease and lung function. *American Journal of Respiratory and Critical Care Medicine, 171*(9), 966–971.

Meeker, M. A., Finnell, D., & Othman, A. K. (2011). Family caregivers and cancer pain management: A review. *Journal of Family Nursing, 17,* 29–60.

Minozzi, S., Amato, L., & Davoli, M. (2013). Development of dependence following treatment with opioid analgesics for pain relief: A systematic review. *Addiction, 108,* 688–698.

Onen, S. H., Onen, F., Courpron, P., & Dubray, C. (2005). How pain and analgesics disturb sleep. *Clinical Journal of Pain Childhood Abuse and Pain in Adulthood, 21*(5), 422–431.

Chapter 24: Pharmacotherapy of Local and General Anesthesia

Bosslet, G. T., Devito, M. L., Lahm, T., Sheski, F. D., & Mathur, P. N. (2010). Nurse-administered propofol sedation: Feasibility and safety in bronchoscopy. *Respiration, 79*(4), 315–321.

Dillane, D., & Finucane, B. T. (2010). Local anesthetic systemic toxicity. *Canadian Journal of Anesthesia/Journal canadien d'anesthésie, 57,* 368–380.

Evered, L., Scott, D. A., Silbert, B., & Maruff, P. (2011). Postoperative cognitive dysfunction is independent of type of surgery and anesthetic. *Anesthesia & Analgesia, 112,* 1179–1185.

Health Canada. (2016). *Drug product database.* Retrieved from http://www.hc-sc.gc.ca/dhp-mps/prodpharma/databasdon/index-eng.php

Kanaya, N., Satoh, H., Seki, S., Nakayama, M., & Namiki, A. (2002). Propofol anesthesia enhances the pressor response to intravenous ephedrine. *Anesthesia & Analgesia, 94*(5), 1207–1211.

Kids Health for Parents. (2003). *Your child's anesthesia.* Retrieved from http://www.kidshealth.org

Mayo Clinic. (2013). *Anesthesia.* Retrieved from http://www.mayoclinic.com/health/anesthesia/MY00100

Stoelting, R. K. (2014). *Pharmacology and physiology in anesthetic practice* (5th ed.). Philadelphia, PA: Wolters Kluwer.

Visolu, M., Young, M. C., Wieland, K., & Brandom, B. W. (2014). Anesthetic drugs and onset of malignant hyperthermia. *Anesthesia & Analgesia, 118,* 388–396.

Chapter 25: Pharmacotherapy in Substances of Abuse and Addiction

Alameida, M. D., Harrington, C., LaPlante, M., & Kang, T. (2010). Factors associated with alcohol use and its consequences. *Journal of Addictions Nursing, 21,* 194–206.

American Psychiatric Association. (2013). *Diagnostic and statistical manual of mental disorders* (5th ed.). Washington, DC: Author.

Ashton, H. (2005). The diagnosis and management of benzodiazepine dependence. *Current Opinion in Psychiatry, 18*(3), 249–255.

Brust, J. C. M. (2004). Abused agents: Acute effects, withdrawal, and treatment. *CONTINUUM: Lifelong Learning in Neurology. Neurologic Complications of Substance Abuse, 10*(5), 14–47.

Cahill, K., Stead, L. F., & Lancaster, T. (2012). Nicotine receptor partial agonists for smoking cessation. *Cochrane Database of Systematic Reviews, 4,* CD006103.

Canadian Centre on Substance Abuse (CCSA). (2016). http://www.ccsa.ca/Pages/default.aspx

Cohen, L. M., Collins Jr., F. L., Young, A. M., McChargue, D. E., Leffingwell, T. R., & Cook, K. L. (2009). *Pharmacology and treatment of substance abuse.* New York, NY: Taylor & Francis.

Health Canada. (2016). *Federal drug legislation.* Retrieved from http://laws-lois.justice.gc.ca/eng/acts/c-38.8/

Health Canada. (2016). *National Native Alcohol and Drug Abuse Program.* Retrieved from http://www.hc-sc.gc.ca/fniah-spnia/pubs/substan/_ads/1998_rpt-nnadap-pnlaada/index-eng.php

Jason, L. A., Davis, M. I., Ferrari, J. R., & Bishop, P. D. (2001). A review of research and implications for substance abuse recovery and community research. *Journal of Drug Education, 31*(1), 1–28.

Kandel, D. B. (2003). Does marijuana use cause the use of other drugs? *Journal of the American Medical Association, 289*(4), 482–483.

National Institute on Drug Abuse. (2014). *Drug facts: High school and youth trends.* Retrieved from http://www.drugabuse.gov/publications/drugfacts/high-school-youth-trends

O'Malley, P. (2010). Prescription and over-the-counter drug and substance abuse: Something available for every age, anytime and anywhere: Update for the clinical nurse specialist. *Clinical Nurse Specialist, 24,* 286–288.

Peterson, K. (2004/2005). Biomarkers for alcohol use. *Alcohol Research and Health, 28*(1), 1–28.

Statistics Canada. (2016). http://www.statscan.ca

Chapter 26: Brief Review of the Endocrine System

Colbert, J. B., Ankney, J., & Lee, K. T. (2011). *Anatomy and physiology for health professionals: An interactive journey* (2nd ed.). Upper Saddle River, NJ: Pearson Education.

Greenstein, B., & Wood, D. (2011). *The endocrine system at a glance* (3rd ed.). Malden, MA: Wiley-Blackwell.

Krogh, D. (2011). *Biology: A guide to the natural world* (5th ed.). San Francisco, CA: Benjamin Cummings.

Marieb, E. N., & Hoehn, K. (2014). *Human anatomy and physiology* (9th ed.). San Francisco, CA: Benjamin Cummings.

Martini, F. H., Nath, J. L., & Bartholomew, E. F. (2014). *Fundamentals of human anatomy and physiology* (10th ed.). San Francisco, CA: Benjamin Cummings.

Molina, P. (2013). *Endocrine physiology* (4th ed.). Blacklick, OH: McGraw Hill Medical.

Silverthorn, D. U. (2012). *Human physiology: An integrated approach* (6th ed.). San Francisco, CA: Benjamin Cummings.

Chapter 27: Pharmacotherapy of Hypothalamic and Pituitary Disorders

Chernausek, S. D. (2010). Growth and development: How safe is growth hormone therapy for children? *Nature Reviews Endocrinology, 6,* 251–253.

Dehdashti, A. R., & Gentili, F. (2007). Current state of the art in the diagnosis and surgical treatment of Cushing disease: Early experience with a purely endoscopic endonasal technique. *Neurosurgery Focus, 23*(3), E9.

Ferguson, L. A. (2011). Growth hormone use in children: Necessary or designer therapy? *Journal of Pediatric Health Care, 25*(1), 24–30.

Juul, K. V., Klein, B. M., Sandström, R., Erichsen, L., & Nørgaard, J. P. (2011). Gender difference in antidiuretic response to desmopressin. *American Journal of Physiology, Renal Physiology, 300,* F1116–F1122.

Khardori, R. (2014). *Diabetes insipidus.* Retrieved from http://emedicine.medscape.com/article/117648-overview

Marieb, E. N., & Hoehn, K. (2016). *Human anatomy and physiology* (10th ed.), Chapter 16. Upper Saddle River, NJ: Pearson Education.

Molitch, M. E., Clemmons, D. R., Malozowski, S., Merriam, G. R., & Vance, M. L. (2011). Evaluation and treatment of adult growth hormone deficiency: An Endocrine Society clinical practice guideline. *The Journal of Clinical Endocrinology & Metabolism, 96,* 1587–1609.

Sherlock, M., Woods, C., & Sheppard, M. C. (2011). Medical therapy in acromegaly. *Nature Reviews Endocrinology, 7,* 291–300

Simmons, S. (2010). Flushing out the truth about diabetes insipidus. *Nursing Critical Care, 5*(1), 35–39.

Chapter 28: Pharmacotherapy of Diabetes Mellitus

Anguita, M. (2013). Next generation of diabetes drugs arriving, but approach with caution. *Nurse Prescribing, 11,* 59.

Bloomgarden, Z. T. (2006). Aspects of type 2 diabetes and related insulin-resistant states. *Diabetes Care, 29*(3), 732–740.

Boctor, M. A. (2011). Diabetes mellitus. In J. Gray (Ed.), *Therapeutic choices* (6th ed., p. 330). Ottawa, ON: Canadian Pharmacists Association.

Buchanan, T. A., & Xiang, A. H. (2005). Gestational diabetes mellitus. *Journal of Clinical Investigations, 115,* 485–491.

Canadian Diabetes Association. (2013). *Clinical practice guidelines for the prevention and management of diabetes in Canada.* Retrieved from http://guidelines.diabetes.ca/app_themes/cdacpg/resources/cpg_2013_full_en.pdf

Canadian Diabetes Association. (2016). https://www.diabetes.ca/

Canadian Diabetes Association. (2016). *Carbohydrate counting.* Retrieved from http://www.diabetes.ca/diabetes-and-you/healthy-living-resources/diet-nutrition/carbohydrate-counting

Canadian Institute for Health Information. (2016). *Treatment of end-stage organ failure in Canada, 2005-2014.* Retrieved from https://www.cihi.ca/sites/default/files/document/2016_corr_snapshot_enweb.pdf

Chen, S. W. (2002). Editorial: Insulin glargine: Basal insulin of choice? *American Journal of Health-System Pharmacists, 59,* 609, 643.

Chiasson, J. L., Aris-Jilwan, N., Bélanger, R., Bertrand, S., Beauregard, H., Ekoé, J. M., ... Havrankova, J. (2003). Diagnosis and treatment of diabetic ketoacidosis and the hyperglycemic hyperosmolar state. *Canadian Medical Association Journal, 168,* 859–866.

Danne, T., Becker, R. H. A., Heise, T., Bittner, C., Frick, A. D., & Rave, K. (2005). Pharmacokinetics, prandial glucose control, and safety of insulin glulisine in children and adolescents with type 1 diabetes. *Diabetes Care, 28*(9), 2100–2105.

Davis, S. N. (2006). Insulin, oral hypoglycemic agents, and the pharmacology of the endocrine pancreas. In L. L. Brunton, J. S. Lazo, & K. L. Parker (Eds.), *Goodman & Gilman's the pharmacological basis of therapeutics* (11th ed., pp. 1613–1646). New York, NY: McGraw-Hill.

Gates, B. J., & Walker, K. M. (2014). Physiological changes in older adults and their effect on diabetes treatment. *Diabetes Spectrum, 27,* 20–29.

Goulet, S., Trepman, E., Mmath, M. C., Koulack, J., Fong, H., Duerksen, F., ... Embil, J. (2006). Revascularization for peripheral vascular disease in Aboriginal and non-Aboriginal patients. *Journal of Vascular Surgery, 43,* 735–741.

Health Canada. (2016). *Canada's physical activity guide.* Retrieved from http://www.physicalactivityplan.org/resources/CPAG.pdf

Health Canada. (2016). *Eating Well with Canada's Food Guide.* Retrieved from http://www.hc-sc.gc.ca/fn-an/food-guide-aliment/index-eng.php

Hjelm, K., Mufunda, E., Nambozi, G., & Kemp, J. (2003). Preparing nurses to face the pandemic of diabetes mellitus: A literature review. *Journal of Advanced Nursing, 41,* 424–435.

Hovens, M. M., Tamsam, J. T., Beishuizen, E. D., & Huisman, M. V. (2005). Pharmacological strategies to reduce cardiovascular risk in type 2 diabetes mellitus: An update. *Drugs, 65*(4), 433–445.

Inzucchi, S. E. (2006). Management of hyperglycemia in the hospital setting. *New England Journal of Medicine, 355*(18), 1903–1911.

Leiter, L. A., Barr, A., Bélanger, A., Lubin, S., Ross, S. A., Tildesley, H. D., & Fontaine, N. (2001). Diabetes Screening in Canada (DIASCAN) Study: Prevalence of undiagnosed diabetes and glucose intolerance in family physician offices. *Diabetes Care, 24*(6), 1038–1043.

McKnight-Menci, H., Sababu, S., & Kelly, S. D. (2005). The care of children and adolescents with type 2 diabetes. *Journal of Pediatric Nursing, 20*(2), 96–106.

Nathan, D. M. (2014). The diabetes control and complications trial/epidemiology of diabetes interventions and complications study at 30 years: Overview. *Diabetes Care, 37,* 9–16.

Nissen, S. E., & Wolski, K. (2007). Effect of rosiglitazone on the risk of myocardial infarction and death from cardiovascular causes. *New England Journal of Medicine, 356,* 2457–2471.

Norris, S. L., Zhang, X., Avenell, A., Gregg, E., Bowman, B., Schmid, C. H., & Lau, J. (2005). Long-term effectiveness of weight-loss interventions in adults with pre-diabetes: A review. *American Journal of Preventive Medicine, 28*(1), 126–139.

Porth, C. M. (2011). *Essentials of pathophysiology* (3rd ed.). Philadelphia, PA: Lippincott Williams & Wilkins.

Powers, A. C., & D'Alessio, D. (2011). Endocrine pancreas and pharmacotherapy of diabetes mellitus and hypoglycemia. In L. L. Brunton,

B. A. Chabner, & B. C. Knollman (Eds.), *The pharmacological basis of therapeutics* (12th ed., pp. 1237–1274). New York, NY: McGraw-Hill.

Rao, S. S., Disraeli, P., & McGregor, T. (2004). Impaired glucose intolerance and impaired fasting glucose. *American Family Physician, 69*(8), 1961–1968.

Rosenstock, J., Zinman, B., Murphy, L. J., Clement, S. C., Moore, P., Bowering, C. K., … Cefalu, W. T. (2005). Inhaled insulin improves glycemic control when substituted for or added to oral combination therapy in type 2 diabetes: A randomized, controlled trial. *Annals of Internal Medicine, 143*(8), 549–558.

Statistics Canada. (2014). *Canadian community health survey (CCHS).* Retrieved from http://www.statcan.gc.ca/daily-quotidien/150617/dq150617b-eng.htm

Wang, S. S. (2014). *Metabolic syndrome.* Retrieved from http://emedicine.medscape.com/article/165124-overview

Chapter 29: Pharmacotherapy of Thyroid and Parathyroid Disorders

Brent, G. A., & Koenig, R. J. (2011). Thyroid and antithyroid drugs. In L. L. Brunton, B. A. Chabner, & B. C. Knollman (Eds.), *The pharmacological basis of therapeutics* (12th ed., pp. 1129–1162). New York, NY: McGraw-Hill.

Fatourechi, V. (2014). Hyperthyroidism and thyrotoxicosis. In F. Bandeira, H. Gharib, A. Golbert, L. Griz, & M. Faria (Eds.), *Endocrinology and diabetes: A problem-oriented approach* (pp. 9–21). New York, NY: Springer.

Figaro, M. K., Fassler, C. A., Jagasia, S., & Lakhani, V. T. (2013). Thyroid disease: Monitoring and management guidelines. In B. N. Savini (Ed.), *Blood and marrow transplantation long-term management: Prevention and complications* (pp. 225–232). Malden, MA: Wiley-Blackwell.

Hataya, Y., Igarashi, S., Yamashita, T., & Komatsu, Y. (2013). Thyroid hormone replacement therapy for primary hypothyroidism leads to significant improvement of renal function in chronic kidney disease patients. *Clinical and Experimental Nephrology, 17,* 525–531.

Joffe, R. T., Brimacombe, M., Levitt, A. J., & Stagnaro-Green, A. (2007). Treatment of clinical hypothyroidism with thyroxine and triiodothyronine: A literature review and metaanalysis. *Psychosomatics, 48,* 379–384.

Misra, M. (2013). *Thyroid storm.* Retrieved from http://emedicine.medscape.com/article/925147-overview

Pearson, T. (2013). Hypothyroidism: Challenges when treating older adults. *Journal of Gerontological Nursing, 39*(1), 10–14.

Pimentel, L., & Hansen, K. N. (2005). Thyroid disease in the emergency department: A clinical and laboratory review. *Journal of Emergency Medicine, 28*(2), 201–209.

Schori-Ahmed, D. (2003). Defenses gone awry: Thyroid disease. *RN, 66*(6), 38–43.

Simmons, S. (2010). A delicate balance: Detecting thyroid disease. *Nursing, 40*(7), 22–29.

Stan, N. M. (2011). Hyperthyroidism and other causes of thyrotoxicosis: Management guidelines of the American Thyroid Association and American Association of Clinical Endocrinologists. *Thyroid, 21,* 593–646.

Chapter 30: Corticosteroids and Pharmacotherapy of Adrenal Disorders

Adler, G. K. (2014). *Cushing syndrome.* Retrieved from http://emedicine.medscape.com/article/117365-overview

Coureau, B., Bussières, J. F., & Tremblay, S. (2008). Cushing's syndrome induced by misuse of moderate- to high-potency topical corticosteroids. *Annals of Pharmacotherapy, 42*(12), 1903–1907.

Crowther, C. A., McKinlay, C. J. D., Middleton, P., & Harding, J. E. (2011). Intervention review: Repeat doses of prenatal corticosteroids for women at risk of preterm birth for improving neonatal health outcomes. *Cochrane Database of Systematic Reviews, 6,* CD003935.

Falorni, A., Minarelli, V., & Morelli, S. (2013). Therapy of adrenal insufficiency: An update. *Endocrine, 43,* 514–528.

Gardner, D. G., & Shoback, D. (Eds.). (2011). *Greenspan's basic and clinical endocrinology* (9th ed.). New York, NY: McGraw-Hill.

Griffing, G. T. (2014). *Addison disease clinical presentation.* Retrieved from http://emedicine.medscape.com/article/116467-clinical

Mazereeuw, G., Lanctôt, K. L., Chau, S. A., Swardfager, W., & Herrmann, N. (2012). Effects of omega-3 fatty acids on cognitive performance: A meta-analysis. *Neurobiology of Aging, 33*(7), 1482.e17–29.

Robinson, P. D., & Van Asperen, P. (2013). Update in paediatric asthma management: Where is evidence challenging current practice? *Journal of Paediatrics and Child Health, 49,* 346–352.

Tritos, N. A., & Biller, B. M. (2012). Advances in medical therapies for Cushing's syndrome. *Discovery Medicine, 13*(69), 171–179.

Chapter 31: Pharmacotherapy of Disorders of the Female Reproductive System

Aggarwal, R. S., Gujarant, I., Mishra, V. V., & Aggarwal, S. V. (2013). Oral contraceptive pills: A risk factor for retinal vascular occlusion in in-vitro fertilization patients. *Journal of Human Reproductive Sciences, 6,* 79–81.

Bhagavath, B., & Carson, S. A. (2012). Ovulation induction in women with polycystic ovary syndrome: An update. *American Journal of Obstetrics and Gynecology, 206*(3), 195–198.

Brown, J., & Fortier, M. (2006). Canadian consensus conference on osteoporosis, 2006 update. *Society of Obstetricians and Gynaecologists of Canada, 172,* S95–S112.

Davidson, M. R., London, M. L., & Ladewig, P. L. (2012). *Maternal newborn nursing and women's health across the lifespan* (9th ed.). Upper Saddle River, NJ: Pearson Prentice Hall.

deVilliers, T. J., Gass, M. L., Haines, C. J., Hall, J. E., Lobo, R. A., Pierroz, D. D., & Rees, M. (2013). Global consensus statement on menopausal hormone therapy. *Climacteric, 16,* 203–204.

Estephan, A. (2012). *Dysfunctional uterine bleeding in emergency medicine.* Retrieved from http://emedicine.medscape.com/article/795587-overview

Freeman, S., & Schulman, L. P. (2010). Considerations for the use of progestin-only contraceptives. *Journal of the American Academy of Nurse Practitioners, 22,* 81–91.

Levin, E. R., & Hammes, S. R. (2011). Estrogens and progestins. In L. L. Brunton, B. A. Chabner, & B. C. Knollman (Eds.), *The pharmacological basis of therapeutics* (12th ed., pp. 1163–1194). New York, NY: McGraw-Hill.

Lopez, L. M., Grimes, D. A., Chen, M., Otterness, C., Westhoff, C., Edelman, A., & Helmerhorst, F. M. (2013). Hormonal contraceptives for contraception in overweight or obese women. *Cochrane Database of Systematic Reviews, 4,* CD008452.

Mansour, D., Gemzell-Danielsson, K., & Jensen, J. T. (2011). Fertility after discontinuation of contraception: A comprehensive review of the literature. *Contraception, 84,* 465–477.

Schimmer, B. P., & Parker, K. L. (2011). Contraception and the pharmacotherapy of obstetrical and gynecological disorders. In L. L. Brunton, B. A. Chabner, & B. C. Knollman (Eds.), *The pharmacological basis of therapeutics* (12th ed., pp. 1833–1852). New York, NY: McGraw-Hill.

Chapter 32: Pharmacotherapy of Disorders of the Male Reproductive System

Bent, S., Kane, C., Shinohara, K., Neuhaus, J., Hudes, E. S., Goldberg, H., & Avins, A. L. (2006). Saw palmetto for benign prostatic hyperplasia. *New England Journal of Medicine, 354*(6), 557–566.

Brock, G. B. (2003). Tadalafil: A new agent for erectile dysfunction. *Canadian Journal of Urology, 10*(Suppl. 1), 17–22.

Bruzziches, R., Francomano, D., Gareri, P., Lenzi, A., & Aversa, A. (2013). An update on pharmacological treatment of erectile dysfunction with phosphodiesterase type 5 inhibitors. *Expert Opinion on Pharmacotherapy, 14*, 1333–1344.

Bullock, T. L., & Andriole, G. L. (2006). Emerging drug therapies for benign prostatic hyperplasia. *Expert Opinion on Emergency Drugs, 11*(1), 111–123.

Canadian Prostate Health Council. (2016). http://www.canadian-prostate.com

Canadian Urological Association. (2016). http://www.cua.org.

Filson, C. P., Wei, J. T., & Hollingsworth, J. M. (2013). Trends in medical management of men with lower urinary tract symptoms suggestive of benign prostatic hyperplasia. *Urology, 82*(6), 1386–1392.

Grover, S. A., Lowensteyn, I., Kaouache, M., Marchand, S., Coupal, L., DeCarolis, E., … Defoy, I. (2006). The prevalence of erectile dysfunction in the primary care setting: Importance of risk factors for diabetes and vascular disease. *Archives of Internal Medicine, 166*, 213–219.

Hellstrom, W. J., Douglass, L. M., & Powers, M. K. (2012). *How does avanafil compare for erectile dysfunction?* Retrieved from http://www.medscape.com/viewarticle/768904

Kim, E. D. (2014). *Erectile dysfunction.* Retrieved from http://emedicine.medscape.com/article/444220-overview

Roehrborn, C. G. (2011). Male lower urinary tract symptoms (LUTS) and benign prostatic hyperplasia (BPH). *Medical Clinics of North America, 95*, 87–100. doi:10.1016/j.mcna.2010.08.013

Samplaski, M. K., Loai, Y., Wong, K., Lo, K. C., Grober, E. D., & Jarvi, K. A. (2014). Testosterone use in the male infertility population: Prescribing patterns and effects on semen and hormonal parameters. *Fertility and Sterility, 101*, 64–69.

Ullah, M. I., Riche, D. M., & Koch, C. A. (2014). Transdermal testosterone replacement therapy in men. *Drug Design, Development and Therapy, 8*, 101.

Winters, B. R., & Walsh, T. J. (2014). The epidemiology of male infertility. *Urologic Clinics of North America, 41*, 195–204.

Chapter 33: Brief Review of the Gastrointestinal System

Bouchez, C. (n.d.). *9 surprising facts about your stomach.* Retrieved from http://www.webmd.com/women/features/stomach-problems

Farrell, S. E. (2014). *Acetaminophen toxicity.* Retrieved from http://emedicine.medscape.com/article/820200-overview

Krogh, D. (2011). *Biology: A guide to the natural world* (5th ed.). San Francisco, CA: Benjamin Cummings.

Martini, F. H., Nath, J. L., & Bartholomew, E. F. (2012). *Fundamentals of human anatomy and physiology* (9th ed.). San Francisco, CA: Benjamin Cummings.

Seifert, S. M., Schaechter, J. L., Hershorin, E. R., & Lipshultz, S. E. (2011). Health effects of energy drinks on children, adolescents, and young adults. *Pediatrics, 127*, 511–528.

Silverthorn, D. U. (2012). *Human physiology: An integrated approach* (5th ed.). San Francisco, CA: Benjamin Cummings.

Chapter 34: Pharmacotherapy of Peptic Ulcer Disease

Anand, B. S. (2012). *Peptic ulcer disease.* Retrieved from http://emedicine.medscape.com/article/181753-overview#a0101

Barletta, J. F., El-Ibiary, S. Y., Davis, L. E., Nguyen, B., & Raney, C. R. (2013). Proton pump inhibitors and the risk for *Clostridium dificile* infection. *Mayo Clinic Proceedings, 88*, 1085–1090.

Bavishi, C., & Dupont, H. L. (2011). Systematic review: The use of proton pump inhibitors and increased susceptibility to enteric infection. *Alimentary Pharmacology & Therapeutics, 34*, 1269–1281.

Fraser, L. A., Leslie, W. D., Targownik, L. E., Papaioannou, A., & Adachi, J. D. (2013). The effect of proton pump inhibitors on fracture risk: Report from the Canadian multicentre osteoporosis study. *Osteoporosis International, 24*, 1161–1168.

Gatta, L., Vakil, N., Vaira, D., & Scarpignato, C. (2013). Global eradication rates for *Helicobacter pylori* infection: Systematic review and meta-analysis of sequential therapy. *BMJ (Clinical Research Ed.), 347*, f4587.

Gill, J. M., Player, M. S., & Metz, D. C. (2011). Balancing the risks and benefits of proton pump inhibitors. *Annals of Family Medicine, 9*, 200–202.

Gurney, S., Carvalho, L., Gonzalez, C., Galaviz, E., & Sonstein, F. (2014). An efficacious and cost-effective pharmacologic treatment for *Helicobacter pylori. The Journal for Nurse Practitioners, 10*, 22–29.

Hart, A. M. (2013). Evidence-based recommendations for GERD treatment. *The Nurse Practitioner, 38*(8), 26–34.

Hernández-Díaz, S., Martín-Merino, E., & Rodríguez, L. A. G. (2013). Risk of complications after a peptic ulcer diagnosis: Effectiveness of proton pump inhibitors. *Digestive Diseases and Sciences, 58*, 1653–1662.

Marmo, R., Bucci, C., Rea, M., & Rotondano, G. (2013). Treat the patient, not just the source of bleeding. *The American Journal of Gastroenterology, 108*(9), 1533–1534.

Patti, M. G. (2014). *Gastroesophageal reflux disease.* Retrieved from http://emedicine.medscape.com/article/176595-overview

Chapter 35: Pharmacotherapy of Bowel Disorders and other Gastrointestinal Alterations

Apotex. (2016). *Prescribing information: Lactulose solution USP.* Retrieved from http://www.apotexcorp.com

Bharucha, A. E., Pemberton, J. H., & Locke, G. R., III. (2013). American Gastroenterological Association technical review on constipation. *Gastroenterology, 144*(1), 218–238.

Crohn's and Colitis Foundation of Canada. (2016). http://www.ccfc.ca

Ford, A. C., Brenner, D. M., & Schoenfeld, P. S. (2013). Efficacy of pharmacological therapies for the treatment of opioid-induced constipation: Systematic review and meta-analysis. *The American Journal of Gastroenterology, 108*, 1566–1574.

Golembiewski, J., Chernin, E., & Chopra, T. (2005). Prevention and treatment of postoperative nausea and vomiting. *American Society of Health-System Pharmacists, 62*(12), 1247–1260.

Grundmann, O., & Yoon, S. L. (2014). Complementary and alternative medicines in irritable bowel syndrome: An integrative view. *World Journal of Gastroenterology, 20*, 346–362.

Kumar, A., & Kumar, A. (2013). Antiemetics: A review. *International Journal of Pharmaceutical Sciences & Research, 4*(1), 113–123.

Lehrer, J. K. (2014). *Irritable bowel syndrome.* Retrieved from http://emedicine.medscape.com/article/180389-overview

Peyrin-Biroulet, L., Fiorino, G., Buisson, A., & Danese, S. (2013). First-line therapy in adult Crohn's disease: Who should receive anti-TNF agents? *Nature Reviews Gastroenterology and Hepatology, 10*, 345–351.

Rowe, W. A. (2014). *Inflammatory bowel disease.* Retrieved from http://emedicine.medscape.com/article/179037-overview #a0156

Sharkey, K. A., & Wallace, J. L. (2011). Treatment of disorders of bowel motility and water flux; antiemetics; agents used in biliary and pancreatic disease. In L. L. Brunton, B. A. Chabner, & B. C. Knollman (Eds.), *The pharmacological basis of therapeutics* (12th ed., pp. 1323–1350). New York, NY: McGraw-Hill.

Wallace, J. L., & Sharkey, K. A. (2011). Pharmacotherapy of inflammatory bowel disease. In L. L. Brunton, B. A. Chabner, & B. C. Knollman (Eds.), *The pharmacological basis of therapeutics* (12th ed., pp. 1351–1362). New York, NY: McGraw-Hill.

Whelan, K., & Quigley, E. M. (2013). Probiotics in the management of irritable bowel syndrome and inflammatory bowel disease. *Current Opinion in Gastroenterology, 29*, 184–189.

Chapter 36: Pharmacotherapy of Obesity and Weight Management

Clark, A., Franklin, J., Pratt, I., & McGrice, M. (2010). Overweight and obesity: Use of portion control in management. *Australian Family Physician, 39*(6), 407–411. Retrieved from http://www.racgp.org.au/afp/201006/37655

Derosa, G., & Maffioli, P. (2012). Anti-obesity drugs: A review about their effects and their safety. *Expert Opinion on Drug Safety, 11*, 459–471.

Greenway, F. L., & Bray, G. A. (2010). Combination drugs for treating obesity. *Current Diabetes Reports, 10*, 108–115.

Grove, K. A., & Lambert, J. D. (2010). Laboratory, epidemiological, and human intervention studies show that tea (*Camellia sinensis*) may be useful in the prevention of obesity. *The Journal of Nutrition, 140*, 446–453.

Halford, J. C., Boyland, E. J., Blundell, J. E., Kirkham, T. C., & Harrold, A. (2010). Pharmacological management of appetite expression in obesity. *Nature Reviews Endocrinology, 6*, 255–269.

Jurgens, T. M., Whelan, A. M., Killian, L., Doucette, S., Kirk, S., & Foy, E. (2012). Green tea for weight loss and weight maintenance in overweight or obese adults. *Cochrane Database of Systematic Reviews, 12*, CD008650.

Kang, J. G., & Park, C. Y. (2012). Anti-obesity drugs: A review about their effects and safety. *Diabetes & Metabolism Journal, 36*, 13–25.

Kaplan, L. M. (2010). Pharmacologic therapies for obesity. *Gastroenterology Clinics of North America, 39*, 69–79.

Katout, M., Zhu, H., Rutsky, J., Shah, P., Brook, R. D., Zhong, J., & Rajagopalan, S. (2014). Effects of GLP-1 mimetics on blood pressure and relationship to weight loss and glycemic lowering: Results of a systematic meta-analysis and meta-regression. *American Journal of Hypertension, 27*, 130–139.

Powell, A. G., Apovian, C. M., & Aronne, L. J. (2011). New drug targets for the treatment of obesity. *Clinical Pharmacology & Therapeutics, 90*, 40–51.

Schwarz, S. (2011). *Obesity in children.* Retrieved from http://emedicine.medscape.com/article/985333-overview

Chapter 37: Pharmacotherapy of Nutritional Disorders

Bistrian, B. R. (2012). The who, what, where, when, why, and how of early enteral feeding. *The American Journal of Clinical Nutrition, 95*, 1303–1304.

Campbell, S. M. (2006). An anthology of advances in enteral tube feeding formulations. *Nutrition in Clinical Practice, 21*(4), 411–415.

Canadian Parenteral-Enteral Nutrition Association (CPENA). (2016). http://www.cpena.ca

Dibb, M., Teubner, A., Theis, V., Shaffer, J., & Lal, S. (2013). Review article: The management of long-term parenteral nutrition. *Alimentary Pharmacology & Therapeutics, 37*, 587–603.

Hark, L., Ashton, K., & Deen, D. (Eds.). (2012). *The nurse practitioner's guide to nutrition* (2nd ed.). Oxford, UK: Wiley-Blackwell.

Hise, M. E., Kattelmann, K., & Parkhurst, M. (2005). Evidence-based clinical practice: Dispelling the myths. *Nutrition in Clinical Practice, 20*(3), 294–302.

Martínez, R. A., Ortega, E. R., Munuera, C. C., Medina, J. M. F., Vinuesa, M. D. S., & Barrado-Narvión, M. J. (2014). Effectiveness of continuous enteral nutrition versus intermittent enteral nutrition in intensive care patients: A systematic review. *JBI Database of Systematic Reviews and Implementation Reports, 12*(1), 281–317.

Padayatty, S. J., Katz, A., Wang, Y., Eck, P., Kwon, O., Lee, J. H., … Levine, M. (2003). Vitamin C as an antioxidant: Evaluation of its role in disease prevention. *Journal of the American College of Nutrition, 22*(1), 18–35.

Rampersaud, G. C., Kauwell, G. P., & Bailey, L. B. (2003). Folate: A key to optimizing health and reducing disease risk in the elderly. *Journal of the American College of Nutrition, 22*(1), 1–8.

Rollins, C. J. (2010). Drug–nutrient interactions in patients receiving enteral nutrition. In J. I. Boullata & V. T. Armenti (Eds.), *Handbook of drug–nutrient interactions.* New York, NY: Humana.

Seres, D. S., Valcarcel, M., & Guillaume, A. (2013). Advantages of enteral nutrition over parenteral nutrition. *Therapeutic Advances in Gastroenterology, 6*, 157–167.

Tucker, S., & Dauffenbach, V. (2011). *Nutrition and diet therapy.* Upper Saddle River, NJ: Pearson.

Walmsley, R. S. (2013). Refeeding syndrome: Screening, incidence, and treatment during parenteral nutrition. *Journal of Gastroenterology and Hepatology, 28*(Suppl. 4), 113–117.

Chapter 38: Pharmacotherapy of Asthma, Common Cold, and Other Pulmonary Disorders

Albertson, T. E., Schivo, M., Gidwani, N., Kenyon, N. J., Sutter, M. E., Chan, A. L., & Louie, S. (2015). Pharmacotherapy of critical asthma syndrome: Current and emerging therapies. *Clinical Reviews in Allergy & Immunology, 48*(1), 7–30.

Becker, A., Lemiere, C., Berube, D., Boulet, L., Ducharme, F., Fitgerald, M., & Kovesi, T. (2006). 2003 Canadian Asthma Consensus

Guidelines Executive Summary. *Allergy, Asthma and Clinical Immunology, 2*(24), 24–38.

Bjerg, A., Lundbäck, B., & Lötvall, J. (2012). The future of combining inhaled drugs for COPD. *Current Opinion in Pharmacology, 12,* 252–255.

Canadian Thoracic Society. (2010). *Canadian Thoracic Society recommendations for management of chronic obstructive pulmonary disease—2007 update.* Retrieved from http://www.respiratoryguidelines.ca/guideline/chronic-obstructive-pulmonary-disease

Colbert, B. J., Gonzales, L. S., & Kennedy, B. J. (2012). *Integrated cardiopulmonary pharmacology* (3rd ed.). Upper Saddle River, NJ: Pearson Education.

Ferry-Rooney, R. (2013). Asthma in primary care: A case-based review of pharmacotherapy. *Nursing Clinics of North America, 48,* 25–34.

Greiner, A. N., Hellings, P. W., Rotiroti, G., & Scadding, G. K. (2011). Allergic rhinitis. *The Lancet, 378,* 2112–2122.

Hemilä, H., & Chalker, E. (2013). Vitamin C for preventing and treating the common cold. *Cochrane Database of Systematic Reviews, 1,* CD000980.

Isbister, G. K., Prior, F., & Kilham, H. A. (2012). Restricting cough and cold medicines in children. *Journal of Paediatrics and Child Health, 48,* 91–98.

Kaufman, G. (2012). Asthma: Assessment, diagnosis, and treatment adherence. *Nurse Prescribing, 10,* 331–338.

Lareau, S. C., & Hodder, R. (2012). Teaching inhaler use in chronic obstructive pulmonary disease patients. *Journal of the American Academy of Nurse Practitioners, 24,* 113–120.

Mascitelli, L. & Pezzetta, F. (2007). Treatment of chronic respiratory diseases in obese people. *Canadian Medical Association Journal, 176,* 1130–1130a.

Paul, I. M. (2012). Therapeutic options for acute cough due to upper respiratory infections in children. *Lung, 190*(1), 41–44.

Slavin, R. G. (2010). Special considerations in treatment of allergic rhinitis in the elderly: Role of intranasal corticosteroids. *Allergy and Asthma Proceedings, 31,* 179–184.

Smith, S. M., Schroeder, K., & Fahey, T. (2012). Over-the-counter medications for acute cough in children and adults in ambulatory settings. *Cochrane Database of Systematic Reviews, 8,* CD001831.

Turner, P. J., & Kemp, A. S. (2012). Allergic rhinitis in children. *Journal of Paediatrics and Child Health, 48,* 302–310.

Vega, C. (2005). Budesonide/formoterol may be effective for maintenance and acute relief of asthma. *American Journal of Respiratory Critical Care Medicine, 171,* 129–136.

Wooltorton, E. (2005). Long-acting ß2-agonists in asthma: Safety concerns. *Canadian Medical Association Journal, 173,* 1030–1031.

Yanai, K., Rogala, B., Chugh, K., Paraskakis, E., Pampura, A. N., & Boev, R. (2012). Safety considerations in the management of allergic diseases: Focus on antihistamines. *Current Medical Research & Opinion, 28*(4), 623–642.

Chapter 39: Brief Review of Body Defences and the Immune System

DiPiro, J. T., Talbert, R. L., Yee, G. C., Matzke, G. R., Wells, B. G., & Posey, L. M. (Eds.). (2012). *Pharmacotherapy: A pathophysiologic approach* (7th ed.). New York, NY: McGraw-Hill.

Kim, H., Kataru, R. P., & Koh, G. Y. (2012). Regulation and implications of inflammatory lymphangiogenesis. *Trends in Immunology, 33,* 350–356.

Krogh, D. (2011). *Biology: A guide to the natural world* (5th ed.). San Francisco, CA: Benjamin Cummings.

Madigan, M. T., Martinko, J. M., Stahl, D. A., & Clark, D. P. (2012). *Brock biology of microorganisms* (13th ed.). Upper Saddle River, NJ: Pearson Prentice Hall.

Martini, F. H., Nath, J. L., & Bartholomew, E. F. (2012). *Fundamentals of human anatomy and physiology* (9th ed.). San Francisco, CA: Benjamin Cummings.

Silverthorn, D. U. (2013). *Human physiology: An integrated approach* (6th ed.). San Francisco, CA: Benjamin Cummings.

Chapter 40: Pharmacotherapy with Immunostimulants and Immunosupressants

Agnew, L. L., Guffogg, S. P., Matthias, A., Lehmann, R. P., Bone, K. M., & Watson, K. (2005). Echinacea intake induces an immune response through altered expression of leucocyte hsp70, increased white cell counts, and improved erythrocyte antioxidant defences. *Journal of Clinical Pharmacy and Therapeutics, 30*(4), 363–369.

Coelho, T., Tredger, M., & Dhawan, A. (2012). Current status of immunosuppressive agents for solid organ transplantation in children. *Pediatric Transplantation, 16,* 106–122.

Gabardi, S., & Tichy, E. M. (2012). Overview of immunosuppressive therapies in renal transplantation. In A. Chandraker, M. H. Sayegh, & A. K. Singh (Eds.), *Core concepts in renal transplantation* (pp. 97–127). New York, NY: Springer.

Kaufman, C. (2011). The secret life of lymphocytes. *Nursing, 41*(6), 50–54.

Krensky, A. M., Bennett, W. M., & Vincenti, E. (2011). Immunosuppressants, tolerogens, and immunostimulants. In L. L. Brunton, B. A. Chabner, & B. C. Knollman (Eds.), *The pharmacological basis of therapeutics* (12th ed., pp. 1005–1030). New York, NY: McGraw-Hill.

Linde, K., Barrett, B., Bauer, R., Melchart, D., & Woelkart, K. (2006). Echinacea for preventing and treating the common cold. *Cochrane Database of Systematic Reviews, 1,* CD000530.

Pelligrino, B. (2013). Immunosuppression. *Medscape Reference.* Retrieved from http://emedicine.medscape.com/article/432316-overview#a1

Sharma, M., Arnason, J. T., Burt, A., & Hudson, J. B. (2006). Echinacea extracts modulate the pattern of chemokine and cytokine secretion in rhinovirus-infected and uninfected epithelial cells. *Phytotherapy Research, 20*(2), 147–152.

Chapter 41: Pharmacotherapy of Immune System Modulation and Immunization

Ball, J. W., & Bindler, R. C. (2011). *Pediatric nursing: Caring for children* (5th ed.). Upper Saddle River, NJ: Pearson.

Canadian Nursing Coalition on Immunization (CNCI). (2016). *National surveys of provincial and territorial immunization programs.* Retrieved from http://www.phac-aspc.gc.ca/naci-ccni/index-eng.php

Centers for Disease Control and Prevention. (2014). *Genital HPV infection fact sheet.* Retrieved from http://www.cdc.gov/std/HPV/STD-Fact-HPV.htm#a5

Janniger, C. K. (2013). *Herpes zoster.* Retrieved from http://emedicine.medscape.com/article/1132465-overview

Kessels, S. J., Marshall, H. S., Watson, M., Braunack-Mayer, A. J., Reuzel, R., & Tooher, R. L. (2012). Factors associated with HPV vaccine uptake in teenage girls: A systematic review. *Vaccine, 30,* 3546–3556.

Luthy, K. E., Beckstrand, R. L., Callister, L. C., & Cahoon, S. (2012). Reasons parents exempt children from receiving immunizations. *The Journal of School Nursing, 28,* 153–160.

Markowitz, L. E., Tsu, V., Deeks, S. L., Cubie, H., Wang, S. A., Vicari, A. S., & Brotherton, J. M. (2012). Human papillomavirus vaccine introduction—the first five years. *Vaccine, 30*(Suppl. 5), F139–F148.

Music, T. (2012). Protecting patients, protecting healthcare workers: A review of the role of influenza vaccination. *International Nursing Review, 59,* 161–167.

The National Advisory Committee on Immunization. (2016). Statement on influenza vaccination for the 2015–2016 season. Retrieved from http://www.phac-aspc.gc.ca/naci-ccni/flu-2015-grippe-eng.php

Public Health Agency of Canada. (2006). *Canadian national report on immunization.* Retrieved from http://www.phac-aspc.gc.ca/im/natreports-eng.php

Public Health Agency of Canada. (2015). *Canada Communicable Disease Report (CCDR).* Retrieved from http://www.phac-aspc.gc.ca/publicat/ccdr-rmtc/15vol41/index-eng.php

Public Health Agency of Canada. (2015–2016). *Vaccine updates: National Advisory Committee on Immunization (NACI).* Retrieved from http://www.phac-aspc.gc.ca/naci-ccni/assets/pdf/flu-2015-grippe-eng.pdf

Public Health Agency of Canada. (2016). *Canadian Adverse Event Following Immunization Surveillance System (CAEFISS).* Retrieved from http://www.phac-aspc.gc.ca/im/vs-sv/index-eng.php

Public Health Agency of Canada. (2016). *Canadian Immunization Awareness Program (CIAP).* Retrieved from http://www.immunize.cpha.ca

Public Health Agency of Canada. (2016). *Canadian immunization guide.* Retrieved from http://www.phac-aspc.gc.ca/publicat/cig-gci/index-eng.php

Public Health Agency of Canada. (2016). *National immunization strategy.* Retrieved from http://www.phac-aspc.gc.ca/im/nis-sni/

Chapter 42: Pharmacotherapy of Inflammation, Fever, and Allergies

Abramson, S. B. (2011). Clinical guidelines: Expert recommendations for NSAID use: A user-friendly model? *Nature Reviews Rheumatology, 7,* 133–134.

Agnew, L. L., Guffogg, S. P., Matthias, A., Lehmann, R. P., Bone, K. M., & Watson, K. (2005). Echinacea intake induces an immune response through altered expression of leucocyte hsp70, increased white cell counts, and improved erythrocyte antioxidant defences. *Journal of Clinical Pharmacy and Therapeutics, 30*(4), 363–369.

Bachert, C., Chuchalin, A. G., Eisebitt, R., Netayzhenko, V. Z., & Voelker, M. (2005). Aspirin compared with acetaminophen in the treatment of fever and other symptoms of upper respiratory tract infection in adults: A multicenter, randomized, double-blind, double-dummy, placebo-controlled, parallel-group, single-dose, 6-hour dose-ranging study. *Clinical Therapeutics, 27*(7), 993–1003.

Barkin, R. L., Beckerman, M., Blum, S. L., Clark, F. M., Koh, E. K., & Wu, D. S. (2010). Should nonsteroidal anti-inflammatory drugs (NSAIDs) be prescribed to the older adult? *Drugs and Aging, 27*(10), 775–789.

Botting, R., & Ayoub, S. S. (2005). COX-3 and the mechanism of action of paracetamol/acetaminophen. *Prostaglandins, Leukotrienes and Essential Fatty Acids, 72*(2), 85–87.

Braunstahl, G., & Hellings, P. W. (2003). Allergic rhinitis and asthma: The link further unraveled. *Current Opinion in Pulmonary Medicine, 9*(1), 46–51.

Farrell, S. E. (2013). *Acetaminophen toxicity.* Retrieved from http://emedicine.medscape.com/article/820200-overview#aw2aab6b2b4

Grosser, T., Smythe, E., & Fitzgerald, G. A. (2010). In L. L. Brunton, B. A. Chabner, & B. C. Knollman (Eds.), *The pharmacological basis of therapeutics* (12th ed., pp. 1067–1100). New York, NY: McGraw-Hill.

Marshall, S. F., Bernstein, L., Anton-Culver, H., Deapen, D., Horn-Ross, P. L., Mohrenweiser, H., … Ross, R. K. (2005). Nonsteroidal anti-inflammatory drug use and breast cancer risk by stage and hormone receptor status. *Journal of the National Cancer Institute, 97,* 805–812.

Pierce, C. A., & Voss, B. (2010). Efficacy and safety of ibuprofen and acetaminophen in children and adults: A meta-analysis and qualitative review. *The Annals of Pharmacotherapy, 44,* 489–506.

Rothwell, P. M., Wilson, M., Elwin, C. E., Norrving, B., Algra, A., Warlow, C. P., & Meade, T. M. (2010). Long-term effect of aspirin on colorectal cancer incidence and mortality: 20-year follow-up of five randomised trials. *The Lancet, 376,* 1741–1750.

Shah, S., & Mehta, V. (2012). Controversies and advances in non-steroidal anti-inflammatory drug (NSAID) analgesia in chronic pain management. *Postgraduate Medical Journal, 88,* 73–78.

Trepanier, C. H., & Milgram, N. W. (2010). Neuroinflammation in Alzheimer's disease: Are NSAIDs and selective COX-2 inhibitors the next line of therapy? *Journal of Alzheimer's Disease, 21*(4), 1089–1099.

Venerito, M., Wex, T., & Malferthiner, P. (2010). Nonsteroidal anti-inflammatory drug–induced gastroduodenal bleeding: Risk factors and prevention strategies. *Pharmaceuticals, 3*(7), 2225–2237.

Wiegand, T. J. (2012). *Nonsteroidal anti-inflammatory agent toxicity.* Retrieved from http://emedicine.medscape.com/article/816117-overview

Chapter 43: Basic Principles of Anti-Infective Pharmacotherapy

Barnes, B. E., & Sampson, D. A. (2011). A literature review on community-acquired methicillin-resistant *Staphylococcus aureus* in the United States: Clinical information for primary care nurse practitioners. *Journal of the American Academy of Nurse Practitioners, 23,* 23–32.

Bauman, R. W. (2012). *Microbiology with diseases by body system* (3rd ed.). San Francisco, CA: Benjamin Cummings.

Custodio, H. T. (2013). *Hospital-acquired infections.* Retrieved from http://emedicine.medscape.com/article/967022-overview#aw2aab6b2b5aa

Gilbert, D. N., Moellering, R. C., & Sande, M. A. (2011). *The Sanford guide to antimicrobial therapy 2011* (41st ed.). Sperryville, VA: Antimicrobial Therapy.

Gumbo, T. (2011). General principles of antimicrobial therapy. In L. L. Brunton, B. A. Chabner, & B. C. Knollman (Eds.), *The pharmacological basis of therapeutics* (12th ed., pp. 1365–1382). New York, NY: McGraw-Hill.

Gurusamy, K. S., Koti, R., Toon, C. D., Wilson, P., & Davidson, B. R. (2013). Antibiotic therapy for the treatment of methicillin-resistant *Staphylococcus aureus* (MRSA) infections in surgical wounds. *Cochrane Database of Systematic Reviews, 8,* CD009726.

Kee, V. R. (2012). *Clostridium difficile* infection in older adults: A review and update on its management. *The American Journal of Geriatric Pharmacotherapy, 10*(1), 14–24.

Madigan, M. T., Martinko, J. M., Stahl, A. A., & Clark, D. P. (2012). *Brock biology of microorganisms* (13th ed.). San Francisco, CA: Benjamin Cummings.

Rice, L. B. (2012). Mechanisms of resistance and clinical relevance of resistance to β-lactams, glycopeptides, and fluoroquinolones. *Mayo Clinic Proceedings, 8,* 198–208. doi.org/10.1016/j.mayocp.2011.12.003

Spellberg, B., Bartlett, J. G., & Gilbert, D. N. (2013). The future of antibiotics and resistance. *New England Journal of Medicine, 368,* 299–302.

Tortora, G. J., Funke, B. R., & Case, C. L. (2012). *Microbiology: An introduction* (11th ed.). San Francisco, CA: Benjamin Cummings.

Chapter 44: Pharmacotherapy of Bacterial Infections

Albertson, T. E., Dean, N. C., El Solh, A. A., Gotfried, M. H., Kaplan, C., & Niederman, M. S. (2010). Fluoroquinolones in the management of community-acquired pneumonia. *International Journal of Clinical Practice, 64,* 378–388.

Anderson, R. J., Groundwater, P. W., Todd, A., & Worsley, A. J. (2012). Macrolide antibiotics. In *Antibacterial agents: Chemistry, mode of action, mechanisms of resistance and clinical applications* (pp. 173–196). Chichester, UK: John Wiley & Sons, Ltd.

Andresen, M. (2007). Macrolides resistance rising. *Canadian Medical Association Journal, 176,* 159.

Centers for Disease Control and Prevention. (2013). *Get smart: Know when antibiotics work. Antibiotic resistance questions and answers.* Retrieved from http://www.cdc.gov/getsmart/antibiotic-use/anitbiotic-resistance-faqs.html

Chang, C., Mahmood, M. M., Teuber, S. S., & Gershwin, M. E. (2012). Overview of penicillin allergy. *Clinical Reviews in Allergy & Immunology, 43*(1–2), 84–97.

Chen, L. F., Chopra, T., & Kaye, K. S. (2010). Pathogens resistant to antibacterial agents. *Medical Clinics of North America, 95,* 647–676.

Dalhoff, A. (2012). Global fluoroquinolone resistance epidemiology and implications for clinical use. *Interdisciplinary Perspectives on Infectious Diseases,* Article ID 976273, 37 pages.

Dancer, S. J. (2007). Attention prescribers: Be careful with antibiotics. *Lancet, 369*(9560), 442.

Davey, P., Sneddon, K., & Nathwani, D. (2010). Overview of strategies for overcoming the challenge of antimicrobial resistance. *Expert Review of Clinical Pharmacology, 3,* 667–686.

Karras, G., Giannakaki, V., Kotsis, V., & Miyakis, S. (2012). Novel antimicrobial agents against multi-drug-resistant gram-negative bacteria: An overview. *Recent Patents on Anti-Infective Drug Discovery, 7*(3), 175–181.

Labby, K. J., & Garneau-Tsodikova, S. (2013). Strategies to overcome the action of aminoglycoside-modifying enzymes for treating resistant bacterial infections. *Future Medicinal Chemistry, 5,* 1285–1309.

Madigan, M. T., Martinko, J. M., Stahl, D. A., & Clark, D. P. (2012). *Brock biology of microorganisms* (13th ed.). San Francisco, CA: Benjamin Cummings.

Malhotra-Kumar, S., Lammens, C., Coenen, S., Van Herck, K., & Goossens, H. (2007). Effect of azithromycin and clarithromycin therapy on pharyngeal carriage of macrolide-resistant streptococci in healthy volunteers: A randomised, double-blind, placebo-controlled study. *Lancet, 369,* 482.

Matteo, B., Ginocchio, F., Giacobbe, D. R., & Malgorzata, M. (2011). Development of antibiotics for gram-negatives: Where now? *Clinical Investigation, 1,* 221–227.

Ofner-Agostini, M., Simor, A. E., Mulvey, M., Bryce, E., Loeb, M., McGeer, A., … Paton, S. (2006). Methicillin-resistant *Staphylococcus aureus* in Canadian Aboriginal people. *Infection Control & Hospital Epidemiology, 27*(2), 204–207.

Paitan, Y., & Ron, E. Z. (2014). Gram-negative pathogens: Overview of novel and emerging resistant pathogens and drugs. In F. Marinelli & O. Genilloud (Eds.), *Antimicrobials* (pp. 29–56). Berlin, Germany: Springer.

Public Health Agency of Canada. (2013). *Canadian Integrated Program for Antimicrobial Resistance Surveillance 2013: Annual report.* Retrieved from http://www.phac-aspc.gc.ca/cipars-picra/2013/annu-report-rapport-eng.php

Sheff, B. (2001). Taking aim at antibiotic-resistant bacteria. *Nursing, 31*(11), 62–68.

Somasundaram, S., & Manivannan, K. (2013). An overview of fluoroquinolones. *Annual Review & Research in Biology, 3,* 296–313.

Sousa, J., Alves, G., Fortuna, A., & Falcão, A. (2014). Third- and fourth-generation fluoroquinolone antibacterials: A systematic review of safety and toxicity profiles. *Current Drug Safety, 9,* 89–105.

Chapter 45: Pharmacotherapy of Fungal, Protozoan, and Helminthic Infections

Alangaden, G. J. (2011). Nosocomial fungal infections: Epidemiology, infection control, and prevention. *Infectious Disease Clinics of North America, 25,* 201–225.

Auberger, J., Lass-Flörl, C., Aigner, M., Clausen, J., Gastl, G., & Nachbaur, D. (2012). Invasive fungal breakthrough infections, fungal colonization and emergence of resistant strains in high-risk patients receiving antifungal prophylaxis with posaconazole: Real-life data from a single-centre institutional retrospective observational study. *Journal of Antimicrobial Chemotherapy, 67,* 2268–2273.

Baird, J. K. (2012). Elimination therapy for the endemic malarias. *Current Infectious Disease Reports, 14,* 227–237.

Bennet, J. E. (2011). Antifungal agents. In L. L. Brunton, B. A. Chabner, & B. C. Knollman (Eds.), *The pharmacological basis of therapeutics* (12th ed.). New York, NY: McGraw-Hill.

Dickson, R., Awasthi, S., Dimellweek, C., & Williamson, P. (2000). Antihelminthic drugs for treating worms in children: Effects on growth and cognitive performance. *Cochrane Database of Systematic Reviews, 2,* CD000371.

Fleckenstein, J. M., Bartels, S. R., Drevets, P. D., Bronze, M. S., & Drevets, D. A. (2010). Infectious agents of food- and water-borne illnesses. *The American Journal of the Medical Sciences, 340,* 238–246.

Gould, D. (2011). Diagnosis, prevention and treatment of fungal infections. *Nursing Standard, 25*(33), 38–48.

Huang, Y. C., Su, C. C., & Wang, H. P. (2013). Hookworm infestation, an old but not vanished disease. *Journal of Acute Medicine, 3*(1), 26–28.

Madigan, M. T., Martinko, J. M., Stahl, A. A., & Clark, D. P. (2012). *Brock biology of microorganisms* (13th ed.). San Francisco, CA: Benjamin Cummings.

Oh, R. (2005). Practical applications of fish oil (omega-3 fatty acids) in primary care. *Journal of American Board of Family Practice, 18*(1), 28–36.

Pfaller, M. A. (2012). Antifungal drug resistance: Mechanisms, epidemiology, and consequences for treatment. *The American Journal of Medicine, 125*(Suppl. 1), S3–S13.

Phillips, M. A., & Stanley, S. L. (2011). Chemotherapy of protozoal infections: Amebiasis, giardiasis, trichomoniasis, trypanosomiasis, leishmaniasis and other protozoal infections. In L. L. Brunton, B. A. Chabner, & B. C. Knollman (Eds.), *The pharmacological basis of therapeutics* (12th ed., pp. 1419–1442). New York, NY: McGraw-Hill.

Rotta, I., Sanchez, A., Gonçalves, P. R., Otuki, M. F., & Correr, C. J. (2012). Efficacy and safety of topical antifungals in the treatment of dermatomycosis: A systematic review. *British Journal of Dermatology, 166*, 927–933.

van Lieshout, L., & Jaco, J. (2010). Newer diagnostic approaches to intestinal protozoa. *Current Opinion in Infectious Diseases, 23*, 488–493.

Vinetz, J. M., Clain, J., Bounkeua, V., Eastman, R. T., & Fidock, D. T. (2011). Chemotherapy of malaria. In L. L. Brunton, B. A. Chabner, & B. C. Knollman (Eds.), *The pharmacological basis of therapeutics* (11th ed., pp. 1383–1418). New York, NY: McGraw-Hill.

World Health Organization. (2013). *World malaria report 2013 shows major progress in fight against malaria, calls for sustained financing.* Retrieved from http://www.who.int/mediacentre/news/releases/2013/world-malaria-report-20131211/en/

Chapter 46: Pharmacotherapy of Non-HIV Viral Infections

Acosta, E. P., & Flexner, C. (2011). Antiviral agents (nonretroviral). In L. L. Brunton, B. A. Chabner, & B. C. Knollman (Eds.), *The pharmacological basis of therapeutics* (12th ed., pp. 1593–1622). New York, NY: McGraw-Hill.

Buggs, A. M. (2012). *Viral hepatitis.* Retrieved from http://emedicine.medscape.com/article/775507-overview

Chou, R., Hartung, D., Rahman, B., Wasson, N., Cottrell, E. B., & Fu, R. (2013). Comparative effectiveness of antiviral treatment for hepatitis C virus infection in adults: A systematic review. *Annals of Internal Medicine, 158*, 114–123.

Derlet, R. W. (2014). *Influenza.* Retrieved from http://emedicine.medscape.com/article/219557-overview

Fiore, A. E., Fry, A., Shay, D., Gubareva, L., Bresee, J. S., & Uyeki, T. M. (2011). Antiviral agents for the treatment and chemoprophylaxis of influenza. *Morbidity and Mortality Weekly Report, 60*(RR1), 1–24.

Kiser, J. J., & Flexner, C. (2013). Direct-acting antiviral agents for hepatitis C virus infection. *Annual Review of Pharmacology and Toxicology, 53*, 427–449.

Kroger, A. T., Sumaya, C. V., Pickering, L. K., & Atkinson, W. L. (2011). General recommendations on immunization, recommendations of the Advisory Committee on Immunization Practices (ACIP). *Morbidity and Mortality Weekly Report, 60*(RR2), 1–24.

Lee, H., Park, W., & You, K. S. (2010). Management of hepatitis B infection. *Gastroenterology Nursing, 33*(2), 120–126.

Muir, P. (2014). Management of herpes simplex and varicella-zoster infections. *Prescriber, 25*(3), 14–23.

Public Health Agency of Canada. (2007). *Notifiable diseases online.* Retrieved from http://dsol-smed.phac-aspc.gc.ca/dsol-smed/ndis/index-eng.php

Public Health Agency of Canada. (2016). *Influenza updates.* Retrieved from http://www.phac-aspc.gc.ca/im/influenza-eng.php

Pyrsopoulos, N. T. (2013). *Hepatitis B.* Retrieved from http://emedicine.medscape.com/article/177632-overview

Salvaggio, M. R. (2012). *Herpes simplex.* Retrieved from http://emedicine.medscape.com/article/218580-overview

World Health Organization. (2016). *Influenza updates.* Retrieved from http://www.who.int/influenza/surveillance_monitoring/updates/latest_update_GIP_surveillance/en/

Chapter 47: Pharmacotherapy of HIV-AIDS

Center for Infectious Disease Prevention and Control, Public Health Agency of Canada. (2016). *HIV and AIDS in Canada surveillance report to December 31, 2014.* Retrieved from http://healthycanadians.gc.ca/publications/diseases-conditions-maladies-affections/hiv-aids-surveillance-2014-vih-sida/index-eng.php

Centers for Disease Control and Prevention. (2013). Update to interim guidance for preexposure prophylaxis (PrEP) for the prevention of HIV infection: PrEP for injecting drug users. *Morbidity and Mortality Weekly Report, 62*(23), 463–465.

Hankins, C. (2013). Overview of the current state of the epidemic. *Current HIV/AIDS Reports, 10*, 113–123.

Hoyle, B. (2011). *2- or 3-drug regimen lessens intrapartum HIV transmission.* Retrieved from http://www.medscape.com/viewarticle/738814

Kulkarni, S. P., Shah, K. R., Sarma, K. V., & Mahjan, A. P. (2013). Clinical uncertainties, health service challenges, and ethical complexities of HIV "test-and-treat": A systematic review. *American Journal of Public Health, 103*(6), e14–e23.

Kuritzkes, D. R., Boyle, B. A., Gallant, J. E., Squires, K. E., & Zolopa, A. (2003). Current management challenges in HIV: Antiretroviral resistance. *AIDS Reader, 13*(3), 133–135, 138–142.

Lowes, R. (2011). Peril, progress and promise: 30 years of HIV/AIDS. *Medscape Medical News.* Retrieved from http://www.medscape.com/viewarticle/743927

Madigan, M. T., Martinko, J. M., Stahl, D. A., & Clark, D. P. (2012). *Brock biology of microorganisms* (13th ed.). Upper Saddle River, NJ: Prentice Hall.

National Institute of Allergy and Infectious Diseases. (2011). *NIH news: Treating HIV-infected people with antiretrovirals protects partners from infections: Findings result from NIH-funded international study.* Retrieved from http://www.niaid.nih.gov/news/newsreleases/2011/Pages/HPTN052.aspx

Panel on Treatment of HIV-Infected Pregnant Women and Prevention of Perinatal Transmission. (2014). *Recommendations for use of antiretroviral drugs in pregnant HIV-1-infected women for maternal health and interventions to reduce perinatal HIV transmission in the United States.* Retrieved from http://aidsinfo.nih.gov/contentfiles/lvguidelines/perinatalgl.pdf

Public Health Agency of Canada. (2016). *Federal initiative to address HIV/AIDS in Canada.* Retrieved from http://www.phac-aspc.gc.ca/aids-sida/fi-if/index-eng.php

Public Health Agency of Canada. (2016). *HIV/AIDS epidemiology reports and updates.* Retrieved from http://www.phac-aspc.gc.ca/aids-sida/publication/epi/2010/1-eng.php

Rathburn, R. C. (2013). *Antiretroviral therapy for HIV infection.* Retrieved from http://emedicine.medscape.com/article/1533218-overview

Tissot, F., Erard, V., Dang, T., & Cavassini, M. (2010). Nonoccupational HIV post-exposure prophylaxis: A 10-year retrospective analysis. *HIV Medicine, 11*, 584–592.

Chapter 48: Brief Review of the Cardiovascular System

D'Amico, D., & Barbarito, C. (2012). *Health and physical assessment in nursing* (2nd ed.). Upper Saddle River, NJ: Pearson.

Krogh, D. (2011). *Biology: A guide to the natural world* (5th ed.). San Francisco, CA: Benjamin Cummings.

Marieb, E. N., & Hoehn, K. (2013). *Human anatomy and physiology* (9th ed.). San Francisco, CA: Benjamin Cummings.

Martini, F. H., Nath, J. L., & Bartholomew, E. F. (2012). *Fundamentals of human anatomy and physiology* (9th ed.). San Francisco, CA: Benjamin Cummings.

Silverthorn, D. U. (2013). *Human physiology: An integrated approach* (6th ed.). Upper Saddle River, NJ: Pearson.

Chapter 49: Pharmacotherapy of Lipid Disorders

Berglund, L., Brunzell, J. D., Goldberg, A. C., Goldberg, I. J., Sacks, F., Murad, M. H., & Stalenhoef, A. F. (2012). Evaluation and treatment of hypertriglyceridemia: An Endocrine Society clinical practice guideline. *Journal of Clinical Endocrinology & Metabolism, 97*(9), 2969–2989.

Bersot, T. P. (2011). Drug therapy for hypercholesterolemia and dyslipidemia. In L. L. Brunton, B. A. Chabner, & B. C. Knollman (Eds.), *The pharmacological basis of therapeutics* (12th ed., pp. 877–908). New York, NY: McGraw-Hill.

Canadian Cardiovascular Society. (2016). Canadian Cardiovascular Society position statement: Recommendations for the diagnosis and treatment of dyslipidemia and prevention of cardiovascular disease. Retrieved from http://www.ccs.ca/en/guidelines/guidelines-library

Citkowitz, E. (2013). Familial hypercholesterolemia. *Medscape Reference.* Retrieved from http://emedicine.medscape.com/article/121298-overview

Eiland, L. S., & Luttrell, P. K. (2010). Use of statins for dyslipidemia in the pediatric population. *Journal of Pediatric Pharmacology and Therapeutics, 15,* 160–172.

Meagher, E. A. (2004). Addressing cardiovascular disease in women: Focus on dyslipidemia. *Journal of the American Board of Family Practice, 17*(6), 424–437.

Ray, K. K., Seshasai, S. R., Erqou, S., Sever, P., Jukema, J. W., Ford, I., & Sattar, N. (2010). Statins and all-cause mortality in high-risk primary prevention: A meta-analysis of 11 randomized controlled trials involving 65,229 participants. *JAMA Internal Medicine, 170,* 1024–1031.

Smith, R. J., & Hiatt, W. R. (2013). Two new drugs for homozygous familial hypercholesterolemia: Managing benefits and risks in a rare disorder. *JAMA Internal Medicine, 173,* 1491–1492.

Spratt, K. A. (2010). Treating dyslipidemia: Re-evaluating the data using evidence-based medicine. *The Journal of the American Osteopathic Association, 110*(4, Suppl. 5), 6–11.

Taylor, F., Ward, K., Moore, T. H. M., Burke, M., Davey-Smith, G., Casas, J. P., & Ebrahim, S. (2011). Statins for the primary prevention of cardiovascular disease. *Cochrane Database of Systematic Reviews, 1,* CD004816.

Chapter 50: Pharmacotherapy of Angina Pectoris, Myocardial Infarction, and Cerebrovascular Accident

Alaeddini, J. (2014). *Angina pectoris.* Retrieved from http://emedicine.medscape.com/article/150215-overview

Bhat, D. L. (2010). Acute coronary syndrome update for hospitalists. *Journal of Hospital Medicine, 5*(Suppl. 4), S15–S21.

Jayasekara, R. (2010). Effect of early treatment with antihypertensive drugs on short- and long-term mortality in patients with an acute cardiovascular event. *International Journal of Evidence-Based Healthcare, 8,* 41.

Kee, J. L. (2014). *Laboratory and diagnostic tests with nursing implications* (9th ed.). Upper Saddle River, NJ: Pearson Education.

Manuel, D. G., Kwong, K., Tanuseputro, P., Lim, J., Mustard, C. A., Anderson, G. M., ... Laupacis, A. (2006). Effectiveness and efficiency of different guidelines on statin treatment for preventing deaths from coronary heart disease: Modelling study. *British Medical Journal, 332*(7555), 1419.

Maron, B. A., & Rocco, T. P. (2011). Pharmacotherapy of heart failure. In L. L. Brunton, B. A. Chabner, & B. C. Knollman (Eds.), *The pharmacological basis of therapeutics* (12th ed., pp. 789–814). New York, NY: McGraw-Hill.

McDonald, M. A., Simpson, S. H., Ezekowitz, J. A., Gyenes, G., & Tsuyuki, R. T. (2005). Angiotensin receptor blockers and risk of myocardial infarction: Systematic review. *British Medical Journal, 331*(7521), 873–879.

Norton, C., Georgiopoulou, V., Kalogeropoulos, A., & Butler, J. (2011). Chronic stable angina: Pathophysiology and innovations in treatment. *Journal of Cardiovascular Medicine, 12,* 218–219.

Shah, A., & Fox, K. (2013). Stable angina: Current guidelines and advances in management. *Prescriber, 24*(17), 35–44.

Sharma, V., Bell, R. M., & Yellon, D. M. (2012). Targeting reperfusion injury in acute myocardial infarction: A review of reperfusion injury pharmacotherapy. *Expert Opinion on Pharmacotherapy, 13,* 1153–1175.

Sloan, M. A. (2005). Use of anticoagulant agents for stroke prevention. *Continuum: Lifelong Learning in Neurology Stroke Prevention, 11*(4), 97–127.

University of Maryland Medical Center. (2013). *Omega-3 fatty acids.* Retrieved from http://umm.edu/health/medical/altmed/supplement/omega3-fatty-acids

Zafari, A. M. (2014). *Myocardial infarction.* Retrieved from http://emedicine.medscape.com/article/155919-overview

Chapter 51: Pharmacotherapy of Hypertension

Clark, C. E., Smith, L. F., Taylor, R. S., & Campbell, J. L. (2010). Nurse led interventions to improve control of blood pressure in people with hypertension: Systematic review and meta-analysis. *British Medical Journal, 341,* c3995.

Colbert, B. J., & Mason, B. J. (2012). *Integrated cardiopulmonary pharmacology* (3rd ed.). Upper Saddle River, NJ: Pearson.

Cook, N. R., Cutler, J. A., Obarzanek, E., Buring, J. E., Rexrode, K. M., Kumanyika, S. K., ... Whelton, P. K. (2007). Long term effects of dietary sodium reduction on cardiovascular disease outcomes: Observational follow-up of the trials of hypertension prevention (TOHP). *British Medical Journal, 334*(7599), 885–888.

Heart and Stroke Foundation. (2016) High blood pressure. Retrieved from http://www.heartandstroke.com/site/c.ikIQLcMWJtE/b.3484023/k.2174/Heart_disease__High_blood_pressure.htm

Hermida, R. C., Ayala, D. E., Mojón, A., & Fernández, J. R. (2011). Bedtime dosing of antihypertensive medications reduces cardiovascular risk in CKD. *Journal of the American Society of Nephrology, 22,* 2313–2321.

Hill, M. N., Miller, N. H., & DeGeest, S. (2011). Adherence and persistence with taking medication to control high blood pressure. *Journal of the American Society of Hypertension, 5,* 56–63.

Hopkins, C. (2013). *Hypertensive emergencies.* Retrieved from http://emedicine.medscape.com/article/1952052-overview

Hypertension Canada. (2015). *Canadian Hypertension Education Program (CHEP) guidelines.* Retrieved from http://guidelines.hypertension.ca/

James, P. A., Oparil, S., Carter, B. L., Cushman, W. C., Dennison-Himmelfarb, C., Handler, J., ... Ortiz, E. (2014). 2014 evidence-based guideline for the management of high blood pressure in adults: Report from the panel members appointed to the Eighth Joint National Committee (JNC 8). *JAMA, 311,* 507–520.

Michel, T., & Hoffman, B. B. (2011). Treatment of myocardial ischemia and hypertension. In L. L. Brunton, B. A. Chabner, & B. C. Knollman (Eds.), *The pharmacological basis of therapeutics* (12th ed., pp. 745–788). New York, NY: McGraw-Hill.

Sabanayagam, C., & Shankar, A. (2010). Sleep duration and cardiovascular disease: Results from the National Health Interview Survey. *Sleep, 33*(8), 1037–1042.

Touyz, R. M. (2011). Advancement in hypertension pathogenesis: Some new concepts. *Current Opinion in Nephrology and Hypertension, 20,* 105–106.

University of Maryland Medical Center. (2013). *Grape seed.* Retrieved from http://umm.edu/health/medical/altmed/herb/grape-seed

Chapter 52: Diuretic Therapy and Pharmacotherapy of Renal Failure

Alfie, J., Aparicio, L. S., & Waisman, G. D. (2011). Current strategies to achieve further cardiac and renal protection through enhanced renin-angiotensin-aldosterone system inhibition. *Reviews on Recent Clinical Trials, 6*(2), 134.

Brandimarte, F., Mureddu, G. F., Boccanelli, A., Cacciatore, G., Brandimarte, C., Fedele, F., & Gheorghiade, M. (2010). Diuretic therapy in heart failure: Current controversies and new approaches for fluid removal. *Journal of Cardiovascular Medicine, 11,* 563–570.

Cadwallader, A. B., De La Torre, X., Tieri, A., & Botrè, F. (2010). The abuse of diuretics as performance-enhancing drugs and masking agents in sports doping: Pharmacology, toxicology and analysis. *British Journal of Pharmacology, 161,* 1–16.

Glover, M., & Clayton, J. (2012). Thiazide-induced hyponatraemia: Epidemiology and clues to pathogenesis. *Cardiovascular Therapeutics, 30*(5), e219–e226.

Kidney Foundation of Canada. (2013). *Facing the facts.* Retrieved from http://www.kidney.ca/document.doc?id=4083

Martin, R. K. (2010). Acute kidney injury: Advances in definition, pathophysiology, and diagnosis. *AACN Advanced Critical Care, 21,* 350–356.

Reilly, R. F., & Jackson, E. K. (2011). *Diuretics.* In L. L. Brunton, B. A. Chabner, & B. C. Knollman (Eds.), *The pharmacological basis of therapeutics* (12th ed., pp. 671–720). New York, NY: McGraw-Hill.

St. Peter, W. L. (2010). Improving medication safety in chronic kidney disease patients on dialysis through medication reconciliation. *Advances in Chronic Kidney Disease, 17,* 413–419.

Verbalis, J. G., Goldsmith, S. R., Greenberg, A., Schrier, R. W., & Sterns, R. H. (2007). Hyponatremia treatment guidelines 2007: Expert panel recommendations. *American Journal of Medicine, 120*(11, Suppl. 1), S1–S21.

Wassertheil-Smoller, S., Psaty, B., Greenland, P., Oberman, A., Kotchen, T., Mouton, C., ... Trevisan, M. (2004). Association between cardiovascular outcomes and antihypertensive drug treatment in older women. *Journal of the American Medical Association, 292,* 2849–2859.

Chapter 53: Pharmacotherapy of Fluid and Electrolyte Imbalances and Acid-Base Disorders

Adrogue, H. J. (2006). Metabolic acidosis: Pathophysiology, diagnosis and management. *Journal of Nephrology, 19*(Suppl. 9), S62–S69.

Bhananker, S. M., Paek, R., & Vavilala, M. S. (2004). Water intoxication and symptomatic hyponatremia after outpatient surgery. *Anesthesia & Analgesia, 98*(5), 1294–1296.

Bunn, F., & Trivedi, D. (2012). Colloid solutions for fluid resuscitation. *Cochrane Database of Systematic Reviews, 6,* CD001319.

Coyle, J. D., Joy, M. S., & Hladik, G. A. (2011). Disorders of sodium and water homeostasis. In J. T. DiPiro, R. L. Talbert, C. Y. Yee, G. R. Matzke, B. G. Wells, & L. M. Posey (Eds.), *Pharmacotherapy: A pathophysiologic approach* (8th ed.). New York, NY: McGraw-Hill.

Huang, L. H. (2012). *Dehydration.* Retrieved from http://emedicine.medscape.com/article/906999-overview

James, M. F. M. (2010). Magnesium in obstetrics. *Best Practice & Research Clinical Obstetrics & Gynaecology, 24,* 327–337.

Lehnhardt, A., & Kemper, M. J. (2011). Pathogenesis, diagnosis and management of hyperkalemia. *Pediatric Nephrology, 26,* 377–384.

Matzke, G. R., Devlin, J. W., & Palevsky, P. M. (2011). Acid-base disorders. In J. T. DiPiro, R. L. Talbert, C. Y. Yee, G. R. Matzke, B. G. Wells, & L. M. Posey (Eds.), *Pharmacotherapy: A pathophysiologic approach* (8th ed.). New York, NY: McGraw-Hill.

Metheny, N. (2011). *Fluid and electrolyte balance: Nursing considerations.* Sudbury, MA: Jones & Bartlett.

Myburgh, J. A., & Mythen, M. G. (2013). Resuscitation fluids. *New England Journal of Medicine, 369,* 1243–1251.

Perel, P., Roberts, I., & Ker, K. (2013). Colloids versus crystalloids for fluid resuscitation in critically ill patients. *Cochrane Database of Systematic Reviews, 2,* CD000567.

Rizoli, S. (2011). PlasmaLyte. *The Journal of Trauma and Acute Care Surgery, 70*(Suppl. 5), S17–S18.

Rosanoff, A., Weaver, C. M., & Rude, R. K. (2012). Suboptimal magnesium status in the United States: Are the health consequences underestimated? *Nutrition Reviews, 70,* 153–164.

Sterns, R. H., Hix, J. K., & Silver, S. (2010). Treatment of hyponatremia. *Current Opinion in Nephrology and Hypertension, 19*(5), 493–498.

Chapter 54: Pharmacotherapy of Heart Failure

Ahmed, A., Rich, M. W., Love, T. E., Lloyd-Jones, D. M., Aban, I. B., Colucci, W. S., ... Gheorghiade, M. (2006). Digoxin and reduction in mortality and hospitalization in heart failure: A comprehensive post hoc analysis of the DIG trial. *European Heart Journal, 27,* 178–186.

Allen, L. A., & O'Connor, C. M. (2007). Management of acute decompensated heart failure. *Canadian Medical Association Journal, 176*(6), 797–805.

Al-Mohammad, A., & Mant, J. T. (2011). The diagnosis and management of chronic heart failure: Review following the publication of the NICE guidelines. *Heart, 97,* 411–416.

Canadian Cardiovascular Society. (2012). *Canadian Cardiovascular Society consensus conference guidelines on heart failure 2008.* Retrieved from http://www.onlinecjc.ca/article/S0828-282X(12)01379-7/pdf

Corotto, P. S., McCarey, M. M., Adams, S., Khazanie, P., & Whellan, D. J. (2013). Heart failure patient adherence: Epidemiology, cause, and treatment. *Heart Failure Clinics, 9*(1), 49–58.

DeFelice, P., Masucci, M., McLoughlin, J., Salvatore, S., Shane, M., & Wong, D. (2010). Congestive heart failure: Redefining health care and nursing. *Journal of Continuing Education in Nursing, 41*(9), 390–391.

Dobre, D., van Veldhuisen, D. J., DeJongste, M. J., Lucas, C., Cleuren, G., Sanderman, R., ... Haaijer-Ruskamp, F. M. (2007). Prescription of beta-blockers in patients with advanced heart failure and preserved left ventricular ejection fraction: Clinical implications and survival. *European Journal of Heart Failure, 9*(3), 280–286.

Dumitru, I. (2014). *Heart failure.* Retrieved from http://emedicine.medscape.com/article/163062-overview

Dungan, K. M., Osei, K., Nagaraja, H. N., Schuster, D. P., & Binkley, P. (2010). Relationship between glycemic control and readmission rates in patients hospitalized with congestive heart failure during implementation of hospital-wide initiatives. *Endocrine Practice, 16*(6), 945–951.

Dupree, C. S. (2010). Primary prevention of heart failure: An update. *Current Opinion in Cardiology, 25,* 478–483.

Kee, J. L. (2014). *Laboratory and diagnostic tests with nursing implications* (9th ed.). Upper Saddle River, NJ: Pearson Education.

Krum, H., & Driscoll, A. (2013). Management of heart failure. *The Medical Journal of Australia, 199,* 334–339. doi:10.5694/mja12.10993

Lam, C., & Smeltzer, S. C. (2013). Patterns of symptom recognition, interpretation, and response in heart failure patients: An integrative review. *Journal of Cardiovascular Nursing, 28,* 348–359.

Maron, B. A., & Rocco, T. P. (2011). Pharmacotherapy of congestive heart failure. In L. L. Brunton, B. A. Chabner, & B. C. Knollman (Eds.), *The pharmacological basis of therapeutics* (12th ed., pp. 789–814). New York, NY: McGraw-Hill.

Owan, T. E., Hodge, D. O., Herges, R. M., Jacobsen, S. J., Roger, V. L., & Redfield, M. M. (2006). Trends in prevalence and outcome of heart failure with preserved ejection fraction. *New England Journal of Medicine, 355,* 251–259.

Rich, M. W. (2012). Pharmacotherapy of heart failure in the elderly: Adverse events. *Heart Failure Reviews, 17,* 589–595.

Stewart, S. (2013). What is the optimal place for heart failure treatment and care: Home or hospital? *Current Heart Failure Reports, 10,* 227–231.

Tankanow, R., Tamer, H. R., Streetman, D. S., Smith, S. G., Welton, J. L., Annesley, T., … Bleske, B. (2003). Interaction study between digoxin and a preparation of hawthorn (*Crataegus oxyacantha*). *Journal of Clinical Pharmacology, 43*(6), 637–642.

Wakefield, B. J., Boren, S. A., Groves, P. S., & Conn, V. S. (2013). Heart failure care management programs: A review of study interventions and meta-analysis of outcomes. *Journal of Cardiovascular Nursing, 28,* 8–19.

Chapter 55: Pharmacotherapy of Dysrhythmias

Antzelevitch, C., & Burashnikov, A. (2011). Overview of basic mechanisms of cardiac arrhythmia. *Cardiac Electrophysiology Clinics, 3*(1), 23–45.

Atwood, S., Stanton, C., & Storey-Davenport, J. (2011). *Introduction to basic cardiac dysrhythmias.* Burlington, MA: Jones & Bartlett.

Canadian Cardiovascular Society. (2005). *2004 consensus conference: Atrial fibrillation.* Retrieved from http://www.ccs.ca/images/Guidelines/Guidelines_POS_Library/AF_CC_2004.pdf

Chang, Q., Zhong, Z., Walter, K. & Moses, S. (2005). Comparison of the pharmacokinetics of hawthorn phenolics in extract versus individual pure compound. *The Journal of Clinical Pharmacology, 45*(1), 106-112.

Dagres, N., Sommer, P., Anastasiou-Nana, M., & Hindricks, G. (2011). Treating arrhythmias: An expert opinion. *Expert Opinion on Pharmacotherapy, 12,* 1359–1367.

Dorian, P., & Connors, S. P. (2005). Pharmacological and nonpharmacological methods for rate control. *Canadian Journal of Cardiology, 21*(Suppl. B), 26B–30B.

Goyal, S. K. (2014). *Ventricular fibrillation.* Retrieved from http://emedicine.medscape.com/article/158712-overview

Ismail, H., & Lewin, R. J. (2013). The role of a new arrhythmia specialist nurse in providing support to patients and caregivers. *European Journal of Cardiovascular Nursing, 12,* 177–183.

Jie, W., Xingjiang, X., & Bo, F. (2013). Effect of *Crataegus* usage in cardiovascular disease prevention: An evidence-based approach. *Evidence-based Complementary and Alternative Medicine, 2013,* Article ID 149363, 16 pages. Retrieved from https://www.hindawi.com/journals/ecam/2013/149363/

Kaneko, M., Yoshihara, A., & Miyazaki, H. (2011). Relationship between root caries and cardiac dysrhythmia. *Gerodontology, 28,* 289–295.

Knapp, E., & Watson, K. (2011). Medication management of atrial fibrillation: Emerging therapies for rhythm control and stroke prevention. *Pharmacy and Therapeutics, 36,* 518–528.

Mary, C. T., Rosari, K., Deirdra, G., Mary, L., & Ambrose, F. (2010). Hawthorn (*Cretaegus spp*) in the treatment of cardiovascular disease. *Pharmacology Review, 4*(7), 32-41.

Pittler, M. H., Schmidt, K., & Ernst, E. (2003). Hawthorn extract for treating chronic heart failure: Meta-analysis of randomized trials. *American Journal of Medicine, 114*(8), 665-674.

Sampson, K. J., & Kaas, R. S. (2011). Anti-arrhythmic drugs. In L. L. Brunton, B. A. Chabner, & B. C. Knollman (Eds.), *The pharmacological basis of therapeutics* (12th ed., pp. 815–848). New York, NY: McGraw-Hill.

Sullivan, S. D., Orme, M. E., Morais, E., & Mitchell, S. A. (2013). Interventions for the treatment of atrial fibrillation: A systematic literature review and meta-analysis. *International Journal of Cardiology, 165,* 229–236.

Tsiperfall, A., Ottoboni, L. K., Beheiry, S., Al-Ahmad, A., Natale, A., & Wang, P. (2011). *Cardiac arrhythmia management: A practical guide for nurses and allied professionals.* Ames, IA: Wiley-Blackwell.

Chapter 56: Pharmacotherapy of Coagulation Disorders

Abad, R., Pitarch, J., & Rocha, E. (2010). Overview of venous thromboembolism. *Drugs, 70*(Suppl. 2), 3–10.

Connolly, S. J., & Gillis, A. M. (2005). Therapies for the prevention of stroke and other vascular events in atrial fibrillation and atrial flutter. *Canadian Journal of Cardiology, 21*(Suppl. B), 71B–73B.

Ernst, E., & Posadzki, P. (2012). Can garlic intake reduce the risk of cancer? A systematic review of randomised controlled trials. *Focus on Alternative and Complementary Therapies, 17,* 192–196.

Franchini, M., & Mannucci, P. M. (2011). Inhibitors of propagation of coagulation (factors VIII, IX and XI): A review of current therapeutic practice. *British Journal of Clinical Pharmacology, 72,* 553–562.

Goldhaber, S. Z., & Bounameaux, H. (2012). Pulmonary embolism and deep vein thrombosis. *The Lancet, 379*(9828), 1835–1846.

Health Canada. (2016). *Warfarin.* Retrieved from http://healthy-canadians.gc.ca/drugs-products-medicaments-produits/buying-using-achat-utilisation/products-canada-produits/drugs-devices-medicaments-instruments/warfarin-eng.php

Lin, Y., Stanworth, S., Birchall, J., Doree, C., & Hyde, C. (2011). Use of recombinant factor VIIa for the prevention and treatment of bleeding in patients without hemophilia: A systematic review and meta-analysis. *Canadian Medical Association Journal, 183*(1), 223–247.

Mantha, S., Bauer, K. A., & Zwicker, J. I. (2009). Low molecular weight heparin to achieve live birth following unexplained pregnancy loss: A systematic review. *Journal of Thrombosis and Haemostasis, 8,* 263–268.

Patel, K. (2014). *Deep venous thrombosis.* Retrieved from http://emedicine.medscape.com/article/1911303-overview

Pereira, J. A., Holbrook, A. M., Dolovich, L., Goldsmith, C., Thabane, L., Douketis, J. D., … Ginsberg, J. S. (2005). Are brand-name and generic warfarin interchangeable? A survey of Ontario patients and physicians. *Canadian Journal of Clinical Pharmacology, 12*(3), e240–e245.

Pilote, L., Dasgupta, K., Guru, V., Humphries, K. H., McGrath, J., Norris, C., … Tagalakis, V. (2007). A comprehensive view of sex-specific issues related to cardiovascular disease. *Canadian Medical Association Journal, 176*(6), S1–S44.

Thrombosis Interest Group of Canada. (2016). http://thrombosis-canada.ca/

Weltz, D. S., & Weltz, J. I. (2010). Update on heparin: What do we need to know? *Journal of Thrombosis and Thrombolysis, 29*, 199–207.

Wiltink, E. H. (2014). Anticoagulant therapy: We have to do better! A systematic review. *European Journal of Hospital Pharmacy, 21*, 108–112.

Chapter 57: Pharmacotherapy of Hematopoietic Disorders

Fishbane, S., & Nissenson, A. R. (2010). Anemia management in chronic kidney disease. *Kidney International, 78*(Suppl. 117), S3–S9.

Flores, I. Q., & Ershler, W. (2010). Managing neutropenia in older patients with cancer receiving chemotherapy in a community setting. *Clinical Journal of Oncology Nursing, 14*, 81–86.

Freburger, J. K., Ng, L. J., Bradbury, B. D., Kshirsagar, A. V., & Brookhart, M. A. (2012). Changing patterns of anemia management in US hemodialysis patients. *The American Journal of Medicine, 125*, 906–914.

Health Canada. (2013). *Dietary reference intakes.* Retrieved from http://www.hc-sc.gc.ca/fn-an/nutrition/reference/index-eng.php

Kaushansky, K., & Kipps, T. J. (2011). Hematopoietic agents: Growth factors, minerals and vitamins. In L. L. Brunton, B. A. Chabner, & B. C. Knollman (Eds.), *The pharmacological basis of therapeutics* (12th ed., pp. 1067–1100). New York, NY: McGraw-Hill.

Khan, M., & Mikhael, J. (2010). A review of immune thrombocytopenic purpura: Focus on the novel thrombopoietin agonists. *Journal of Blood Medicine, 1*, 21–31.

Sabol, V. K., Resnick, B., Galik, E., Gruber-Baldini, A., Morton, P. G., & Hicks, G. E. (2010). Anemia and its impact on function in nursing home residents: What do we know? *Journal of the American Academy of Nurse Practitioners, 22*, 3–16.

Scialdone, L. (2012). Overview of supportive care in patients receiving chemotherapy antiemetics, pain management, anemia, and neutropenia. *Journal of Pharmacy Practice, 25*, 209–221. doi:10.1177/0897190011431631

Statistics Canada. (2016). *Vitamin D blood levels of Canadians.* Retrieved from http://www.statcan.gc.ca/pub/82-624-x/2013001/article/11727-eng.htm

Tucker, B. B., & Dauffenbach, V. (2011). *Nutrition and diet therapy for nurses.* Upper Saddle River, NJ: Pearson Education.

Chapter 58: Pharmacotherapy of Shock

Dellinger, R. P. (2003). Cardiovascular management of septic shock. *Critical Care Medicine, 31*(3), 946–955.

Hasdai, D., Berger, P. B., Battler, A., & Holmes, D. R. (2002). *Cardiogenic shock: Diagnosis and treatment.* Totowa, NJ: Humana Press.

Menon, V., & Fincke, R. (2003). Cardiogenic shock: A summary of the randomized SHOCK trial. *Congestive Heart Failure, 9*(1), 35–39.

Thiele, H., Ohman, E., Desch, S., Eitel, I., & de Waha, S. (2015). Management of cardiogenic shock. *European Heart Journal, 36*, 1223–1230.

Chapter 59: Basic Principles of Antineoplastic Therapy

Bruce, S. D. (2013). Before you press that button: A look at chemotherapy errors. *Clinical Journal of Oncology Nursing, 17*(1), 31–32.

Cassileth, B. R., & Keefe, F. J. (2010). Integrative and behavioral approaches to the treatment of cancer-related neuropathic pain. *The Oncologist, 15*(Suppl. 2), 19–23.

Chen, R. (2011). Cochrane review summary for cancer nursing: Drug therapy for the management of cancer-related fatigue. *Cancer Nursing, 34*, 250–251.

Esper, P. (2013). Identifying strategies to optimize care with oral cancer therapy. *Clinical Journal of Oncology Nursing, 17*(6), 629–636.

Given, B. A., Spoelstra, S. L., & Grant, M. (2011). The challenges of oral agents as antineoplastic treatments. *Seminars in Oncology Nursing, 27*, 93–103.

Kee, J. L. (2013). *Laboratory and diagnostic tests with nursing implications* (9th ed.). Upper Saddle River, NJ: Pearson.

Lemone, P., Burke, K., & Bauldoff, G. (2011). *Medical-surgical nursing: Critical thinking in client care* (5th ed.). Upper Saddle River, NJ: Pearson.

Simmons, C. (2010). Oral chemotherapeutic drugs: Handle with care. *Nursing, 40*(7), 44–47.

Yarbro, C. H., Wujcik, D., & Gobel, B. H. (2011). *Cancer nursing: Principles and practice* (7th ed.). Sudbury, MA: Jones-Bartlett.

Chapter 60: Pharmacotherapy of Neoplasia

Birner, A. (2003). Safe administration of oral chemotherapy. *Clinical Journal of Oncological Nursing, 2*, 158–162.

Buzdar, A. U. (2000). Tamoxifen's clinical applications: Old and new. *Archives of Family Medicine, 9*, 906–912.

Chabner, B. A., Bertino, J., Cleary, J., Ortiz, T., Lane, A., Supko, J. G., & Ryan, D. (2011). Cytotoxic agents. In L. L. Brunton, B. A. Chabner, & B. C. Knollman (Eds.), *The pharmacological basis of therapeutics* (12th ed., pp. 1677–1730). New York, NY: McGraw-Hill.

Halfdanarson, T. R., & Jatoi, A. (2010). Oral cancer chemotherapy: The critical interplay between patient education and patient safety. *Current Oncology Reports, 12*, 247–252.

Hung, A., & Mullins, C. D. (2013). Relative effectiveness and safety of chemotherapy in elderly and nonelderly patients with stage III colon cancer: A systematic review. *The Oncologist, 18*, 54–63.

Levine, M. N., & Whelan, T. (2006). Adjuvant chemotherapy for breast cancer—30 years later. *New England Journal of Medicine, 355*(18), 1920–1922.

Lizée, G., Overwijk, W. W., Radvanyi, L., Gao, J., Sharma, P., & Hwu, P. (2013). Harnessing the power of the immune system to target cancer. *Annual Review of Medicine, 64*, 71–90.

Mendelsohn, J. (2013). Personalizing oncology: Perspectives and prospects. *Journal of Clinical Oncology, 31*, 1904–1911.

Montagna, E., Cancello, G., & Colleoni, M. (2013). The aromatase inhibitors (plus ovarian function suppression) in premenopausal breast cancer patients: Ready for prime time? *Cancer Treatment Reviews, 39*, 886–890.

Moy, B., Lee, R. J., & Smith, M. (2011). Natural products in cancer chemotherapy: Hormones and related agents. In L. L. Brunton, B. A. Chabner, & B. C. Knollman (Eds.), *The pharmacological basis of therapeutics* (12th ed., pp. 1755–1770). New York, NY: McGraw-Hill.

Seitz, S., Hohla, F., Schally, A. V., Moder, A., Engel, J. B., Horn, F., ... Buchholz, S. (2008). Inhibition of estrogen receptor positive and negative breast cancer cell lines with a growth hormone-releasing hormone antagonist. *Oncology Reports, 20,* 1289–1294.

Versteeg, K. S., Konings, I. R., Lagaay, A. M., van de Loosdrecht, A. A., & Verheul, H. M. (2014). Prediction of treatment related toxicity and outcome with geriatric assessment in elderly patients with solid malignancies treated with chemotherapy: A systematic review. *Annals of Oncology, 25*(10), 1914–1918.

Watts, R. G., & Parsons, K. (2013). Chemotherapy medication errors in a pediatric cancer treatment center: Prospective characterization of error types and frequency and development of a quality improvement initiative to lower the error rate. *Pediatric Blood & Cancer, 60,* 1320–1324.

Yarbro, C. H., Wujcik, D., & Gobel, B. H. (2011). *Cancer nursing: Principles and practice* (7th ed.). Sudbury, MA: Jones-Bartlett.

Chapter 61: Pharmacotherapy of Bone and Joint Disorders

Allaart, C. F., & Huizinga, T. (2011). Treatment strategies in recent onset rheumatoid arthritis. *Current Opinion in Rheumatology, 23,* 241–244.

The Arthritis Society. (2016). Getting a grips on arthritis: Online OA and RA modules. Retrieved from http://arthritis.ca/healthcare-professionals/getting-a-grip-on-arthritis-online-oa-and-ra-modules

Black, D. M., Bauer, D. C., Schwartz, A. V., Cummings, S. R., & Rosen, C. J. (2012). Continuing bisphosphonate treatment for osteoporosis—for whom and for how long? *New England Journal of Medicine, 366,* 2051–2053.

Britton, C., & Walsh, J. (2012). Paget disease of bone: An update. *Australian Family Physician, 41*(3), 100–103.

Buch, M. H., & Emery, P. (2011). New therapies in the management of rheumatoid arthritis. *Current Opinion in Rheumatology, 23,* 245–251.

Clegg, D. O., Reda, D. J., Harris, C. L., Klein, M. A., O'Dell, J. R., Hooper, M. M., ... Williams, H. J. (2006). Glucosamine, chondroitin sulfate, and the two in combination for painful knee osteoarthritis. *New England Journal of Medicine, 354*(8), 795–808.

Eriksen, E. F., Díez-Pérez, A., & Boonen, S. (2014). Update on long-term treatment with bisphosphonates for postmenopausal osteoporosis: A systematic review. *Bone, 58,* 126–135.

Jacobs-Kosmin, D. (2013). *Osteoporosis.* Retrieved from http://emedicine.medscape.com/article/330598-overview#a0156

Levis, S., & Theodore, G. (2012). AHRQ's comparative effectiveness review of treatments to prevent fractures in men and women with low bone density or osteoporosis: A summary of key findings. *Journal of Managed Care Pharmacy, 18*(4, Suppl. B), S1–S15.

Love, C. (2003). Dietary needs for bone health and the prevention of osteoporosis. *British Journal of Nursing, 12*(1), 12–21.

Osteoporosis Canada. (2016). *2010 osteopososis clinical guidelines.* Retrieved http://www.osteoporosis.ca/health-care-professionals/guidelines/

Temprano, K. (2014). *Rheumatoid arthritis.* Retrieved from http://emedicine.medscape.com/article/331715-overview

Vieth, R., Cole, D. E., Hawker, G. A., Trang, H. M., & Rubin, L. A. (2001). Wintertime vitamin D insufficiency is common in young Canadian women, and their vitamin D intake does not prevent it. *European Journal of Clinical Nutrition, 55,* 1091–1097.

Warriner, A. H., & Saag, K. G. (2013). Osteoporosis diagnosis and medical treatment. *Orthopedic Clinics of North America, 44,* 125–135.

Chapter 62: Pharmacotherapy of Dermatological Disorders

Banasikowska, A. K. (2013). *Rosacea.* Retrieved from http://emedicine.medscape.com/article/1071429-overview

Canadian Dermatology Association. (2016). http://www.dermatology.ca

Hall, B. J., & Hall, J. C. (2010). *Sauer's manual of skin diseases* (10th ed.). Philadelphia, PA: Lippincott, Williams & Wilkins.

Meffert, J. (2014). *Psoriasis.* Retrieved from http://emedicine.medscape.com/article/1943419-overview

Psoriasis Society of Canada. (2016). http://www.psoriasissociety.org

Rustin, M. H. A. (2012). Long-term safety of biologics in the treatment of moderate-to-severe plaque psoriasis: Review of current data. *British Journal of Dermatology, 167*(Suppl. 3), 3–11.

Samarasekera, E. J., Sawyer, L., Wonderling, D., Tucker, R., & Smith, C. H. (2013). Topical therapies for the treatment of plaque psoriasis: Systematic review and network meta-analyses. *British Journal of Dermatology, 168,* 954–967.

Stanley, M. C., Ifeanyi, O. E., & Eziokwu, O. G. (2014). Antimicrobial effects of aloe vera on some human pathogens. *International Journal of Current Microbiology and Applied Science, 3*(3), 1022–1028.

Treat, J. R. (2012). Skin signs of severe systemic medication reactions. *Current Problems in Pediatric and Adolescent Health Care, 42*(8), 193–197.

Wehner, M. R., Shive, M. L., Chren, M. M., Han, J., Qureshi, A. A., & Linos, E. (2012). Indoor tanning and non-melanoma skin cancer: Systematic review and meta-analysis. *BMJ: British Medical Journal, 345,* e5909.

Williams, H. C., Dellavalle, R. P., & Garner, S. (2012). Acne vulgaris. *The Lancet, 379*(9813), 361–372.

Chapter 63: Pharmacotherapy of Eye and Ear Disorders

Academy of Family Physicians. (2004). Diagnosis and management of acute otitis media. *Pediatrics, 113,* 1451–1465.

Boston, M. E. (2012). *Labyrinthitis.* Retrieved from http://emedicine.medscape.com/article/856215-overview

De, M., McDonald, P., & Vaughan-Jones, R. (2007). Variability of ear drops in normal population: An accurate delivery device required. *The Internet Journal of Otorhinolaryngology, 6*(1), 143–147.

Huber, M., Kölzsch, M., Stahlmann, R., Hofmann, W., Bolbrinker, J., Dräger, D., & Kreutz, R. (2013). Ophthalmic drugs as part of polypharmacy in nursing home residents with glaucoma. *Drugs & Aging, 30,* 31–38.

Kaufman, P. L., & Rasmussen, C. A. (2012). Advances in glaucoma treatment and management: Outflow drugs. *Investigative Ophthalmology & Visual Science, 53,* 2495–2500.

Oron, Y., Zwecker-Lazar, I., Levy, D., Kreitler, S., & Roth, Y. (2010). Cerumen removal: Comparison of cerumenolytic agents and effect on cognition among the elderly. *Archives of Gerontology and Geriatrics, 52*(2), 228–232.

Pappas, S., Nikolopoulos, T. P., Korres, S., Papacharalampous, G., Tzangarulakis, A., & Ferekidis, E. (2006). Topical antibiotic ear drops: Are they safe? *International Journal of Clinical Practice, 60,* 1115–1119.

Razeghinejad, M. R., & Katz, L. J. (2011). Steroid-induced iatrogenic glaucoma. *Ophthalmic Research, 47,* 66–80.

Saito, M., & Nakada, T. (2013). Contact urticarial syndrome from eye drops: Levofloxacin hydrate ophthalmic solution. *The Journal of Dermatology, 40*(2), 130–131.

Saxby, C., Williams, R., & Hickey, S. (2013). Finding the most effective cerumenolytic. *The Journal of Laryngology & Otology, 127*, 1067–1070.

Shields, M. B. (2010). *Textbook of glaucoma* (6th ed.). Philadelphia, PA: Lippincott, Williams and Wilkins.

Shim, S. H., Kim, J. M., Choi, C. Y., Kim, C. Y., & Park, K. H. (2012). Ginkgo biloba extract and bilberry anthocyanins improve visual function in patients with normal tension glaucoma. *Journal of Medicinal Food, 15*, 818–823.

Venekamp, R. P., Sanders, S., Glasziou, P. P., Del Mar, C. B., & Rovers, M. M. (2013). Antibiotics for acute otitis media in children. *Cochrane Database Systematic Reviews, 1*, CD000219.

Yumori, J. W., & Cadogan, M. P. (2011). Primary open-angle glaucoma: Clinical update. *Journal of Gerontological Nursing, 37*(3), 10–15.

Chapter 64: Toxicology, Bioterrorism, and Emergency Preparedness

Biddinger, P. D., Savoia, E., Massin-Short, S. B., Preston, J., & Stoto, M. A. (2010). Public health emergency preparedness exercises: Lessons learned. *Public Health Reports, 125*(Suppl. 5), 100–106.

Blendon, R. J., Des Roches, C. M., Benson, J. M., Herrmann, M. J., Taylor-Clark, K., & Weldon, K. J. (2003). The public and the smallpox threat. *New England Journal of Medicine, 348*(5), 426–432.

Canadian Nurses Association. (2008). Nurses' ethical considerations in a pandemic or other emergency. Retrieved from https://www.cna-aiic.ca/~/media/cna/page-content/pdf-en/ethics_in_practice_august_2008_e.pdf?la=en

Cao, Y., Skaug, M. A., Andersen, O., & Aaseth, J. (2014). Chelation therapy in intoxications with mercury, lead and copper. *Journal of Trace Elements in Medicine and Biology, 31*.

Chandran, L., & Cataldo, R. (2010). Lead poisoning: Basics and new developments. *Pediatrics in Review, 31*, 399–406.

Danzig, R. (2012). A decade of countering bioterrorism: Incremental progress, fundamental failings. *Biosecurity and Bioterrorism: Biodefense Strategy, Practice, and Science, 10*, 49–54.

Elder, G. M. (2010). Activated charcoal: To give or not to give? *International Emergency Nursing, 18*, 154–157.

McHugh, M. (2010). Hospital nurse staffing and public health emergency preparedness: Implications for policy. *Public Health Nursing, 27*, 442–449.

Mitchell, C. J., Kernohan, W. G., & Higginson, R. (2012). Are emergency care nurses prepared for chemical, biological, radiological, nuclear or explosive incidents? *International Emergency Nursing, 20*, 151–161.

Mortimer, P. P. (2003). Can postexposure vaccination against smallpox succeed? *Clinical Infectious Diseases, 36*(5), 622–629.

Public Health Agency of Canada. (2016). *Centre for Emergency Preparedness and Response (CEPR)*. Retrieved from http://www.phac-aspc.gc.ca/cepr-cmiu/index-eng.php

Public Health Agency of Canada. (2016). *National Emergency Stockpile System (NESS)*. Retrieved from http://www.phac-aspc.gc.ca/ep-mu/ness-eng.php

Spain, K. M., Clements, P. T., DeRanieri, J. T., & Holt, K. (2012). When disaster happens: Emergency preparedness for nurse practitioners. *The Journal for Nurse Practitioners, 8*, 38–44.

Stokes, E., Gilbert-Palmer, D., Skorga, P., Young, C., & Persell, D. (2004). Chemical agents of terrorism: Preparing nurse practitioners. *The Nurse Practitioner Journal, 29*(5), 30–39.

Stokowski, L. A. (2012). *Ready, willing and able: Preparing nurses to respond to disasters*. Retrieved from http://www.medscape.com/viewarticle/579888_8

Strangeland, P. A. (2010). Disaster nursing: A retrospective review. *Critical Care Nursing Clinics of North America, 22*(4), 421–436.

World Health Organization. (2016). *Epidemic and pandemic alert and response (EPR)*. Retrieved from http://www.afro.who.int/en/clusters-a-programmes/dpc/epidemic-a-pandemic-alert-and-response.html

World Health Organization. (2016). *Health aspects of biological and chemical weapons*. Retrieved from http://www.who.int/csr/en/

Index